Melanoma

Adam I. Riker
Editor

Melanoma

A Modern Multidisciplinary Approach

Springer

Editor
Adam I. Riker
Louisiana State University
New Orleans
Louisiana
USA

ISBN 978-3-030-08670-1 ISBN 978-3-319-78310-9 (eBook)
DOI 10.1007/978-3-319-78310-9

Softcover re-print of the Hardcover 1st edition 2018

Printed on acid-free paper

This Springer imprint is published by the registered company Springer International Publishing AG part of Springer Nature.
The registered company address is: Gewerbestrasse 11, 6330 Cham, Switzerland

Preface

This book has been a labor of love, really beginning with my surgical oncology fellowship at the National Cancer Institute, Surgery Branch, under the leadership of Dr. Steven Rosenberg. During this time, we learned just about every aspect of treating melanoma, from the treatment of the primary and locoregional recurrence to the treatment of widespread metastatic disease with various forms of immunotherapy. I have been interested in this formidable cancer ever since this time, incorporating the management of melanoma into my clinical practice for almost two decades now. I remain an "immunotherapist" at heart, still asking basic questions about our immune system and how we can maximize our own bodies potential to fight cancer.

My impetus for writing this book has been the rapidity of progress and change in how we currently manage melanoma, further highlighted by the impressive recent advances in our treatment paradigm for treating metastatic melanoma with immunotherapy. Many of you have likely participated as an investigator of basic science and translational research, clinical trials, and the immunotherapy of melanoma. Others may find this book useful as a nice overview of melanoma and its current overall management. I believe it will be useful for almost anyone with an interest in melanoma.

I have done my best to include what I feel are the essentials of melanoma, ranging from the early detection and prevention of melanoma through the surgical and medical management of this disease. We have included several chapters focused upon complex wound reconstruction options. Other chapters are focused upon more common, non-melanoma skin cancers and rare tumors, such as Merkel cell carcinoma.

I have gathered together a phenomenal group of internationally renowned authors, all of whom are highly respected, committed, and experienced individuals in their areas of expertise. It has been an honor and a privilege to be able to collaborate with such a fine group of individuals, many of whom I have known for years, while others I have come to appreciate as respected colleagues throughout this process.

Finally, I would like to thank all of the folks at Springer, especially Tracy Marton, for providing the support and direction to keep this project on track and on time.

New Orleans, LA, USA Adam I. Riker

Contents

Contributors

Sanjiv S. Agarwala Department of Hematology and Oncology, St. Luke's University Health Network, Bethlehem, PA, USA

Corin Agoris Morsani College of Medicine, University of South Florida, Tampa, FL, USA

Bardia Amirlak Department of Plastic Surgery, UT Southwestern Medical Center, Dallas, TX, USA

Pramila R. Anne Department of Radiation Oncology, Sidney Kimmel Medical College, Thomas Jefferson University, Philadelphia, PA, USA

Marjan E. Askarian-Amiri Auckland Cancer Society Research Centre, University of Auckland, Grafton, Auckland, New Zealand

Department of Molecular Medicine and Pathology, School of Medical Sciences, University of Auckland, Grafton, Auckland, New Zealand

Bruce C. Baguley Auckland Cancer Society Research Centre, University of Auckland, Grafton, Auckland, New Zealand

Mihaela Balu Department of Surgery, Beckman Laser Institute and Medical Clinic, University of California, Irvine, CA, USA

Lea J. Bellomo Department of Dermatology, Stony Brook Medicine, Stony Brook, NY, USA

Marianne Berwick Department of Internal Medicine and Dermatology, University of New Mexico, Albuquerque, NM, USA

Fernando Cassinello Department of Anesthesiology, Fundación Jiménez Díaz, Madrid, Spain

John Wen-Cheng Chang Division of Hematology and Oncology, Department of Internal Medicine, Chang Gung Memorial Hospital at Linkou, Taoyuan, Taoyuan, Taiwan

Aniruddha Chatterjee Department of Pathology, Dunedin School of Medicine, University of Otago, Dunedin, New Zealand

Maurice Wilkins Centre for Molecular Biodiscovery, Auckland, New Zealand

Suephy C. Chen Department of Dermatology, Emory University and Atlanta VA Medical Center, Atlanta, GA, USA

Basil Cherpelis Department of Dermatology and Cutaneous Surgery, Morsani College of Medicine, University of South Florida, Tampa, FL, USA

Ann Y. Chung Division of Surgical Oncology, Department of Surgery, East Carolina University Brody School of Medicine, Greenville, NC, USA

G. Travis Clifton Department of General Surgery, San Antonio Military Medical Center, Fort Sam Houston, TX, USA

Brendon J. Coventry Department of Surgery, Royal Adelaide Hospital, University of Adelaide, Adelaide, SA, Australia

Clara Curiel-Lewandrowski Department of Medicine and Dermatology, University of Arizona, Tucson, AZ, USA

Department of Dermatology, The University of Arizona, Tucson, AZ, USA

Cutaneous Oncology Program, University of Arizona, Tucson, AZ, USA

Skin Cancer Institute, University of Arizona, Tucson, AZ, USA

Julian D'Achille Division of Plastic and Reconstructive Surgery, Department of Surgery, Louisiana State University Health Sciences Center, New Orleans, LA, USA

Anthony B. Daniels Department of Ophthalmology and Visual Sciences, Department of Radiation Oncology, Vanderbilt-Ingram Cancer Center, Vanderbilt University Medical Center, Nashville, TN, USA

Program in Cancer Biology, Vanderbilt University, Nashville, TN, USA

Phillip Darcy Research Division, Peter MacCallum Cancer Centre, Melbourne, VIC, Australia

Adil Daud Department of Medicine, University of California, San Francisco, San Francisco, CA, USA

Amir Dehdashtian Department of Medicine, School of Medicine, School of Public Health, Tehran University of Medical Sciences, Tehran, Iran

Keith A. Delman Department of Surgical Oncology, Emory University Hospital, Atlanta, GA, USA

Shaun Desai Division of Facial Plastic and Reconstructive Surgery, Department of Otolaryngology—Head & Neck Surgery, Johns Hopkins Hospital, Baltimore, MD, USA

Charles L. Dupin Division of Plastic and Reconstructive Surgery, Department of Surgery, Louisiana State University Health Sciences Center, New Orleans, LA, USA

Michael E. Egger Department of Surgical Oncology, University of Texas MD Anderson Cancer Center, Houston, TX, USA

Department of Surgery, University of Louisville, Louisville, KY, USA

Paul Elmslie Healthcert International, Singapore, Singapore

National Skin Cancer Centres, Adelaide, SA, Australia

Kevin Emerick Department of Otolaryngology—Head & Neck Surgery, Massachusetts Eye and Ear Infirmary, Harvard Medical School, Boston, MA, USA

Karim Essani Laboratory of Virology, Department of Biological Sciences, Western Michigan University, Kalamazoo, MI, USA

Clara R. Farley Department of Surgical Oncology, Emory University Hospital, Atlanta, GA, USA

Neil Alan Fenske Department of Dermatology and Cutaneous Surgery, Morsani College of Medicine, University of South Florida, Tampa, FL, USA

Beatriz Castelo Department of Medical Oncology, Hospital Universitario La Paz, Madrid, Spain

Laura K. Ferris Department of Dermatology, University of Pittsburgh Medical Center, Pittsburgh, PA, USA

Graeme Finlay Auckland Cancer Society Research Centre, University of Auckland, Grafton, Auckland, New Zealand

Department of Molecular Medicine and Pathology, School of Medical Sciences, University of Auckland, Grafton, Auckland, New Zealand

Pedram Gerami Skin Cancer Institute of Northwestern Medicine (SCIN-Med), Chicago, IL, USA

Melanoma Program of SCIN-Med, Department of Dermatology, Northwestern Hospital, Chicago, IL, USA

Jeffrey E. Gershenwald Department of Surgical Oncology, University of Texas MD Anderson Cancer Center, Houston, TX, USA

Department of Cancer Biology, University of Texas MD Anderson Cancer Center, Houston, TX, USA

Melanoma and Skin Center, The University of Texas MD Anderson Cancer Center, Houston, TX, USA

Adele C. Green Population Health, Herston, QLD, Australia

QIMR Berghofer Medical Research Institute and CRUK Manchester Institute, University of Manchester, Manchester, UK

David E. Gyorki Division of Cancer Surgery, Peter MacCallum Cancer Centre, Melbourne, VIC, Australia

Department of Surgery, University of Melbourne, Parkville, VIC, Australia

Katja Harbst Faculty of Medicine, Department of Clinical Sciences Lund, Oncology and Pathology, Lund University, Lund, Sweden

Steffen Heegaard Eye Pathology Section, Department of Pathology and Department of Ophthalmology, Rigshospitalet, University of Copenhagen, Copenhagen, Denmark

Lucie Heinzerling Department of Dermatology, University Hospital Erlangen, Erlangen, Germany

Garth S. Herbert Department of General Surgery, San Antonio Military Medical Center, Fort Sam Houston, TX, USA

Eddy C. Hsueh Department of surgery, Saint Louis University, St. Louis, MO, USA

Anna M. Huismans Melanoma Institute Australia, The University of Sydney, Sydney, NSW, Australia

Chia-Yen Hung Hematology and Oncology Division, Internal Medicine Department, Mackay Memorial Hospital, Taipei, New Taipei, Taiwan

Division of Hematology and Oncology, Department of Internal Medicine, Chang Gung Memorial Hospital at Linkou, Taoyuan, Taoyuan, Taiwan

Sheila Jalalat Department of Dermatology and Cutaneous Surgery, Morsani College of Medicine, University of South Florida, Tampa, FL, USA

Rahel A. John Department of Pathology, Lutheran General Hospital, Park Ridge, IL, USA

Mariah M. Johnson Department of Dermatology, Oregon Health & Science University, Portland, OR, USA

Göran Jönsson Faculty of Medicine, Department of Clinical Sciences Lund, Oncology and Pathology, Lund University, Lund, Sweden

Yutaka Kawakami Division of Cellular Signaling, Institute for Advanced Medical Research, Keio University School of Medicine, Tokyo, Japan

Richard Kefford Westmead Hospital, Westmead, NSW, Australia

Melanoma Institute Australia, The University of Sydney, Sydney, NSW, Australia

Faculty of Medicine and Health Sciences, Macquarie University, North Ryde, NSW, Australia

Michael Constantin Kirchberger Department of Dermatology, University Hospital Erlangen, Erlangen, Bavaria, Germany

Hidde M. Kroon Melanoma Institute Australia, The University of Sydney, Sydney, NSW, Australia

Department of General Surgery, Flinders Medical Centre, Adelaide, SA, Australia

Department of Surgery, Royal Adelaide Hospital, University of Adelaide, Adelaide, SA, Australia

George Kroumpouzos Department of Dermatology, The Warren Alpert Medical School of Brown University, Providence, RI, USA

Department of Dermatology, Medical School of Jundiai, Sao Paulo, Brazil

Division of Dermatology, Veterans Affairs Medical Center, Providence, RI, USA

Radhika Sreeraman Kumar Radiation Oncology Services, Riverdale, GA, USA

Joy Kunishige Department of Plastic Surgery, Zitelli & Brodland Skin Cancer Center, University of Pittsburgh Medical Center, Pittsburgh, PA, USA

Shachar Laks Department of Surgery, University of North Carolina at Chapel Hill, Chapel Hill, NC, USA

Jonathan S. Lam Section of Surgical Oncology, Department of Surgery, School of Medicine, Louisiana State University, New Orleans, LA, USA

Stephen L. Lambert Department of Family Medicine, Health Science Center, Louisiana State University, New Orleans, LA, USA

Sancy A. Leachman Department of Dermatology, Oregon Health & Science University, Portland, OR, USA

Alex M. Lin Frank H. Netter MD School of Medicine at Quinnipiac University, Hamden, CT, USA

Konstantinos Liopyris Department of Medicine, Dermatology Service, Memorial Sloan Kettering Cancer Center, New York, NY, USA

Lois J. Loescher The University of Arizona, College of Nursing, Tucson, AZ, USA

Mary E. Logue School of Medicine, University of New Mexico, Albuquerque, NM, USA

Kimberly Loo Department of Hematology/Oncology, Melanoma, University of California, San Francisco, San Francisco, CA, USA

Josep Malvehy Department of Dermatology, Hospital Clinic of Barcelona, Barcelona, Catalonia, Spain

Ashfaq A. Marghoob Division of Dermatology, Department of Medicine, Memorial Sloan Kettering Cancer Center, New York, NY, USA

Kathryn Martires Stanford University School of Medicine, Department of Dermatology, Palo Alto, CA, USA

M. Susana Medina Department of Dermatology, Príncipe de Asturias University Hospital, Madrid, Spain

Jane L. Messina Departments of Anatomic Pathology and Cutaneous Oncology, Moffitt Cancer Center, Tampa, FL, USA

Departments of Pathology and Cell Biology and Dermatology, University of South Florida Morsani College of Medicine, Tampa, FL, USA

Lauge Hjorth Mikkelsen Eye Pathology Section, Department of Pathology and Department of Ophthalmology, Rigshospitalet, University of Copenhagen, Copenhagen, Denmark

Ronald W. Milam Department of Ophthalmology and Visual Sciences, Vanderbilt University Medical Center, Vanderbilt Eye Institute, Nashville, TN, USA

Jane Mills Division of Cancer Surgery, Peter MacCallum Cancer Center, Melbourne, VIC, Australia

David Esteban Moreno Department of Radiation Oncology, Fundación Jiménez Díaz, Madrid, Spain

Catalina Mosquera Division of Surgical Oncology, Department of Surgery, East Carolina University Brody School of Medicine, Greenville, NC, USA

Euphemia W. Mu Ronald O. Perelman Department of Dermatology, NYU, New York, NY, USA

Sowmiya Murali University of New Mexico, Albuquerque, NM, USA

David W. Ollila Department of Surgery, University of North Carolina at Chapel Hill, Chapel Hill, NC, USA

Shukan Patel Department of Plastics and Reconstructive Surgery, Louisiana State University Health Science Center—New Orleans, New Orleans, LA, USA

Elisabeth Eapen Paul Department of Hematology and Oncology, St. Luke's University Health Network, Bethlehem, PA, USA

Kaitlin M. Peace Department of General Surgery, San Antonio Military Medical Center, Fort Sam Houston, TX, USA

Giovanni Pellacani Department of Dermatology, University of Modena and Reggio Emilia, Modena, Italy

George E. Peoples Cancer Insight, LLC, San Antonio, TX, USA

Teresa Pérez-de-la-Fuente Department of Plastic Surgery, Fundación Jiménez Díaz, Madrid, Spain

Tracy Petrie Department of Dermatology, Oregon Health & Science University, Portland, OR, USA

Isabel Prieto Department of Radiation Oncology, Fundación Jiménez Díaz, Madrid, Spain

Susana Puig Department of Dermatology, Hospital Clinic Barcelona, Barcelona, Catalonia, Spain

Marco Antonio Rajo Section of Surgical Oncology, Department of Surgery, School of Medicine, Louisiana State University, New Orleans, LA, USA

Damon R. Reed Departments of Cutaneous Oncology and Sarcoma Oncology, Moffitt Cancer Center, Tampa, FL, USA

Pediatric Cancer and Blood Disorders Institute, Johns Hopkins All Children's Hospital, St Petersburg, FL, USA

Adam I. Riker Section of Surgical Oncology, Department of Surgery, Louisiana State University, School of Medicine, LSU Health-New Orleans, New Orleans, LA, USA

Euan J. Rodger Department of Pathology, Dunedin School of Medicine, University of Otago, Dunedin, Dunedin, New Zealand

Maurice Wilkins Centre for Molecular Biodiscovery, Auckland, New Zealand

Michael Saco Department of Dermatology and Cutaneous Surgery, University of South Florida, Tampa, FL, USA

Inga Saknite Vanderbilt University Medical Center, Department of Medicine, Vanderbilt Health, One Hundred Oaks, Nashville, TN, USA

Nuria Rodriguez Salas Department of Medical Oncology, Hospital Universitario La Paz, Madrid, Spain

Richard Scolyer Melanoma Institute Australia, The University of Sydney, Sydney, NSW, Australia

Sydney Medical School, The University of Sydney, Sydney, NSW, Australia

Royal Prince Alfred Hospital, Camperdown, NSW, Australia

Ladan Shahabi The Ronald O. Perelman Department of Dermatology, NYU Langone Medical Center, New York, NY, USA

Wenyin Shi Department of Radiation Oncology, Sidney Kimmel Medical College, Thomas Jefferson University, Philadelphia, PA, USA

David I. Silverstein Department of Dermatology, Stony Brook Medicine, Stony Brook, NY, USA

Brittany Simone Department of Radiation Oncology, Sidney Kimmel Medical College, Thomas Jefferson University, Philadelphia, PA, USA

Taylor Smith Louisiana State University Health Sciences Center, New Orleans, LA, USA

Vernon K. Sondak Department of Cutaneous Oncology, Moffitt Cancer Center, Tampa, FL, USA

Departments of Oncologic Sciences and Surgery, University of South Florida Morsani College of Medicine, Tampa, FL, USA

Clara Stemwedel Department of Dermatology, Oregon Health & Science University, Portland, OR, USA

Graham Stevens Western Sydney University, Bathurst Clinical School, Orange, NSW, Australia

Orange Hospital, Bathurst, NSW, Australia

Thomas P. Stringer Department of Dermatology, NYU Langone School of Medicine, New York, NY, USA

Per Svedenhag SciBase, Stockholm, Sweden

Susan M. Swetter Stanford University Medical Center and Cancer Institute, Stanford, CA, USA

VA Palo Alto Health Care System, Palo Alto, CA, USA

Department of Dermatology/Cutaneous Oncology, Stanford Dermatology/ Cutaneous Oncology, Stanford, CA, USA

Yvonne Talamantes CRTC Population Science Academic Unit, Albuquerque, NM, USA

Oren Tessler Department of Surgery, University Medical Center, New Orleans, New Orleans, LA, USA

John F. Thompson Melanoma Institute Australia, The University of Sydney, Sydney, NSW, Australia

Sydney Medical School, The University of Sydney, Sydney, NSW, Australia

Royal Prince Alfred Hospital, Camperdown, NSW, Australia

Faculty of Medicine and Health Sciences, Macquarie University, North Ryde, NSW, Australia

Eric R. Tkaczyk Cutaneous Imaging Clinic, Vanderbilt University Medical Center, Department of Medicine, One Hundred Oaks—Dermatology, Nashville, TN, USA

Nasreen A. Vohra Division of Surgical Oncology, Department of Surgery, Brody School of Medicine, East Carolina University, Greenville, NC, USA

Soraya A. Voigt Division of Surgical Oncology, Department of Surgery, Brody School of Medicine, East Carolina University, Greenville, NC, USA

Timothy J. Vreeland Department of General Surgery, Womack Army Medical Center, Fort Bragg, NC, USA

Joanna L. Walker Department of Dermatology, The Warren Alpert Medical School of Brown University, Providence, RI, USA

Division of Dermatology, Veterans Affairs Medical Center, Providence, RI, USA

Annie Wang Department of Dermatology, Hawaii Permanente Medical Group, Honolulu, HI, USA

Abby Joan Warren Department of Plastic Surgery, UT Southwestern Medical Center, Dallas, TX, USA

Cindy Wassef Department of Dermatology, Stony Brook Medicine, Stony Brook, NY, USA

Martin A. Weinstock Department of Dermatology, The Warren Alpert Medical School of Brown University, Providence, RI, USA

Division of Dermatology, Veterans Affairs Medical Center, Providence, RI, USA

Noelle Williams Department of Radiation Oncology, Sidney Kimmel Medical College, Thomas Jefferson University, Philadelphia, PA, USA

Oliver J. Wisco Department of Dermatology, Oregon Health & Science University, Portland, OR, USA

Ian R. Wisecarver Louisiana State University Health Sciences Center, New Orleans, LA, USA

Zachary J. Wolner Department of Medicine, Dermatology Service, Memorial Sloan Kettering Cancer Center, New York, NY, USA

Jan H. Wong Division of Surgical Oncology, Department of Surgery, East Carolina University, Greenville, NC, USA

Helene Woyczesczyk Laboratory of Virology, Department of Biological Sciences, Western Michigan University, Kalamazoo, MI, USA

Clinton Wu Department of Melanoma Oncology, University of California, San Francisco, San Francisco, CA, USA

Oriol Yélamos Department of Medicine, Dermatology Service, Memorial Sloan Kettering Cancer Center, New York, NY, USA

Joseph Zenga Department of Otolaryngology—Head & Neck Surgery, Massachusetts Eye and Ear Infirmary, Harvard Medical School, Boston, MA, USA

John Zitelli Departments of ENT and Plastic Surgery, Zitelli & Brodland Skin Cancer Center, University of Pittsburgh Medical Center, Pittsburgh, PA, USA

History of Melanoma

1

John F. Thompson, Richard Kefford, Graham Stevens, and Richard Scolyer

Melanoma in Antiquity and Through the Ages

Melanoma classically occurs in fair-skinned individuals of European origin. It is therefore surprising that the earliest evidence of melanoma has been found in the skeletons and skin of pre-Columbian, non-European mummies discovered in the foothills of the Peruvian Andes [1]. As well as widespread metastases in bone, rounded melanotic masses were identified in the skin of these mummies. Carbon dating has indicated that these individuals died around 2400 years ago.

At about the same time in Europe, in the fifth century BC, the Greek physician Hippocrates described a condition that he referred to as the "fatal black tumor," almost certainly melanoma. This condition was subsequently reported in the writings of Rufus of Ephesus in the first century AD, but there was no further mention of it until references were made to "fatal black tumor," and "black fluid in the body" in European reports from the seventeenth and eighteenth centuries, including the writings of Highmore in 1651 [1], Bartholin in 1677 [2], Bonet in 1679, and Henrici and Nothnagel in 1757 [2]. In 1804, René Laennec, inventor of the stethoscope, used the term "melanose" to describe a distinct disease entity [3]. Laennec's mentor in Paris was an anatomist and surgeon Baron Guillaume Dupuytren, and in 1812 they published detailed descriptions of "la melanose". Jean Cruveilhier, author of the

J. F. Thompson, M.D. (✉)
Melanoma Institute Australia, The University of Sydney, Sydney, NSW, Australia

Sydney Medical School, The University of Sydney, Sydney, NSW, Australia

Royal Prince Alfred Hospital, Camperdown, NSW, Australia

Faculty of Medicine and Health Sciences, Macquarie University, North Ryde, NSW, Australia
e-mail: john.thompson@melanoma.org.au

R. Kefford
Westmead Hospital, Westmead, NSW, Australia

Melanoma Institute Australia, The University of Sydney, Sydney, NSW, Australia
e-mail: richard.kefford@mq.edu.au

G. Stevens
Western Sydney University, Bathurst Clinical School, Bathurst, NSW, Australia

Orange Hospital, Orange, NSW, Australia
e-mail: graham.stevens@health.nsw.gov.au

R. Scolyer
Melanoma Institute Australia, The University of Sydney, Sydney, NSW, Australia

Sydney Medical School, The University of Sydney, Sydney, NSW, Australia

Royal Prince Alfred Hospital, Camperdown, NSW, Australia
e-mail: richard.scolyer@sswahs.nsw.gov.au

A. I. Riker (ed.), *Melanoma*, https://doi.org/10.1007/978-3-319-78310-9_1

famous treatise *Anatomie pathologique du corps humain*, was another student of Dupuytren, and published the earliest descriptions of melanoma of the hand, foot, and vulva [2].

In 1858, Oliver Pemberton, a surgeon from Birmingham, England, reported a series of 60 patients with metastatic melanoma treated over a 37-year period, describing their clinical features and the sites to which metastasis occurred. Based on Greek words "melas" (dark) and "oma" (tumor), the English word "melanoma" is believed to have been first introduced by a Scottish pathologist, Robert Carswell, in 1838 [4, 5]. Carswell produced a monograph entitled *Illustrations of the Elementary Forms of Disease,* in which he depicted examples of melanomas. However, in the mid-1900s, this disease was often referred to as "melanoblastoma" [6], presumably because it was observed to behave more like a sarcoma than a skin cancer [4, 5].

Melanoma Pathology: Classical and Modern

The first illustrated descriptions of both primary and metastatic melanomas, notably those of Cruveilhier in 1829, were derived from autopsies. In 1853, a surgeon at St Bartholomew's Hospital in London, James Paget, published a report documenting 25 cases of melanoma, and he appears to have been the first to point out that melanoma can progress from a radial growth phase to a vertical growth phase [7]. In 1894, one of the first pathological descriptions of an excised melanoma was published by the British surgeon, Jonathan Hutchinson. He described a case of lentigo maligna melanoma in which an excised amelanotic nodule was examined pathologically by his son (Jonathan Hutchinson, Jr.), who identified a malignant tumor composed of spindle-shaped cells resembling a sarcoma and which he therefore called "melanotic sarcoma."

It was not until the 1900s that detailed descriptions of the histopathological features of melanoma were published. In 1948, a monograph entitled *Biology of Melanomas* was published by the New York Academy of Sciences detailing the state of knowledge at the time. In early 1967 a committee of Australian pathologists, led by the eminent melanoma researcher Vincent McGovern, published recommendations for melanoma classification and terminology [8]. Additionally, in 1967, the US pathologist, Dr. Wallace Clark, published his landmark paper on the histogenetic classification of melanoma that became the basis of previous and current versions of the *WHO Classification of Melanoma* [9]. He described three types of melanoma (lentigo maligna melanoma, superficial spreading melanoma, and nodular melanoma), and also suggested that they had differing prognoses. Subsequent studies provided some evidence in support of this assertion [10–12]. However, in their 1969 publication, Clark et al. showed that the prognosis of melanoma was primarily related to the depth of invasion, which they categorized according to five levels of the skin (now known as Clark-McGovern levels, reflecting the contributions that both these pathology doyens made to establishing level of invasion as an important prognostic factor for patients with primary melanomas) [10–12].

Although it had been documented as early as 1953 that the depth of invasion appeared to be associated with prognosis [13], it was not until the publication in 1970 of Alexander Breslow's landmark paper on the prognostic significance of tumor thickness that the vertical (Breslow's) tumor thickness was established as a very strong prognostic factor [14]. Breslow defined tumor thickness as the vertical depth from the top of the granular layer of the epidermis to the deepest invasive cell. Melanomas <0.76 mm thick and Clark level II tumors were noted to be associated with a more favorable prognosis. The pioneering work of Breslow remains relevant today, with tumor thickness now confirmed in multiple studies to be the strongest predictor of outcome in patients with clinically localized primary melanomas. It has been, and remains, an important factor in successive versions of the internationally accepted American Joint Committee on Cancer (AJCC) Melanoma Staging System [15].

At the International Pigment Cell Conference and the International Cancer Conference held concurrently in Sydney in 1972, an international group of pathologists, chaired by Vincent McGovern, met to develop a consensus on the classification and histopathological reporting of melanoma. The classification, published in 1973 [16], was based on Clark's original proposal and listed two forms of noninvasive "in situ" melanoma (Hutchinson's melanotic freckle and superficial spreading melanoma), and three forms of invasive melanoma (invasive melanoma with adjacent intraepidermal component of Hutchinson's melanotic freckle type, invasive melanoma with an adjacent intraepidermal component of superficial spreading type, and invasive melanoma without an adjacent intraepidermal component).

In 1977 Arrington, Reed et al. described the features of melanomas involving acral skin as a distinct subtype of melanoma that has subsequently become known as acral lentiginous melanoma [17].

The 1972 Sydney classification was revised at an international workshop held in Sydney in 1982 [18]. The original categories were retained (albeit with some slightly different terminologies) but new categories were added: melanoma with an adjacent component of acral lentiginous type, melanoma with an adjacent component of mucosal lentiginous type, and melanoma of unclassifiable histogenetic type.

In the 1960s, and for the next 25–30 years, the disease was usually referred to as "malignant" melanoma, but use of this adjective is now strongly discouraged because it is confusing to patients and to many physicians because there is no nonmalignant form of invasive melanoma. In 2013, Bahmer and Bahmer referred to melanoma in more dramatic terms, describing it as "the black death of modern times"! [19].

In the early years of the twenty-first century, great technological advances facilitated a new understanding of the molecular pathogenesis of a wide variety of diseases, including melanoma [20]. In 2005, Boris Bastian and colleagues published their landmark study showing the presence of common oncogenic somatic gene mutations in BRAF, NRAS, and CKIT in many melanomas. They also showed associations of these mutations with the anatomical site of the primary tumor and the degree of chronic sun damage [21]. These discoveries paved the way for the development of a molecular classification of melanoma that was subsequently expanded into four major melanoma molecular subclasses by The Cancer Genome Atlas Melanoma Project: BRAF mutant, NRAS mutant, NF1 mutant, and triple-wild-type tumors [22]. These advances also led to the development of new therapies that targeted specific gene mutations in melanoma patients, resulting in new treatment options for those with advanced-stage disease.

Recognition of Genetic and Environmental Factors Predisposing to Melanoma

Hereditary Predisposition to Melanoma

In 1820, William Norris, a British general practitioner, noted that satellite lesions frequently occurred around a primary cutaneous melanoma (which he referred to as "fungoid disease"), and observed that spread could occur to distant sites including the lungs, liver, brain, and bone [23]. Norris also appears to have been the first to point out that patients with melanoma sometimes have a family history of melanoma, suggesting that there was an inherited predisposition [24]. Norris later commented on the fact that most of his patients with the condition had a fair complexion and light hair. He based this observation on his clinical experience that a father of one of his melanoma patients later died of an apparently similar disease. Furthermore, the patient's children had multiple nevi on their bodies, as did the patient himself. (It seems likely that they had the atypical multiple mole syndrome, now a well-recognized entity partially attributed to germline CDKN2A mutations; we now know that melanoma occurs by 80 years of age in 58–92% of individuals with these mutations [25]). Thus, Norris appears to have been the first to propose that melanomas could develop from preexisting nevi. Although Norris had suggested that melanomas typically occurred in individuals with fair skin and light hair, a rare case of what we now know as melanoma occurring in a patient with dark skin, a native of Madagascar, was reported by Pemberton in 1858 [26].

The Role of Exposure to Sunshine in Melanoma Development

Sun worshippers have existed for millennia [27]. In some ancient civilizations, sun gods were regarded as the source of all goodness and life, and "Sunday" was designated the special day to worship the sun. For the Greeks, Apollo was the god of the sun and his son Asclepius the god of medicine. It is therefore not surprising that sun bathing was widely practiced in the Asclepian health clinics in the first century BC.

It was not until the late nineteenth century that there was any suggestion that sunshine might not always be beneficial to health. The first documented proposal that sunshine could be harmful is attributed to Unna [28], who in 1893 described severe damage to the skin of sailors caused by prolonged and intense solar exposure. In the early twentieth century, it was specifically noted that skin cancer was more common in geographical areas where there was much sunshine, particularly in outdoor workers.

In 1956, a landmark report was published by the Australian researcher H.O. Lancaster [29], containing data supporting the concept that sunshine was involved in the initiation of cutaneous melanoma. Lancaster indicated that his studies had been undertaken to test the earlier proposal by AGS Cooper, director of the Queensland Radium Institute in Brisbane, that sunlight was an important predisposing factor for all forms of skin cancer. He had observed that skin cancer was far more common in northern Queensland than southern Queensland. Cooper did not publish his results until 1959 [30]. In this article, he noted that a similar observation about latitude and skin cancer incidence had been made in the United States, in the southern cities of New Orleans and Dallas, respectively, and published by Sarnat and Schour in 1950 [31].

A subsequent paper by Lancaster and Nelson, published in 1957 [32], explored in more detail the concept as it applied specifically to melanoma. They noted that those most commonly affected by melanoma in Australia had a fair complexion and did not tan readily, but instead sunburned easily and developed freckles. Lancaster and Nelson clearly documented the fact that melanoma, as well as other types of skin cancer, developed more often in white Australians who lived in the northern state of Queensland than in the southern states of New South Wales and Victoria, with a remarkable latitudinal gradient correlation with melanoma incidence rates. Population-based incidence data for cutaneous melanoma have been collected in Australia and most other developed countries since the 1960s, with a steady increase in observed incidence worldwide. This is attributed mainly to increased UV exposure, mainly from sunshine but also from artificial sources of UV including skin tanning equipment.

Recognition of Melanoma as a Treatable Entity in the Eighteenth and Nineteenth Centuries

In 1844 Samuel Cooper, a London surgeon, recommended early surgical removal of malignant pigmented tumors, but as Norris had done previously he emphasized the apparently untreatable situation of patients with locally advanced and metastatic disease [1, 2, 33]. Subsequently, Norris discussed treatment options in more detail, recommending wide excision of the skin and subcutaneous tissue around a primary melanoma to minimize the risk of recurrence [23].

The first known surgical resection of metastatic melanoma appears to have been undertaken in 1787 [4] by a British surgeon, John Hunter, in London [2]. He reported resection of a recurrent tumor mass behind the angle of the mandible of a 35-year-old man, and described it as a "cancerous fungus excrescence" [34]. It is not clear whether Hunter knew what condition he was dealing with, but the preserved tumor is still on display in the Hunterian Museum of the Royal College of Surgeons in London, subsequently confirmed to be melanoma [35]. The fate of the patient is unknown. The first reported groin dissection for melanoma was in 1851 by Ferguson [36]. Shortly afterwards, in 1857, Jonathan Hutchinson provided the first definite description of subungual melanoma, and stated that early amputation was required [37].

Establishment of Surgical Treatment Paradigms for Melanoma in the Late Nineteenth and Early Twentieth Centuries

Herbert Snow, of the Marsden Hospital in London, was the first to propose surgical clearance of the regional lymph nodes as part of the initial management of patients with primary cutaneous melanoma (which he called "melanotic cancerous disease"). Snow suggested that the regional lymph nodes functioned as "traps" (filters) to prevent the spread of cancer cells into the bloodstream. What is today referred to as an elective lymph node dissection (ELND) was described by Snow as "anticipatory gland dissection" in 1892 [38]. In 1903 Frederick Eve [39] also recommended excision of regional lymph nodes as well as wide excision of the primary melanoma site, whether or not there was any clinical evidence of metastatic disease in the nodes. In 1907, William Sampson Handley emphasized that generous wide excision of primary melanomas (which he referred to as "melanotic growths") was required for effective treatment, in combination with surgical clearance of the regional lymph nodes, and amputation in selected cases [40]. Handley noticed the lymphatic spread of melanoma at the time of autopsy in the leg of a woman who had apparently died of advanced metastatic melanoma. Based on this single case, he recommended not only removal of two inches of skin around the primary melanoma site, with an even wider excision of subcutaneous tissue down to the level of muscle fascia, but also removal of the regional lymph nodes. This treatment plan went unchallenged for the subsequent 50 years.

Pringle, in 1908, extended Handley's concept of lymphatic spread of melanoma, and proposed wide excision of the primary melanoma site and in continuity excision of a generous strip of skin, subcutaneous tissue, and fascia between the primary site and involved regional lymph nodes, all as a single operative specimen [41].

ELND, as part of the primary definitive treatment of melanomas more than 1.5 mm in Breslow's thickness, continued to be performed at many major melanoma treatment centers worldwide. This did not come under debate until the mid-1980s, when its value had become a matter of ongoing controversy. Those who advocated ELND based their recommendation mainly on retrospective studies that may have been subject to selection bias. Prospective clinical trials had not been performed at this point, with little evidence of a true benefit. There were two large, randomized, multicenter clinical trials led by Charles Balch in the United States and Pino Cascinelli in Italy (the Intergroup Melanoma Surgical Trial [42] and the WHO Melanoma Group Trial Number 14 [43]), both failing to demonstrate a statistically significant overall survival benefit. However, both studies showed a nonsignificant trend in favor of ELND.

The History of Radiation Therapy for Melanoma

The use of radiation therapy in the treatment of melanoma has a checkered history, with periods of enthusiasm alternating with bouts of skepticism. Following the discovery of radiation and radioactivity by Roentgen [44], Becquerel [45], and the Curies [46] in 1895–1896, radiation was applied enthusiastically to a wide range of medical conditions, including cancers [47]. However, its inappropriate use and the occurrence of late complications led to disrepute. Early reports of radiation treatment for melanoma were particularly disappointing, leading to the conclusion that melanomas responded poorly to radiation. In retrospect, many of these early treatments were for advanced, incurable melanomas for which meaningful responses would have been unlikely.

The concept that melanoma was a radioresistant tumor was strengthened by in vitro studies of the response of melanoma cell lines by Dewey and Barranco [48, 49]. Both reported that fewer melanoma cells than non-melanoma cells were killed by low doses of radiation. However, enhanced cell killing occurred for higher radiation doses than the usual daily amounts administered. This response to radiation was viewed as an intrinsic characteristic of melanoma cells, which had a high capacity for repair of radiation damage, but which could be overcome by delivering higher daily doses of radiation. A large number of in vivo studies ensued, indicating that high response rates resulted from a hypofractionated treatment schedule (a small number of large fractions of radiation). This became the prevailing methodology for both therapeutic and adjuvant radiation therapy in the late twentieth century [50].

There was, however, growing evidence of a marked heterogeneity in melanoma response to radiation therapy from both in vitro and in vivo studies. In vitro cell line and xenograft studies showed that melanomas had a wide range of radiation sensitivities, from highly sensitive to highly resistant types. A randomized clinical trial failed to show an improvement for an extreme hypofractionated treatment schedule (8 Gray × 4 fractions) compared with a mildly hypofractionated schedule (2.5 Gray × 20 fractions). It has now become clear that most melanomas are somewhat less sensitive to radiation than other common cancer types, such that mildly hypofractionated schedules are appropriate. These have become the most common treatment schedules for adjuvant radiation therapy following resection of primary melanomas with desmoplastic features or positive margins, and following regional lymph node dissection. A Phase III clinical trial clearly showed evidence of substantially lower node field recurrence rates (18% vs. 31%) in patients at high risk of regional recurrence [51].

Novel strategies to improve the response of melanomas have included the combination of radiation with hyperthermia [52]; however, uniform and selective heating of deeply placed tumors was difficult. This was complicated by the lack of specialized equipment being readily available except for a few institutions. Other methods have included selective targeting of melanoma cells using boron neutron capture therapy (BNCT) [53] or alpha-emitting isotopes attached to melanoma-selective probes (TAT-targeted alpha therapy) [54]. None of these approaches has become widely available for clinical practice. By contrast, proton therapy has been used with great success for uveal melanomas for several decades in selected institutions [55, 56].

The modern era of radiation therapy is dominated by continued improvements in the delivery of radiation from linear accelerators. Dose rates have increased, reducing concerns regarding tumor and organ motion; multileaf collimators (MLCs) have replaced single-square apertures, allowing greater conformality of tumor shape from different angles; "onboard" imaging devices (plain X-ray, CT, or MRI scans) allow real-time imaging of tumors and normal anatomy. Inverse treatment planning allows dose sculpting around critical normal tissues, and dynamic motion of all moving components permits safety margins around tumors to be reduced. This allows for higher radiation doses to be delivered to the tumors without causing unacceptable complications.

The availability of these advances has led to the development of "stereotactic" radiation therapy, in which very high radiation doses, delivered as single treatments, or as a highly hypofractionated schedule with great precision, are used to ablate tumors. This technology was used initially for the treatment of intracranial metastases, called stereotactic radiosurgery (SRS), and is delivered using linear accelerators, the Gamma Knife or the CyberKnife. Studies indicated that the differing radiosensitivities observed for conventionally fractionated treatments did not persist following ablative therapy, with high response rates for all tumor types, including melanoma [57]. This technology is increasingly applied to tumors throughout the body, called "stereotactic body radiation therapy (SBRT)."

With the recent availability of effective systemic therapies for locally recurrent and metastatic melanoma, a new role for radiation therapy is emerging. The success of immunotherapy depends on the activation of cytotoxic T lymphocytes. Priming doses of radiation are used to disrupt melanoma cells, releasing melanoma antigens and thereby facilitating the antitumor immune response to immunotherapy or as an abscopal radiation response at distant sites [58].

The Evolution of Locoregional Techniques for Treating Melanoma Metastases: Isolated Limb Perfusion, Isolated Limb Infusion, Intralesional and Topical Therapies

Until the mid-twentieth century, patients with locally advanced or extensive metastatic melanoma involving a limb were usually treated by amputation. This dramatic and disabling surgery was able to be avoided in most cases after the introduction, in 1958, of the isolated limb perfusion (ILP) technique by Creech and Krementz et al. in Louisiana [59]. This procedure involved temporary isolation of the limb vasculature from the general circulation, and then perfusion of the "isolated" limb with cytotoxic drugs via large-bore catheters inserted surgically into the major vessels of the groin or axilla and connected to a modified heart-lung external circuit. Overall response rates of around 80% were achieved with ILP, and use of the technique meant that limb amputation was able to be avoided in most patients [60].

The ILP technique was complex and technically challenging. Consequently, it was only performed in a few specialized centers. In 1994, Thompson et al. in Sydney described a similar but much simpler technique that they called isolated limb infusion (ILI) [61]. Percutaneously inserted arterial and venous catheters were used, and after inflating a pneumatic tourniquet around the proximal limb the infused drug was circulated using a syringe and a three-way tap via a simple external circuit containing a heating device without an oxygenator. The results obtained by ILI were similar to those achieved by ILP, and ILI is now being used at many melanoma treatment centers around the world [62].

Another form of treatment that has been used to treat melanoma in transit metastases is intratumoral injection. A wide variety of agents have been injected. Reports dating as far back as 1896 [63] have documented intratumoral injection of bacillus prodigiosus, BCG, and the cytotoxic drug thiotepa [64–67]. In the 1980s, there were reports of intralesional injection of interleukin-2 [68], and more recently of Rose Bengal (PV-10) [69] and talimogene laherparepvec (TVEC, "Imlygic") [70]. Good local control of injected lesions has been reported for each of the latter three agents. Involution of nearby, non-injected lesions can also occur, and occasionally there is an abscopal effect on distant metastatic disease. These effects on non-injected tumor deposits are attributed to an antitumoral immune response enhanced by the release of antigens from tumor cells damaged or killed by the intratumoral injection.

Another local therapy technique for melanoma recurrences is electrochemotherapy (electroporation) [71–75]. First reported in 1987 [76], this technique involves intratumoral or systemic administration of a cytotoxic drug (usually bleomycin), and then application of an electrical field to tumor deposits using an array of needle electrodes. Transient permeability of the tumor cell membrane to the drug occurs, resulting in cell death [72]. Yet another form of local therapy for recurrent melanoma involves the topical application of diphencyprone. This was first reported by Damian and Thompson in 2007 [77] and is often effective in controlling or eliminating extensive but superficial melanoma recurrences, sometimes with an abscopal effect on metastases at remote sites.

Early Studies of Lymphatic Anatomy and Physiology Leading to Understanding of the Sentinel Node Concept

In 280 BC, the existence of the lymphatic system was first noted by Erasistratus, who described vessels that contained milky fluid and terminated in mesenteric lymph nodes, and considered them to be a form of blood vessel. Nearly two centuries later, lymphatic vessels in the mesentery were rediscovered by Gasparo Aselli in Italy. He too proposed that they were lacteal "veins." In the early part of the seventeenth century, several investigators including Vessling, Folius, Tulp, Wallee, and Pecquet confirmed the existence of lymphatic vessels [78]. The Danish polymath Thomas Bartholin reported the existence of the thoracic duct in 1652, and appears to have been the first to clearly state that the lymphatic system was separate from the vascular system [79]. He proposed (correctly) that lymph originated from the blood by filtration. He was also the first to introduce the term "lymphatic", referring to the lymph vessels that he observed as "vasa lymphatica." Subsequently, a number of investigators attempted to map the lymphatic system, including Nuck (1650–1692), a professor of anatomy in the Netherlands, who injected mercury mixed with tin and lead into lymphatics to demonstrate their course towards lymph nodes [80].

The function of lymphatics and lymph nodes was essentially unknown until the studies of the famous German pathologist, Rudolf Ludwig Carl Virchow, in the mid-nineteenth century. In 1863, he proposed that lymph from any particular body site drained through lymphatics to specific lymph nodes, and then onwards to other lymph nodes [81]. This proposal was based on autopsy findings in a sailor who had a tattoo on the skin of his arm and was found to have obvious carbon pigment in a single axillary lymph node. The sentinel node concept is thus at least 150 years old!

Sentinel Lymph Node Biopsy: A New Gold Standard for Melanoma Staging

As previously discussed, "elective" lymph node dissection was widely practiced in patients with melanomas >1.5 mm in thickness until the 1980s. It was known that only about 20% of patients could possibly benefit, because only this percentage had metastatic disease in their regional nodes, but there was no way of identifying them. In 1992, Morton and Cochran et al. published a landmark article [82] describing the technique of sentinel node biopsy (SNB). This was practice-changing, and allowed the 20% of node-positive patients to be identified and offered a completion lymph node dissection. In 1994, a large international study, the first Multicenter Selective Lymphadenectomy Trial (MSLT-I), was commenced [83], and 2001 patients were randomized. The final results, published in 2014 [84] with 10 years minimum follow-up, showed no overall survival benefit for SN biopsy. However, there was a substantial survival benefit (compared with patients who were simply observed) in the subgroup of patients who had a positive SN followed by an immediate completion lymph node dissection (CLND). The great advantage of SN biopsy for all patients, however, was that it provided much better staging than had been possible previously, and allowed more accurate estimates of prognosis to be made. Consequently, SN status has become an essential part of the AJCC/UICC Melanoma Staging System. Whether CLND is necessary in all patients found to be SN positive is being assessed in another trial designed by Morton, the Second Multicenter Selective Lymphadenectomy Trial (MSLT-II). Initial results indicate that routine CLND in SN-positive patients does not improve survival outcome [85].

Reliable SN identification requires careful lymphatic mapping, and although Morton's initial studies were with blue dye only, the importance of high-quality lymphoscintigraphy soon became apparent. Detailed lymphoscintigraphic studies by Uren, Thompson et al. in the 1990s, undertaken in the course of SN mapping for melanoma and breast cancer, provided important new insights into lymphatic anatomy that had major implications for melanoma surgery [86, 87].

Treatment of Metastatic Melanoma with Conventional Systemic Therapies: 1960 to 2010

Chemotherapy

For half a century, following the introduction of cytotoxic chemotherapy for solid human cancers in the 1950s, efforts in treating metastatic melanoma focused largely on attempts to use this class of drugs to achieve standard clinical endpoints: tumor shrinkage (response), durable response, improved progression-free survival, and prolonged overall survival. Clinical trialists recognized early that, as with other solid cancers, the most relevant of these was overall survival. Metastatic melanoma is relatively resistant to treatment with cytotoxic drugs, with no convincing evidence from randomized, controlled trials that any form of chemotherapy prolongs overall survival. Partial responses to single agents occurred in less than 25% of treated patients, and complete responses in less than 5% [88]. The median duration of response was 5–6 months. Although other cytotoxic drugs had similar or possibly slightly superior response rates, the standard of care throughout this period was single-agent dacarbazine (DTIC), yet in only 2% of patients treated with DTIC were long-term complete responses observed [89].

Immunotherapy

Adoptive immunotherapy using expanded pools of autologous tumor-infiltrating lymphocytes, when infused into selected immune-conditioned patients, showed clear activity against metastatic melanoma and, in a subgroup of selected patients, long-term disease control was observed [90]. This work by Steven Rosenberg at the National Cancer Institute, Surgery Branch in Bethesda, Maryland, as well as many others, clearly and convincingly established the proof of principle that immunotherapy had a central role in the treatment of metastatic melanoma. However, the intensive and costly nature of the original protocols and its associated toxicity led to its utilization only in highly selected centers.

Trials with interleukin-2, reported by Atkins et al., showed long-term disease control in a subgroup of patients with metastatic melanoma, leading to FDA approval of this cytokine [91]. Toxicity and lack of randomized, phase 3 data resulted in the regimen being confined to just a few centers, mostly in the United States. Other cytokines, like interferon-alpha, had limited activity as single agents, and when interferon-alpha and interleukin-2 were combined with chemotherapy ("biochemotherapy") there was no survival advantage over single-agent dacarbazine [92], despite substantially greater toxicity.

The Early-Twenty-First-Century Revolution in Melanoma Treatment: Targeted Therapies and Immune Checkpoint Inhibitors

The frequency and potential importance of driver BRAF mutations in melanoma were known from the late 1990s, together with the fact that the MAP kinase pathway was constitutively activated in more than 90% of cases. Early attempts to use small molecules to block MAP kinase activation were made with fairly nonspecific "pan"-RAF inhibitors, such as sorafenib. These showed minimal single-agent clinical activity and a brief signal of synergy between sorafenib with other cytotoxic drugs failed to stand up to phase 3 testing [93]. It took a decade to develop potent, selective drugs to target and inhibit mutant BRAF and its downstream substrate kinase, MEK. The first of these selective agents, vemurafenib, was a landmark development, with the results of a phase 1 trial first presented in 2010 [94]. Its spectacular induction of rapid metabolic responses in metastatic melanoma resulted in front-page headlines in the *New York Times*. In around 80% of patients with a specific point mutation within the BRAF gene, there was substantial or even complete regression of bulky metastatic disease, far superior to dacarbazine, and a significant improvement in all clinical endpoints, including overall survival [95].

Subsequent refinements in MAP kinase targeting included the development of other effective mutant BRAF inhibitors like dabrafenib and encorafenib, with similar activity to vemurafenib, but with markedly different toxicity profiles. It was also demonstrated that dabrafenib was active against brain metastases [96], and that there was an extension of progression-free and overall survival when MEK inhibitors were combined with inhibitors of mutant BRAF [97]. The combination of BRAF and MEK inhibitors had the additional advantage of abrogating premalignant and malignant keratopathy from single-agent BRAF inhibitors. However, despite the massive progress achieved with the introduction of MAPK inhibitors, nearly all treated patients eventually developed resistance to them, with >50% showing disease progression within 12 months. This was due to reactivation of the MAPK pathway via alternative pathways. It was immediately recognized by clinicians and researchers worldwide that another strategy was clearly required.

Fortunately, in parallel developments, clinical trials were under way using monoclonal antibodies targeting the complex synapse between, on the one hand, T cells and antigen-presenting cells (the afferent arm of the immune response) and, on the other hand, T cells and melanoma cells (the efferent arm). The first of these so-called immune checkpoint inhibitors, ipilimumab, targeted the CTLA4 receptor, a cell surface molecule on T cells which mediates inhibition of T-cell activation in the afferent immune response. Despite achieving only low levels of RECIST tumor response, long-term disease control was achieved in a subset of patients with metastatic melanoma treated with ipilimumab. Phase 3 trials confirmed an overall survival benefit over dacarbazine, and pooled trial results showed a plateau on the Kaplan-Meier curve, with around 26% of treatment-naïve patients exhibiting progression-free survival at up to 10 years of follow-up [98].

A further landmark discovery was the demonstration that monoclonal antibodies inhibiting the synapse between the programmed death receptor 1(PD1) on T cells and its ligand, PDL1 on tumor cells, resulted in profound T-cell activation in many patients, with substantial consequent tumor cell death. The first two anti-PD1 drugs to be approved by the FDA were pembrolizumab (initially named lambrolizumab) and nivolumab (reviewed by Lee et al. [99]). Both drugs showed RECIST tumor responses in 30–40% of treated melanoma patients, with significant improvements in progression-free and overall survival in phase 3 trials. Patients achieving a complete response to therapy rarely relapsed within 3 years of follow-up. Further improvements in response rates and other clinical endpoints were obtained with combinations of the checkpoint inhibitors, ipilimumab/nivolumab and ipilimumab/pembrolizumab. Many more immune checkpoint inhibitors are in clinical development, with a vast array of potential combinations in the pipeline.

Summary and Conclusions

Cutaneous melanoma has been recognized as an entity for more than two millennia. Once considered to be an uncommon disease, its incidence worldwide has increased substantially since detailed population-based statistics began to be collected in the 1960s, and continues to increase. Surgery was the mainstay of treatment throughout the twentieth century, and even today 80% of patients are still cured by surgery alone. The extent of surgical intervention is clearly less invasive than previously, minimizing the potential for serious postsurgical side effects and complications. Whereas previously the outlook was dismal for those who developed inoperable metastatic disease, effective systemic therapies in the form of immunotherapy and checkpoint inhibitors have revolutionized our current approach to patients with metastatic melanoma. It is now a reality that a select group of patients with metastatic melanoma can achieve long-term, often lifetime, disease-free survival after such treatment. The history of melanoma continues to be written, as incredible advances in our treatment of this disease continue to be made.

References

1. Rebecca VW, Sondak VK, Smalley KS. A brief history of melanoma: from mummies to mutations. Melanoma Res. 2012;22:114–22.
2. Rotte A, Bhandaru M. Melanoma—introduction, history and epidemiology. Immunotherapy of melanoma. Cham: Springer International Publishing AG; 2016. p. 3–20.
3. Laennec RTH. Extrait au memoire de M Laennec, sur les melanoses. Paris: Bull L'Ecole Societie de Medicine; 1812; p. 24.
4. Gorantla VC, Kirkwood JM. State of melanoma: an historic overview of a field in transition. Hematol Oncol Clin North Am. 2014;28:415–35.

5. Urteaga O, Pack GT. On the antiquity of melanoma. Cancer. 1966;19:607–10.
6. McGovern VJ. Melanoblastoma. Med J Aust. 1952;1:139–42.
7. Paget J. Lectures on surgical pathology. In: Turner W, editor. . London: Longman, Brown, Green and Longman; 1853. p. 639.
8. Moles and malignant melanoma: terminology and classification. Med J Aust. 1967;1:123–5.
9. de Vries E, Bray F, Coebergh JW, et al. Melanocytic tumours. In: PE LB, Burg G, Weedon D, Sarasin A, editors. World Health Organisation classification of tumours: pathology and genetics of skin tumours. Lyon: International Agency for Research on Cancer (IARC) Press; 2006. p. 49–120.
10. Clark WH Jr, From L, Bernardino EA, et al. The histogenesis and biologic behavior of primary human malignant melanomas of the skin. Cancer Res. 1969;29:705–27.
11. McGovern VJ. The classification of melanoma and its relationship with prognosis. Pathology. 1970;2:85–98.
12. Mihm MC Jr, Clark WH Jr, From L. The clinical diagnosis, classification and histogenetic concepts of the early stages of cutaneous malignant melanomas. N Engl J Med. 1971;284:1078–82.
13. Allen AC, Spitz S. Malignant melanoma; a clinicopathological analysis of the criteria for diagnosis and prognosis. Cancer. 1953;6:1–45.
14. Breslow A. Thickness, cross-sectional areas and depth of invasion in the prognosis of cutaneous melanoma. Ann Surg. 1970;172:902–8.
15. Gershenwald JE, Scolyer RA, Hess KR, et al. for members of the American Joint Committee on Cancer Melanoma Expert P, the International Melanoma D, Discovery P. Melanoma staging: Evidence-based changes in the American Joint Committee on Cancer eighth edition cancer staging manual. CA Cancer J Clin 2017;67:472–492
16. McGovern VJ, Mihm MC Jr, Bailly C, et al. The classification of malignant melanoma and its histologic reporting. Cancer. 1973;32:1446–57.
17. Arrington JH 3rd, Reed RJ, Ichinose H, et al. Plantar lentiginous melanoma: a distinctive variant of human cutaneous malignant melanoma. Am J Surg Pathol. 1977;1:131–43.
18. McGovern VJ, Cochran AJ, Van der Esch EP, et al. The classification of malignant melanoma, its histological reporting and registration: a revision of the 1972 Sydney classification. Pathology. 1986;18:12–21.
19. Bahmer FA, Bahmer JA. Cutaneous melanoma—"black death" of modern times? Traces in contemporary literature. Hautarzt. 2013;64:864–7.
20. Thompson JF, Scolyer RA, Kefford RF. Cutaneous melanoma in the era of molecular profiling. Lancet. 2009;374:362–5.
21. Curtin JA, Fridlyand J, Kageshita T, et al. Distinct sets of genetic alterations in melanoma. N Engl J Med. 2005;353:2135–47.
22. Cancer Genome Atlas Network. Genomic classification of cutaneous melanoma. Cell. 2015;161:1681–96.
23. Norris W. Eight cases of melanosis with pathological and therapeutic remarks on that disease. London: Longman and Robarts; 1857.
24. Norris W. Case of fungoid disease. Edinburgh Med Surg J. 1820;16:562–5.
25. Begg CB, Orlow I, Hummer AJ, et al. Lifetime risk of melanoma in CDKN2A mutation carriers in a population-based sample. J Natl Cancer Inst. 2005;97:1507–15.
26. Pemberton O. On melanosis. Observations on the history, pathology and treatment of cancerous disease. London: John Churchill; 1858. p. 1–38.
27. Davis NC, Shaw HM, McCarthy WH. Melanoma: an historical perspective. In: Thompson JF, Morton DL, Kroon BBR, editors. Textbook of melanoma. London, UK: Martin Dunitz; 2004. p. 1–12.
28. Randle HW. Suntanning: differences in perceptions throughout history. Mayo Clin Proc. 1997;72:461–6.
29. Lancaster HO. Some geographical aspects of the mortality from melanoma in Europeans. Med J Aust. 1956;43:1082–7.
30. Cooper AGS. The contribution of radiotherapy to the problem of skin cancer in Queensland. Acta Radiol Suppl. 1959;188:61–70.
31. Sarnat BG, Schour I. Oral and facial cancer. Chicago: The Yearbook Publishers, Inc.; 1950.
32. Lancaster HO, Nelson J. Sunlight as a cause of melanoma; a clinical survey. Med J Aust. 1957;44:452–6.
33. Cooper S. The first lines of the theory and practice of surgery. London: Longman; 1840.
34. Home E. Observations on cancer, connected with histories of the disease. London: W. Bulmer and Co.; 1805.
35. Bodenham DC. A study of 650 observed malignant melanomas in the south-west region. Ann R Coll Surg Engl. 1968;43:218–39.
36. Fergusson A. Recurrence of a melanotic tumour: removal. Lancet. 1851;57:622.
37. McCarthy WH, Shaw HM. The surgical treatment of primary melanoma. Hematol Oncol Clin North Am. 1998;12:797–805.
38. Snow H. Melanotic cancerous disease. Lancet. 1892;140:872–4.
39. Eve F. A lecture on melanoma. Practitioner. 1903;70:165–74.
40. Handley WS. The pathology of melanotic growths in relation to their operative treatment. Lancet. 1907;169:927–33.
41. Pringle JH. A method of operation in melanotic tumours of the skin. Edinb Med J. 1908;23:496–9.
42. Balch CM, Soong S, Ross MI, et al. Long-term results of a multi-institutional randomized trial comparing prognostic factors and surgical results for intermediate thickness melanomas (1.0 to 4.0 mm). Intergroup Melanoma Surgical Trial. Ann Surg Oncol. 2000;7:87–97.
43. Cascinelli N, Morabito A, Santinami M, et al. Immediate or delayed dissection of regional nodes in patients with melanoma of the trunk: a randomised trial. WHO Melanoma Programme. Lancet. 1998;351:793–6.

44. Röntgen WC, Stokes GGB, Thomson JJ. Röntgen rays—memoirs by Röntgen, Stokes and JJ Thomson. New York and London: Harper & Brothers Publishers; 1899.
45. Becquerel H. Sur les radiations émises par phosphorescence. C R Acad Sci. 1896;122:420–1.
46. Curie P, Curie M, Bémont MG. Sur une nouvelle substance fortement redio-active, contenue dans la pechblende. C R Acad Sci. 1898;127:1215–7.
47. Coutard H. The results and methods of treatment of cancer by radiation. Ann Surg. 1937;106:584–98.
48. Dewey DL. The radiosensitivity of melanoma cells in culture. Br J Radiol. 1971;44:816–7.
49. Barranco SC, Romsdahl MM, Humphrey RM. The radiation response of human malignant melanoma cells grown in vitro. Cancer Res. 1971;31:830–3.
50. Johanson CR, Harwood AR, Cummings BJ, et al. 0-7-21 radiotherapy in nodular melanoma. Cancer. 1983;51:226–32.
51. Burmeister BH, Henderson MA, Ainslie J, et al. Adjuvant radiotherapy versus observation alone for patients at risk of lymph-node field relapse after therapeutic lymphadenectomy for melanoma: a randomised trial. Lancet Oncol. 2012;13:589–97.
52. Overgaard J, Gonzalez Gonzalez D, Hulshof MC, et al. Hyperthermia as an adjuvant to radiation therapy of recurrent or metastatic malignant melanoma. A multicentre randomized trial by the European Society for Hyperthermic Oncology. Int J Hyperth. 1996;12:3–20.
53. Larsson BS, Larsson B, Roberto A. Boron neutron capture therapy for malignant melanoma: an experimental approach. Pigment Cell Res. 1989;2:356–60.
54. Raja C, Graham P, Abbas Rizvi SM, et al. Interim analysis of toxicity and response in phase 1 trial of systemic targeted alpha therapy for metastatic melanoma. Cancer Biol Ther. 2007;6:846–52.
55. Lawton AW. Proton beam therapy for uveal melanoma. Ophthalmology. 1989;96:138–9.
56. Marucci L, Ancukiewicz M, Lane AM, et al. Uveal melanoma recurrence after fractionated proton beam therapy: comparison of survival in patients treated with reirradiation or with enucleation. Int J Radiat Oncol Biol Phys. 2011;79:842–6.
57. Yaeh A, Nanda T, Jani A, et al. Control of brain metastases from radioresistant tumors treated by stereotactic radiosurgery. J Neuro-Oncol. 2015;124:507–14.
58. Okwan-Duodu D, Pollack BP, Lawson D, et al. Role of radiation therapy as immune activator in the era of modern immunotherapy for metastatic malignant melanoma. Am J Clin Oncol. 2015;38:119–25.
59. Creech O Jr, Krementz ET, Ryan RF, et al. Chemotherapy of cancer: regional perfusion utilizing an extracorporeal circuit. Ann Surg. 1958;148:616–32.
60. Kapma MR, Vrouenraets BC, Nieweg OE, et al. Major amputation for intractable extremity melanoma after failure of isolated limb perfusion. Eur J Surg Oncol. 2005;31:95–9.
61. Thompson JF, Waugh RC, Saw RPM, et al. Isolated limb infusion with melphalan for recurrent limb melanoma: a simple alternative to isolated limb perfusion. Regional Cancer Treatment. 1994;7:188–92.
62. Kroon HM, Coventry BJ, Giles MH, et al. Australian multicenter study of isolated limb infusion for melanoma. Ann Surg Oncol. 2016;23:1096–103.
63. Coley WB. The therapeutic value of the mixed toxins of the streptococcus of erysipelas and bacillus prodigiosus in the treatment of inoperable malignant tumors. With a report of 160 cases. Am J Med Sci. 1896;112:251–81.
64. Nathanson L, Schoenfeld D, Regelson W, et al. Prospective comparison of intralesional and multipuncture BCG in recurrent intradermal melanoma. Cancer. 1979;43:1630–5.
65. Krown SE, Hilal EY, Pinsky CM, et al. Intralesional injection of the methanol extraction residue of bacillus Calmette-Guerin (MER) into cutaneous metastases of malignant melanoma. Cancer. 1978;42:2648–60.
66. Mastrangelo MJ, Sulit HL, Prehn LM, et al. Intralesional BCG in the treatment of metastatic malignant melanoma. Cancer. 1976;37:684–92.
67. Oratz R, Hauschild A, Sebastian G, et al. Intratumoral cisplatin/adrenaline injectable gel for the treatment of patients with cutaneous and soft tissue metastases of malignant melanoma. Melanoma Res. 2003;13:59–66.
68. Adler A, Stein JA, Kedar E, et al. Intralesional injection of interleukin-2-expanded autologous lymphocytes in melanoma and breast cancer patients: a pilot study. J Biol Response Mod. 1984;3:491–500.
69. Thompson JF, Hersey P, Wachter E. Chemoablation of metastatic melanoma using intralesional rose Bengal. Melanoma Res. 2008;18:405–11.
70. Andtbacka RH, Kaufman HL, Collichio F, et al. Talimogene Laherparepvec improves durable response rate in patients with advanced melanoma. J Clin Oncol. 2015;33:2780–8.
71. Allen BJ, Raja C, Rizvi S, et al. Intralesional targeted alpha therapy for metastatic melanoma. Role of electrochemotherapy in the treatment of metastatic melanoma and other metastatic and primary skin tumors [Review]. Cancer Biol Ther. 2006;5:118–9.
72. Byrne CM, Thompson JF, Johnston H, et al. Treatment of metastatic melanoma using electroporation therapy with bleomycin (electrochemotherapy). Melanoma Res. 2005;15:45–51.
73. Campana LG, Testori A, Mozzillo N, et al. Treatment of metastatic melanoma with electrochemotherapy. J Surg Oncol. 2014;109:301–7.
74. Dolinsek T, Prosen L, Cemazar M, et al. Electrochemotherapy with bleomycin is effective in BRAF mutated melanoma cells and interacts with BRAF inhibitors. Radiol Oncol. 2016;50:274–9.
75. Kunte C, Letule V, Gehl J, et al. Electrochemotherapy in the treatment of metastatic malignant melanoma: a prospective cohort study by InspECT. Br J Dermatol. 2017;176(6):1475–85.
76. Okino M, Mohri H. Effects of a high-voltage electrical impulse and an anticancer drug on in vivo growing tumors. Jpn J Cancer Res. 1987;78:1319–21.
77. Damian DL, Thompson JF. Treatment of extensive cutaneous metastatic melanoma with topical diphencyprone. J Am Acad Dermatol. 2007;56:869–71.

78. Delamere G, Poirier P, Charpy A. The lymphatics: general anatomy of the Lymphatics, with special study of the Lymphatics in different parts of the body. Westminster: Archibald Constable & Co. Ltd; 1903.
79. Bartholin T. De lacteis thoracicis in homine brutisque nuperrime observatis, historia anatomica. Martzan, M: Copenhagen, Denmark; 1652.
80. Nieweg OE, Uren RF, Thompson JF. The history of sentinel lymph node biopsy. Cancer J. 2015;21:3–6.
81. Virchow R. Die Krankhaften Geschwulste. Berlin, Germany: Hirschwald; 1863.
82. Morton DL, Wen DR, Wong JH, et al. Technical details of intraoperative lymphatic mapping for early stage melanoma. Arch Surg. 1992;127:392–9.
83. Morton DL, Thompson JF, Cochran AJ, et al. Sentinel-node biopsy or nodal observation in melanoma. N Engl J Med. 2006;355:1307–17.
84. Morton DL, Thompson JF, Cochran AJ, et al. Final trial report of sentinel-node biopsy versus nodal observation in melanoma. N Engl J Med. 2014;370:599–609.
85. Faries MB, Thompson JF, Cochran AJ, et al. Completion Dissection or Observation for Sentinel-Node Metastasis in Melanoma. N Engl J Med. 2017;376:2211–2222.
86. Thompson JF, Uren RF, Shaw HM, et al. Location of sentinel lymph nodes in patients with cutaneous melanoma: new insights into lymphatic anatomy. J Am Coll Surg. 1999;189:195–204.
87. Uren RF, Howman-Giles RB, Shaw HM, et al. Lymphoscintigraphy in high-risk melanoma of the trunk: predicting draining node groups, defining lymphatic channels and locating the sentinel node. J Nucl Med. 1993;34:1435–40.
88. Hill GJ 2nd, Krementz ET, Hill HZ. Dimethyl triazeno imidazole carboxamide and combination therapy for melanoma. IV. Late results after complete response to chemotherapy (Central Oncology Group protocols 7130, 7131, and 7131A). Cancer. 1984;53:1299–305.
89. Coates AS, Segelov E. Long term response to chemotherapy in patients with visceral metastatic melanoma. Ann Oncol. 1994;5:249–51.
90. Dudley ME, Yang JC, Sherry R, et al. Adoptive cell therapy for patients with metastatic melanoma: evaluation of intensive myeloablative chemoradiation preparative regimens. J Clin Oncol. 2008;26:5233–9.
91. Atkins MB, Lotze MT, Dutcher JP, et al. High-dose recombinant interleukin 2 therapy for patients with metastatic melanoma: analysis of 270 patients treated between 1985 and 1993. J Clin Oncol. 1999;17:2105–16.
92. Atkins MB, Hsu J, Lee S, et al. Phase III trial comparing concurrent biochemotherapy with cisplatin, vinblastine, dacarbazine, interleukin-2, and interferon alfa-2b with cisplatin, vinblastine, and dacarbazine alone in patients with metastatic malignant melanoma (E3695): a trial coordinated by the eastern cooperative oncology group. J Clin Oncol. 2008;26:5748–54.
93. Flaherty KT, Lee SJ, Zhao F, et al. Phase III trial of carboplatin and paclitaxel with or without sorafenib in metastatic melanoma. J Clin Oncol. 2013;31:373–9.
94. Flaherty KT, Puzanov I, Kim KB, et al. Inhibition of mutated, activated BRAF in metastatic melanoma. N Engl J Med. 2010;363:809–19.
95. Chapman PB, Hauschild A, Robert C, et al. Improved survival with vemurafenib in melanoma with BRAF V600E mutation. N Engl J Med. 2011;364:2507–16.
96. Falchook GS, Long GV, Kurzrock R, et al. Dabrafenib in patients with melanoma, untreated brain metastases, and other solid tumours: a phase 1 dose-escalation trial. Lancet. 2012;379:1893–901.
97. Flaherty KT, Robert C, Hersey P, et al. Improved survival with MEK inhibition in BRAF-mutated melanoma. N Engl J Med. 2012;367:107–14.
98. Schadendorf D, Hodi FS, Robert C, et al. Pooled analysis of long-term survival data from phase II and phase III trials of Ipilimumab in unresectable or metastatic melanoma. J Clin Oncol. 2015;33:1889–94.
99. Lee J, Kefford R, Carlino M. PD-1 and PD-L1 inhibitors in melanoma treatment: past success, present application and future challenges. Immunotherapy. 2016;8:733–46.

Anatomy and Physiology of the Skin

2

Amir Dehdashtian, Thomas P. Stringer, Abby Joan Warren, Euphemia W. Mu, Bardia Amirlak, and Ladan Shahabi

Basic Anatomy of the Skin, Associated Structures, and Their Relationship to the Development of Melanoma

Though delivering a deeper and more nuanced understanding of melanoma is the goal of this text, a brief review of the function and structures of the skin is necessary before narrowing its focus to pigmented lesions.

The epidermis, a stratified squamous keratinized epithelium, is the outermost layer of the skin, lying closest to the external environment (Fig. 2.1). As such, its primary function is that of a self-renewing barrier. The epidermis denies entry to pathogens and other foreign objects, protects the body from DNA damage wrought by ultraviolet (UV) radiation, and retains water. The epidermis is divided into five layers: the stratum corneum, stratum lucidum, stratum granulosum, stratum spinosum, and stratum basale.

Perched atop the dermo-epidermal junction that divides dermis from epidermis (Fig. 2.1), the stratum basale (also known as the stratum germinativum) is the epidermal layer furthest from the external environment. It contains the germinating keratinocytes, the fundamental epidermal cells which allow the epidermis to constantly replenish itself [1]. The journey of a keratinocyte from this germinal layer to the skin's surface ranges from 15 to 30 days in duration. In addition to keratinocyte precursors, the stratum basale is also home to more specialized cells such as melanocytes, Langerhans cells, and Merkel cells. Respectively, these cells function as protection from UV light, antigen-presenting cells (APCs), and traffickers of neuroendocrine peptides. The stratum basale also projects pillars of tissue into the subjacent dermis. These are known as rete ridges, which help safeguard the epidermis against shear trauma [2].

Within the cells of the stratum spinosum, keratinocytes begin to produce cytokeratin. Out of this raw material, they manufacture intermediate tonofilaments, which in turn form the basis of tonofibrils. The name of the stratum spinosum is derived from the spiny appearance of intercellular connections comprised of tonofibrils, which are in turn fastened by desmosomes [3]. Through the alignment of tonofilaments and tonofibrils, the keratinocytes of the stratum spinosum transition from the cuboi-

A. Dehdashtian, M.D., M.P.H.
School of Medicine, School of Public Health, Tehran University of Medical Sciences, Tehran, Iran
e-mail: Dehdashtian.am@gmail.com

T. P. Stringer, M.D., M.S.
Ronald O. Perelman Department of Dermatology, NYU School of Medicine, New York, NY, USA
e-mail: thomas.stringer89@gmail.com

A. J. Warren, M.D. · B. Amirlak, M.D., F.A.C.S. (✉)
Department of Plastic Surgery, UT Southwestern Medical Center, Dallas, TX, USA
e-mail: abby.warren@phhs.org; bardia.amirlak@utsouthwestern.edu

E. W. Mu, M. D. · L. Shahabi, M.D., F.A.A.D.
Ronald O. Perelman Department of Dermatology, NYU Langone Medical Center, New York, NY, USA
e-mail: euphemia.mu@nyumc.org; ladanshahabi@gmail.com

A. I. Riker (ed.), *Melanoma*, https://doi.org/10.1007/978-3-319-78310-9_2

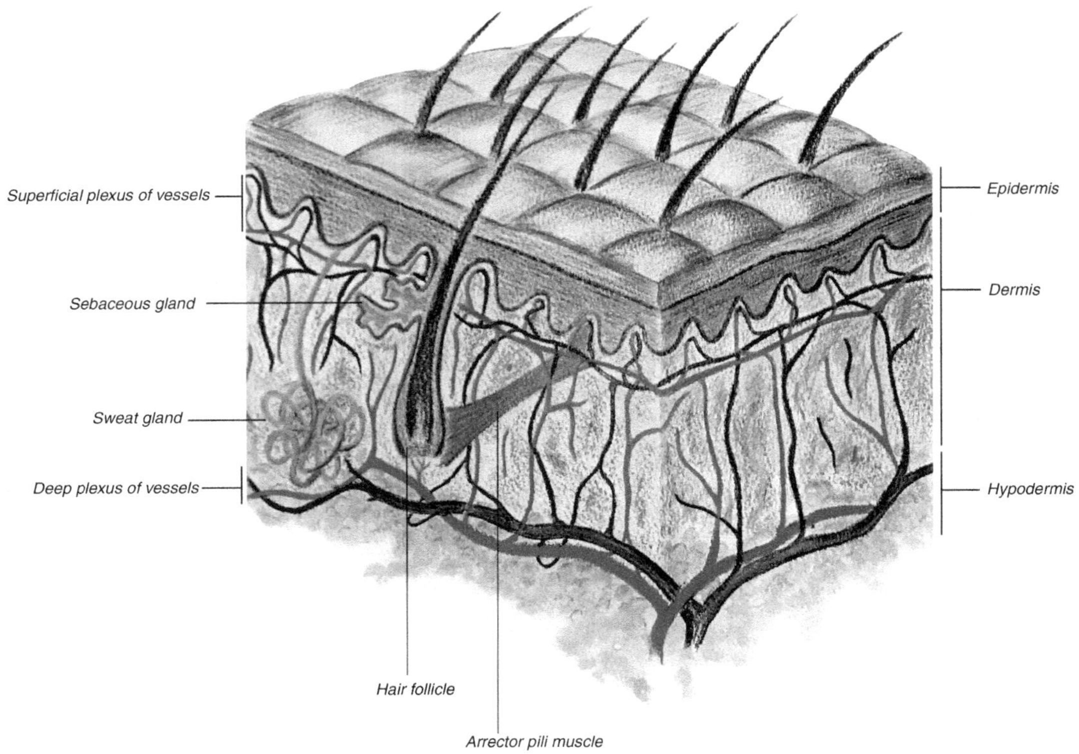

Fig. 2.1 Anatomy of the skin

dal and polyhedral forms of the stratum basale to the flattened cells of upper strata. Langerhans cells, which help to initiate the cascade of adaptive immunity by presenting foreign antigens to T-cells, localize primarily to this epidermal layer [4].

At the stratum granulosum, the final layer of transition between the strata spinosum and corneum, nucleated keratinocytes secrete lamellar bodies containing lipid granules which comprise the major permeability barrier of the epidermis [5]. This layer gains its name from the abundant cytoplasmic granules filled with cytoskeletal proteins evident on histological and immunohistochemical examination.

The stratum lucidum, considered to be a subdivision of the supervening stratum corneum, is only present in areas of thick skin. Thick skin is present in regions of the body such as the palms and soles that are subject to a high degree of shear stress [6]. It is so named because its cells appear translucent with thickened cell membranes on histological examination [7].

The stratum corneum is comprised of terminally differentiated, enucleate skin cells known as corneocytes. The most common metaphor employed in the description of the stratum corneum is that of a "brick and mortar" system, in which the corneocytes are bricks and intercellular lipids mortar. These lipids, synthesized by the stratum granulosum beneath, serve as the permeability barrier for the skin. Corneocytes are joined together by desmosomes, and their degradation by proteolytic enzymes causes the sloughing off of corneocytes known as desquamation. The thickness of stratum corneum accounts for the greater epidermal depth of thick skin [8]. Though the stratum corneum was initially thought to be a passive and inert deposition of cells, recent studies suggest that this epidermal layer may be more metabolically active than previously thought, particularly in its crosstalk with the stratum granulosum [9].

The dermis receives the preponderance of the skin's blood supply as well as the deeper extensions of skin features such as eccrine glands, apocrine glands, and hair follicles (Fig. 2.1). Rather than keratinocytes, it contains fibroblasts, dendritic cells, and mast cells. The fibroblasts synthesize a great number of collagen, reticular, and elastic fibers which interweave to increase dermal resilience and optimize its protection of the epidermis [10]. A ground substance composed of glycoproteins and proteoglycans provides the medium in which the cellular and fibrillar elements of the dermis contend.

The dermis is subdivided into two layers: the superficial or papillary dermis, and the deep or reticular dermis. True to its name, the superficial dermis covers papillary dermal projections which interlock with the rete ridges of the stratum basale for greater protection against shear forces. Due to its interface with the avascular epidermis, it is the point of inflection for looped capillaries which exchange oxygen and waste products with the epidermis. Meanwhile, the deeper dermis contains the encapsulated bodies of mechanoreceptors such as Ruffini and Pacinian corpuscles [11].

Traditionally, the white adipose and loose connective tissues underlying the dermis have been considered under the aegis of encompassing terms such as "hypodermis" or "subcutis." However, studies have indicated that depots of dermal adipose have genetic and morphological profiles distinct from subcutaneous white adipose tissue [12]. Researchers are even now attempting to elucidate the precise role of this adipose tissue in the signaling of metabolic processes such as hair growth cycling [13].

We now turn our attention to the melanocyte, the cellular clou of melanoma. Melanocytes produce melanin, the compound which serves as pigment in the skin of vertebrates. Dysregulation of these cells can give rise to malignancy.

The primordium of the melanocyte lies in the embryologic structure known as the neural tube. As development progresses, the dorsal eminence of this tube shifts from epithelial to mesenchymal tissue, thereby becoming the neural crest. Neural crest cells (NCCs) are multipotent stem cells that migrate throughout the body to form derivatives such as craniofacial cartilage, peripheral nerves, endocrine cells, and melanocytes. In this embryologic diaspora, the neural crest cells that will become melanocytes originate in the truncal province of the neural crest and exit dorsolaterally to sites throughout the nascent epidermis, inner ear, iris, and choroid [14]. Studies in chicks have demonstrated that an additional population of melanocytes derived from Schwann cells migrate ventrally, though whether this is recapitulated in mammals is not yet known [15]. Recent work further suggests that genes which govern signaling pathways essential to melanocyte ontogeny may also play a role in melanoma [16, 17].

Following their migration to the epidermis, cutaneous melanocytes are positioned by external molecular signals into hair follicles, whereupon they assume their primary function: the manufacture of melanin and its transport to keratinocytes [18]. Within the melanocyte, melanin is produced from tyrosine, a progenitor shared with dopamine, in a specialized lysosome known as a melanosome. Through sharing pigment with several dozen keratinocytes, melanocytes are integrated into an epidermal-melanin unit; this functional linkage represents a rare occasion in which an organelle is transferred from a cell of one histologic subtype to another [19, 20].

Melanin itself is subdivided into two types: pheomelanin, which is alkali soluble and light red/yellow in coloration, and eumelanin, an alkali-insoluble, dark brown/blue compound [21]. Its functions are diverse and a subject of fervent investigation. Most apparent is its determination of skin pigmentation, which is derived from the activity of melanocytes and the type of melanin they produce rather than the strength of their numbers [22]. Further, melanin helps to protect skin against damage from UV light. Acutely, UV radiation may induce erythema, photodamage, and immunosuppression; chronically, it has been shown to cause photoaging and photocarcinogenesis [23]. The effect of UV radiation on human skin and the mechanisms by which melanin mitigates photodamage will be covered in a later section.

Melanosomes are the vehicle through which melanocytes transfer melanin to keratinocytes and produce pigmentation of the skin. The biogenesis and maturation of the melanosome as it travels towards a keratinocyte have been subdivided into four stages based on early work with electron microscopy. The origins of the melanosome are much speculated upon; some studies suggest that it is a product of the endoplasmic reticulum, while others maintain that its provenance lies in later secretory pathways. A melanosome in stage I is a perinuclear, membrane-bound vesicle resembling an early lysosome [24]. Stage II melanosomes, or pre-melanosomes, are defined as containing fibrous striations but lacking pigment. EM studies in melanoma cell lines have demonstrated that the protein, Pmel17, is in large part responsible for the formation of melanosomal striations, though the intricacies of its manufacture and localization have yet to be elucidated [25]. In stage III melanosomes, melanin is observed to be deposited upon these fibrous striations, and in stage IV the organelle is filled with pigment.

It is necessary for a melanocyte to transfer melanosomes to neighboring keratinocytes to effect skin pigmentation. This is accomplished through dendrite processes that extend from the melanocytes. Melanosomes are translocated towards the plus or minus ends of a dendritic microtubule by kinesin and dynesin, respectively. Once reaching the tip of a microtubule, they are captured by the keratinocyte through the complexion of actin with myosin type-Va.

Though a variety of mechanisms have been described, evidential consensus presently centers on two hypotheses: the "shedding-phagocytosis" model and the "exocytosis-endocytosis" model [26]. The former describes a sequence of events wherein a melanocyte extrudes membrane-bound packets of melanosomes that are subsequently phagocytosed by the receiving keratinocyte. The latter refers to a process in which the melanin core of the melanosome is exocytosed into the extracellular space by a melanocyte and then taken up by a keratinocyte. It remains to be seen which of the two takes place in humans—indeed, the two may not be mutually exclusive.

The ultimate function of the melanocyte and melanin is to interact with sunlight. Ultraviolet radiation emanates from our sun and exerts pleiotropic effects upon human cells, particularly those of the skin. The UVR which reaches the earth's surface is divided into two subtypes: long-wavelength (320–400 nm) UVA and short-wavelength (200–280 nm) UV-B [27]. Of these, UVB, though comprising only 5% of terrestrial UVR, has been demonstrated to be a far more potent provocateur of erythema, melanogenesis, and DNA damage [28, 29]. Humanity's first line of protection against UVB is the ozone layer, though it is thought that anthropogenic climate change may be weakening this natural defense [30]. By contrast, UVA is not filtered even by window glass and penetrates deeper into the dermis than its short-wave coeval. Both play a distinct role in the DNA-damaging properties of sunlight. UVA is thought to generate reactive oxygen species (ROS) which induce single-strand breaks in DNA, while UVB has been demonstrated to be directly toxic to genetic material, generating cyclobutane pyrimidine dimers and pyrimidine-pyrimidone photoproducts [31–33]. It is principally through these mechanisms that ultraviolet light initiates carcinogenesis.

What role does melanin play in the protection of skin from UV damage and the ensuing risk of melanoma? Epidemiological and empirical evidence alike has long demonstrated that darker pigmented skin is better protected from the consequences of solar radiation than light skin. Eumelanin, which is far more abundant in dark skin, performs multiple functions to safeguard the skin from UVR, acting to block and disperse UVR as well as scavenge associated free radicals [27, 34].

Lymphatic Anatomy and Its Relation to Specific Draining Patterns for a Primary Melanoma

Malignant melanoma is considered one of the most aggressive neoplasms. Ninety percent of local metastasis occurs via lymphatic vessels, and the tumor tends to metastasize early in regional lymph nodes. Hematogenous dissemination of tumor cells is also possible; however, this is less common and more difficult to assess and treat [35, 36].

As hydrostatic pressure causes plasma proteins and fluid to escape the circulation of the skin, blind-ended lymphatic capillaries are responsible for their return to the circulation. These capillaries form in the interstitial spaces of papillary dermis as unvalved vessels, and drain into deep dermal and subcutaneous plexuses. In this area, these vessels are larger and have valves. These large-caliber vessels then merge together and create lymphatic collectors, which are in turn filtered by multiple lymph nodes before connecting to the venous system.

Melanoma metastasis happens through three main pathways which influence the prognostic staging of primary melanoma [37]. These include satellite or in-transit metastasis, lymph node metastasis, and distant metastasis. Satellite metastasis is the presence of skin or subcutaneous metastases within two centimeters of the primary lesion, while in-transit metastasis is defined as the presence of metastases in a lymphatic drainage area before involving the sentinel lymph node [38, 39].

Evidence suggests that early detection and removal of lymph nodes with micrometastasis (i.e., infiltration with melanoma cells regardless of metastatic pathway) will improve the prognosis of patients with primary melanoma [40, 41]. To achieve this, accurate location of the responsible regional lymph nodes is mandatory. In 1874, Sappey conducted experiments in which he cannulated the lymphatic vessels and injected them with mercury, thereby mapping lymphatic circulation. He then postulated that lymphatic drainage between the two sides of the body is symmetric and that lymphatic vessels neither cross the assumptive vertical midline nor the horizontal line around the waist at the level of the umbilicus [42]. These boundaries, dividing the body into four areas, were thereafter called Sappey's lines. He concluded that lymphatics of any of these areas drain to the corresponding axillary or groin lymph nodes.

Sappey's results were widely accepted until the 1970s, when Sugarbaker and McBride used lymphoscintigraphy to reveal an ambiguous area of 2.5 cm on each side of Sappey's lines with unpredictable lymphatic drainage [43]. In 1991, Norman et al. showed that lymphatic drainage is also unpredictable in the head and neck and therefore suggested an expansion of the ambiguous area to 11 cm on either side of Sappey's lines [44]. Further study has shown that Sappey's demarcation of lymphatic drainage may not be useful in 30% of patients, in which an individual pattern for lymphatic drainage was found in comparable areas of the skin. The most recent comprehensive review, which used lymphoscintigraphy data from 5232 melanoma patients, revealed that most of the body has symmetric lymphatic drainage and the asymmetry assumed in previous studies might be due to lack of sufficient lymphoscintigraphy data. Given this recently discovered anatomic variability, it is still rational to consider lymphoscintigraphy preoperatively because of the importance of lymphatic involvement in the prognosis of these patients [45].

Vascular Anatomy as It Relates to the Skin and Its Importance to the Development and Possibly the Metastasis of Melanoma

Although melanoma may involve the regional lymph nodes before the development of distant metastasis, this is not always true. It is not absolutely clear whether spreading of malignant cells through lymphatics is required before systemic dissemination, but direct entry through the venous return may also be possible [46].

Indeed, skin has a rich blood supply which is necessary for dermal and epidermal nutrition as well as thermoregulation. Michel Salmon stated in 1936 that blood vessels supply branches to each type of tissue they adjoin, including bones, nerves, muscle, fascia, and fat [47].

The concept of the angiosome is widely accepted in the field of cutaneous vascular anatomy and is vital to our current understanding of hematogenous spread in melanoma. An angiosome is a segment of soft tissue spanning from bone to skin supplied by a main source vessel. There are connections between adjacent angiosomes either via identical caliber (true) or reduced caliber (choke) anastomotic vessels. Source vessels give rise to perforator arteries directly (septocutaneous and fasciocutaneous vessels) or indirectly (musculocutaneous, or terminal branches of muscular vessels) serving the skin [48, 49]. These perforator arteries pass through the intermuscular or intramuscular septa or even proximally to tendons to form a deep plexus of vessels within the dermo-hypodermal junction (Fig. 2.1). Deep plexuses connect to superficial plexuses via ascending arterioles perpendicular to the skin surface. Superficial plexuses, also known as sub-papillary plexuses, lie between papillary and reticular dermis and create small capillary loops extending into dermal papillae. These capillaries allow transportation of materials to the epidermal cells. Drainage occurs through descending limbs of these loops, called postcapillary venules, from which blood flows into sub-papillary plexuses and thereafter the descending venules. This eventually reaches the deep plexuses and collecting veins (Fig. 2.1) [50–52].

There have been numerous studies investigating the relation of vascular invasion, melanoma relapse, lymph node involvement, and distant metastasis. They have shown that vascular invasion may influence the prognosis of melanoma, similar to that of ulceration [53]. Furthermore, it has been suggested that melanoma cells can even spread along the external surface of vessels without intravasation. This mechanism is known as extravascular migratory metastasis [54].

Tumor cells are also capable of acquiring endothelial-like features and stimulating angiogenesis to supply the requisite oxygen and nutrients to the growing tumor mass. These new vessels play an important role in the spread of melanoma cells and the vertical growth phase described with melanoma growth patterns [55, 56].

The Tumor Microenvironment of the Skin and Its Relationship with the Progression of Melanoma

At one time, melanoma growth was considered to be an isolated cellular event. However, it is now known that the development, invasion, and spread of melanoma largely depend upon its interactions with the surrounding microenvironment. The melanoma microenvironment is complex and consists of the malignant cells and supporting stroma including fibroblasts, endothelial cells, immune cells, soluble molecules, and extracellular matrix (ECM) [57–59]. This microenvironment influences the development and progression of melanoma either favorably or adversely. In the following section, we discuss this microenvironment and its relation to the progression of melanoma.

Melanocytes are located on the stratum basale of the epidermis and hair follicles. The primary regulators of melanocytes are keratinocytes. Keratinocytes govern melanocytes through the secretion of cytokines and growth factors as well as cell adhesion. When this regulation is disrupted, a transformation from melanocyte to melanoma is thought to take place in a stepwise fashion. The exact cellular or genetic events that result in such transformation have been the focus of much research over the last decade. The melanoma cells are thought to transition to a radial growth phase, followed by vertical growth and possibly distant metastases.

Keratinocytes regulate melanocytes through both paracrine growth factors and intracellular communication with cell adhesion molecules. Cadherins are a family of transmembrane proteins that promote cell-to-cell adhesion through the interaction of the cadherin's extracellular domain with similar cadherins of adjacent cells. Cell adhesion molecules involved in regulation of melanocytes include epithelial cadherin (E-cadherin), membranous placental cadherin (P-cadherin), and desmoglein-1. Hepatocyte growth factor, secreted by melanoma cells, downregulates E-cadherin and desmoglein-1, and melanomas often have reduced or absent E-cadherin, P-cadherin, and/or desmoglein-1 [60]. E-cadherin acts by downregulating β-catenin and providing tight junctions with surrounding cells. β-Catenin promotes proliferation of melanocytes by inducing transcription of growth and survival genes including c-Myc, cyclin D1, and MITF. In melanoma cells, E-cadherin is downregulated, allowing for increased β-catenin activity and therefore proliferation and survival of melanocytes [61]. P-cadherin and desmoglein-1 promote melanocyte-keratinocyte adhesion and prevent invasion of melanoma cells. The loss of P-cadherin and desmoglein-1 allows for invasion and spread of the malignant cells [60, 62]. In contrast, neural cadherin (N-cadherin) promotes melanocyte growth and survival. Melanoma cells upregulate N-cadherin, which allows interaction with other N-cadherin cells including fibroblasts and endothelial cells. This results in increased motility secondary to looser interactions among melanocytes with adjacent cells. N-cadherin also represses pro-apoptotic factors, further promoting melanoma growth and survival [57].

Melanomas secrete growth factors that have both autocrine and paracrine effects. HGF, PDGF-A, FGF, and IL-8 secreted by melanoma cells promote growth and survival of melanoma cells. VEGF and β FGF secreted by melanomas induce proliferation of endothelial cells and angiogenesis, and TGF-β and PDGF activate fibroblasts. PDGF plays a role in organizing the ECM and stimulating additional growth factors [63]. Fibroblasts become associated with the melanoma and play a large part in promoting its growth and survival by secreting paracrine growth factors such as bFGF, IGF-1, HGF, and endothelin [63, 64]. Melanoma-associated fibroblasts can also differentiate into pericytes and promote angiogenesis. Interestingly, TGF-β has an inhibitory effect on melanocytes; however, the melanoma cells themselves are resistant. Melanoma-secreted TGF-β promotes ECM deposition, angiogenesis, survival, immunosuppression, and transition to more aggressive melanoma phenotypes [57].

Integrin proteins mediate cell cytoskeletal adhesion to the extracellular matrix and influence proliferation, migration, invasion, and survival of melanocytes as well as angiogenesis for tumor survival and spread. Integrins are proteins consisting of alpha- and beta-subunits that form transmembrane heterodimers. Conformational changes and decreased expression of integrins promote melanoma cell dissociation from the primary tumor, migration through surrounding stroma, and eventually metastasis. Integrins lack kinase activity, but they are able to activate intracellular signaling cascades including MAPK, PI3K, and nuclear factor kappa B (NF-κ). They can also influence cell signaling through growth factors by acting as a co-receptor, directly interacting with the receptor, or by indirectly changing a growth factor's function. Through these mechanisms, characteristics of the invasive edge of a melanoma include proteolysis of collagen and elastin and infiltration of lymphocytes [57].

Special Insight into the Development of a Melanoma from a Skin Lesion, Such as a Mole or Atypical Nevus

We now purpose to deepen our probe of melanoma's ontogeny and explore whether and to what extent it might arise from a preexisting nevus versus bursting into existence de novo (that is, from a single aberrant melanocyte). Though this may appear to be a simple, dichotomous question, it is one that tests the limits of the field's methods of knowing and description.

Melanocytic nevi are defined as a focal proliferation of melanocytes, and are subclassified into dysplastic and common (i.e., nondysplastic) nevi. Forms of nevus include junctional, dermal, and compound. Junctional nevi are proliferations of melanocytes at the basal epidermal layer in which they normally reside. A compound nevus connotes joint proliferation of both basal epidermal melanocytes and melanocytes which have descended into the dermis, while the waning of basal epidermal proliferation in these nests signals transition to a dermal nevus. Clark et al. maintained that proliferations of melanocytes, though benign in histological appearance, may represent a quiescent, primordial step in the tumorigenesis of melanoma [65].

The term "dysplasia," which Ackerman [66] defines as "cytologic atypia, disordered growth, or some combination thereof," has been a subject of great contention when applied to melanocytic nevi, as many authors believe that it incorrectly implies an inevitable progression towards malignancy. The term "nevus with architectural disorder" was suggested by the NIH Consensus Conference in 1992, but is uncommonly applied in practice among non-dermatopathologists. Therefore, in keeping with the argument of Duffy and Grossman [67], this text will distinguish between the clinical finding of atypical nevus and the histopathological diagnosis of dysplastic nevus.

When first disclosed clinically, suspicious nests of melanocytes are termed atypical nevi (Fig. 2.2). The Dutch Working Group's criteria for atypical nevi include a diameter >5 mm, vague border, asymmetric shape, irregular pigmentation, and red hue [68]. Only through histopathologic examination may a diagnosis of dysplastic nevus be rendered (Fig. 2.3). The World Health Organization defines the major criteria for diagnosis of a dysplastic nevus thusly: "(1) basilar proliferation of atypical melanocytes which must extend beyond three rete ridges beyond the dermal component and (2) organization of this proliferation in a lentiginous or epithelioid cell pattern [69]." Though dysplastic nevi may bear close phenotypic resemblance to melanoma, its presumed risk of malignant transformation has fluctuated over the past half-century.

Seminal work by Clark, Lynch, and Elder in the description of patients with both familial and nonfamilial forms of a dysplastic nevus syndrome represented the first associations between atypical nevi and malignant melanoma [70–72]. However, Clark and his group noted that the presence of atypical nevi in these patients was not necessary for the development of melanoma, and that the majority of these lesions often regressed or became stable [73]. Moreover, early studies in this area were hamstrung by the lack of histopathological confirmation that these atypical nevi were, indeed, dysplastic [74, 75]. Multiple subsequent investigations have demonstrated a poor-to-fair correlation between clinical atypia and histologic dysplasia [76, 77]. In counterpoint,

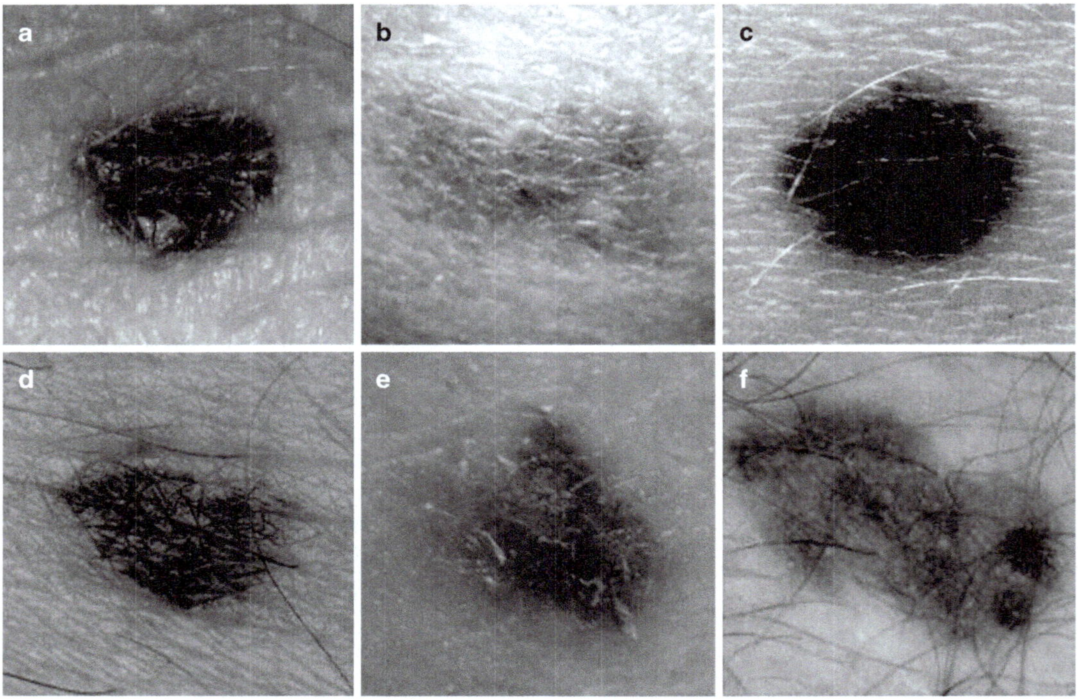

Fig. 2.2 Clinical features of atypical nevi, including indistinct borders (**a**–**c**), and variable pigmentation (**b**–**f**). Reprinted from Duffy K, Grossman D. The dysplastic nevus: from historical perspective to management in the modern era: part I. Historical, histologic, and clinical aspects. Journal of the American Academy of Dermatology. 2012;67(1):1. e-. e16 with permission from Elsevier

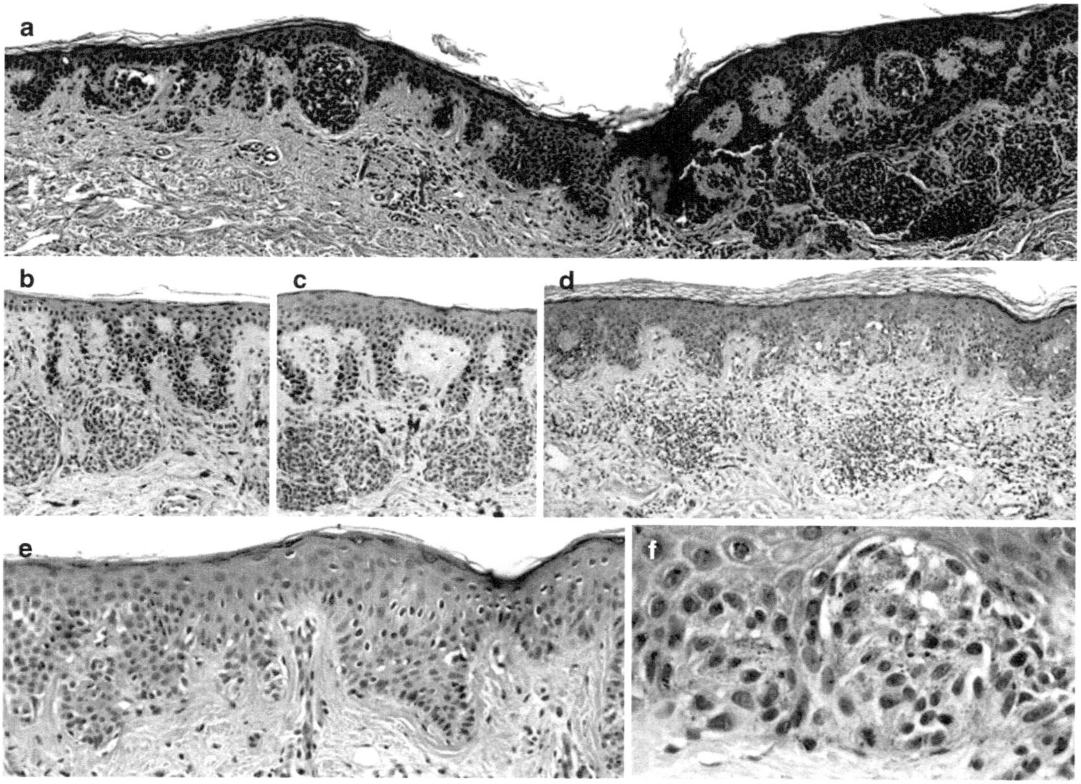

Fig. 2.3 Histologic features of dysplastic nevi. (**a**) Architectural disorder demonstrated by lateral asymmetry and "shouldering" (original magnification ×40). (**b**) Lentiginous melanocytic hyperplasia with bridging of rete ridges (original magnification ×200) and (**c**) cellular atypia (original magnification ×200). (**d**) Patchy lymphocytic host response (original magnification ×100). (**e**) Prominent eosinophilic fibroplasias (original magnification ×200). (**f**) Variable and "random" cytologic atypia and mitotic junctional activity (original magnification ×600). Reprinted from Duffy K, Grossman D. The dysplastic nevus: from historical perspective to management in the modern era: part I. Historical, histologic, and clinical aspects. Journal of the American Academy of Dermatology. 2012;67(1):1. e-. e16 with permissions from Elsevier

Crucioli and Stilwell [78] averred that if serial sections of the malignant lesion are not taken, the probability of finding an associated nevus decreases even further. Taken together, these findings call into question the proposition that atypical and/or dysplastic nevi confer greater risk of malignant transformation than their common counterparts.

As such, a great number of contemporary studies have been undertaken to discern the proportion of malignant melanoma which arises from a nevus, whether dysplastic or common. In extant literature, melanoma has been histopathologically demonstrated to contain a neval component in about 20–30% of cases, though in many instances the distinction between cancer and melanocytic nevus is far from clear. Further investigations have attempted to assess the proportion of melanomas that are derived from a dysplastic as opposed to a common nevus. Here, there is evidential concordance: Grossly, common nevi are more often associated with melanoma than dysplastic nevi [59, 79, 80]. Since there has been little study anent the ratios of histologically dysplastic versus common nevi in the populace, it is difficult to extrapolate which of the two carries the greater proportionate risk of associated melanoma.

Part of the issue lies in the epistemological limitations of histopathology itself. A pathological section captures but a single instant of time and so lacks the temporal breadth to detect the transition from nevus to malignant melanoma, if indeed such a transition does occur. Duffy and Grossman point out that any conclusions derived from these techniques may be confounded by the malignancy's usurpation of the nevus or, alternatively, the proximate formation of melanoma and nevus. In the absence of a reliable model for melanoma development, dermatologists are left in an evidential twilight of retrospective studies and expert opinion.

This text would be remiss if it elided the entity of congenital melanocytic nevus. Though they appear quite similar to benign common nevi, congenital nevi have been found to exhibit multiple histologic patterns which may distinguish them from their parvenu-acquired brethren [81]. These nevi are most commonly subclassified as small (<1.5 cm at largest diameter), medium (1.5–19.9 cm), or giant (≥20 cm). The risk of malignant development in giant lesions is estimated to be from 5 to 30%, great enough that they are often excised prophylactically [59]. Malignant transformation of small or medium lesions is less well characterized, and therefore no clear guidelines exist.

Due to the present limitations of the field, the question of melanoma's origin remains open. Though current oncogene-expressing murine models of the disease are thought to represent poor histopathologic correlates, improved models may strengthen our ability to observe the progression of malignancy, whether from an extant lesion or a single cell. Novel imaging technologies may also represent a way forward. Regardless of modality, continuing the investigations of melanoma's provenance is our best way forward in combating this oft-fatal disease.

References

1. Sen GL. Remembering one's identity: the epigenetic basis of stem cell fate decisions. FASEB J. 2011;25(7):2123–8.
2. Gantwerker EA, Hom DB. Skin: histology and physiology of wound healing. Facial Plast Surg Clin North Am. 2011;19(3):441–53.
3. Brody I. The ultrastructure of the tonofibrils in the keratinization process of normal human epidermis. J Ultrastruct Res. 1960;4(3):264–97.
4. Stingl G, Wolff-Schreiner EC, Pichler W, Gschnait F, Knapp W. Epidermal Langerhans cells bear Fc and C3 receptors. Nature. 1977;268:245–6.
5. Elias PM. Structure and function of the stratum corneum extracellular matrix. J Investig Dermatol. 2012;132(9):2131–3.
6. Arda O, Göksügür N, Tüzün Y. Basic histological structure and functions of facial skin. Clin Dermatol. 2014;32(1):3–13.
7. Mescher AL. Junqueira's basic histology: text and atlas: McGraw-Hill; 2013.
8. Hwang K, Kim H, Kim DJ. Thickness of skin and subcutaneous tissue of the free flap donor sites: a histologic study. Microsurgery. 2016;36(1):54–8.
9. Menon GK, Cleary GW, Lane ME. The structure and function of the stratum corneum. Int J Pharm. 2012;435(1):3–9.
10. Kanitakis J. Anatomy, histology and immunohistochemistry of normal human skin. Eur J Dermatol. 2001;12(4):390–9. quiz 400-1
11. Ross M, Pawlina W. Histology a text and atlas. Baltimore: Lippincott Williams & Wilkins, a Wolters Kluwer Business; 2011.
12. Driskell RR, Jahoda CA, Chuong CM, Watt FM, Horsley V. Defining dermal adipose tissue. Exp Dermatol. 2014;23(9):629–31.
13. Schmidt B, Horsley V. Unravelling hair follicle–adipocyte communication. Exp Dermatol. 2012;21(11):827–30.
14. Mayor R, Theveneau E. The neural crest. Development. 2013;140(11):2247–51.
15. Nitzan E, Pfaltzgraff ER, Labosky PA, Kalcheim C. Neural crest and Schwann cell progenitor-derived melanocytes are two spatially segregated populations similarly regulated by Foxd3. Proc Natl Acad Sci. 2013;110(31):12709–14.
16. White RM, Zon LI. Melanocytes in development, regeneration, and cancer. Cell Stem Cell. 2008;3(3):242–52.
17. Shakhova O. Neural crest stem cells in melanoma development. Curr Opin Oncol. 2014;26(2):215–21.
18. Mort RL, Jackson IJ, Patton EE. The melanocyte lineage in development and disease. Development. 2015;142(4):620–32.
19. Fitzpatrick TB, Breathnach A. The epidermal melanin unit system. Dermatol Wochenschr. 1963;147:481–9.
20. Joly-Tonetti N, Wibawa JI, Bell M, Tobin DJ. Melanin fate in the human epidermis: a re-assessment of how best to detect and analyze histologically. Exp Dermatol. 2016;
21. Thody AJ, Higgins EM, Wakamatsu K, Ito S, Burchill SA, Marks JM. Pheomelanin as well as eumelanin is present in human epidermis. J Investig Dermatol. 1991;97(2):340–4.
22. Pathak M, Jimbow K. Fitzpatrick T, editors. Sendai, Japan: Photobiology of pigment cell phenotypic expression in pigment cells. Proceedings of the Xth International Pigment Cell Conference; 1980.
23. Brenner M, Hearing VJ. The protective role of melanin against UV damage in human skin. Photochem Photobiol. 2008;84(3):539–49.

24. Kushimoto T, Valencia JC, Costin GE, Toyofuku K, Watabe H, Yasumoto KI, et al. The melanosome: an ideal model to study cellular differentiation. Pigment Cell Res. 2003;16(3):237–44.
25. Dell'Angelica EC. Melanosome biogenesis: shedding light on the origin of an obscure organelle. Trends Cell Biol. 2003;13(10):503–6.
26. Wu X, Hammer JA. Melanosome transfer: it is best to give and receive. Curr Opin Cell Biol. 2014;29:1–7.
27. Gilchrest BA, Eller MS, Geller AC, Yaar M. The pathogenesis of melanoma induced by ultraviolet radiation. N Engl J Med. 1999;340(17):1341–8.
28. Young AR, Chadwick CA, Harrison GI, Nikaido O, Ramsden J, Potten CS. The similarity of action spectra for thymine dimers in human epidermis and erythema suggests that DNA is the chromophore for erythema. J Investig Dermatol. 1998;111(6):982–8.
29. Hölzle E, Hönigsmann H. [UV-radiation--sources, wavelength, environment]. Journal der Deutschen Dermatologischen Gesellschaft= Journal of the German Society of Dermatology: JDDG. 2005;3:S3-10.
30. De Fabo EC. Arctic stratospheric ozone depletion and increased UVB radiation: potential impacts to human health. International journal of circumpolar health. 2005;64(5).
31. Fisher GJ, Kang S, Varani J, Bata-Csorgo Z, Wan Y, Datta S, et al. Mechanisms of photoaging and chronological skin aging. Arch Dermatol. 2002;138(11):1462–70.
32. Vink AA, Roza L. Biological consequences of cyclobutane pyrimidine dimers. J Photochem Photobiol B Biol. 2001;65(2):101–4.
33. Kvam E, Tyrrell RM. Induction of oxidative DNA base damage in human skin cells by UV and near visible radiation. Carcinogenesis. 1997;18(12):2379–84.
34. Kaidbey KH, Agin PP, Sayre RM, Kligman AM. Photoprotection by melanin—a comparison of black and Caucasian skin. J Am Acad Dermatol. 1979;1(3):249–60.
35. Mervic L. Time course and pattern of metastasis of cutaneous melanoma differ between men and women. PLoS One. 2012;7(3):e32955.
36. Streit M, Detmar M. Angiogenesis, lymphangiogenesis, and melanoma metastasis. Oncogene. 2003;22(20):3172–9.
37. León P, Daly JM, Synnestvedt M, Schultz DJ, Elder DE, Clark WH. The prognostic implications of microscopic satellites in patients with clinical stage I melanoma. Arch Surg. 1991;126(12):1461–8.
38. Leiter U, Meier F, Schittek B, Garbe C. The natural course of cutaneous melanoma. J Surg Oncol. 2004;86(4):172–8.
39. Meier F, Will S, Ellwanger U, Schlagenhauff B, Schittek B, Rassner G, et al. Metastatic pathways and time courses in the orderly progression of cutaneous melanoma. Br J Dermatol. 2002;147(1):62–70.
40. Cascinelli N, Morabito A, Santinami M, MacKie R, Belli F. Immediate or delayed dissection of regional nodes in patients with melanoma of the trunk: a randomised trial. Lancet. 1998;351(9105):793–6.
41. Kretschmer L, Hilgers R, Möhrle M, Balda B, Breuninger H, Konz B, et al. Patients with lymphatic metastasis of cutaneous malignant melanoma benefit from sentinel lymphonodectomy and early excision of their nodal disease. Eur J Cancer. 2004;40(2):212–8.
42. Sappey M. Anatomy, physiology and pathology of the lymphatic vessels in man and vertebrates. DeLahaye A, Lecrosnier E (trans-eds) Paris, France. 1874.
43. Sugarbaker E, McBride C. Melanoma of the trunk: the results of surgical excision and anatomic guidelines for predicting nodal metastasis. Surgery. 1976;80(1):22–30.
44. Norman J, Cruse CW, Espinosa C, Cox C, Berman C, Clark R, et al. Redefinition of cutaneous lymphatic drainage with the use of lymphoscintigraphy for malignant melanoma. Am J Surg. 1991;162(5):432–7.
45. Reynolds HM, Walker CG, Dunbar P, O'Sullivan MJ, Uren RF, Thompson JF, et al. Functional anatomy of the lymphatics draining the skin: a detailed statistical analysis. J Anat. 2010;216(3):344–55.
46. Damsky W, Theodosakis N, Bosenberg M. Melanoma metastasis: new concepts and evolving paradigms. Oncogene. 2014;33(19):2413–22.
47. Salmon M. Arteres de la peau: Etude anatomique et chirurgicale; Travail du Laboratoire d'anatomie de la Fac. de Marseille: Masson; 1936.
48. Taylor GI, Palmer J. The vascular territories (angiosomes) of the body: experimental study and clinical applications. Br J Plast Surg. 1987;40(2):113–41.
49. Taylor IG, Pan WR. Angiosomes of the leg: anatomic study and clinical implications. Plast Reconstr Surg. 1998;102(3):599–616.
50. Ryan T. Cutaneous circulation. Biochemistry and physiology of the skin. 1983;2:817–77.
51. Braverman IM, editor The cutaneous microcirculation. Journal of Investigative Dermatology Symposium Proceedings; 2000: Elsevier.
52. Braverman IM, Keh-Yen A. Ultrastructure of the human dermal microcirculation. IV. Valve-containing collecting veins at the dermal–subcutaneous junction. J Investig Dermatol. 1983;81(5):438–42.
53. Fernandez-Flores A. Prognostic factors for melanoma progression and metastasis: from hematoxylin-eosin to genetics. Romanian J Morphol Embryol. 2012;53(3):449–59.
54. Lugassy C, Barnhill RL. Angiotropic melanoma and extravascular migratory metastasis: a review. Adv Anat Pathol. 2007;14(3):195–201.
55. Zbytek B, Carlson JA, Granese J, Ross J, Mihm M, Slominski A. Current concepts of metastasis in melanoma. Expert Rev Dermatol. 2008;3(5):569–85.
56. Bayer-Garner IB, Hough AJ Jr, Smoller BR. Vascular endothelial growth factor expression in malignant melanoma: prognostic versus diagnostic usefulness. Modern pathology: an official journal of the United States and Canadian Academy of Pathology, Inc. 1999;12(8):770–4.

57. Villanueva J, Herlyn M. Melanoma and the tumor microenvironment. Current oncology reports. 2008;10(5):439-46.
58. Brandner JM, Haass NK. Melanoma's connections to the tumour microenvironment. Pathology-Journal of the RCPA. 2013;45(5):443–52.
59. Tannous ZS, Mihm MC, Sober AJ, Duncan LM. Congenital melanocytic nevi: clinical and histopathologic features, risk of melanoma, and clinical management. J Am Acad Dermatol. 2005;52(2):197–203.
60. Li G, Schaider H, Satyamoorthy K, Hanakawa Y, Hashimoto K, Herlyn M. Downregulation of E-cadherin and Desmoglein 1 by autocrine hepatocyte growth factor during melanoma development. Oncogene. 2001;20(56):8125–35.
61. Tang A, Eller MS, Hara M, Yaar M, Hirohashi S, Gilchrest BA. E-cadherin is the major mediator of human melanocyte adhesion to keratinocytes in vitro. J Cell Sci. 1994;107(4):983–92.
62. Van Marck V, Stove C, Van Den Bossche K, Stove V, Paredes J, Vander Haeghen Y, et al. P-cadherin promotes cell-cell adhesion and counteracts invasion in human melanoma. Cancer Res. 2005;65(19):8774–83.
63. Labrousse AL, Ntayi C, Hornebeck W, Bernard P. Stromal reaction in cutaneous melanoma. Crit Rev Oncol Hematol. 2004;49(3):269–75.
64. Li G, Satyamoorthy K, Meier F, Berking C, Bogenrieder T, Herlyn M. Function and regulation of melanoma–stromal fibroblast interactions: when seeds meet soil. Oncogene. 2003;22(20):3162–71.
65. Clark WH, Elder DE, Guerry D, Epstein MN, Greene MH, Van Horn M. A study of tumor progression: the precursor lesions of superficial spreading and nodular melanoma. Hum Pathol. 1984;15(12):1147–65.
66. Ackerman AB, Mihara I. Dysplasia, dysplastic melanocytes, dysplastic nevi, the dysplastic nevus syndrome, and the relation between dysplastic nevi and malignant melanomas. Hum Pathol. 1985;16(1):87–91.
67. Duffy K, Grossman D. The dysplastic nevus: from historical perspective to management in the modern era: part I. Historical, histologic, and clinical aspects. Journal of the American Academy of Dermatology. 2012;67(1):1. e-. e16.
68. Bergman W, van Voorst VP, Ruiter D. Dysplastic nevi and the risk of melanoma: a guideline for patient care. Nederlandse Melanoom Werkgroep van de Vereniging voor Integrale Kankercentra. Ned Tijdschr Geneeskd. 1997;141(42):2010–4.
69. Clemente C, Cochran AJ, Elder DE, Levene A, Mackie RM, Mihm MC, et al. Histopathologic diagnosis of dysplastic nevi: concordance among pathologists convened by the World Health Organization melanoma Programme. Hum Pathol. 1991;22(4):313–9.
70. Lynch HT, Frichot BC, Lynch JF. Familial atypical multiple mole-melanoma syndrome. J Med Genet. 1978;15(5):352–6.
71. Elder DE, Goldman LI, Goldman SC, Greene MH, Clark WH. Dysplastic nevus syndrome: a phenotypic association of sporadic cutaneous melanoma. Cancer. 1980;46(8):1787–94.
72. Clark WH, Reimer RR, Greene M, Ainsworth AM, Mastrangelo MJ. Origin of familial malignant melanomas from heritable melanocytic lesions: the BK mole syndrome. Arch Dermatol. 1978;114(5):732–8.
73. Tucker MA, Fraser MC, Goldstein AM, Struewing JP, King MA, Crawford JT, et al. A natural history of melanomas and dysplastic nevi. Cancer. 2002;94(12):3192–209.
74. Kelly JW, Yeatman JM, Regalia C, Mason G, Henham AP. A high incidence of melanoma found in patients with multiple dysplastic naevi by photographic surveillance. Med J Aust. 1997;167(4):191–4.
75. Greene MH, Clark WH Jr, Tucker MA, Elder DE, Kraemer KH, Guerry D IV, et al. Acquired precursors of cutaneous malignant melanoma: the familial dysplastic nevus syndrome. N Engl J Med. 1985;312(2):91–7.
76. Meyer LJ, Piepkorn M, Goldgar DE, Lewis CM, Cannon-Albright LA, Zone JJ, et al. Interobserver concordance in discriminating clinical atypia of melanocytic nevi, and correlations with histologic atypia. J Am Acad Dermatol. 1996;34(4):618–25.
77. Annessi G, Cattaruzza MS, Abeni D, Baliva G, Laurenza M, Macchini V, et al. Correlation between clinical atypia and histologic dysplasia in acquired melanocytic nevi. J Am Acad Dermatol. 2001;45(1):77–85.
78. Crucioli V, Stilwell J. The Histogenesis of malignant melanoma in relation to pre-existing pigmented lesions. J Cutan Pathol. 1982;9(6):396–404.
79. Sagebiel RW. Melanocytic nevi in histologic association with primary cutaneous melanoma of superficial spreading and nodular types: effect of tumor thickness. J Investig Dermatol. 1993;100(3):322–5.
80. Bevona C, Goggins W, Quinn T, Fullerton J, Tsao H. Cutaneous melanomas associated with nevi. Arch Dermatol. 2003;139(12):1620–4.
81. Barnhill RL, Fleischli M. Histologic features of congenital melanocytic nevi in infants 1 year of age or younger. J Am Acad Dermatol. 1995;33(5):780–5.

Melanoma Epidemiology and Prevention

3

Sowmiya Murali[†], Mary E. Logue[†], Yvonne Talamantes, and Marianne Berwick

Epidemiology

Introduction

The incidence of melanoma is continuing to increase throughout the world in fair-skinned populations. In the United States, melanoma incidence has risen from 8.2 to 9.4 cases per 100,000 within the white population in 1975 (females and males, respectively) to 38.9 and 24.2 cases in 2013. Increased incidence has occurred mainly for thin lesions, those less than 1 mm in Breslow's depth. Reasons for the increased incidence include excessive tanning, potential exposure to chemicals, and a more effective application of diagnostic criteria. Mortality rates have also increased among white males, rising from 2.9 per 100,000 in 1975 to 4.6 in 2013. They have risen very little for white females during the same time period, from 1.7 to 1.9 per 100,000 between 1975 and 2013 [1]. This chapter reviews both causes for and prevention of melanoma.

Risk Factors for Melanoma

The relationship between risk factors and incidence is complex, but increased exposure to UV radiation (UVR) is the major factor responsible for the development of melanoma. In conjunction with UVR, host factors as well as phenotypic and genetic factors are also responsible for an individual's likelihood of developing melanoma.

Phenotypic Factors

Fair Skin Phenotype

It is well established that fair-skinned individuals have an increased risk for melanoma compared to those with darker skin. Phenotypic characteristics such as light eyes, light or red hair, and fair skin color are host factors known to increase the risk of developing melanoma. There appears to be an inverse relationship between darker skinned individuals and the decreased risk of melanoma. In a meta-analysis of 60 studies, individuals with red hair were compared to those with dark hair, finding a relative risk of 3.64 (95% CI, 2.56, 5.37) for developing melanoma. Individuals with blue eyes had a relative risk of 1.47 (95% CI,

[†]Sowmiya Murali and Mary E. Logue contributed equally to this work.

S. Murali
University of New Mexico, Albuquerque, NM, USA
e-mail: somurali1@salud.unm.edu

M. E. Logue
School of Medicine, University of New Mexico, Albuquerque, NM, USA
e-mail: logueme@salud.unm.edu

Y. Talamantes
CRTC Population Science Academic Unit, Albuquerque, NM, USA
e-mail: ytala2@salud.unm.edu

M. Berwick (✉)
Department of Internal Medicine and Dermatology, University of New Mexico, Albuquerque, NM, USA
e-mail: mberwick@salud.unm.edu

A. I. Riker (ed.), *Melanoma*, https://doi.org/10.1007/978-3-319-78310-9_3

1.28, 1.69) compared to those with brown eyes and fair-skinned individuals had a 2.06-fold (95% CI 1.68, 2.52) increased risk [2]. As there is no commonly accepted standard for assessing skin color between studies and populations, some authors feel that a reported inability to tan may be a better risk marker for melanoma and increases risk approximately twofold [3, 4]. Some have developed more quantitative approaches to measure pigmentation such as the extraction and quantification of pheomelanin and eumelanin from undyed hair [5], but these have not been widely adopted due to the difficult assays required.

Freckling

Freckles are benign, ranging in diameter from a few millimeters to a few centimeters, pigmented skin spots that appear with increased sun exposure commonly in fair-skinned individuals. Increased freckling is associated with higher risks of melanoma (RR = 2.10, 95% CI 1.80–2.45) in many studies, and in the meta-analysis by Gandini et al. [2]. Phenotypic characteristics and freckling tendency can be used to identify those at high risk and can be targeted for surveillance.

Nevi

Nevi are a strong risk factor for the development of melanoma. Nevi are benign collections of melanocytes that may be congenital or acquired [6]. The relationship between sun exposure, nevus development, and melanoma risk is still not fully understood. It is theorized that melanocytes within a nevus may be more likely to undergo malignant transformation [2]. A number of studies have shown that melanoma may have arisen from preexisting melanocytic nevi in 30% of cases [7].

Some studies have hypothesized that multiple nevi may be a marker for previous sun exposure suggesting that sun exposure and number of nevi have a multiplicative effect on the risk for melanoma. Children and adolescents who practice sun-protective behaviors have decreased numbers of new developing nevi [8–10]. Sun exposure plays a role in the development of nevi [11]. The risk for melanoma increases as the number of nevi increases, from a risk of 1.47 (95% CI 1.36, 1.59) for fewer than 15 total nevi to a relative risk of 6.89 (95% CI 4.63, 10.25) for more than 100 nevi [12].

The Divergent Pathway to Melanoma Development

Whiteman et al. [13] suggested that melanomas from varied body sites arise through different pathways with different associations with either solar keratosis or nevi. Melanomas located in the head and neck regions are associated with chronic sun exposure, fewer nevi, and more solar keratoses. Melanoma located on the trunk with similar histological features was associated with more intermittent sun exposure, many nevi, and fewer solar keratoses. This suggests that individuals with a greater genetic tendency to form nevi have a lower threshold to UV exposure to induce the melanocytes to proliferate and become neoplastic. In contrast, people with a low genetic tendency to develop nevi require a higher threshold of sun exposure to induce melanocytes to proliferate.

Exposures

Sun Exposure

The cause of melanoma is multifactorial and complex but sun exposure plays a primary role in the development of melanoma. Ultraviolet radiation exposure has been recently classified as a Class I carcinogen [14]; ultraviolet radiation includes UVC (200–280 nm), UVB (280–320 nm), and UVA (320–400 nm). UVC is highly toxic, but very little of it reaches earth as it is screened by the stratospheric ozone layer. UVB rays directly damage DNA through the production of DNA-damaging photoproducts and cyclobutane pyrimidine dimer formation, while UVA indirectly damages DNA through reactive oxygen species production [15]. Analyses in the United Kingdom suggest that 90% of melanoma cases in men and 82% in women are attributable to excess solar irradiation [16] and 68% worldwide [17]. The rising incidence may be due to early detection, increased surveillance, and changes in diagnostic criteria, but the majority are thought to be linked to increased sun exposure through altered patterns of behavior, such as the choice of clothing [18] and outdoor activities.

Sun exposure is classified as "total, intermittent, or chronic" with "sunburn history" as an important component. Intermittent sun exposure refers to intense, short periods of sun exposure experienced on weekends or on vacations in sunny locations. Chronic sun exposure is continuous with less intensity and mostly seen in occupational settings. Total sun exposure is the sum of intermittent and chronic exposures.

A meta-analysis examined 57 studies of sun exposure and melanoma and reported relative risks of 1.34 (95% CI, 1.02, 1.77) for total sun exposure, 1.61 for intermittent sun exposure (95% CI, 1.31, 1.99), 0.95 for chronic sun exposure (95% CI, 0.87, 1.04), and 2.03 for a history of sunburn (95% CI, 1.73, 2.37) [19]. It is unclear whether, in fact, chronic sun exposure decreases the risk for melanoma. Certainly, those with chronic sun exposure have adapted to the UV and thus are less likely to be harmed by it. Similar results have been found when looking at the risk of sun exposure on multiple primary melanomas [20].

Current evidence does not clearly show a critical period during life where risk from sun exposure is highest [21, 22]. For example, the increased risk for more than five sunburns during childhood was 2.0 (95% CI, 1.2, 3.5) and during adulthood was 2.1 (95% CI, 1.4, 3.3) [21]. Sunburns during any period of life, whether it is childhood, adolescence, or adulthood, increase the risk for melanoma. Due to the fact that sunburns are based on self-report and memory is fallible, there is no strong evidence for any specific "number" of sunburns and increased risk for melanoma. Although many experts purport that various specific numbers increase risk, there is no validity to a specific number.

Indoor Tanning

Approximately 7.8 million women and 1.9 million men use tanning beds each year [23], and the International Agency for Research on Cancer [14] has identified ultraviolet radiation (UVR) emitted from tanning beds as carcinogenic. Indoor tanning beds emit both UVA and UVB rays in amounts 2–4 times stronger than the midday sun during the summer in Washington, DC [24]. The longer a person uses indoor tanning beds and the earlier that someone begins using them, the more likely that one is to develop melanoma in the future [25]. A dose-response relationship was also noted between total hours ($P < 0.0001$), number of sessions ($P = 0.0002$) or years ($P < 0.006$), and melanoma risk [26]. Shifting trends in anatomic location of melanoma also appear to demonstrate the influence of indoor tanning on the risk for melanoma. There was a significant rise in truncal melanomas in women after 2002 in Iceland that coincided with rapidly expanding sunbed use after 1985 [27].

Occupation and Melanoma

Most studies of melanoma have focused on the relationship between host factors, UV radiation, and melanoma risk, but a number of relatively small studies have found links to polycyclic aromatic hydrocarbons, benzene, and other chemicals used in the printing industry [28–32]. Studies of electrical and electronics workers have demonstrated an increased risk for melanoma [33]. It must be noted that not all studies have shown positive associations. It is likely that the various occupational workers are also exposed to additional agents and many of the studies did not have appropriate control for confounders. For example, cosmic radiation, such as that received by pilots and airline attendants, has often been associated with increased melanoma risk. However, the lifestyle of these occupations may confound the association [34, 35]—whether due to circadian rhythm disruption [36] or opportunities for intense intermittent sun exposure. Multiple small studies have looked at issues related to occupation and due to the small number of subjects and incomplete control for confounding they are unable to determine strong links.

Polychlorinated Biphenyls

PCBs may affect melanomagenesis. PCBs are chlorinated compounds previously used as coolants in electrical apparatus and which, as now discarded, leak into the environment. When that happens, meat, fish, milk, and water often contain PCBs [37–39]. There has been little research in dietary PCB exposure and melanoma risk, but one cohort study reported that exposure to dietary PCBs was associated with a fourfold increased risk of malignant melanoma [40]. A small pilot study conducted in British Columbia found strong associations between the risk of melanoma and plasma levels of non-dioxin-like PCBs (OR 7.02, 95% CI, 2.30, 21.43) [41]. This study is now being validated in a larger cohort.

Chromium

Chromium may play a major role in the pathogenesis of cutaneous melanoma [42]. Textile industries, which can often contain chemicals that are potentially harmful to skin, are known to contain the following chemicals: formaldehyde, nickel, and hexavalent chromium [43]. Cells exposed to chromium changed their shape and developed chromosomal abnormalities. Hexavalent chromium is a toxic form of the element, chromium. It can be used in electroplating, steel production, and metal plating. Tantalizing data [44–46] demonstrate an association between risk or mortality and melanoma after hip replacement with metal implants.

Genetic Factors

Melanoma is a heterogeneous disease with multiple signaling pathways associated with its pathogenesis. Insight into the pathways responsible for melanoma initiation and progression has come from current next-generation sequencing studies. It is beyond the scope of this chapter to fully elucidate the exciting developments in genetics that are leading to new understanding of the mechanisms of melanoma development. Excellent reviews of inherited and somatic mutations are by Hill et al. and Zhang et al. [47, 48].

Family History

A family history of melanoma is a strong risk factor for the development of melanoma, accounting for 10% of all melanoma cases [49]. Individuals with a first-degree relative with melanoma have a twofold increased risk for developing melanoma compared with those without a family history [50]. This assessment can be somewhat complex, as several family members with melanoma may have acquired the tumor due to genetic susceptibility or to common exposures, or possibly both. Mutations in the CDKN2A gene are the most common genetic mutations among families, with CDK4 occurring very much less frequently. Population-based studies have demonstrated the rarity of CDKN2A mutations among sporadic cases of melanoma [51]. Patients with a genetic predisposition acquire melanoma at a younger age, generally have thinner melanomas, and often have a history of dysplastic nevi or precursor lesions [52]. They also have a significantly higher risk for developing multiple primary melanomas [53]. It is not well known that melanoma can also arise in conjunction with familial cancer syndromes such as Li-Fraumeni, familial retinoblastoma, and Lynch syndrome type 2 [49].

Inherited Genetic Factors, Single-Nucleotide Polymorphisms

Pigmentation pathways clearly contribute to the risk of developing melanoma, with genetic loci at MC1R (melanocortin-1 receptor) and OCA2 identified in relation to facial freckling and total nevi [54] as well as red hair and fair skin [55]. MC1R mediates pigmentation and is expressed on the surface of melanocytes as a G protein-coupled receptor. It signals to downstream effectors to regulate skin pigmentation and control apoptosis and cell proliferation [56]. MC1R has also been shown to initiate the DNA repair process, increase phosphorylation of DNA repair proteins, and activate survival pathways [57, 58]. Mutations in the MC1R gene are therefore linked to inefficient DNA repair and melanocyte apoptosis [59]. Several recent studies have examined the role of MC1R in melanoma risk, finding that carriers of MC1R variants are at a significantly higher risk of melanoma, independent of sun exposure [60, 61].

Somatic Mutations

The Cancer Genome Atlas (TCGA) is currently the largest analysis of somatic aberrations in melanoma to date, including 333 cutaneous melanomas (80% of which were metastatic), and providing valuable insight into mutations that drive melanoma [48]. Whole-exome sequencing studies have shown that melanoma carries one of the highest mutation burdens compared to most other cancers [62, 63]. Identifying the specific mutations involved with the development of melanoma may not only improve our understanding of molecular pathogenesis, but also recognize therapeutic options as well as link clinical characteristics to genetic subtypes. To date, most studies have generally been small and come up with different sets of somatic mutations associated with survival.

Tumor Subtypes

Melanoma has a variety of histological subtypes with multifaceted epidemiology. Different patterns have been noted including differences in anatomical site and age-specific incidence, leading to the idea that more than one pathway may be responsible for the development of melanoma. Different genotypes have been associated with various clinical and histological subtypes. Previous evidence indicates that melanoma arising from chronically sun-exposed skin compared to non-chronically sun-exposed skin differs in terms of location of primary tumor, histological and clinical presentation, age at onset, and speed of progression. BRAF gene mutations were commonly found in tumors arising from intermittently sun-exposed skin. These mutations tend to be found more commonly in melanoma arising from the trunk, which is exposed during intermittent sun exposure [64]. Data show that the BRAF V600E mutation occurred in significantly younger patients who had increased nevi and fewer actinic keratoses and were more likely to have a family history of melanoma [65]. BRAF V600E mutations have been significantly associated with the presence of ulceration, increased tumor thickness, and reduced survival [66]. NRAS mutations occur more commonly in melanoma arising from chronically sun-exposed sites such as the head and neck and extremities [47].

Hacker et al. [65] conducted a study analyzing 414 patients with newly diagnosed cutaneous melanoma and found mutually exclusive mutations in BRAF V600E (26%), BRAF V600 K (8%), BRAF wild type (5%), and NRAS (9%), as did Thomas et al. [67]. Data shows that BRAF V600E mutations occurred in significantly younger patients, those with increased nevi, fewer actinic keratoses, and those with a family history of melanoma [65]. Both Hugdahl et al. [66] and Thomas et al. [67] found that BRAF V600E mutations significantly associated with the presence of ulceration, increased tumor thickness, and reduced survival. BRAF V600 K and NRAS gene mutations occurred more commonly with increased nevi, increasing age, and less overall sun exposure [67].

Prevention of Melanoma

Melanoma is caused by a set of different combinations of excessive sun exposure and genetic factors. Until we understand the genetic factors and interactions more precisely, preventing melanoma generally means preventing excessive sunburn. Genetic testing can give us some indication of risk, but such testing is not yet ready for general population use. New studies are evaluating the use of chemopreventive agents. These are, however, still in the pipeline and are not quite ready for use by the general population [68]. Vitamin D supplements have been proposed as a way to reduce melanoma incidence and mortality, but there is little direct evidence that these will be effective [69].

Prevention of Excessive Sun Exposure: Primary Prevention

As sunburn at any life stage, including childhood, increases the risk of melanoma [70], there are multiple prevention programs that aim to prevent sunburns. Most individuals, particularly children, may not use adequate sun protection [71–73]. There has been a very strong emphasis on the use of sunscreens to prevent sunburns and skin cancer of all types. Green et al. [74] performed a randomized trial demonstrating that in Queensland, over a long period of time, the use of sunscreen decreased the incidence of melanoma. Additionally, a population-based case–control study showed that the use of sunscreens was significantly more common among the control group [75]. However, the same study has found that other forms of sun protection, such as seeking shade and wearing long sleeves and hats, had an even stronger effect on risk reduction of melanoma. The Ontario Sun Safety Working Group [76] recently developed an update to recommendations for sun safety and recommended, in this order: protecting your skin, seeking shade or bring your own, wearing clothing and a wide-brimmed hat, and using sunscreen labeled "broad spectrum" and "water resistant" with a sun protection factor (SPF) of 30. Apply and reapply frequently. Don't use UV tanning equipment and avoid getting a sunburn while protecting your eyes with sunglasses.

Educational Efforts at Prevention Around the World and Within the United States

Recently, school-based sun safety educational programs and policies have been developed to teach sun safety, which when taught at an early age can influence a lifetime of healthy habits. The caveat is that such educational efforts must be implemented frequently and over a long period of time [77–79]. In 2012, the Community Prevention Services Task Force at CDC [78] reviewed 33 sun safety educational and policy interventions within schools between 1966 and 2011. They concluded that such programs "increased sun-protective behaviors and decreased ultraviolet exposure, sunburn incidence, and formation of new moles" [80].

As Australia and New Zealand have the highest rates of melanoma in the world, Australia developed the 1988 "Slip! Slop! Slap!" campaign that evolved into a comprehensive, multi-setting, multi-approach program that includes a voluntary "Sun Smart" school accreditation program [81]. Resources are provided for early childhood, primary and secondary schools, as well as workplaces, local government, sports groups, events, festivities, and families.

Examples of Sun Smart criteria include mandatory hat wearing, encouraging shade seeking, avoiding peak UVR hours, and positive sun-protective behavioral role modeling. A total of 90% of schools in Victoria, Australia, are registered with Sun Smart, reaching an estimated 430,000 children. Only 17% of Victorian primary schools had sun protection policies in 1993; 20 years later, 89% have policies in place. Australia's "no hat, no play" policy (recently promoted in Hawaii, USA) was shown to significantly increase hat wearing among children on the playground [82]. Only 2% of Victorian preschools reported hats available to preschoolers in 1988; 20 years later, 91% now have hats available [83].

In the United States and other countries like Sweden, Norway, and the UK, projected melanoma incidence will continue to rise [84]. Multiple skin cancer prevention programs are available on the Web [85]. In 2008, the SunWise program in the United States was estimated to prevent more than 11,000 cases of skin cancer and 50 premature deaths by 2015 and found that "every federal dollar invested in SunWise would save $2-4 in public health costs" [86]. Critically, the implementation of policy leads to increased practice [87]. Sun safety education campaigns have also been developed and adopted by a number of other countries such as South Africa, New Zealand, Canada, France, Germany, Northern Ireland, and Israel [85], although later in time compared to the Australian Sun Smart campaign and more sporadic implementation [84].

The success of sun safety education programs is in large part dependent upon the comprehensive nature of their implementation. Extracurricular programs such as aquatic centers, summer camps, and parks have been excellent scaffolding for the dissemination of sun safety knowledge and encouragement of sun safety behaviors. For example, the CDC-funded "Pool Cool" campaign was developed in order to increase UVR risk awareness and teach sun-protective behaviors before swimming lessons. The program was designed to target children, parents, patrons, and staff. The eight-lesson curriculum consists of a 5-min lesson on sun safety by lifeguards and/or instructors before swim practice. As part of the program, centers receive shade structures, signage, and sunscreen dispensers for the promotion of a sun safe pool environment. An increase in sun-protective behaviors was reported in one randomized study and a decrease in sunburns reported in another observational study [88, 89].

Effectiveness of Skin Cancer Screening by Individuals and Physicians: Secondary Prevention

Skin cancer screening is still considered controversial, despite the seemingly intuitive advantages of being able to visually identify a skin cancer in its early stages by performing a full-body skin exam. In 2016, the United States Preventive Services Task Force (USPSTF) concluded that evidence was still insufficient for the recommendation of clinical skin cancer screening guidelines for asymptomatic adults without a history of prior malignant or premalignant skin conditions [90]. In 2003, a melanoma screening program piloted in the state of Schleswig-Holstein after intensive public awareness campaigns and skin cancer detection training for general health practitioners. The initial 5-year results showed an almost 50% reduction in melanoma rates compared to surrounding states [91]. Unfortunately, after nationwide implementation, 5-year data has yet to show any measurable reduction; in fact, mortality has since returned to baseline levels in Schleswig-Holstein [92, 93]. After reviewing tumor-stage distribution and malignant melanoma survival in Germany between 2002 and 2011, neither Schoffer et al. nor Boniol et al. found any direct influence on mortality from the introduction of this national skin cancer screening program [94, 95].

Preliminary data from a University of Pittsburgh screening program [96] and a Queensland study [97] have shown that finding a melanoma with decreased tumor thickness was associated with the screened group versus unscreened population. Most recently, a 2017 systematic review of 15 studies found the most current evidence, though low, showing some benefit to a skin cancer screening program [98]. Specialized surveillance for high-risk individuals has also been shown to result in lower treatment costs and fewer invasive procedures compared to standard community care [99] and has been recommended by a group of melanoma experts at the Society for Melanoma Research [100].

A study from Belgium found "lesion-directed skin exams" to have similar detection rates as total-body skin exams, which are six times more time consuming [101]. Public education on warning features and proper self-exam techniques are building blocks for successful lesion-directed skin exams, as these factors prompt physician follow-up for concerning moles [102]. There is insufficient data to elucidate the long-term effects of skin cancer screening on mortality. However, primary physician skin exams, particularly lesion directed, could be beneficial. These, in conjunction with specialized exams for high-risk populations, may offer the most potential for capturing benefits such as decreased tumor thickness and cost savings.

Guidelines and Recommendations for Melanoma Prevention and Screening

Multiple groups have made valuable recommendations for the prevention and screening for melanoma. Most suggest that effective prevention lies in the general population awareness of their skin and any changes. For example, Berwick and Paddock reported that among those who reported being aware of their skin, defined as aware of it for medical or cosmetic reasons, there was a 50% reduction in mortality from melanoma [103]. Furthermore, there is a need to assess the benefits of targeted screening to those at highest risk, such as males that are older than 50 years of age. In the meantime, the messages that may help to reduce melanoma incidence include the following: (1) protect the skin when the UV index is 3 or higher, (2) seek shade, (3) wear clothing and (4) a wide-brimmed hat as well as (5) generously apply sunscreen labeled "broad spectrum" and reapply after 2 h in the sun to skin not covered by clothing, and finally (6) see your healthcare provider if you notice any suspicious-looking lesions.

Conclusions

Understanding the basic biology of melanoma has recently led to new therapies. Clearly, more work in this area is critical to understanding fully how melanoma develops and how to prevent it. Furthermore, there is a great deal more research needed to refine the definition of high-risk individuals for targeted education and screening in order to prevent melanoma.

References

1. Howlader N, Noone AM, Krapsho M, Miller D, Bishop K, Altekruse SF, et al., editors. SEER cancer statistics review, 1975–2013. Bethesda, MD., http://seer.cancer.gov/csr/1975-2013/, based on November 2015 SEER data submission, to the SEER web site, April: National Cancer Institute; 2016.
2. Gandini S, Sera F, Cattaruzza MS, Pasquini P, Zanetti R, Masini C, et al. Meta-analysis of risk factors for cutaneous melanoma: III: family history, actinic damage and phenotypic factors. Eur J Cancer. 2005;41:2040–59.
3. Armstrong BK, Kricker A. The epidemiology of UV induced skin cancer. J Photochem Photobiol B. 2001;63:8–18.
4. Fears TR, Bird CC, Guerry D, Sagebiel RW, Gail MH, Elder DE, et al. Average midrange ultraviolet radiation flux and time outdoors predict melanoma risk. Cancer Res. 2002;62:3992–6.
5. Zanetti R, Prota G, Napolitano A, Martinez C, Sancho-Garnier H, Østerlind A, et al. Development of an integrated method of skin phenotype measurement using the melanins. Melanoma Res. 2001;11:551–7.
6. Goldstein AM, Tucker MA. Dysplastic nevi and melanoma. Cancer Epidemiol Biomark Prev. 2013;22:528–32.
7. Marks R. Epidemiology of melanoma. Clin Exp Dermatol. 2000;25:459–63.
8. Gallagher RP, Rivers JK, Lee TK, Bajdik CD, McLean DI, Coldman AJ. Broad-spectrum sunscreen use and the development of new nevi in white children: a randomized controlled trial. JAMA. 2000;283:2955–60.
9. Milne E, Johnston R, Cross D, Giles-Corti B, English DR. Effect of a school-based sun-protection intervention on the development of melanocytic nevi in children. Am J Epidemiol. 2002;155:739–45.
10. Autier P, Boniol M, Severi G, Pedeux R, Grivegnée AR, Doré JF. Sex differences in numbers of nevi on body sites of young European children: implications for the etiology of cutaneous melanoma. Cancer Epidemiol Biomark Prev. 2004;13:2003–5.
11. Stierner U, Augustsson A, Rosdahl I, Suurküla M. Regional distribution of common and dysplastic naevi in relation to melanoma site and sun exposure. A case-control study. Melanoma Res. 1992;1:367–75.
12. Gandini S, Sera F, Cattaruzza MS, Pasquini P, Abeni D, Boyle P, Melchi CF. Meta-analysis of risk factors for cutaneous melanoma: I. Common and atypical naevi. Eur J Cancer. 2005a;41:28–44.
13. Whiteman DC, Watt P, Purdie DM, Hughes MC, Hayward NK, Green AC. Melanocytic nevi, solar keratoses, and divergent pathways to cutaneous melanoma. J Natl Cancer Inst. 2003;95:806–12.
14. International Agency for Research on Cancer Working Group on artificial ultraviolet (UV) light and skin cancer. The association of use of sunbeds with cutaneous malignant melanoma and other skin cancers: a systematic review. Int J Cancer. 2007;120:1116–22.
15. Matsumura Y, Ananthaswamy HN. Toxic effects of ultraviolet radiation on the skin. Toxicol Appl Pharmacol. 2004;195:298–308.
16. Parkin DM, Mesher D, Sasieni P. Cancers attributable to solar (ultraviolet) radiation exposure in the UK in 2010. Br J Cancer. 2011;105:66–9.
17. Armstrong BK, Kricker A. How much melanoma is caused by sun exposure? Melanoma Res. 1993;3:395–401.
18. Chang C, Murzaku EC, Penn L, Abbasi NR, Davis PD, Berwick M, et al. More skin, more sun, more tan, more melanoma. Am J Public Health. 2014;104:92–9.
19. Gandini S, Sera F, Cattaruzza M, Pasquini P, Picconi O, Boyle P, et al. Meta-analysis of risk factors for cutaneous melanoma: II. Sun exposure. Eur J Cancer. 2005b;41:45–60.
20. Kricker A, Armstrong BK, Goumas C, Litchfield M, Begg CB, Hummer AJ, et al. Ambient UV, personal sun exposure and risk of multiple primary melanomas. Cancer Causes Control. 2007;18:295–304.
21. Pfahlberg A, Kölmel KF, Gefeller O. Timing of excessive ultraviolet radiation and melanoma: epidemiology does not support the existence of a critical period of high susceptibility to solar ultraviolet radiation- induced melanoma. Br J Dermatol. 2001;144(3):471–5.
22. Whiteman DC, Whiteman CA, Green AC. Childhood sun exposure as a risk factor for melanoma: a systematic review of epidemiologic studies. Cancer Causes Control. 2001;12:69–82.
23. Guy GP, Berkowitz Z, Holman DM, Hartman AM. Recent changes in the prevalence of and factors

associated with frequency of indoor tanning among US adults. JAMA Dermatol. 2015;151:1256–9.
24. Hornung RL, Magee KH, Lee WJ, Hansen LA, Hsieh YC. Tanning facility use: are we exceeding Food and Drug Administration limits? J Am Acad Dermatol. 2003;49:655–61.
25. Lazovich D, Vogel RI, Weinstock MA, Nelson HH, Ahmed RL, Berwick M. Association between indoor tanning and melanoma in younger men and women. JAMA Dermatol. 2016;152:268–75.
26. Lazovich D, Vogel RI, Berwick M, Weinstock MA, Anderson KE, Warshaw EM. Indoor tanning and risk of melanoma: a case-control study in a highly exposed population. Cancer Epidemiol Biomark Prev. 2010;19:1557–68.
27. Héry C, Tryggvadóttir L, Sigurdsson T, Ólafsdóttir E, Sigurgeirsson B, Jonasson JG, et al. A melanoma epidemic in Iceland: possible influence of sunbed use. Am J Epidemiol. 2010;172:762–7.
28. Bulbulyan MA, Ilychova SA, Zahm SH, Astashevsky SV, Zaridze DG. Cancer mortality among women in the Russian printing industry. Am J Ind Med. 1999;36:166–71.
29. Nielsen H, Henriksen L, Olsen JH. Malignant melanoma among lithographers. Scand J Work Environ Health. 1996;22:106–11.
30. Linet MS, Malker HS, Chow WH, McLaughlin JK, Weiner JA, Stone BJ, et al. Occupational risks for cutaneous melanoma among men in Sweden. J Occup Environ Med. 1995;37:1127–35.
31. McLaughlin JK, Malker HS, Blot WJ, Ericsson JL, Gemne G, Fraumeni JF, JR. Malignant melanoma in the printing industry. Am J Ind Med. 1988;13:301–4.
32. Dubrow R. Malignant melanoma in the printing industry. Am J Ind Med. 1986;10:119–26.
33. Robinson CF, Petersen M, Palu S. Mortality patterns among electrical workers employed in the U.S. construction industry. Am J Ind Med. 1999;36:630–7.
34. DeTrolio R, Di Lorenzo G, Fumo B, Ascierto PA. Cosmic radiation and cancer: is there a link? JAMA Dermatol. 2015;151:51–8.
35. Sanlorenzo M, Wehner MR, Linos E, Kornak J, Kainz W, Posch C, et al. The risk of melanoma in airline pilots and cabin crew: a meta-analysis. Occup Environ Med. 2014;71:398–404.
36. Pukkala E, Martinsen JI, Weiderpass E, Kjaerheim K, Lynge E, Tryggvadottir L, et al. Cancer incidence among firefighters: 45 years of follow-up in five Nordic countries. Occup Environ Med. 2014;71:398–404.
37. Wang L, Ding G, Zhou Z, Liu X, Wang Y, Xie HQ, et al. Patterns and dietary intake of polychlorinated dibenzo-p-dioxins and polychlorinated dibenzofurans in food products in China. J Environ Sci (China). 2017;51:165–72.
38. Wood SA, Armitage JM, Binnington MJ, Wania F. Deterministic modeling of the exposure of individual participants in the National Health and Nutrition Examination Survey (NHANES) to polychlorinated biphenyls. Environ Sci Process Impacts. 2016;18:1157–68.
39. Fromberg A, Granby K, Hajgard A, Fagr S, Larsen JC. Estimation of dietary intake of PCB and organochlorine pesticides for children and adults. Food Chem. 2011;125:1179–87.
40. Donat-Vargas C, Berglund M, Glynn A, Wolk A, Åkesson A. Dietary polychlorinated biphenyls, long-chain n-3 polyunsaturated fatty acids and incidence of malignant melanoma. Eur J Cancer. 2017;72:137–43.
41. Gallagher RP, Macarthur AC, Lee TK, Weber JP, Leblanc A, Elwood MJ, et al. Plasma levels of polychlorinated biphenyls and risk of cutaneous malignant melanoma: a preliminary study. Int J Cancer. 2011;128:1872–80.
42. Meyskens FL, Yang S. Thinking about the role (largely ignored) of heavy metals in cancer prevention: hexavalent chromium and melanoma as a case in point. Recent Results Cancer Res. 2011;188:65–74.
43. Rizzi M, Cravello B, Renò F. Textile industry manufacturing by-products induce human melanoma cell proliferation via ERK1/2 activation. Cell Prolif. 2014;47:578–86.
44. Visuri TI, Pukkala E, Pulkkinen P, Paavolainen P. Cancer incidence and causes of death among total hip replacement patients: a review based on Nordic cohorts with a special emphasis on metal-on-metal bearings. Proc Inst Mech Eng H. 2006;220:399–407.
45. Onega T, Baron J, MacKenzie T. Cancer after total joint arthroplasty: a meta-analysis. Cancer Epidemiol Biomark Prev. 2006;15:1532–7.
46. Nyren O, McLaughlin JK, Gridley G, Ekborn A, Johnell O, Fraumeni JR Jr, Adami HO. Cancer risk after hip replacement with metal implants: a population-based cohort study in Sweden. J Natl Cancer Inst. 1995;87:28–33.
47. Hill VK, Gartner JJ, Samuels Y, Goldstein AM. The genetics of melanoma: recent advances. Annu Rev Genomics Hum Genet. 2013;14:257–79.
48. Zhang T, Dutton-Regester K, Brown KM, Hayward NK. The genomic landscape of cutaneous melanoma. Pigment Cell Melanoma Res. 2016;29:266–83.
49. Markovic SN, Erickson LA, Rao RD, Weenig RH, Pockaj BA, Bardia A, et al. Malignant melanoma in the 21st century, Part 1: Epidemiology, risk factors, screening, prevention, and diagnosis. Mayo Clin Proc. 2007;82:364–80.
50. Cho E, Rosner BA, Colditz GA. Risk factors for melanoma by body site. Cancer Epidemiol Biomark Prev. 2005;14:1241–4.
51. Berwick M, Orlow I, Hummer AJ, Armstrong BK, Kricker A, Marrett LD, et al. The prevalence of CDKN2A germ-line mutations and relative risk for cutaneous malignant melanoma: an international population-based study. Cancer Epidemiol Biomark Prev. 2006;15:1520–5.
52. Barnhill RL, Roush GC, Titus-Ernstoff L, Ernstoff MS, Duray PH, Kirkwood JM. Comparison of

nonfamilial and familial melanoma. Dermatology. 1992;184:2–7.
53. Ferrone CR, Ben Porat L, Panageas KS, Berwick M, Halpern AC, Patel A, et al. Clinicopathological features of and risk factors for multiple primary melanomas. JAMA. 2005;294:1647–54.
54. Barón AE, Asdigian NL, Gonzalez V, Aalborg J, Terzian T, Stiegmann RA. Interactions between ultraviolet light and MC1R and OCA2 variants are determinants of childhood nevus and freckle phenotypes. Cancer Epidemiol Biomark Prev. 2014;23:2829–39.
55. Beaumont KA, Shekar SN, Cook AL, Duffy DL, Sturm RA. Red hair is the null phenotype of MC1R. Hum Mutat. 2008;29:88–94.
56. García-Borrón JC, Abdel-Malek Z, Jiménez-Cervantes C. MC1R, the cAMP pathway, and the response to solar UV: extending the horizon beyond pigmentation. Pigment Cell Melanoma Res. 2014;27:699–720.
57. Cassidy PB, Abdel-Malek Z, Leachman SA. Beyond red hair and sunburns: uncovering the molecular mechanisms of MC1R signaling and repair of UV-induced DNA damage. J Invest Dermatol. 2015;135:2918–21.
58. Jarrett SG, Wolf Horrell EM, Boulanger MC, D'Orazio JA. Defining the contribution of MC1R physiological ligands to ATR phosphorylation at Ser435, a predictor of DNA repair in melanocytes. J Invest Dermatol. 2015;135:3086–95.
59. Denat L, Kadekaro AL, Marrot L, Leachman SA, Abdel-Malek ZA. Melanocytes as instigators and victims of oxidative stress. J Invest Dermatol. 2014;134:1512–8.
60. Wendt J, Rauscher S, Burgstaller-Muehlbacher S, Fae I, Fischer G, Pehamberger H, et al. Human determinants and the role of melanocortin-1 receptor variants in melanoma risk independent of UV radiation exposure. JAMA Dermatol. 2016;152:776–82.
61. Pasquali E, Garcia-Borron JC, Fargnoli MC, Gandini S, Maisonneuve P, Bagnardi V, et al. MC1R variants increased the risk of sporadic cutaneous melanoma in darker-pigmented Caucasians: a pooled-analysis from the M-SKIP project. Int J Cancer. 2015;136:618–31.
62. Hodis E, Watson IR, Kryukov GV, Arold ST, Imielinski M, Theurillat JP, et al. A landscape of driver mutations in melanoma. Cell. 2012;150:251–63.
63. Krauthammer M, Kong Y, Ha BH, Evans P, Bacchiocchi A, McCusker JP, et al. Exome sequencing identifies recurrent somatic RAC1 mutations in melanoma. Nat Genet. 2012;44(9):1006–14.
64. Thomas NE, Kanetsky PA, Edmiston SN, Alexander A, Begg CB, Groben PA, et al. Relationship between germline MC1R variants and BRAF-mutant melanoma in a North Carolina population-based study. J Invest Dermatol. 2010;130:1463–5.
65. Hacker E, Olsen CM, Kvaskoff M, Pandeya N, Yeo A, Green AC. Histologic and phenotypic factors and MC1R status associated with BRAFV600E, BRAFV600K, and NRAS mutations in a community-based sample of 414 cutaneous melanomas. J Invest Dermatol. 2016;136:829–37.
66. Hugdahl E, Kalvenes MB, Puntervoll HE, Ladstein RG, Akslen LA. BRAF-V600E expression in primary nodular melanoma is associated with aggressive tumour features and reduced survival. Br J Cancer. 2016;114:801–8.
67. Thomas NE, Edmiston SN, Alexander A, Groben PA, Parrish E, Kricker A, et al. Association between NRAS and BRAF mutational status and melanoma-specific survival among patients with higher-risk primary melanoma. JAMA Oncol. 2015;1:359–68.
68. Mounessa J, Buntinx-Krieg T, Qin R, Dunnick CA, Dellavalle RP. Primary and secondary chemoprevention of malignant melanoma. Am J Clin Dermatol. 2016;17:625–34.
69. Moyer VA, U.S. Preventive Services Task Force. Vitamin, mineral, and multivitamin supplements for the primary prevention of cardiovascular disease and cancer: US Preventive Services Task Force recommendation statement. Ann Intern Med. 2014;160:558–64.
70. Dennis LK, Vanbeek MJ, Freeman LEB, Smith BJ, Dawson DV, Coughlin JA. Sunburns and risk of cutaneous melanoma: does age matter? A comprehensive meta-analysis. Ann Epidemiol. 2008;18:614–27.
71. Rouhani P, Parmet Y, Bessell AG, Peay T, Weiss A, Kirsner RS. Knowledge, attitudes, and behaviors of elementary school students regarding sun exposure and skin cancer. Pediatr Dermatol. 2009;26:529–35.
72. Hall HI, Jorgensen CM, McDavid K, Kraft JM, Breslow R. Protection from sun exposure in US white children ages 6 months to 11 years. Public Health Rep. 2001;116:353–61.
73. Buller DB, Cokkinides V, Hall HI, Hartman AM, Saraiya M, Miller E, et al. Prevalence of sunburn, sun protection, and indoor tanning behaviors among Americans: review from national surveys and case studies of 3 states. J Am Acad Dermatol. 2011;65:114–23.
74. Green AC, Williams GM, Logan V, Strutton GM. Reduced melanoma after regular sunscreen use: randomized trial follow-up. J Clin Oncol. 2011;29:257–63.
75. Lazovich D, Vogel RI, Berwick M, Weinstock MA, Warshaw EM, Anderson KE. Melanoma risk in relation to use of sunscreen or other sun protection methods. Cancer Epidemiol Biomark Prev. 2011;20:2583–93.
76. Marrett LD, Chu MB, Atkinson J, Nuttall R, Bromfield G, Hershfield L, et al. An update to the recommended core content for sun safety messages for public eduction in Canada: a consensus report. Can J Public Health. 2016;207:473–9.
77. García-Romero MT, Geller AC, Kawachi I. Using behavioral economics to promote healthy behavior toward sun exposure in adolescents and young adults. Prev Med. 2015;81:184–8.
78. Ettridge KA, Bowden JA, Rayner JM, Wilson CJ. The relationship between sun protection policy

and associated practices in a national sample of early childhood services in Australia. Health Educ Res. 2011;26:53–62.
79. Wright CY, Reeder AI, Albers PN. Knowledge and practice of sun protection in schools in South Africa where no national sun protection programme exists. Health Educ Res. 2016;31:247–59.
80. Community Preventive Services Task Force. Preventing skin cancer: primary and middle school-based interventions; 2012. https://www.thecommunityguide.org/sites/default/files/assets/Skin-Cancer-Primary-and-Middle-School.pdf. Accessed: 20 Jan 2017.
81. Montague M, Borland R, Sinclair C. Slip! slop! slap! and SunSmart, 1980–2000: skin cancer control and 20 years of population-based campaigning. Health Educ Behav. 2001;28:290–305.
82. Giles-Corti B, English DR, Costa C, Milne E, Cross D, Johnston R. Creating sunsmart schools. Health Educ Res. 2004;19:98–109.
83. Cancer Council Victoria: History of Sun Smart. http://www.sunsmart.com.au/about/history. Accessed 18 Feb 2017.
84. Whiteman DC, Green AC, Olsen CM. The growing burden of invasive melanoma: projections of incidence rates and numbers of new cases in six susceptible populations through 2013. J Invest Dermatol. 2016;136:1164–71.
85. World Health Organization. Sun Protection and schools: How to make a difference. World Health Organization, 2003. http://www.who.int/uv/publications/en/sunprotschools.pdf. Accessed 20 Jan 2017.
86. Kyle JW, Hammett JK, Lim HW, Geller AC, Hall-Jordan LH, Maibach EW, et al. Economic evaluation of the US Environmental Protection Agency's SunWise program: sun protection education for young children. Pediatrics. 2008;121:e1074–84.
87. Dono J, Ettridge KA, Sharplin GR, Wilson CJ. The relationship between sun protection policies and practices in schools with primary-age students: the role of school demographics, policy comprehensiveness and SunSmart membership. Health Educ Res. 2014;29:1–12.
88. Geller AC, Glanz K, Shigaki D, Isnec MR, Sun T, Maddock J. Impact of skin cancer prevention on outdoor aquatics staff: the pool cool program in Hawaii and Massachusetts. Prev Med. 2001;33:155–61.
89. Glanz K, Geller AC, Shigaki D, Maddock JE, Isnec MR. A randomized trial of skin cancer prevention in aquatics settings: the pool cool program. Health Psychol. 2002;21:579–87.
90. US Preventive Services Task Force, Bibbins-Domingo K, Grossman DC, Curry SJ, Davidson KW, Ebell M, et al. Screening for skin cancer: US preventive services task force recommendation statement. JAMA. 2016;316:429–35.
91. Katalinic A, Waldmann A, Weinstock MA, Geller AC, Eisemann N, Greinert R, et al. Does skin cancer screening save lives? An observational study comparing trends in melanoma mortality in regions with and without screening. Cancer. 2012;118:5395–402.
92. Stang A, Garbe C, Autier P, Jockel KH. The many unanswered questions related to the German skin cancer screening programme. Eur J Cancer. 2016;64:83–8.
93. Stang A, Jockel KH. Does skin cancer screening save lives? A detailed analysis of mortality time trends in Schleswig-Holstein and Germany. Cancer. 2016;122:432–7.
94. Schoffer O, Schülein S, Arand G, Arnholdt H, Baaske D, Bargou RC, et al. Tumour stage distribution and survival of malignant melanoma in Germany 2002–2011. BMC Cancer. 2016;16:936.
95. Boniol M, Autier P, Gandini S. Melanoma mortality following skin cancer screening in Germany. BMJ Open. 2015;5:e008158.
96. Ferris LK, Saul MI, Lin Y, Deng F, Weinstock MA, Geller AC, et al. A large skin cancer screening quality initiative. Description and first-year outcomes. JAMA Oncol. 2017.; [Epub ahead of print]
97. Aitken JF, Elwood M, Baade PD, Youl P, English D. Clinical whole-body skin examination reduces the incidence of thick melanomas. Int J Cancer. 2010;126:450–8.
98. Brunssen A, Waldmann A, Eisemann N, Katalinic A. Impact of skin cancer screening and secondary prevention campaigns on skin cancer incidence and mortality: a systematic review. J Am Acad Dermatol. 2017;76:129–39.
99. Watts CG, Cust AE, Menzies SW, Mann GJ, Morton RL. Cost-effectiveness of skin surveillance through a specialized clinic for patients at high risk of melanoma. J Clin Oncol. 2017;35:63–71.
100. Merlino G, Herlyn M, Fisher DE, Bastian BC, Flaherty KT, Davies MA, et al. The state of melanoma: challenges and opportunities. Pigment Cell Melanoma Res. 2016;29:404–16.
101. Hoorens I, Vossaert K, Pil L, Boone B, De Schepper S, Ongenae K, et al. Total-body examination vs lesion-directed skin cancer screening. JAMA Dermatol. 2016;152:27–34.1.
102. Weinstock MA, Risica PM, Martin RA, Rakowski W, Smith KJ, Berwick M, et al. Reliability of assessment and circumstances of performance of thorough skin self-examination for the early detection of melanoma in the Check-It-Out Project. Prev Med. 2004;38:761–5.
103. Paddock LE, Lu SE, Bandera EV, Rhoads GG, Fine J, Paine S, et al. Skin self-examination and long-term melanoma survival. Melanoma Res. 2016;26:401–8.

Methods of Melanoma Detection

4

Clara Curiel-Lewandrowski, Clara Stemwedel, Mihaela Balu, Suephy C. Chen, Laura K. Ferris, Pedram Gerami, Adele C. Green, Mariah M. Johnson, Lois J. Loescher, Josep Malvehy, Ashfaq A. Marghoob, Kathryn Martires, Giovanni Pellacani, Tracy Petrie, Susana Puig, Inga Saknite, Susan M. Swetter, Per Svedenhag, Eric R. Tkaczyk, Oliver J. Wisco, and Sancy A. Leachman

Clara Curiel-Lewandrowski and Sancy A. Leachman contributed equally to this work.

C. Curiel-Lewandrowski, M.D. (✉)
Department of Dermatology, The University of Arizona, Tucson, AZ, USA
e-mail: ccuriel@email.arizona.edu

C. Stemwedel, M.L.S. · M. M. Johnson, M.D.
T. Petrie, Ph.D. · O. J. Wisco, D.O.
S. A. Leachman, M.D., Ph.D. (✉)
Department of Dermatology, Oregon Health & Science University, Portland, OR, USA
e-mail: stemwedc@ohsu.edu; johmaria@ohsu.edu; petrie@ohsu.edu; wisco@ohsu.edu; leachmas@ohsu.edu

M. Balu, Ph.D.
Department of Surgery, Beckman Laser Institute and Medical Clinic, University of California, Irvine, CA, USA
e-mail: mbalu@uci.edu

S. C. Chen, M.D.
Department of Dermatology, Emory University and Atlanta VA Medical Center, Atlanta, GA, USA
e-mail: schen2@emory.edu

L. K. Ferris, M.D., Ph.D.
Department of Dermatology, University of Pittsburgh Medical Center, Pittsburgh, PA, USA
e-mail: ferrislk@upmc.edu

P. Gerami, M.D.
Skin Cancer Institute of Northwestern Medicine (SCIN-Med), Chicago, IL, USA

Melanoma Program of SCIN-Med, Department of Dermatology, Northwestern Hospital, Chicago, IL, USA
e-mail: pedram.gerami@nm.org

A. C. Green, M.B.B.S., Ph.D., F.A.H.M.S.
Population Health, Herston, QLD, Australia

QIMR Berghofer Medical Research Institute and CRUK Manchester Institute, University of Manchester, Manchester, UK
e-mail: Adele.Green@qimrberghofer.edu.au

L. J. Loescher, Ph.D., R.N., F.A.A.N.
The University of Arizona, College of Nursing, Tucson, AZ, USA
e-mail: loescher@email.arizona.edu

J. Malvehy, M.D., Ph.D. · S. Puig, M.D., Ph.D.
Department of Dermatology, Hospital Clinic Barcelona, Barcelona, Catalonia, Spain

A. A. Marghoob, M.D.
Division of Dermatology, Department of Medicine, Memorial Sloan Kettering Cancer Center, New York, NY, USA
e-mail: marghooa@mskcc.org

K. Martires, M.D.
Stanford University School of Medicine, Department of Dermatology, Palo Alto, CA, USA
e-mail: martires@stanford.edu

G. Pellacani, M.D.
Department of Dermatology, University of Modena and Reggio Emilia, Modena, Italy
e-mail: Giovanni.pellacani@unimore.it

A. I. Riker (ed.), *Melanoma*, https://doi.org/10.1007/978-3-319-78310-9_4

I. Saknite, Ph.D.
Vanderbilt University Medical Center, Department of Medicine, Vanderbilt Health, One Hundred Oaks, Nashville, TN, USA
e-mail: inga.saknite@vanderbilt.edu

S. M. Swetter, M.D.
Stanford University Medical Center and Cancer Institute, Stanford, CA, USA

VA Palo Alto Health Care System, Palo Alto, CA, USA

Department of Dermatology/Cutaneous Oncology, Stanford Dermatology/Cutaneous Oncology, Stanford, CA, USA
e-mail: sswetter@stanford.edu

P. Svedenhag, M.Sc.E.E.
SciBase, Stockholm, Sweden
e-mail: per.svedenhag@scibase.com

E. R. Tkaczyk, M.D., Ph.D.
Cutaneous Imaging Clinic, Vanderbilt University Medical Center, Department of Medicine, One Hundred Oaks—Dermatology, Nashville, TN, USA
e-mail: eric.tkaczyk@vanderbilt.edu

Background and Introduction

Principles of Melanoma Early Detection

Diagnosing melanoma early, before it develops the capacity to metastasize and kill, has the potential to reduce morbidity and mortality from the disease and its treatment. In turn, this will also result in a decrease in the cost of care for individuals and society, as a whole. Delay of diagnosis and treatment may lead to the need for wider local excisions, additional procedures to sample and/or remove lymph nodes or other organs, and therapeutic interventions that can have substantial side effects. These side effects may subsequently result in the further need for care, treatment, and hospitalization [1]. Additionally, although as many as 50% of patients may achieve long-term remission with therapy for advanced melanoma [2], the disfigurement and long-term sequelae of therapy can be quite significant (e.g., chronic lymphedema, cognitive impairment, lifelong endocrinopathies). As a result, survivors will often have a diminished quality of life and even a reduced duration of life relative to what they would have experienced in the setting of effective primary prevention and early detection.

The costs of treating melanoma increase as the patient presents with more advanced disease. The American Academy of Dermatology (AAD) has recently commissioned an analysis of the cost burden of skin cancer in the United States, finding that 1,073,875 Americans received a diagnosis of melanoma in 2013. The average cost of treatment for melanoma, per person, is $1366.08, with an estimated 9.5 years of life lost, and a loss of $88 million of productivity secondary to life lost from melanoma [3]. A recent systematic review by Rubio-Rodriguez and colleagues concludes that it is currently not possible to determine which therapy among BRAF inhibitors, MEK inhibitors, or immunotherapies is the most cost-effective relative to chemotherapy [4].

However, the new targeted immunotherapies are expensive and range from $169,320 for a full course of treatment with nivolumab, and to $228,352 for combination therapy with nivolumab and ipilimumab [5]. When modeling the cost-effectiveness of nivolumab, ipilimumab, and nivolumab-ipilimumab combination as first-line therapy for patients with metastatic melanoma, nivolumab-ipilimumab combination therapy was shown to be a cost-effective choice. The total costs are significant, with an amount of $454,092 per progression-free survival quality-adjusted life year compared with nivolumab monotherapy [5]. It is anticipated that the cost of treating advanced melanoma will continue to increase in the foreseeable future. Additional long-term clinical trial results and cost-effectiveness studies are needed in order to guide sensitive and responsible guideline recommendations for treatment of advanced melanoma.

Thus, from the perspective of morbidity, mortality, quality of life, and cost, there is a compelling need to improve the early detection of melanoma. Fortunately, because melanoma is usually visible on the surface of the skin, it is well suited for the application of early detection approaches and noninvasive technologies. The purpose of this chapter is to present a broad spectrum of approaches for melanoma detection, ranging from improvements in standard clinical assessment with "naked eye" examination (examination of the skin without the assistance of other devices) to the use of advanced imaging technologies and molecular assays that establish an earlier, and more accurate, diagnosis and prognosis of melanoma.

The Importance of Valid Endpoints and Accurate Statistics

Prior to embarking upon a discussion of the various methods of melanoma detection, it is important to briefly reflect upon the importance of how the success of these methods can be ascertained and measured. As with all areas of rigorous methodological investigation, it is critical to demonstrate that a particular method, approach, or technology improves patient outcomes. In the case of melanoma, desired outcomes include reduced morbidity and mortality, improved quality of life, and decreased cost. The reproducibility and reliability of any given method or test, as well as its sensitivity and specificity, must be demonstrated, with the clinical context and appropriate patient population clearly defined. However, the ultimate impact of early melanoma detection methods on our society, particularly the cost-benefit analysis, can only be determined by accurately measuring changes in incidence, prevalence, and mortality. This is not only true within a particular study setting, but also across the general population and among specific risk cohort groups.

Measurements of incidence, prevalence, and mortality rely upon registry data. The quality of population-based cancer registries is variable, and largely defined by the completeness, accuracy, and timeliness of incident cases and reported demographics. Both Surveillance, Epidemiology, and End Results (SEER) cancer registries and non-SEER population-based state cancer registries have been regularly relied upon to examine whether interventions to reduce incidence and mortality have been effective. However, while the quality of data in SEER cancer registries has often been examined and improved, the quality of reporting data in non-SEER state registries has rarely been assessed [6].

Studies measuring the magnitude of underreporting of melanoma have identified a concerning rate in non-SEER active registry sites that range from 50–78% [7, 8]. The potential for underreporting can be especially high with melanoma, because it is frequently diagnosed and treated in outpatient settings that are not subjected to centralized pathology review by the cancer registries. It is likely that this limitation will worsen with the increasing decentralization of melanoma diagnosis and outpatient treatment. Thus, a concerted effort needs to be implemented at the state level to overcome this important limitation, but this is frequently cost prohibitive for many state registries. Thus, our review of the opportunities to enhance our current screening efforts and methods of detection must be interpreted in the context of our limited understanding of accurate incidence rates for melanoma.

A Rational Approach to Implementation of Early Detection Methodologies

It would be ideal to implement screening approaches and exciting emerging technologies in a rational manner. Provider-based screening of the entire general population is unlikely to result in a cost-effective intervention or impact overall survival, primarily due to the large numbers of individuals who would need to be screened in order to identify a relatively small number of melanomas [9]. However, if a stratified approach to screening can be developed, whereby high-risk individuals receive screening based upon their increased likelihood of developing melanoma, then it would be possible to establish a cost-effective screening program. Fifty melanoma subspecialists recently published guidelines for melanoma screening based upon the risk level [10]. The guidelines include screening of individuals between the ages of 35 and 75 who have the following risk factors: a personal or family history of melanoma, a personal history of skin cancer, a vulnerable constitutional makeup (light skin, hair, or eye color; numerous or atypical moles; freckles), immunosuppression, or substantial UV exposure (blistering sunburns; chronic exposure to ultraviolet light; tanning-booth exposure) [10] (Table 4.1). These guidelines create a first pass at identification of higher risk populations that can benefit the most from screening, but will necessarily involve an educational campaign among primary care providers and the lay population to achieve maximal success.

Table 4.1 Risk factors indicating annual screening

Risk category	Risk factor
Personal history	
	History of skin cancer or actinic keratosis
	High-penetrance gene mutation carrier [225–227]
	Immunocompromised status due to disease or medication
Family history	
	Melanoma in one or more family members
	Known or suspected hereditary predisposition to melanoma
Physical features	
	Light skin (Fitzpatrick skin types I–III) [228]
	Blonde or red hair
	>40 total nevi
	Two or more atypical nevi [58]
	Extensive freckling
	Severely sun-damaged skin
UVR overexposure	
	History of blistering or peeling sunburns
	History of indoor tanning

Adults aged 35–75 years with one or more of the following risk factors should be screened at least annually with a total-body skin examination (includes evaluation of entire skin surface, eyes, oral mucosa, hair, and nails) [10]

A complementary approach to provider-based screening of high-risk populations is through empowerment of the general population to perform better self-screening examinations for melanoma. This empowerment could include public educational campaigns that focus on early detection, "telehealth" approaches to expand the number of individuals that can be screened per provider, and mobile health technologies that can allow individuals to self-identify suspicious lesions. By combining a risk-based, selective approach to provider-based screening with empowerment of the general population to identify concerning lesions themselves, it may be possible to produce a comprehensive program to detect melanoma earlier.

The explosion of non-invasive diagnostic devices for melanoma over the past 5 years has opened up new opportunities to decrease the benign-to-malignant skin biopsy ratio while maintaining a reasonably high sensitivity rate. It is currently estimated that 10–20 biopsies are performed (depending on the provider expertise) for every diagnosed melanoma, resulting in a large number of benign lesions being biopsied unnecessarily [11]. Therefore, reducing morbidity and maximizing the chance of accurate melanoma diagnosis is a worthwhile goal, from both the patient-care and fiscal-responsibility perspectives.

In addition to implementing rational, systematic screening efforts, it is also essential to perform studies to confirm the value of current and emergent noninvasive diagnosis-enhancing devices. Only after adequate comparative studies have been performed can we determine which technologies are effective and cost effective for particular patient populations. In particular, understanding how each emerging technology can impact decision-making of providers is critical. Ideally, experts in the field should propose specific milestones and expectations for a technology prior to launch of the product, rather than waiting for the expectations set forth by the United States Food and Drug Administration (FDA) in a post-market setting. It is likely that a combination, rather than a single technological approach, will be necessary in order to achieve the level of sensitivity and specificity that is needed in real practice for early melanoma detection. In this chapter, we systematically review several state-of-the-art methods for melanoma detection, from screening processes of populations and individuals to screening of suspicious lesions with novel technologies.

Methods of Early Detection

Visual Examination by Physicians, Nonphysician Providers, and Self-Skin Examination

Clinician skin examination, including self-examination, represents a basic and fundamental means of detecting melanoma early in its course. Studies have demonstrated the associations between patient or provider skin examination, earlier melanoma detection, and reduced mortality [9]. This is especially true for men over the age of 60, those with Fitzpatrick skin types I and II, and/or those reporting a changing mole [12].

The prevalence of annual clinician skin examination ranges from 8 to 32% [13, 14]. While dermatologists perform skin examinations more commonly than primary care providers, a significant proportion of physician-detected melanomas are found and biopsied by primary care providers [15]. The role of advanced practice providers (nurse practitioners and physician assistants) in melanoma detection is less clear. There is currently a nationwide shortage of dermatologists; thus, the role of advanced practice providers and primary care physicians will become even more important in the future if a widespread skin cancer screening program is to be successful [16].

Several barriers currently exist to routine clinician skin examination in the primary care setting, including time constraints, lack of reimbursement for such services, competing comorbidities, and a lack of clinician confidence and education in the ability to detect skin cancer [17]. Educational methods to address knowledge gaps in performance of clinician skin examination have demonstrated success in improving primary care provider accuracy, confidence, and proper triage for a suspected skin cancer [15]. One validated method is INFORMED (INternet-based program FOR Melanoma Early Detection, available at www.skinsight.com/info/for_professionals/skin-cancer-detection-informed/skin-cancer-education), an interactive, Web-based training program [18].

Skin self-examination represents an integral part of skin cancer detection and surveillance and is complementary to clinician skin examination. Melanoma detection occurs more frequently in patients reporting a change in a skin lesion, with studies demonstrating decreased Breslow's depth at first detection and reduced mortality in those who performed skin self-examination [19]. However, the prevalence of thorough skin self-examination is estimated to be only 10–25% among adults in the United States, though rates are improved by public education and clinician teaching [20].

A consistent, systematic approach to both clinician skin examination and skin self-examination is likely to improve their efficiency and efficacy at detecting melanoma. A "look-and-see" approach has been suggested, involving first to look, and then to recognize potentially problematic lesions requiring intervention. Focusing on high-risk anatomical sites and populations, such as the back in older white men, may represent a more efficient means to promote primary care provider performance of clinician skin examination.

Despite the potential benefits to melanoma detection and mortality, the US Preventive Services Task Force (USPSTF) issued an "insufficient" (I) statement for clinician skin examination and excluded skin self-examination in their overall recommendations for 2016 [21]. The reasons cited include lack of controlled studies conclusively demonstrating a reduction in mortality and morbidity and failure of current studies to address the associated potential harms of routine screening [22]. The USPSTF focused on the Skin Cancer Research to Provide Evidence for Effectiveness of Screening in Northern Germany (SCREEN) study, which demonstrated a 50% reduction in melanoma mortality 5 years post-intervention, [23] but without observance of further reduction in the subsequent nationwide screening program. The SCREEN intervention included intensive provider education, public outreach, visual inspection by primary care providers, and subsequent referral to a dermatologist based upon the level of suspicion. This study resulted in the elimination of the public outreach and dermatologic referral aspects of the program. The SCREEN study was criticized as an ecological study, preventing inference of a causal relationship, and it remains unclear whether removal of the public education campaign and dermatologic referral component of the program contributed to the differences in outcome observed in the regional versus national study.

Since the USPSTF statement, the preliminary results of a 3-year, population-based melanoma screening initiative by INFORMED-trained primary care providers in Western Pennsylvania (through the University of Pittsburgh Medical Center) have demonstrated no substantial increase in potential harms of screening, including over-referral to dermatology, over-biopsy, and increased skin cancer surgeries [24]. The lack of harm was likely attributed to improvement in the diagnosis and management of benign lesions by primary care providers, as well as earlier detection of both melanoma and non-melanoma skin cancers, allowing for less invasive and less costly therapy. This study has also preliminarily shown a reduction in melanoma thickness upon initial diagnosis.

Given the potential benefits of clinician skin examination and skin self-examination and early data demonstrating a lack of harm associated with skin cancer screening, we conclude that the current USPSTF recommendations should not preclude performance of visual skin inspection, especially for high-risk individuals, in the primary care setting.

Visual Examination by Skin Service Providers

Routine examinations by physicians often do not include thorough visual skin examination [13]. Conclusions from studies on patterns of melanoma detection indicate that patients and their partners detect the majority (61–86%) of all melanomas [25, 26]; however, adherence to skin examination recommendations and detection of suspicious lesions are suboptimal [27–29]. Therefore, it is not unreasonable to add more "eyes on the skin" by involving personal service workers such as massage therapists, cosmetologists (estheticians and hair professionals), and tattoo artists, in skin cancer counseling and visual skin examination, particularly targeting clients with known skin cancer risk factors.

Massage therapists are well positioned to conduct casual or thorough visual skin examination. The American Massage Therapy Association estimates that there are 325,000–375,000 massage therapists in the United States, with 43.8–57.6 million adult Americans having at least one massage per year [30]. These professionals have unique access to nearly all of a client's skin, providing the potential to perform visual skin examination. During a typical full-body massage, the client is unclothed under a drape. Massage therapists systematically undrape and view each anatomical area, allowing near-total-body visual skin examination. This process allows massage therapists to assess skin cancer risk factors such as sunburn, tanning lines, high mole counts, or suspicious lesions. Compared to primary care providers or dermatologists, massage therapists are more likely to have repeated and longer appointments that are more oriented towards health promotion [31–33], thereby providing greater opportunities to see potential lesions on the skin over time. Massage therapists report comfort with discussing skin cancer with clients but do this inconsistently, and are therefore not confident in identifying suspicious lesions [34].

Less is known about the potential for visual skin examination by cosmetologists. In the United States, there are approximately 55,000 estheticians, with numbers projected to grow 12% by 2024, faster than the average for all other occupations [35]. Estheticians may or may not view the entire skin; however, many treatments involve close inspection of skin cancer high-risk areas such as the head, neck, face, hands, and feet

[36]. Hair professionals (hairstylists and barbers) numbered 656,400 in 2014 and are increasing at a rate of 10% per year [37]. Hair professionals routinely view a client's scalp, neck, and face and consequently are in a unique position to detect skin cancers on those areas. They typically see their clients regularly and frequently discuss a variety of health-related topics, including medical care [38, 39]. A survey of 203 hair professionals in the greater Houston, Texas, area found that they looked for abnormal moles on the following skin areas for more than 50% of their clients: 37.1% looked at scalps, 28.8% looked at necks, and 15.3% looked at the face during a preceding month. Frequency of their observation of clients' lesions was significantly associated with self-reported health communication and personal skin protection practices but was not significantly associated with their skin cancer knowledge [40].

Tattoo artists are vastly understudied as potential performers of visual skin examination. Most literature focuses on the public health implications of tattoos rather than integrating health-oriented surveillance into tattoo artists' practice. Over 45 million Americans have at least one tattoo on their bodies, likely done at one of the 21,000 licensed tattoo parlors in the United States [41]. In a public campaign sponsored by Ogilvy Brazil, tattoo artists throughout Brazil were trained by skin cancer specialists to check their clients for signs of skin cancer [42]. According to a personal communication from Dr. João Pedreira Duprat Neto, the campaign director, 450 tattoo artists saw 6 clients a day, providing visual skin examination to 18,900 persons each week; several clients referred to dermatologists by their tattoo artists had a skin cancer diagnosis. Only one survey of tattoo artists and skin care has been published. About half (55.2%) of the 90 tattoo artists surveyed reported always looking for atypical moles on customers' skin while performing a tattoo [43].

The primary barrier to the performance of a visual skin examination by these professional service workers is education about visual skin examination. While massage therapists receive some skin cancer education (60% during, and 25% after, primary professional education) [34], its content, duration, source, and depth vary. Similarly, basic training programs for cosmetologists lack uniformity from state to state and have limited skin cancer content. Estheticians learn about sun damage and wrinkles, but not typically in the context of skin cancer. Estheticians who work in medical fields (e.g., dermatology) may have advanced training that often includes skin anatomy, physiology, chemistry, and pathology [36]. The few skin cancer-focused, in-person workshops (and one online course) available to massage therapists have not been evaluated, and do not include training for skin lesion assessment or skin cancer prevention education [34]. The Associated Skin Care Professionals website lists no continuing education for estheticians, though the American Society for Dermatologic Surgery has recently launched Stylists Against Skin Cancer, a dermatologist-led educational campaign for hair professionals that focuses on detection and prevention of scalp skin cancer [44].

Lack of training may affect confidence in performing visual skin examination and hence reduce opportunities for these service professionals to perform it during a client visit. There is a need to establish efficacy of visual skin examination training and assist with the boundaries between recommendations and diagnosis for them, particularly given popular press stories of their involvement in detecting melanoma [34, 45, 46]. A potential implication early on in the training process of these professionals will be an increased number of unnecessary referrals or inaccurate recommendations. Therefore, optimally designed studies evaluating and standardizing the educational approach of skin service providers need to be undertaken.

Stratifying the Approach to Melanoma Screening/Detection Efforts

Introduction

Despite significant progress in our research and understanding of the risk factors for melanoma, there is little consensus in the medical community regarding the segments of the population that may benefit from melanoma screening. This disagreement may be partly due to the paucity of high-quality data demonstrating a reduction in mortality associated with screening (see Section "Visual Examination by Physicians, Nonphysician Providers, and Self-Skin Examination"). This may also be impacted by the likelihood that a significant proportion of individuals who die from melanoma do not neatly fall into "high-risk" categories. In addition, a significant minority of primary melanomas are not amenable to population-based screening efforts (e.g., nodular, acral lentiginous, and amelanotic types). Further, there is ongoing ambiguity regarding the potential for screening-associated overdiagnosis and morbidity, particularly among individuals with phenotypes that complicate early detection efforts through naked-eye examination (e.g., individuals with multiple clinically atypical nevi or a large number of seborrheic keratosis that mimic nevi) or whose absolute risk of death is low.

Genetic, phenotypic, and environmental risk factors for melanoma are well established. Approximately 5–10% of melanoma cases occur in strong familial clusters, suggesting the inheritance of a mutation in a high-penetrance predisposition gene [47, 48]. Up to 40% of strong family clusters have germline mutations in the cyclin-dependent kinase inhibitor 2A (*CDKN2A*) gene [49]. By the age of 80, the penetrance for melanoma development in *CDKN2A* gene mutation carriers has been estimated to range from 58 to 91% [50] in a strong familial setting, and approximately 30% in a general population-based setting [51]. Depending on the specific mutation, there may be a relatively high penetrance of over 20% for pancreatic cancer as well, with studies suggesting that there may be some benefit to screening with imaging studies for pancreatic cancer in these high-risk populations [52, 53]. Additional high-penetrance melanoma susceptibility genes have been identified, including *CDK4, BAP1, MITF, POT1*, and *TERT*, but are considered rare. For about 50% of familial melanoma clusters, a germline mutation cannot be detected [54, 55]. It is becoming increasingly apparent that additional cancer predisposition genes (e.g., *BRCA2*, *PTEN*, and *TP53*) may predispose to melanoma, but with lower penetrance than they predispose to other cancers. Conversely, strong melanoma predisposition genes may predispose to other cancers with less penetrance, such as *BAP1*-mediated predisposition to uveal melanoma and mesothelioma [55]. The overarching goals of germline genetic characterization are (1) to identify individuals at risk of developing cancer and the cancers to which they may be predisposed and (2) to implement screening regimens before the cancer becomes life threatening.

In non-hereditary pattern melanoma, a meta-analysis demonstrated that the relative risk for melanoma in an individual with a single relative with a melanoma diagnosis is approximately 1.74 [56]. This is likely an underestimate because up to 50% of self-reported first-degree family histories of melanoma are inaccurate [57]. Total body melanocytic nevus counts and clinically atypical nevi are the most important and robust phenotypic risk factors for melanoma. For example, the presence of 101–120 nevi on the body compared with <15 nevi is associated with a relative risk of 6.89 for melanoma. Furthermore, having any atypical nevi compared to none at all is associated with a relative risk of 10.12 [58].

Additional phenotypic markers for melanoma risk are comparatively modest, relative to nevus phenotype, such as skin type (I vs. IV: =2.09), freckling (=2.10), skin color (fair vs. dark: =2.06), eye color (green, hazel, blue vs. dark: =1.61, 1.52, and 1.47, respectively), hair color (red, blonde vs. dark: =3.64 and 1.96, respectively), and premalignant and non-melanoma skin cancer lesions (=4.28) [56]. Yet, these lower relative risk levels are comparable to those for other conditions that have received positive screening recommendations by the USPSTF (e.g., lipid laboratory screening is recommended for obese patients with a relative risk of 1.9) [10]. Early detection efforts based on phenotype risk stratification are complicated by the fact that individuals at highest risk (i.e., many nevi, atypical nevi, actinic damage) are often the most challenging to screen without technologies, such as total-body photography and dermoscopy, due to an abundance of benign lesions on their skin that can simulate a melanoma on naked-eye examination alone.

The principal environmental risk factor for melanoma is the overexposure to ultraviolet radiation, either from the sun or indoor tanning devices, which are both considered class I carcinogens by the World Health Organization [59]. Indoor tanning is associated with early-onset melanoma, particularly in women, with the risk increasing with greater exposure and earlier ages of initiation [60, 61]. In a meta-analysis, intermittent exposure to solar radiation and a history of sunburn are associated with a relative risk of 1.61 and 2.03, respectively, for melanoma development [62].

Important to any discussion of screening for melanoma is the relationship between age, gender, and race with melanoma incidence and mortality (Table 4.2). For example, the incidence and mortality rates of melanoma are 1.7-fold and 2.4-fold higher in men than women; 23.5-fold and 7.75-fold higher in whites than blacks; and 7.0-fold and 12.4-fold higher in individuals ≥65 years of age (vs. <65 years), respectively [60]. The consequence of these mortality trends is that half of all melanoma deaths are estimated to occur in white males aged 50 years and older [63]. Therefore, it is critically important to account for both absolute and relative risks for melanoma (onset and death) when developing guidelines for stratified melanoma screening based on risk factors.

Table 4.2 SEER Incidence[a] and US death rates[b], age adjusted, by race and sex, 2009–2013 [229]

	Melanoma incidence	Melanoma mortality
Black females <65 years	0.5	0.1
Black males <65 years	0.5	0.2
White females <65 years	14.9	1.0
White males <65 years	15.4	1.8
Black females ≥65 years	4.6	1.9
Black males ≥65 years	5.4	2.6
White females ≥65 years	58.5	8.6
White males ≥65 years	158.0	24.4
Males, all races, all ages	28.5	4.1
Females, all races, all ages	16.9	1.7
Blacks, all ages, males and females	1.1	0.4
Whites, all ages, males and females	25.9	3.1
<65 years, all races, males and females	12.4	1.1
≥65 years, all races, males and females	86.5	13.6
Total, all races, all ages, males and females	21.8	2.7

[a]SEER 18 areas. Rates are per 100,000 and are age adjusted to the 2000 US Std Population (19 age groups—Census P25-1130)
[b]US Mortality Files, National Center for Health Statistics, Centers for Disease Control and Prevention. Rates are per 100,000 and are age adjusted to the 2000 US Std Population (19 age groups—Census P25-1130)

Potential harms associated with melanoma cancer screening include inaccuracy in melanoma management as a result of (1) *overdiagnosis* of a true melanoma without relevant lethal potential, (2) *over-treatment* of lesions that have an equivocal histological diagnosis, and (3) *over-interpretation* of melanoma due to shifting diagnostic criteria. This is distinct from risks associated with over-screening of populations with low absolute numbers of deaths, such as children and dark-skinned individuals. In fact, a recent study estimated that approximately 1035 biopsies are currently performed for every melanoma detected in individuals 19 years and younger in the United States, leading to a positive predictive value of 0.001% [64]. Among dark-skinned individuals, most melanomas that occur are of the acral lentiginous subtype, for which there are no studies associating screening with improved mortality and no known risk factors that could guide targeted screening. Finally, screening of populations with the highest risk of melanoma death (e.g., white males and females ≥65 years) would be expected to lead to an increased detection and treatment of non-melanoma skin cancers (see Section "Visual Examination by Physicians, Nonphysician Providers, and Self-Skin Examination").

Detection Methods Vary in Cost and Impact: How Can Screening Be Stratified to Take Cost-Effectiveness into Account?

To deploy melanoma screening on a population level, both clinicians and policy makers must take into account the realities of having a finite amount of healthcare resources. Cost-effectiveness analyses have attempted to combine costs with outcomes, namely life expectancy (life year saved) and remaining quality of life (quality-adjusted life year). Such analyses can thus inform both clinicians and policy makers as to the value of the intervention in question. Just as one would take into account the fuel efficiency prior to buying a new car, good stewards of healthcare dollars should take into account the value of the medical intervention they are about to deploy. To utilize cost-effectiveness analyses data, consumers should realize that the results are reported as incremental cost-effectiveness, comparing the intervention of interest to the accepted standard of care. Given the low rates of skin cancer screening in the general population and in primary care settings, the current standard of care may be "no screening." The typical monetary standard for a "cost-effective intervention" is a cost of less than $50,000 per life year saved [65]. Lastly, cost-effectiveness analyses rely on the robustness of the data that are utilized. To date, there are no randomized controlled trials published on melanoma screening, particularly not for heterogeneous populations. Thus, melanoma screening cost-effectiveness analyses are dependent on data parsed from published literature and reasonable assumptions.

Nonetheless, three melanoma cost-effectiveness analyses have been published. In 1996, Girgis and colleagues [66] published a cost-effectiveness model examining primary care providers that performed melanoma screening for a population aged 50 years and older. They utilized gender-specific data from the Australian population in order to characterize age-specific distributions of mortality from melanoma. The authors assumed 30–60% sensitivity and 98% specificity in the diagnostic accuracy of melanoma. They found a cost-effectiveness of AUS$6853 per life year saved for men, if the screening were performed every 5 years, and AUS$12,137 if screening were performed every 2 years. For women, the cost-effectiveness was AUS$11,102 and AUS$20,877 per life year saved for 5- and 2-year intervals, respectively. They concluded that an every-fifth-year screening program could be cost effective for men older than 50 years if performed by family practitioners.

In 1999, Freedberg and colleagues [67] performed a cost-effectiveness analysis comparing a single skin cancer screening by a dermatologist to no screening. Their population consisted of adults older than 20 years who were considered to be at a high risk for developing a skin cancer. They found an incremental cost-effectiveness of $29,170 per life year saved with screening. Their sensitivity analysis showed that the cost-effectiveness ratio remained below the $50,000/life year saved, if the prevalence of melanoma was at least 0.0009 and was localized (94.8% of the cases) or the cost of each screen was below $57.

Losina and colleagues [68] published a cost-effectiveness analysis in 2007 that evaluated one-time screening, annual screening, and screening every 2 years, compared to background screening in a hypothetical cohort of a general population aged 50 years and older. They derived the prevalence, incidence, and mortality data from the SEER data program and found an incremental cost-effectiveness ratio of $10,100/quality-adjusted life year, $80,700/quality-adjusted life year, and $586,800/quality-adjusted life year for screening one time, every 2 years, and annually, respectively. For siblings of patients with melanoma, they found incremental cost-effectiveness ratios of $4000/quality-adjusted life year, $35,500/quality-adjusted life year, and $257,800/quality-adjusted life year, in one-time, every 2 years, and annually screened populations, respectively. They concluded that a one-time melanoma screening of the general population older than 50 years old, as well as screening siblings of melanoma patients every 2 years, would be cost effective.

The three cost-effectiveness analyses are informative in both their conclusions and their limitations, but they need to be interpreted with caution. The published cost-effectiveness analyses are careful to focus on certain risk characteristics, such as gender [66] and age greater than 50 years. However, the populations studied were skewed towards high-risk or self-selected populations. The Australian population in the Girgis study is known to be at particularly high risk, given an overall more homogeneous, lighter complexioned population and a higher intensity of sun exposure. The population of the United States is very heterogeneous for melanoma risk, and thus evaluation of screening strategies should take into account the risk profile, whether it is race, age, gender, or a combination of factors. The screened population in the Freedberg study was derived from the people who went to skin cancer screenings conducted by the AAD, and thus people who either were at higher risk or simply worry more compared to those who did not go to an AAD screening. Registries such as SEER, as used in the Losina study, are dependent upon accurate reporting by tumor registries. Melanomas treated exclusively in outpatient settings are usually lower staged melanomas and tend not to be reported to state cancer registries, and are therefore not captured in SEER (see Section "The Importance of Valid Endpoints and Accurate Statistics") [69].

The assumed prevalence in the Freedberg study needed to be at least 90 per 100,000, which may not be true in all populations. According to SEER, in 2013, there were an estimated 1,034,460 people living with melanoma of the skin in the United States, which is above the Freedberg study prevalence threshold. The gender, race, and age-specific SEER data reported are incidences, and not prevalence, but one may expect that the prevalence for non-Caucasians and women may fall below the 90 per 100,000 threshold.

Lastly, the screenings in the cost-effectiveness analyses were performed by either dermatologists [67, 68] or primary care providers [66] in face-to-face settings with total-body skin examinations. Alternative screening modalities such as teledermatology [70] and lesion-directed skin cancer screening [71] may become more acceptable in healthcare systems with limited budgets or longer waiting times. Implementation of these methods could dramatically affect the cost-effectiveness estimates. Costs are population costs, with effectiveness measured in life years saved and weighted by quality of life, not by the number of cases ascertained. New interventions need to be compared to the standard of care, and the incremental cost-effectiveness ratio should be less than $50,000/life year saved. As new detection devices and methods are introduced, the cost and effectiveness need to be measured in a standard, systematic manner similar to that of the three cost-effectiveness analyses described above.

Proposal for a Stratified Approach to Melanoma Screening Efforts

Public Education

Despite the prior discussion of populations at highest risk for the development of melanoma, a substantial absolute number of fatal melanomas occurs in individuals who do not have these risk factors (i.e., young individuals without a large number of nevi, a family or personal history of melanoma, or an underlying vulnerability to ultraviolet radiation exposure or sunburn). For those at low risk, education of community members is important as to the causes of melanoma, prevention, and clinical recognition through broad-based public health campaigns. Such education is considered to be the first fundamental step in a stratified screening program, because it aims to bring needed attention to suspicious pigmented lesions in those whose skin would not normally be under surveillance. Building a foundation of community members and practitioners who are "melanoma-aware" leads to an earlier presentation of potentially fatal lesions [72] that may otherwise be missed in detection programs restricted to people with classic high-risk profiles.

The value of a broad, public health campaign is supported by the apparent success of long-standing Australian public awareness programs that have reduced the melanoma incidence while maintaining relatively low mortality rates in a high-incidence setting [73–75]. Indeed, the net worth of increased melanoma awareness can be seen in white populations in the Northern Hemisphere, both in the decrease in average tumor thickness of melanomas over recent decades. Today, the majority of melanomas diagnosed at the initial presentation are <1 mm at diagnosis [76], with a projected long-term decline in mortality worldwide [77]. Public awareness can now be further enhanced by encouraging community members to use validated risk prediction tools [78, 79] online, or in clinical practice settings, to self-identify as being at high risk, and to present to their healthcare providers for skin examination.

Defining High-Risk Groups

In the context of screening, the approach can be maximized by targeting a population at most risk for the development of melanoma (see Sections "Introduction" and "Detection Methods Vary in Cost and Impact: How Can Screening Be Stratified to Take Cost-Effectiveness into Account?"). An additional step is to identify a cohort of individuals who are at risk of increased mortality. Combining the knowledge of the demographic groups in the population whose mortality is high, with selection of the strongest individual risk factors, will help to identify those who are prime candidates for regular skin cancer screening examinations.

Towards Cost-Effective Stratified Screening

As noted above, there are no stratified intervention data, and only limited evidence to date on cost-effective approaches to population-based melanoma screening. It is therefore difficult to guide the frequency and method of total-body skin examination for those most susceptible to developing fatal melanoma. It should be noted that while approaches like skin self-examination result in increased detection of melanomas [80], relatively few of these are likely to be fatal. Previous estimations of cost-effective screening by primary care practitioners of the older (>50 years) Australian population every 5 years provide a starting point [66]. No study to date has shown that annual screening is cost effective, but screening intervals shorter than 5 years, e.g., every 2 years, may be warranted for those in the highest risk stratum. Annual screening may be warranted for older men who have phenotypic risk factors, given their increased propensity for fast-growing, more aggressive nodular melanomas [81].

Regarding persons to best perform total-body skin examination, the evidence suggests that any skilled clinical examiner could be deployed, cost-effectively, to regularly inspect the skin of older susceptible persons with acceptable results. However, deploying dermatologists as the primary screeners is neither feasible, due to the limited size of the available workforce, nor cost effective. The only competency required is expertise in total-body skin examination, and trained nurse specialists, nurse practitioners, or physician assistants may be more suitable skin examiners in a targeted screening program [70]. Other modalities such as teledermatology [82] and automated skin cancer detection [83] using sophisticated mobile devices for triage or diagnosis of suspicious lesions encountered by other practitioners lacking specialized training also hold promise for containing costs [84]. Finally, stratified screening for melanoma will be most efficient when incorporated as a policy into existing healthcare services [63].

Technical Modalities for Screening

Aided Examination: Role of Clinical Photography and Dermoscopy in the Identification of Typical and Atypical Melanocytic Neoplasms

Advances in Total-Body Photography Systems in the Surveillance of Melanoma (Acquisition, Registration, and Change Detection)

Total-body photography alone, or in combination with sequential digital dermoscopy, has been shown to be a particularly useful method as an aid in the early detection of melanoma in patients with atypical mole syndrome [85–87] or other high-risk cohorts (i.e., xeroderma pigmentosum, carriers of high-penetrance mutated melanoma genes, or patients under B-Raf inhibitor treatment) [88, 89]. In addition to early identification of melanoma, total-body photography has demonstrated a reduction in the number of unnecessary skin biopsies, thereby decreasing the morbidity experienced by patients with complex nevi phenotypes [90].

Even if the method is proven to be useful in high-risk patient surveillance, it may not be universally utilized due to logistical and time constraints in most cases [91]. To solve this limitation, total-body photography has recently shown technological advances in acquisition, quality of images, and software solutions to detect changes in the potentially suspicious skin lesions in patients. However, some technical gaps are still evident in terms of the lack of standardization of images (i.e., color calibration), nomenclature, and minimal development of standards for image-associated metadata and Digital Imaging and Communications in Medicine (DICOM) formatting [92–94].

Two-dimensional systems recently introduced to the market incorporate body mapping systems with high-resolution reflex cameras and fast automatized acquisition that can reduce the time of the procedure to just a few minutes. Some of these devices use polarized light to create total-body photography with better resolution, or even low-resolution total-body dermoscopic images [95]. New three-dimensional systems for skin mapping have high resolution and a whole representation of the body that has the potential advantage to accurately represent volumetric and textural features of lesions [96]. This procedure has the potential to change the paradigm of total-body photography with many applications in skin diseases, including inflammatory and pigmentary disorders. Superimposition of other diagnostic methods, such as confocal reflectance microscopy or electrical spectroscopy, may also be used on changing lesions detected by total-body photography to improve the diagnostic specificity for detecting a melanoma [97, 98].

Computer vision can be incorporated in total-body photography to detect changes in existing and new lesions in patients. Some companies provide software with this aim, but clinical validation of these tools has not yet been proven. At present, there are no computer vision systems that allow for an accurate differentiation of changes that occur in banal lesions (i.e., banal nevi or seborrheic keratoses) relative to those changes associated with skin cancer. In the future, new computer-aided algorithms based in deep learning, artificial intelligence, and other methodologies may substantially contribute to the automatized detection of skin cancer in patients with total-body photography [83].

Dermoscopy

The introduction of the ABCD mnemonic and the "ugly duckling sign" to describe the clinical/morphologic features of melanoma has been quite useful for many to identify potentially suspicious skin lesions. This can be followed by the use of photography to identify biologically dynamic lesions, enhancing our ability to differentiate nevi from melanoma and improving our competency for identifying early melanoma [99, 90, 100, 101]. However, the greatest impact to date for improving our ability to discriminate benign nevi from melanoma has been the introduction of dermoscopy into clinical practice [102–104]. The ability to directly visualize and discern cutaneous subsurface structures and correlate them with histopathology findings has greatly facilitated our ability to correctly identify melanomas and nevi, essentially transforming the way in which we assess cutaneous lesions (Figs. 4.1 and 4.2).

In 2001, the first meta-analysis evaluating the diagnostic power of dermoscopy showed that it is more accurate than the naked-eye examination alone for the diagnosis of melanoma [105]. Two additional meta-analyses have since reinforced these findings [102, 106]. The most recent meta-analysis, by Vestergaard and colleagues, included only prospective studies performed in clinical settings, and thus most accurately reflects the routine day-to-day dermoscopy use by clinicians [102]. A total of 8487 suspicious lesions, most of which were melanocytic tumors, were included,

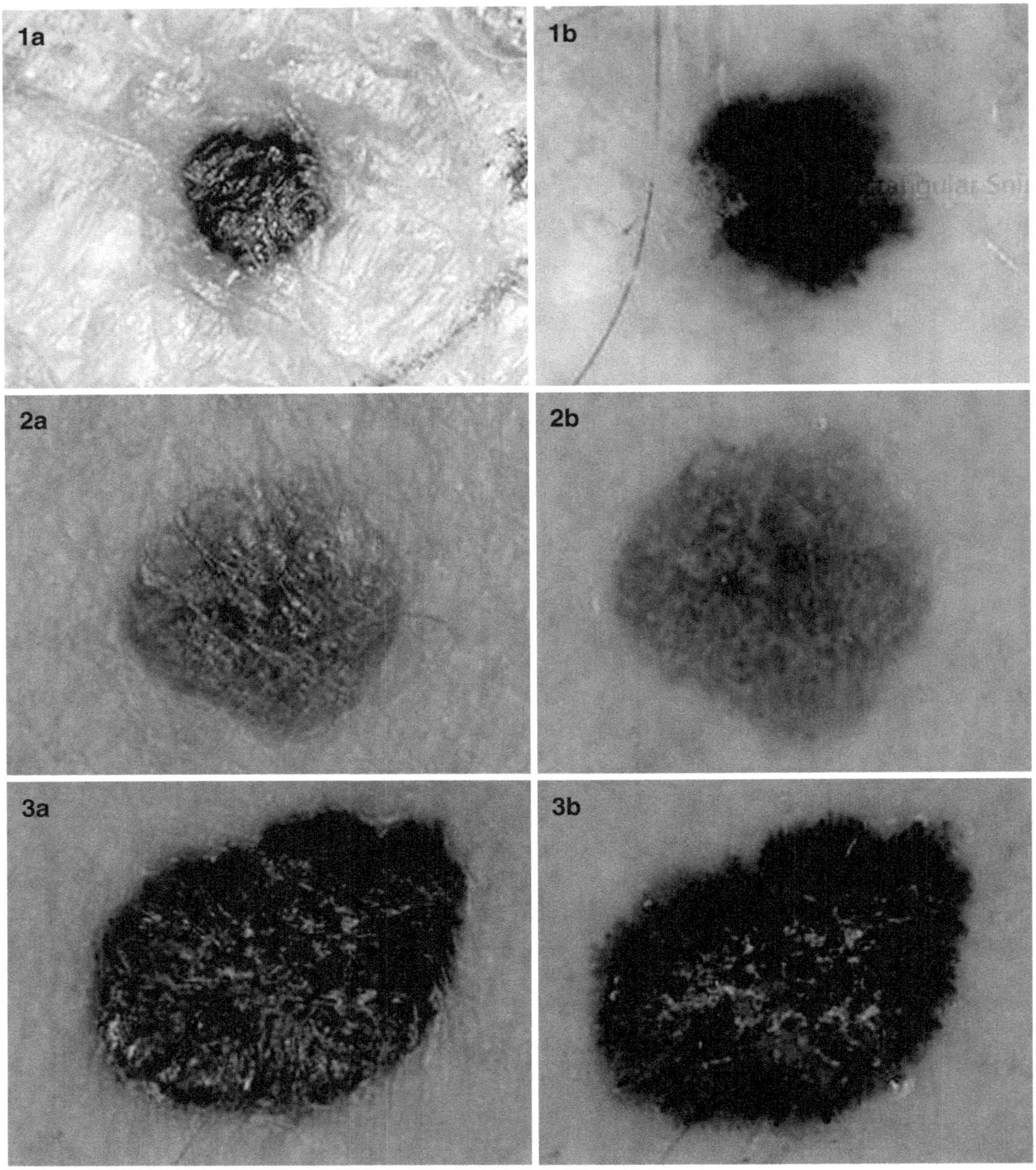

Fig. 4.1 (**1.1a–b** to **1.3a–b**): The set of three invasive melanomas highlight how dermoscopy can improve sensitivity for melanoma detection. **1.1a** is a 3 mm in diameter lesion that does not have any of the ABCD features of melanoma. On dermoscopy (**1.1b**) the diagnosis of melanoma can be made based on the disorganized architecture and the presence of multiple colors and a blue-white veil. **1.2A** is a 5 mm in diameter lesion without the ABCD features of melanoma. On dermoscopy (**1.2b**) the presence of a negative network raises concern that the lesion may be a melanoma. Biopsy of this lesion revealed this lesion to be an invasive spitzoid melanoma. **1.3a** is a 7 mm lesion that had the clinical appearance and feel of a seborrheic keratosis. On dermoscopy (**1.3b**) there are no seborrheic keratosis-associated structures present. Instead, the lesion manifests a disorganized architecture with atypical dots and globules, all features predictive of melanoma

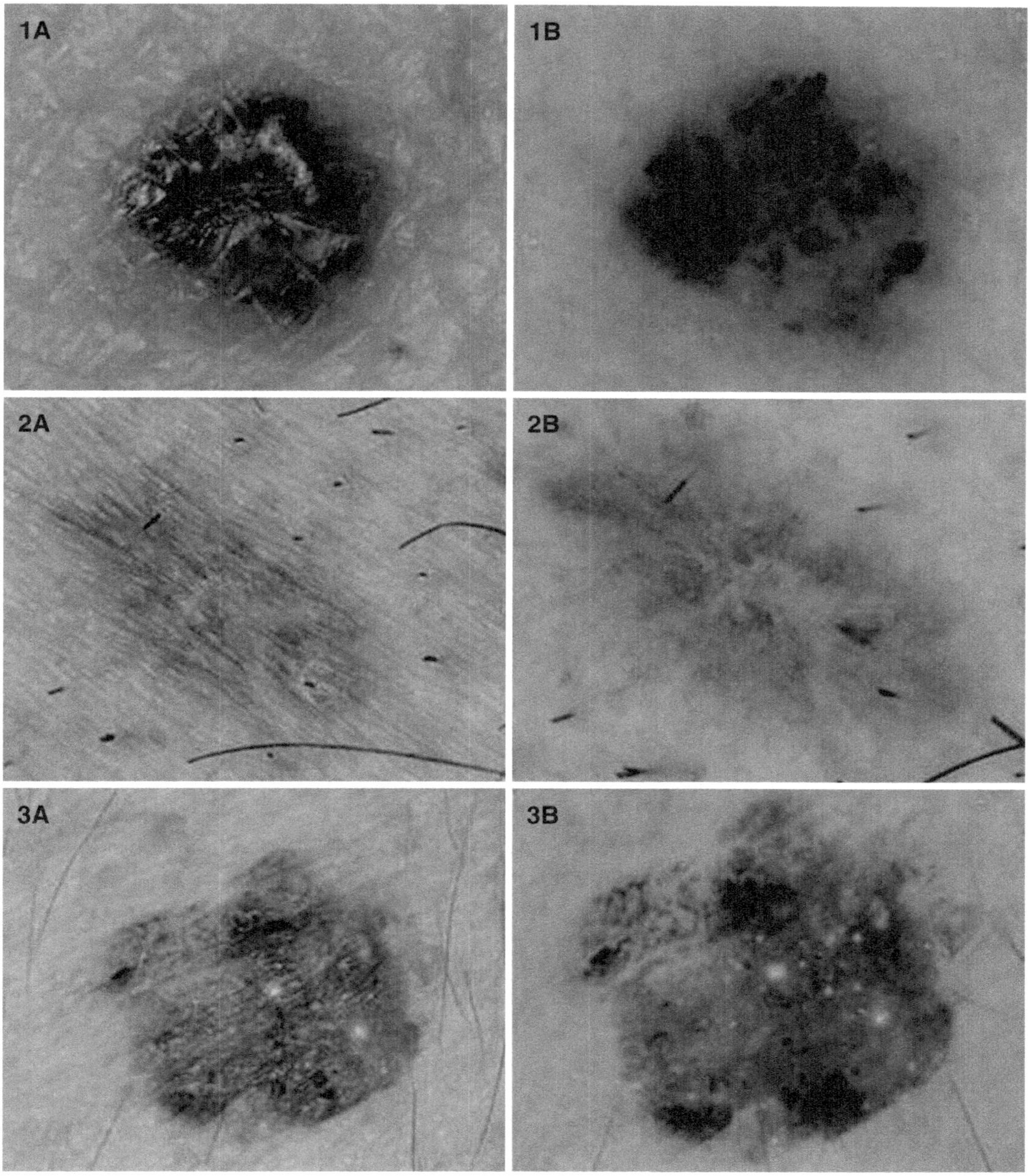

Fig. 4.2 (**2.1a–b** to **2.3a–b**): Showcased here are three benign melanoma mimickers that are often biopsied to rule out melanoma. Dermoscopy can help identify these as benign lesions, reassuring the clinician and thereby obviating the need for a biopsy. **2.1a** is a raised asymmetric blue papule with irregular borders. While the differential diagnosis includes melanoma and pigmented basal cell carcinoma, dermoscopy (**2.1b**) reveals lacunae, which are features diagnostic of an angioma. **2.2a** is a 7 mm asymmetric lesion with irregular borders. The differential diagnosis includes a hypomelanotic melanoma. Dermoscopy (**2.2b**) reveals a pattern composed of a thin peripheral network with central scar-like area; these features are consistent with the diagnosis of a dermatofibroma. In addition, the lesion "dimpled" when lateral pressure was applied to it. **2.3a** is an 8 mm asymmetric lesion with irregular borders, which are features concerning for melanoma. On dermoscopy (**2.3b**) there are no melanoma-specific structures evident. Instead, there are gyri and sulci and numerous milia-like cysts and comedo-like openings. The constellation of findings is diagnostic of a seborrheic keratosis

with a melanoma prevalence ranging from 0.5 to 21.1% and a Breslow's thickness depth ranging from 0.35 to 0.95 mm. Dermoscopic and clinical accuracy were evaluated through the diagnostic odds ratio, which was found to be 15.6 times higher for dermoscopy compared to a naked-eye examination (CI: 2.9–83.7, $p = 0.016$). A summary estimate of sensitivity was also higher with dermoscopy (0.90, CI: 0.80–0.95) versus naked-eye examination (0.71, CI: 0.59–82, $p = 0.002$). It is important to appreciate that this improvement in sensitivity did not occur at the cost of a lower specificity; that is, while the sensitivity for detecting melanoma improved with dermoscopy, there was no statistical difference in specificity between naked eye- and dermoscopy-based examinations (0.90, CI: 0.57–98 vs. 0.81, CI: 0.48–0.95, $p = 0.18$).

As expected, the aforementioned meta-analyses found that the diagnostic accuracy was dependent on the experience of the examiner. Terushkin and colleagues found, through assessment of the benign-to-malignant biopsy ratio, that a dermatologist who was new to adopting dermoscopy into their practice experienced a learning curve [107]. Initially, benign-to-malignant biopsy ratio of the study participant increased compared to naked-eye examination, but with time and experience their biopsy ratio approached the level of pigmented lesion specialists. Several other studies have demonstrated that short dermoscopy training modules can improve the diagnostic performance of inexperienced dermatologists, general practitioners, and even medical students [108–110]. However, the training modalities have varied widely among studies, with the ideal teaching method for beginners still unclear [111].

The benign-to-malignant biopsy ratio can vary widely, and while it is influenced by the clinician's sensitivity and specificity, it is also influenced by the prevalence and incidence of melanoma in the overall patient population. Improvements in this ratio suggest that the increased sensitivity seen with dermoscopy does not result in an increase in the number of unnecessary biopsies, and thus an increase in morbidity. Carli and colleagues retrospectively examined two dermoscopy users before and after the introduction of dermoscopy and compared them to four dermoscopy nonusers [103]. They showed a significant improvement in the benign-to-malignant biopsy ratio over a 4-year study period in the dermoscopy arm (18:1–4.3:1, $p = 0.037$). The benign-to-malignant biopsy ratio for dermoscopy nonusers had no significant difference at the beginning and the end of the study (11.8:1–14.8:1).

The use of dermoscopy in melanoma screening allows for the earlier detection of melanoma and improves clinical management. Several studies have shown that dermoscopic monitoring of lesions enables the detection of thinner melanomas. In a meta-analysis with a mean follow-up of 30 months, Salerni and colleagues showed that dermoscopy allowed for the detection of a greater number of thinner melanomas compared to naked-eye examination (mean Breslow's depth of 0.77 vs. 1.43 mm, $p \leq 0.05$) [112]. Haenssle and colleagues found that participation in specialized dermoscopic screening programs and dermoscopic examinations at the time of diagnoses were also significantly associated with the detection of thinner melanomas ($p \leq 0.01$) [104].

In summary, dermoscopy has been shown to increase the diagnostic sensitivity for skin cancer detection, decrease the benign-to-malignant biopsy ratio, and allow for the diagnosis of thinner melanomas compared to naked-eye examination. What does the future have in store when it comes to dermoscopy? The patterns and dermoscopy criteria useful in identifying the various subtypes of melanoma and differentiating them from nevi will continue to be refined [113, 114]. In addition, computer vision designed to augment the clinician's cognition will likely become a reality within the next decade. While many researchers have attempted to develop computer vision algorithms to analyze pigmented skin lesions [115], their efforts were hampered by small image data sets and computing power that had not reached the level of the deep learning neural networks currently being developed and utilized [83, 116]. New developments are occurring at an increasingly rapid pace, with the increasing availability of large and ever-expanding open-access image databases such as the International Skin Imaging Collaboration and MoleMapper, ushering in a new era of computer-assisted diagnosis that will be accessible not only by clinicians, but also by patients directly via their mobile phone computers [83, 84, 117, 118].

Teledermatology and the Early Detection of Melanoma

Melanoma awareness and concern, along with access-to-care issues, have prompted an increase in the number of digital tools available to assist healthcare providers and patients. Clinicians currently perform two types of teledermatology visits: (1) direct patient-to-dermatologist virtual visits and (2) consultative visits where the patient's non-dermatology provider makes virtual contact with the dermatologist. Teledermatology visits that utilize store-and-forward images are typically preferred over real-time video systems, as the current video resolution in the real-time systems is not high enough to adequately capture the precise detail needed to thoroughly evaluate a pigmented lesion. With the expanding use of these virtual systems, teledermatology has improved access to dermatology specialists and increased the knowledge and skill set of primary care providers with regard to melanoma detection [119]. One study showed the potential to reduce overall mortality from melanoma by detecting invasive melanoma earlier [120]. Teledermatology for pigmented lesions has also led to reduced overall healthcare costs by decreasing unnecessary referrals [121].

Despite the potential advantages of teledermatology for melanoma detection, there are a few limitations with the current virtual systems. Teledermatology is based on two-dimensional image evaluation, with inherent limitations relative to a three-dimensional physical examination. Image-based evaluations also eliminate the ability to palpate the lesion, which can provide additional information to the practitioner. However, with the addition of teledermoscopy, virtual evaluation, compared to face-to-face evaluation, has shown comparable diagnostic accuracy [122, 123].

The ability to identify a melanoma virtually is also dependent upon the capacity of the non-dermatologist clinician (or patient) to identify which lesions need to be further evaluated. This is particularly significant in patient-to-dermatologist virtual visits, because hard-to-see areas tend to be overlooked by the patient [124]. With regard to primary care provider-to-dermatologist visits, one study calculated that the frequency of missed melanomas by primary care clinicians was 10.1 per 10,000 virtual consultations [125].

Teledermatology has demonstrated its benefit in the evaluation of patients with concerning pigmented lesions. The upsurge of mobile medical applications ("apps"), along with the improvement of imaging technology and the use of dermatoscope accessories, is driving the evolution of an alternate care delivery system for patients with pigmented lesions (see Section "Aided Examination: Role of Other Noninvasive Technologies in the Identification of Typical and Atypical Melanocytic Neoplasms").

There are still several limitations, and clear regulation is needed, but those limitations are being addressed and will eventually be overcome. As imaging and analysis technology continues to improve, particularly in the realm of artificial intelligence and machine learning, melanoma early detection will hopefully be streamlined, enabling lowered costs and decreased mortality and morbidity.

Consumer-Based Technologies for Early Detection of Melanoma

As smartphones have rapidly gained popularity, there are now thousands of apps available, including those that evaluate lesions suspicious for skin cancer. Such apps have the potential to reach a large number of patients, provide educational information, and overcome geographic barriers associated with access to dermatologists. Currently, however, they are not subject to regulatory oversight.

Categories of Apps Available

Most apps aimed at melanoma detection serve primarily as an educational resource, providing information about melanoma identification, sun protection recommendations, UV index, and instruction on skin self-examination [126, 127]. Such apps also provide patients with self-monitoring capabilities, including tools to log, organize, and track concerning moles using their device's built-in camera. These apps have the potential to allow patients to communicate with healthcare providers about potentially concerning lesions. Some apps allow patients to store full-body images to use as an aid in skin self-examination.

Mole mapping has been shown to be a useful tool for dermatologists and patients to improve the accuracy of melanoma detection [87]. These apps have the advantage of providing patients with an inexpensive way to create their own images. However, the quality of patient-generated images can be variable, and given the sensitive nature of these photos, privacy and security of such images is a concern [128]. MoleMapper™, an open-source mole tracking app, takes advantage of the ResearchKit (iOS) and ResearchStack (Android) platforms and allows users to participate in research projects to further the field [84].

Mobile apps are a logical platform to deliver direct-to-patient teledermatology, and some mobile apps primarily focus on skin lesions that are suspicious for cancer. While this may enhance access for patients, a recent study found that many of these apps did not provide the identity and/or credentials of the consulting physician, or used physicians who were not licensed to practice medicine in the state of the patient (or even in the United States) and that these consulting physicians incorrectly diagnosed a nodular melanoma in 3/14 cases [129].

With the advent of inexpensive dermatoscopes that can attach to a smartphone, patient-directed teledermoscopy is also possible. Studies have shown that this technique can be easily learned by most patients, but with one study finding that patient-selected lesions often did not encompass skin cancers present on clinical skin examination. Thus, this technique has limited utility as a standalone modality, although it may be helpful for monitoring single lesions together with a dermatologist [82, 124]. Some apps assess lesions using a mathematical algorithm and provide an assessment using risk stratification (low vs. high), giving guidance for how essential it is to seek medical attention for that lesion. However, these apps are more likely than dermatologists to misclassify melanomas as a low-risk lesion [130, 131]. Inaccurate risk assessment has the potential to cause harm by delaying patients from seeking medical attention for melanoma, potentially missing the opportunity to benefit from early intervention.

Regulatory Oversight and Ethical Concerns

With the rapid proliferation of medical apps, it has become clear that guidelines for regulatory oversight need to be updated in order to keep pace with advances in technology. On February 9, 2015, the FDA published "Mobile Medical Applications Guidance for Industry and Food and Drug Administration Staff" [132], a document that contains non-binding recommendations. This document states that regulatory oversight will be enforced on mobile apps that meet the definition of a medical device. Specifically, this document states that the FDA will exercise enforcement discretion (i.e., will not plan to regulate) "(a)pps specifically intended for medical uses that utilize the mobile device's built-in camera or a connected camera for purposes of documenting or transmitting pictures (e.g., photos of a patient's skin lesions or wounds) to supplement or augment what would otherwise be a verbal description in a consultation between healthcare providers or between healthcare providers and patients/caregivers [132]." However, this document also states that "(m)obile apps that analyze an image of a skin lesion using mathematical algorithms, such as fractal analysis, and provide the user with an assessment of the risk of the lesion" [132] are an example of apps that transform a smartphone into a regulated medical device, and thus will fall under the FDA's regulatory oversight.

The increasingly widespread use of mobile apps has also posed new ethical challenges that need to be addressed if this new technology is to be fully developed with minimal risk of harm to patients. There are important ethical concerns regarding patient confidentiality, informed consent, transparency of data ownership, and data privacy protection. According to one 2014 report, only ~12% of mobile applications are HIPAA compliant [133]. Many apps require users to consent to their data policies, but how the patient's data are mined, used, and externally shared is often not transparent. The potential misuse of sensitive digital total-body images is an area of vulnerability related to information safety and privacy. It has become a growing area of concern, particularly when patient anonymity is not always possible. The challenge for the field of dermatology will be to balance the potential benefits of melanoma and skin cancer detection apps, including the ability to inexpensively provide education to the public, additionally to provide access to dermatologists for patients who may otherwise go without expert care, with the potential harms they may pose, particularly the potential to provide false reassurance with a possible delay in the diagnosis of skin cancer.

Aided Examination: Role of Other Noninvasive Technologies in the Identification of Typical and Atypical Melanocytic Neoplasms

Hyperspectral/Multispectral Imaging

In the standard total-body skin examination, lesion color plays an important role in a dermatologist's accuracy for detecting a melanoma. Indeed, a crucial visual feature leading to timely clinical diagnosis of a melanoma is the variation in absorption and reflection of different wavelengths (colors) of visible light by blood and melanin at varying depths within the skin. Already evident to the naked eye, this phenomenon is central to many electro-optical systems designed to assist in early melanoma detection. Multispectral imaging is the acquisition of simultaneous images of a single object at several discrete wavelength bands of the electromagnetic spectrum (typically on the order of 3–10 or more). The term, hyperspectral, is often used if the wavelength bands are contiguous and sufficiently narrow to permit a greater number of simultaneous images (typically a hundred or more) [134]. Dermatology implementations of multispectral and hyperspectral imaging have benefited greatly from machine vision, satellite remote sensing, military, and other applications developed several decades ago.

Each multispectral "image" of a skin lesion is, in fact, a set of several two-dimensional images (data cube). These collectively provide unique information that is derived from the wavelength-dependent interactions of light with matter (Fig. 4.3). For pigmented lesions, red light provides clean maps of melanin because most other skin chromophores are rather transparent (have low absorption and scattering) at red (long) wavelengths of light. By comparison, because of high absorption by hemoglobin, green wavelengths provide excellent images of blood and even oxygenation (Fig. 4.4). In particular, oxyhemoglobin absorption peaks at 540 and 575 nm, whereas the peak is 555 nm in the deoxygenated state [135]. Furthermore, light scattering depends strongly on wavelength, which means that longer (red) wavelengths penetrate tissue deeper and short (blue) wavelengths are more highly scattered (Fig. 4.5). One result is the clinically blue appearance of deep melanin, with another possibility for the ability to calculate the exact melanin depth [136].

Currently, there are two multispectral devices (Fig. 4.6) that are approved by the FDA with the ability to provide information on pigmented lesions of the skin, both of which are evolved digital dermatoscopes: the SIAscope (MedX Health Corp, Mississauga, ON, Canada; 510(k) [137] in 2003) and the MelaFind™ (MELA Sciences, Inc., now STRATA Skin Sciences, Inc., Horsham Township, PA; pre-market approval [138] in 2011). These devices are similar, acquiring images in eight and ten, respectively, narrow bands from blue visible (~400 nm) to the near infrared (~1000 nm), but they differ in output. The SIAscope and accompanying software (SIMSYS-MoleMate™) displays approximate distribution maps of melanin, hemoglobin, and collagen in the

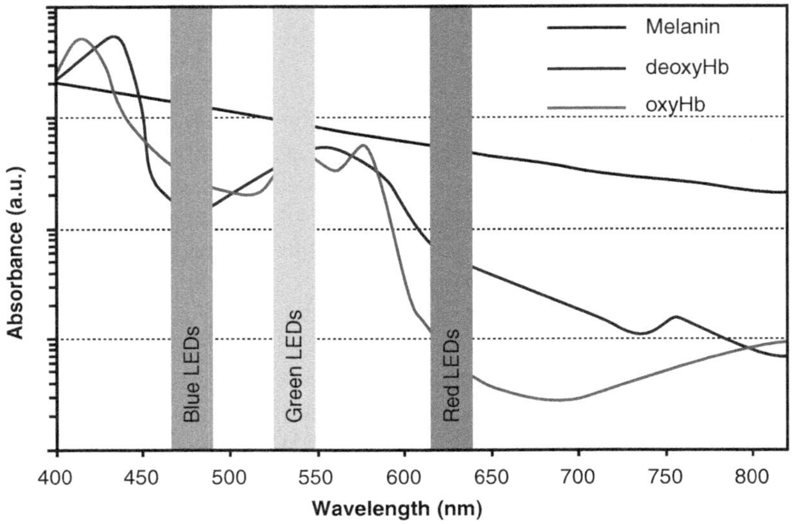

Fig. 4.3 Melanin, oxy-, and deoxyhemoglobin are seen with different relative brightness at blue, green, and red wavelengths of light due to their unique absorption spectra shown here [152]

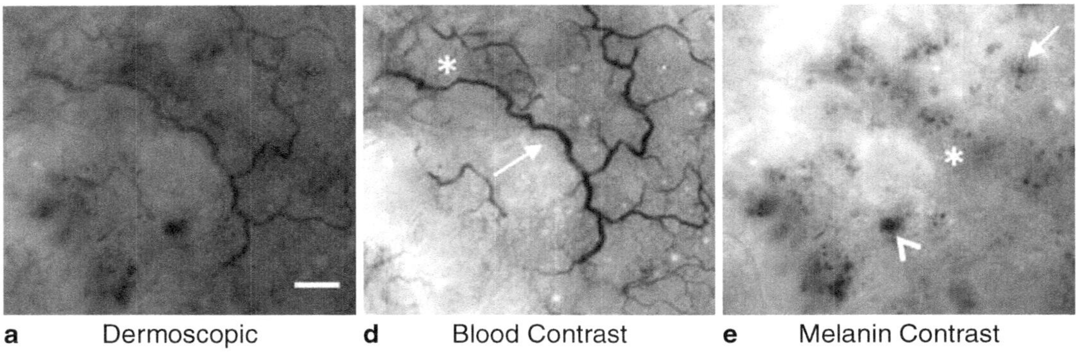

Fig. 4.4 Relative to dermoscopy (**a**), multispectral images enable separation of hemoglobin (**d**) and melanin (**e**) in a single-pigmented lesion [152]

epidermis and dermis [139, 140]. In contrast, the MelaFind™ uses proprietary analysis software to give an automated, "yes/no" biopsy recommendation based on a classifier score that quantifies the level or amount of disorganization. In 2016, there were approximately 500–1000 SIAscopes and 100 MelaFind™ units in use worldwide. The MelaFind™ is the only multispectral device to receive Current Procedural Terminology (CPT) codes: two Category III codes were awarded in 2016, a year after manufacturing, marketing, and follow-up research studies were halted. STRATA Skin Sciences is no longer making, selling, or marketing any new MelaFind units, but is continuing to offer support to existing users.

The SIAscope and MelaFind™ experiences provide useful lessons for upcoming devices attempting to enter the market. Validated performance for the intended user is critical, as is the comparison to alternative approaches in terms of accuracy, efficiency, necessary training, initial investment, and physician reimbursement. For example, although expert SIAscope users may have a sensitivity and specificity as high as 80% [141–143], it has been contested whether diagnostic accuracy is improved for trained dermoscopists [144]. The SIAscope now is mostly used for primary care screening prior to dermatology referral. However, triage decisions are similar following best practice guidelines (clinical history, naked-eye examination, and seven-point checklist) [145]. Additional lessons come from the MelaFind™'s large, multicenter trials. The results challenged expert histopathology as the

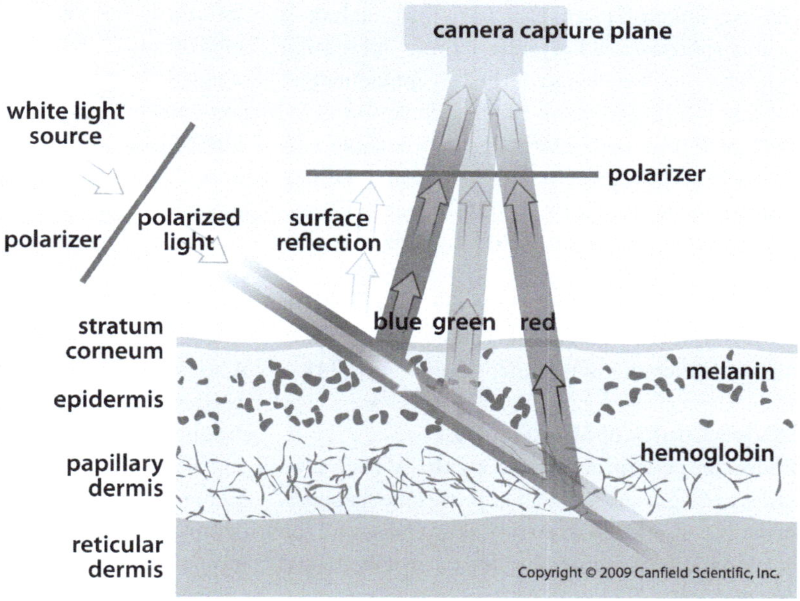

Fig. 4.5 Short (blue) wavelengths of light are more highly scattered than longer (red) wavelengths, enabling imaging from different depths with different spectral bands (courtesy of Dennis O'Neal, Canfield Scientific, Inc, [231])

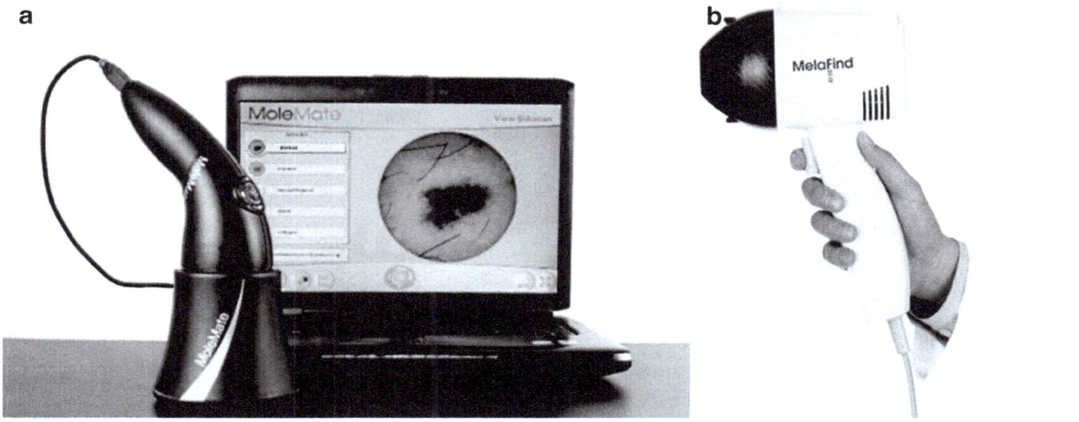

Fig. 4.6 FDA-approved multispectral devices. A. SIAscope with SIMSYS-MoleMate™ software (MedX Health Corp). B. MelaFind™ device [232]

gold standard for melanoma diagnosis [146]. They also demonstrated that device accuracy estimates can change when increasingly large populations are studied. MelaFind™ sensitivity and specificity estimates fell from 100% and 85%, initially [147], to 98% and 10% in the landmark 2011 study by Monheit and colleagues [148]. The resulting high rate of excision recommendations has drawn criticism [149], but this was the trade-off for high sensitivities accompanying automated diagnosis thresholds set to avoid any risk of false reassurance. Such studies cannot be directly compared to interventions, such as the SIAscope or confocal microscopy, that incorporate a clinician's interpretation. Subsequent studies examining the MelaFind™'s effect on clinical assessment suggest increased dermatologist sensitivity for melanoma but lower specificity relative to unaided evaluation [150].

The SIAscope and MelaFind™ are certainly not the final word for multispectral techniques in dermatology. Many groups have developed multispectral digital dermatoscope prototypes and accompanying algorithms for single-pigmented lesion evaluation [141, 151, 152–155], including a smartphone-based system [156]. Increasing numbers of wavelengths, better mathematical models [157], and more precise detection [158, 159] of light-tissue interaction may enable significantly higher specificities while maintaining exquisitely high sensitivity [160]. Further, non-contact implementations [161] may result in sufficient sensitivity and specificity for incorporation into total-body/regional imaging systems for truly high-throughput screening and more informed melanoma treatment decisions [134].

In Vivo Confocal Microscopy

Reflectance confocal microscopy (RCM) is a noninvasive diagnostic tool that improves the diagnosis of neoplastic and inflammatory skin lesions and can be used routinely during the clinical visit by trained practitioners. RCM provides high-resolution, magnified images of the skin, permitting examination of the epidermis and the papillary dermis at the cellular level [162]. RCM devices use a low-power laser (830 nm) that penetrates the skin and is reflected from subcellular structures at a desired focal point within the skin to pass back through a gating pinhole and enter the detector. This process allows grayscale horizontal images of the epidermis and papillary dermis up to an imaging depth of about 250 μm to be obtained, with lateral resolution of approximately 1 μm (Fig. 4.7). Highly reflective organelles or structures appear bright/white, while non-reflective structures appear dark. Melanin, keratin, collagen, and some activated organelles (e.g., Birbeck granules) have a high reflection index, thus appearing light gray to white. At a cellular level, melanocytes, pigmented keratinocytes, melanin-containing histiocytes (melanophages), and metabolically activated inflammatory cells strongly reflect 830 nm laser light and appear bright. Acquisition of the images requires approximately 3–10 minutes, depending on the device used and the dimension of the lesion. Output images are horizontal sections, parallel to the surface of the skin, giving a forward-facing representation of the epidermis/dermis at the selected scanning depth. The most widely used RCM device (VivaScope 1500; CaliberID, Rochester, NY) stitches single images of 0.5 × 0.5 mm into larger mosaic images, allowing the acquisition of up to an 8 × 8 mm area. A handheld RCM device (VivaScope 3000; CaliberID) is able to rapidly image lesions located on concave or convex surfaces (e.g., the tip of the nose) by obtaining 1 × 1 mm horizontal virtual sections. Ex vivo RCM imaging of excised tissue (VivaScope 2500; CaliberID) is opening a novel and promising field of application of the RCM tech-

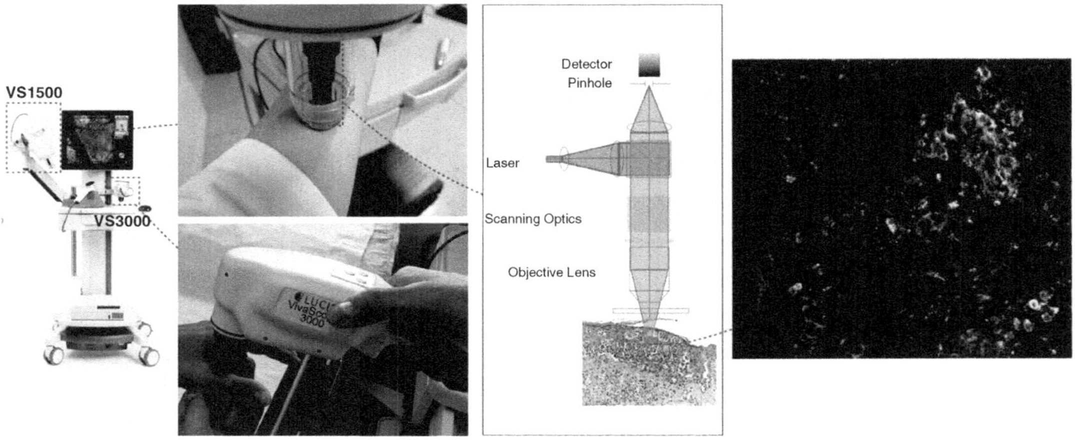

Fig. 4.7 Description of RCM technology. From left to right: The combo device, holding both VivaScope 1500 (on the left) and VivaScope 3000 (on the right), with dermoscopic camera in the center. Highlight of VivaScope 1500 (on the top) and VivaScope 3000 positioned on the skin for image acquisition. Technical scheme of image generation with laser light (830 nm) entering the tissue and reflected light is detected by a sensor after filtered through a pinhole to ensure a sharply in-focus image. Example of confocal microscopy image showing atypical melanocytes aggregated into a nest at the dermal-epidermal junction in a melanoma (MAVIG GmbH)

nique, allowing the reliable assessment of the surgical margins and resulting in faster and more feasible management during surgical intervention [163].

Confocal criteria for melanocytic and non-melanocytic lesions show high sensitivity and specificity for the diagnosis of nevi, melanomas, and other benign or malignant skin neoplasms [164]. In detail, typical nevi are usually characterized by preserved dermal-epidermal junction architecture, usually composed of ringed and meshwork pattern, with irregular junctional nests and atypical junctional cells at the center of the lesion [165]. The presence of cytologic atypia in association with atypical junctional nests (showing short interconnections or characterized by nonhomogeneous cellularity) is suggestive of histologic atypia ("dysplastic" nevus) [166], while widespread pagetoid cells scattered along the whole epidermis or atypical cells diffused throughout the junction (associated with non-edged papillae) are typically found in melanoma [167] (Fig. 4.8).

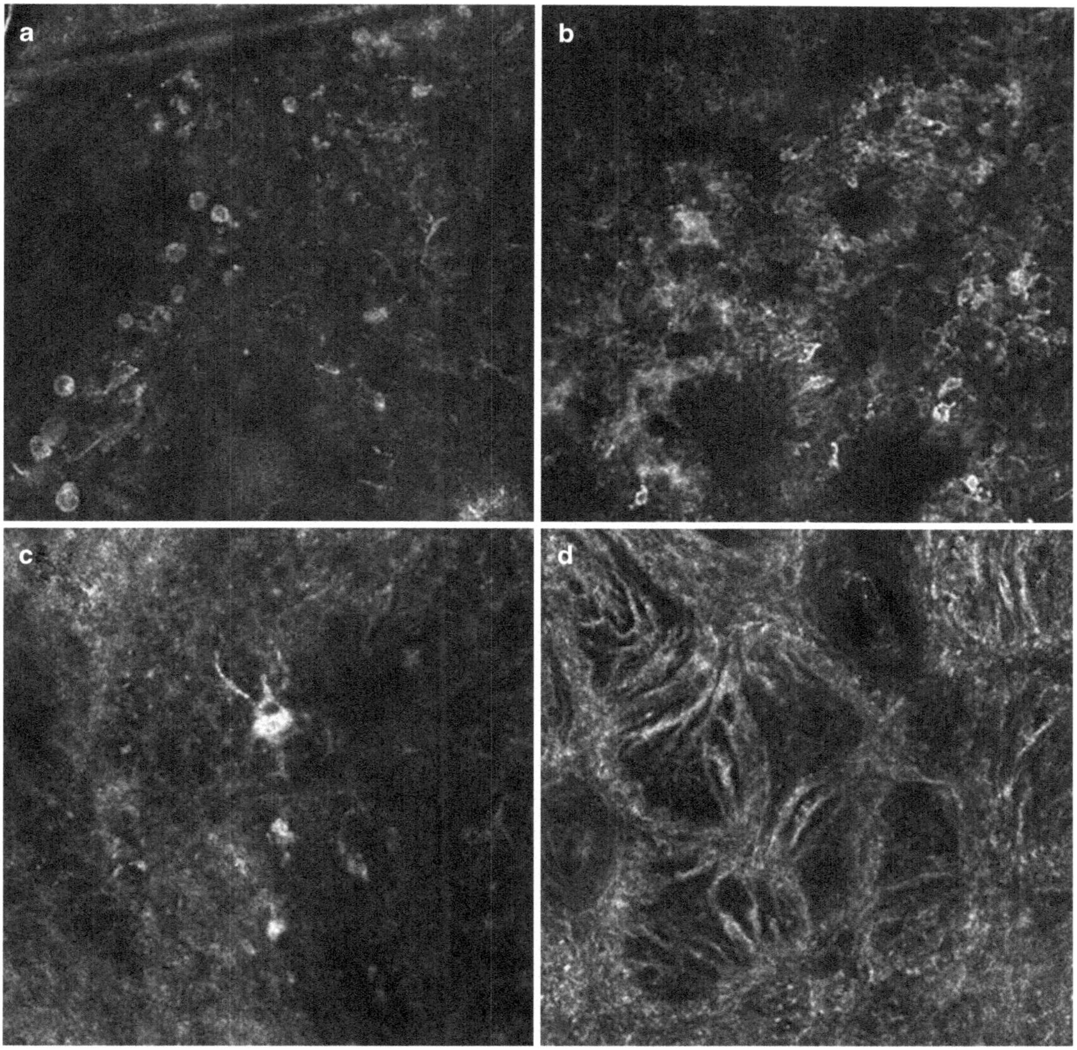

Fig. 4.8 Examples of different melanoma types. **A** and **B** represent a "pagetoid-type" melanoma, constituted by large, roundish pleomorphic cells in the epidermis (**a**) and atypical cells mostly clustered into nests at the junction (**b**). **C** and **D** represent "dendritic cell-type" melanoma, characterized by dendritic cells in the epidermis (**c**) and junction (**d**) displayed as numerous tangled lines

Pagetoid cells, mild-to-moderate cytological atypia, and non-edged papillae are described in thin/in situ melanomas. With increasing Breslow's thickness depth, epidermal disorder, cellular pleomorphism, papillary infiltration by atypical cells, and presence of atypical dermal nests (i.e., cerebriform nests) are observed (Fig. 4.8). With respect to RCM characteristics, melanomas can be classified into different subgroups [168], such as a superficial spreading melanoma associated with intermittent sun exposure and melanomas associated with chronic sun damage. Superficial spreading melanomas associated with intermittent sun exposure occur mainly on the trunk of adults with a history of intermittent solar exposure, often showing abundant pagetoid cells, mainly of roundish shape, distributed throughout the lesion. The dermal-epidermal junction is predominantly characterized by meshwork architecture with some atypical cells. Melanomas that occur on sun-damaged skin and lentigo maligna are characterized by dendritic pagetoid cells, mainly located around the hair follicle, in the context of a disordered epidermis. At the dermal-epidermal junction, ringed, meshwork, or uneven patterns can be observed in association with atypical cells. The upper dermis is predominantly characterized by collagen alterations and solar elastosis.

The identification of characteristic RCM features enables identification of early melanomas and discrimination with improved accuracy between benign and malignant lesions. The RCM imaging technique can be used as a diagnostic aid for lesions that display equivocal clinical and dermoscopic features. Even though histopathology remains the gold standard for the diagnosis of skin cancers, dermoscopy and RCM analysis can improve early recognition of dangerous skin lesions by clinicians. Recent studies demonstrate that the application of RCM as a second-level skin examination improves cutaneous melanoma diagnostic accuracy [169, 170]. In fact, the routine application of RCM by expert confocalists greatly improves specificity (ranging between 50 and 70%, with average sensitivity of approximately 90%) compared with dermoscopy, suggesting its effectiveness in sparing unnecessary excisions [171].

Moreover, in prospective interventional studies, characterized by the measurement of accuracy in real-world clinical practice, excellent sensitivity, without dramatically lower specificity, has been achieved. The main outcome was a significant reduction in the number of benign lesions excised in order to detect one melanoma, which averaged about 50% in all studies. In a more conservative setting, limiting the use of RCM to influence the decision of whether to excise moderately equivocal lesions only (i.e., all suspicious lesions were excised) resulted in over 50% of benign lesions being eligible for non-excision. This reduced the benign-to-malignant ratio from 15 to ~7 nevi for every one melanoma, and no melanoma was missed [172]. In the same setting, the introduction of RCM in the diagnostic workflow for melanoma showed the possibility of cost savings, since the expense of RCM examination was much lower than surgical and histopathologic procedures [173]. Moreover, implementation of RCM in cohorts of dermoscopically positive lesions reached the target of 1–2 benign lesions excised for every melanoma [169, 170]. Of note, on a large sample, the achievement of such an excellent performance resulted in a sensitivity of 95%, with 1 out of 20 melanomas only detected during digital follow-up. Thus, published data shows that RCM in the clinical setting is a powerful and cost-effective tool, able to reduce unnecessary excisions, while demonstrating very low risk of missing melanomas, especially when applied on moderately atypical lesions following dermoscopic evaluation [170].

The major limitations for introduction of RCM into clinical practice include the need for a trained expert confocalist and the slow speed of image acquisition. The latter can be solved with technical improvements. Concerning the need for training of expert confocalists, variable accuracy values are achieved depending on the evaluators' expertise [174]. The ability to rapidly implement RCM reading in clinical practice will also likely be adaptable to telemedicine application in the future [175].

Electrical Impedance Spectroscopy

Electrical impedance spectroscopy (EIS) is an innovative method that allows objective information to be drawn from atypical lesions. EIS is a measure of a material's overall resistance to the flow of alternating electric currents of various frequencies. Electrical impedance of biological materials can reflect the clinical status of the tissue under study. Normal and abnormal tissues differ with regard to cell size, shape, orientation, compactness, and structure of cell membranes. These different properties influence the ability of the cells to conduct and store electricity, meaning that these properties will also be reflected in an EIS measurement.

A harmless, imperceptible alternating electrical current is applied between two electrodes at the probe tip (Figs. 4.9 and 4.10). In order to cover the lesion both in width and in depth, the measurement is performed with 35 frequencies (1 kHz–2.5 MHz) and 4 depth settings for a total of 10 permutations over the entire lesion. In general, EIS measurements at low frequencies are related to the resistive properties of the extracellular environments, whereas impedance at high frequencies is related both to the resistive properties of the intra- and extracellular environments and the capacitive properties (reactance) of the cell membranes (Fig. 4.11).

This method measures and analyzes atypical lesions and produces an EIS score between 0 and 10, as well as a dichotomous result (EIS negative/positive) at a fixed cutoff. The fixed threshold is set at 4. This means that EIS scores less than 4 are EIS negative (−), with scores 4 or greater considered EIS positive (+). In this way, additional information is available to the examining clinician for melanoma detection. The accuracy of the EIS method has been tested in multiple clinical studies using the Nevisense system from the company SciBase (Stockholm, Sweden). The accuracy of the system was validated in an international, multicenter, prospective, blinded clinical trial including 1951 subjects, which yielded a sensitivity of 97% and a specificity of 34% on lesions destined for excision based on a clinical suspicion of melanoma [176].

The Nevisense system and the EIS method can be used in clinical practice as a diagnostic support tool to detect melanomas or rule out benign lesions. Nevisense is intended for use on cutaneous lesions with one or more clinical or historical characteristics of melanoma. The system is optimally designed for use when a clinician chooses to obtain additional information by considering excision. The Nevisense EIS score becomes an additional element of the overall clinical assessment of a lesion. Not only the negative or positive EIS outcome, but also the actual EIS score (0–10), as the score value is associated with the stage and severity of a lesion, can be incorporated into the assessment.

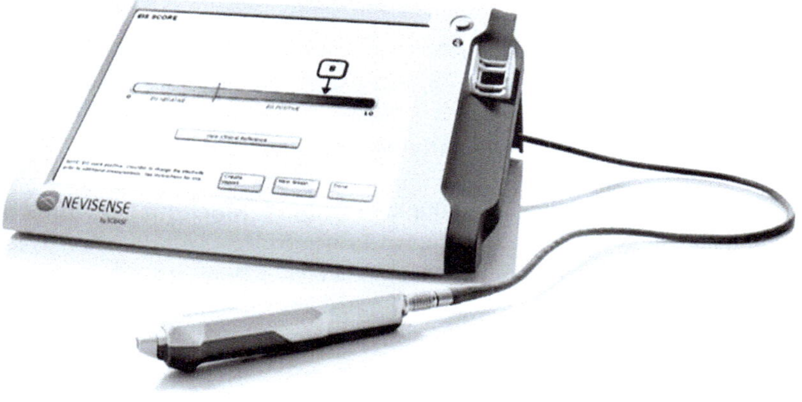

Fig. 4.9 Nevisense control unit, probe, and probe cable

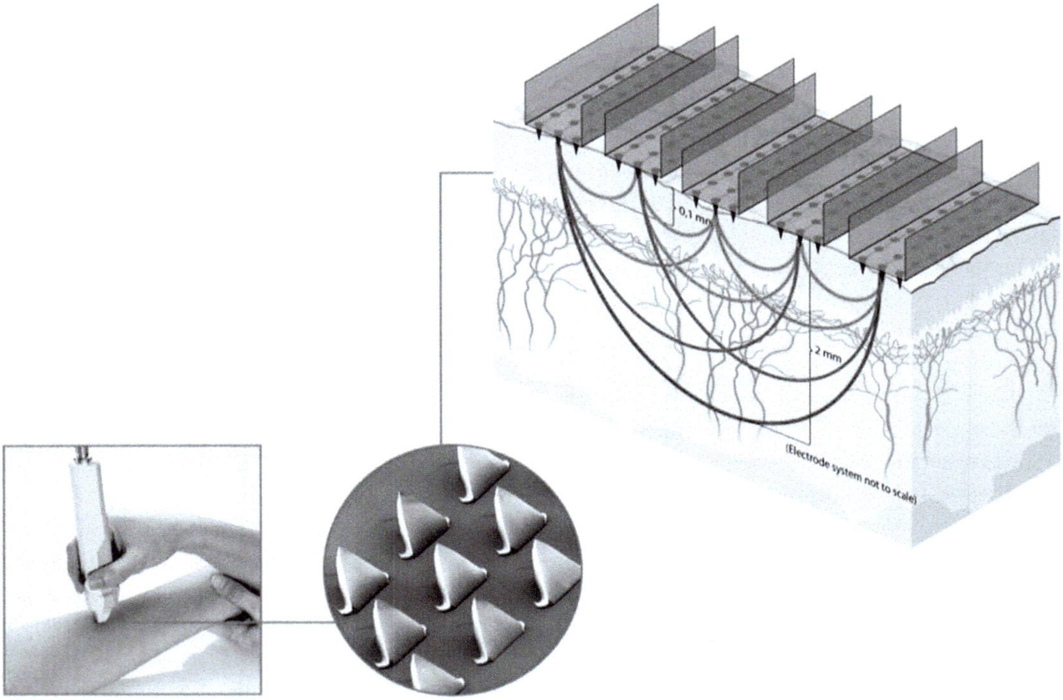

Fig. 4.10 Principle of operation

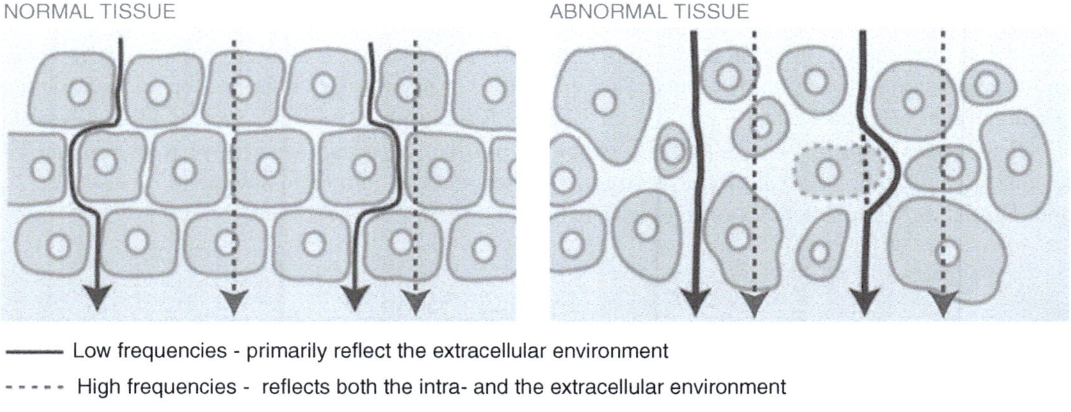

Fig. 4.11 Properties of low- and high-frequency impedance

In summary, the EIS method implemented in the Nevisense system has been shown to be an accurate and safe device that can be used in conjunction with clinical risk assessment for patients with suspicion of melanoma. Nevisense has regulatory approvals in Europe and Australia, also receiving PMA approval from the FDA in 2017 for clinical use in all major markets.

Machine Learning

Premature Promises

Beginning in the 1980s, several advances in the field of artificial intelligence enabled artificial neural networks to overcome early design flaws [177–179], as the closely related field of computer vision emerged with the advent of inexpensive hardware in the form of scanners, printers, and computers with new graphical user interfaces [180]. A significant achievement from this period was the demonstration that machines could learn from the data sets presented to them, rather than having to be programmed on how to think. This is the key idea behind machine learning.

One of the areas in which machine learning showed early success and therefore generated premature optimism was in the field of dermatology. From the mid-1990s, computer scientists were touting diagnostic tools for melanoma [181–183]. These claims were met with appropriate skepticism as demonstrated by the fact that by mid-2017, over two decades later, we still do not have an approved, accepted computer diagnostic system for any skin disease. Recently, Brewer and colleagues identified both the potential and risks of using mobile technology, including those of technologies making diagnostic claims [184]. Wolf and colleagues were straightforward about the actual dangers of using smartphones to try to classify melanomas [130]. Nevertheless, a review of almost 40 apps [126] reveals that work in this area is continuing unabated.

The replacement of artificial neural networks with new machine learning techniques continued to show promise through the mid-2000s, but the pace of improvements substantially slowed [185]. At the same time, further improvements to artificial neural network architectures and training algorithms [186, 179] coincided with the proliferation of a new kind of device, the general-purpose graphics processing unit (GP-GPU). These devices provided a critical hardware capability that researchers were quick to take advantage of, and were especially useful for, problems involving images, such as the classification and location of objects in images [116]. The new bottleneck evolved into actually having too few images to develop a training set on, further developed with new data sets (e.g., ImageNet [187] and MS-COCO [188]) and consistent improvement in object recognition on the order of 1–2% improvement each year. In 2012, deep convolutional neural networks were introduced and showed an improvement of over 11%, dropping the error rate to 15.3% [189], launching a mini-revolution in object detection and recognition in images (as well as additional problems); by 2016, the error rate had dropped to 3.0% [190].

Current Successes and Challenges

The impact of deep learning, a new field of machine learning, will be felt broadly and quickly and has already become normative in devices we talk to that respond with relevant information. Dermatology stands to be positively impacted by these advances. Much of the "Is it melanoma?" image research has shifted to work on dermoscopy images, which include several more features for computers to learn about. In late 2016, Codella and colleagues published preprint work [118] on dermoscopy images, demonstrating a computer system capable of outperforming eight expert dermatologists on a test set of images, both in terms of accuracy and specificity. Yet by modern data set standards, the size of their data set was relatively small, despite being the largest publicly available to date. In early 2017, Esteva and colleagues published results of a skin cancer classification system that demonstrated the ability to compete with board-certified dermatologists, at least at the task of classifying static images of lesions [83]. The promise of deep learning is that the capability will only improve with larger data sets, with results leading to interesting and effective new tools in the clinic, in teledermatology, and eventually in the hands of ordinary users on mobile devices.

Perspective on Emerging Technologies

Melanoma diagnostic techniques are evolving alongside imaging innovations driven both by worldwide consumer demands and advances in science. Among the increasingly diverse array of physical phenomena applied in dermatologic diagnosis (Table 4.3) are three noteworthy examples: Raman spectroscopy, multiphoton microscopy, and photoacoustic imaging.

Raman spectroscopy (Fig. 4.12) measures molecular vibrations by detecting energy shifts in light (spontaneous Raman scattering). In the-

Table 4.3 2016 overview of available and novel dermatologic noninvasive imaging devices [230]

Fundamental technique and synonyms or variations	*Most likely user,* examples of CE devices **(bold for FDA-approved and price range)**	Clinical uses and highest quality in vivo clinical trial result	Features typically visualized and imaging time	Advantages and unique technologic capabilities	Limitations of currently available devices	Technological developments and anticipations
Polarization techniques (dermoscopy, polarimetry)	*All dermatologists,* DermLite (3Gen), EpiScope (Welch Allyn), NevoScope (TransLite), Dermascope (American Diagnostic Corp), MoleMax (Derma Medical Systems), Derma Medical Systems, DermoGenius (Dermoscan), handyscope (Fotofinder), Canfield; $0.1 k to $2 k	Assistance of dermatologic physical exam, especially for cancer screening; melanoma vs. benign nevi (sens 89%, spec 84%[a])	Modestly magnified subsurface morphology including vessels; melanin distribution and other skin cancer features; instantaneous images	Rapid skin cancer screening; wide base of experienced dermoscopy users; significant improvement in sensitivity and specificity relative to unaided clinical exam; devices do not require FDA approval (class I)	Added value highly user and training dependent; low-resolution images; top-view image (no cross-sectional images at depth)	Mobile phone mounts and apps; advanced polarimetry techniques will extend possibilities, e.g., automatic evaluation of average nuclear morphology or tissue heterogeneity; www.demoscopy-ids.org
Total-body digital photography (TBDP), regional imaging	*Pigmented lesion experts*, Dermspectra, Canfield, FotoFinder, MoleMax, MoleSave, MoleMap, MelanoScan, Dermoscan, Visiomed; $10 k to $250 k	Monitoring melanocytic neoplasms in high-risk pigmented lesion clinics, NMSC, and inflammation diseases	Generally same features as clinical exam; 10 min for total body	Rapidly acquire and monitor large portion of skin surface; computer algorithms help track changes and suspicious features	Challenging to rapidly present and interpret resulting large data set in clinical setting	Increasing number of commercial devices with automated image acquisition; comprehensive resource at http://isdis.net/imaging-modalities/total-body-photography/

Confocal microscopy (LSCM, CSLM, RCM)	*All dermatologists willing to invest in necessary training,* six category 1 CPT reimbursement codes; **VivaScope** (CaliberID and Mavig, formerly Lucid), **Stratum** (Optiscan); $100 k	Identify diverse lesions for which biopsy can be avoided; preoperative mapping of malignancies including lentigo maligna for reduced surgical defects; melanoma vs. benign nevi (sens 97%, spec 83%[a]) diagnosis of equivocal lesions vs. BCC (sens 100%, spec 89%[a])	Microscopic structures as in H&E but only in horizontal (en face) sections; 25 min for 6 × 6 mm image stack (including prep time described in CPT 96932)	Highest accuracy; only imaging technology with Medicare reimbursement; video-rate single-lesion, histology-grade (<1 mm) resolution of cellular components based on scattered light; able to view dendrites on melanocytes (unachievable with standard H&E)	En face views best interpreted by experienced confocalist difficult-to-detect invasion through dermal-epidermal junction and other depth-resolved features such as melanoma stage or HAK vs. SCC; unable to image beneath papillary dermis (limited to 0.25 mm depth)	Intraoperative use, e.g., coupled to laser ablation; combination with fluorescent techniques; working group at http://www.confocal-icwg.com/
Spectral (multispectral, hyperspectral, RGB, infrared thermography imaging)	*Few dermatologists,* category 3 CPT codes for research use; **MelaFind** (Melasciences) $30 k; **SIAscope** (MedX) with SIMSYS or MoleMate software $6 k–$8 k; Dermlite II MS (3gen) $1 k; TiVi (WheelsBridge) $20 k	Help triage pigmented lesions for biopsy; for melanoma vs. nevus, MelaFind (sens 98.3%, spec 9.9%[c]) (sens 80%, spec 76% [d]); clinical research with TiVi	Erythema and blanching, oxy- and deoxyhemoglobin and melanin; Siascope 5 s for single 11 × 11 mm image; MelaFind 45 s for single image up to 22 × 22 mm; TiVi 30fps wide field or single lesion	Mapping of some chemical component through the entire thickness of skin (to 2.5 mm deep) based on light collection at numerous frequencies; often combined with polarization technique	Large data set interpretation highly dependent on training set that computer algorithms use; top-view image (no cross-sectional images at depth)	Research needed correlating spectral properties of skin to disease; handheld spectral polarization camera probes operating on tablets
Optical coherence tomography (low-coherence interferometry, FF-OCT, GD-OCT)	*Few academic dermatologists,* **Vivosight** (Michelson Diagnostics), Light-CT (LL Tech), **Skintell** (Agfa), Nitid (DermaLumics), SkinDex300 (ISIS Optronics); $130–$180 k	Depth demarcation and reduction of presurgical biopsy rate for BCCs; dynamic blood flow imaging; as adjunct to expert dermoscopy exam, sens not significantly improved, but spec for BCC improved from 54 to 75%[c])	Macroscopic structures (e.g. blood vessels, DEJ, BCC border); Vivosight 20 s for 6 × 6 mm image stack; Skintell <2 s for 1.8 × 1.5 × 1 mm 3D volume; Light-CT 1 min for 10 × 10 mm image	Optical analogue of ultrasound; images relatively deep in dermis (~1 mm), able to image flow with speckle variance or Doppler; images in same plane of view (vertical) as traditional H&E	Diagnostic accuracy limited by lateral resolution (Vivosight 8 mm, Skintell 3 mm with adaptive optics). FF-OCT OVERCOMES THIS (Light-CT resolution 1 mm) but in excised tissue and limited to 0.2 mm depth	Intraoperative Mohs margins with FF-OCT; OCT elastography; molecular imaging; polarization-sensitive OCT; potential resolution improvement with Gabor domain liquid lens or Mirau interferometer

Table 4.3 (continued)

Fundamental technique and synonyms or variations	*Most likely user,* examples of CE devices **(bold for FDA-approved and price range)**	Clinical uses and highest quality in vivo clinical trial result	Features typically visualized and imaging time	Advantages and unique technologic capabilities	Limitations of currently available devices	Technological developments and anticipations
Interferometry (dynamic light scattering, laser Doppler flowmetry, LDPI, laser speckle imaging, LSPI, LSFG, LASCA, MESI)	*Research centers*, FluxExplorer (Microvascular Imaging), Moor, Perimed, Lisca	Skin grafts, vascular lesion treatment monitoring, patch test quantification, Raynaud's scoring, scar evaluation; in detection of active morphea (sens 80% spec 77% in single-center trial[f])	Color-coded perfusion image reflecting blood flow level or velocity; imaged area adjustable; 1 s for 50 × 50 mm	Low cost, noncontact; rapidly evaluates blood flow over a large area (up to 500 × 500 mm)	Low resolution (>100 mm)	Combination with OCT
Vibrational spectroscopy (Raman, FTIR)	*Research centers;* gen2-SCA (rIVERd) $100 K TO $250 K; Aura (Verisante) $65 k	Determining skin hydration, antioxidant levels, and distribution of cosmetics and other topical treatment; diagnostically, benign (including SK) vs. malignant (including AK) lesions had sens 90–99%, spec 75–20% in single-center trial[g]	Molecular composition and biochemical information; single-point or depth-resolved spectra acquired in seconds but without yielding actual images	Quantitative measurements of many known compounds already available, e.g., carotenoid antioxidants, NMF, urea, lactate; theoretically any molecule will have unique Raman signature	Rapid high-resolution volumetric imaging impractical as Raman effect (inelastic scattering) several orders of magnitude weaker than reflectance (elastic scattering) or fluorescence; spectra are difficult to interpret for unknown compounds	Research needed correlating Raman signatures to disease; more complex nonlinear implementations (e.g., CARS, stimulated Raman) enable rapid imaging for some specific chemical signature lines

Fluorescence (autofluorescence lifetime imaging, photodynamic diagnosis, fluorescence videomicroscopy)	*Research centers,* SkinSpect (Spectral Molecular Imaging)	Presently early research phase; not used as single modality; primarily used to enhance confocal images, especially in perioperative imaging	Images of added or intrinsic fluorescent compounds	Fluorescent agents can improve contrast of other modalities; fluorescence lifetime measurements, when used, are sensitive to microenvironment of detected compounds	Little dermatologic clinical data; limited by width of fluorescence absorption and emission lines and few FDA-approved exogenous fluorescent compounds (fluorescein, indocyanine green, methylene blue)	Much R&D needed
Diffuse optics (spatial frequency domain imaging)	*Research centers and wound care physicians;* Ox-Imager (Modulated Imaging) $100 k	Presently early research phase; preliminary data in wound monitoring, burn thickness assessment, and surgical flap viability prediction based on blood supply	Hemoglobin total concentration and oxygenation; optical properties of skin (scattering, absorption); 1 s for two frequency scan, 25 s for full scan	Non-contact imaging of large area (size adjustable up to 200 × 150 mm)	Little dermatologic clinical data; low resolution (>100 mm)	Much R&D needed

[a]Langley RG. Dermatology 2007;215(4):365–72—(125 patients single center)
[b]Guitera P. J Invest Dermatol. 2012;(132(10):2386–94—(663 patients multicenter)
[c]Mnheit G. Arch Dermtol. 2011;147(2):188–94—(1251 patients multicenter)
[d]Tomatis S. Phys Med Biol. 2005;21(50(8):1675–87—(1278 patients single center)
[e]Ulrich M. Br J Dermatol. 2015;173(2):428–35—(250 patients multicenter)
[f]Weibel L. et al. Arthritis Rheum. 2007;56(10:3489–95—(111 lesions)
[g]Zhao J. et al. Analyst 2016;7:141(3):1034–43—(127 lesions tested)

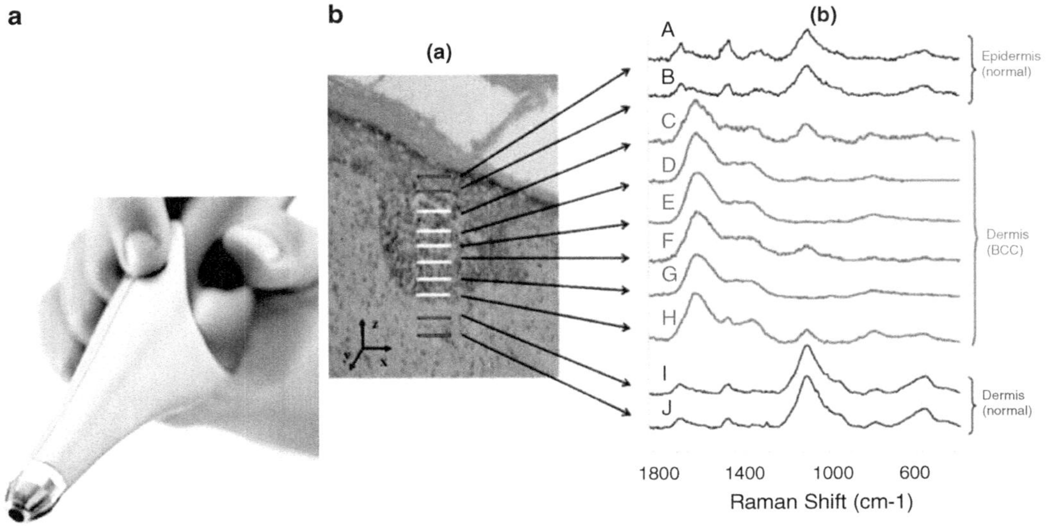

Fig. 4.12 **A.** Verisante Aura, a commercial Raman spectroscopy device [233]. **B.** Difference in Raman spectra between basal cell carcinoma and normal surrounding skin [234]

ory, every molecule has a unique Raman spectrum. This has enabled the development of commercial devices by RiverD (Rotterdam, The Netherlands) and Biozoom (Kassel, Germany) that noninvasively measure concentrations of compounds ranging from natural moisturizing factor to antioxidants, even in neonate skin [191]. However, the *in vivo* Raman spectra of involved biomolecules are not known for melanoma detection. Instead, large known data sets are used to train computer algorithms to differentiate benign from malignant, analogous to automated multispectral imaging technologies similar to MelaFind™. With this approach, a commercial device, the Aura™, has been developed by Verisante (Vancouver, Canada). HealthCanada approved the Verisante Aura for the early detection of skin cancer, following the results of a study that predicted 90% sensitivity and 68% specificity to differentiate benign pigmented lesions (286 cases) from melanoma (44 cases) within its training set [192].

No device to date has been able to produce practical skin images with spontaneous Raman signals, mainly because they are at least one million fold weaker than the elastic light scattering background. However, nonlinear implementations employing high-peak-power laser systems are an active area of research, demonstrating video-rate preclinical imaging via coherent Raman scattering [193]. Cutaneous malignancies are only beginning to be explored [194], but unique insights might be obtained through the ability to measure changes in biomolecule distributions and active cell metabolism [195].

Multiphoton Microscopy

Multiphoton microscopy (Fig. 4.13) provides submicron image resolution (superior to confocal microscopy) through nonlinear light-matter interactions created by femtosecond lasers. The most important signals are (1) two-photon fluorescence, which depends upon several biomolecules including melanin and NADH in different oxidation states, and 2) second harmonic generation (SHG), which is particularly sensitive to collagen. As a result, subcellular morphological details can be visualized, as can the relation of melanocytes and keratinocytes to dermal collagen. The largest multiphoton study to date showed a 75% sensitivity and 80% specificity to discriminate melanoma from benign nevi among 53 suspicious pigmented lesions in vivo [196]. A

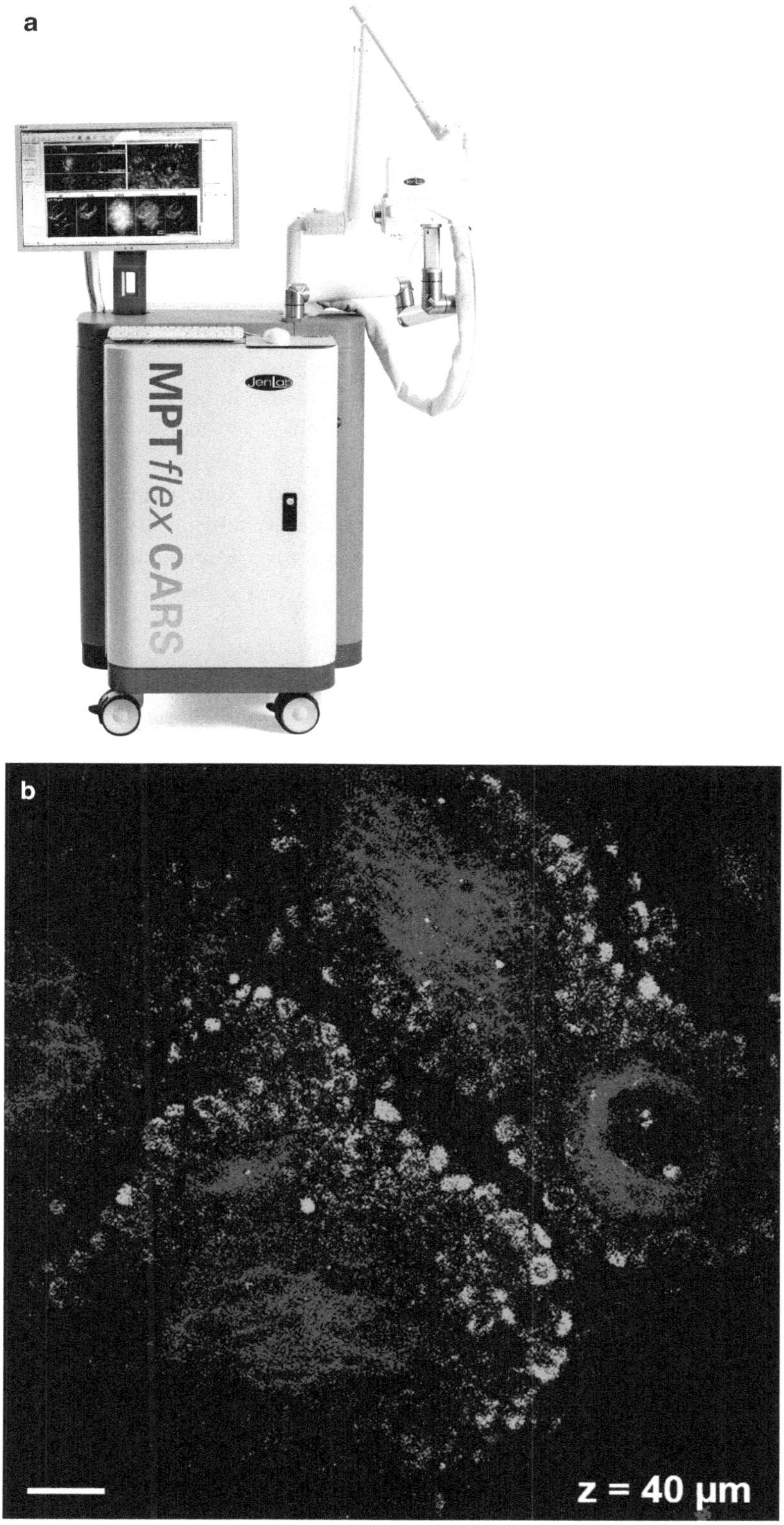

Fig. 4.13 **A.** MPTflex, a commercial clinical multiphoton microscope [235]. **B.** Multiphoton view of a pigmented lesion at a depth of 40 microns in skin: second harmonic generation (SHG—blue) from dermal collagen surrounded by pigmented keratinocytes visualized by two-photon fluorescence (green). Image taken at the Beckman Laser Institute, University of California, Irvine. Scale bar = 50 µm

more recent pilot study has suggested higher accuracy when the nonlinear signal strengths are incorporated into the assessment [197]. Jenlab (Berlin, Germany) has commercialized the DermaInspect and MPTFlex devices, which provide high-resolution images along with label-free biochemical information from fluorescence lifetime [198] and nonlinear Raman measurements. However, dissemination has been limited by the high price (€400,000) and smaller field of view (a 0.35 × 0.35 mm image at a single depth acquired in several seconds). Beyond multiphoton microscopy, femtosecond lasers enable several other related nonlinear optical techniques that may impact melanoma detection. Pump-probe ultrafast spectroscopy in particular has demonstrated high sensitivity for ex vivo melanoma detection through label-free measurement of eumelanin-to-pheomelanin ratios [199].

Photoacoustic Imaging

Photoacoustic imaging (Fig. 4.14) is a hybrid technology that measures sound waves resulting from the absorption of light. Thus, it marries the resolution and molecular specificity of optical imaging with the depth advantages of ultrasound. It is exquisitely sensitive to light-absorbing molecules such as hemoglobin and melanin. This enables label-free, noninvasive detection of melanoma with more than a 50-fold higher contrast when compared to optical microscopy [200]. When multiple wavelengths are used, oxygenation changes in single capillary loops can be visualized in the human cuticle and elsewhere [201]. The Mutispectral Opto-acoustic Tomography Acuity is a commercial device available from iThera Medical (Munich, Germany). Capitalizing on photo-acoustic depth capabilities, it enabled 100% sensitive detection of nodal mel-

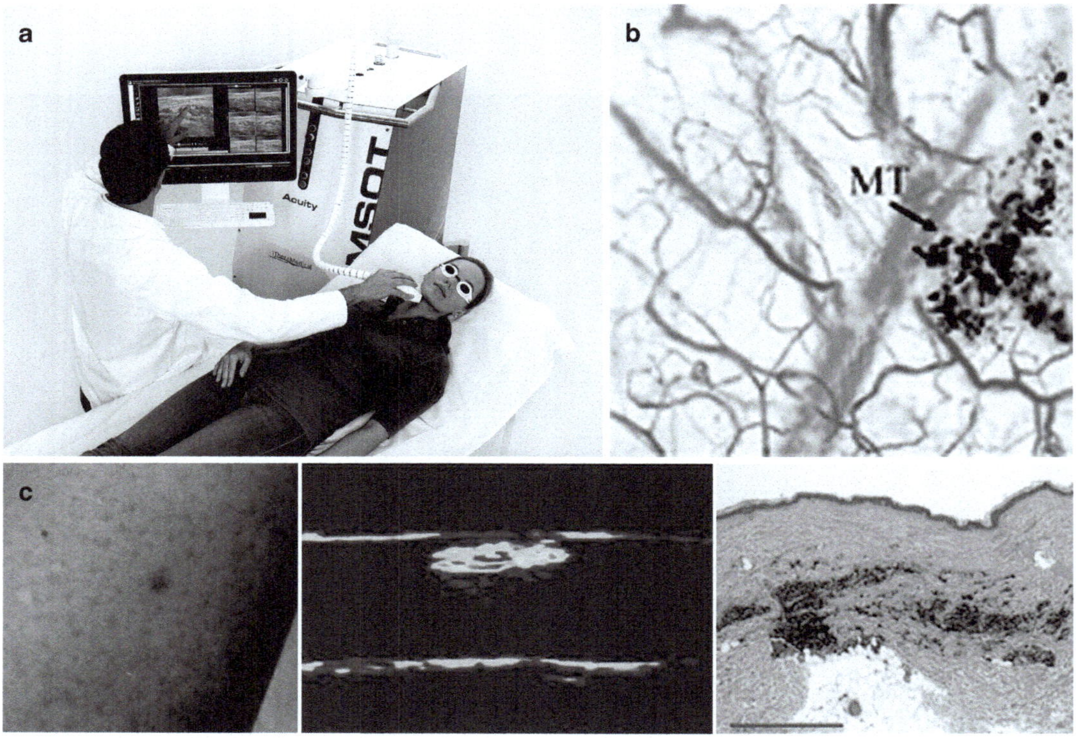

Fig. 4.14 **A.** MSOT Acuity, a commercial clinical photoacoustic imaging device used to detect melanoma in lymph nodes [courtesy of iThera Medical]. **B.** Photoacoustic microscopy enables label-free imaging of blood and individual melanosomes of a 4-day-old melanoma metastasis in a mouse ear [200]. **C.** Noninvasive depth measurement of a patient's 1.67 mm melanoma (left) via photo-acoustics (center) and confirmed by histopathology (right) [203]

anoma metastases prior to sentinel lymph node biopsy. Specificity was only 49%, due to false positives from nodal melanin and hemorrhage, with no false negatives detected [202]. More recently, a handheld clinical device has enabled noninvasive measurements of melanoma tumor thickness in good agreement with measured Breslow's depth [203], which may alleviate staging inaccuracies from partial biopsies [204]. Photo-acoustics may even have a therapeutic role, as evidenced by noninvasive enumeration and real-time intravascular destruction of circulating melanoma cells in mice [205]. These early results collectively suggest that photoacoustics may have a significant role in several aspects of melanoma management in the future.

Perspective on Technological Advances

As mounting clinical experience reveals their practical utility and limitations, emerging diagnostic techniques will be refined in new and unexpected ways. This is foreshadowed by the leaps reported in the optics literature for established technologies such as optical coherence tomography (OCT). The lofty goal of individual skin cell resolution has been achieved in multiple variations, including full-field OCT [206], Mirau interferometry [207], Gabor-domain OCT [208], and with adaptive optics and liquid lenses [209]. At the other end of the spectrum, wide-field OCT has been developed to provide fast volumetric images of hundreds of square centimeters of skin [210].

While it is currently possible to categorize most large imaging studies into one of 11 different modalities (Table 4.3), boundaries are beginning to blur as multimodal devices emerge that synergistically couple individual strengths to overcome limitations. A combined fluorescence and Raman device has demonstrated rapid margin mapping and assessment for Mohs surgery [211]. Spectral and fluorescence imaging are also being explored as potential diagnostic enhancements to established techniques like dermoscopy [153] and confocal microscopy [212]. The inventors of the VivaScope (see Section "In Vivo Confocal Microscopy") have recently developed a system of co-registering confocal microscopy and OCT images [213], overcoming the depth and resolution limitations of either technique alone. An integrated photoacoustic OCT device has also been developed [214]. This trend indicates that a combination modality will likely be the optimal approach to achieve meaningful clinical implementation.

Molecular Assays for Detection of Melanoma and Lethal Melanoma

Evaluation of mRNA expression profiles originally identified by microarrays, and then further refined to qRT-PCR, has emerged as a method of diagnostic confirmation and prognostication for melanoma. There are currently three commercially available qRT-PCR assays, two that focus on diagnosis and one upon prognosis. DermTech International, Inc. (La Jolla, CA) has developed a non-invasive technique that isolates mRNA from corneocytes removed by tape stripping the surface of pigmented lesions. In principle, it is believed that the corneocytes contain mRNA from melanosomes transferred to them from melanocytes. The assay then uses qRT-PCR to look for expression of either *LINC00518* or *PRAME*. The identification of either renders a positive score, raising concern for the possibility of melanoma. The sensitivity and specificity of the assay in a combination of serially collected and archival samples were 91% and 69%, respectively. In an exclusive set of serially collected samples, the respective sensitivity and specificity were 79% and 80% [215]. The non-invasive nature of the assay is clearly the strength of the technique. It is most ideal for lesions that have some concerning features, but are considered able to be monitored with dermoscopy; that is, the test would not replace a biopsy for lesions clearly atypical enough to warrant histologic assessment. The limitation of the technique is that lesions must be at least 6 mm in diameter and on a body surface that allows optimal application of the adhesive. Mucosal and acral lesions are excluded.

Myriad Genetics, Inc. (Salt Lake City, UT) has developed a qRT-PCR assay that assesses mRNA expression levels of 23 distinct genes from formalin-fixed, paraffin-embedded (FFPE) tissue in order to better classify histologically controversial or difficult-to-diagnose cases [216]. The 23 genes include *PRAME*, which encodes a known melanoma tumor antigen, and is the same gene utilized in the DermTech tape stripping assay; 5 *S100A* genes known as the S100A9 component; 8 immune-related genes; and 9 housekeeping genes. In a validation set of 1400 melanocytic lesions, the test performed with a sensitivity of 91.5% and specificity of 92.5% [217]. The strength of this assay is that it can be performed on relatively paucicellular processes and has been studied in relatively large validation cohorts. Alternatively, there have been no studies assessing the test's ability to classify truly histologically ambiguous cases with long-term follow-up, so it is unknown how well the assay would perform on those cases that would be of greatest value to the field.

A prognostic assay based on mRNA expression profiling of 31 genes has been developed by Castle Biosciences (Friendswood, TX) for prognostication of histologically confirmed melanoma [218]. Genes related to tissue development, epithelial differentiation, and cell junction-related genes are highly represented in the gene set. Since the initial development of the assay, in an independent validation study of 523 patients, the recurrence-free survival (RFS) rates for class 1 (good prognostic signature) and class 2 (poor prognostic signature) were 88% and 52%, respectively, with distant metastasis-free survival (DMFS) rates of 93% versus 60%, respectively ($p < 0.001$). The gene class signature was a significant predictor in multivariate analyses (RFS HR = 2.1, $p = 0.003$; DMFS HR = 2.7, $p = 0.002$) with thickness and sentinel lymph node (SLN) status. The strength of this assay, as shown from the validation study with 523 patients, was its ability to identify 70% of SLN-negative patients who ultimately developed metastatic disease. The Kaplan-Meier curves have shown particularly strong separation in the 5-year RFS and DMFS of stage II and IIIa melanoma patients. Among the stage I patients, the 5-year RFS survival for class 1 patients was 96%, compared to 85% in class 2 patients, which was a statistically significant difference but not of the same magnitude as seen with stage II and IIIa patients [219].

Liquid biopsy with assessment of either circulating tumor cells, cell-free circulating tumor DNA, or cell-free circulating microRNA has been investigated as a potential prognostic tool. In a meta-analysis of nine studies looking at the prognostic value of liquid biopsy, Khoja and colleagues showed that the studies have markedly different rates of tumor detection, based on the technique being utilized and the time at which the samples are obtained. Taken together, these results have been highly variable and inconclusive as to the prognostic value of the assays [220].

The patient population in which liquid biopsy seemed most promising was in the assessment of stage III melanoma patients. Scoggins and colleagues assessed 820 patients who were part of the Sunbelt Melanoma Trial before they underwent lymphadenectomy [221]. After the sentinel lymph node biopsy, tyrosinase, MelanA/MART1, MAGE3, and gp-100 were serially assessed with qRT-PCR in 820 patients before the completion dissection. It was determined that stage III melanoma patients with a positive PCR test for >1 marker at any time point showed worse disease-free survival ($p = 0.006$) and overall survival ($p = 0.0012$) compared with patients with only one positive marker. However, there were only seven stage III patients with a positive PCR test for >1 marker, which makes it difficult to draw any definitive conclusions. Validation studies on greater numbers of stage III patients would be of value. Additionally, since there are now so many possible circulating factors that may be assessed, including BRAFV600E, miRNAs, and others, it may take some time to determine which markers, and what time periods, would give optimal results [222, 223].

A number of studies have utilized mass spectroscopy as a method of studying the proteomics of melanoma tumors. Byrum and colleagues showed 171 proteins that were differentially expressed in comparison of FFPE samples of benign nevi, primary melanomas, and metastatic tumors [224]. These broader studies may allow the identification of smaller groups of proteins that may be investigated by immunohistochemistry as potential biomarkers. Overall, validation studies using algorithms developed by proteomic analysis of training sets, and then applied to large validation sets of patients with known outcomes, have not yet been performed and hence are still in their infancy.

Conclusions

Of all lethal cancers, melanoma is perhaps the "poster child" for the benefits that can be derived from its early detection. It is an aggressive cancer that when detected early has great potential for cure. Unfortunately, when detected late, it has a very high mortality rate, despite recent therapeutic advances. Its primary localization in the skin offers a distinct advantage for early detection from the perspective of naked-eye examinations, assessment with technologies such as dermoscopy, *in vivo* confocal microscopy, and other advanced non-invasive technologies. The ease of accessibility also makes sampling and histologic evaluation simple, and allows for the implementation of genetic and genomic technologies applied towards melanocytic tumors for the purpose of improved diagnostic and prognostic information. Technologies that capitalize on the cutaneous location of melanoma are rapidly evolving to reach the right populations with mobile devices, to identify the individuals in greatest need of screening, and to apply the right technologies to identify melanoma before it reaches metastatic competency.

Furthermore, beyond all of these technological advances is the potential to apply deep learning and artificial intelligence to the challenge of early detection. Perhaps the final frontier that remains is how to couple and extend the clinical knowledge we have gained over the years with exciting and evolving technologies into the public health realm. The problem of reaching the right individuals, convincing them of their vulnerability, and persuading them to seek attention if they have a concerning lesion remains. Bridging this gap between medical science, responsible adoption of technology, public health challenges, and behavior modifications will be critical, especially if we are to take advantage of all the progress that has been made with respect to melanoma early detection. Success in this arena will certainly minimize melanoma deaths and will also serve as a model for other cancers and disease types that can benefit from early detection.

References

1. Coit DG, Thompson JA, Andtbacka R, Anker CJ, Bichakjian CK, Carson WE 3rd, et al. Melanoma, version 4.2014. J Natl Compr Cancer Netw. 2014;12(5):621–9.
2. Hodi FS, Chesney J, Pavlick AC, Robert C, Grossmann KF, McDermott DF, et al. Combined nivolumab and ipilimumab versus ipilimumab alone in patients with advanced melanoma: 2-year overall survival outcomes in a multicentre, randomised, controlled, phase 2 trial. Lancet Oncol. 2016;17(11):1558–68. https://doi.org/10.1016/S1470-2045(16)30366-7.
3. Skin cancer by the numbers. In: Skin disease briefs: American Academy of Dermatology; 2017.
4. Rubio-Rodriguez D, De Diego BS, Perez M, Rubio-Terres C. Cost-effectiveness of drug treatments for advanced melanoma: a systematic literature review. PharmacoEconomics. 2017. https://doi.org/10.1007/s40273-017-0517-1.
5. Oh A, Tran DM, McDowell LC, Keyvani D, Barcelon JA, Merino O, et al. Cost effectiveness of nivolumab-ipilimumab combination therapy compared with monotherapy for first-line treatment of metastatic melanoma in the United States. J Manag Care Spec Pharm. 2017;23(6):653–64. https://doi.org/10.18553/jmcp.2017.23.6.653.
6. Silva A, Rauscher GH, Ferrans CE, Hoskins K, Rao R. Assessing the quality of race/ethnicity, tumor, and breast cancer treatment information in a non-SEER state registry. J Registry Manag. 2014;41(1):24–30.
7. Harris RB, Koch SM, Newton C, Silvis NG, Curiel-Lewandroski C, Giancola J, et al. Underreporting of melanoma in Arizona and strategies for increasing reporting: a public health partnership approach. Public Health Rep. 2015;130(6):737–44. https://doi.org/10.1177/003335491513000624.
8. Cockburn M, Swetter SM, Peng D, Keegan TH, Deapen D, Clarke CA. Melanoma underreporting: why does it happen, how big is the problem, and how do we fix it? J Am Acad Dermatol. 2008;59(6):1081–5. https://doi.org/10.1016/j.jaad.2008.08.007.
9. Brunssen A, Waldmann A, Eisemann N, Katalinic A. Impact of skin cancer screening and secondary prevention campaigns on skin cancer incidence and mortality: a systematic review. J Am Acad Dermatol. 2017;76(1):129–39. e10. https://doi.org/10.1016/j.jaad.2016.07.045.

10. Johnson MM, Leachman SA, Aspinwall LG, Cranmer LD, Curiel-Lewandrowski C, Sondak VK, et al. Skin cancer screening: recommendations for data-driven screening guidelines and a review of the US preventive services task force controversy. Melanoma Manage. 2017;4(1):13–37.
11. Byrnes P, Ackermann E, Williams ID, Mitchell GK, Askew D. Management of skin cancer in Australia--a comparison of general practice and skin cancer clinics. Aust Fam Physician. 2007;36(12):1073–5.
12. Swetter SM, Johnson TM, Miller DR, Layton CJ, Brooks KR, Geller AC. Melanoma in middle-aged and older men: a multi-institutional survey study of factors related to tumor thickness. Arch Dermatol. 2009;145(4):397–404. https://doi.org/10.1001/archdermatol.2008.603.
13. LeBlanc WG, Vidal L, Kirsner RS, Lee DJ, Caban-Martinez AJ, McCollister KE, et al. Reported skin cancer screening of US adult workers. J Am Acad Dermatol. 2008;59(1):55–63. https://doi.org/10.1016/j.jaad.2008.03.013.
14. Miller KA, Langholz BM, Zadnick J, Hamilton AS, Cozen W, Mack TM, et al. Prevalence and predictors of recent skin examination in a population-based twin cohort. Cancer Epidemiol Biomark Prev. 2015;24(8):1190–8. https://doi.org/10.1158/1055-9965.EPI-14-1389.
15. Goulart JM, Quigley EA, Dusza S, Jewell ST, Alexander G, Asgari MM, et al. Skin cancer education for primary care physicians: a systematic review of published evaluated interventions. J Gen Intern Med. 2011;26(9):1027–35. https://doi.org/10.1007/s11606-011-1692-y.
16. Martires KJ, Kurlander DE, Minwell GJ, Dahms EB, Bordeaux JS. Patterns of cancer screening in primary care from 2005 to 2010. Cancer. 2014;120(2):253–61. https://doi.org/10.1002/cncr.28403.
17. Oliveria SA, Heneghan MK, Cushman LF, Ughetta EA, Halpern AC. Skin cancer screening by dermatologists, family practitioners, and internists: barriers and facilitating factors. Arch Dermatol. 2011;147(1):39–44. https://doi.org/10.1001/archdermatol.2010.414.
18. Eide MJ, Asgari MM, Fletcher SW, Geller AC, Halpern AC, Shaikh WR, et al. Effects on skills and practice from a web-based skin cancer course for primary care providers. J Am Board Fam Med. 2013;26(6):648–57. https://doi.org/10.3122/jabfm.2013.06.130108.
19. Berwick M, Armstrong BK, Ben-Porat L, Fine J, Kricker A, Eberle C, et al. Sun exposure and mortality from melanoma. J Natl Cancer Inst. 2005;97(3):195–9. https://doi.org/10.1093/jnci/dji019.
20. Weinstock MA, Risica PM, Martin RA, Rakowski W, Dube C, Berwick M, et al. Melanoma early detection with thorough skin self-examination: the "check it out" randomized trial. Am J Prev Med. 2007;32(6):517–24. https://doi.org/10.1016/j.amepre.2007.02.024.
21. Preventive Services Task Force US, Bibbins-Domingo K, Grossman DC, Curry SJ, Davidson KW, Ebell M, et al. Screening for skin cancer: US Preventive Services Task Force recommendation statement. JAMA. 2016;316(4):429–35. https://doi.org/10.1001/jama.2016.8465.
22. Wernli KJ, Henrikson NB, Morrison CC, Nguyen M, Pocobelli G, Whitlock EP. Screening for skin cancer in adults: An updated systematic evidence review for the U.S. Preventive Services Task Force. Rockville, MD: U.S. Preventive Services Task Force Evidence Syntheses, formerly Systematic Evidence Reviews; 2016.
23. Katalinic A, Waldmann A, Weinstock MA, Geller AC, Eisemann N, Greinert R, et al. Does skin cancer screening save lives? An observational study comparing trends in melanoma mortality in regions with and without screening. Cancer. 2012;118(21):5395–402. https://doi.org/10.1002/cncr.27566.
24. Weinstock MA, Ferris LK, Saul MI, Geller AC, Risica PM, Siegel JA, et al. Downstream consequences of melanoma screening in a community practice setting: first results. Cancer. 2016;122(20):3152–6. https://doi.org/10.1002/cncr.30177.
25. Goulart JM, Malvehy J, Puig S, Martin G, Marghoob AA. Dermoscopy in skin self-examination: a useful tool for select patients. Arch Dermatol. 2011;147(1):53–8. https://doi.org/10.1001/archdermatol.2010.387.
26. Titus LJ, Clough-Gorr K, Mackenzie TA, Perry A, Spencer SK, Weiss J, et al. Recent skin self-examination and doctor visits in relation to melanoma risk and tumour depth. Br J Dermatol. 2013;168(3):571–6. https://doi.org/10.1111/bjd.12003.
27. Greaney ML, Puleo E, Geller AC, Hu SW, Werchniak AE, DeCristofaro S, et al. Patient follow-up after participating in a beach-based skin cancer screening program. Int J Environ Res Public Health. 2012;9(5):1836–45. https://doi.org/10.3390/ijerph9051836.
28. Hamidi R, Peng D, Cockburn M. Efficacy of skin self-examination for the early detection of melanoma. Int J Dermatol. 2010;49(2):126–34. https://doi.org/10.1111/j.1365-4632.2009.04268.x.
29. Pollitt RA, Geller AC, Brooks DR, Johnson TM, Park ER, Swetter SM. Efficacy of skin self-examination practices for early melanoma detection. Cancer Epidemiol Biomark Prev. 2009;18(11):3018–23. https://doi.org/10.1158/1055-9965.EPI-09-0310.
30. American Massage Therapy Association. Massage therapy industry fact sheet 2017. 2017. https://www.amtamassage.org/infocenter/economic_industry-fact-sheet.html.
31. Nahin RL, Barnes PM, Stussman BJ, Bloom B. Costs of complementary and alternative medicine (CAM) and frequency of visits to CAM practitioners: United States, 2007. Natl Health Stat Rep. 2009(18):1–14.
32. Cherkin DC, Deyo RA, Sherman KJ, Hart LG, Street JH, Hrbek A, et al. Characteristics of visits

to licensed acupuncturists, chiropractors, massage therapists, and naturopathic physicians. J Am Board Fam Pract. 2002;15(6):463–72.
33. Heiligers PJ, de Groot J, Koster D, van Dulmen S. Diagnoses and visit length in complementary and mainstream medicine. BMC Complement Altern Med. 2010;10:3. https://doi.org/10.1186/1472-6882-10-3.
34. Campbell SM, Louie-Gao Q, Hession ML, Bailey E, Geller AC, Cummins D. Skin cancer education among massage therapists: a survey at the 2010 meeting of the American massage therapy association. J Cancer Educ. 2013;28(1):158–64. https://doi.org/10.1007/s13187-012-0403-7.
35. US Department of Labor, Bureau of Labor Statistics. Skincare Specialists. In: Occupational outlook handbook, 2016–17 edition. December 17, 2015. https://www.bls.gov/ooh/personal-care-and-service/skin-care-specialists.htm. Accessed March 19, 2017.
36. Beauty Schools Marketing Group. Esthetician, Skin Care & Medical Esthetician job Description. In: Beauty Schools Directory. 2017. http://www.beautyschoolsdirectory.com/faq/esthetician.php. Accessed March 20, 2017.
37. US Department of Labor, Bureau of Labor Statistics . Barbers, hairdressers, and cosmetologists. In: Occupational outlook handbook, 2016–17 edition. December 17, 2015. https://www.bls.gov/ooh/personal-care-and-service/barbers-hairdressers-and-cosmetologists.htm. Accessed March 20, 2017.
38. Linnan LA, Kim AE, Wasilewski Y, Lee AM, Yang J, Solomon F. Working with licensed cosmetologists to promote health: results from the North Carolina BEAUTY and health pilot study. Prev Med. 2001;33(6):606–12. https://doi.org/10.1006/pmed.2001.0933.
39. Solomon FM, Linnan LA, Wasilewski Y, Lee AM, Katz ML, Yang J. Observational study in ten beauty salons: results informing development of the North Carolina BEAUTY and Health Project. Health Educ Behav. 2004;31(6):790–807. https://doi.org/10.1177/1090198104264176.
40. Bailey EE, Marghoob AA, Orengo IF, Testa MA, White VR, Geller AC. Skin cancer knowledge, attitudes, and behaviors in the salon: a survey of working hair professionals in Houston. Texas Arch Dermatol. 2011;147(10):1159–65. https://doi.org/10.1001/archdermatol.2011.184.
41. Statistics Brain. Tattoo statistics. August 13, 2016. http://www.statisticbrain.com/tattoo-statistics/. Accessed March 20, 2017.
42. Beltrone G. Sunscreen brand trains Tattoo Artists to look for signs of skin cancer. In: Adweek May 13, 2014. http://www.adweek.com/creativity/sun-screen-brand-trains-tattoo-artists-look-signs-skin-cancer-157639/. Accessed March 20, 2017.
43. Rosenbaum BE, Milam EC, Seo L, Leger MC. Skin care in the tattoo parlor: a survey of tattoo artists in New York City. Dermatology. 2016;232(4):484–9. https://doi.org/10.1159/000446345.
44. American Society for Dermatologic Surgery. Stylists against skin cancer: program overview. https://www.asds.net/SHADE/. Accessed July 27, 2017.
45. Neufeld BS, Anderson SK. Massage therapists and the detection of skin cancer in clients. Massage Today. 2013 2013/02.
46. La Plante C. Early detection of skin cancer by massage therapists can save lives. In: Merican massage therapy association, reflections - first line of defense. March 21, 2008. https://www.amtamassage.org/articles/3/MTJ/detail/1641. Accessed March 20, 2017.
47. Potrony M, Badenas C, Aguilera P, Puig-Butille JA, Carrera C, Malvehy J, et al. Update in genetic susceptibility in melanoma. Ann Transl Med. 2015;3(15):210. https://doi.org/10.3978/j.issn.2305-5839.2015.08.11.
48. Soura E, Eliades PJ, Shannon K, Stratigos AJ, Tsao H. Hereditary melanoma: update on syndromes and management: genetics of familial atypical multiple mole melanoma syndrome. J Am Acad Dermatol. 2016;74(3):395–407.; quiz 8-10. https://doi.org/10.1016/j.jaad.2015.08.038.
49. Florell SR, Boucher KM, Garibotti G, Astle J, Kerber R, Mineau G, et al. Population-based analysis of prognostic factors and survival in familial melanoma. J Clin Oncol. 2005;23(28):7168–77. https://doi.org/10.1200/JCO.2005.11.999.
50. Bishop DT, Demenais F, Goldstein AM, Bergman W, Bishop JN, Bressac-de Paillerets B, et al. Geographical variation in the penetrance of CDKN2A mutations for melanoma. J Natl Cancer Inst. 2002;94(12):894–903.
51. Orlow I, Begg CB, Cotignola J, Roy P, Hummer AJ, Clas BA, et al. CDKN2A germline mutations in individuals with cutaneous malignant melanoma. J Invest Dermatol. 2007;127(5):1234–43. https://doi.org/10.1038/sj.jid.5700689.
52. Parker JF, Florell SR, Alexander A, DiSario JA, Shami PJ, Leachman SA. Pancreatic carcinoma surveillance in patients with familial melanoma. Arch Dermatol. 2003;139(8):1019–25. https://doi.org/10.1001/archderm.139.8.1019.
53. Vasen HF, Gruis NA, Frants RR, van Der Velden PA, Hille ET, Bergman W. Risk of developing pancreatic cancer in families with familial atypical multiple mole melanoma associated with a specific 19 deletion of p16 (p16-Leiden). Int J Cancer. 2000;87(6):809–11.
54. Read J, Wadt KA, Hayward NK. Melanoma genetics. J Med Genet. 2016;53(1):1–14. https://doi.org/10.1136/jmedgenet-2015-103150.
55. Leachman SA, Lucero OM, Sampson JE, Cassidy P, Bruno W, Queirolo P, et al. Identification, genetic testing, and management of hereditary melanoma. Cancer Metastasis Rev. 2017;36(1):77–90. https://doi.org/10.1007/s10555-017-9661-5.
56. Gandini S, Sera F, Cattaruzza MS, Pasquini P, Zanetti R, Masini C, et al. Meta-analysis of risk factors for cutaneous melanoma: III. Family history, actinic damage and phenotypic factors. Eur J Cancer.

2005;41(14):2040–59. https://doi.org/10.1016/j.ejca.2005.03.034.
57. Weinstock MA, Brodsky GL. Bias in the assessment of family history of melanoma and its association with dysplastic nevi in a case-control study. J Clin Epidemiol. 1998;51(12):1299–303.
58. Gandini S, Sera F, Cattaruzza MS, Pasquini P, Abeni D, Boyle P, et al. Meta-analysis of risk factors for cutaneous melanoma: I. Common and atypical naevi. Eur J Cancer. 2005;41(1):28–44. https://doi.org/10.1016/j.ejca.2004.10.015.
59. El Ghissassi F, Baan R, Straif K, Grosse Y, Secretan B, Bouvard V, et al. A review of human carcinogens—Part D: Radiation. Lancet Oncol. 2009;10(8):751–2.
60. Cust AE, Armstrong BK, Goumas C, Jenkins MA, Schmid H, Hopper JL, et al. Sunbed use during adolescence and early adulthood is associated with increased risk of early-onset melanoma. Int J Cancer. 2011;128(10):2425–35. https://doi.org/10.1002/ijc.25576.
61. Lazovich D, Isaksson Vogel R, Weinstock MA, Nelson HH, Ahmed RL, Berwick M. Association between indoor tanning and melanoma in younger men and women. JAMA Dermatol. 2016;152(3):268–75. https://doi.org/10.1001/jamadermatol.2015.2938.
62. Gandini S, Sera F, Cattaruzza MS, Pasquini P, Picconi O, Boyle P, et al. Meta-analysis of risk factors for cutaneous melanoma: II. Sun exposure. Eur J Cancer. 2005;41(1):45–60. https://doi.org/10.1016/j.ejca.2004.10.016.
63. Geller AC, Miller DR, Swetter SM, Demierre MF, Gilchrest BA. A call for the development and implementation of a targeted national melanoma screening program. Arch Dermatol. 2006;142(4):504–7. https://doi.org/10.1001/archderm.142.4.504.
64. Oliveria SA, Selvam N, Mehregan D, Marchetti MA, Divan HA, Dasgeb B, et al. Biopsies of nevi in children and adolescents in the United States, 2009 through 2013. JAMA Dermatol. 2015;151(4):447–8. https://doi.org/10.1001/jamadermatol.2014.4576.
65. Russell LB, Gold MR, Siegel JE, Daniels N, Weinstein MC. The role of cost-effectiveness analysis in health and medicine. Panel on Cost-Effectiveness in Health and Medicine. JAMA. 1996;276(14):1172–7.
66. Girgis A, Clarke P, Burton RC, Sanson-Fisher RW. Screening for melanoma by primary health care physicians: a cost-effectiveness analysis. J Med Screen. 1996;3(1):47–53. https://doi.org/10.1177/096914139600300112.
67. Freedberg KA, Geller AC, Miller DR, Lew RA, Koh HK. Screening for malignant melanoma: a cost-effectiveness analysis. J Am Acad Dermatol. 1999;41(5 Pt 1):738–45.
68. Losina E, Walensky RP, Geller A, Beddingfield FC 3rd, Wolf LL, Gilchrest BA, et al. Visual screening for malignant melanoma: a cost-effectiveness analysis. Arch Dermatol. 2007;143(1):21–8. https://doi.org/10.1001/archderm.143.1.21.
69. Salopek TG, Slade JM, Marghoob AA, Rigel DS, Kopf AW, Bart RS, et al. Management of cutaneous malignant melanoma by dermatologists of the American Academy of Dermatology. II. Definitive surgery for malignant melanoma. J Am Acad Dermatol. 1995;33(3):451–61.
70. Robinson JK, Halpern AC. Cost-effective melanoma screening. JAMA Dermatol. 2016;152(1):19–21. https://doi.org/10.1001/jamadermatol.2015.2681.
71. Hoorens I, Vossaert K, Pil L, Boone B, De Schepper S, Ongenae K, et al. Total-body examination vs lesion-directed skin cancer screening. JAMA Dermatol. 2016;152(1):27–34. https://doi.org/10.1001/jamadermatol.2015.2680.
72. Aitken JF, Elwood M, Baade PD, Youl P, English D. Clinical whole-body skin examination reduces the incidence of thick melanomas. Int J Cancer. 2010;126(2):450–8. https://doi.org/10.1002/ijc.24747.
73. Whiteman DC, Green AC, Olsen CM. The growing burden of invasive melanoma: projections of incidence rates and numbers of new cases in six susceptible populations through 2031. J Invest Dermatol. 2016;136(6):1161–71. https://doi.org/10.1016/j.jid.2016.01.035.
74. Baade P, Coory M. Trends in melanoma mortality in Australia: 1950-2002 and their implications for melanoma control. Aust N Z J Public Health. 2005;29(4):383–6.
75. Iannacone MR, Green AC. Towards skin cancer prevention and early detection: evolution of skin cancer awareness campaigns in Australia. Melanoma Manage. 2014;1(1):75–84. https://doi.org/10.2217/mmt.14.6.
76. Criscione VD, Weinstock MA. Melanoma thickness trends in the United States, 1988–2006. J Invest Dermatol. 2010;130(3):793–7. https://doi.org/10.1038/jid.2009.328.
77. Autier P, Koechlin A, Boniol M. The forthcoming inexorable decline of cutaneous melanoma mortality in light-skinned populations. Eur J Cancer. 2015;51(7):869–78. https://doi.org/10.1016/j.ejca.2015.01.056.
78. Olsen CM, Neale RE, Green AC, Webb PM, The QSkin Study, The Epigene Study, et al. Independent validation of six melanoma risk prediction models. J Invest Dermatol. 2015;135(5):1377–84. https://doi.org/10.1038/jid.2014.533.
79. Vuong K, Armstrong BK, Weiderpass E, Lund E, Adami HO, Veierod MB, et al. Development and external validation of a melanoma risk prediction model based on self-assessed risk factors. JAMA Dermatol. 2016. https://doi.org/10.1001/jamadermatol.2016.0939.
80. Robinson JK, Wayne JD, Martini MC, Hultgren BA, Mallett KA, Turrisi R. Early detection of new melanomas by patients with melanoma and their partners using a structured skin self-examination skills training intervention: a randomized clinical trial. JAMA Dermatol. 2016;152(9):979–85. https://doi.org/10.1001/jamadermatol.2016.1985.

81. Liu W, Dowling JP, Murray WK, McArthur GA, Thompson JF, Wolfe R, et al. Rate of growth in melanomas: characteristics and associations of rapidly growing melanomas. Arch Dermatol. 2006;142(12):1551–8. https://doi.org/10.1001/archderm.142.12.1551.
82. Wu X, Oliveria SA, Yagerman S, Chen L, DeFazio J, Braun R, et al. Feasibility and efficacy of patient-initiated mobile teledermoscopy for short-term monitoring of clinically atypical nevi. JAMA Dermatol. 2015;151(5):489–96. https://doi.org/10.1001/jamadermatol.2014.3837.
83. Esteva A, Kuprel B, Novoa RA, Ko J, Swetter SM, Blau HM, et al. Dermatologist-level classification of skin cancer with deep neural networks. Nature. 2017;542(7639):115–8. https://doi.org/10.1038/nature21056.
84. Webster DE, Suver C, Doerr M, Mounts E, Domenico L, Petrie T, et al. The Mole Mapper Study, mobile phone skin imaging and melanoma risk data collected using ResearchKit. Sci Data. 2017;4:170005. https://doi.org/10.1038/sdata.2017.5.
85. Salerni G, Carrera C, Lovatto L, Marti-Laborda RM, Isern G, Palou J, et al. Characterization of 1152 lesions excised over 10 years using total-body photography and digital dermatoscopy in the surveillance of patients at high risk for melanoma. J Am Acad Dermatol. 2012;67(5):836–45. https://doi.org/10.1016/j.jaad.2012.01.028.
86. Feit NE, Dusza SW, Marghoob AA. Melanomas detected with the aid of total cutaneous photography. Br J Dermatol. 2004;150(4):706–14. https://doi.org/10.1111/j.0007-0963.2004.05892.x.
87. Banky JP, Kelly JW, English DR, Yeatman JM, Dowling JP. Incidence of new and changed nevi and melanomas detected using baseline images and dermoscopy in patients at high risk for melanoma. Arch Dermatol. 2005;141(8):998–1006. https://doi.org/10.1001/archderm.141.8.998.
88. Perier-Muzet M, Thomas L, Poulalhon N, Debarbieux S, Bringuier PP, Duru G, et al. Melanoma patients under vemurafenib: prospective follow-up of melanocytic lesions by digital dermoscopy. J Invest Dermatol. 2014;134(5):1351–8. https://doi.org/10.1038/jid.2013.462.
89. Green WH, Wang SQ, Cognetta AB Jr. Total-body cutaneous examination, total-body photography, and dermoscopy in the care of a patient with xeroderma pigmentosum and multiple melanomas. Arch Dermatol. 2009;145(8):910–5. https://doi.org/10.1001/archdermatol.2009.87.
90. Truong A, Strazzulla L, March J, Boucher KM, Nelson KC, Kim CC, et al. Reduction in nevus biopsies in patients monitored by total body photography. J Am Acad Dermatol. 2016;75(1):135–43. e5. https://doi.org/10.1016/j.jaad.2016.02.1152.
91. Leachman SA, Cassidy PB, Chen SC, Curiel C, Geller A, Gareau D, et al. Methods of melanoma detection. Cancer Treat Res. 2016;167:51–105. https://doi.org/10.1007/978-3-319-22539-5_3.
92. Marghoob AA, International Skin Imaging Collaboration Melanoma Project Working Group. Standards in dermatologic imaging. JAMA Dermatol. 2015;151(8):819–21. https://doi.org/10.1001/jamadermatol.2015.32.
93. Katragadda C, Finnane A, Soyer HP, Marghoob AA, Halpern A, Malvehy J, et al. Technique standards for skin lesion imaging: a Delphi consensus statement. JAMA Dermatol. 2016. https://doi.org/10.1001/jamadermatol.2016.3949.
94. Finnane A, Curiel-Lewandrowski C, Wimberley G, Caffery L, Katragadda C, Halpern A, et al. Proposed technical guidelines for the acquisition of clinical images of skin-related conditions. JAMA Dermatol. 2017;153(5):453–7. https://doi.org/10.1001/jamadermatol.2016.6214.
95. Korotkov K, Quintana J, Puig S, Malvehy J, Garcia R. A new total body scanning system for automatic change detection in multiple pigmented skin lesions. IEEE Trans Med Imaging. 2015;34(1):317–38. https://doi.org/10.1109/TMI.2014.2357715.
96. Bogo F, Romero J, Peserico E, Black MJ. Automated detection of new or evolving melanocytic lesions using a 3D body model. Med Image Comput Comput Assist Interv. 2014;17(Pt 1):593–600.
97. Lovatto L, Carrera C, Salerni G, Alos L, Malvehy J, Puig S. In vivo reflectance confocal microscopy of equivocal melanocytic lesions detected by digital dermoscopy follow-up. J Eur Acad Dermatol Venereol. 2015;29(10):1918–25. https://doi.org/10.1111/jdv.13067.
98. Ceder H, Hylen AS, Larko AW, Paoli J. Evaluation of electrical impedance spectroscopy as an adjunct to dermoscopy in short-term monitoring of atypical melanocytic lesions. Dermatol Pract Concept. 2016;6(4):1–6. https://doi.org/10.5826/dpc.0604a01.
99. American Academy of Dermatology Ad Hoc Task Force for the ABCDEs of Melanoma, Tsao H, Olazagasti JM, Cordoro KM, Brewer JD, Taylor SC, et al. Early detection of melanoma: reviewing the ABCDEs. J Am Acad Dermatol. 2015;72(4):717–23. https://doi.org/10.1016/j.jaad.2015.01.025.
100. Moloney FJ, Guitera P, Coates E, Haass NK, Ho K, Khoury R, et al. Detection of primary melanoma in individuals at extreme high risk: a prospective 5-year follow-up study. JAMA Dermatol. 2014;150(8):819–27. https://doi.org/10.1001/jamadermatol.2014.514.
101. Gaudy-Marqueste C, Wazaefi Y, Bruneu Y, Triller R, Thomas L, Pellacani G, et al. Ugly duckling sign as a major factor of efficiency in melanoma detection. JAMA Dermatol. 2017. https://doi.org/10.1001/jamadermatol.2016.5500.
102. Vestergaard ME, Macaskill P, Holt PE, Menzies SW. Dermoscopy compared with naked eye examination for the diagnosis of primary melanoma: a meta-analysis of studies performed in a clinical setting. Br J Dermatol. 2008;159(3):669–76. https://doi.org/10.1111/j.1365-2133.2008.08713.x.

103. Carli P, De Giorgi V, Crocetti E, Mannone F, Massi D, Chiarugi A, et al. Improvement of malignant/benign ratio in excised melanocytic lesions in the "dermoscopy era": a retrospective study 1997–2001. Br J Dermatol. 2004;150(4):687–92. https://doi.org/10.1111/j.0007-0963.2004.05860.x.
104. Haenssle HA, Hoffmann S, Holzkamp R, Samhaber K, Lockmann A, Fliesser M, et al. Melanoma thickness: the role of patients' characteristics, risk indicators and patterns of diagnosis. J Eur Acad Dermatol Venereol. 2015;29(1):102–8. https://doi.org/10.1111/jdv.12471.
105. Bafounta ML, Beauchet A, Aegerter P, Saiag P. Is dermoscopy (epiluminescence microscopy) useful for the diagnosis of melanoma? Results of a meta-analysis using techniques adapted to the evaluation of diagnostic tests. Arch Dermatol. 2001;137(10):1343–50.
106. Kittler H, Pehamberger H, Wolff K, Binder M. Diagnostic accuracy of dermoscopy. Lancet Oncol. 2002;3(3):159–65.
107. Terushkin V, Warycha M, Levy M, Kopf AW, Cohen DE, Polsky D. Analysis of the benign to malignant ratio of lesions biopsied by a general dermatologist before and after the adoption of dermoscopy. Arch Dermatol. 2010;146(3):343–4. https://doi.org/10.1001/archdermatol.2010.12.
108. Argenziano G, Puig S, Zalaudek I, Sera F, Corona R, Alsina M, et al. Dermoscopy improves accuracy of primary care physicians to triage lesions suggestive of skin cancer. J Clin Oncol. 2006;24(12):1877–82. https://doi.org/10.1200/JCO.2005.05.0864.
109. Binder M, Puespoeck-Schwarz M, Steiner A, Kittler H, Muellner M, Wolff K, et al. Epiluminescence microscopy of small pigmented skin lesions: short-term formal training improves the diagnostic performance of dermatologists. J Am Acad Dermatol. 1997;36(2 Pt 1):197–202.
110. Chen LL, Liebman TN, Soriano RP, Dusza SW, Halpern AC, Marghoob AA. One-year follow-up of dermoscopy education on the ability of medical students to detect skin cancer. Dermatology. 2013;226(3):267–73. https://doi.org/10.1159/000350571.
111. Rogers T, Marino ML, Dusza SW, Bajaj S, Usatine RP, Marchetti MA, et al. A clinical aid for detecting skin cancer: The Triage Amalgamated Dermoscopic Algorithm (TADA). J Am Board Fam Med. 2016;29(6):694–701. https://doi.org/10.3122/jabfm.2016.06.160079.
112. Salerni G, Teran T, Puig S, Malvehy J, Zalaudek I, Argenziano G, et al. Meta-analysis of digital dermoscopy follow-up of melanocytic skin lesions: a study on behalf of the International Dermoscopy Society. J Eur Acad Dermatol Venereol. 2013;27(7):805–14. https://doi.org/10.1111/jdv.12032.
113. Rose SE, Argenziano G, Marghoob AA. Melanomas difficult to diagnose via dermoscopy. G Ital Dermatol Venereol. 2010;145(1):111–26.
114. Carrera C, Marchetti MA, Dusza SW, Argenziano G, Braun RP, Halpern AC, et al. Validity and reliability of dermoscopic criteria used to differentiate nevi from melanoma: a web-based international Dermoscopy Society Study. JAMA Dermatol. 2016;152(7):798–806. https://doi.org/10.1001/jamadermatol.2016.0624.
115. Ali A-RA, Deserno TM. A systematic review of automated melanoma detection in dermatoscopic images and its ground truth data. In: Proc. SPIE 8318, medical imaging 2012: Image perception, observer performance, and technology assessment, 83181I. Feburary 29, 2012. https://doi.org/10.1117/12.912389.
116. He KZ, Zhang X, Ren S, Sun J. Deep residual learning for image recognition. arXivorg. December 10, 2015. doi:arXiv:1512.03385.
117. Collaboration ISI. ISIC Archive: International skin imaging collaboration: melanoma project. https://isic-archive.com/. Accessed March 20, 2017.
118. Codella NN, Nguyen QB, Pankanti S, Gutman D, Helba B, Halpern A, Smith JR. Deep Learning Ensembles for Melanoma Recognition in Dermoscopy Images. arXivorg. October 18, 2016. doi:arXiv:1610.04662.
119. Moreno-Ramirez D, Ferrandiz L, Nieto-Garcia A, Carrasco R, Moreno-Alvarez P, Galdeano R, et al. Store-and-forward teledermatology in skin cancer triage: experience and evaluation of 2009 teleconsultations. Arch Dermatol. 2007;143(4):479–84. https://doi.org/10.1001/archderm.143.4.479.
120. Ferrandiz L, Ruiz-de-Casas A, Martin-Gutierrez FJ, Peral-Rubio F, Mendez-Abad C, Rios-Martin JJ, et al. Effect of teledermatology on the prognosis of patients with cutaneous melanoma. Arch Dermatol. 2012;148(9):1025–8. https://doi.org/10.1001/archdermatol.2012.778.
121. Griffiths WA. Improving melanoma diagnosis in primary care--A tele-dermatoscopy project. J Telemed Telecare. 2010;16(4):185–6. https://doi.org/10.1258/jtt.2010.004005.
122. Arzberger E, Curiel-Lewandrowski C, Blum A, Chubisov D, Oakley A, Rademaker M, et al. Teledermoscopy in high-risk melanoma patients: a comparative study of face-to-face and teledermatology visits. Acta Derm Venereol. 2016;96(6):779–83. https://doi.org/10.2340/00015555-2344.
123. Warshaw EM, Gravely AA, Nelson DB. Reliability of store and forward teledermatology for skin neoplasms. J Am Acad Dermatol. 2015;72(3):426–35. https://doi.org/10.1016/j.jaad.2014.11.001.
124. Janda M, Loescher LJ, Banan P, Horsham C, Soyer HP. Lesion selection by melanoma high-risk consumers during skin self-examination using mobile teledermoscopy. JAMA Dermatol. 2014;150(6):656–8. https://doi.org/10.1001/jamadermatol.2013.7743.
125. Gendreau JL, Gemelas J, Wang M, Capulong D, Lau C, Bratten DM, et al. Unimaged melanomas in store-and-forward teledermatology. Telemed J E Health. 2016. https://doi.org/10.1089/tmj.2016.0170.
126. Kassianos AP, Emery JD, Murchie P, Walter FM. Smartphone applications for melanoma detection

by community, patient and generalist clinician users: a review. Br J Dermatol. 2015;172(6):1507–18. https://doi.org/10.1111/bjd.13665.
127. Hamilton AD, Brady RR. Medical professional involvement in smartphone "apps" in dermatology. Br J Dermatol. 2012;167(1):220–1. https://doi.org/10.1111/j.1365-2133.2012.10844.x.
128. Marek AJ, Chu EY, Ming ME, Kovarik CL. Assessment of smartphone applications for total body digital photography-guided skin exams by patients. J Am Acad Dermatol. 2016;75(5):1063–4.e1. https://doi.org/10.1016/j.jaad.2016.06.005.
129. Resneck JS Jr, Abrouk M, Steuer M, Tam A, Yen A, Lee I, et al. Choice, transparency, coordination, and quality among direct-to-consumer telemedicine websites and apps treating skin disease. JAMA Dermatol. 2016;152(7):768–75. https://doi.org/10.1001/jamadermatol.2016.1774.
130. Wolf JA, Moreau JF, Akilov O, Patton T, English JC 3rd, Ho J, et al. Diagnostic inaccuracy of smartphone applications for melanoma detection. JAMA Dermatol. 2013;149(4):422–6. https://doi.org/10.1001/jamadermatol.2013.2382.
131. Maier T, Kulichova D, Schotten K, Astrid R, Ruzicka T, Berking C, et al. Accuracy of a smartphone application using fractal image analysis of pigmented moles compared to clinical diagnosis and histological result. J Eur Acad Dermatol Venereol. 2015;29(4):663–7. https://doi.org/10.1111/jdv.12648.
132. U.S. Department of Health and Human Services Food and Drug Administration. Mobile medical applications: Guidance for industry and Food and Drug Administration staff. February 9, 2015. https://www.fda.gov/downloads/MedicalDevices/.../UCM263366.pdf. Accessed December 8, 2016.
133. Anastasiou A, Giokas K, Koutsouris D. Monitoring of compliance on an individual treatment through mobile innovations. Conf Proc IEEE Eng Med Biol Soc. 2015;2015:7320–3. https://doi.org/10.1109/EMBC.2015.7320082.
134. Neittaanmaki N, Salmivuori M, Polonen I, Jeskanen L, Ranki A, Saksela O, et al. Hyperspectral imaging in detecting dermal invasion in lentigo maligna melanoma. Br J Dermatol. 2016. https://doi.org/10.1111/bjd.15267.
135. Robles FE, Chowdhury S, Wax A. Assessing hemoglobin concentration using spectroscopic optical coherence tomography for feasibility of tissue diagnostics. Biomed Opt Express. 2010;1(1):310–7. https://doi.org/10.1364/boe.1.000310/.
136. Gareau D, Jacques S, Krueger J. Monte Carlo modeling of pigmented lesions. In: Proc. SPIE 8926, photonic therapeutics and diagnostics X, 89260V. March 4, 2014. https://doi.org/10.1117/12.2040473.
137. U.S. Food and Drug Administration. SIASCOPE II 510(k) Premarket Notifications. 2003. http://www.accessdata.fda.gov/scripts/cdrh/cfdocs/cfPMN/pmn.cfm?ID=K023729. Accessed December 29, 2016.
138. U.S. Food and Drug Administration. MELAFIND Premarket Approval (PMA). 2011. http://www.accessdata.fda.gov/scripts/cdrh/cfdocs/cfpma/pma.cfm?id=p090012. Accessed December 29, 1976.
139. Claridge E, Cotton S, Hall P, Moncrieff M. From colour to tissue histology: physics-based interpretation of images of pigmented skin lesions. Med Image Anal. 2003;7(4):489–502.
140. Terstappen K, Suurkula M, Hallberg H, Ericson MB, Wennberg AM. Poor correlation between spectrophotometric intracutaneous analysis and histopathology in melanoma and nonmelanoma lesions. J Biomed Opt. 2013;18(6):061223. https://doi.org/10.1117/1.JBO.18.6.061223.
141. Moncrieff M, Cotton S, Claridge E, Hall P. Spectrophotometric intracutaneous analysis: a new technique for imaging pigmented skin lesions. Br J Dermatol. 2002;146(3):448–57.
142. Emery JD, Hunter J, Hall PN, Watson AJ, Moncrieff M, Walter FM. Accuracy of SIAscopy for pigmented skin lesions encountered in primary care: development and validation of a new diagnostic algorithm. BMC Dermatol. 2010;10:9. https://doi.org/10.1186/1471-5945-10-9.
143. Tomatis S, Carrara M, Bono A, Bartoli C, Lualdi M, Tragni G, et al. Automated melanoma detection with a novel multispectral imaging system: results of a prospective study. Phys Med Biol. 2005;50(8):1675–87. https://doi.org/10.1088/0031-9155/50/8/004.
144. Haniffa MA, Lloyd JJ, Lawrence CM. The use of a spectrophotometric intracutaneous analysis device in the real-time diagnosis of melanoma in the setting of a melanoma screening clinic. Br J Dermatol. 2007;156(6):1350–2. https://doi.org/10.1111/j.1365-2133.2007.07932.x.
145. Walter FM, Morris HC, Humphrys E, Hall PN, Prevost AT, Burrows N, et al. Effect of adding a diagnostic aid to best practice to manage suspicious pigmented lesions in primary care: randomised controlled trial. BMJ. 2012;345:e4110. https://doi.org/10.1136/bmj.e4110.
146. Braun RP, Gutkowicz-Krusin D, Rabinovitz H, Cognetta A, Hofmann-Wellenhof R, Ahlgrimm-Siess V, et al. Agreement of dermatopathologists in the evaluation of clinically difficult melanocytic lesions: how golden is the “gold standard”? Dermatology. 2012;224(1):51–8. https://doi.org/10.1159/000336886.
147. Elbaum M, Kopf AW, Rabinovitz HS, Langley RG, Kamino H, Mihm MC Jr, et al. Automatic differentiation of melanoma from melanocytic nevi with multispectral digital dermoscopy: a feasibility study. J Am Acad Dermatol. 2001;44(2):207–18. https://doi.org/10.1067/mjd.2001.110395.
148. Monheit G, Cognetta AB, Ferris L, Rabinovitz H, Gross K, Martini M, et al. The performance of MelaFind: a prospective multicenter study. Arch Dermatol. 2011;147(2):188–94. https://doi.org/10.1001/archdermatol.2010.302.
149. Cukras AR. On the comparison of diagnosis and management of melanoma between dermatologists

and MelaFind. JAMA Dermatol. 2013;149(5):622–3. https://doi.org/10.1001/jamadermatol.2013.3405.
150. March J, Hand M, Grossman D. Practical application of new technologies for melanoma diagnosis: Part I. Noninvasive approaches. J Am Acad Dermatol. 2015;72(6):929–41.; quiz 41-2. https://doi.org/10.1016/j.jaad.2015.02.1138.
151. Gutkowicz-Krusin D, Elbaum M, Jacobs A, Keem S, Kopf AW, Kamino H, et al. Precision of automatic measurements of pigmented skin lesion parameters with a MelaFind(TM) multispectral digital dermoscope. Melanoma Res. 2000;10(6):563–70.
152. Kapsokalyvas D, Bruscino N, Alfieri D, de Giorgi V, Cannarozzo G, Cicchi R, et al. Spectral morphological analysis of skin lesions with a polarization multispectral dermoscope. Opt Express. 2013;21(4):4826–40. https://doi.org/10.1364/OE.21.004826.
153. Vasefi F, MacKinnon N, Saager RB, Durkin AJ, Chave R, Lindsley EH, et al. Polarization-sensitive hyperspectral imaging in vivo: a multimode dermoscope for skin analysis. Sci Rep. 2014;4:4924. https://doi.org/10.1038/srep04924.
154. Spigulis J, Uldis Rubins EK, Rubenis O. SkImager: a concept device for in-vivo skin assessment by multimodal imaging. P Est Acad Sci. 2014;63(3):301–8.
155. Delpueyo X, Vilaseca M, Royo S, Ares M, Rey-Barroso L, Sanabria F, et al. Multispectral imaging system based on light-emitting diodes for the detection of melanomas and basal cell carcinomas: a pilot study. J Biomed Opt. 2017;22(6):65006. https://doi.org/10.1117/1.JBO.22.6.065006.
156. Kim S, Cho D, Kim J, Kim M, Youn S, Jang JE, et al. Smartphone-based multispectral imaging: system development and potential for mobile skin diagnosis. Biomed Opt Express. 2016;7(12):5294–307. https://doi.org/10.1364/BOE.7.005294.
157. Vasefi F, McKinnon N, Farkas DL. Hyperspectral and multispectral imaging in dematology. In: Hamblin M, Avici P, Gupta G, editors. Imaging in dermatology: Elsevier Academic Press; 2016. p. 187–201.
158. Alenin AS, Morrison L, Curiel C, Tyo JS. Hyperspectral measurement of the scattering of polarized light by skin. In: Proc. SPIE 8160, polarization science and remote sensing V, 816014. September 10 2011. https://doi.org/10.1117/12.895552.
159. Gareau DS, Correa da Rosa J, Yagerman S, Carucci JA, Gulati N, Hueto F et al. Digital imaging biomarkers feed machine learning for melanoma screening. Exp Dermatol. 2016. doi:https://doi.org/10.1111/exd.13250.
160. Martin J, Krueger J, Gareau D, editors. Hyperspectral imaging for melanoma screening. In: Proc. SPIE 8926, photonic therapeutics and diagnostics X, 892611. March 4, 2014. https://doi.org/10.1117/12.2040396.
161. Kuzmina I, Diebele I, Jakovels D, Spigulis J, Valeine L, Kapostinsh J, et al. Towards noncontact skin melanoma selection by multispectral imaging analysis. J Biomed Opt. 2011;16(6):060502. https://doi.org/10.1117/1.3584846.
162. Rajadhyaksha M, Grossman M, Esterowitz D, Webb RH, Anderson RR. In vivo confocal scanning laser microscopy of human skin: melanin provides strong contrast. J Invest Dermatol. 1995;104(6):946–52.
163. Longo C, Rajadhyaksha M, Ragazzi M, Nehal K, Gardini S, Moscarella E, et al. Evaluating ex vivo fluorescence confocal microscopy images of basal cell carcinomas in Mohs excised tissue. Br J Dermatol. 2014;171(3):561–70. https://doi.org/10.1111/bjd.13070.
164. Guitera P, Menzies SW, Longo C, Cesinaro AM, Scolyer RA, Pellacani G. In vivo confocal microscopy for diagnosis of melanoma and basal cell carcinoma using a two-step method: analysis of 710 consecutive clinically equivocal cases. J Invest Dermatol. 2012;132(10):2386–94. https://doi.org/10.1038/jid.2012.172.
165. Pellacani G, Scope A, Farnetani F, Casaretta G, Zalaudek I, Moscarella E, et al. Towards an in vivo morphologic classification of melanocytic nevi. J Eur Acad Dermatol Venereol. 2014;28(7):864–72. https://doi.org/10.1111/jdv.12181.
166. Pellacani G, Farnetani F, Gonzalez S, Longo C, Cesinaro AM, Casari A, et al. In vivo confocal microscopy for detection and grading of dysplastic nevi: a pilot study. J Am Acad Dermatol. 2012;66(3):e109–21. https://doi.org/10.1016/j.jaad.2011.05.017.
167. Pellacani G, Guitera P, Longo C, Avramidis M, Seidenari S, Menzies S. The impact of in vivo reflectance confocal microscopy for the diagnostic accuracy of melanoma and equivocal melanocytic lesions. J Invest Dermatol. 2007;127(12):2759–65. https://doi.org/10.1038/sj.jid.5700993.
168. Pellacani G, De Pace B, Reggiani C, Cesinaro AM, Argenziano G, Zalaudek I, et al. Distinct melanoma types based on reflectance confocal microscopy. Exp Dermatol. 2014;23(6):414–8. https://doi.org/10.1111/exd.12417.
169. Alarcon I, Carrera C, Palou J, Alos L, Malvehy J, Puig S. Impact of in vivo reflectance confocal microscopy on the number needed to treat melanoma in doubtful lesions. Br J Dermatol. 2014;170(4):802–8. https://doi.org/10.1111/bjd.12678.
170. Borsari S, Pampena R, Lallas A, Kyrgidis A, Moscarella E, Benati E, et al. Clinical indications for use of reflectance confocal microscopy for skin cancer diagnosis. JAMA Dermatol. 2016;152(10):1093–8. https://doi.org/10.1001/jamadermatol.2016.1188.
171. Stevenson AD, Mickan S, Mallett S, Ayya M. Systematic review of diagnostic accuracy of reflectance confocal microscopy for melanoma diagnosis in patients with clinically equivocal skin lesions. Dermatol Pract Concept. 2013;3(4):19–27. https://doi.org/10.5826/dpc.0304a05.
172. Pellacani G, Pepe P, Casari A, Longo C. Reflectance confocal microscopy as a second-level examination

in skin oncology improves diagnostic accuracy and saves unnecessary excisions: a longitudinal prospective study. Br J Dermatol. 2014;171(5):1044–51. https://doi.org/10.1111/bjd.13148.
173. Pellacani G, Witkowski A, Cesinaro AM, Losi A, Colombo GL, Campagna A, et al. Cost-benefit of reflectance confocal microscopy in the diagnostic performance of melanoma. J Eur Acad Dermatol Venereol. 2016;30(3):413–9. https://doi.org/10.1111/jdv.13408.
174. Farnetani F, Scope A, Braun RP, Gonzalez S, Guitera P, Malvehy J, et al. Skin cancer diagnosis with reflectance confocal microscopy: reproducibility of feature recognition and accuracy of diagnosis. JAMA Dermatol. 2015;151(10):1075–80. https://doi.org/10.1001/jamadermatol.2015.0810.
175. Rao BK, Mateus R, Wassef C, Pellacani G. In vivo confocal microscopy in clinical practice: comparison of bedside diagnostic accuracy of a trained physician and distant diagnosis of an expert reader. J Am Acad Dermatol. 2013;69(6):e295–300. https://doi.org/10.1016/j.jaad.2013.07.022.
176. Malvehy J, Hauschild A, Curiel-Lewandrowski C, Mohr P, Hofmann-Wellenhof R, Motley R, et al. Clinical performance of the Nevisense system in cutaneous melanoma detection: an international, multicentre, prospective and blinded clinical trial on efficacy and safety. Br J Dermatol. 2014;171(5):1099–107. https://doi.org/10.1111/bjd.13121.
177. Fukushima K. Neocognitron--a self-organizing neural network model for a mechanism of pattern recognition unaffected by shift in position. NHK 放送科学基礎研究所報告. 1981;15:p106–15.
178. Hinton GE, Sejnowski TJ. Learning and releaming in Boltzmann machines. Parallel Distrilmted Process. 1986;1
179. Rumelhart DE, Hinton GE, Williams RJ. Learning representations by back-propagating errors. Nature. 1986;323(6088):533–6.
180. Forsyth DPJ, Computer vision: a modern approach. Prentice Hall Professional Technical Reference; 2002.
181. Hintz-Madsen M, Hansen LK, Larsen J, Olesen E, Drzewiecki KT, editors. Detection of malignant melanoma using neural classifiers. In: Proceedings of international conference on engineerings applications on neural networks; 1996.
182. Binder M, Kittler H, Seeber A, Steiner A, Pehamberger H, Wolff K. Epiluminescence microscopy-based classification of pigmented skin lesions using computerized image analysis and an artificial neural network. Melanoma Res. 1998;8(3):261–6.
183. Maglogiannis I, Pavlopoulos S, Koutsouris D. An integrated computer supported acquisition, handling, and characterization system for pigmented skin lesions in dermatological images. IEEE Trans Inf Technol Biomed. 2005;9(1):86–98.
184. Brewer AC, Endly DC, Henley J, Amir M, Sampson BP, Moreau JF, et al. Mobile applications in dermatology. JAMA Dermatol. 2013;149(11):1300–4. https://doi.org/10.1001/jamadermatol.2013.5517.
185. Goodfellow I, Bengio Y, Courville A. Deep learning: MIT Press; 2016.
186. LeCun Y, Bottou L, Bengio Y, Haffner P. Gradient-based learning applied to document recognition. Proc IEEE. 1998;86(11):2278–324.
187. ImageNet. 2016. http://www.image-net.org/.
188. Lin T-Y, Maire M, Belongie S, Hays J, Perona P, Ramanan D, et al., editors. Microsoft coco: Common objects in context. In: European conference on computer vision: Springer; 2014.
189. Krizhevsky A, Sutskever I, Hinton GE, editors. Imagenet classification with deep convolutional neural networks. Advances in neural information processing systems; 2012.
190. Large Scale Visual Recognition Challenge 2016 (ILSVRC2016). 2016. http://image-net.org/challenges/LSVRC/2016/results. Accessed March 21, 2017.
191. O'Regan GM, Kemperman PM, Sandilands A, Chen H, Campbell LE, Kroboth K, et al. Raman profiles of the stratum corneum define 3 filaggrin genotype-determined atopic dermatitis endophenotypes. J Allergy Clin Immunol. 2010;126(3):574–80. e1. https://doi.org/10.1016/j.jaci.2010.04.038.
192. Lui H, Zhao J, McLean D, Zeng H. Real-time Raman spectroscopy for in vivo skin cancer diagnosis. Cancer Res. 2012;72(10):2491–500. https://doi.org/10.1158/0008-5472.CAN-11-4061.
193. Liao CS, Slipchenko MN, Wang P, Li J, Lee SY, Oglesbee RA, et al. Microsecond scale vibrational spectroscopic imaging by multiplex stimulated Raman scattering microscopy. Light Sci Appl. 2015;4. https://doi.org/10.1038/lsa.2015.38.
194. Legesse FB, Medyukhina A, Heuke S, Popp J. Texture analysis and classification in coherent anti-stokes Raman scattering (CARS) microscopy images for automated detection of skin cancer. Comput Med Imaging Graph. 2015;43:36–43. https://doi.org/10.1016/j.compmedimag.2015.02.010.
195. Yue S, Cheng JX. Deciphering single cell metabolism by coherent Raman scattering microscopy. Curr Opin Chem Biol. 2016;33:46–57. https://doi.org/10.1016/j.cbpa.2016.05.016.
196. Dimitrow E, Ziemer M, Koehler MJ, Norgauer J, Konig K, Elsner P, et al. Sensitivity and specificity of multiphoton laser tomography for in vivo and ex vivo diagnosis of malignant melanoma. J Invest Dermatol. 2009;129(7):1752–8. https://doi.org/10.1038/jid.2008.439.
197. Balu M, Kelly KM, Zachary CB, Harris RM, Krasieva TB, Konig K, et al. Distinguishing between benign and malignant melanocytic nevi by in vivo multiphoton microscopy. Cancer Res. 2014;74(10):2688–97. https://doi.org/10.1158/0008-5472.CAN-13-2582.
198. Dimitrow E, Riemann I, Ehlers A, Koehler MJ, Norgauer J, Elsner P, et al. Spectral fluorescence lifetime detection and selective melanin imaging by multiphoton laser tomography for melanoma

diagnosis. Exp Dermatol. 2009;18(6):509–15. https://doi.org/10.1111/j.1600-0625.2008.00815.x.
199. Matthews TE, Piletic IR, Selim MA, Simpson MJ, Warren WS. Pump-probe imaging differentiates melanoma from melanocytic nevi. Sci Transl Med. 2011;3(71):71ra15. https://doi.org/10.1126/scitranslmed.3001604.
200. Zhang C, Maslov K, Wang LV. Subwavelength-resolution label-free photoacoustic microscopy of optical absorption in vivo. Opt Lett. 2010;35(19):3195–7. https://doi.org/10.1364/OL.35.003195.
201. Hu S, Wang LV. Optical-resolution photoacoustic microscopy: auscultation of biological systems at the cellular level. Biophys J. 2013;105(4):841–7. https://doi.org/10.1016/j.bpj.2013.07.017.
202. Stoffels I, Morscher S, Helfrich I, Hillen U, Leyh J, Burton NC, et al. Metastatic status of sentinel lymph nodes in melanoma determined noninvasively with multispectral optoacoustic imaging. Sci Transl Med. 2015;7(317):317ra199. https://doi.org/10.1126/scitranslmed.aad1278.
203. Zhou Y, Tripathi SV, Rosman I, Ma J, Hai P, Linette GP, et al. Noninvasive determination of melanoma depth using a handheld photoacoustic probe. J Invest Dermatol. 2017. https://doi.org/10.1016/j.jid.2017.01.016.
204. Ng JC, Swain S, Dowling JP, Wolfe R, Simpson P, Kelly JW. The impact of partial biopsy on histopathologic diagnosis of cutaneous melanoma: experience of an Australian tertiary referral service. Arch Dermatol. 2010;146(3):234–9. https://doi.org/10.1001/archdermatol.2010.14.
205. Galanzha EI, Shashkov EV, Spring PM, Suen JY, Zharov VP. In vivo, noninvasive, label-free detection and eradication of circulating metastatic melanoma cells using two-color photoacoustic flow cytometry with a diode laser. Cancer Res. 2009;69(20):7926–34. https://doi.org/10.1158/0008-5472.CAN-08-4900.
206. Federici A, Dubois A. Full-field optical coherence microscopy with optimized ultrahigh spatial resolution. Opt Lett. 2015;40(22):5347–50. https://doi.org/10.1364/OL.40.005347.
207. Tsai C-C, Wang Y-T, Ho T-S, Lin M-Y, Tjiu J-W, Hsu K-Y, et al. Mirau-based full-field time-domain optical coherence tomography using Ce3+ : YAG crystal fiber light source. In: Proc. SPIE 8802, optical coherence tomography and coherence techniques VI, 880209. June 18, 2013. https://doi.org/10.1117/12.2032478.
208. Lee KS, Zhao H, Ibrahim SF, Meemon N, Khoudeir L, Rolland JP. Three-dimensional imaging of normal skin and nonmelanoma skin cancer with cellular resolution using Gabor domain optical coherence microscopy. J Biomed Opt. 2012;17(12):126006. https://doi.org/10.1117/1.JBO.17.12.126006.
209. Murali S, Meemon P, Lee KS, Kuhn WP, Thompson KP, Rolland JP. Assessment of a liquid lens enabled in vivo optical coherence microscope. Appl Opt. 2010;49(16):D145–56. https://doi.org/10.1364/AO.49.00D145.
210. Song S, Xu J, Wang RK. Long-range and wide field of view optical coherence tomography for in vivo 3D imaging of large volume object based on akinetic programmable swept source. Biomed Opt Express. 2016;7(11):4734–48. https://doi.org/10.1364/BOE.7.004734.
211. Kong K, Rowlands CJ, Varma S, Perkins W, Leach IH, Koloydenko AA, et al. Diagnosis of tumors during tissue-conserving surgery with integrated autofluorescence and Raman scattering microscopy. Proc Natl Acad Sci U S A. 2013;110(38):15189–94. https://doi.org/10.1073/pnas.1311289110.
212. Wang Z. Multiwavelength reflectance confocal microscopy for immune cell identification. Rochester: University of Rochester; 2008.
213. Iftimia N, Peterson G, Chang EW, Maguluri G, Fox W, Rajadhyaksha M. Combined reflectance confocal microscopy-optical coherence tomography for delineation of basal cell carcinoma margins: an ex vivo study. J Biomed Opt. 2016;21(1):16006. https://doi.org/10.1117/1.JBO.21.1.016006.
214. Zhang EZ, Povazay B, Laufer J, Alex A, Hofer B, Pedley B, et al. Multimodal photoacoustic and optical coherence tomography scanner using an all optical detection scheme for 3D morphological skin imaging. Biomed Opt Express. 2011;2(8):2202–15. https://doi.org/10.1364/BOE.2.002202.
215. Gerami P, Yao Z, Polsky D, Jansen B, Busam K, Ho J, et al. Development and validation of a noninvasive 2-gene molecular assay for cutaneous melanoma. J Am Acad Dermatol. 2017;76(1):114–20. e2. https://doi.org/10.1016/j.jaad.2016.07.038.
216. Clarke LE, Warf MB, Flake DD. 2nd, Hartman AR, Tahan S, Shea CR et al. clinical validation of a gene expression signature that differentiates benign nevi from malignant melanoma. J Cutan Pathol. 2015;42(4):244–52. https://doi.org/10.1111/cup.12475.
217. Clarke LE, Flake DD 2nd, Busam K, Cockerell C, Helm K, McNiff J, et al. An independent validation of a gene expression signature to differentiate malignant melanoma from benign melanocytic nevi. Cancer. 2017;123(4):617–28. https://doi.org/10.1002/cncr.30385.
218. Gerami P, Cook RW, Wilkinson J, Russell MC, Dhillon N, Amaria RN, et al. Development of a prognostic genetic signature to predict the metastatic risk associated with cutaneous melanoma. Clin Cancer Res. 2015;21(1):175–83. https://doi.org/10.1158/1078-0432.CCR-13-3316.
219. Zager JS, Messina SJ, Sondak VK, Ferris L, Cook RW, Middlebrook B, et al. Performance of a 31-gene expression profile in a previously unreported cohort of 334 cutaneous melanoma patients. J Clin Oncol. 2016;(34, Suppl):9581.
220. Khoja L, Lorigan P, Dive C, Keilholz U, Fusi A. Circulating tumour cells as tumour biomarkers in melanoma: detection methods and clinical relevance. Ann Oncol. 2015;26(1):33–9. https://doi.org/10.1093/annonc/mdu207.

221. Scoggins CR, Ross MI, Reintgen DS, Noyes RD, Goydos JS, Beitsch PD, et al. Prospective multi-institutional study of reverse transcriptase polymerase chain reaction for molecular staging of melanoma. J Clin Oncol. 2006;24(18):2849–57. https://doi.org/10.1200/JCO.2005.03.2342.
222. Ashida A, Sakaizawa K, Mikoshiba A, Uhara H, Okuyama R. Quantitative analysis of the BRAF V600E mutation in circulating tumor-derived DNA in melanoma patients using competitive allele-specific TaqMan PCR. Int J Clin Oncol. 2016;21(5):981–8. https://doi.org/10.1007/s10147-016-0976-y.
223. Schreuer M, Meersseman G, Van Den Herrewegen S, Jansen Y, Chevolet I, Bott A, et al. Quantitative assessment of BRAF V600 mutant circulating cell-free tumor DNA as a tool for therapeutic monitoring in metastatic melanoma patients treated with BRAF/MEK inhibitors. J Transl Med. 2016;14:95. https://doi.org/10.1186/s12967-016-0852-6.
224. Byrum SD, Larson SK, Avaritt NL, Moreland LE, Mackintosh SG, Cheung WL, et al. Quantitative proteomics identifies activation of hallmark pathways of cancer in patient melanoma. J Proteomics Bioinform. 2013;6(3):43–50. https://doi.org/10.4172/jpb.1000260.
225. Ribero S, Longo C, Glass D, Nathan P, Bataille V. What is new in melanoma genetics and treatment. Dermatology. 2016. https://doi.org/10.1159/000445767.
226. Breast Cancer Linkage Consortium. Cancer risks in BRCA2 mutation carriers. J Natl Cancer Inst. 1999;91(15):1310–6.
227. Bubien V, Bonnet F, Brouste V, Hoppe S, Barouk-Simonet E, David A, et al. High cumulative risks of cancer in patients with PTEN hamartoma tumour syndrome. J Med Genet. 2013;50(4):255–63. https://doi.org/10.1136/jmedgenet-2012-101339.
228. Fitzpatrick TB. The validity and practicality of sun-reactive skin types I through VI. Arch Dermatol. 1988;124(6):869–71.
229. Howlader N, Noone AM, Krapcho M, Miller D, Bishop K, Altekruse SF, et al., editors. SEER Cancer Statistics Review (CSR) 1975–2013. Bethsda, MD: National Cancer Institute; 2016. Accessed March 20, 2017
230. Tkaczyk E. Innovations and developments in dermatologic non-invasive optical imaging and potential clinical applications. Acta Derm Venereol. 2017. https://doi.org/10.2340/00015555-2717.
231. Demirli R, Otto P,Viswanathan R, Patwardhan S, Larkey J. RBX® Technology Overview. n.d. http://www.canfieldsci.com/FileLibrary/RBX%20tech%20overview-LoRz1.pdf. Accessed January 18, 2017.
232. . Learn about MelaFind and Melanoma. Strata Skin Sciences. http://www.melafind.com/melafind/. Accessed January 2, 2017.
233. Verisante Technology, Inc. Aura http://www.verisante.com/aura/medical_professional/. Accessed January 16, 2017.
234. Choi J, Choo J, Chung H, Gweon DG, Park J, Kim HJ, et al. Direct observation of spectral differences between normal and basal cell carcinoma (BCC) tissues using confocal Raman microscopy. Biopolymers. 2005;77(5):264–72. https://doi.org/10.1002/bip.20236.
235. MPTflex Multiphoton Laser Tomography. JenLab GmbH. http://www.jenlab.de/MPTflex.114.0.html. Accessed January 16, 2017.

Staging and Classification of Melanoma

5

Michael E. Egger and Jeffrey E. Gershenwald

Introduction

Cutaneous melanoma is staged according to the American Joint Committee on Cancer (AJCC) melanoma staging system. The AJCC employs a TNM-based system according to tumor (T), regional nodal (N), and distant metastasis (M) categories. The TNM designations are based on the primary tumor pathological characteristics (T), number of regional lymph node metastases or non-nodal regional metastases (N), and presence and site of distant metastases (M). As our understanding of the relevant risk factors for melanoma has improved, and staging techniques have evolved, our understanding of the biology of melanoma has also advanced. These insights have prompted changes in the staging system over time, included in the most recent 8th Edition AJCC melanoma staging system [1].

A goal of cancer staging is to classify patients into groups of generally similar risk; it requires a balance between parsing patients into more defined groups with fewer numbers of patients with relatively homogenous survival outcomes versus limiting the number of groups to foster relative simplicity. Thus, staging systems, per se, may not be the optimal tool to provide an individual patient risk profile assessment. Rather, stage groupings are useful to broadly risk stratify patients into relatively homogenous groups that are used for clinical decision-making and to compare patients across different treatment centers and geographic regions. Stage groups are also used to define inclusion/exclusion and stratification criteria for patients enrolled in clinical trials. Overall, accurate and detailed staging allows clinicians to "speak the same language." This chapter introduces the 8th Edition AJCC melanoma staging system, discusses the rationale for its revisions, and discusses future directions in the staging of cutaneous melanoma.

TNM Criteria

The 8th Edition AJCC melanoma staging system (summarized in Table 5.1) was published in October 2016, with its use recommended and considered as an important part of clinical care.

M. E. Egger
Department of Surgical Oncology, The University of Texas MD Anderson Cancer Center, Houston, TX, USA

Department of Surgery, University of Louisville, Louisville, KY, USA
e-mail: michael.egger@louisville.edu

J. E. Gershenwald (✉)
Department of Surgical Oncology, The University of Texas MD Anderson Cancer Center, Houston, TX, USA

Department of Cancer Biology, The University of Texas MD Anderson Cancer Center, Houston, TX, USA

Melanoma and Skin Center, The University of Texas MD Anderson Cancer Center, Houston, TX, USA
e-mail: jgershen@mdanderson.org

A. I. Riker (ed.), *Melanoma*, https://doi.org/10.1007/978-3-319-78310-9_5

Table 5.1 TNM-based 8th Edition AJCC staging system for cutaneous melanoma

T category	Thickness	Ulceration status
TX: Primary tumor thickness cannot be assessed (e.g., diagnosis by curettage)	Not applicable	Not applicable
T0: No evidence of primary tumor (e.g., unknown primary or completely regressed melanoma)	Not applicable	Not applicable
Tis (melanoma in situ)	Not applicable	Not applicable
T1	≤1.0 mm	Unknown or unspecified
T1a	<0.8 mm	Without ulceration
T1b	<0.8 mm 0.8–1.0 mm	With ulceration With or without ulceration
T2	>1.0–2.0 mm	Unknown or unspecified
T2a	>1.0–2.0 mm	Without ulceration
T2b	>1.0–2.0 mm	With ulceration
T3	>2.0–4.0 mm	Unknown or unspecified
T3a	>2.0–4.0 mm	Without ulceration
T3b	>2.0–4.0 mm	With ulceration
T4	>4.0 mm	Unknown or unspecified
T4a	>4.0 mm	Without ulceration
T4b	>4.0 mm	With ulceration
N category	**Number of tumor-involved regional lymph nodes**	**Presence of in-transit, satellite, and/or microsatellite metastases**
NX	Regional nodes not assessed (e.g., SLN biopsy not performed, regional nodes previously removed for another reason). **Exception:** Pathological N category is not required for T1 melanomas, use cN.	No
N0	No regional metastases detected	No
N1	One tumor-involved node or in-transit, satellite, and/or microsatellite metastases with no tumor-involved nodes	
N1a	One clinically occult (i.e., detected by SLN biopsy)	No
N1b	One clinically detected	No
N1c	No regional lymph node disease	Yes
N2	Two or three tumor-involved nodes or in-transit, satellite, and/or microsatellite metastases with one tumor-involved node	
N2a	Two or three clinically occult (i.e., detected by SLN biopsy)	No
N2b	Two or three, at least one of which was detected clinically	No
N2c	One clinically occult or clinically detected	Yes
N3	Four or more tumor-involved nodes or in-transit, satellite, and/or microsatellite metastases with two or more tumor-involved nodes, or any number of matted nodes without or with in-transit, satellite, and/or microsatellite metastases	
N3a	Four or more clinically occult (i.e., detected by SLN biopsy)	No

Table 5.1 (continued)

T category	Thickness	Ulceration status
N3b	Four or more, at least one of which was clinically detected, or presence of any number of matted nodes	No
N3c	Two or more clinically occult or clinically detected and/or presence of any number of matted nodes	Yes
M category	**Anatomic site**	**LDH level**
M0	No evidence of distant metastases	Not applicable
M1	Evidence of distant metastasis	See below
M1a	Distant metastasis to skin, soft tissue including muscle, and/or non-regional lymph node	Not recorded or unspecified
M1a(0)		Not elevated
M1a(1)		Elevated
M1b	Distant metastasis to lung with or without M1a sites of disease	Not recorded or unspecified
M1b(0)		Not elevated
M1b(1)		Elevated
M1c	Distant metastasis to non-CNS visceral sites with or without M1a or M1b sites of disease	Not recorded or unspecified
M1c(0)		Not elevated
M1c(1)		Elevated
M1d	Distant metastasis to CNS with or without M1a, M1b, or M1c sites of disease	Not recorded or unspecified
M1d(0)		Normal
M1d(1)		Elevated

Suffixes for M category: (0) LDH not elevated, (1) LDH elevated. No suffix is used if LDH is not recorded or is unspecified

This updated version was formally adopted for national registry reporting requirements beginning in January 2017. The 8th Edition contains several revisions to the T, N, and M category criteria, as well as changes to the stage groupings.

T Category

Breslow's thickness and ulceration continue to constitute the two primary tumor characteristics that inform the T category. Breslow's thickness, or primary tumor thickness, is defined as the distance from the top of the granular layer of epidermis to the deepest invasive cell across the broad base of the tumor [2]. Since the 7th Edition AJCC melanoma staging system, this measurement has supplanted Clark level (a primary tumor-based schema based on the extent of invasion of melanoma relative to the papillary and reticular dermis) as the principal T category criterion, as it provides a more objective and reproducible measure of tumor thickness and more accurately risk stratifies patients compared to Clark level [3, 4]. Primary tumor thickness cut points of 1.0, 2.0, and 4.0 mm continue to define T1, T2, T3, and T4 category melanomas in the 8th Edition, and are unchanged from the 7th edition [1]. New to the 8th Edition is the subcategorization of T1 melanomas by tumor thickness. T1a lesions are defined as a non-ulcerated primary melanoma that is <0.8 mm in tumor thickness. A T1b lesion is a non-ulcerated lesion with a primary tumor thickness of 0.8–1.0 mm, or any ulcerated lesion ≤1.0 mm in primary tumor thickness. Additionally, new to the 8th Edition AJCC, primary tumor thickness measurements should be recorded to the nearest 0.1 mm, rather than the nearest 0.01 mm. Reasons for this change include general measurement imprecision as well as a goal to avoid clustering of reported measurements around T category cut points (1.0, 2.0, and 4.0 mm), the latter of which has been demonstrated to bias overall tumor staging [5].

Mitotic rate, defined as the number of mitoses per mm^2 using the dermal "hot spot" method, was previously used to subcategorize T1 lesions in the 7th edition AJCC, but is no longer used as a T category criterion in the 8th Edition [6]. Primary tumor thickness and ulceration are the only pathologic factors needed to determine the T category. The 8th Edition AJCC melanoma expert panel strongly recommends that mitotic rate continue to be recorded for all patients with cutaneous melanoma. Research using the AJCC database has identified that increasing mitotic rate, measured along its continuum, is independently associated with a worse survival in patients, with or without nodal micrometastasis [7, 8]. The mitotic rate is an important component of overall risk assessment for patients with cutaneous melanoma and will likely continue to be incorporated into risk-assessing clinical tools to better inform clinical decision-making.

N Category

N category criteria include the number of tumor-involved regional lymph nodes as well as the presence of microsatellites, in-transit metastases, and/or satellite metastases. The number of positive lymph nodes used as cut points to define N1, N2, and N3 disease generally remain as 1, 2, and 4, respectively. Tumor-involved sentinel lymph nodes (SLN) and tumor-involved non-SLN (i.e., from a completion lymph node dissection) are added together to determine the total number of positive lymph nodes and appropriate N category. In the 8th Edition, N category criteria include the suffix "a" to denote clinically occult regional nodes (e.g., identified by SLN biopsy), the suffix "b" to denote clinically detected regional nodal disease, (e.g., palpable disease detected on clinical exam or by radiographic imaging), and the suffix "c" to denote the presence of non-nodal regional disease that includes in-transit, satellite, and/or microsatellite metastases. The nomenclature for SLN-positive disease in the 8th Edition has been changed and is now termed "clinically occult" rather than "microscopic." Likewise, palpable nodal disease is termed "clinically detected" rather than "macroscopic." Patients with non-nodal regional disease are categorized as N1c, N2c, or N3c depending on the number of tumor-involved regional lymph nodes. Satellite metastases are cutaneous or subcutaneous metastases classically defined as within 2 cm of the primary tumor, with in-transit metastases defined as cutaneous or subcutaneous metastases located >2 cm from the primary tumor site; both are usually located between the primary tumor and draining nodal basin. From a staging perspective, both are considered equivalent with similar clinical outcomes. Microsatellites, defined pathologically as the presence of discontinuous nests of melanoma cells >0.05 mm in diameter, are separated from the primary tumor by at least 0.3 mm of intervening normal dermal or subcutaneous tissue. This is another example of non-nodal regional metastases. Microsatellite disease is associated with an increased risk of regional nodal metastases and survival rates comparable to those associated with satellite or in-transit metastases [9, 10]. The stratification of non-nodal regional disease by extent of regional nodal disease burden is new to the 8th Edition; in the 7th Edition, all non-nodal regional disease was classified as N2c and considered either stage IIIB or stage IIIC based on the absence or presence of concomitant regional nodal disease, respectively [6].

According to the 8th Edition AJCC melanoma staging system, SLN biopsy is required for AJCC pathological classification in order to complete N categorization of T2, T3, and T4 primary melanomas without clinical evidence of metastatic disease. Selective consideration of SLN biopsy for patients with T1 primary tumors is at the discretion of the clinician. This procedure is not requisite for AJCC pathological classification of T1 primary melanomas. SLN tumor burden, while not incorporated directly into the 8th Edition N category, is an important prognostic factor that should be collected for all patients who have positive SLNs. Sentinel node tumor burden may be incorporated into future prognostic models and clinical tools as further guidance for uniform reporting becomes available.

M Category

The presence or absence of distant metastatic disease for cutaneous melanoma is designated as M1 or M0, respectively. In the 8th Edition AJCC melanoma staging system, characterization of the M subcategory is based on two factors: anatomic location of the distant metastasis and serum lactate dehydrogenase (LDH) level. M1a denotes distant metastasis confined to distant skin, subcutaneous tissue, or distant (non-regional) nodal metastases. A non-regional nodal basin is one that is not in the usual drainage pattern for a particular primary tumor. For example, the axilla is a non-regional basin for a primary tumor on the lower extremity, but would be considered a regional nodal basin for a primary tumor on the trunk or upper extremity. Distant metastatic disease confined to the skin, subcutaneous tissues, or non-regional lymph nodes is associated with a more favorable survival compared to other sites of metastasis [6, 11–13]. M1b denotes metastatic disease confined to the lung, with such patients having an intermediate overall survival risk that is worse than M1a disease, but more favorable than non-pulmonary visceral metastases [6, 11, 12].

The 8th Edition AJCC melanoma staging system includes the stratification of non-pulmonary visceral metastases (previously designated as M1c regardless of the presence or absence of CNS metastasis in the 7th Edition) into noncentral nervous system (CNS) visceral metastases (categorized as M1c) and CNS metastases (classified as M1d). This new designation of CNS disease into its own subcategory was incorporated because patients with CNS metastasis have worse prognosis than those without CNS metastasis, with median survival rates historically reported to be <1 year, and 5-year survival rates of <10% [11, 12]. The M1d designation is also pragmatic, in that CNS involvement is frequently an inclusion or exclusion criterion for clinical trial eligibility, as well as a component of clinical trial stratification and analysis. For all four subcategories, the highest M1 subcategory corresponding to the anatomic site(s) of distant metastasis is used for staging purposes. The 8th Edition AJCC staging system preserves the use of an LDH level in M1, but its designation has been slightly modified. Rather than designating all patients with elevated LDH levels and metastatic disease as M1c regardless of the anatomic site of metastatic disease, the 8th Edition provides a new suffix designation of (0) or (1), to represent the absence or presence of an elevated LDH level, respectively. This designation can be used across all four M1 subcategories. For example, a patient with M1c(1) disease has distant non-pulmonary, non-CNS visceral metastasis with an elevated LDH level.

Metastatic Melanoma of Unknown Primary Site

Staging of metastatic melanoma of an unknown primary site is specifically addressed in the 8th Edition AJCC melanoma staging system [1]. In a population-based study from the Netherlands, 2.6% of all patients diagnosed with melanoma had an unknown primary site [14]. In most single-center reports on metastatic melanoma of unknown primary, the most common sites of metastatic disease are the lymph node basins (~60%) [15, 16]. The recent population-based study from the Netherlands reported that the most common site of diagnosis of melanoma of unknown primary was distant metastases (which included subcutaneous metastases in their study) [14]. After an exhaustive search for a primary tumor, with care taken to examine mucosal or ocular primary sites, these patients should be staged according to the same criteria for patients with known primary tumors. For example, patients with disease limited to lymph node basins should be considered stage III. Several studies have shown that patients with lymph node metastases from an unknown primary have similar, if not more favorable, outcomes compared to patients with stage III disease from a known primary melanoma [17–21].

Table 5.2 Stage groupings for cutaneous melanoma, 8th Edition AJCC melanoma staging system

Clinical stage				Pathological stage			
T	N	M	Stage group	T	N	M	Stage group
Tis	N0	M0	0	Tis	N0	M0	0
T1a	N0	M0	IA	T1a	N0	M0	IA
T1b	N0	M0	IB	T1b	N0	M0	IA
T2a	N0	M0	IB	T2a	N0	M0	IB
T2b	N0	M0	IIA	T2b	N0	M0	IIA
T3a	N0	M0	IIA	T3a	N0	M0	IIA
T3b	N0	M0	IIB	T3b	N0	M0	IIB
T4a	N0	M0	IIB	T4a	N0	M0	IIB
T4b	N0	M0	IIC	T4b	N0	M0	IIC
Any T, Tis	≥ N1	M0	III	T0	N1b, N1c	M0	IIIB
				T0	N2b, N2c, N3b or N3c	M0	IIIC
				T1a/b-T2a	N1a or N2a	M0	IIIA
				T1a/b-T2a	N1b/c or N2b	M0	IIIB
				T2b/T3a	N1a-N2b	M0	IIIB
				T1a-T3a	N2c or N3a/b/c	M0	IIIC
				T3b/T4a	Any N ≥ N1	M0	IIIC
				T4b	N1a-N2c	M0	IIIC
				T4b	N3a/b/c	M0	IIID
Any T	Any N	M1	IV	Any T, Tis	Any N	M1	IV

AJCC Stage Groupings

Stage groupings for the 8th Edition AJCC melanoma staging system for melanoma are summarized in Table 5.2. As in prior editions, clinical and pathological classifications are included. The clinical classification can be used after the biopsy of the primary tumor has been performed with clinical or biopsy assessment of the regional lymph nodes. For clinical classification, the only assessment of the lymph nodes required is a thorough physical examination. In clinically node-negative patients, primary tumor pathological features (primary tumor thickness and ulceration) define stages IA, IB, IIA, IIB, and IIC. Clinically evident regional lymph node or non-nodal regional disease designates a patient as stage III, without further subcategorization. Clinical stage IV includes all patients with distant metastases at the time of diagnosis, regardless of anatomic location.

AJCC pathological classification is determined after the regional lymph nodes are assessed by either SLN biopsy or regional lymph node dissection in patients with T2, T3, and T4 primary tumors; for patients with T1 primary tumors no further assessment of the regional lymph nodes beyond clinical exam is required, but if SLN biopsy is performed the pathological status of the SLN is also incorporated into the pathological classification. Pathological classification uses additional information obtained from the wide excision of the primary tumor, as well as from the assessment of the regional nodal basin by either SLN biopsy or therapeutic lymph node dissection. Pathologically staged groups I and II remain those patients with disease confined to the primary tumor, without evidence of nodal, non-nodal regional, or distant metastasis. Primary tumor thickness and ulceration define pathological stages IA, IB, IIA, IIB, and IIC. Patients with clinical T1bN0 tumors are clinical stage IB. If SLN biopsy is performed and found to be negative, such patients are stage IA. Pathological stage III disease consists of patients with nodal or non-nodal regional disease. In the 8th Edition, there are four stage III groups, based on both T and N category criteria. Primary tumor thickness and ulceration remain important risk factors for survival across the different N subcategories, and are included in the definition of stage III groupings. Pathological stage IV remains the only stage grouping for patients with metastatic disease regardless of M1 subcategory.

Risk Factors Not Used in AJCC Staging

Pathological assessment of the primary tumor generally includes many more features than are required to define the T category. Although not currently included in the AJCC melanoma staging system, the AJCC melanoma expert panel recommends assessment of these factors for clinical care. Some of these factors include mitotic rate as a continuous variable, level of invasion (Clark level), regression, lymphovascular invasion, tumor-infiltrating lymphocytes, and neurotropism. These factors may contribute relevant information towards the risk assessment for an individual patient, but their influence on overall survival, independent of more established pathological prognostic factors like primary tumor thickness or ulceration, has not been unequivocally established. The 8th Edition AJCC melanoma staging system recommends that these factors be reported in registry data, although they are not explicitly required for staging.

Primary tumor regression is pathologically defined as the replacement of tumor cells by lymphocytic infiltration [22]. It is an immune-related process by which either a portion or the entire tumor is destroyed by an immune response. Lymphovascular invasion is defined as the presence of melanoma cells within the lumen of blood or lymphatic vessels and is associated with an adverse prognosis [23–28]. Tumor-infiltrating lymphocytes (TILs) are defined as the presence of lymphocytes infiltrating and disrupting tumor nests and/or directly opposing tumor cells. TILs are usually graded in a semiquantitative fashion as absent, non-brisk, or brisk. The presence of tumor-infiltrating lymphocytes is a favorable prognostic factor that is believed to signify a robust immune response. In some studies, it has been associated with a decreased risk of SLN metastasis [29–33]. Neurotropism, defined as the presence of melanoma cells abutting nerve sheaths either circumferentially or within nerves, is recorded as being present or absent. If present, neurotropism has been associated with an increased risk of local recurrence [34].

Regional Nodal Disease: Assessment and Management

Determining the pathological status of the regional lymph nodes is a critical component of the staging process for cutaneous melanoma. Regional lymph node status is a powerful prognostic factor with important implications for consideration of treatment, follow-up recommendations, and clinical trial eligibility. The SLN biopsy technique has revolutionized the assessment of regional nodal disease in cutaneous melanoma and is an essential part of the staging process for clinically node-negative patients without evidence of distant metastasis at the time of initial assessment.

The technique of lymphatic mapping and SLN biopsy was introduced by Morton and colleagues in 1992 [35]. The prognostic significance of the technique was validated in a multi-institutional study by Gershenwald and colleagues [36]. The rationale for the SLN biopsy is based on the concept that for a primary tumor in any given anatomic area, there is at least one regional lymph node that receives direct afferent lymphatic drainage from the tumor site, termed the "sentinel node," prior to the remaining regional nodal basin. The SLN is the most likely first site of metastasis to the regional nodal basin if any lymph nodes are involved. If the SLN is negative, the remaining nodes within the regional nodal basin are unlikely to harbor microscopic melanoma metastasis [37–39]. The technique's accuracy has been validated in multiple multi-institutional studies, and has been incorporated into the AJCC melanoma staging system since 2002 (6th Edition) [36, 40, 41]. The pathological status of the SLN is of critical importance for the accurate assessment of patients with at-risk melanoma who have clinically negative regional lymph nodes.

From a staging perspective, the purpose of lymphatic mapping and SLN biopsy is to identify microscopic regional lymph node metastases in clinically node-negative patients; the presence of tumor-involved SLNs upstages a patient to stage III disease. The predicted risk of clinically occult regional disease informs the decision to perform lymphatic mapping and SLN biopsy for staging. Primary tumor factors, including Breslow's thickness, ulceration, and mitotic rate, can be used to identify patients at high or low risk of clinically occult regional lymph node metastases [42–45]. Based on the associations of these primary tumor factors with microscopic regional lymph node metastases, the 8th Edition AJCC staging system requires that SLN biopsy be performed for patients with T2, T3, and T4 primary tumors with clinically negative regional lymph node basins in order to report AJCC pathological stage group. Selective consideration of SLN biopsy for patients with T1 melanoma is permitted, and if performed SLN biopsy results are included in the pathological classification of such patients. Several studies have reported that for patients with a "thin" melanoma, i.e., <1.0 mm tumor thickness, patient and primary tumor factors such as ulceration, decreased age, increased primary tumor thickness, advanced Clark level and mitotic rate that is $\geq 1/\text{mm}^2$ can be used to identify patients at higher risk of SLN metastases [42, 46–49]. The surgeon may consider these factors when counseling patients with thin melanomas regarding the utility of SLN biopsy.

Consistent with how the SLN biopsy technique was originally conceived, a completion lymph node dissection (CLND) of the involved regional nodal basin has been classically performed after a positive SLN biopsy. From a staging perspective, CLND allows for a more accurate, complete assessment of the regional nodal basin and has been included in the N category assessment to date. Two randomized clinical trials have been designed to address the potential survival benefit of CLND (MSLT-2 and DeCOG-SLT) [50, 51]. The DeCOG-SLT study failed to meet original accrual goals; nonetheless, at a median follow-up of 35 months, there were no overall significant differences in 5-year relapse-free-, distant metastasis free-, or melanoma specific-survival. The initial results of the MSLT-2 trial were recently published. Similar to the initial findings of the smaller DECOG-SLT trial, the larger MSLT-2 trial, at a median follow up of 43 months, did not demonstrate a survival benefit for patients who had CLND following a positive SLN biopsy compared to patients with a positive SLN who had active surveillance of the SLN positive nodal basin. Nonetheless, from a staging standpoint, the pathological information from CLND may identify some patients with high risk disease in whom adjuvant therapy might otherwise not be considered [52–54]. Formal discussion of the clinical decision-making regarding CLND and its relative therapeutic benefit is beyond the scope of this chapter. When a patient has not undergone a completion lymph node dissection after a positive SLN biopsy, the use of a (sn) designation for the N category has been introduced into 8th Edition AJCC melanoma staging system to identify such patients.

Only 10–20% of patients with positive SLNs will have tumor-involved non-SLNs when a CLND is performed in the regional nodal basin. This suggests that, in theory, up to 80–90% of patients are not capable of deriving a therapeutic benefit from a CLND because no additional metastatic melanoma is removed [55–58]. However, there is powerful prognostic information gained from determining the pathological status of the non-SLNs. Multiple studies have demonstrated that patients who have clinically occult disease confined to the SLNs have a favorable survival compared to those with additional disease identified in the non-SLNs. The reported hazard ratio for survival in these studies ranges from 2 to 3, compared to patients with SLN disease alone [56, 57, 59–61]. Non-SLN pathological status is not incorporated directly into the 8th Edition AJCC melanoma staging system; rather, it is indirectly accounted for as a component of the total number of tumor-involved regional lymph nodes. Similar to the 7th Edition, the 8th Edition distinguishes clinically occult (a) from clinically detected (b) lymph node disease, as there are both differences in survival and in relevant clinical and pathological risk factors between patients with clinically occult and clinically detected lymph node disease [8].

Efforts to identify SLN-positive patients with a high and low risk for non-SLN metastases based on the likelihood of finding additional microscopic metastatic nodal disease have relied on patient, tumor, and SLN factors to risk stratify patients. The goal has been to identify low-risk groups, for whom a CLND may be electively omitted, or high-risk groups in which the benefit of a CLND may outweigh concerns about operative morbidity and patient comorbidities. This risk stratification, based on data available after SLN biopsy, is very important in the current post-MSLT-2 era in which fewer CLNDs are likely to be performed. Investigators found that patient and primary tumor factors such as increased age, increasing tumor thickness, and male gender were associated with an increased risk of non-SLN metastases. This suggests that these factors may guide clinical decision-making regarding CLND [62, 63]. Other investigators, using patient and primary tumor factors, were unable to identify risk factors predictive of non-SLN metastases, prompting recommendations for routine CLND with a positive SLN biopsy [64, 65]. Efforts that have focused on assessing SLN tumor burden to predict non-SLN metastases have also been promising to predict non-SLN metastases. The SLN tumor burden can be assessed by a variety of measures, including measurement of the diameter of the largest metastatic focus, the depth of invasion of the SLN tumor deposit, or the anatomic distribution of the metastases within the SLN [66–71]. Some authors have reported that single measurements of metastatic SLN tumor burden are predictive of non-SLN metastases [72–74]. Others have used composite measures, sometimes including several different assessments of SLN tumor burden measures, with or without clinical and primary tumor data, to predict the risk of non-SLN metastases [55, 75, 76]. Comparisons across different SLN tumor burden measures have generally confirmed that most measures can identify high- and low-risk patients. Linear measurement of the maximum diameter of the largest SLN metastatic deposit has generally been favored, due to reproducibility and overall consistent predictive ability for both non-SLN metastases and survival [77–80]. Recognizing the prognostic importance and potential clinical utility of SLN tumor burden assessment, the 8th Edition AJCC staging system recommends that at a minimum, the single largest maximum diameter of the largest discrete metastatic deposit in the SLN be measured by an ocular micrometer to the nearest 0.1 mm for reporting purposes [1].

The presence of non-nodal regional disease, i.e., microsatellite, satellite, or in-transit metastases, is associated with poor prognosis and designated as N(c) in the N category of the 8th Edition AJCC melanoma staging system [81–84]. The regional lymph nodes should be assessed for evidence of metastatic disease when non-nodal regional disease is identified. In the 8th Edition, patients with non-nodal regional disease are further subcategorized according to the number of tumor-positive regional lymph nodes (Table 5.1).

Future Directions

Classification and staging criteria for cutaneous melanoma continue to evolve. The AJCC continues to develop and mature a framework by which additional known or putative prognostic elements can be assessed and considered for use in the development of predictive clinical tools. Indeed, the AJCC melanoma expert panel recommends that additional clinicopathological factors be collected beyond those needed for AJCC melanoma staging. Some of the factors recommended for routine collection have been discussed above, including additional primary tumor characteristics and measurements of SLN tumor burden. Our technology and understanding of melanoma continue to move forward, as well as our ability to capture molecular-based information and insight. Genetic mutational patterns, gene expression, epigenetic changes, immune response changes, and other novel tumor markers may also be incorporated into the clinical arena as these develop [85, 86]. These changes can be focused on assessments of the host, primary tumor, regional metastasis, or distant metastatic disease burden. Though not a formal part of staging at this time, such factors may become more relevant in the development of an individualized risk assessment profile for each patient. Such "profiles" may allow for more precise risk stratification and may inform therapeutic decision-making.

Primary Tumor Assessment

Researchers are beginning to understand the molecular underpinnings of the transition from a benign melanocytic lesion to melanoma. Mutations within the BRAF and N-RAS genes are more commonly found in lesions not associated with chronic sun exposure, suggesting alternative paths to malignancy based on ultraviolet light damage or BRAF/N-RAS derangement [87]. Promoter mutations in the TERT gene are associated with both familial and sporadic melanoma, and may be part of the pathway to malignancy via ultraviolet light damage [88]. The succession of genetic alterations involved in the evolution of melanoma from benign precursor lesions has been described and includes, among others, BRAF and N-RAS, TERT promoter, PTEN, TP53, and CDKN2A mutations, along with ultraviolet radiation damage [89]. Many of these mutations are already targetable or may be targets for future therapy.

Cutaneous melanoma has been classically divided into five histological subtypes: superficial spreading, nodular, lentigo maligna, acral lentiginous, and desmoplastic. The most common subtype is superficial spreading. Currently, the 8th Edition AJCC melanoma staging system does not incorporate histological subtypes for staging purposes, as other factors have generally been shown to be prognostically more significant. The histological subtype should be recorded in the cutaneous melanoma registry data for classification purposes. However, more rational, genomic-based classification of melanoma subtypes based upon driver mutations and actionable mutation profiles are still needed.

Exploratory studies have attempted to classify primary melanoma tumors by differential gene expression [90–94]. Driver mutations have been identified that are potentially targetable and provide insight into the molecular drivers of oncogenesis in both BRAF wild-type and mutant melanoma [95]. The Cancer Genome Atlas Network has molecularly classified melanoma into four subtypes based on genomic profiles that can also inform rational therapies for the individual subtypes [96]. The four subtypes reported were BRAF, RAS, NF1, and triple wild type. A unique immune signature was also identified by RNAseq analysis, independent of the four subtypes, that carries potential implications with regard to the use of immunotherapy. Gene sequencing may be used not only to identify actionable mutations for targeted therapy (e.g., N-RAS and BRAF mutations), but also to some extent for risk stratification to inform decision-making regarding additional targeted or immune therapies [94, 97, 98]. The genomic classification of melanoma is analogous to that of breast cancer, the latter being based on hormone status and Her2-neu receptor status. The classification is not only rationally based on the underlying genetic profile of each tumor, but also guides potential therapies.

Current research efforts are attempting to identify unique gene signatures, epigenetic profiles, or immune response markers in both primary tumors and in metastatic disease. Researchers have identified microRNAs, stress markers, and epithelial-mesenchymal transition markers in primary tumors that are associated with survival [99–101]. Immune profiles in primary tumors have been described that predict SLN positivity and survival [102]. Other investigators have identified specific gene profiles in primary tumors that may predict survival [93]. Gene signature changes in primary tumors compared to SLN metastases have been described that provide some insight into the genetic alterations associated with metastases [92].

Lymph Node Assessment

Molecular profiling of melanoma-containing lymph nodes has yielded insight into potential markers of risk of progression. While efforts to quantify SLN tumor burden (described above) have improved our ability to risk stratify SLN patients beyond the binary positive (i.e., tumor-involved) or negative (i.e., tumor-free), improved molecular understanding may ultimately inform next-generation individualized risk models. Immune profiles of positive SLNs have been identified that are associated with increased risk of progression and decreased survival [103–105]. A specific gene signature in positive SLNs was found to outperform the AJCC 7th Edition staging system with regard to predicting overall survival [106]. In the future, a more robust understanding of the molecular profile of the primary melanoma, lymph node metastasis, or both may provide meaningful individualized prognostic information beyond that which is already possible with classical TNM-based staging.

Evaluation of Metastatic Disease

Traditionally, metastatic disease has been assessed with physical exam and cross-sectional imaging. Serum LDH levels are known to be associated with prognosis in stage IV melanoma and are incorporated into staging. More recently, novel tumor markers, immunologic profiles, and assessment of levels of circulating melanoma cells have been studied in an effort to identify occult metastatic disease or monitor response to therapy. One recent advance is the so-called "liquid biopsy" approach that is able to identify circulating tumor cells, cell-free circulating DNA, or cell-free circulating microRNA. This approach appears to correlate with survival and metastatic disease burden, proving to be a promising advance in surveillance and diagnosis for melanoma and other solid tumors. This may profoundly impact how melanoma patients are assessed, and treated, in the near future [107].

Hematologic profiles that correlate with immune response, such as the neutrophil-to-lymphocyte ratio or receptor expression on CD4+ and CD8+ T lymphocytes may be associated with survival in patients with metastatic melanoma [108–110]. Exosomes, small (50–100 nm) secreted vesicles formed from the cellular membrane, may actively participate in signaling and microenvironment manipulation directly related to oncogenesis [111]. Circulating exosomes in peripheral serum contain minute concentrations of putative melanoma biomarkers, such as MIA and S100B, that can be detected and quantified for diagnostic and prognostic purposes [112]. Circulating melanoma tumor cells can be detected and have been associated with prognosis in patients with stage II–IV melanoma [113–115].

Melanoma-specific serum markers have also been explored in an effort to provide additional prognostic information beyond serum LDH levels. For example, in some studies, serum levels of MIA, S100, and YKL-40 have been shown to predict survival and non-SLN tumor involvement in patients with stage II–IV disease [116–118]. Changes in LDH and S100 may also be associated with tumor response to targeted and immune therapies in patients with stage IV disease [116, 119, 120]. Elevated LDH levels were shown to correlate with poor survival in patients treated with the anti-CTLA-4 immunotherapy drug ipilimumab [121].

Personalized Risk Assessment

The complex interplay among multiple known or putative risk factors in host and tumor, the wide range of prognosis within stage groups, and the power of computer-based analysis together provide unparalleled opportunities to further refine individualized risk assessment beyond TNM-based AJCC staging. Personalized risk assessment can complement the initial risk stratification that is accomplished with initial staging. Current AJCC staging is necessarily constrained under the TNM-based system, and does not allow for the consideration of numerous risk factors that can provide a more personalized individual risk assessment. Instead, individualized risk assessment is more likely in the context of clinically validated prognostic tools that can more comprehensively incorporate additional informative elements [122, 123]. These prognostic tools estimate a single individual's risk of melanoma recurrence or death based on a number of clinical and pathological features. The tools use mathematical modeling of the marginal risk contributed by each negative or positive risk factor considered to create a comprehensive, individualized risk assessment. This assessment is often presented in terms of survival, either with an estimated hazard ratio or a 5-year survival estimate. The tools can also offer estimates of the a priori odds of SLN or non-SLN metastases. Estimates are often reported with confidence intervals to better inform the clinician and patient about its precision.

Risk calculators have been developed that provide patients and clinicians with personalized risk assessment [124, 125]. In principle, such models can be useful clinical tools to improve clinical decision-making and risk assessment; however, one must be mindful of the shortcomings of currently available clinical prognostic tools and discuss such limitations with patients. A recent review of available clinical prognostic tools for melanoma found that many of them were developed based on relatively old data (pre-2006), internal validity was not rigorously performed, and fewer than half were externally validated [126]. This review concluded that there was opportunity for improvement in the currently available melanoma clinical prognostic tools.

The AJCC Precision Medicine Core has developed criteria by which clinical prognostic tools can be critically assessed in an effort to inform both professional and lay users of these tools [123]. The criteria can be used to objectively and critically evaluate the utility of a prognostic tool for potential clinical use. For example, legacy prognostic models have sometimes been built upon data that are somewhat dated and/or may not take into account contemporary treatment strategies. This core group has put forth a series of inclusion and exclusion criteria to critically evaluate a prognostic tool. The model should use relevant, clinically accessible predictors, and should clearly report the inclusion and exclusion criteria of the populations used to develop and/or validate the model. Users of the model can use these criteria to determine whether the model is appropriate for use in their specific population of interest. The actual mathematical form of the model should be published and accessible. Some measure of discrimination of the model should be reported and published in peer-review literature.

Conclusions

The current 8th Edition AJCC melanoma staging system uses a TNM-based assessment of the primary tumor, nodal and non-nodal regional metastases, and distant metastases. Primary tumor thickness and ulceration are factors by which the T category is determined, with these factors useful for both prognosis and treatment decision-making in localized and regional disease. The status of the regional lymph nodes, most commonly assessed by the SLN biopsy technique, is the most powerful predictor of prognosis in patients with cutaneous melanoma. Patients with distant metastatic disease can be risk stratified according to the anatomic location of their disease and serum LDH levels. Clinicians must continue to collect data on clinical and pathological risk factors so that predictive models and staging systems can be continuously reassessed and revised in an evidence-based fashion. The future of staging for cutaneous melanoma will likely incorporate molecular characteristics in addition to contemporary clinical and pathological factors. These classifications may inform targeted treatment decisions in addition to providing survival stratification. In the future, validated clinical tools will augment staging to provide more precise estimates of individual prognosis.

References

1. Gershenwald JE, Scolyer RA, Hess KR, Thompson JF, Long GV, Ross MI, et al. Melanoma of the skin. In: Amin MB, Edge SB, Greene FL, Byrd DR, Brookland RK, Washington MK, et al., editors. AJCC cancer staging manual. 8th ed. New York: Springer; 2017.
2. Breslow A. Thickness, cross-sectional areas and depth of invasion in the prognosis of cutaneous melanoma. Ann Surg. 1970;172(5):902–8.
3. Clark WH Jr, From L, Bernardino EA, Mihm MC. The histogenesis and biologic behavior of primary human malignant melanomas of the skin. Cancer Res. 1969;29(3):705–27.
4. Breslow A. Tumor thickness, level of invasion and node dissection in stage I cutaneous melanoma. Ann Surg. 1975;182(5):572–5.

5. Ge L, Vilain RE, Lo S, Aivazian K, Scolyer RA, Thompson JF. Breslow thickness measurements of melanomas around American Joint Committee on Cancer staging cut-off points: imprecision and terminal digit bias have important implications for staging and patient management. Ann Surg Oncol. 2016;23(8):2658–63.
6. Balch CM, Gershenwald JE, Soong SJ, Thompson JF, Atkins MB, Byrd DR, et al. Final version of 2009 AJCC melanoma staging and classification. J Clin Oncol. 2009;27(36):6199–206.
7. Thompson JF, Soong SJ, Balch CM, Gershenwald JE, Ding S, Coit DG, et al. Prognostic significance of mitotic rate in localized primary cutaneous melanoma: an analysis of patients in the multi-institutional American Joint Committee on Cancer melanoma staging database. J Clin Oncol. 2011;29(16):2199–205.
8. Balch CM, Gershenwald JE, Soong SJ, Thompson JF, Ding S, Byrd DR, et al. Multivariate analysis of prognostic factors among 2313 patients with stage III melanoma: comparison of nodal micrometastases versus macrometastases. J Clin Oncol. 2010;28(14):2452–9.
9. Kimsey TF, Cohen T, Patel A, Busam KJ, Brady MS. Microscopic satellitosis in patients with primary cutaneous melanoma: implications for nodal basin staging. Ann Surg Oncol. 2009;16(5):1176–83.
10. Bartlett EK, Gupta M, Datta J, Gimotty PA, Guerry D, Xu X, et al. Prognosis of patients with melanoma and microsatellitosis undergoing sentinel lymph node biopsy. Ann Surg Oncol. 2014;21(3):1016–23.
11. Balch CM, Soong SJ, Murad TM, Smith JW, Maddox WA, Durant JR. A multifactorial analysis of melanoma. IV. Prognostic factors in 200 melanoma patients with distant metastases (stage III). J Clin Oncol. 1983;1(2):126–34.
12. Barth A, Wanek LA, Morton DL. Prognostic factors in 1521 melanoma patients with distant metastases. J Am Coll Surg. 1995;181(3):193–201.
13. Bowen GM, Chang AE, Lowe L, Hamilton T, Patel R, Johnson TM. Solitary melanoma confined to the dermal and/or subcutaneous tissue: evidence for revisiting the staging classification. Arch Dermatol. 2000;136(11):1397–9.
14. de Waal AC, Aben KK, van Rossum MM, Kiemeney LA. Melanoma of unknown primary origin: a population-based study in the Netherlands. Eur J Cancer. 2013;49(3):676–83.
15. Velez A, Walsh D, Karakousis CP. Treatment of unknown primary melanoma. Cancer. 1991;68(12):2579–81.
16. Anbari KK, Schuchter LM, Bucky LP, Mick R, Synnestvedt M, Guerry D, et al. Melanoma of unknown primary site: presentation, treatment, and prognosis--a single institution study. University of Pennsylvania Pigmented Lesion Study Group. Cancer. 1997;79(9):1816–21.
17. Cormier JN, Xing Y, Feng L, Huang X, Davidson L, Gershenwald JE, et al. Metastatic melanoma to lymph nodes in patients with unknown primary sites. Cancer. 2006;106(9):2012–20.
18. Prens SP, van der Ploeg AP, van Akkooi AC, van Montfort CA, van Geel AN, de Wilt JH, et al. Outcome after therapeutic lymph node dissection in patients with unknown primary melanoma site. Ann Surg Oncol. 2011;18(13):3586–92.
19. Lee CC, Faries MB, Wanek LA, Morton DL. Improved survival after lymphadenectomy for nodal metastasis from an unknown primary melanoma. J Clin Oncol. 2008;26(4):535–41.
20. Weide B, Faller C, Elsasser M, Buttner P, Pflugfelder A, Leiter U, et al. Melanoma patients with unknown primary site or nodal recurrence after initial diagnosis have a favourable survival compared to those with synchronous lymph node metastasis and primary tumour. PLoS One. 2013;8(6):e66953.
21. van der Ploeg AP, Haydu LE, Spillane AJ, Scolyer RA, Quinn MJ, Saw RP, et al. Melanoma patients with an unknown primary tumor site have a better outcome than those with a known primary following therapeutic lymph node dissection for macroscopic (clinically palpable) nodal disease. Ann Surg Oncol. 2014;21(9):3108–16.
22. Smoller BR, Balch CB, Balzer BL, Crowson AN, Didolkar M, Lazar A, et al. Protocol for the examination of specimens from patients with melanoma of the skin: College of American Pathologists; 2016 [updated January 2016; cited 2016 4/12/2016]. 3.4.0.0. http://www.cap.org/web/home/resources/cancer-reporting-tools/cancer-protocol-templates.
23. Kashani-Sabet M, Sagebiel RW, Ferreira CM, Nosrati M, Miller JR 3rd. Vascular involvement in the prognosis of primary cutaneous melanoma. Arch Dermatol. 2001;137(9):1169–73.
24. Straume O, Akslen LA. Lymphatic vessel density and prognosis in cutaneous melanoma. Br J Cancer. 2004;91(6):1224–5.
25. Nagore E, Oliver V, Botella-Estrada R, Moreno-Picot S, Insa A, Fortea JM. Prognostic factors in localized invasive cutaneous melanoma: high value of mitotic rate, vascular invasion and microscopic satellitosis. Melanoma Res. 2005;15(3):169–77.
26. Egger ME, Gilbert JE, Burton AL, McMasters KM, Callender GG, Quillo AR, et al. Lymphovascular invasion as a prognostic factor in melanoma. Am Surg. 2011;77(8):992–7.
27. Storr SJ, Safuan S, Mitra A, Elliott F, Walker C, Vasko MJ, et al. Objective assessment of blood and lymphatic vessel invasion and association with macrophage infiltration in cutaneous melanoma. Mod Pathol. 2012;25(4):493–504.
28. Xu X, Chen L, Guerry D, Dawson PR, Hwang WT, VanBelle P, et al. Lymphatic invasion is independently prognostic of metastasis in primary cutaneous melanoma. Clin Cancer Res. 2012;18(1):229–37.
29. Taylor RC, Patel A, Panageas KS, Busam KJ, Brady MS. Tumor-infiltrating lymphocytes predict sentinel lymph node positivity in patients with cutaneous melanoma. J Clin Oncol. 2007;25(7):869–75.

30. Burton AL, Roach BA, Mays MP, Chen AF, Ginter BA, Vierling AM, et al. Prognostic significance of tumor infiltrating lymphocytes in melanoma. Am Surg. 2011;77(2):188–92.
31. Azimi F, Scolyer RA, Rumcheva P, Moncrieff M, Murali R, McCarthy SW, et al. Tumor-infiltrating lymphocyte grade is an independent predictor of sentinel lymph node status and survival in patients with cutaneous melanoma. J Clin Oncol. 2012;30(21):2678–83.
32. Thomas NE, Busam KJ, From L, Kricker A, Armstrong BK, Anton-Culver H, et al. Tumor-infiltrating lymphocyte grade in primary melanomas is independently associated with melanoma-specific survival in the population-based genes, environment and melanoma study. J Clin Oncol. 2013;31(33):4252–9.
33. Schatton T, Scolyer RA, Thompson JF, Mihm MC Jr. Tumor-infiltrating lymphocytes and their significance in melanoma prognosis. Methods Mol Biol. 2014;1102:287–324.
34. Quinn MJ, Crotty KA, Thompson JF, Coates AS, O'Brien CJ, McCarthy WH. Desmoplastic and desmoplastic neurotropic melanoma: experience with 280 patients. Cancer. 1998;83(6):1128–35.
35. Morton DL, Wen DR, Wong JH, Economou JS, Cagle LA, Storm FK, et al. Technical details of intraoperative lymphatic mapping for early stage melanoma. Arch Surg. 1992;127(4):392–9.
36. Gershenwald JE, Thompson W, Mansfield PF, Lee JE, Colome MI, Tseng CH, et al. Multi-institutional melanoma lymphatic mapping experience: the prognostic value of sentinel lymph node status in 612 stage I or II melanoma patients. J Clin Oncol. 1999;17(3):976–83.
37. Ross MI, Reintgen D, Balch CM. Selective lymphadenectomy: emerging role for lymphatic mapping and sentinel node biopsy in the management of early stage melanoma. Semin Surg Oncol. 1993;9(3):219–23.
38. Reintgen D, Cruse CW, Wells K, Berman C, Fenske N, Glass F, et al. The orderly progression of melanoma nodal metastases. Ann Surg. 1994;220(6):759–67.
39. Thompson JF, McCarthy WH, Bosch CM, O'Brien CJ, Quinn MJ, Paramaesvaran S, et al. Sentinel lymph node status as an indicator of the presence of metastatic melanoma in regional lymph nodes. Melanoma Res. 1995;5(4):255–60.
40. Balch CM, Buzaid AC, Soong SJ, Atkins MB, Cascinelli N, Coit DG, et al. Final version of the American Joint Committee on Cancer staging system for cutaneous melanoma. J Clin Oncol. 2001;19(16):3635–48.
41. Morton DL, Thompson JF, Essner R, Elashoff R, Stern SL, Nieweg OE, et al. Validation of the accuracy of intraoperative lymphatic mapping and sentinel lymphadenectomy for early-stage melanoma: a multicenter trial. Multicenter Selective Lymphadenectomy Trial Group. Ann Surg. 1999;230(4):453–63. discussion 63-5
42. Kesmodel SB, Karakousis GC, Botbyl JD, Canter RJ, Lewis RT, Wahl PM, et al. Mitotic rate as a predictor of sentinel lymph node positivity in patients with thin melanomas. Ann Surg Oncol. 2005;12(6):449–58.
43. Rousseau DL Jr, Ross MI, Johnson MM, Prieto VG, Lee JE, Mansfield PF, et al. Revised American Joint Committee on cancer staging criteria accurately predict sentinel lymph node positivity in clinically node-negative melanoma patients. Ann Surg Oncol. 2003;10(5):569–74.
44. McMasters KM, Wong SL, Edwards MJ, Ross MI, Chao C, Noyes RD, et al. Factors that predict the presence of sentinel lymph node metastasis in patients with melanoma. Surgery. 2001;130(2):151–6.
45. Sondak VK, Taylor JM, Sabel MS, Wang Y, Lowe L, Grover AC, et al. Mitotic rate and younger age are predictors of sentinel lymph node positivity: lessons learned from the generation of a probabilistic model. Ann Surg Oncol. 2004;11(3):247–58.
46. Cecchi R, Buralli L, Innocenti S, De Gaudio C. Sentinel lymph node biopsy in patients with thin melanomas. J Dermatol. 2007;34(8):512–5.
47. Faries MB, Wanek LA, Elashoff D, Wright BE, Morton DL. Predictors of occult nodal metastasis in patients with thin melanoma. Arch Surg. 2010;145(2):137–42.
48. Han D, Zager JS, Shyr Y, Chen H, Berry LD, Iyengar S, et al. Clinicopathologic predictors of sentinel lymph node metastasis in thin melanoma. J Clin Oncol. 2013;31(35):4387–93.
49. White RL Jr, Ayers GD, Stell VH, Ding S, Gershenwald JE, Salo JC, et al. Factors predictive of the status of sentinel lymph nodes in melanoma patients from a large multicenter database. Ann Surg Oncol. 2011;18(13):3593–600.
50. Faries MB, Thompson JF, Cochran AJ, Andtbacka RH, Mozzillo N, Zager JS, et al. Completion Dissection or Observation for Sentinel-Node Metastasis in Melanoma. N Engl J Med. 2017;376(23):2211–22.
51. Leiter U, Stadler R, Mauch C, Hohenberger W, Brockmeyer N, Berking C, et al. Complete lymph node dissection versus no dissection in patients with sentinel lymph node biopsy positive melanoma (DeCOG-SLT): a multicentre, randomised, phase 3 trial. Lancet Oncol. 17(6):757–67.
52. Bilimoria KY, Balch CM, Bentrem DJ, Talamonti MS, Ko CY, Lange JR, et al. Complete lymph node dissection for sentinel node-positive melanoma: assessment of practice patterns in the United States. Ann Surg Oncol. 2008;15(6):1566–76.
53. Wong SL, Morton DL, Thompson JF, Gershenwald JE, Leong SP, Reintgen DS, et al. Melanoma patients with positive sentinel nodes who did not undergo completion lymphadenectomy: a multi-institutional study. Ann Surg Oncol. 2006;13(6):809–16.

54. van der Ploeg AP, van Akkooi AC, Rutkowski P, Cook M, Nieweg OE, Rossi CR, et al. Prognosis in patients with sentinel node-positive melanoma without immediate completion lymph node dissection. Br J Surg. 2012;99(10):1396–405.
55. Gershenwald JE, Andtbacka RH, Prieto VG, Johnson MM, Diwan AH, Lee JE, et al. Microscopic tumor burden in sentinel lymph nodes predicts synchronous nonsentinel lymph node involvement in patients with melanoma. J Clin Oncol. 2008;26(26):4296–303.
56. Ghaferi AA, Wong SL, Johnson TM, Lowe L, Chang AE, Cimmino VM, et al. Prognostic significance of a positive nonsentinel lymph node in cutaneous melanoma. Ann Surg Oncol. 2009;16(11):2978–84.
57. Ariyan C, Brady MS, Gonen M, Busam K, Coit D. Positive nonsentinel node status predicts mortality in patients with cutaneous melanoma. Ann Surg Oncol. 2009;16(1):186–90.
58. Egger ME, Callender GG, McMasters KM, Ross MI, Martin RC 2nd, Edwards MJ, et al. Diversity of stage III melanoma in the era of sentinel lymph node biopsy. Ann Surg Oncol. 2013;20(3):956–63.
59. Jakub JW, Huebner M, Shivers S, Nobo C, Puleo C, Harmsen WS, et al. The number of lymph nodes involved with metastatic disease does not affect outcome in melanoma patients as long as all disease is confined to the sentinel lymph node. Ann Surg Oncol. 2009;16(8):2245–51.
60. Brown RE, Ross MI, Edwards MJ, Noyes RD, Reintgen DS, Hagendoorn LJ, et al. The prognostic significance of nonsentinel lymph node metastasis in melanoma. Ann Surg Oncol. 2010;17(12):3330–5.
61. Reintgen M, Murray L, Akman K, Giuliano R, Lozicki A, Shivers S, et al. Evidence for a better nodal staging system for melanoma: the clinical relevance of metastatic disease confined to the sentinel lymph nodes. Ann Surg Oncol. 2013;20(2):668–74.
62. Sabel MS, Griffith K, Sondak VK, Lowe L, Schwartz JL, Cimmino VM, et al. Predictors of nonsentinel lymph node positivity in patients with a positive sentinel node for melanoma. J Am Coll Surg. 2005;201(1):37–47.
63. Cadili A, Smylie M, Danyluk J, Dabbs K. Prediction of nonsentinel lymph node metastasis in malignant melanoma. J Surg Res. 2009;154(2):324–9.
64. McMasters KM, Wong SL, Edwards MJ, Chao C, Ross MI, Noyes RD, et al. Frequency of nonsentinel lymph node metastasis in melanoma. Ann Surg Oncol. 2002;9(2):137–41.
65. Page AJ, Carlson GW, Delman KA, Murray D, Hestley A, Cohen C. Prediction of nonsentinel lymph node involvement in patients with a positive sentinel lymph node in malignant melanoma. Am Surg. 2007;73(7):674–8. discussion 8-9
66. Ranieri JM, Wagner JD, Azuaje R, Davidson D, Wenck S, Fyffe J, et al. Prognostic importance of lymph node tumor burden in melanoma patients staged by sentinel node biopsy. Ann Surg Oncol. 2002;9(10):975–81.
67. Carlson GW, Murray DR, Lyles RH, Staley CA, Hestley A, Cohen C. The amount of metastatic melanoma in a sentinel lymph node: does it have prognostic significance? Ann Surg Oncol. 2003;10(5):575–81.
68. Dewar DJ, Newell B, Green MA, Topping AP, Powell BW, Cook MG. The microanatomic location of metastatic melanoma in sentinel lymph nodes predicts nonsentinel lymph node involvement. J Clin Oncol. 2004;22(16):3345–9.
69. Starz H, Siedlecki K, Balda BR. Sentinel lymphonodectomy and s-classification: a successful strategy for better prediction and improvement of outcome of melanoma. Ann Surg Oncol. 2004;11(3 Suppl):162S–8S.
70. Debarbieux S, Duru G, Dalle S, Beatrix O, Balme B, Thomas L. Sentinel lymph node biopsy in melanoma: a micromorphometric study relating to prognosis and completion lymph node dissection. Br J Dermatol. 2007;157(1):58–67.
71. van Akkooi AC, Nowecki ZI, Voit C, Schafer-Hesterberg G, Michej W, de Wilt JH, et al. Sentinel node tumor burden according to the Rotterdam criteria is the most important prognostic factor for survival in melanoma patients: a multicenter study in 388 patients with positive sentinel nodes. Ann Surg. 2008;248(6):949–55.
72. Scolyer RA, Li LX, McCarthy SW, Shaw HM, Stretch JR, Sharma R, et al. Micromorphometric features of positive sentinel lymph nodes predict involvement of nonsentinel nodes in patients with melanoma. Am J Clin Pathol. 2004;122(4):532–9.
73. Frankel TL, Griffith KA, Lowe L, Wong SL, Bichakjian CK, Chang AE, et al. Do micromorphometric features of metastatic deposits within sentinel nodes predict nonsentinel lymph node involvement in melanoma? Ann Surg Oncol. 2008;15(9):2403–11.
74. Cadili A, Scolyer RA, Brown PT, Dabbs K, Thompson JF. Total sentinel lymph node tumor size predicts nonsentinel node metastasis and survival in patients with melanoma. Ann Surg Oncol. 2010;17(11):3015–20.
75. Satzger I, Volker B, Meier A, Kapp A, Gutzmer R. Criteria in sentinel lymph nodes of melanoma patients that predict involvement of nonsentinel lymph nodes. Ann Surg Oncol. 2008;15(6):1723–32.
76. van der Ploeg AP, van Akkooi AC, Rutkowski P, Nowecki ZI, Michej W, Mitra A, et al. Prognosis in patients with sentinel node-positive melanoma is accurately defined by the combined Rotterdam tumor load and Dewar topography criteria. J Clin Oncol. 2011;29(16):2206–14.
77. Murali R, Cochran AJ, Cook MG, Hillman JD, Karim RZ, Moncrieff M, et al. Interobserver reproducibility of histologic parameters of melanoma deposits in sentinel lymph nodes: implications for management of patients with melanoma. Cancer. 2009;115(21):5026–37.

78. Fink AM, Weihsengruber F, Duschek N, Schierl M, Wondratsch H, Jurecka W, et al. Value of micromorphometric criteria of sentinel lymph node metastases in predicting further nonsentinel lymph node metastases in patients with melanoma. Melanoma Res. 2011;21(2):139–43.
79. Egger ME, Bower MR, Czyszczon IA, Farghaly H, Noyes RD, Reintgen DS, et al. Comparison of sentinel lymph node micrometastatic tumor burden measurements in melanoma. J Am Coll Surg. 2014;218(4):519–28.
80. van der Ploeg AP, van Akkooi AC, Haydu LE, Scolyer RA, Murali R, Verhoef C, et al. The prognostic significance of sentinel node tumour burden in melanoma patients: an international, multicenter study of 1539 sentinel node-positive melanoma patients. Eur J Cancer. 2014;50(1):111–20.
81. Day CL Jr, Harrist TJ, Gorstein F, Sober AJ, Lew RA, Friedman RJ, et al. Malignant melanoma. Prognostic significance of "microscopic satellites" in the reticular dermis and subcutaneous fat. Ann Surg. 1981;194(1):108–12.
82. Leon P, Daly JM, Synnestvedt M, Schultz DJ, Elder DE, Clark WH Jr. The prognostic implications of microscopic satellites in patients with clinical stage I melanoma. Arch Surg. 1991;126(12):1461–8.
83. Buzaid AC, Ross MI, Balch CM, Soong S, McCarthy WH, Tinoco L, et al. Critical analysis of the current American joint committee on cancer staging system for cutaneous melanoma and proposal of a new staging system. J Clin Oncol. 1997;15(3):1039–51.
84. Read RL, Haydu L, Saw RP, Quinn MJ, Shannon K, Spillane AJ, et al. In-transit melanoma metastases: incidence, prognosis, and the role of lymphadenectomy. Ann Surg Oncol. 2015;22(2):475–81.
85. Castiglione R, Ihle MA, Heydt C, Schultheis AM, Merkelbach-Bruse S, Mauch C, et al. The impact of sequencing on diagnosis and treatment of malignant melanoma. Expert Rev Mol Diagn. 2016;16(4):423–33.
86. Lee CY, Gerami P. Molecular techniques for predicting behaviour in melanocytic neoplasms. Pathology. 2016;48(2):142–6.
87. Curtin JA, Fridlyand J, Kageshita T, Patel HN, Busam KJ, Kutzner H, et al. Distinct sets of genetic alterations in melanoma. N Engl J Med. 2005;353(20):2135–47.
88. Horn S, Figl A, Rachakonda PS, Fischer C, Sucker A, Gast A, et al. TERT promoter mutations in familial and sporadic melanoma. Science. 2013;339(6122):959–61.
89. Shain AH, Yeh I, Kovalyshyn I, Sriharan A, Talevich E, Gagnon A, et al. The genetic evolution of melanoma from precursor lesions. N Engl J Med. 2015;373(20):1926–36.
90. Bittner M, Meltzer P, Chen Y, Jiang Y, Seftor E, Hendrix M, et al. Molecular classification of cutaneous malignant melanoma by gene expression profiling. Nature. 2000;406(6795):536–40.
91. Jaeger J, Koczan D, Thiesen HJ, Ibrahim SM, Gross G, Spang R, et al. Gene expression signatures for tumor progression, tumor subtype, and tumor thickness in laser-microdissected melanoma tissues. Clin Cancer Res. 2007;13(3):806–15.
92. Koh SS, Wei JP, Li X, Huang RR, Doan NB, Scolyer RA, et al. Differential gene expression profiling of primary cutaneous melanoma and sentinel lymph node metastases. Mod Pathol. 2012;25(6):828–37.
93. Gerami P, Cook RW, Russell MC, Wilkinson J, Amaria RN, Gonzalez R, et al. Gene expression profiling for molecular staging of cutaneous melanoma in patients undergoing sentinel lymph node biopsy. J Am Acad Dermatol. 2015;72(5):780–5. e3
94. Rajkumar S, Watson IR. Molecular characterisation of cutaneous melanoma: creating a framework for targeted and immune therapies. Br J Cancer. 2016;115(2):145–55.
95. Hodis E, Watson IR, Kryukov GV, Arold ST, Imielinski M, Theurillat JP, et al. A landscape of driver mutations in melanoma. Cell. 2012;150(2):251–63.
96. Akbani R, Akdemir Kadir C, Aksoy BA, Albert M, Ally A, Amin Samirkumar B, et al. Genomic classification of cutaneous melanoma. Cell. 2015;161(7):1681–96.
97. Rutkowski P, Gos A, Jurkowska M, Switaj T, Dziewirski W, Zdzienicki M, et al. Molecular alterations in clinical stage III cutaneous melanoma: correlation with clinicopathological features and patient outcome. Oncol Lett. 2014;8(1):47–54.
98. Thomas NE, Edmiston SN, Alexander A, Groben PA, Parrish E, Kricker A, et al. Association between NRAS and BRAF mutational status and melanoma-specific survival among patients with higher-risk primary melanoma. JAMA Oncol. 2015;1(3):359–68.
99. Saldanha G, Elshaw S, Sachs P, Alharbi H, Shah P, Jothi A, et al. microRNA-10b is a prognostic biomarker for melanoma. Mod Pathol. 2016;29(2):112–21.
100. Shimizu A, Kaira K, Yasuda M, Asao T, Ishikawa O. Clinical and pathological significance of ER stress marker (BiP/GRP78 and PERK) expression in malignant melanoma. Pathol Oncol Res. 2017;23(1):111–6.
101. Pieniazek M, Donizy P, Halon A, Leskiewicz M, Matkowski R. Prognostic significance of immunohistochemical epithelial-mesenchymal transition markers in skin melanoma patients. Biomark Med. 2016;10(9):975–85.
102. Ma MW, Medicherla RC, Qian M, Vega-Saenz de Miera E, Friedman EB, Berman RS, et al. Immune response in melanoma: an in-depth analysis of the primary tumor and corresponding sentinel lymph node. Mod Pathol. 2012;25(7):1000–10.
103. Mohos A, Sebestyen T, Liszkay G, Plotar V, Horvath S, Gaudi I, et al. Immune cell profile of sentinel lymph nodes in patients with malignant melanoma—FOXP3+ cell density in cases with positive

sentinel node status is associated with unfavorable clinical outcome. J Transl Med. 2013;11:43.
104. Vallacchi V, Vergani E, Camisaschi C, Deho P, Cabras AD, Sensi M, et al. Transcriptional profiling of melanoma sentinel nodes identify patients with poor outcome and reveal an association of CD30(+) T lymphocytes with progression. Cancer Res. 2014;74(1):130–40.
105. Vallacchi V, Camisaschi C, Dugo M, Vergani E, Deho P, Gualeni A, et al. microRNA expression in sentinel nodes from progressing melanoma patients identifies networks associated with dysfunctional immune response. Genes. 2016;7(12):124.
106. Hao H, Xiao D, Pan J, Qu J, Egger M, Waigel S, et al. Sentinel lymph node genes to predict prognosis in node-positive melanoma patients. Ann Surg Oncol. 2017;24(1):108–16.
107. Huang SK, Hoon DS. Liquid biopsy utility for the surveillance of cutaneous malignant melanoma patients. Mol Oncol. 2016;10(3):450–63.
108. Gandini S, Ferrucci PF, Botteri E, Tosti G, Barberis M, Pala L, et al. Prognostic significance of hematological profiles in melanoma patients. Int J Cancer. 2016;139(7):1618–25.
109. Jacquelot N, Enot DP, Flament C, Vimond N, Blattner C, Pitt JM, et al. Chemokine receptor patterns in lymphocytes mirror metastatic spreading in melanoma. J Clin Invest. 2016;126(3):921–37.
110. Toia F, Buccheri S, Anfosso A, Moschella F, Dieli F, Meraviglia S, et al. Skewed differentiation of circulating Vgamma9Vdelta2 T lymphocytes in melanoma and impact on clinical outcome. PLoS One. 2016;11(2):e0149570.
111. Thery C, Ostrowski M, Segura E. Membrane vesicles as conveyors of immune responses. Nat Rev Immunol. 2009;9(8):581–93.
112. Alegre E, Zubiri L, Perez-Gracia JL, Gonzalez-Cao M, Soria L, Martin-Algarra S, et al. Circulating melanoma exosomes as diagnostic and prognosis biomarkers. Clin Chim Acta. 2016;454:28–32.
113. Hoshimoto S, Shingai T, Morton DL, Kuo C, Faries MB, Chong K, et al. Association between circulating tumor cells and prognosis in patients with stage III melanoma with sentinel lymph node metastasis in a phase III international multicenter trial. J Clin Oncol. 2012;30(31):3819–26.
114. Hida T, Yoneta A, Wakamatsu K, Yanagisawa K, Ishii-Osai Y, Kan Y, et al. Circulating melanoma cells as a potential biomarker to detect metastasis and evaluate prognosis. Australas J Dermatol. 2016;57(2):145–9.
115. Hoshimoto S, Faries MB, Morton DL, Shingai T, Kuo C, Wang HJ, et al. Assessment of prognostic circulating tumor cells in a phase III trial of adjuvant immunotherapy after complete resection of stage IV melanoma. Ann Surg. 2012;255(2):357–62.
116. Egberts F, Kotthoff EM, Gerdes S, Egberts JH, Weichenthal M, Hauschild A. Comparative study of YKL-40, S-100B and LDH as monitoring tools for stage IV melanoma. Eur J Cancer. 2012;48(5):695–702.
117. Damude S, Hoekstra HJ, Bastiaannet E, Muller Kobold AC, Kruijff S, Wevers KP. The predictive power of serum S-100B for non-sentinel node positivity in melanoma patients. Eur J Surg Oncol. 2016;42(4):545–51.
118. Nikolin B, Djan I, Trifunovic J, Dugandzija T, Novkovic D, Djan V, et al. MIA, S100 and LDH as important predictors of overall survival of patients with stage IIb and IIc melanoma. J BUON. 2016;21(3):691–7.
119. Abusaif S, Jradi Z, Held L, Pflugfelder A, Weide B, Meier F, et al. S100B and lactate dehydrogenase as response and progression markers during treatment with vemurafenib in patients with advanced melanoma. Melanoma Res. 2013;23(5):396–401.
120. Diem S, Kasenda B, Spain L, Martin-Liberal J, Marconcini R, Gore M, et al. Serum lactate dehydrogenase as an early marker for outcome in patients treated with anti-PD-1 therapy in metastatic melanoma. Br J Cancer. 2016;114(3):256–61.
121. Kelderman S, Heemskerk B, van Tinteren H, van den Brom RR, Hospers GA, van den Eertwegh AJ, et al. Lactate dehydrogenase as a selection criterion for ipilimumab treatment in metastatic melanoma. Cancer Immunol Immunother. 2014;63(5):449–58.
122. Collins GS, Reitsma JB, Altman DG, Moons KG. Transparent reporting of a multivariable prediction model for Individual Prognosis or Diagnosis (TRIPOD): the TRIPOD statement. Br J Surg. 2015;102(3):148–58.
123. Kattan MW, Hess KR, Amin MB, Lu Y, Moons KG, Gershenwald JE, et al. American Joint Committee on cancer acceptance criteria for inclusion of risk models for individualized prognosis in the practice of precision medicine. CA Cancer J Clin. 2016;66(5):370–4.
124. Soong SJ, Ding S, Coit D, Balch CM, Gershenwald JE, Thompson JF, et al. Predicting survival outcome of localized melanoma: an electronic prediction tool based on the AJCC Melanoma Database. Ann Surg Oncol. 2010;17(8):2006–14.
125. Callender GG, Gershenwald JE, Egger ME, Scoggins CR, Martin RC 2nd, Schacherer CW, et al. A novel and accurate computer model of melanoma prognosis for patients staged by sentinel lymph node biopsy: comparison with the American Joint Committee on Cancer model. J Am Coll Surg. 2012;214(4):608–17. discussion 17-9
126. Mahar AL, Compton C, Halabi S, Hess KR, Gershenwald JE, Scolyer RA, et al. Critical assessment of clinical prognostic tools in melanoma. Ann Surg Oncol. 2016;23(9):2753–61.

The Genetic Evolution of Melanoma

6

Katja Harbst and Göran Jönsson

Abbreviations

cAMP	Cyclic adenosine monophosphate
CDK	Cyclin-dependent kinase
COSMIC	Catalogue of Somatic Mutations in Cancer
CSD	Chronic sun damage
DNA	Deoxyribonucleic acid
EMA	European Medicines Agency
FDA	US Food and Drug Administration
ITH	Intratumor heterogeneity
MAPK	Mitogen-activated protein kinase
TCGA	The Cancer Genome Atlas
UVB	Ultraviolet B radiation
UVR	Ultraviolet radiation

Genetic Changes in Melanoma Tumors

Introduction

Malignant melanoma originates from a transformed melanocyte, the cell type in the human body that produces melanin pigment. Melanocytes are primarily located within the basal membrane of the skin, with the melanin distributed to its neighboring cells, mainly keratinocytes. These pigment-laden cells are important for protection of the nuclear DNA that can become damaged from the harmful effects of overexposure to ultraviolet radiation (UVR). As with any other cancer type, melanoma harbors a set of characteristic genetic aberrations that highlight its dependence upon particular cellular pathways and functions. In this chapter, we explore the landscape of genetic aberrations and transcriptional changes that drive the transformation, development, and progression of melanoma. We also discuss the current model of temporal progression that is typical for this malignancy.

Molecular Pathways Affected by Genetic Aberrations

Melanoma is dependent on several cellular signalling pathways, which is demonstrated by the high frequency of observed genetic alterations in these pathways. In particular, the mitogen-activated protein kinase (MAPK) pathway is affected in most tumors at a very early stage (Fig. 6.1). The Cancer Genome Atlas (TCGA) melanoma study investigated 333 melanomas and identified mutations in either *BRAF*, *NF1*, or *RAS* genes (all key members of the MAPK signalling chain) in 86% of melanomas [1]. A recent study compiling four cohorts

K. Harbst, M.Sc., Ph.D. · G. Jönsson, Ph.D. (✉)
Faculty of Medicine, Department of Clinical Sciences Lund, Oncology and Pathology, Lund University, Lund, Sweden
e-mail: katja.harbst@med.lu.se

A. I. Riker (ed.), *Melanoma*, https://doi.org/10.1007/978-3-319-78310-9_6

that total 870 tumors has found similar aberration frequency [2]. Therefore, melanomas can be divided further based upon the main genetic aberrations in one of these genes: BRAF (45–50%), RAS (28%), NF1 (8%), or none of these (so-called *triple-wild-type* tumors, 14–19%). The majority of BRAF mutations encode the Val600Glu (V600E) amino acid change, which was identified in several human cancer types in 2002 [3]. Soon thereafter, it was found to be the most frequent somatic genetic aberration in melanoma. The findings have prompted the development of multiple inhibitors of mutant BRAF. Of these, vemurafenib was approved by the US Food and Drug Administration (FDA) in 2011 and by the European Medicines Agency (EMA) in 2012. It is widely used today for the treatment of patients with a BRAF-mutant melanoma in the clinical setting. Another inhibitor, dabrafenib, was approved by the FDA in 2013, for use as a single agent in BRAF V600 mutant melanoma. On the other hand, inhibitors of MEK target the MAPK pathway one step downstream of the BRAF gene. One such agent, trametinib, was approved by the FDA in 2013 for the treatment of BRAF V600 mutant melanoma. Since resistance commonly arises to the BRAF and MEK inhibitors when they are used as single agents, combination therapy with trametinib and dabrafenib is more commonly used (approved by the FDA in 2014).

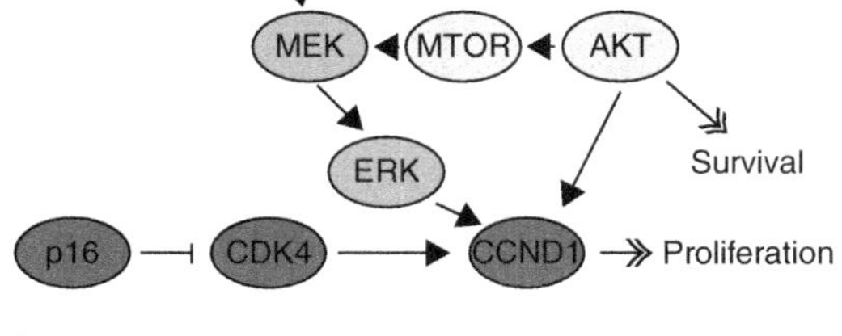

Fig. 6.1 Members of the MAPK signaling pathway frequently affected by genetic alterations in melanoma tumors.

Among RAS gene mutations, the majority affect *NRAS* and cause the substitution of glutamine at position 61 for an arginine, a lysine, or a leucine (Q61R/K/L), but can also affect *HRAS* and *KRAS*. Today, there are no agents targeting mutant RAS, and MEK inhibitors are not used for treatment of RAS mutant melanoma.

Unlike these hotspot mutations transforming the activity of the BRAF and RAS oncogenes, *NF1* harbors loss-of-function (nonsense, splice-site, or frameshift) mutations. These mutations are dispersed throughout the length of the gene and are characteristic of the inactivation pattern seen with tumor suppressors. Lastly, the triple-wild-type group appears to be molecularly heterogeneous, as no single driver has been identified for this group. Mutations in *KIT* and *GNA11*/*GNAQ* are typical for non-sun-induced and uveal melanomas, respectively. Frequent copy number aberrations are typically characteristic for this group.

The constitutive activation of the MAPK pathway caused by mutations in *BRAF*, *RAS*, or *NF1* genes fuels the cell cycle through the expression of cyclins and cyclin-dependent kinases (CDKs). However, CDKs are regulated by certain inhibitors; one of these is $p16^{INK4A}$, which is encoded by the *cyclin-dependent kinase inhibitor 2A* (*CDKN2A*) gene. *CDKN2A* is altered in 50% of melanomas by mutation, hyper-methylation, or deletion of chromosome locus 9p21. The gene also encodes the $p14^{ARF}$ protein, an inhibitor of mouse double minute 2 (MDM2), which targets p53 for degradation, thus abrogating its function. The *CDKN2A* mutations provide a mechanism to abrogate p53 function in melanoma, whereby *TP53* gene mutations are rare.

The cell survival and growth pathway regulated by phosphoinositide 3-kinase (PI3K) and serine/threonine kinase AKT is not targeted by *PIK3CA* mutations, as can be found in some of the major solid cancers, such as breast and colorectal carcinoma. Instead, it is targeted through a phosphatase and tensin homolog (*PTEN*) gene mutation, deletion of whole chromosome 10 (50% of melanomas), or overexpression of *AKT3* (20%). The recently described telomerase reverse transcriptase (*TERT*) promoter mutations [4, 5] leading to modest upregulation of telomerase have been found to be the most frequent somatic event in melanoma. Although they are identified in 70–80% of BRAF/RAS/NF1 melanomas, they are absent in triple-wild-type lesions, where TERT is instead targeted by gene amplification.

Interestingly, *BRAF* mutations tend to occur together with amplifications of the *MITF* gene and *PTEN* deletions, while such a tendency is not observed in *NRAS* mutant tumors. This may be due to efficient activation of both PI3K/AKT and MAPK pathways by a single genetic aberration in the latter case (e.g., *NRAS* mutation), which is indeed upstream of both PI3K/AKT and MEK/ERK signalling.

Ultraviolet Radiation and Mutational Load

Most melanomas arise on sun-exposed skin, and the contribution of the sun to melanoma etiology has been established through decades of research. Therefore, it is not surprising that the genomes of melanoma tumors are dominated by mutations that arise as a consequence of DNA damage caused by UVB radiation. This has been elegantly shown through whole-genome and whole-exome sequencing of melanoma-based studies over the past decade. Such mutations can represent up to 80–90% of all mutations in the genome of a cutaneous melanoma. This "UVB mutation signature" is characterized by the cytosine (C) to thymine (T) transition at di-pyrimidine sites (sites that are typically preceded by another C or a T at the 5′ end), as well as CC to TT tandem base substitutions [6].

With its average mutation rate of 16.8 mutations/Mb, melanoma has long been considered to be the most highly mutated cancer type. However, a recent study of basal cell carcinoma (BCC) of the skin showed an even higher mutation rate of 65 mutations/Mb. It also had a similar UVB signature that was comparable to that seen with melanoma [7].

In light of these findings, it is intriguing that UVR may not be necessary to acquire the genetic event that often lays the ground for melanoma initiation. Indeed, neither BRAF V600E (BRAF c.1799 T > A) nor NRAS Q61R (NRAS c.182A > G) are typical UVB-induced DNA changes. In addition, BRAF V600E and NRAS Q61R mutations are recurrent in other cancers, not associated with UVB radiation, such as papillary thyroid carcinoma [8] and colorectal carcinoma [9] (Catalogue of Somatic Mutations in Cancer, COSMIC, http://cancer.sanger.ac.uk/cosmic).

Progression from Nevus to Primary to Metastatic Melanoma and Genetic Changes Associated with It

The nature of the precursor lesion to the full-blown primary malignant melanoma has long been debated. Previously, it was thought that a melanoma originates from a benign nevus, that undergoes malignant transformation accompanied by unlimited proliferation, independency from growth factors, and other hallmark features of cancer [10]. This theory is supported by the observation that most common acquired nevi (~80%) carry the BRAF V600E mutation, which is a recurrent and clonal mutation in melanoma, and therefore an early event in its development. Another piece of evidence comes from the observation of an associated nevus found within, or as a part of, many primary melanomas upon pathological examination. This observation has lent support to the idea that the tumor developed from a cell within the nevus. Melanomas that originate within a nevus have a moderate mutation load, and arise on intermittently sun-exposed skin (e.g., trunk and extremities) in younger individuals (median 50 years).

However, as discussed above, many melanomas do not carry a *BRAF* V600E mutation, and instead are initiated by an *NRAS*, an *NF1*, or a *BRAF* non-V600E mutation. Such melanomas arise on skin that has been exposed to sun for many years, and carry signs of chronic sun damage (CDS), such as solar elastosis [11]. Such lesions arise with no benign precursor, such as a benign nevus. However, intermediate precursors may exist, as well as a melanoma in situ (MIS) represented by a lentigo maligna. This type of lesion arises on the skin of elderly people, and is located mainly on chronically exposed areas of the skin, such as the face, head and neck, and dorsum of hand and forearms. Dysplastic nevus can also serve as a precursor lesion, arising as a result of a genetic predisposition and typically harboring *NRAS* or *BRAF* non-V600E mutations. Melanomas that arise on such a background typically arise in older individuals and carry frequent cyclin D1 (*CCND1*) amplifications, KIT proto-oncogene receptor tyrosine kinase (*KIT*) mutations or copy number gains and *NF1* mutations, along with a high mutation load with a large contribution of the UVB signature.

The third type of melanoma arises on sun-protected body sites, e.g., acral lentiginous melanoma on glabrous skin (e.g., palms of the hands, soles of the feet), and mucosal melanoma on mucosal surfaces (most commonly those of the head and neck region, the anorectal region, and the female genital tract). These melanomas are characterized by the absence of *BRAF* and *NRAS* mutations, generally few mutations, and virtually no contribution of the UVB mutation signature. However, they carry many genomic copy number aberrations, including broad and focal chromosomal changes targeting *KIT*, *CDK4*, and other genes.

Different stages of melanoma progression are characterized by distinct, recurrent mutations that probably signify the acquirement of a trait necessary at that particular stage [12]. Benign nevi carry no recurrent alterations other than the *BRAF* V600E mutation. The *BRAF* V600E mutation, by itself, is insufficient for the establishment of a melanoma, and nevus cells remain within the defined boundaries of a nevus. However, nevi have the propensity to change in appearance over time, often regressing as we age. They proliferate when influenced by certain conditions, such as immunosuppressive treatment and pregnancy. Therefore, their state is not an irreversible arrest of proliferation. Intermediate lesions, such as those melanocytic proliferations that are difficult to classify as either benign or malignant, are often characterized by *BRAF*, *NRAS*, *TERT*, and heterozygous alterations of the *CDKN2A* gene [12]. Indeed, this set of alterations is the same observed in lesions classified as an MIS, arguing in favor of their true distinction from the benign cases.

Established invasive primary melanoma is also characterized by a biallelic inactivation of *CDKN2A*, *PTEN*, or *TP53* loss, and mutations in the SWI/SNF chromatin remodelling complex (ARID2, ARID1A). In addition, a high frequency of DNA copy number aberrations appears at this stage. The comparatively late entrance of this class of genetic alterations may indicate that it is a consequence of genomic instability caused by one of the mutations, such as those affecting the SWI/SNF complex. At this stage, the contribution of the UVB signature has reached its maximum, and UVB-induced mutations are not acquired at high frequency any longer. This may possibly be associated with the melanoma cells invading into deeper tissues away from body surface and UV radiation. Indeed, sequencing of multiple regions of the same metastasis has revealed diminished UVB signature among branch mutations, in this case mutations that are acquired in parts of the tumor (also called subclonal mutations) [13].

Gene Expression Characteristics of Melanoma Tumors

Main Drivers of Classification

Transcriptomics-based (i.e., the study of transcription levels of all genes) classification of bulk tumor tissue can provide valuable insight into the predominant biological cellular processes at work and identify weak points for therapeutic targeting. Since the pioneering study by Bittner and colleagues in 2000 [14], a number of independent studies have attempted to identify biological patterns and to classify melanoma tumors by means of investigation of the transcriptomic profile. Among these, the TCGA [1] classification with "keratin," "immune," and "MITF-low" subtypes and the Lund [15–17] classification with "pigmentation/MITF-high," "proliferative/MITF-low," "high-immune," and "normal-like" subtypes exist. The main driving forces of such classification systems converge on the same features, namely *pigmentation, immune response, proliferative*, and *invasive* processes [18].

Pigmentation, Proliferation, and Tissue Invasion

Pigmentation is the main function and feature of the differentiated melanocyte. It is governed by the transcription factor, MITF, which is the master regulator of both the melanocyte fate and function. The recurrent germline mutation, MITF E318K, confers a genetic predisposition to melanoma [19, 20]. MITF induces the transcription for a plethora of genes, including those within the pigmentation pathway. This pathway is activated in normal melanocytes by the alpha-melanocyte-stimulating hormone (alpha-MSH), secreted locally by keratinocytes in response to UVR exposure. Alpha-MSH binds and activates the melanocortin 1 receptor (MC1R), which signals through cyclic adenosine monophosphate (cAMP) and MITF, and induces the transcription of Melan-A (MLANA), melanocyte protein PMEL (homolog of mouse *silver* locus) and tyrosinase (TYR), necessary for the synthesis of melanin.

According to the rheostat model, MITF activity in the cell is tightly regulated, since very low activity levels induce senescence, while very high levels result in cell differentiation. Intermediate levels appear to regulate the balance between proliferation and invasion, two properties that are two opposing states of a melanocyte or melanoma cell [21]. Indeed, melanoma cell lines have been found to be either proliferative (i.e., MITF-high) with high expression of MITF, SOX10, and pigmentation pathway genes or invasive (i.e., MITF-low) with high expression of AXL, WNT5A, TGF-beta, and TCF/LEF [22–24].

In patient-derived tumors, these phenotypes have been difficult to recapitulate.

This may be due to the fact that tumors are communities of heterogeneous cells (some malignant, some not), with each cell possessing its own transcriptional profile. Moreover, the malignant cells within a tumor lesion may display different phenotypes [25]. However, tumor invasiveness and proliferation appear to define a certain phenotype and drive classification, with MITF-high ("keratin" subgroup in TCGA classification, "pigmentation" and "normal-like" subgroups in Lund notation) and MITF-low ("MITF-low" by TCGA, "proliferative" by Lund) cases clearly separated.

Immune System

Immune response signatures have been found that distinguish a subgroup of melanoma tumors in multiple, independent studies utilizing global gene expression profiling, further associated with a "good prognosis" signature in both primary and metastatic disease [26–28]. Both TCGA and the Lund classification systems have identified a cluster of genes, characterized by the overexpression of immune response-related genes ("immune" in TCGA, "high-immune" in Lund). These signatures contain cytokines and chemokines, markers of antigen-presenting cells and interferon pathway genes. More importantly, they represent the presence of immune cells, as confirmed by immunohistochemical (IHC) CD3 staining, demonstrating T-cell infiltration.

Melanoma has long been recognized as an immunogenic disease, due to the high proportion of immune cells that infiltrate the tumor. Additionally, there are several reported cases of spontaneous tumor regression, estimated to occur in 15–50% of primary melanomas [29, 30]. Spontaneous systemic immune response may ensue against cells expressing tumor-associated antigens (TAAs), such as Melan-A/MART-1, tyrosinase, MAGE, gp100, and NY-ESO-1. At the same time, it will cause the destruction of normal cells of the same phenotype. This phenomenon is illustrated clinically in patients who develop vitiligo, which is the appearance of white patches on the skin due to the destruction of cutaneous melanocytes [31, 32].

However, despite clinical signs of spontaneous (i.e., nontreatment-induced) tumor regression, the disease may still result in death [31]. Ultimately, the high mutational load that is characteristic of sun-induced melanoma provides a possible explanation for its immunogenicity. This assumes that the chances of creating an immunogenic neo-antigen will increase with the number of somatic mutations. Studies have shown that tumor-infiltrating immune cells may not react to tumor cells due to immunosuppressive microenvironment created by the latter. Mechanisms may include the recruitment of tumor-associated macrophages and regulatory T cells which inhibit the activity of the cytotoxic cells [33]. Other reasons may be due to the downregulation of antigen presentation by the tumor cells [34, 35]. This vulnerability has been used by investigators to target immune checkpoints for inhibition, such as anti-CTLA-4 and PD-1/PD-L1 antibodies. Intriguingly, in a fraction of patients, these agents induce vitiligo, with some studies suggesting a positive correlation between its development and an improved outcome to therapy [36].

Association to Mutations

The transcriptomic subtypes are not recapitulated by the classification based on mutations in the MAPK pathway. Therefore, there is no association to BRAF, NRAS, and NF1 mutations and these are equally distributed across gene expression subtypes [1, 15, 16]. This may indicate that the transcriptional subtypes arise independently of genetic driver events. This is also corroborated by the absence of prognostic significance for *BRAF* and *NRAS* gene mutations. However, some differences exist between the subtypes. For instance, the MITF-low/proliferative tumors more commonly comprise *BRAF* or *NRAS* mutations, with homozygous *CDKN2A* deletions and downregulation of p16 mRNA enriched within this subtype. On the other hand, mutations in beta-catenin (*CTNNB1*) and amplifications of cyclin D1 (*CCND1*) and MITF prevail among tumors of the MITF-high/pigmentation subtype [15, 16].

Association to Disease Stage

Since the transcriptional subtypes, to some extent, reflect the tumor microenvironment, they are unequally represented across the stages of disease. In particular, a large proportion of primary tumors belong to the normal-like/keratin subtype and only a few are found to be proliferative [1, 17]. In contrast, proliferative subtypes are overrepresented among both regional and distant metastases, while the normal-like subtype is almost nonexistent [15]. In addition, the signatures for a primary melanoma strongly correlate with a tumor Breslow's thickness [37], with pigmentation and proliferative subtypes enriched for thicker tumors, and normal-like and high-immune signatures seen with thinner tumors [17].

Progression

Heterogeneity and Clonal Evolution

Cancer is a result of an evolutionary process that acts at each cell division through selection of the cells with the highest fitness, a process acting on random mutations. This process may create multiple genetic clones of cells that coexist within the same tumor, defining intratumoral heterogeneity (ITH). Comprehensive methodology is essential for studies aiming at describing the diversity of cells within a tumor. Such methodology has only recently become available, with multi-region sampling of a tumor lesion followed by sequencing (currently mostly whole exome, but in some studies whole genome). The extent of ITH is quite complex, with our current understanding still in its infancy, highlighted further in the landmark study by Gerlinger and colleagues [38]. This study showed that between 63 and 69% of all mutations in a primary renal cell carcinoma are heterogeneous and spatially oriented within the tumor.

These results were later confirmed in another publication [39]. However, the range of mutation-based heterogeneity spanned between 28 and 92% among the ten tumor lesions. Studies of other primary cancers have followed, all showing a diverse degree of ITH, such as multifocal prostate cancer (~100%) [40, 41], esophageal adenocarcinoma (55%) [42], ovarian cancer (49%) [43], and lung cancer (24–30%) [44, 45]. In lung cancer, the TRACERx study examined 100 primary tumors, showing a large variation of ITH among tumors [46].

Within melanoma, such assessment of primary tumors is lacking, due to the unavailability of technology for comprehensive and reliable delineation of genetic alterations within small lesions. However, assessment of ITH within metastatic melanoma tumors has revealed that between 3 and 21% of all mutations are restricted to certain areas within a tumor [13]. This lower extent of heterogeneity may be specific for melanoma, or may signify the more homogeneous composition of metastases compared to that of primary tumors. Interestingly, while the ubiquitous mutations seen within a melanoma tumor are dominated by the UVB signature, the heterogeneous mutations represented all types of nucleotide substitution. This may indicate a diminished role of UVB in diversification mutagenesis within a metastatic lesion after its establishment. The degree of ITH may also have implications for multiple areas, in particular high levels of ITH have been associated with poor prognosis in several cancer types [47].

At the transcriptional level, ITH also exists, reflecting the specific contribution of the tumor microenvironment, as discussed above. Instead, it would be more interesting to assess transcriptional ITH among singular melanoma cells. Although this is technologically challenging, one such study has been performed, showing that melanoma tumors harbor cells that span the expression continuum between MITF-high and MITF-low subtypes. This appears to be irrespective of the main subtype (MITF-high or -low) assigned to the tumor that is based on the analysis of bulk tissue [25]. These results confirm predictions based on mathematical models of phenotypic states within a tumor [48].

In melanoma cell line models, a proliferative (MITF-high) and an invasive (MITF-low) state are thought to be plastic, with cells having the capacity to assume one, or the other, state. This plasticity is primarily due to the influences of the tumor microenvironment, such as cellular factors and signals [49]. Moreover, malignant cells are thought to oscillate between these two states, sought to be a driving force of tumor progression [50], with multiple cycles of "invade-proliferate" stages. In breast cancer, it has been demonstrated that different cancer cell clones cooperate with each other in order to establish a viable tumor deposit [51]. Clinically, an MITF-low state has been shown to confer resistance to multiple therapeutic modalities [52, 53]. Altogether, this may indicate that (a) tumors are composed of cells in different phenotypic states that are defined by their transcriptional profile; (b) some of these states may be resistant to anticancer therapies; and (c) plasticity of the phenotypic state may pose a serious challenge for therapy.

Diversity Between Metastases

Genetic and phenotypic diversity may also be observed between multiple metastatic lesions that have formed from the same primary melanoma. Generally, such lesions are very similar genomically and display only minor differences in mutations and DNA copy number aberrations [54]. In some cases, a single metastasis may acquire additional mutations, indicating a mutagenic effect, or a genetic event, leading to genome destabilization [54]. Phenotypically, MITF loss appears to be irreversible, as metastatic lesions classified as MITF-low at the transcriptional level are terminal in a sequence of multiple metastases, supported by the fact that subsequent lesions do not regain MITF expression [54]. It is unclear how the malignant cells within such lesions avoid senescence associated with MITF loss. The mechanisms underlying these observations remain to be elucidated.

Future Insight into the Molecular Pathology of Melanoma

During the past decade, our understanding of the molecular evolution of melanoma has increased. Further development of single-cell sequencing technologies applied to benign nevi, intermediate lesions, and invasive melanoma will provide us with an increased understanding of the molecular mechanisms underlying the development of melanocytic tumors.

References

1. Cancer Genome Atlas N. Genomic classification of cutaneous melanoma. Cell. 2015;161(7):1681–96. https://doi.org/10.1016/j.cell.2015.05.044.
2. Cirenajwis H, Lauss M, Ekedahl H, Torngren T, Kvist A, Saal LH, et al. NF1-mutated melanoma tumors harbor distinct clinical and biological characteristics. Mol Oncol. 2017;11(4):438–51. https://doi.org/10.1002/1878-0261.12050.
3. Davies H, Bignell GR, Cox C, Stephens P, Edkins S, Clegg S, et al. Mutations of the BRAF gene in human cancer. Nature. 2002;417(6892):949–54. https://doi.org/10.1038/nature00766. nature00766 [pii].
4. Huang FW, Hodis E, Xu MJ, Kryukov GV, Chin L, Garraway LA. Highly recurrent TERT promoter mutations in human melanoma. Science. 2013;339(6122):957–9. https://doi.org/10.1126/science.1229259.
5. Horn S, Figl A, Rachakonda PS, Fischer C, Sucker A, Gast A, et al. TERT promoter mutations in familial and sporadic melanoma. Science. 2013;339(6122):959–61. https://doi.org/10.1126/science.1230062.
6. Alexandrov LB, Nik-Zainal S, Wedge DC, Aparicio SA, Behjati S, Biankin AV, et al. Signatures of mutational processes in human cancer. Nature. 2013;500(7463):415–21. https://doi.org/10.1038/nature12477.
7. Bonilla X, Parmentier L, King B, Bezrukov F, Kaya G, Zoete V, et al. Genomic analysis identifies new drivers and progression pathways in skin basal cell carcinoma. Nat Genet. 2016;48(4):398–406. https://doi.org/10.1038/ng.3525.
8. Cancer Genome Atlas Research N. Integrated genomic characterization of papillary thyroid carcinoma. Cell. 2014;159(3):676–90. https://doi.org/10.1016/j.cell.2014.09.050.
9. Cancer Genome Atlas N. Comprehensive molecular characterization of human colon and rectal cancer. Nature. 2012;487(7407):330–7. https://doi.org/10.1038/nature11252.
10. Hanahan D, Weinberg RA. Hallmarks of cancer: the next generation. Cell. 2011;144(5):646–74. https://doi.org/10.1016/j.cell.2011.02.013.
11. Shain AH, Bastian BC. From melanocytes to melanomas. Nat Rev Cancer. 2016;16(6):345–58. https://doi.org/10.1038/nrc.2016.37.
12. Shain AH, Yeh I, Kovalyshyn I, Sriharan A, Talevich E, Gagnon A, et al. The genetic evolution of melanoma from precursor lesions. N Engl J Med. 2015;373(20):1926–36. https://doi.org/10.1056/NEJMoa1502583.
13. Harbst K, Lauss M, Cirenajwis H, Isaksson K, Rosengren F, Torngren T, et al. Multiregion whole-exome sequencing uncovers the genetic evolution and mutational heterogeneity of early-stage metastatic melanoma. Cancer Res. 2016;76(16):4765–74. https://doi.org/10.1158/0008-5472.CAN-15-3476.
14. Bittner M, Meltzer P, Chen Y, Jiang Y, Seftor E, Hendrix M, et al. Molecular classification of cutaneous malignant melanoma by gene expression profiling. Nature. 2000;406(6795):536–40. https://doi.org/10.1038/35020115.
15. Jonsson G, Busch C, Knappskog S, Geisler J, Miletic H, Ringner M, et al. Gene expression profiling-based identification of molecular subtypes in stage IV melanomas with different clinical outcome. Clin Cancer Res. 2010;16(13):3356–67. https://doi.org/10.1158/1078-0432.CCR-09-2509.
16. Cirenajwis H, Ekedahl H, Lauss M, Harbst K, Carneiro A, Enoksson J, et al. Molecular stratification of metastatic melanoma using gene expression profiling: prediction of survival outcome and benefit from molecular targeted therapy. Oncotarget. 2015;6(14):12297–309.
17. Harbst K, Staaf J, Lauss M, Karlsson A, Masback A, Johansson I, et al. Molecular profiling reveals low- and high-grade forms of primary melanoma. Clin Cancer Res. 2012;18(15):4026–36. https://doi.org/10.1158/1078-0432.CCR-12-0343.
18. Lauss M, Nsengimana J, Staaf J, Newton-Bishop J, Jonsson G. Consensus of melanoma gene expression subtypes converges on biological entities. J Invest Dermatol. 2016;136(12):2502–5. https://doi.org/10.1016/j.jid.2016.05.119.
19. Bertolotto C, Lesueur F, Giuliano S, Strub T, de Lichy M, Bille K, et al. A SUMOylation-defective MITF germline mutation predisposes to melanoma and renal carcinoma. Nature. 2011;480(7375):94–8. https://doi.org/10.1038/nature10539.
20. Yokoyama S, Woods SL, Boyle GM, Aoude LG, MacGregor S, Zismann V, et al. A novel recurrent mutation in MITF predisposes to familial and sporadic melanoma. Nature. 2011;480(7375):99–103. https://doi.org/10.1038/nature10630.
21. Wellbrock C, Arozarena I. Microphthalmia-associated transcription factor in melanoma development and MAP-kinase pathway targeted therapy. Pigment Cell Melanoma Res. 2015;28(4):390–406. https://doi.org/10.1111/pcmr.12370.
22. Hoek KS, Schlegel NC, Brafford P, Sucker A, Ugurel S, Kumar R, et al. Metastatic potential of melanomas defined by specific gene expression profiles with no BRAF signature. Pigment Cell Res. 2006;19(4):290–302. https://doi.org/10.1111/j.1600-0749.2006.00322.x.
23. Widmer DS, Cheng PF, Eichhoff OM, Belloni BC, Zipser MC, Schlegel NC, et al. Systematic classification of melanoma cells by phenotype-specific gene expression mapping. Pigment Cell Melanoma Res. 2012;25(3):343–53. https://doi.org/10.1111/j.1755-148X.2012.00986.x.

24. Howlin J, Cirenajwis H, Lettiero B, Staaf J, Lauss M, Saal L, et al. Loss of CITED1, an MITF regulator, drives a phenotype switch in vitro and can predict clinical outcome in primary melanoma tumours. Peer J. 2015;3:e788. https://doi.org/10.7717/peerj.788.
25. Tirosh I, Izar B, Prakadan SM, Wadsworth MH 2nd, Treacy D, Trombetta JJ, et al. Dissecting the multicellular ecosystem of metastatic melanoma by single-cell RNA-seq. Science. 2016;352(6282):189–96. https://doi.org/10.1126/science.aad0501.
26. Mandruzzato S, Callegaro A, Turcatel G, Francescato S, Montesco MC, Chiarion-Sileni V, et al. A gene expression signature associated with survival in metastatic melanoma. J Transl Med. 2006;4:50. https://doi.org/10.1186/1479-5876-4-50.
27. Bogunovic D, O'Neill DW, Belitskaya-Levy I, Vacic V, Yu YL, Adams S, et al. Immune profile and mitotic index of metastatic melanoma lesions enhance clinical staging in predicting patient survival. Proc Natl Acad Sci U S A. 2009;106(48):20429–34. https://doi.org/10.1073/pnas.0905139106.
28. Mann GJ, Pupo GM, Campain AE, Carter CD, Schramm SJ, Pianova S, et al. BRAF mutation, NRAS mutation, and the absence of an immune-related expressed gene profile predict poor outcome in patients with stage III melanoma. J Invest Dermatol. 2013;133(2):509–17. https://doi.org/10.1038/jid.2012.283.
29. Maio M. Melanoma as a model tumour for immuno-oncology. Ann Oncol. 2012;23(Suppl 8):viii10–viii4. https://doi.org/10.1093/annonc/mds257.
30. Wenzel J, Bekisch B, Uerlich M, Haller O, Bieber T, Tuting T. Type I interferon-associated recruitment of cytotoxic lymphocytes: a common mechanism in regressive melanocytic lesions. Am J Clin Pathol. 2005;124(1):37–48. https://doi.org/10.1309/4EJ9KL7CGDENVVLE.
31. Redondo P, Del Olmo J. Images in clinical medicine. Vitiligo and cutaneous melanoma. N Engl J Med. 2008;359(3):e3. https://doi.org/10.1056/NEJMicm053764.
32. Nordlund JJ, Kirkwood JM, Forget BM, Milton G, Albert DM, Lerner AB. Vitiligo in patients with metastatic melanoma: a good prognostic sign. J Am Acad Dermatol. 1983;9(5):689–96.
33. Kitamura T, Qian BZ, Pollard JW. Immune cell promotion of metastasis. Nat Rev Immunol. 2015;15(2):73–86. https://doi.org/10.1038/nri3789.
34. Thor Straten P, Garrido F. Targetless T cells in cancer immunotherapy. J Immunother Cancer. 2016;4:23. https://doi.org/10.1186/s40425-016-0127-z.
35. Shukla SA, Rooney MS, Rajasagi M, Tiao G, Dixon PM, Lawrence MS, et al. Comprehensive analysis of cancer-associated somatic mutations in class I HLA genes. Nat Biotechnol. 2015;33:1152–8. https://doi.org/10.1038/nbt.3344.
36. Teulings HE, Limpens J, Jansen SN, Zwinderman AH, Reitsma JB, Spuls PI, et al. Vitiligo-like depigmentation in patients with stage III–IV melanoma receiving immunotherapy and its association with survival: a systematic review and meta-analysis. J Clin Oncol. 2015;33(7):773–81. https://doi.org/10.1200/JCO.2014.57.4756.
37. Riker AI, Enkemann SA, Fodstad O, Liu S, Ren S, Morris C, et al. The gene expression profiles of primary and metastatic melanoma yields a transition point of tumor progression and metastasis. BMC Med Genet. 2008;1:13. https://doi.org/10.1186/1755-8794-1-13.
38. Gerlinger M, Rowan AJ, Horswell S, Larkin J, Endesfelder D, Gronroos E, et al. Intratumor heterogeneity and branched evolution revealed by multiregion sequencing. N Engl J Med. 2012;366(10):883–92. https://doi.org/10.1056/NEJMoa1113205.
39. Gerlinger M, Horswell S, Larkin J, Rowan AJ, Salm MP, Varela I, et al. Genomic architecture and evolution of clear cell renal cell carcinomas defined by multiregion sequencing. Nat Genet. 2014;46(3):225–33. https://doi.org/10.1038/ng.2891.
40. Boutros PC, Fraser M, Harding NJ, de Borja R, Trudel D, Lalonde E, et al. Spatial genomic heterogeneity within localized, multifocal prostate cancer. Nat Genet. 2015;47(7):736–45. https://doi.org/10.1038/ng.3315.
41. Cooper CS, Eeles R, Wedge DC, Van Loo P, Gundem G, Alexandrov LB, et al. Analysis of the genetic phylogeny of multifocal prostate cancer identifies multiple independent clonal expansions in neoplastic and morphologically normal prostate tissue. Nat Genet. 2015;47(4):367–72. https://doi.org/10.1038/ng.3221.
42. Murugaesu N, Wilson GA, Birkbak NJ, Watkins TB, McGranahan N, Kumar S, et al. Tracking the genomic evolution of esophageal adenocarcinoma through neoadjuvant chemotherapy. Cancer Discov. 2015;5(8):821–31. https://doi.org/10.1158/2159-8290.CD-15-0412.
43. Bashashati A, Ha G, Tone A, Ding J, Prentice LM, Roth A, et al. Distinct evolutionary trajectories of primary high-grade serous ovarian cancers revealed through spatial mutational profiling. J Pathol. 2013;231(1):21–34. https://doi.org/10.1002/path.4230.
44. Zhang J, Fujimoto J, Zhang J, Wedge DC, Song X, Zhang J, et al. Intratumor heterogeneity in localized lung adenocarcinomas delineated by multiregion sequencing. Science. 2014;346(6206):256–9. https://doi.org/10.1126/science.1256930.
45. de Bruin EC, McGranahan N, Mitter R, Salm M, Wedge DC, Yates L, et al. Spatial and temporal diversity in genomic instability processes defines lung cancer evolution. Science. 2014;346(6206):251–6. https://doi.org/10.1126/science.1253462.
46. Jamal-Hanjani M, Wilson GA, McGranahan N, Birkbak NJ, Watkins TBK, Veeriah S, et al. Tracking the evolution of non-small-cell lung cancer. N Engl J Med. 2017;376(22):2109–21. https://doi.org/10.1056/NEJMoa1616288.
47. Morris LG, Riaz N, Desrichard A, Senbabaoglu Y, Hakimi AA, Makarov V, et al. Pan-cancer analysis of intratumor heterogeneity as a prognostic determinant

of survival. Oncotarget. 2016;7(9):10051–63. https://doi.org/10.18632/oncotarget.7067.
48. Li Q, Wennborg A, Aurell E, Dekel E, Zou JZ, Xu Y, et al. Dynamics inside the cancer cell attractor reveal cell heterogeneity, limits of stability, and escape. Proc Natl Acad Sci U S A. 2016;113(10):2672–7. https://doi.org/10.1073/pnas.1519210113.
49. Eichhoff OM, Weeraratna A, Zipser MC, Denat L, Widmer DS, Xu M, et al. Differential LEF1 and TCF4 expression is involved in melanoma cell phenotype switching. Pigment Cell Melanoma Res. 2011;24(4):631–42. https://doi.org/10.1111/1755-148X.2011.00871.x.
50. Hoek KS, Eichhoff OM, Schlegel NC, Dobbeling U, Kobert N, Schaerer L, et al. In vivo switching of human melanoma cells between proliferative and invasive states. Cancer Res. 2008;68(3):650–6. https://doi.org/10.1158/0008-5472.CAN-07-2491.
51. Cleary AS, Leonard TL, Gestl SA, Gunther EJ. Tumour cell heterogeneity maintained by cooperating subclones in Wnt-driven mammary cancers. Nature. 2014;508(7494):113–7. https://doi.org/10.1038/nature13187.
52. Muller J, Krijgsman O, Tsoi J, Robert L, Hugo W, Song C, et al. Low MITF/AXL ratio predicts early resistance to multiple targeted drugs in melanoma. Nat Commun. 2014;5:5712. https://doi.org/10.1038/ncomms6712.
53. Konieczkowski DJ, Johannessen CM, Abudayyeh O, Kim JW, Cooper ZA, Piris A, et al. A melanoma cell state distinction influences sensitivity to MAPK pathway inhibitors. Cancer Discov. 2014;4(7):816–27. https://doi.org/10.1158/2159-8290.CD-13-0424.
54. Harbst K, Lauss M, Cirenajwis H, Winter C, Howlin J, Torngren T, et al. Molecular and genetic diversity in the metastatic process of melanoma. J Pathol. 2014;233(1):39–50. https://doi.org/10.1002/path.4318.

Epigenetics in Melanoma

7

Marjan E. Askarian-Amiri, Euan J. Rodger, Aniruddha Chatterjee, Graeme Finlay, and Bruce C. Baguley

Introduction

Melanoma is the deadliest form of skin cancer and originates from the malignant transformation of melanocytes, the pigment-producing cells of the epidermis. Lysosome-like organelles called melanosomes, inside melanocytes, synthesise and store melanin pigments. A variety of melanocyte-specific enzymatic and structural proteins, as well as proteins important for trafficking and sorting of melanin, are required for the normal physiological function of melanocytes. Figure 7.1 illustrates the key pathways in melanin production [1].

Melanoblasts, the precursor cells of melanocytes, are derived from the embryonic neural crest, and migrate to the epidermis during embryogenesis. Melanoblasts reside predominately in the basal layer of the epidermis where they are in contact with keratinocytes [2, 3]. Melanocyte function is tightly regulated by keratinocytes, secreting α-melanocyte-stimulating hormone (α-MSH) upon environmental stimulation such as UV irradiation. In turn, this binds to the melanocortin 1 receptor (MC1R) on melanocytes (Fig. 7.1).

Stimulation of melanogenesis induces the production of melanins, which in vertebrates is formed from a family of closely related molecules derived from L-tyrosine. There are two types of melanin in mammals: dark/black 'eumelanin' and reddish/yellow 'phaeomelanin' (Fig. 7.1). After melanin pigments are produced they are packaged into melanosomes and subsequently transferred to keratinocytes and distributed there. They are strategically localised over the sun-exposed side of nuclei to protect the DNA by forming cap-like structures [2, 4, 5].

Melanoma

Most deaths from skin cancer are attributable to melanoma, which is known as the most aggressive form of skin cancer. Melanoma is highly curable if

M. E. Askarian-Amiri, Ph.D. (✉) · G. Finlay
Department of Molecular Medicine and Pathology, School of Medical Sciences, University of Auckland, Grafton, Auckland, New Zealand

Auckland Cancer Society Research Centre, University of Auckland, Grafton, Auckland, New Zealand
e-mail: m.askarian-amiri@auckland.ac.nz; g.finlay@auckland.ac.nz

E. J. Rodger · A. Chatterjee
Department of Pathology, Dunedin School of Medicine, University of Otago, Dunedin, New Zealand

Maurice Wilkins Centre for Molecular Biodiscovery, Auckland, New Zealand
e-mail: euan.rodger@otago.ac.nz; aniruddha.chatterjee@otago.ac.nz

B. C. Baguley
Auckland Cancer Society Research Centre, University of Auckland, Grafton, Auckland, New Zealand
e-mail: b.baguley@auckland.ac.nz

A. I. Riker (ed.), *Melanoma*, https://doi.org/10.1007/978-3-319-78310-9_7

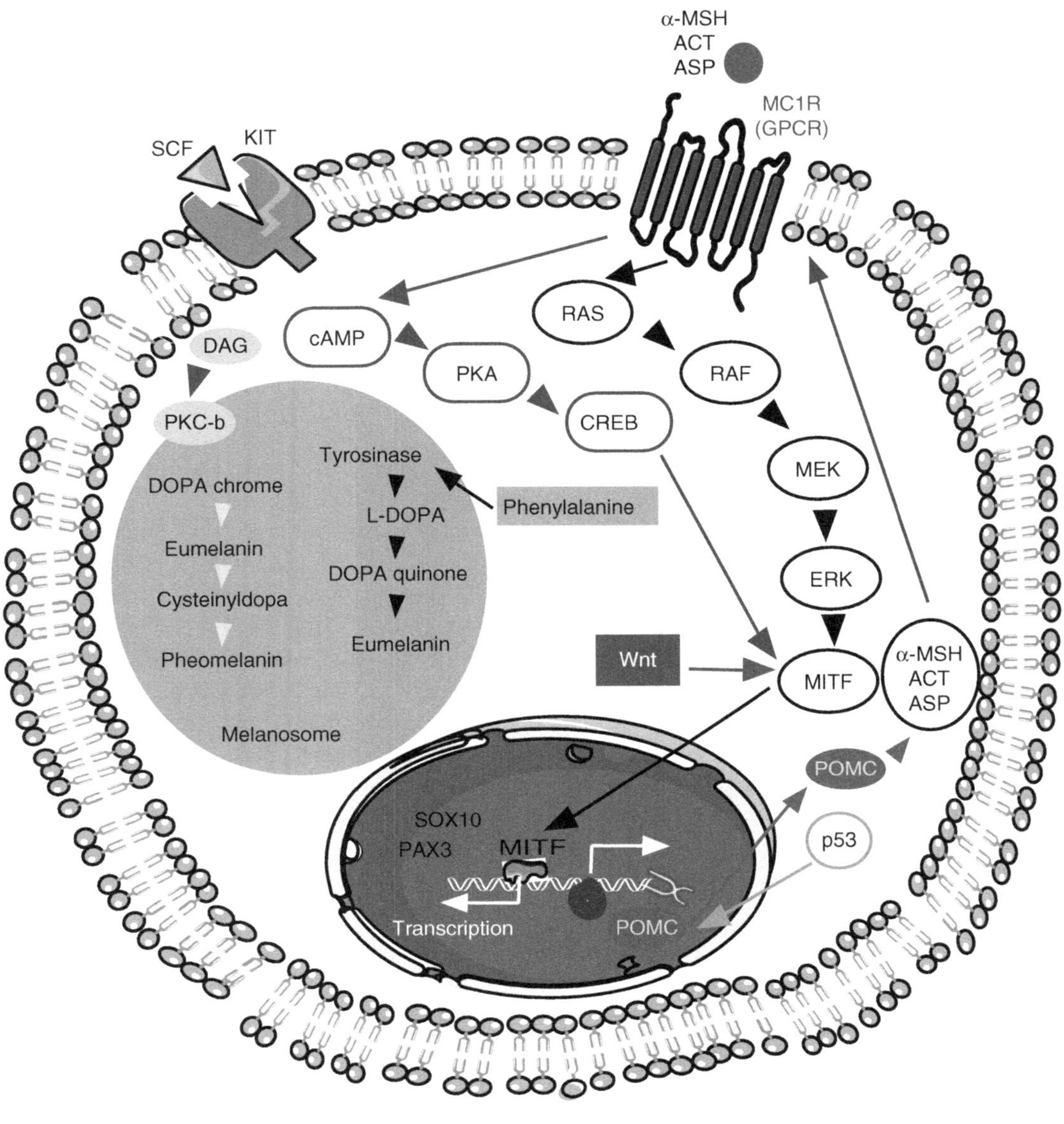

Fig. 7.1 Pathways in melanogenesis. A series of reactions within melanosomes of melanocytes produce eumelanin and phaeomelanin. Production of the enzymes involved in melanin synthesis is driven by the MITF transcription factor. MITF activity itself is regulated by a number of signalling pathways including protein kinase C, cyclic AMP, MEK and WNT. Receptors such as KIT (ligand: SCF) and MC1R (ligands: α-MSH, ACTH and ASP) activate these signalling pathways. The expression of genes such as *PAX3* and *SOX10* is also driven by MITF

detected during the early stages of disease; however, metastatic disease becomes very difficult to treat despite improved recent treatment options. Identifying the exact mechanisms of initiation and progression of human melanoma would greatly help to identify molecular targets for early detection, treatment and prognosis of this malignancy. About 5–12% of all worldwide melanoma is caused by germline mutations; therefore about 10% of patients present with a family history of melanoma [6]. The genetic factors involved in melanoma have been studied extensively [7–9].

Although the identification of new susceptibility genes may shed light on the complexity of the genetic landscape of melanoma, the specific cellular mechanisms as to how these genes influence patient phenotypes seem to be much more complex.

Epigenetics

Despite the genetic contribution to melanoma progression, its development is also attributed to diverse epigenetic factors [10]. Epigenetic factors are normally heritable [11], and neoplastic phenotypes may be manifested when there are reversible changes in gene regulation, without the sequence of the genome being changed. Epigenetic changes include aberrant DNA methylation, histone modifications and expression of variants, chromatin remodelling and nucleosome re-positioning as well as deregulation of small and long non-coding RNAs (ncRNAs) [10, 12]. Among epigenetic factors, DNA methylation followed by chromatin modification are the best studied. However, the roles of ncRNAs in recent years have become apparent. Since epigenetic changes normally occur prior to malignant transformation and genetic aberration, their characterisation may help us to identify biomarkers and use them for the early detection and treatment of melanoma.

DNA Methylation

Methylation of cytosine (5mC) is a stable and mitotically heritable epigenetic marker that is established and maintained by DNA methyltransferase (DNMT) enzymes [13]. If 5mC marks are not maintained, they are passively erased in a replication-dependent manner or they can be actively removed in a process mediated by TET enzymes [14]. These marks are found almost exclusively in the context of CpG dinucleotides, of which there are 28 million across the human genome. DNA methylation is critical for genomic imprinting, X chromosome inactivation, tissue differentiation and regulation of transcriptional activity. Most protein-coding genes have small CpG-rich regions (~1 kb), called CpG islands (CGIs), in their promoter regions [15]. These regions are typically unmethylated, which makes the chromatin structure more accessible for transcription factor (TF) binding and hence permits transcription of the associated genes.

Aberrant changes in DNA methylation have a well-established role in contributing to tumorigenesis [16]. Promoter hypermethylation (i.e. an increase in 5mC marks) of so-called tumour-suppressor genes that regulate critical cellular pathways is by far the most studied epigenetic feature in cancer [17]. In melanoma, the most frequently hypermethylated tumour-suppressor genes include *TNFRSF10D* (~80% of melanomas) [18], *COL1A2* (~80%) [19], *RARB* (up to 70%) [20], *PTEN* (~60%) [21], *RASSF1A* (~55%) [20], *MGMT* (~34%) [20] and *SYK* (30%) [19]. Advances in genome-wide techniques over the last decade have provided the opportunity to investigate methylation changes at an unprecedented scale [22, 23]. A recent analysis of 458 melanomas (99 primary tumours and 358 metastatic tumours) identified hypermethylation in the promoter regions of the *HOXD12*, *TNFRSF10C*, *FGFR2* and *TERT* genes [24]. It is interesting to mention that hypermethylation of genes such as *TERT* is associated with the increased expression in melanoma patients [25]. Furthermore, genome-wide studies have identified methylation signatures that are beneficial for diagnosis [26–29] and prognosis [30–33].

In addition to site-specific gain of methylation at gene promoters, genomic hypomethylation is an established feature of most cancers. Indeed, compared to their wild-type counterparts, melanoma cells are typically globally hypomethylated; that is, genome-wide there are fewer 5mC marks [34, 35]. This hypomethylation is potentially due to dysregulation of the de novo methyltransferase DNMT3A, especially for tumours harbouring the recurrent BRAF driver mutation V600E [35]. Highlighting prognostic importance, further global hypomethylation occurs upon metastatic progression [30, 36].

The global loss of methylation primarily occurs in repeat regions, such as satellite DNAs, Alu elements and long interspersed elements (LINEs). Expression of normally inactivated transposable elements within these regions results in genomic instability, which contributes to tumour progression [37]. It has been shown that hypomethylation of LINE1 elements in primary melanomas is associated with decreased relapse-free survival and increased metastatic potential [38]. Furthermore, in melanoma and other cancers, hypomethylation has been shown to activate cancer-testis (CT) genes such as *MAGE* (melanoma antigen family) [39] and *BAGE* (B melanoma antigen) [40]. As the aberrant expression of CT genes is highly tumour specific and higher levels are correlated with poorer outcome [41], they have been an attractive target for immunotherapy [42].

The site-specific gain of promoter methylation and global loss of methylation in intergenic regions described above have mainly been studied in the context of primary cancers. In comparison, fewer studies have focused on epigenetic changes associated with the metastatic cascade. However, the role of aberrant methylation in metastasis is just starting to be appreciated. In a recent genome-wide DNA methylation analysis of cell lines derived from primary melanomas and their matched metastases, hypomethylation was shown to activate a cryptic 47 kDa transcript of *TBC1D16*. This transcript generated an isoform of a Rab GTPase-activating protein, expression of which promoted melanoma growth and metastasis, and was associated with poorer prognosis [33].

Interestingly, although DNA methylation has been strongly established as a gene-silencing mechanism, in an analysis of paired primary and metastatic cell lines, a gene has been identified (*EBF3*) of which high promoter methylation facilitates mRNA expression. Treatment of these cells with DNA methylation inhibitors decreased *EBF3* mRNA levels, which implies that the methylation level is likely to have a causal role in regulating this gene [36]. It was proposed that methylation of the *EBF3* promoter impedes binding of a transcriptional repressor and that this results in elevated expression of *EBF3* in metastatic melanoma.

It was also observed that, compared to the paired primary cell lines, the metastatic cell lines were globally hypomethylated, with regions of site-specific hypermethylation enriched for active chromatin marks. In contrast, the hypomethylated regions were enriched for repetitive elements (particularly SINE elements) and silenced chromatin marks. Hypomethylation of otherwise repressed regions could result in their reactivation in melanoma metastasis [43]. Indeed, another study has shown that hypomethylation of transposable elements was associated with metastatic capacity of primary melanomas [38]. Further, other studies have recently reported methylation-mediated deregulation of HOX family (in particular *HOXD9*) [30], *RASSF6*, [44] and *TFAP2A* [45] genes in metastatic melanoma.

Transcriptional activity can also be modulated by methylation of enhancer elements, which are perturbed in cancer [46]. Enhancers can be difficult to identify as (a) they are often up to 1 Mbp away from transcription start sites (TSSs), (b) a single enhancer can regulate more than one gene and (c) multiple enhancers can regulate a single gene [47]. In an integrated analysis of over 6200 DNA methylation profiles from melanoma patients' tumour and normal tissue, Bell et al. [48] discovered that enhancers have a higher proportion of differentially methylated regions (DMRs) than any other region. These tumour-associated DMRs were more commonly hypomethylated and were enriched for central pluripotent TFs. Furthermore, they also found that enhancer DMRs were often specific to a single metastasis site and were the best genomic predictor of prognosis. Very little work has been done so far to understand the regulation of genes by these long-range interactions in melanoma and this is likely to be an area that will be explored in more depth in the future.

Histone Modification

DNA molecules are tightly wrapped around highly basic histone proteins, which consist of H2, H2B, H3 and H4 as well as other variants. Covalent post-translational modifications of histone proteins have been known for more than a half century and identified as key mechanisms for regulating the function of these proteins.

Histones can be modified by addition of chemical groups to their tails. The proteins that mediate the addition of these chemical groups are known as writer proteins, and eraser proteins remove these marks. These modifications act as templates for reader proteins, which recruit transcription factors (or repress their activities) to modulate gene expression. Besides the modifications of histones, alterations of nucleosome structure can affect gene expression [49].

Histone modification can either induce or suppress transcription, depending on the nature and location of the modification that dictates the accessibility of DNA to the transcriptional machinery. More than 100 post-translational modifications are known for human histones. The best known post-translational modifications of histones include methylation, acetylation, phosphorylation, ubiquitylation, sumoylation, ADP ribosylation, deamination and proline isomerisation [50]. These modifications affect diverse biological processes such as transcriptional regulation, DNA damage response and chromosome packaging [50]. Table 7.1 summarises different modifications, and identifies the residues modified and the enzymes involved in the modification. The use of antibodies against the modified histones in chromatin immunoprecipitation assays has revolutionised the understanding of the global distribution of histone modifications. This understanding of chromatin modifications has revealed that they are not uniformly distributed, that common features such as acetylation at the 5′ end of genes are associated with actively transcribed regions of the genome and that there is a basic blueprint of modification patterns [50].

Aberrant patterns of histone modifications have been associated with a large number of human malignancies including melanoma. Here, we discuss our understanding of the mechanisms

Table 7.1 Modifications of histones

Modification	Residues modified	Enzymes involved in modification
Acetylation	Lysine	HAT1, CBP/P300, PCAF/GCN5, TIP60. HB01, ScSAS2, ScSAS3, ScRTT109
Deacetylation	Lysine	SirT2, HDAC1-11 [142]
Methylation	Lysine; K-me1, K-me2, K-me3	SUV39H1, SUV39H2, G9a, ESET/SETDB1, EuHMTase/GLP, CLL8, SpClr4, MLL1, MLL2, MLL3, MLL4, MLL5, SET1A, SET1B, ASH1, Sc/Sp SET1, Sc/Sp SET2, NSD1, SYMD2, DOT1, Sc/Sp DOT1, Pr-SET 7/8, SUV2 20H1, SUV4 20H2, SpSet9, EZH2, RIZ1
Demethylation	Lysine; K-me1, K-me2, K-me3	LSD1/BHC110, JHDM1a, JHDM1b, JHDM2a, JHDM2b, JMJD2A/JHDM3A, JMJD2B, JMJD2C/GASC1, JMJD2D
Methylation	Arginine; R-me1, R-me2, R-me3	CARM1, PRMT4, PRMT5
Phosphorylation	Serine, tyrosine	Haspin, MSK1, MSK2, CKII, Mst1
Ubiquitylation	Lysine	Bmi/Ring1A, RNF20/RNF40
Sumoylation	Lysine	UBC9 [143]
ADP ribosylation	Glutamic acid	ARH1, ARH2, ARH3, PARGs [144, 145]
Deimination[a]	Arginine	
Proline isomerisation	Proline-cis or trans	SCFPR4

The process of deimination has been correlated with the disappearance of methyl-arginine, indicating that deimination has the potential to antagonise arginine methylation. The data are derived from [50] except for the references given in the table that control and maintain the histone marks and show how disruptions of these modifications contribute towards the pathogenesis of melanoma.

Histone Acetylation/Methylation

The transfer of acetyl groups from acetyl-CoA to the amino groups of lysine side chains leads to histone lysine (K) acetylation. The process of acetylation/deacetylation is catalysed by histone acetyl transferases (HATs) and histone deacetylases (HDACs), respectively [49–51]. The acetylation of lysine residues suppresses their positive charges and their interaction with negatively charged DNA leads to the formation of open or euchromatin that facilitates transcription and induces gene expression. The best studied targets for histone acetylation are the lysine residues in the tails of H3 and H4, although other residues such as K56 in H3 are internally acetylated. To change the status of euchromatin to heterochromatin (closed form) the acetyl groups on histones must be removed to facilitate the deposition of activating or repressive marks, such as H3K9me3 and H3K27me3, respectively [49].

Histone modifications are dynamic processes. For most modifications, enzymes have been identified that remove the modification. Although enzymes actively remove methyl groups from lysine residues (Table 7.1), methyl groups can be removed from arginine residues by deimination, a reaction that is antagonistic to arginine methylation. The most well-characterised modification is methylation, since methyltransferases are the enzymes most specific to histone modification [52]. Despite kinases being specific for histone modification, they have not been studied as extensively as have enzymes responsible for methylation. This is due to the activation of distinct signalling pathways that are required for phosphorylation of histones [53].

The recruitment of enzymes essential for modifications requires the disruption of the contacts among nucleosomes in order for the proteins to access the histones. Acetylation and phosphorylation are among the modifications that have impact on chromatin compaction via changes in ionic charges [54–57].

A complex cross talk between modifications arises from the abundance of modifications [50]. Cross talk occurs since several modifications that are antagonistic to each other take place on histone lysine residues. They are mutually exclusive and a modification may disturb the binding of proteins to adjacent sites on the histone [54]. This results in the compromise of the enzyme's catalytic activity [58], or its substrate recognition enhanced [59]. The cross talk of modifications also occurs between different histone tails [50].

The differential acetylation of histones during melanogenesis has been reported. For instance, deacetylation of histones and methylation of the same residues in the *CDKN2A* locus downregulate the expression of the tumour-suppressor genes $p14^{ARF}$ and $p16^{INK4a}$ [49, 60]. Despite extensive studies performed on HDACs, not much is known about their functions in melanoma. However, the expression of HDAC8 is related to improved survival rates, and HDAC1 and -8 increase the phosphorylation of the NF-κB p65 subunit that is associated with resistance to MAPK inhibitors [61, 62].

On the other hand, histone methyltransferases have been shown to have effects on melanoma progression. For instance, enhancer of zeste homologue 2 (EZH2), the catalytic subunit of polycomb repressor complex 2 (PRC2), methylates H3K27 and represses transcription [63]. Activating mutations of EZH2 have also been reported [64]. It has been shown that the histone marks H3K9me3 and H3K27me3 were not changed significantly in the promoter region of the $p16^{INK4a}$ gene when skin keratinocytes were exposed to UV irradiation, but an H3K4me3 mark was reduced when cells were treated with UVA chronically [65]. The H3K4me3 mark was also enriched at the promoter of the *KLF4* gene in the UVA-irradiated cells. A decreased H3K9me3 mark (70% reduction) was observed for *P21WAF1/CIP1* after 15 weeks of UVA treatment. Cells treated for 15 weeks with UVA also revealed a 40% reduction of the H3K27me3 mark at the *hTERT* promoter [66].

Reader Proteins

Apart from histone-modifying proteins, reader proteins also can affect gene expression. Reader proteins contain a variety of domains that bind to specific modifications. Histone reader proteins regulate gene expression by recruiting enzymes such as transcription elongation factors, by causing further modification or by inherent catalytic activities. The involvement of reader proteins such as the bromodomain and extra terminal (BET) family in melanoma has been reported. BRD2 and BRD4 from this family are overexpressed in melanoma. Also it has been shown that ING1 protein, that contains a plant homology domain (PHD) that binds to acetylated lysine, is overexpressed in melanoma and that its expression induced upon UV irradiation [67].

It has been reported that a variable number of nucleotides are localised in each nucleosome. The SWI/SNF proteins constitute chromatin-remodelling complexes that determine nucleosome positioning. Components of the SWI/SNF complex [68] including ARID2 [69–71] and ARID1A, and ARID1B and SMARCA4 [72], are mutated in melanoma, suggesting that the deregulation of chromatin-remodelling proteins features in melanoma progression.

Histone Variants

The replacement of canonical histones by variant histones, which have different sequences and properties, has been reported. Among these, variants of H2A and H3 are the most common. The expression of variants results in altered chromatin structure, post-translational modifications and changes to gene expression [73]. Histone variant H2A.Z, which is increased in melanoma, consists of the two subforms H2A.Z.1 and H2A.Z.2 that differ by three amino acids and are transcribed from distinct genomic regions [74]. H2A.Z.2 is highly expressed in melanoma and results in the activation of genes, especially E2F targets that promote cell cycle progression [74]. Expression of macroH2A, another variant of H2, suppresses melanoma progression via suppression of *CDK8* expression and it is generally lost with the development of melanoma [74]. The histone 3 variants H3.3 are also associated with *E2F* target gene expression. Its over-expression leads to suppression of *E2F* target genes and senescence [75]. The variants of histones or the chaperones that direct them to specific regions of chromatin can be targeted to change the sensitivity of melanoma cells to MAPK inhibitors or immunotherapy [49].

Non-coding RNA

The role of RNA in cells has been undergoing revision since the demonstration that only about 1.5–2% of the human genome is transcribed into protein-coding RNAs, while the vast majority is transcribed as non-coding RNAs (ncRNAs) [76]. The higher abundance of non-coding as compared to protein-coding genes in eukaryotes suggests that ncRNAs may contribute to their complex physiology and development [77]. This finding evinces the biological relevance to these molecules and points to their contribution to the genetic and physiological complexity of higher eukaryotes. NcRNAs function as housekeeping RNAs such as ribosomal RNAs (rRNAs), transfer RNAs (tRNAs), small nuclear and small nucleolar RNAs (snRNAs and snoRNAs, respectively), as well as regulatory RNAs.

Regulatory RNAs act as epigenetic modulators and are classified into small and long ncRNAs based on their lengths [78]. Short ncRNAs are those with less than 200 nucleotides and long ncRNAs (lncRNAs) with sizes ranging from 200 nucleotides to several kilobases (kb). The identities and functions of short ncRNAs such as microRNA (miRNA) and short interfering RNA (siRNA) are well studied [79]. These ncRNAs regulate various pathways that are crucial to development and that are perturbed in disease [76, 79].

On the other hand, with the exception of a few well-studied transcripts, the identities and functions of the vast majority of lncRNAs are yet to be characterised. The range of cellular processes that are in one way or another governed by ncRNAs is beyond estimation since they regulate gene transcription, RNA processing such as splicing and modification, and stability and translation of mRNA as well as act as scaffold and signalling molecules [80]. Therefore, they are capable of acting at multiple levels to control cellular functions and contribute towards the aetiology of diseases including cancer.

Long Non-coding RNA

LncRNAs are emerging as important regulatory molecules, the function of which is altered in cancer progression and have the potential to be used as novel diagnostic and prognostic markers as well as therapeutic targets. The expression of lncRNAs is more tissue specific than that of protein-coding transcripts, with many regulated during development and growth and showing altered regulation in disease progression [81–84]. Recent transcriptome analysis has revealed that the expression of many lncRNAs is dysregulated in cancer, and that their expression can be used as signatures that distinguish cancer cells from normal matched tissues [85].

The nuclear-enriched *MALAT1* is one of the best studied cancer-causing lncRNAs [86]. *MALAT1* is involved in RNA alternative splicing and transcriptional control. It contains sequence that is conserved across 33 mammalian species [87] and more recently has been found in the nuclear speckles which are sites of association of splicing factors and pre-mRNA splicing complexes [88]. Following these studies, many lncRNAs have been presented as a new class of cancer-related genes with potential to be used for diagnostic or therapeutic purposes.

Long Non-coding RNA in Melanoma

Recent transcriptome analysis has revealed that a large number of lncRNAs are expressed differentially in melanoma when compared to normal tissues. The potential roles of some of these lncRNAs are summarised in Table 7.2 [10, 89]. The regulatory role of lncRNAs as epigenetic modulators is well established. However their

Table 7.2 List of lncRNAs involved in melanoma

Long ncRNA	Function	Ref
ANRIL	Correlated with p16	[146]
BANCR	Tumour suppressor	[100]
CASC15	Oncogene	[147]
HOTAIR	Oncogene	[148]
LIMe23	Oncogene	[149]
MALAT1	Oncogene	[97]
MIR31HG	Anti-correlated with p16	[94]
PAUPAR	Tumour suppressor	[95]
PTENP1	Tumour suppressor	[150]
SAMMSON	Oncogene	[102]
SLNCR1	Oncogene	[151]
SPRY4-IT1	Oncogene	[152]
UCA1	Oncogene	[97]

functions are diverse, depending on their subcellular localisation and binding partners. NcRNAs are able to target chromatin architecture to facilitate the modification of various proteins in chromatin. LncRNAs such as *HOTAIR* [90], *ANRIL* [91–93] and *MIR31HG* [94] have been reported to interact with polycomb repressor complexes (PRC) to suppress the expression of target genes.

It is also suggested that *PAUPAR* lncRNA may interact with histone-modifying complexes to inhibit histone H3K4 methylation and modulate the expression of the transcription factor *HES1* [95] (Fig. 7.2a). However, the interaction of lncRNAs with PRC complexes has been reported to be promiscuous [96]. Other lncRNAs such as *UCA1* and *MALAT1* contribute to cell migration. Knockdown of these lncRNAs affects cell migration in cultures of melanoma cells [97]. *UCA1* interacts with heterogeneous nuclear ribonucleoprotein (hnRNP) complexes and increases p27 translation in melanoma. *UCA1* can also be targeted by *miR-507* in melanoma cells. *miR-507* on the other hand can target *FOXM1* [98], a transcription factor that is elevated and activated in malignant melanoma [99]. Therefore, *FOXM1* can be down-regulated by either up-regulation of *miR-507* or depletion of *UCA1* (Fig. 7.2b).

The up-regulation of the lncRNA *SLNCR1* in melanoma has been reported. The brain-specific homeobox protein 3a (Brn3a) and the androgen receptor (AR) bind within and adjacent to *SLNCR1*'s conserved region, respectively. The transcriptional activation of matrix metalloprotein-

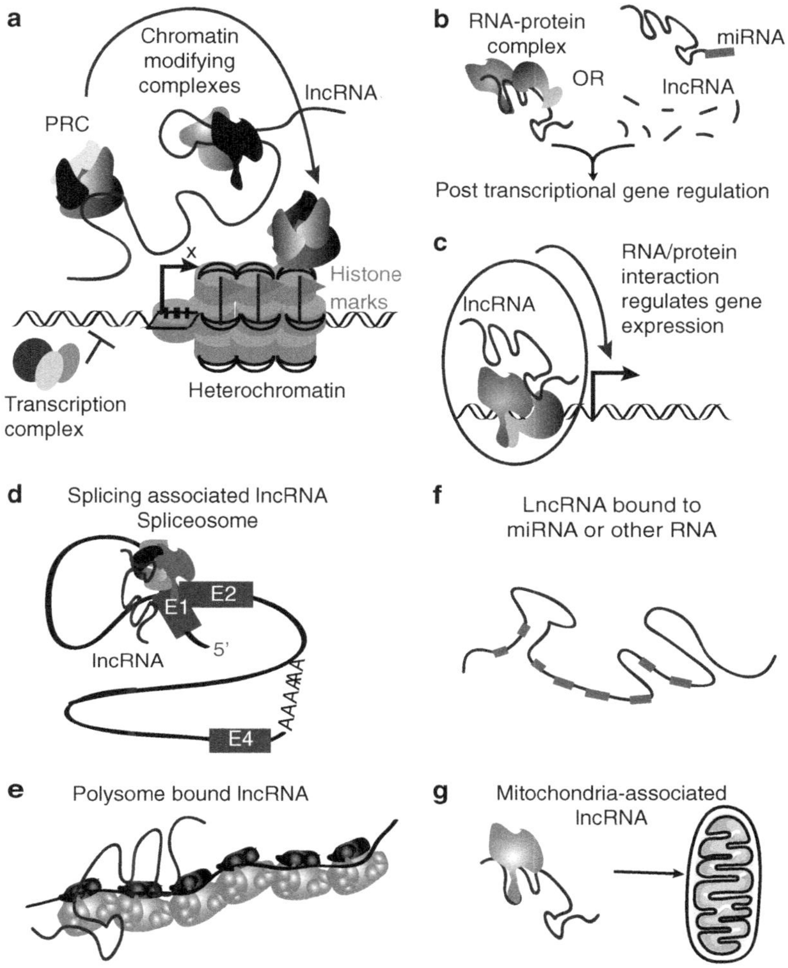

Fig. 7.2 Regulatory roles of lncRNA in melanoma. (**a**) LncRNAs interact with PRCs to suppress gene transcription. (**b**) LncRNAs interact with hnRNP, which regulates the translation of mRNAs. Alternatively, a regulatory lncRNA is targeted by a miRNA that leads to its degradation resulting in gene regulation. (**c**) LncRNAs interact with proteins to regulate gene expression. (**d**) LncRNAs interact with splicing factors to regulate the splicing of pre-mRNAs. (**e**) LncRNAs interact with polysomes to regulate the translation of certain mRNAs. (**f**) LncRNAs can bind to small RNAs such as miRNAs and suppress their function. (**g**) LncRNAs interact with proteins to regulate mitochondrial function

ase 9 (MMP9) that increases melanoma invasion requires assembly of the *SLNCR1*, Brn3a and AR complex (Fig. 7.2c). Other nuclear lncRNAs such as Llme23 are exclusively expressed in melanoma cells and regulate splicing. Llme23 knockdown has significant effects on cell growth (Fig. 7.2d).

On the other hand, cytoplasmic lncRNAs such as *SPRY4-IT* and *PTENP1* have diverse functions. *SPRY4-IT* is a polysome-associated RNA and regulates the abundance of the lipid phosphatase lipin 2 (Fig. 7.2e), while *PTENP1* acts as a positive regulator of *PTEN* mRNA by binding to *PTEN*-targeted miRNA and suppressing the binding of the miRNA to its target site (Fig. 7.2f). The *BANCR* transcript is up-regulated in BRAF^{V600E} mutant primary melanoma and acts in trans to regulate the expression of genes involved in cell migration [100]. *BANCR* also activates the ERK1/2 and JNK MAPK pathways to promote proliferation in melanoma [101], although the mechanism of action is not fully understood.

The lncRNA *SAMMSON* gene is amplified consistently with the melanoma-specific oncogene *MITF*. These two genes are both located in 3p13–3p14 and their amplification had been reported in more than 10% of melanoma cases [102]. *SAMMSON* is also a target of the transcription factor SOX10 and its expression is detected in more than 90% of human melanomas. Knockdown of *SAMMSON* reduces melanoma cell viability and clonogenicity regardless of whether the *BRAF*, *NRAS*, or *TP53* genes are mutated. Knockdown of *SAMMSON* also further reduces the viability of melanoma cells treated with BRAF^{V600E}- and

MEK-targeted agents (vemurafenib and pimasertib, respectively). The interaction of *SAMMSON* and p32, a regulator of mitochondrial homeostasis and metabolism, reveals evidence for *SAMMSON* silencing and perturbation of mitochondrial function (Fig. 7.2g) [102].

Other lncRNAs such as *CASC5* regulate gene expression in melanoma cells, although the mechanism of action of this transcript remains to be clarified. Figure 7.2 summarises the various mechanisms by which lncRNA can regulate gene expression in melanoma.

Small Nucleolar RNA

The small nucleolar RNAs (snoRNAs) are relatively small RNAs in the range of 70–200 nucleotides involved in ribosomal RNA (rRNA) modifications. There are two major classes of snoRNAs: box C/D and H/ACA [103, 104]. This classification is based on the conserved sequences in each family. SnoRNAs from the C/D box family share sequence motifs UGAUGA (box C) and CUGA (box D) at the 5′ and 3′ ends, respectively. The 5′ and 3′ ends of C/D box snoRNAs normally base-pair and expose the C and D boxes (Fig. 7.3) to form a K-turn that creates a motif that is bound to specific proteins to make ribonucleoproteins (snoRNPs).

Most of the C/D box snoRNAs contain C- and D-like motifs called C′ and D' boxes that are separated by a short spacer sequence (Fig. 7.3). C/D box snoRNAs normally process rRNAs by guiding snoRNPs to evolutionarily conserved complementary sequences of rRNA and methylating particular bases in rRNA (Fig. 7.3) [105]. The H/ACA box snoRNA family on the other hand is characterised by the ANANNA motif (box H) and is a highly conserved ACA (ACA box) motif. Most of the H/ACA snoRNAs fold into a hairpin-hinge-hairpin-tail structure. The hinge and tail, which are single-stranded regions, contain the H and ACA motifs, respectively (Fig. 7.3). Box ACA is always positioned three nucleotides upstream from the 3′ end, shown as NNN in the ACA box in Fig. 7.3. The internal loops located close to the base of the hairpins usually contain short sequences that are complementary to rRNA sequences that undergo base modification (pseudouridylation Ψ) [103, 106] (Fig. 7.3).

The functions of snoRNAs in recent years have been expanded and shown to be involved in the modification of small nuclear or snRNAs that mediate mRNA splicing [107]. Also snoRNA

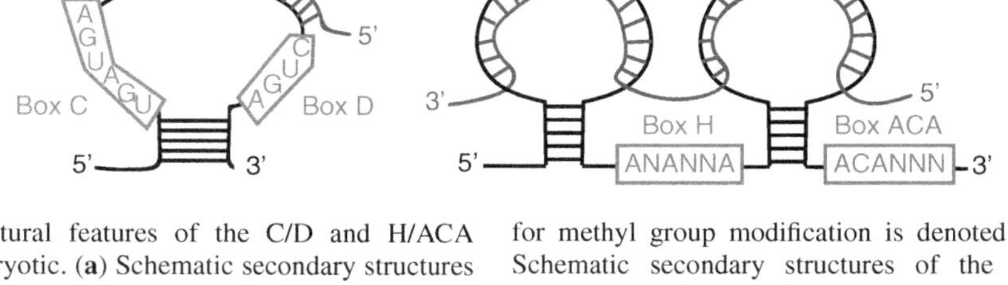

Fig. 7.3 Structural features of the C/D and H/ACA classes of eukaryotic. (**a**) Schematic secondary structures of the C/D box snoRNA. The 5′–3′ terminal stem allowing the formation of the box C/D structural motif. Box C and D conserved motifs are shown in green and blue, respectively. The sequence tracts complementary to the RNA target are depicted in red. The nucleotide targeted for methyl group modification is denoted by CH_3. (**b**) Schematic secondary structures of the H/ACA box snoRNA. Box H and ACA conserved motifs are shown in green and blue, respectively. The sequence tracts complementary to the RNA target are depicted in red. The nucleotide targeted for modification by pseudouridylation is denoted by N Ψ

transcripts can serve as the precursors of miRNA-like small RNAs and regulate alternative splicing [108, 109]. It was also found that 20–25-nucleotide-long RNAs could be produced by the processing of the H/ACA box snoRNA species, known as ACA45.

The processed RNA is associated with Argonaut proteins and targets specific mRNAs, including *CDK11* [108]. A subset of miRNAs also share functional H/ACA box snoRNA characteristics and it has been suggested that these miRNAs might have evolved from snoRNAs [110]. Moreover, it was shown that some snoRNAs could be processed to produce smaller RNAs, of which some have similar functions to miRNAs. Since miRNAs play crucial role in different functions, such as cell survival and proliferation, such processing of snoRNAs could be of crucial importance.

SnoRNA in Melanoma

The first report of down-regulation of snoRNA in human meningioma was reported by Chang et al. in 2002 [111]. Following this finding, the differential expression of snoRNA in hepatocellular carcinoma [112], prostate cancer [113, 114] and B-cell lymphoma was shown [115]. Many genes hosting snoRNA sequences are deregulated in cancer [116–120]. The *SNHG5* gene specifies a 524 bp lncRNA hosting *snoRNA50A/B*. It is located on chromosome 6q15 at the breakpoint of the chromosomal translocation t(3,6)(q27;q15); this site is involved in human B-cell lymphoma [115]. Recently, somatic *SNORD50A/B* deletions in melanoma have been reported and are associated with reduced survival rates [121].

SNORD50A/B specifies two C/D box snoRNAs that target *28S* rRNA, although this housekeeping function of these snoRNAs has no link to their carcinogenic effects. Both of these snoRNAs bind to K-Ras4A and K-Ras4B, with residues involved in RNA binding. These are widely distributed in K-Ras while a 7-nucleotide oligo derived from the C box largely abolishes this binding. This finding not only indicated the involvement of snoRNA in melanoma but also showed that snoRNAs are located both in the nucleolus and outside the nucleus. The phenotype consequent upon the deletion of *snoRNA50A* is the result of snoRNA deletion rather than that of its host gene [121]. On the other hand, up-regulation of *SNHG5* in the serum of melanoma patients has been reported [122]. This suggests that *SNHG5* may play some role in melanogenesis and/or melanoma metastasis independent of *snoRNA50A/B* although further investigations are required to fully address this question.

MicroRNA

MicroRNA (miRNA) is categorized as single-stranded small (~22 nucleotide) ncRNAs that target the 3′-untranslated region of mRNA to inhibit their expression. The number of identified functional roles of miRNA in various cancers has grown immensely over the past decade. miRNA genes are transcribed either independently or coexpressed from an intron of another gene by RNA polymerase II. The primary transcript of individual or coexpressed miRNAs is processed in the nucleus to generate precursor miRNAs of about 70 nucleotides. The precursor miRNAs are actively transported into the cytoplasm by exportin-5. In the cytoplasm, they bind to an RNase III-type endonuclease Dicer that processes the precursor miRNAs to mature miRNAs (Fig. 7.4). Single-stranded mature miRNAs then bind to the RNA-induced silencing complex (RISC), which guides them to their target sites [123].

miRNA in Melanoma

Melanoma-associated miRNAs are known to deregulate the expression of important genes in signalling pathways involved in different aspects of melanin synthesis and metastasis. Understanding the role of miRNA in melanoma progression and its metastasis will help us to develop miRNA-targeted therapy. More than 80% of melanoma cell lines have copy number

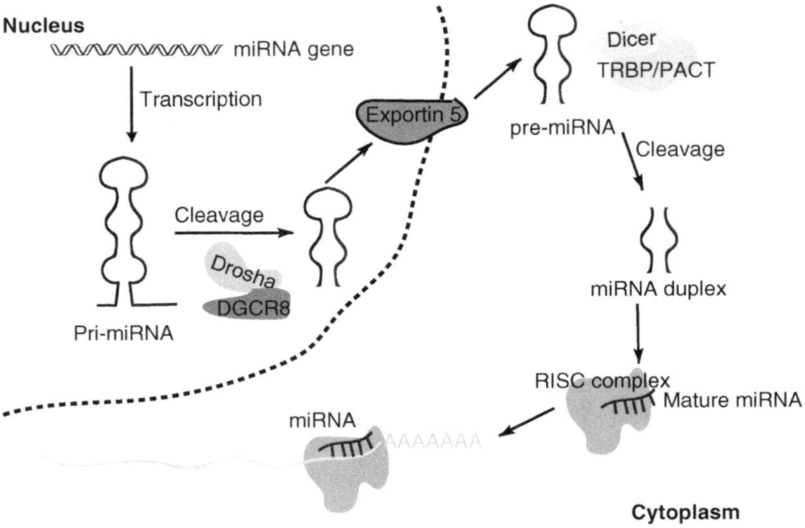

Fig. 7.4 Pathway involved in miRNA synthesis. miRNA is transcribed in the nucleus as primary miRNA (Pri-miRNA). It is then processed by the Drosha/DCGR8 complex to pre-miRNA and actively exported to the cytoplasm. In the cytoplasm, pre-miRNA is processed to miRNA duplexes by the Dicer complex. Single-stranded mature miRNA then is loaded on the RISC complex and binds to the 3' UTR of mRNAs

variation in genomic regions containing miRNA genes and some of these are melanoma specific [124]. Some of the differentially expressed miRNAs can be used as diagnostic markers as they are unique to melanoma cells (reviewed in [125]).

MITF plays key roles in cell proliferation and apoptosis and its expression is deregulated in 10–20% of human melanomas. Therefore, miRNAs associated with *MITF* have been studied extensively. Some miRNAs such as *miR-137* are located at the chromosomal region 1p22, which is a melanoma-susceptible region affecting *MITF* regulation. Another miRNA with a significant role in melanoma is *miR-182*, located in 7q31-34, and harbours the *c-Met* and *BRAF* genes. Both of these genes are important regulators of the MAPK/ERK signalling pathway [125]. The *miR-148* binds to the *MITF* 3'UTR, and down-regulates this transcript [126]. *MITF* also regulates the expression of many miRNAs [127] and the functional significance of some of these has been investigated extensively (reviewed in [125]).

A more recent study has shown that melanosomes carry miRNAs into fibroblasts, which lead to increased proliferation, migration, and proinflammatory gene expression. Among melanosomal miRNAs, *miR-211* targets *IGF2R* and activates the MAPK signalling pathway [128].

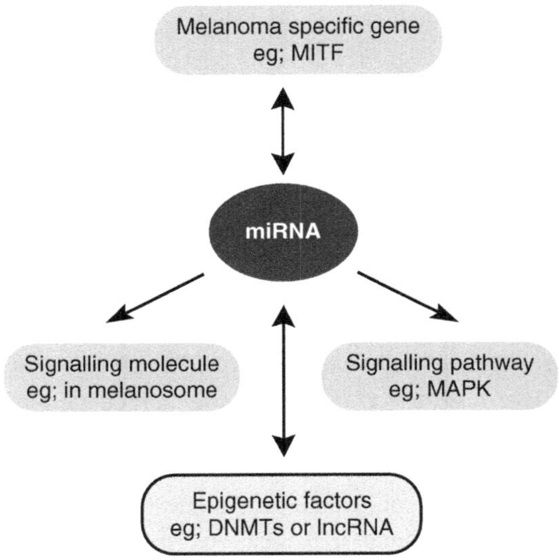

Fig. 7.5 Functions of miRNA in melanoma. miRNA can target melanoma-specific genes such as *MITF*, signalling pathways involved in melanogenesis and pathways inside melanosomes. miRNAs also regulate and are regulated by epigenetic factors. Differential expression of miRNA would regulate target genes accordingly

The epigenetic regulation of miRNAs can influence the development of melanoma. On the other hand, miRNAs can regulate the expression of epigenesis-related genes such as *DNMT3* [126]. The functions of miRNA in melanoma are summarised in Fig. 7.5 and have been reviewed extensively [10, 124, 125].

Targeting Epigenetic Factors for Therapy

Epigenetic alterations in cancer are potentially mediated by genetic changes. However, there is limited understanding of the extent and impact of genetic mutations on the cancer epigenome. Recent extensive genome sequencing of cancer genomes (mainly by international consortia such as The Cancer Genome Atlas) has provided meaningful insight into genetic mutation of epigenetic modulators (EM). It is now clear that in many cancers, a high proportion of EM genes become mutated. A targeted analysis of 275 genes (including 41 epigenetic regulator genes) in 38 treatment-naïve melanoma samples revealed a high EM mutation rate (92.1% of the patients harboured at least one mutation in an EM gene) [129].

This list of EM genes included histone modification-related genes (*MECOM, MLL2, SETD2*), major chromatin-remodelling genes (*ARID1B, ARID2*) and DNA methylation (*DNMTs*) and demethylation regulator genes (*TET2, IDH1*) [129]. However, the role of these EM mutations in shaping the cancer cell phenotype is yet to be explored. This has substantial therapeutic potential as several drugs are available or in clinical trial that can specifically target these EM genes.

After years of seemingly minimal progress, cancer immunotherapies have recently come to the forefront of therapy for patients with metastatic melanoma. Such immunotherapeutic approaches have clearly demonstrated both durable and long-lasting complete responses in patients with stage 4 disease. Immune checkpoint molecules act as 'brakes' to suppress an excessive immune response when required. However, in cancer, up-regulation of these immune checkpoint molecules allows the tumour cell to evade the host immune response. Monoclonal antibodies targeting immune checkpoints can reactivate antitumour immunity [130]. Two of these antibodies (nivolumab and pembrolizumab) block the activity of one of the most important checkpoints, mediated by the programmed death-ligand-1 or PD-L1 protein.

Although these therapies can be very effective, a large proportion (60–70%) of melanoma patients do not respond to these treatments or many suffer relapse and side effects of these drugs [131]. However, the combination of DNA methylation inhibitors with an anti-PD-L1 antibody has remarkably improved patient responses in clinical trials. This suggests that different epigenetic profiles exist between responding and non-responding patients [132–135]. There is substantial interest in understanding how epigenetic therapy could enhance the efficacy of immunotherapies. The current understanding is that if DNA methylation inhibitors are given first, specific immune signatures are activated, creating an environment in which immunotherapies can act more effectively [136]. Although much more work is required to understand the key regulators of these combinatorial therapies, they hold a tremendous promise to improve patient outcome and survival [134].

New drugs targeting DNA methylation and histone modifications have already been tested and some have been approved by the US Food and Drug Administration (FDA) [137]. Table 7.3 summarises the FDA-approved drugs targeting DNA methylation and histone

Table 7.3 List of drugs targeting epigenetic modulator approved by the FDA [137]

Target	Function	Drug	Cancer type
DNMT	Inhibition of DNA methylation	Azacitidine (Vidaza)	MDS
		Decitabine (Dacogen)	MDS, AML
		Guadecitabine	AML
HDAC	Inhibition of histone deacetylation	Belinostat (Beleodaq)	Peripheral T-cell lymphoma
		Panobinostat (Farydak)	Multiple myeloma
		Romidepsin (Istodax)	Cutaneous T-cell lymphoma
		Vorinostat (Zolinza)	Cutaneous T-cell lymphoma

MDS myelodysplastic syndrome, *AML* acute myeloid leukaemia modification. However, none of these target solid tumours including melanoma.

Single targeted therapies for BRAF and EGFR bearing particular mutations have been used in melanoma and size reductions of tumours detected [138], although in almost all cases drug-resistant cells eventually emerge. Currently combinational therapy with different drugs is being tested, and the future for epigenetic therapies for solid tumours is also relying on a combination of drugs based.

Different histone-modifying enzymes are also being targeted for therapy. EZH2, a catalytic subunit of PRC2 involved in tri-methylation of lysine 27 on histone 3, plays important roles in melanomagenesis. Targeting EZH2 via small-molecule inhibition has been used in preclinical and clinical studies. Although EZH2 inhibitors reduced histone methylation, none of them provided a promising result in melanoma [63].

The use of oligonucleotides as potential drugs for cancer therapy has been investigated extensively in recent years. Diverse classes of oligonucleotides have been used as drugs. These include antisense oligonucleotides (ASOs), siRNAs, miRNAs and aptamers. Several ASOs have been approved by the FDA, although none of them has been offered for cancer therapy yet. A great challenge in using oligonucleotides as drugs is the optimisation of their structures for safety as well as delivery.

The success of using oligonucleotides as drugs similar to small molecules is dependent upon their effects on target sites, and their pharmacokinetics (as defined by absorption, distribution, metabolism and excretion) [139]. Oligonucleotides in targeted therapy either up-regulate [140] or down-regulate gene expression as well as modify RNA splicing [141]. This phenomenon is not limited to targeting mRNA and can be applied to lncRNA. Therefore, using oligonucleotides could be a promising procedure for targeting ncRNAs in cancer therapy.

Conclusion

Epigenetic factors are key elements in cancer progression including that of melanoma. Better understanding of epigenetic processes and alteration of their states in melanoma will provide opportunities to study the disease. It is well established that epigenetic factors are key players in gene regulation and many epigenetic modifier genes themselves can act as tumour suppressor or oncogenes. Therefore, they could be targeted for better diagnosis, therapy and prognosis. Most epigenetic alterations in neoplasia take place prior to genetic alterations and therefore they could be used as early diagnostic markers or therapeutic targets.

References

1. D'Mello SA, et al. Signaling pathways in Melanogenesis. Int J Mol Sci. 2016;17(7)
2. Besaratinia A, Tommasi S. Epigenetics of human melanoma: promises and challenges. J Mol Cell Biol. 2014;6(5):356–67.
3. Miller AJ, Mihm MC Jr. Melanoma. N Engl J Med. 2006;355(1):51–65.
4. Gray-Schopfer V, Wellbrock C, Marais R. Melanoma biology and new targeted therapy. Nature. 2007;445(7130):851–7.
5. Tsao H, et al. Melanoma: from mutations to medicine. Genes Dev. 2012;26(11):1131–55.
6. Ransohoff KJ, et al. Familial skin cancer syndromes: increased melanoma risk. J Am Acad Dermatol. 2016;74(3):423–34. quiz 435-6
7. Law MH, et al. Genome-wide meta-analysis identifies five new susceptibility loci for cutaneous malignant melanoma. Nat Genet. 2015;47(9):987–95.
8. Skolnick MH, Cannon-Albright LA, Kamb A. Genetic predisposition to melanoma. Eur J Cancer. 1994;30A(13):1991–5.
9. Wangari-Talbot J, Chen S. Genetics of melanoma. Front Genet. 2012;3:330.
10. Sarkar D, et al. Epigenetic regulation in human melanoma: past and future. Epigenetics. 2015;10(2):103–21.
11. Youngson NA, Whitelaw E. Transgenerational epigenetic effects. Annu Rev Genomics Hum Genet. 2008;9:233–57.
12. Portela A, Esteller M. Epigenetic modifications and human disease. Nat Biotechnol. 2010;28(10):1057–68.
13. Bestor T, et al. Cloning and sequencing of a cDNA encoding DNA methyltransferase of mouse cells. The carboxyl-terminal domain of the mammalian enzymes is related to bacterial restriction methyltransferases. J Mol Biol. 1988;203(4):971–83.
14. Rodger EJ, Chatterjee A, Morison IM. 5-hydroxymethylcytosine: a potential therapeutic target in cancer. Epigenomics. 2014;6(5):503–14.

15. Jones PA. Functions of DNA methylation: islands, start sites, gene bodies and beyond. Nat Rev Genet. 2012;13(7):484–92.
16. Vogelstein B, et al. Cancer genome landscapes. Science. 2013;339(6127):1546–58.
17. Kulis M, Esteller M. DNA methylation and cancer. Adv Genet. 2010;70:27–56.
18. Liu S, et al. Identification of novel epigenetically modified genes in human melanoma via promoter methylation gene profiling. Pigment Cell Melanoma Res. 2008;21(5):545–58.
19. Muthusamy V, et al. Epigenetic silencing of novel tumor suppressors in malignant melanoma. Cancer Res. 2006;66(23):11187–93.
20. Hoon DS, et al. Profiling epigenetic inactivation of tumor suppressor genes in tumors and plasma from cutaneous melanoma patients. Oncogene. 2004;23(22):4014–22.
21. Lahtz C, et al. Methylation of PTEN as a prognostic factor in malignant melanoma of the skin. J Invest Dermatol. 2010;130(2):620–2.
22. Chatterjee A, et al. Tools and strategies for analysis of genome-wide and gene-specific DNA methylation patterns. Methods Mol Biol. 2017;1537:249–77.
23. Stockwell PA, et al. DMAP: differential methylation analysis package for RRBS and WGBS data. Bioinformatics. 2014;30(13):1814–22.
24. Chatterjee, A., et al., *scan_tcga tools for integrated epigenomic and transcriptomic analysis of tumor subgroups*. Epigenomics, 2016.
25. Seynnaeve B, et al. Genetic and epigenetic alterations of TERT are associated with inferior outcome in adolescent and young adult patients with melanoma. Sci Rep. 2017;7:45704.
26. Koga Y, et al. Genome-wide screen of promoter methylation identifies novel markers in melanoma. Genome Res. 2009;19(8):1462–70.
27. Conway K, et al. DNA-methylation profiling distinguishes malignant melanomas from benign nevi. Pigment Cell Melanoma Res. 2011;24(2):352–60.
28. Gao L, et al. Promoter CpG island hypermethylation in dysplastic nevus and melanoma: CLDN11 as an epigenetic biomarker for malignancy. J Invest Dermatol. 2014;134(12):2957–66.
29. Jin SG, et al. The DNA methylation landscape of human melanoma. Genomics. 2015;106(6):322–30.
30. Marzese DM, et al. Epigenome-wide DNA methylation landscape of melanoma progression to brain metastasis reveals aberrations on homeobox D cluster associated with prognosis. Hum Mol Genet. 2014;23(1):226–38.
31. Lauss M, et al. DNA methylation subgroups in melanoma are associated with proliferative and immunological processes. BMC Med Genet. 2015;8:73.
32. Sigalotti L, et al. Whole genome methylation profiles as independent markers of survival in stage IIIC melanoma patients. J Transl Med. 2012;10:185.
33. Vizoso M, et al. Epigenetic activation of a cryptic TBC1D16 transcript enhances melanoma progression by targeting EGFR. Nat Med. 2015;21(7):741–50.
34. Feinberg AP, Vogelstein B. Hypomethylation distinguishes genes of some human cancers from their normal counterparts. Nature. 1983;301(5895):89–92.
35. Guo X, Xu Y, Zhao Z. In-depth genomic data analyses revealed complex transcriptional and epigenetic dysregulations of BRAFV600E in melanoma. Mol Cancer. 2015;14:60.
36. Chatterjee A, et al. Genome-wide methylation sequencing of paired primary and metastatic cell lines identifies common DNA methylation changes and a role for EBF3 as a candidate epigenetic driver of melanoma metastasis. Oncotarget. 2017;8(4):6085–101.
37. Ross JP, Rand KN, Molloy PL. Hypomethylation of repeated DNA sequences in cancer. Epigenomics. 2010;2(2):245–69.
38. Ecsedi SI, et al. Transposable hypomethylation is associated with metastatic capacity of primary melanomas. Int J Clin Exp Pathol. 2013;6(12):2943–8.
39. Sigalotti L, et al. Promoter methylation controls the expression of MAGE2, 3 and 4 genes in human cutaneous melanoma. J Immunother. 2002;25(1):16–26.
40. Grunau C, et al. Frequent DNA hypomethylation of human juxtacentromeric BAGE loci in cancer. Genes Chromosomes Cancer. 2005;43(1):11–24.
41. Barrow C, et al. Tumor antigen expression in melanoma varies according to antigen and stage. Clin Cancer Res. 2006;12(3 Pt 1):764–71.
42. Gjerstorff MF, Andersen MH, Ditzel HJ. Oncogenic cancer/testis antigens: prime candidates for immunotherapy. Oncotarget. 2015;6(18):15772–87.
43. Baylin SB, Jones PA. A decade of exploring the cancer epigenome - biological and translational implications. Nat Rev Cancer. 2011;11(10):726–34.
44. Mezzanotte JJ, et al. RASSF6 exhibits promoter hypermethylation in metastatic melanoma and inhibits invasion in melanoma cells. Epigenetics. 2014;9(11):1496–503.
45. Hallberg AR, et al. Aberrant CpG methylation of the TFAP2A gene constitutes a mechanism for loss of TFAP2A expression in human metastatic melanoma. Epigenetics. 2014;9(12):1641–7.
46. Aran D, Sabato S, Hellman A. DNA methylation of distal regulatory sites characterizes dysregulation of cancer genes. Genome Biol. 2013;14(3):R21.
47. Coppola CJ. C.R. R, and E.M. Mendenhall, *Identification and function of enhancers in the human genome*. Hum Mol Genet. 2016;25(R2):R190–7.
48. Bell RE, et al. Enhancer methylation dynamics contribute to cancer plasticity and patient mortality. Genome Res. 2016;26(5):601–11.
49. Gallagher SJ, Tiffen JC, Hersey P. Histone modifications, modifiers and readers in melanoma resistance to targeted and immune therapy. Cancers (Basel). 2015;7(4):1959–82.
50. Kouzarides T. Chromatin modifications and their function. Cell. 2007;128(4):693–705.

51. Bannister AJ, Kouzarides T. Regulation of chromatin by histone modifications. Cell Res. 2011;21(3):381–95.
52. Zhang Y, Reinberg D. Transcription regulation by histone methylation: interplay between different covalent modifications of the core histone tails. Genes Dev. 2001;15(18):2343–60.
53. Lee MG, et al. An essential role for CoREST in nucleosomal histone 3 lysine 4 demethylation. Nature. 2005;437(7057):432–5.
54. Fischle W, et al. Regulation of HP1-chromatin binding by histone H3 methylation and phosphorylation. Nature. 2005;438(7071):1116–22.
55. Krishnamoorthy T, et al. Phosphorylation of histone H4 Ser1 regulates sporulation in yeast and is conserved in fly and mouse spermatogenesis. Genes Dev. 2006;20(18):2580–92.
56. Shogren-Knaak M, et al. Histone H4-K16 acetylation controls chromatin structure and protein interactions. Science. 2006;311(5762):844–7.
57. Shogren-Knaak M, Peterson CL. Switching on chromatin - mechanistic role of histone H4-K16 acetylation. Cell Cycle. 2006;5(13):1361–5.
58. Nelson CJ, Santos-Rosa H, Kouzarides T. Proline isomerization of histone H3 regulates lysine methylation and gene expression. Cell. 2006;126(5):905–16.
59. Clements A, et al. Structural basis for histone and phosphohistone binding by the GCN5 histone acetyltransferase. Mol Cell. 2003;12(2):461–73.
60. Zhao R, et al. Implications of genetic and epigenetic alterations of CDKN2A (p16(INK4a)) in cancer. EBioMedicine. 2016;8:30–9.
61. Konieczkowski DJ, et al. A melanoma cell state distinction influences sensitivity to MAPK pathway inhibitors. Cancer Discov. 2014;4(7):816–27.
62. Wilmott JS, et al. Expression of the class 1 histone deacetylases HDAC8 and 3 are associated with improved survival of patients with metastatic melanoma. Mod Pathol. 2015;28(7):884–94.
63. Tiffen J, Gallagher SJ, Hersey P. EZH2: an emerging role in melanoma biology and strategies for targeted therapy. Pigment Cell Melanoma Res. 2015;28(1):21–30.
64. Barsotti AM, et al. Epigenetic reprogramming by tumor-derived EZH2 gain-of-function mutations promotes aggressive 3D cell morphologies and enhances melanoma tumor growth. Oncotarget. 2015;6(5):2928–38.
65. Chen IP, et al. UVA-induced epigenetic regulation of P16(INK4a) in human epidermal keratinocytes and skin tumor derived cells. Photochem Photobiol Sci. 2012;11(1):180–90.
66. Mahmoud F, et al. Role of EZH2 histone methyltrasferase in melanoma progression and metastasis. Cancer Biol Ther. 2016;17(6):579–91.
67. Campos EI, et al. The novel tumour suppressor gene ING1 is overexpressed in human melanoma cell lines. Br J Dermatol. 2002;146(4):574–80.
68. Ondrusova L, et al. MITF-independent pro-survival role of BRG1-containing SWI/SNF complex in melanoma cells. PLoS One. 2013;8(1):e54110.
69. Nikolaev SI, et al. A single-nucleotide substitution mutator phenotype revealed by exome sequencing of human colon adenomas. Cancer Res. 2012;72(23):6279–89.
70. Stark MS, et al. Frequent somatic mutations in MAP 3K5 and MAP 3K9 in metastatic melanoma identified by exome sequencing. Nat Genet. 2012;44(2):165–9.
71. Wei XM, et al. Exome sequencing identifies GRIN2A as frequently mutated in melanoma. Nat Genet. 2011;43(5):442–+.
72. Hodis E, et al. A landscape of driver mutations in melanoma. Cell. 2012;150(2):251–63.
73. Vardabasso C, et al. Histone variants: emerging players in cancer biology. Cell Mol Life Sci. 2014;71(3):379–404.
74. Kapoor A, et al. The histone variant macroH2A suppresses melanoma progression through regulation of CDK8. Nature. 2010;468(7327):1105–9.
75. Duarte, L.F., et al., *Histone H3.3 and its proteolytically processed form drive a cellular senescence programme.* Nat Commun, 2014. 5: p. 5210.
76. Mattick, J.S. and I.V. Makunin, *Non-coding RNA.* Hum Mol Genet, 2006. **15 Spec No 1**: p. R17-29.
77. Mattick JS. Non-coding RNAs: the architects of eukaryotic complexity. EMBO Rep. 2001;2(11):986–91.
78. Ponting CP, Oliver PL, Reik W. Evolution and functions of long noncoding RNAs. Cell. 2009;136(4):629–41.
79. Carthew RW, Sontheimer EJ. Origins and mechanisms of miRNAs and siRNAs. Cell. 2009;136(4):642–55.
80. Cech TR, Steitz JA. The noncoding RNA revolution-trashing old rules to forge new ones. Cell. 2014;157(1):77–94.
81. Cabili MN, et al. Integrative annotation of human large intergenic noncoding RNAs reveals global properties and specific subclasses. Genes Dev. 2011;25(18):1915–27.
82. Derrien T, et al. The GENCODE v7 catalog of human long noncoding RNAs: analysis of their gene structure, evolution, and expression. Genome Res. 2012;22(9):1775–89.
83. Hung T, et al. Extensive and coordinated transcription of noncoding RNAs within cell-cycle promoters. Nat Genet. 2011;43(7):621–9.
84. Mercer TR, et al. Specific expression of long noncoding RNAs in the mouse brain. Proc Natl Acad Sci U S A. 2008;105(2):716–21.
85. Yan X, et al. Comprehensive genomic characterization of long non-coding RNAs across human cancers. Cancer Cell. 2015;28(4):529–40.
86. Yoshimoto R, et al. MALAT1 long noncoding RNA in cancer. Biochim Biophys Acta. 2016;1859(1):192–9.

87. Ji P, et al. MALAT-1, a novel noncoding RNA, and thymosin beta4 predict metastasis and survival in early-stage non-small cell lung cancer. Oncogene. 2003;22(39):8031–41.
88. Spector, D.L. and A.I. Lamond, *Nuclear speckles*. Cold Spring Harb Perspect Biol, 2011. **3**(2).
89. Leucci E, et al. The emerging role of long noncoding RNAs in cutaneous melanoma. Pigment Cell Melanoma Res. 2016;29(6):619–26.
90. Wu L, et al. Binding interactions between long noncoding RNA HOTAIR and PRC2 proteins. Biochemistry. 2013;52(52):9519–27.
91. Kotake Y, et al. Long non-coding RNA ANRIL is required for the PRC2 recruitment to and silencing of p15(INK4B) tumor suppressor gene. Oncogene. 2011;30(16):1956–62.
92. Sato K, et al. ANRIL is implicated in the regulation of nucleus and potential transcriptional target of E2F1. Oncol Rep. 2010;24(3):701–7.
93. Yap KL, et al. Molecular interplay of the noncoding RNA ANRIL and methylated histone H3 lysine 27 by polycomb CBX7 in transcriptional silencing of INK4a. Mol Cell. 2010;38(5):662–74.
94. Montes M, et al. The lncRNA MIR31HG regulates p16(INK4A) expression to modulate senescence. Nat Commun. 2015;6:6967.
95. Ding X, et al. PAUPAR lncRNA suppresses tumourigenesis by H3K4 demethylation in uveal melanoma. FEBS Lett. 2016;590(12):1729–38.
96. Davidovich C, et al. Toward a consensus on the binding specificity and promiscuity of PRC2 for RNA. Mol Cell. 2015;57(3):552–8.
97. Tian Y, et al. Potential roles of abnormally expressed long noncoding RNA UCA1 and Malat-1 in metastasis of melanoma. Melanoma Res. 2014;24(4):335–41.
98. Wei Y, et al. LncRNA UCA1-miR-507-FOXM1 axis is involved in cell proliferation, invasion and G0/G1 cell cycle arrest in melanoma. Med Oncol. 2016;33(8):88.
99. Kruiswijk F, et al. Targeted inhibition of metastatic melanoma through interference with Pin1-FOXM1 signaling. Oncogene. 2016;35(17):2166–77.
100. Flockhart RJ, et al. BRAFV600E remodels the melanocyte transcriptome and induces BANCR to regulate melanoma cell migration. Genome Res. 2012;22(6):1006–14.
101. Li R, et al. Long non-coding RNA BANCR promotes proliferation in malignant melanoma by regulating MAPK pathway activation. PLoS One. 2014;9(6):e100893.
102. Leucci E, et al. Melanoma addiction to the long non-coding RNA SAMMSON. Nature. 2016;531(7595):518–22.
103. Bachellerie JP, Cavaille J, Huttenhofer A. The expanding snoRNA world. Biochimie. 2002;84(8):775–90.
104. Weinstein LB, Steitz JA. Guided tours: from precursor snoRNA to functional snoRNP. Curr Opin Cell Biol. 1999;11(3):378–84.
105. Cavaille J, Bachellerie JP. SnoRNA-guided ribose methylation of rRNA: structural features of the guide RNA duplex influencing the extent of the reaction. Nucleic Acids Res. 1998;26(7):1576–87.
106. Ganot P, Caizergues-Ferrer M, Kiss T. The family of box ACA small nucleolar RNAs is defined by an evolutionarily conserved secondary structure and ubiquitous sequence elements essential for RNA accumulation. Genes Dev. 1997;11(7):941–56.
107. Kishore S, Stamm S. The snoRNA HBII-52 regulates alternative splicing of the serotonin receptor 2C. Science. 2006;311(5758):230–2.
108. Ender C, et al. A human snoRNA with microRNA-like functions. Mol Cell. 2008;32(4):519–28.
109. Kishore S, et al. The snoRNA MBII-52 (SNORD 115) is processed into smaller RNAs and regulates alternative splicing. Hum Mol Genet. 2010;19(7):1153–64.
110. Ono M, et al. Identification of human miRNA precursors that resemble box C/D snoRNAs. Nucleic Acids Res. 2011;39(9):3879–91.
111. Chang LS, et al. Differential expression of human 5S snoRNA genes. Biochem Biophys Res Commun. 2002;299(2):196–200.
112. Donsante A, et al. AAV vector integration sites in mouse hepatocellular carcinoma. Science. 2007;317(5837):477.
113. Dong XY, et al. Implication of snoRNA U50 in human breast cancer. J Genet Genomics. 2009;36(8):447–54.
114. Dong XY, et al. SnoRNA U50 is a candidate tumor-suppressor gene at 6q14.3 with a mutation associated with clinically significant prostate cancer. Hum Mol Genet. 2008;17(7):1031–42.
115. Tanaka R, et al. Intronic U50 small-nucleolar-RNA (snoRNA) host gene of no protein-coding potential is mapped at the chromosome breakpoint t(3;6)(q27;q15) of human B-cell lymphoma. Genes Cells. 2000;5(4):277–87.
116. Askarian-Amiri ME, et al. SNORD-host RNA Zfas1 is a regulator of mammary development and a potential marker for breast cancer. RNA. 2011;17(5):878–91.
117. Liao J, et al. Small nucleolar RNA signatures as biomarkers for non-small-cell lung cancer. Mol Cancer. 2010;9:198.
118. Mourtada-Maarabouni M, et al. Growth arrest in human T-cells is controlled by the non-coding RNA growth-arrest-specific transcript 5 (GAS5). J Cell Sci. 2008;121(Pt 7):939–46.
119. Mourtada-Maarabouni M, et al. GAS5, a non-protein-coding RNA, controls apoptosis and is downregulated in breast cancer. Oncogene. 2009;28(2):195–208.
120. Pickard MR, Mourtada-Maarabouni M, Williams GT. Long non-coding RNA GAS5 regulates apoptosis in prostate cancer cell lines. Biochim Biophys Acta. 2013;1832(10):1613–23.
121. Siprashvili Z, et al. The noncoding RNAs SNORD50A and SNORD50B bind K-Ras and are

recurrently deleted in human cancer. Nat Genet. 2016;48(1):53–8.
122. Ichigozaki Y, et al. Serum long non-coding RNA, snoRNA host gene 5 level as a new tumor marker of malignant melanoma. Exp Dermatol. 2016;25(1):67–9.
123. Valencia-Sanchez MA, et al. Control of translation and mRNA degradation by miRNAs and siRNAs. Genes Dev. 2006;20(5):515–24.
124. Zhang L, et al. microRNAs exhibit high frequency genomic alterations in human cancer. Proc Natl Acad Sci U S A. 2006;103(24):9136–41.
125. Howell PM Jr, et al. MicroRNA in melanoma. Ochsner J. 2010;10(2):83–92.
126. Bemis LT, et al. MicroRNA-137 targets microphthalmia-associated transcription factor in melanoma cell lines. Cancer Res. 2008;68(5):1362–8.
127. Ozsolak F, et al. Chromatin structure analyses identify miRNA promoters. Genes Dev. 2008;22(22):3172–83.
128. Dror, S., et al., *Melanoma miRNA trafficking controls tumour primary niche formation.* Nat Cell Biol, 2016. **18**(9): p. 1006-17.
129. Lee JJ, et al. Targeted next-generation sequencing reveals high frequency of mutations in epigenetic regulators across treatment-naive patient melanomas. Clin Epigenetics. 2015;7:59.
130. Pardoll DM. The blockade of immune checkpoints in cancer immunotherapy. Nat Rev Cancer. 2012;12(4):252–64.
131. Robert C, et al. Pembrolizumab versus Ipilimumab in advanced melanoma. N Engl J Med. 2015;372(26):2521–32.
132. Dear AE. Epigenetic modulators and the new immunotherapies. N Engl J Med. 2016;374(7):684–6.
133. Wrangle J, et al. Alterations of immune response of non-small cell lung cancer with Azacytidine. Oncotarget. 2013;4(11):2067–79.
134. Maio M, et al. Molecular pathways: at the crossroads of cancer epigenetics and immunotherapy. Clin Cancer Res. 2015;21(18):4040–7.
135. Chiappinelli KB, et al. Inhibiting DNA methylation causes an interferon response in cancer via dsRNA including endogenous retroviruses. Cell. 2016;164(5):1073.
136. Chiappinelli KB, et al. Inhibiting DNA methylation causes an interferon response in cancer via dsRNA including endogenous retroviruses. Cell. 2015;162(5):974–86.
137. Jones PA, Issa JP, Baylin S. Targeting the cancer epigenome for therapy. Nat Rev Genet. 2016;17(10):630–41.
138. Poulikakos PI, Rosen N. Mutant BRAF melanomas--dependence and resistance. Cancer Cell. 2011;19(1):11–5.
139. Khvorova A, Watts JK. The chemical evolution of oligonucleotide therapies of clinical utility. Nat Biotechnol. 2017;35(3):238–48.
140. Liang, X.H., et al., *Translation efficiency of mRNAs is increased by antisense oligonucleotides targeting upstream open reading frames.* Nature Biotechnology, 2016. **34**(8): p. 875−+.
141. Lundin KE, Gissberg O, Smith CI. Oligonucleotide therapies: the past and the present. Hum Gene Ther. 2015;26(8):475–85.
142. Witt O, et al. HDAC family: what are the cancer relevant targets? Cancer Lett. 2009;277(1):8–21.
143. Nathan D, Sterner DE, Berger SL. Histone modifications: now summoning sumoylation. Proc Natl Acad Sci U S A. 2003;100(23):13118–20.
144. Koch-Nolte F, et al. Mammalian ADP-ribosyltransferases and ADP-ribosylhydrolases. Front Biosci. 2008;13:6716–29.
145. Moss J. A. Zolkiewska, and I. Okazaki, *ADP-ribosylarginine hydrolases and ADP-ribosyltransferases. Partners in ADP-ribosylation cycles.* Adv Exp Med Biol. 1997;419:25–33.
146. Pasmant E, et al. Characterization of a germ-line deletion, including the entire INK4/ARF locus, in a melanoma-neural system tumor family: identification of ANRIL, an antisense noncoding RNA whose expression coclusters with ARF. Cancer Res. 2007;67(8):3963–9.
147. Lessard L, et al. The CASC15 long Intergenic noncoding RNA locus is involved in melanoma progression and phenotype switching. J Invest Dermatol. 2015;135(10):2464–74.
148. Tang L, et al. Long noncoding RNA HOTAIR is associated with motility, invasion, and metastatic potential of metastatic melanoma. Biomed Res Int. 2013;2013:251098.
149. Wu CF, et al. The non-coding RNA llme23 drives the malignant property of human melanoma cells. J Genet Genomics. 2013;40(4):179–88.
150. Poliseno L, et al. Deletion of PTENP1 pseudogene in human melanoma. J Invest Dermatol. 2011;131(12):2497–500.
151. Schmidt K, et al. The lncRNA SLNCR1 mediates melanoma invasion through a conserved SRA1-like region. Cell Rep. 2016;15(9):2025–37.
152. Khaitan D, et al. The melanoma-upregulated long noncoding RNA SPRY4-IT1 modulates apoptosis and invasion. Cancer Res. 2011;71(11):3852–62.

Immunobiology of the Melanoma Microenvironment

8

Yutaka Kawakami and Adam I. Riker

Introduction

Melanoma has been recognized as one of the cancers that respond to immunotherapies and the best human cancer model to investigate the immunopathology of cancer. The recent analyses on the patients treated with immune checkpoint blockade therapies including PD-1/PD-L1 and CTLA-4 inhibitors led to great progress in our understanding of the immunobiology of human melanoma. The response rate of the PD-1/PD-L1 antibody therapy is ~30%, so that the identification of biomarkers to select appropriate patients who are likely to respond to immunotherapies is essential. Appropriate immunotherapies such as immune checkpoint inhibitors or gene-engineered, high-avidity T-cell-based adoptive immunotherapies are needed to further advance our understanding of the immunobiology of melanoma.

The immune status in tumor-associated microenvironments such as tumor tissue, sentinel lymph nodes, peripheral blood, and bone marrow is different among cancer patients. It is correlated with prognosis following standard therapies in patients with various cancers, including melanoma. The cancer immune status may be defined by cancer cell's genetic characteristics, patients' immune reactivity, and environmental factors. It varies among cancer types, subtypes, and individual patients. In melanoma, there may be differences among disease subtypes (e.g., superficial spreading, acral lentiginous, mucosal melanoma), cancer gene alterations (e.g., DNA mutations generating immunogenic neo-antigens, oncogenes, and somatic copy number alterations causing immune resistance), and environmental factors (e.g., intestinal microbiota). Further understanding of the cancer immunobiology will lead to the identification of new biomarkers for predicting patient outcome, as well as new therapeutic targets for developing effective combination immunotherapy.

Y. Kawakami, M.D., Ph.D. (✉)
Division of Cellular Signaling, Institute for Advanced Medical Research, Keio University School of Medicine, Tokyo, Japan
e-mail: yutakawa@keio.jp

A. I. Riker, M.D., F.A.C.S
Section of Surgical Oncology, Department of Surgery, Louisiana State University, School of Medicine, LSU Health-New Orleans, New Orleans, LA, USA
e-mail: ariker@lsuhsc.edu

T-Cell-Inflamed and Non-inflamed Conditions in Tumors

The initial immunological analyses of tumor tissues prior to initiating treatment within a clinical trial of PD-1/PD-L1 blockade revealed an accumulation of $CD8^+$ T cells at peri- or intratumoral sites. Additionally, IFN-γ production was noted by those $CD8^+$ T cells and PD-L1 expression in melanoma cells or tumor-

A. I. Riker (ed.), *Melanoma*, https://doi.org/10.1007/978-3-319-78310-9_8

infiltrating macrophages were significantly correlated with the response to anti-PD-1 blocking antibody [1–3]. This situation was often referred to as "T-cell inflamed," and about 40% of melanoma patients have such "T-cell-inflamed" tumors [4, 5], with other melanoma patients identified as "T-cell non-inflamed." When immunological changes following PD-1/PD-L1 blockade were evaluated, the peri- and intra-tumor CD8⁺ T cells were found to expand in the tumors and appeared to eradicate melanoma cells. The T-cell repertoire appeared to be skewed, possibly against immunogenic tumor antigens including DNA mutation-derived antigens (neo-antigens). Such phenomenon was not observed in nonresponders (no T-cell infiltration and expansion in tumors and no production of IFN-γ or expression of PD-L1). Therefore, preexisting T-cell immunity, "T-cell inflamed," appeared to be essential for the response to PD-1/PD-L1 therapy in melanoma (Fig. 8.1).

Expansion of Preexisting Partially Exhausted CD8⁺ T Cells Following PD-1/PD-L1 Blockade

Since tumor-infiltrating T lymphocytes (TILs) appear to be important for PD-1/PD-L1 therapy, further characterization of TIL was performed. The high percentage of the partially exhausted PD-1^{hi} CTLA-4^{hi} CD8⁺ T cells producing IFN-γ, but not TNF-α (partially exhausted, loss of multi-functionality), in melanoma tissues prior to therapy was correlated with the response to PD-1 antibody therapy [6]. Interestingly, more completely exhausted T cells through epigenetic changes, such as chromatin remodeling and DNA methylation, may not be reinvigorated by PD-1/PD-L1 blockade. Similarly, other reports indicated that exhausted CD8⁺ T cells (Tex) (e.g., Ki67⁺ CD38⁺ HLA-DR⁺ PD-1^{hi} CTLA-4^{hi} CD45RA^{lo} CD27^{hi} Eomes^{hi} T-bet ^{lo} 2B4^{hi} CD8⁺ T cells) in peripheral blood and tumors expand following PD-1/PD-L1 therapy, and were associated

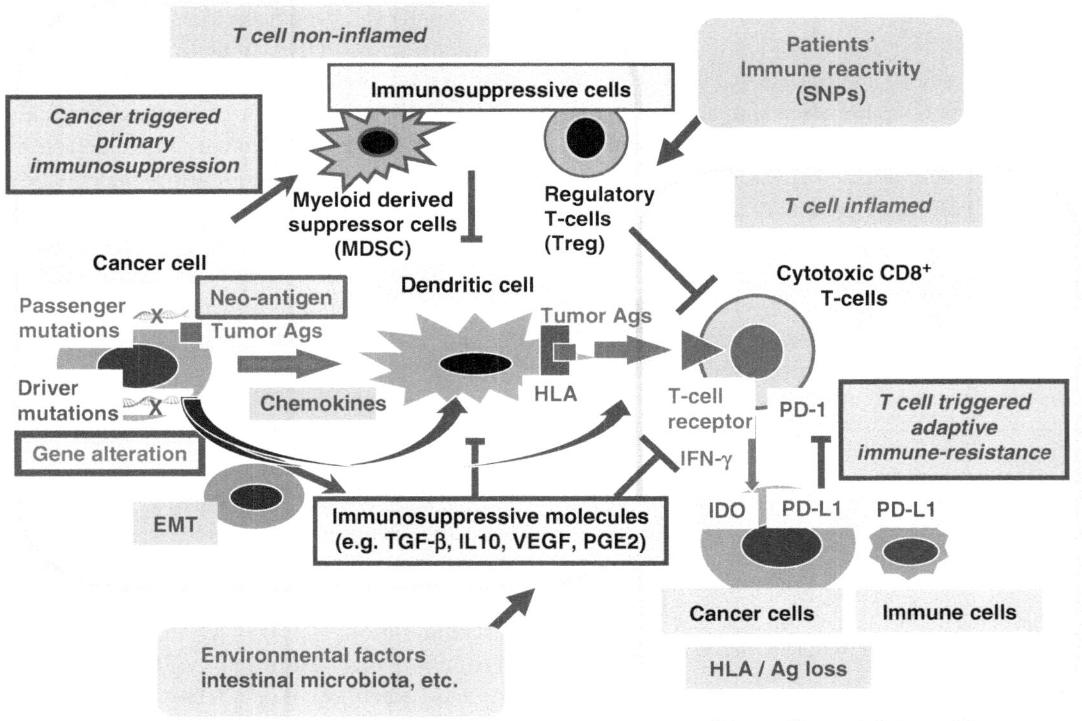

Fig. 8.1 T-cell-inflamed and non-inflamed immune status in melanoma

with responses to PD-1/PD-L1 therapy [7, 8)]. One recent report indicated that the amount of such Tex is proportional to tumor burdens, with the ratio of such expanded Tex cells in peripheral blood and tumor burden correlating with the response of melanoma patients to PD-1/PD-L1 therapy [7]. These results suggest that reinvigorated, expanded Tex may be responsible for eradication of melanoma. However, in murine tumor models, induction of antitumor T cells in lymphoid organs appears to be important for antitumor effects of PD-1/PD-L1 blockade. The involvement of newly induced tumor antigen-specific T cells from naïve T cells (antigen spreading) in the regression of melanoma following MAGE vaccine was previously reported [9]. Therefore, the importance of the induction phase including CD28$^+$ PD-1$^+$ stem cell-like memory T cells in lymph nodes for antitumor activity of PD-1/PD-L1 blockade remains to be further investigated by confirmation of the presence of newly induced tumor antigen-specific T cells in tumors and their antitumor activity after PD-1/PD-L1 blockade.

Tumor Antigens Recognized by Tumor-Infiltrating T Cells and Relation to the Response to Immune Checkpoint Inhibitors

What are the important tumor antigens for TILs to recognize in order to eradicate melanoma cells following PD-1/PD-L1 blockade? We have extensively investigated and identified numerous melanoma antigens that are recognized by TILs [10, 11]. TILs recognize a variety of tumor antigens including neo-antigens derived from DNA mutations, cancer testis antigens (proteins expressed in various cancer cells, but not in normal adult tissues in the exception of special tissues such as testis and placenta), melanocyte lineage differentiation antigens (e.g., melanocyte-related proteins such as MART-1/Melan-A, gp100, tyrosinase, and TRP1/2), and several others.

Among these melanoma antigens, neo-antigens recognized by TILs are generally tumor-specific antigens derived from missense mutations of passenger DNA mutations, considered highly immunogenic and unique to each patient [12]. Melanoma cells, particularly of the superficial spreading subtype, contain a relatively high mutation burden as a result of UV irradiation [13]. Interestingly, patients with higher mutation burdens have significantly better over-survival (OS) following treatment with immune checkpoint blockade with anti-CTLA-4 mAb and anti-PD-1/PD-L1 mAb [14].

The DNA mutations found in a primary melanoma are mainly caused by UV irradiation (UV signature), but other causes may also contribute to the increase in such deleterious mutations. One study showed that the presence of BRCA2 gene mutation that causes hyper-DNA mutation via dysfunction of DNA repair was correlated with a favorable outcome after anti-PD-1 therapy [15]. Other causes include tobacco use, proofreading-related POLE/POLD1, DNA repair-related BRCA1, and DNA mismatch repair (MMR) proteins such as hMLH1. These are all involved in the generation of trunk DNA mutations and are reported to create immunogenic neo-antigens for a subsequent immune response to PD-1/PD-L1 blockade.

Several criteria are necessary for DNA mutations to generate immunogenic neo-antigen epitopes. The antigen molecule should be expressed and translated and epitope peptides should be processed by proteases, including the proteasome complex. The peptides should bind to a patient's own MHC with sufficiently high affinity, and the TCR repertoire for the peptides should be readily present. Neo-antigens may be partly predicted using bioinformatics analysis that considers these factors. In addition, direct identification of HLA-binding neo-antigens using mass spectrometry has recently been reported [16]. Lastly, actual recognition of neo-antigens by TILs can be tested by T-cell functional assays. These technologies are currently being applied for development of novel neo-antigen-specific personalized immunotherapies.

Neo-antigen-specific immunotherapies using the NGS-identified neo-antigens have recently been explored by multiple centers around the world. These neo-antigens are unique for each patient, with the development of specific vaccines (synthetic peptides or RNA virus vectors) or T-cell-based adoptive cell therapy (TIL-derived T cells or neo-antigen-specific TCR-transduced T cells). Clinical trials are already in progress for patients with melanoma and other types of cancers, with some clinically significant tumor responses noted to either neo-antigen vaccine alone or in combination, with PD-1 blockade [17, 18]. These are really personalized immunotherapies potentially without severe immune-related adverse effects that are often observed in the patients treated with immune checkpoint inhibitors.

The presence of TIL within the tumor microenvironment is correlated with the recognition of melanocyte-specific proteins such as MART-1/Melan-A, gp100, tyrosinase, and cancer testis antigens as shared melanoma antigens [19, 20]. The adoptive transfer of T cells specific for MART-1/Melan-A or gp100 resulted in melanoma regression, occasionally resulting in the development of vitiligo, uveitis, and other autoimmune disorders, all of which are signs of normal melanocyte destruction [21]. There is a correlation between the occurrence of autoimmune reactions (irRE: immune-related adverse effect) to melanocytes, vitiligo, and antitumor response as it relates to immune checkpoint blockade therapy in melanoma patients [22].

However, anti-tumor activity of melanocyte-specific T cells for non-mutated self-peptides may not be so high, partially due to the relatively low avidity of the TCR and self-tolerance mechanisms. Neo-antigens, on the other hand, are acquired proteins, and may not be identified through central tolerance mechanisms within the thymus. The role of TILs that are specific for melanocyte proteins in immunotherapy for melanoma remains to be further investigated. The role of the cancer testis antigens, such as MAGE and NY-ESO-1, which are tumor-specific, shared tumor antigens, also remains to be investigated. The adoptive transfer of gene-engineered, high-avidity TCR-T cells that are specific for NY-ESO-1 showed a strong immune response and associated tumor regression without irAE [23]. Furthermore, some reports have suggested the involvement of cancer-testis antigens in tumor infiltration of $CD8^+$ T cells and tumor regression following PD-1/PD-L1 blockade.

Adaptive Immune Resistance

In about 40% of melanoma patients, anti-tumor T cells are already induced and accumulated in tumors before therapies (T-cell inflamed), but tumors continue to grow unless immune interventions are applied because of the presence of immune-resistant mechanisms at local tumor sites including PD-1/PD-L1 interaction (adaptive immune resistance) [24]. In addition to PD-1/PD-L1, other inhibitory co-receptors, such as CTLA4, LAG3, TIM3, BTLA, VISTA, and TIGIT, may also be involved in the adaptive immune resistance [25]. TILs expressing multiple inhibitory co-receptors were reported to be more exhausted T cells [26]. Blocking Abs specific for these inhibitory co-receptors have been developed, with some being evaluated in combination with PD-1/PD-L1 blockade in clinical trials.

In addition to the inhibitory receptors, tryptophan-metabolizing enzyme, indoleamine 2,3-dioxygenase (IDO), is also induced by IFN-γ produced by TILs and involved in the adaptive immune resistance [24]. IDO depletes tryptophan important for T-cell responses, and metabolize tryptophan to kynurenine that has an activity to inhibit T cells. T-cell-induced inflammation and chemokines may also recruit immunosuppressive Tregs and inhibit antitumor T-cell responses. Potential antitumor effects of IDO inhibitors in combination with PD-1/PD-L1 blockade have been shown in clinical trials for melanoma patients.

Primary Immune Resistance

In about 60% of melanoma patients, anti-tumor $CD8^+$ T cells have not been well induced and accumulate in tumors prior to treatment with immunotherapy. An improved understanding of the mechanisms (primary immune resistance) may lead to the further development of new therapeutic strategies, particularly in combination with PD-1/PD-L1 blockade.

CTLA4 is a molecule involved in the negative-feedback mechanisms in priming of naïve T cells by professional antigen-presenting cells, such as dendritic cells (DCs). T cells activated via stimulation of TCR/HLA-Ag complex and CD28/CD80/86 express CTLA4, with CTLA4 having higher binding affinity to CD80/86 than CD28, preferentially blocking the CD28/CD80/86 complex. CTLA4 is also involved in one of the suppression mechanisms of regulatory T cells (Tregs), which are constitutively expressed with CTLA4 and suppress DC function. Therefore, CTLA4 blockade results in enhanced priming and induction of antitumor T cells from naïve T cells.

The combination of anti-CTLA4 ab and anti-PD-1 Ab in melanoma resulted in better ORR (about 60%) than either antibody alone (about 30% ORR) [27], possibly through enhanced induction of antitumor T cells and subsequent infiltration into tumor tissues. The combination therapy prolonged survival of the patients with melanoma not expressing PD-L1 at baseline (likely to be T-cell non-inflamed), but no difference in overall survival was observed between the combination and anti-PD-1 antibody monotherapy. This suggested that CTLA4 blockade promoted induction of anti-tumor T cells and converted T-cell non-inflamed to T-cell-inflamed conditions, which is essential for response to PD-1/PD-L1 blockade [28]. Therefore, CTLA4 blockade may overcome primary resistance in some of the melanoma patients.

Oncogenes Responsible for Immune Resistance

Neo-antigens derived from DNA mutations appear to be one of the major targets for anti-tumor T cells, and may reflect $CD8^+$ T-cell infiltrations in tumors. However, total DNA mutation burden, numbers of predicted neo-antigens, or expression of shared melanoma antigens, such as melanocyte antigens and cancer-testis antigens, are not correlated with $CD8^+$ expression in melanoma tissues [29]. $CD8^+$ T-cell accumulation appears to be affected by other factors (Fig. 8.2).

The mechanism of T-cell non-inflamed status in about a half of melanoma patients may be

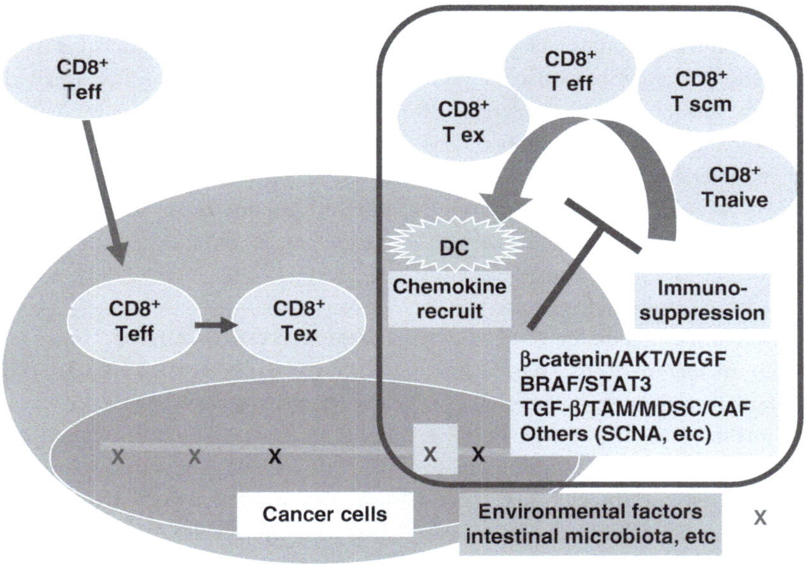

Fig. 8.2 Factors influencing accumulation of antitumor $CD8^+$ T cells in tumors

explained by activated β-catenin signaling in melanoma cells [30]. In the BRAF mutant, PTEN knockout transgenic mouse melanoma model, melanoma cells with activated β-catenin had reduced production of chemokines such as CCL4. They also had reduced recruitment of Batf3-driven CCR5$^+$ CD103$^+$ dendritic cells producing CXCL9/10, and subsequently reduced recruitment of anti-tumor CXCR3$^+$CD8$^+$ T cells into tumors. Similarly in melanoma patients, β-catenin activation may be correlated with reduced Batf3-driven CD141$^+$DC producing CXCL9/10/11 and CXCR3$^+$CD8$^+$ T cells in tumors [31]. We have previously reported intratumoral administration of oncolytic HSV, or partially activated DC, that may restore this type of problems [32, 33]. We have also reported that β-catenin signal activation may also suppress T-cell responses at both induction (partly via IL10-induced suppression of DC) and effector CTL levels. Lastly, it has been shown that a β-catenin inhibitor may restore the DC function of β-catenin-activated melanoma [34].

Melanoma with PTEN loss was also reported to correlate with less CD8$^+$ TILs and poor response to PD-1 blockade therapy [35]. PTEN loss results in AKT signal activation, with one of the AKT downstream molecules identified as VEGF, known to inhibit DC function. An inhibitor for PI3K upstream of AKT signaling or a VEGF inhibitor was shown to restore anti-tumor T cells in murine tumor models. High-serum VEGF was related to a poor response to anti-CTLA4 Ab therapy and combination therapy of anti-VEGF antibody and anti-CTLA4 antibody has been evaluated in several clinical trials [36, 37]. Copy number loss frequently occurs in chromosome 10 that contains the PTEN gene in melanoma, and is inversely correlated with CD8 expression in melanoma [38]. These results indicate that oncogene activation may affect antitumor CD8$^+$ T-cell accumulation into melanoma cells, which have abundant T-cell targets such as neo-antigens. This further indicates that the depletion of these negative factors may enhance CD8$^+$ T-cell infiltration in tumors and may convert non-responders to responders for PD-1/PD-L1 blockade therapies.

BRAF is frequently mutated (common BRAF (V600E) mutation and other mutations) in SSM, and involved in the proliferation and invasion of melanoma cells [39, 40]. Although a BRAF gene mutation is not correlated with the accumulation of CD8$^+$ TILs, it causes MAPK signal activation that may affect T-cell responses [41]. BRAF mutant-selective inhibitors, such as vemurafenib and dabrafenib, inhibit proliferation of melanoma cells with mutant BRAF, but conversely activate T cells with wild-type BRAF through paradoxical activation via CRAF [42]. Along with other mechanisms, such as increased tumor antigen expression, BRAF inhibitors may enhance anti-melanoma T-cell responses. In fact, it is observed that CD8$^+$T cells are significantly increased in regressing melanoma tissues following the administration of BRAF inhibitors [43]. Interestingly, CD8$^+$ T cells disappear and M2-like macrophages increase in tumor microenvironment after drug resistance is acquired for these kinase inhibitors [44]. Thus, target therapy and immunotherapy influenced each other via changes within the tumor microenvironment. Similarly, STAT3 signaling may also be activated in melanoma cells, and may affect immune responses particularly through augmenting STAT3 in various immunosuppressive immune cells such as dendritic cells, macrophages, and Tregs [41, 45].

Other gene alternations, such as somatic copy number alterations (SCNA), particularly aneuploidy, were found to be inversely correlated with CD8 expression in tumors of various cancer types including melanoma, with several possible mechanisms currently being investigated [46]. Since both SCNA and total mutation burden (TMB) are independent, the combination of SCNA and TMB may predict the response to immune checkpoint blockade therapy in melanoma patients better than either alone.

Mesenchymal Tumor Microenvironment Responsible for Immune Resistance

TGF-β is a well-known immunosuppressive factor. We have previously shown that increase of TGF-β within the tumor microenvironment inhibited induction of tumor antigen-specific T cells in draining lymph nodes. It also inhibited subsequent tumor cell accumulation of CD8$^+$ T cells via induction of MDSC and Treg and impairment of DC functions [47]. TGF-β also increases immunosuppressive activity of melanoma cells by promoting the production of immunosuppressive molecules such as IL10, and TSP1 via snail expression, along with causing epithelial to mesenchymal transition (EMT) for metastasis [48]. It was reported that melanoma patients with TGF-β-related mesenchymal tumor microenvironment (increased gene expression related to angiogenesis, would healing, and EMT) did not respond to PD-1 Ab therapy [15]. Inhibitors of immunosuppressive factors, including TGF-β, IL10, IL6, IL8, VEGF, TAM/MDSC, and Tregs in such mesenchymal tumor microenvironments, may also be useful for converting non-responders to responders to PD-1/PD-L1 blockade therapy in melanoma.

Recent Topics in the Immunobiology of Cancers

In addition to cancer cell genetic factors, various factors influencing anti-tumor immune responses have been investigated. As one of the environmental factors, intestinal microbiota were shown to correlate with anti-tumor effects as well as immune-related adverse effects, such as colitis, in anti-CTLA-4 Ab therapy for melanoma [49, 50].

The metabolic conditions within the tumor microenvironment are also one of the major topics in cancer immunology. In tumor tissues, cancer cells preferentially utilize glycolysis (Warburg effect) to produce their energy source via ATP and materials for cell division such as nucleic acids, resulting in hyponutrition, including hypoglucose and hypoxia conditions. In such a unique environment, anti-tumor $CD8^+$ effector T cells for which glycolysis and glutaminolysis are essential for their proliferation and effector functions are weakened, whereas Tregs that utilize fatty acid oxidation survive. Metabolic modulators, such as metformin and fibrates, are improving anti-tumor T-cell survival and functions, additionally synergizing with PD-1/PD-L1 blockade. Energy metabolism may also be related to autophagy involved in processing of tumor antigens for the induction of anti-tumor T-cell responses. Calorie restriction mimetics may enhance anti-tumor T-cell responses partly regulating autophagy.

The metabolic status of various molecules, including amino acids important to the immune response, such as tryptophan, arginine, nucleic acids, and lipids (e.g., prostaglandins generated by COX2, cholesterol, and fatty acids), are also involved in generating tumor-promoting and immunosuppressive conditions in the tumor microenvironment. The specific importance of these molecules as it relates to immune resistance in the tumor microenvironments needs to be investigated in melanoma patients.

Combination Cancer Immunotherapy

Based on the immunopathology evaluated in human melanoma, various combined immunotherapies are being developed by considering the following immunological issues [51]: (1) use of vaccines with appropriate tumor antigens (e.g., neo-antigens), (2) *in situ* tumor destruction to induce immunogenic cancer cell death (e.g., chemotherapy, molecular target therapy, radiation, oncolytic viruses), (3) enhancement of antigen-presenting cells' function (e.g., TLR3/STING/CD40 agonists), (4) in vivo activation of antitumor T cells (e.g., cytokines, agonistic Abs for co-receptors, cultured antitumor T cells), and (5) reversal of immune-resistant mechanism (e.g., primary and adaptive immune resistance). A personalized combination may be important due to unique immune system differences in each patient. In addition to a combination of CTLA4/PD-1 Abs, various new combination immunotherapies, particularly with PD-1/PD-L1 blockade, and combinations with IDO inhibitors and VEGF inhibitors, are currently being evaluated in patients with metastatic melanoma.

Concluding Remarks

The reverse translational research using clinical samples obtained from clinical trials utilizing immune checkpoint blockade and T-cell-based adoptive cellular therapy reveals immunological mechanisms for anti-melanoma T-cell responses in patients. Further understanding of the immunobiology of melanoma, using new technologies such as multi-omics computer analyses and systematic immunological analyses, will lead to the identification of new biomarkers to select appropriate patients and immunotherapies along with new therapeutic targets for effective combination immunotherapies.

In melanoma, about 40% of patients have a T-cell-inflamed tumor microenvironment (antitumor $CD8^+$ T cells specific for various tumor antigens, such as neo-antigens, are induced and accumulated in tumors). However, the adaptive immune-resistant mechanism, such as the PD-1/PD-L1 interaction and tryptophan-metabolizing IDO, does not result in the eradication of melanoma cells by anti-tumor T cells. In other patients, due to primary immune-resistant mechanisms (e.g., low immunogenic tumor antigens, loss of immune cell-recruiting chemokines, cancer cell-producing immunosuppressive molecules and cells), antitumor $CD8^+$ T cells are not efficiently induced and accumulated within tumor tissues.

The presence of immunogenic antigens, including neo-antigens derived from DNA mutations, cancer-testis antigens, and melanocyte antigens, is important in the induction of tumor antigen-specific $CD8^+$ T cells. However, activation of oncogenes such as β-catenin, AKT (loss of PTEN), BRAF, and STAT3; TGF-β-associated mesenchymal conditions; and chromosomal SCNA may affect the induction and accumulation of tumor antigen-specific $CD8^+$ T cells in tumors. In the patients with sufficient immunogenic antigens for T cells, strategies to deplete such negative factors may promote the induction and tumor infiltration of antitumor $CD8^+$ T cells. This improves the antitumor activity of PD-1/PD-L1 blockade through the conversion of T-cell non-inflamed (non-responders) to T-cell-inflamed (responders) conditions within tumor microenvironments.

References

1. Topalian SL, Hodi FS, Brahmer JR, et al. Safety, activity, and immune correlates of anti-PD-1 antibody in cancer. N Engl J Med. 2012;366:2443.
2. Tumeh PC, Harview CL, Yearley JH, et al. PD-1 blockade induces responses by inhibiting adaptive immune resistance. Nature. 2014;515:568.
3. Herbst RS, Soria JC, Kowanetz M, et al. Predictive correlates of response to the anti-PD-L1 antibody MPDL3280A in cancer patients. Nature. 2014;515:563–7.
4. Taube JM, Anders RA, Young GD, et al. Colocalization of inflammatory response with B7-h1 expression in human melanocytic lesions supports an adaptive resistance mechanism of immune escape. Sci Transl Med. 2012;4(127)
5. Gajewski TF, Schreiber H, Fu YX. Innate and adaptive immune cells in the tumor microenvironment. Nat Immunol. 2013;(10):1014–22.
6. Daud AI, Loo K, Pauli ML, Sanchez-Rodriguez R, et al. Tumor immune profiling predicts response to anti-PD-1 therapy in human melanoma. J Clin Invest. 2016;126:3447–52.
7. Huang AC, Postow MA, Orlowski RJ, et al. T-cell invigoration to tumour burden ratio associated with anti-PD-1 response. Nature. 2017;545:60–5.
8. Kamphorst AO, Pillai RN, Yang S, et al. Antigen-specific CD4 T-cell help rescues exhausted CD8 T cells during chronic viral infection. Proc Natl Acad Sci U S A. 2011;108:21182–7.
9. Lurquin C, Lethé B, De Plaen E, et al. Contrasting frequencies of antitumor and anti-vaccine T cells in metastases of a melanoma patient vaccinated with a MAGE tumor antigen. J Exp Med. 2005;201:249–57.
10. Kawakami Y, Fujita T, Matsuzaki Y, et al. Identification of human tumor antigens and its implication for diagnosis and treatment of cancer. Cancer Sci. 2004;95:784–91.
11. Coulie PG, Van den Eynde BJ, van der Bruggen P, et al. Tumour antigens recognized by T lymphocytes: at the core of cancer immunotherapy. Nat Rev Cancer. 2014;14:135–46.
12. Robbins PF, Lu YC, El-Gamil M, et al. Mining exomic sequencing data to identify mutated antigens recognized by adoptively transferred tumor-reactive T cells. Nat Med. 2013;19:747–52.
13. Alexandrov LB, Nik-Zainal S, Wedge DC, et al. Signatures of mutational processes in human cancer. Nature. 2013;500:415–21.
14. Snyder A, Makarov V, Merghoub T, et al. Genetic basis for clinical response to CTLA-4 blockade in melanoma. N Engl J Med. 2014;371:2189.
15. Hugo W, Zaretsky JM, Sun L, et al. Genomic and transcriptomic features of response to anti-PD-1 therapy in metastatic melanoma. Cell. 2016;165:35.
16. Bassani-Sternberg M, Bräunlein E, Klar R, et al. Direct identification of clinically relevant neoepitopes presented on native human melanoma tissue by mass spectrometry. Nat Commun. 2016;7:13404.
17. Sahin U, Derhovanessian E, Miller M, et al. Personalized RNA mutanome vaccines mobilize poly-specific therapeutic immunity against cancer. Nature;547(7662):222–226. 2017.

18. Ott PA, Hu Z, Keskin DB, et al. An immunogenic personal neoantigen vaccine for patients with melanoma. Nature. 2017;547(7662):217–21.
19. Kawakami Y, Eliyahu S, Delgado CH, et al. Cloning of the gene coding for a shared human melanoma antigen recognized by autologous T cells infiltrating into tumor. Proc Natl Acad Sci U S A. 1994;91:3515.
20. Kawakami Y, Eliyahu S, Delgado CH, et al. Identification of human melanoma antigen recognized by tumor infiltrating lymphocytes associated with in vivo tumor rejection. Proc Natl Acad Sci U S A. 1994;91:6458.
21. Johnson LA, Morgan RA, Dudley ME, et al. Gene therapy with human and mouse T-cell receptors mediates cancer regression and targets normal tissues expressing cognate antigen. Blood. 2009;114:535–46.
22. Freeman-Keller M, Kim Y, Cronin H, et al. Nivolumab in resected and Unresectable metastatic melanoma: characteristics of immune-related adverse events and association with outcomes. Clin Cancer Res. 2016;22:886–94.
23. Robbins PF, Morgan RA, Feldman SA, et al. Tumor regression in patients with metastatic synovial cell sarcoma and melanoma using genetically engineered lymphocytes reactive with NY-ESO-1. J Clin Oncol. 2011;29:917–24.
24. Spranger S, Spaapen RM, Zha Y, et al. Up-regulation of PD-L1, IDO, and T(regs) in the melanoma tumor microenvironment is driven by CD8(+) T cells. Sci Transl Med. 2013;5:200ra116.
25. Chen DS, Mellman I. Oncology meets immunology: the cancer-immunity cycle. Immunity. 2013;39:1–10.
26. Inozume T, Yaguchi T, Furuta J. Melanoma cells control antimelanoma CTL responses via interaction between TIGIT and CD155 in the effector phase. J Invest Dermatol. 2016;136:255.
27. Wolchok JD, Kluger H, Callahan MK, et al. Nivolumab plus ipilimumab in advanced melanoma. N Engl J Med. 2013;369:122–33.
28. Postow MA, Chesney J, Pavlick AC, et al. Nivolumab and Ipilimumab versus Ipilimumab in Untreated Melanoma. N Engl J Med. 2015;372:2006–17.
29. Spranger S, Luke JJ, Bao R, et al. Density of immunogenic antigens does not explain the presence or absence of the T-cell-inflamed tumor microenvironment in melanoma. Proc Natl Acad Sci U S A. 2016:113.
30. Spranger S, Bao R, Gajewski TF. Melanoma-intrinsic β-catenin signalling prevents anti-tumour immunity. Nature. 2015;523:231.
31. Spranger S, Dai D, Horton B, et al. Tumor-residing Batf3 dendritic cells are required for effector T cell trafficking and adoptive T cell therapy. Cancer Cell. 2017;31:711–23.
32. Toda M, Iizuka Y, Kawase T, et al. Immuno-viral therapy of brain tumors by combination of viral therapy with cancer vaccination using a replication-conditional HSV. Cancer Gene Ther. 2002;9:356–64.
33. Udagawa M, Kudo-Saito C, Hasegawa G, et al. Enhancement of immunologic tumor regression by intratumoral administration of dendritic cells in combination with cryoablative tumor pretreatment and bacillus Calmette-Guerin Cell Wall skeleton simulation. Clin Cancer Res. 2006;12:7465–75.
34. Yaguchi T, Goto Y, Kido K, et al. Immune suppression and resistance mediated by constitutive activation of Wnt/beta-catenin signaling in human melanoma cells. J Immunol. 2012;189:2110.
35. Peng W, Chen JQ, Liu C, et al. Loss of PTEN promotes resistance to T cell-mediated immunotherapy. Cancer Discov. 2016;6:202.
36. Yuan J, Zhou J, Dong Z, et al. Pretreatment serum VEGF is associated with clinical response and overall survival in advanced melanoma patients treated with ipilimumab. Cancer Immunol Res. 2014;2(2):127–32.
37. Hodi FS, Lawrence D, Lezcano C, et al. Bevacizumab plus ipilimumab in patients with metastatic melanoma. Cancer Immunol Res. 2014;2:632–42.
38. Roh W, Chen PL, Reuben A, et al. Integrated molecular analysis of tumor biopsies on sequential CTLA-4 and PD-1 blockade reveals markers of response and resistance. Sci Transl Med. 2017;9(379):eaah3560.
39. Davies H, Bignell GR, Cox C, et al. Mutations of the BRAF gene in human cancer. Nature. 2002;417:949–54.
40. Sumimoto H, Miyagishi M, Miyoshi H, et al. Inhibition of growth and invasive ability of melanoma by inactivation of mutated BRAF with lentivirus-mediated RNA interference. Oncogene. 2004;23:6031.
41. Sumimoto H, Imabayashi F, Iwata T, et al. The BRAF-MAPK signaling pathway is essential for cancer-immune evasion in human melanoma cells. J Exp Med. 2006;203:1651.
42. Poulikakos PI, Zhang C, Bollag G, et al. RAF inhibitors transactivate RAF dimers and ERK signalling in cells with wild-type BRAF. Nature. 2010;464:427–30.
43. Wilmott JS, Long GV, Howle JR, et al. Selective BRAF inhibitors induce marked T-cell infiltration into human metastatic melanoma. Clin Cancer Res. 2012;18:1386.
44. Hugo W, Shi H, Sun L, et al. Non-genomic and immune evolution of melanoma acquiring MAPKi resistance. Cell. 2015;162:1271–85.
45. Iwata-Kajihara T, Sumimoto H, Kawamura N, et al. Enhanced cancer immunotherapy using STAT3-depleted dendritic cells with high Th1-inducing ability and resistance to cancer cell-derived inhibitory factors. J Immunol. 2011;187:27.
46. Davoli T, Uno H, Wooten EC, et al. Tumor aneuploidy correlates with markers of immune evasion and with reduced response to immunotherapy. Science. 2017;355
47. Nakamura S, Yaguchi T, Kawamura N, et al. TGF-beta1 in tumor microenvironments induces immunosuppression in the tumors and sentinel lymph nodes and promotes tumor progression. J Immunother. 2014;37:63.
48. Kudo-Saito C, Shirako H, Takeuchi T, Kawakami Y. Cancer metastasis is accelerated through

immunosuppression during snail-induced EMT of cancer cells. Cancer Cell. 2009;15:195.44.
49. Vétizou M, Pitt JM, Daillère R, et al. Anticancer immunotherapy by CTLA-4 blockade relies on the gut microbiota. Science. 2015;350:1079–84.
50. Dubin K, Callahan MK, Ren B, et al. Intestinal microbiome analyses identify melanoma patients at risk for checkpoint-blockade-induced colitis. Nat Commun. 2016;7:10391.
51. Kawakami Y, Yaguchi T, Sumimoto H, et al. Improvement of cancer immunotherapy by combining molecular targeted therapy. Front Oncol. 2013;3(136)

9 Dermoscopy of Melanocytic Lesions

Zachary J. Wolner, Oriol Yélamos, Konstantinos Liopyris, and Ashfaq A. Marghoob

Introduction

The diagnosis of skin cancers can be challenging by naked eye examination (NEE) alone. Although the clinical examination is a fundamental component for the diagnosis of skin cancer, NEE alone can miss early skin cancers and clinically symmetric skin cancers (i.e., those lacking the ABCD features), or, conversely, can lead to unnecessary biopsies of benign lesions. To a certain extent, these errors will occur regardless of the diagnostic method utilized; however, the addition of dermoscopy can significantly improve the diagnostic accuracy of both melanoma and non-melanoma skin cancer, reduce the number of unnecessary biopsies, and diagnose thinner and smaller skin cancers [1–3].

Dermoscopy, also referred to as dermatoscopy, uses a handheld device called a dermoscope or dermatoscope that consists of a transilluminating light source and a 10× magnifying lens. When the skin is seen by NEE alone, one can only perceive light reflected off the superficial stratum corneum. Dermoscopes use either polarized or non-polarized light to see beyond the stratum corneum and to identify subsurface features of the epidermis, dermoepidermal junction (DEJ), and papillary dermis unappreciable by NEE [4, 5].

Non-polarized dermoscopy requires the use of a liquid interface, such as ultrasound gel or alcohol, between the dermoscope and the skin surface [6]. Creation of a surface–liquid interface is necessary to visualize structures below the stratum corneum using non-polarized light. Polarized light obviates the need for a liquid interface by filtering out the light reflected off of the stratum corneum. Therefore, polarized dermoscopy can be performed without contacting the skin, resulting in better detection of vascular structures as they are not compressed by the pressure of the dermoscope [7]. Polarized and non-polarized light can also highlight different dermoscopic features due to a difference in light penetration of the skin [7]. Polarized dermoscopy offers improved visualization of structures in the deeper layers of the skin such as blood vessels and alterations of the matrix, such as shiny white structures [7, 8]. In contrast, non-polarized dermoscopy affords improved visualization of superficial structures such as blue-white veil (due to orthokeratosis), milia-like cysts, and comedo-like openings [7].

In the hands of experienced practitioners and novices (with only a few hours of didactic training), dermoscopy can significantly enhance the diagnostic accuracy of skin cancer. In addition, it can reduce the benign-to-malignant biopsy ratio (BMR) and enable users to diagnosis melanomas at an early stage [1–3]. For these reasons, the use

Z. J. Wolner · O. Yélamos · K. Liopyris
A. A. Marghoob, M.D. (✉)
Division of Dermatology, Department of Medicine, Memorial Sloan Kettering Cancer Center, New York, NY, USA
e-mail: wolnerz@mskcc.org; yelamoso@mskcc.org; liopyrik@mskcc.org; marghooa@mskcc.org

A. I. Riker (ed.), *Melanoma*, https://doi.org/10.1007/978-3-319-78310-9_9

of dermoscopy has become an important part of most dermatology practices, further expanding to other specialties such as family medicine [9, 10]. In the following sections, we review the impact of incorporating dermoscopy into clinical practice, describe the dermoscopic structures found in melanocytic neoplasms, discuss the diagnostic and triage algorithms, and highlight the advantages and limitations of dermoscopy.

Utility of Dermoscopy in Diagnosing Melanoma

In multiple meta-analyses, dermoscopy has been shown to improve the diagnostic accuracy for melanoma when compared to NEE alone [2, 11, 12]. Vestergaard et al. analyzed nine prospective clinical studies that included 8487 suspicious pigmented and non-pigmented lesions [2]. Melanoma prevalence among included studies ranged from 0.5 to 21.1% with a Breslow's thickness that ranged from 0.35 to 0.95 mm [2]. Diagnostic accuracy was evaluated through the diagnostic odds ratio (DOR), a function that takes into consideration sensitivity and specificity and their respective trade-offs [2]. Compared to NEE, the DOR for dermoscopy was 15.6 times higher (confidence interval [CI]: 2.9–83.7, $p = 0.016$). A summary estimate of sensitivity was also higher with dermoscopy (0.90, CI: 0.80–0.95) than for NEE (0.71, CI: 0.59–82, $p = 0.002$) [2]. It is important to underscore that this improvement in sensitivity was not associated with a concomitant lowering of specificity. In other words, while the sensitivity for detecting melanoma improved with dermoscopy, there was no statistical difference in specificity between NEE and dermoscopy (0.90, CI: 0.57–98 vs. 0.81, CI: 0.48–0.95, $p = 0.18$) [2].

Another method to investigate the positive impact of dermoscopy is to analyze the number of benign lesions biopsied for each malignant lesion biopsied. This is represented by the benign-to-malignant ratio (BMR). Carli et al. followed this ratio for 4 years with six practitioners, two dermoscopy users, and four nonusers. Dermoscopy users demonstrated an improvement in their BMR from 18:1 to 4.3:1 ($p = 0.037$), whereas dermoscopy nonusers experienced no significant change in their BMR from the beginning (11.8:1) to the end (14.8:1) of the study [1]. Another study compared three groups of dermatologists with and without access to dermoscopy and digital monitoring options. One group had no access to dermoscopy (Group A) while the other did (Group B). The third group had dermoscopy and the option to follow digital dermoscopic images of lesions over time to evaluate for change (Group C). Group A had the highest BMR (10.74:1), followed by Group B (8.14:1), and finally Group C (2.43:1). Therefore, the group that used dermoscopy and had the option to digitally monitor lesions was able to identify melanomas with the fewest biopsied benign lesions. It is important to appreciate that this improved BMR was due to a combination of an increase in the number of melanomas found and reduction in the number of benign lesions biopsied [13]. In yet another study, a 10-year multicenter survey found an improvement in the BMR from 12.8 to 6.8 at clinical sites dedicated to skin cancer treatment. The BMR remained unchanged in clinical sites not dedicated to skin cancer screening. The authors of the study argued that the adoption of dermoscopy was largely responsible for the observed improvement in the BMR [14]. Dermoscopy-led improvement in melanoma detection and reduction of benign biopsies has been associated with a reduction in morbidity and healthcare costs [15].

Another advantage of dermoscopy is that it enables the detection of thinner melanomas. A prospective study of patients with previously diagnosed melanoma evaluated the associations of melanoma tumor thickness at diagnosis with socioeconomic status, clinical factors, behavioral factors, screening strategies, and known melanoma risk factors [16]. Multivariate analysis revealed significant association of thinner melanomas with participation in specialized dermoscopic screening programs ($p < 0.0001$) and performance of dermoscopic examination at diagnosis ($p < 0.04$) [16]. Dermoscopy users identified melanomas with a mean Breslow's thickness of 1.4 mm and dermoscopy nonusers found melanomas with a mean thickness of

2.6 mm, which proved to be a highly significant difference ($p < 0.0001$) [16]. As mentioned previously, the diagnostic power of dermoscopy can be enhanced by the use of digital dermoscopy. In a meta-analysis of digital dermoscopy of melanocytic lesions, including 383 melanomas, greater than 50% of melanomas diagnosed with digital dermoscopy were in situ higher than the expected ratio found in the general population [3]. The likelihood of detecting melanoma increased with lesion surveillance time [3]. In summary, dermoscopy improves diagnostic accuracy, lowers the BMR, and leads to the diagnosis of thinner melanomas. In order to use dermoscopy as a useful skin cancer screening tool, it is necessary to learn the most representative dermoscopic structures that identify skin cancers. In the following sections, we detail the dermoscopic structures associated with melanocytic tumors and we highlight the dermoscopic features specific for the diagnosis of melanoma.

Dermoscopic Structures

Under the lens of dermoscopy, a skin lesion reveals a host of structures and colors unseen by NEE. Most dermoscopic features have unique histologic correlates allowing the user to clinically classify a lesion with high accuracy and even provide the clinician with potential prognostic information [2, 17–21]. Dermoscopy has been in routine use for over 30 years and has resulted in a literature riddled with redundant and ambiguous terminology [22, 23]. In order to standardize the terminology for the most commonly used dermoscopic structures, the International Dermoscopy Society (IDS) has published a consensus paper in 2016 on dermoscopic terms [22]. In this chapter we, with few exceptions, adhere to the IDS 2016 consensus terminology.

Melanocytic Dermoscopic Patterns

When approaching a lesion with dermoscopy, one of the fundamental questions to answer is whether or not the lesion is a melanocytic tumor. A method to help differentiate melanocytic from non-melanocytic lesions was first described after a dermoscopy consensus and is widely known as the two-step algorithm [24]. This algorithm will be fully explained in a later section, but briefly there are three pathways for a lesion to be labeled as melanocytic. The lesion can contain one or more of the nine dermoscopic features that indicate that a lesion is probably melanocytic: pigment network, negative network, angulated lines, streaks, aggregated globules, peripheral rim of globules, homogenous blue pattern, pseudonetwork (facial lesions), and parallel pigment pattern (volar lesions) (Fig. 9.1) [24]. In addition, the lesion can have vasculature indicative of a melanocytic lesion or the lesion is unclassifiable as a non-melanocytic lesion. In the last example, the lesion is then included as a melanocytic lesion in the second step.

Once it has been determined that the lesion is melanocytic, the next step is to determine whether the lesion is a nevus or a melanoma. The lack of dermoscopic structures concerning for malignancy (discussed in "Melanoma-Specific Structures) in conjunction with the identification of a uniform and an organized globular, reticular, starburst, or homogenous blue pattern leads to the diagnosis of a benign melanocytic nevus [25]. The benign melanocytic patterns listed above along with additional benign combinations are summarized and depicted in Fig. 9.2. In contrast, the dermoscopic structures and colors in melanomas are usually distributed in a disorganized and random manner. In addition, several dermoscopic features have been shown to be specific for melanoma. In the following section, we review the melanoma-specific structures. Finally, if the lesion is equivocal, a biopsy or referral to a specialist for further evaluation would be indicated [26].

Melanoma-Specific Structures

Several dermoscopic features are more commonly associated with melanoma than with nevi and these structures are known as the melanoma-specific structures, including atypical pigment network, angulated lines, negative pigment

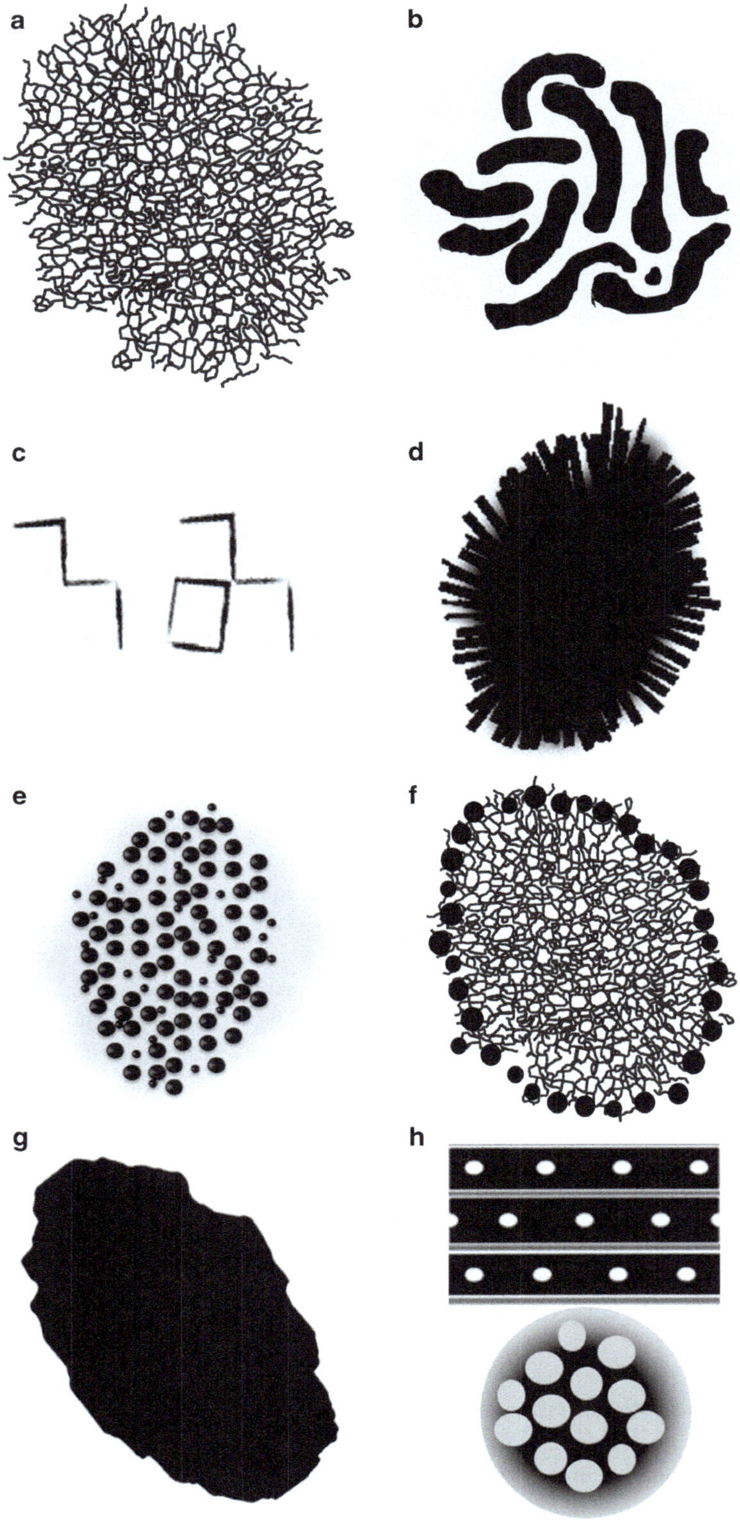

Fig. 9.1 Dermoscopic structures and patterns associated with melanocytic lesions. (**a**) Pigment network. (**b**) Negative network. (**c**) Angulated lines. (**d**) Streak or starburst pattern. (**e**) Globular pattern. (**f**) Peripheral rim of globules. (**g**) Homogeneous blue. (**h**) Top: Parallel pigment pattern (volar sites). Bottom: Pseudonetwork (facial skin)

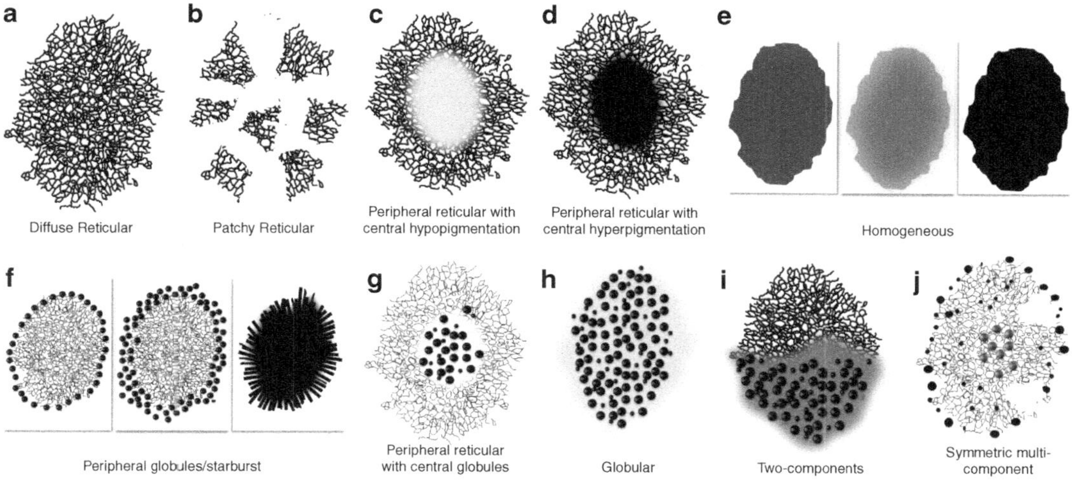

Fig. 9.2 Dermoscopic patterns associated with nevi. (**a**) Diffuse pigment network. (**b**) Patchy pigment network. (**c**) Diffuse pigment network with central hypopigmentation. (**d**) Peripheral pigment network with central hyperpigmentation. (**e**) Homogeneous brown, pink, and blue. (**f**) Diffuse pigment network with a ring of peripheral globules (left), diffuse pigment network with a peripheral ring of tiered globules (middle), and starburst pattern (right). (**g**) Peripheral pigment network with central globules. (**h**) Globular pattern. (**i**) Two-component. (**j**) Symmetric multicomponent

network, atypical dots, atypical globules, irregular streaks, shiny white lines, irregular blotch, blue-white veil, regression structures, polymorphous vasculature, and peripheral tan structureless areas [23]. In this section, we review each melanoma-specific structure and provide representative schematics (Fig. 9.3) and dermoscopic images (Figs. 9.4, 9.5, 9.6, 9.7, and 9.8).

Atypical/irregular pigment network consists of a grid composed of heterogeneous and erratic line thickness, variable size of network holes, and multiple colors ranging from brown to gray to black (Figs. 9.3a and 9.4a). Another sign of atypia is an asymmetrically distributed network with smudging, giving the network the appearance of being out of focus [22]. The network is often distributed in an asymmetric and noncontiguous manner. The presence of an atypical network is associated with superficial spreading melanoma [27]. Histologically, the dark lines of the pigment network correspond to the rete ridges, and the holes of the network correspond to the supra-papillary plates. The lines appear dark due to an increased number of melanized cells in the rete ridges, either melanocytes or pigmented keratinocytes [28]. If a lesion has an atypical pigment network there is a 2.0–9.0 odds ratio (OR) for melanoma [23, 24, 29–31].

Angulated lines consist of straight brown to gray lines that intersect at acute angles to create a zigzag pattern (Figs. 9.3a and 9.4b). These lines can eventually coalesce to form polygonal structures such as rhomboids [22]. The presence of angulated lines is associated with melanoma on sun-damaged skin, such as lentigo maligna [4]. Histologically angulated lines represent confluent atypical melanocytes in the basal layer admixed with dermal melanophages [32]. A lesion with angulated lines has a 1.95 OR for melanoma [33].

Negative pigment network refers to hypopigmented lines that appear to meander around the lesion in a serpiginous pattern (Figs. 9.3b and 9.5a). This can also be described as hypopigmented lines that surround elongated or curvilinear globular structures [22]. Although a negative network can be found in Spitz nevi [34], it is impossible to differentiate Spitz nevi from melanoma with a high degree of certainty. Therefore, its presence should always raise the concern for melanoma arising in a nevus. Although the histological correlate of negative network is not entirely known, it has been suggested

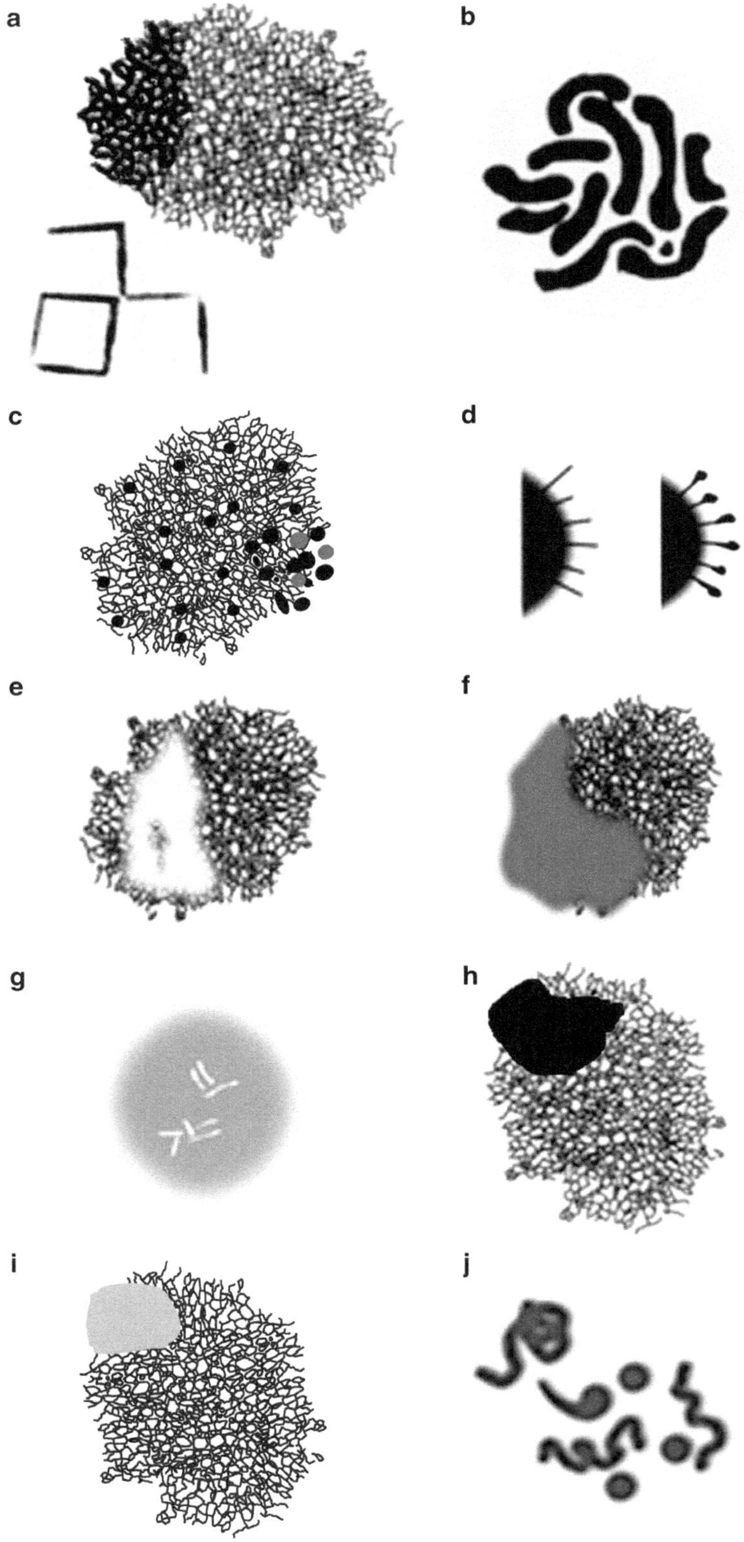

Fig. 9.3 Melanoma-specific dermoscopic structures. (**a**) Atypical pigment network (top) and angulated lines (bottom). (**b**) Negative network. (**c**) Atypical globules and dots. (**d**) Streaks: Radial streaming (left) and pseudopods (right). (**e**) Regression area (scar-like depigmentation and granularity/peppering). (**f**) Blue-white veil. (**g**) Shiny white streaks. (**h**) Atypical blotch. (**i**) Peripheral tan structure. (**j**) Polymorphous vasculature

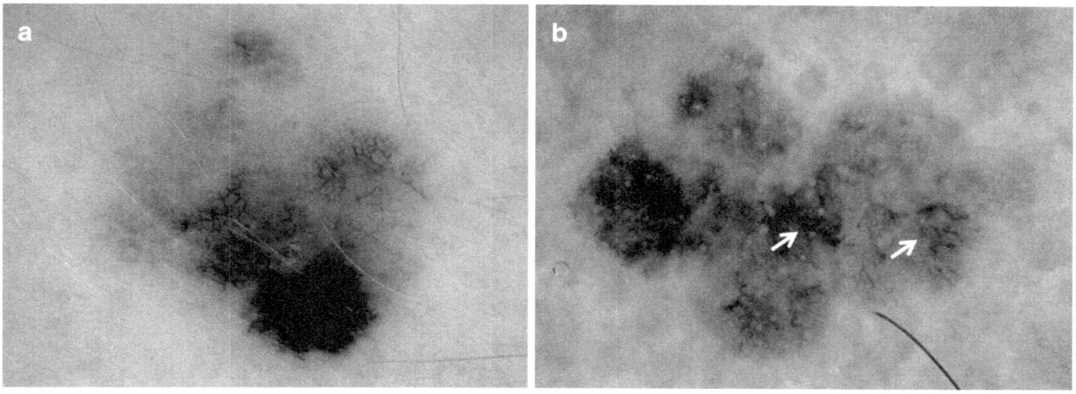

Fig. 9.4 Dermoscopic features of disorganized melanomas. (**a**) Melanoma with atypical network. Lines in the pigment network vary in size and manifest in different colors throughout the lesion. (**b**) Melanoma of the face with atypical network and angulated lines (white arrows) creating a zigzag pattern within the pigment network

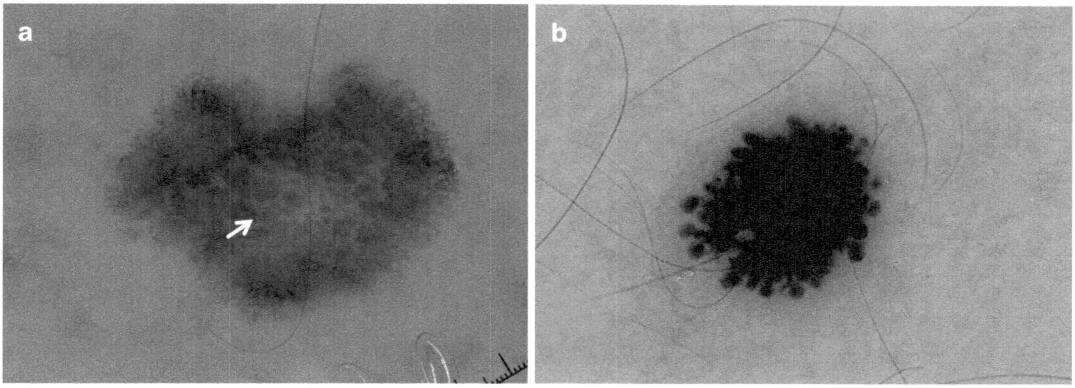

Fig. 9.5 Dermoscopic features of organized melanomas. (**a**) Melanocytic lesion with peripheral regular pigment network with a central area of negative network (arrow) indicative of melanoma arising in a nevus. (**b**) Spitzoid melanoma with pseudopods of different sizes and colors but distributed symmetrically around the entire lesion

that they correspond to bridging of adjacent rete ridges or to elongation of the rete ridges together with the presence of large melanocytic nests in the papillary dermis [35]. The presence of a negative network has been found to have a 1.4–1.8 OR for melanoma [23, 36, 37].

Typical **dots** are located in the center of a lesion, on pigment network lines, or in hole of a pigment network. Dots located in any other distribution are considered atypical. Atypical dots include dots in an asymmetric or a random distribution, in a peripheral location (off center), or unassociated with network lines or holes (Figs. 9.3c, 9.6, and 9.7) [22]. Histologically, brown dots represent dermal-epidermal nests.

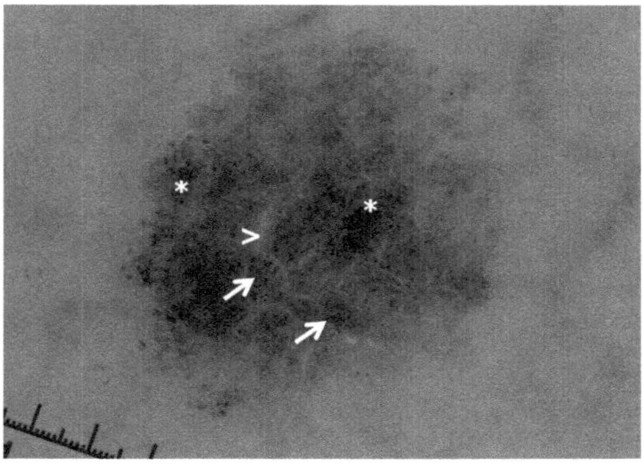

Fig. 9.6 Dermoscopic features of a spitzoid melanoma with irregular dots/globules (asterisks), shiny white streaks (arrowhead), and polymorphous vasculature (arrows)

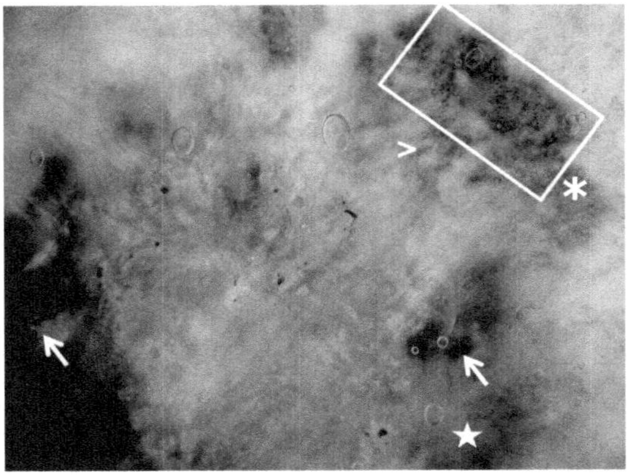

Fig. 9.7 Dermoscopic features of melanoma depicting multiple raised areas with a blue-white veil (white arrows), polymorphous vessels (star), peripheral structureless area (asterisk), irregular dots (rectangle), peppering/granularity (arrowhead), and shiny white streaks (center of the lesion)

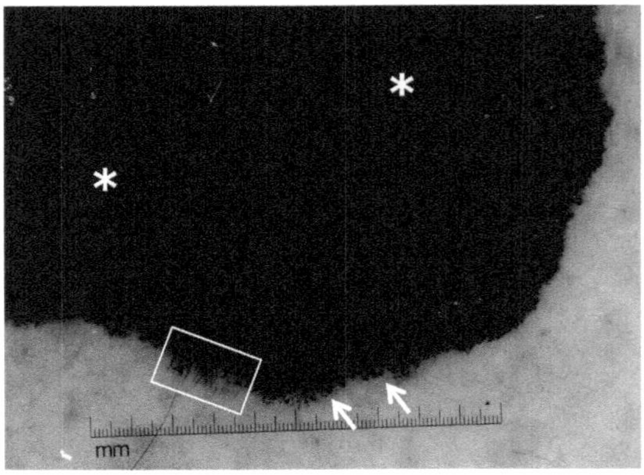

Fig. 9.8 Dermoscopic features of melanoma demonstrating a blue-white veil (asterisk), atypical globules (arrows), and a component of radial streaming (box) corresponding to radial growth

Black dots correspond to nests located in the upper epidermis or stratum corneum [38]. Atypical dots/globules in a lesion have a 1.7–4.8 OR for melanoma [24, 29, 39].

Typical **globules** are of similar size, shape, and color. They tend to be distributed throughout (globular nevus), at the periphery (in growing nevi) or in the center of a lesion (Fig. 9.2). Globules of differing size, shape, and color distributed in an asymmetric and/or random fashion are considered atypical. On histology, brown or black globules correspond to melanocytic nests present at the DEJ or superficial dermis, while blue globules correspond to nests located deeper in the dermis [38]. Atypical dots/globules in a lesion have a 1.7–4.8 OR for melanoma [24, 29, 39]. (Figs. 9.3c, 9.6, and 9.8).

Streaks are linear, pigmented projections that emerge from the perimeter of a lesion and extend into surrounding normal skin. There are two types of streaks: radial streaming and pseudopods. Radial streaming corresponds to linear structures extending from the periphery of a lesion (Fig. 9.3d). Pseudopods are similar to radial streaming but with an added bulbous ending (Fig. 9.5b) [22]. Streaks distributed evenly around the entire periphery of a lesion are typical of a Spitz/Reed nevus [40]. In contrast, when streaks are asymmetrically distributed or limited to a focal area on a lesion then they are considered to be irregular and are indicative of melanoma (Fig. 9.8) [4]. Histologically, streaks have been associated with confluent melanocytic nests located at the DEJ present at the periphery of a lesion [28]. Irregular streaks have an OR 1.5–5.8 for melanoma [23, 24, 29, 30, 39].

Regression structures consist of scar-like depigmentation and granularity/peppering. The areas of regression will be non-palpable and will not contain blood vessels or shiny white structures on polarized dermoscopy [22]. Peppering/granularity is seen as fine blue-gray dots and they correspond with papillary dermal melanophages or free melanin (Fig. 9.7) [17]. Scar-like depigmentation corresponds to dermal fibroplasia that appears dermoscopically as porcelain white structureless areas that are lighter in color compared to adjacent normal skin [22]. Peppering/granularity and scar-like depigmentation often appear together, but they can also present separately, and have an OR 2–18.3 for melanoma [23, 24, 30, 39] (Figs. 9.3e and 9.7).

A **blue-white veil** is a blue to blue-black area covered by a whitish ground-glass haze located in a raised area of the lesion (Figs. 9.3f, 9.7, and 9.8). The bluish color is due to melanin/melanocytes in the dermis and the overlying whitish haze is created by compact orthokeratosis [41]. A homogeneous blue-white veil encompassing the entire lesion can be seen in blue nevi and in epidermotropic melanoma metastasis [42]. A focal blue-white veil with asymmetrical distribution has an OR 1.74–13 for melanoma [23, 24, 30, 39].

Shiny white lines/streaks can only be visualized with polarized light and consist of discrete short white lines that are often oriented in an orthogonal or a parallel configuration (Figs. 9.3g, 9.6, and 9.7). The presence of these lines in a melanocytic lesion narrows the differential diagnosis to between a Spitz nevus and a melanoma [4, 43]. Shiny white streaks correspond to stromal alteration and dermal fibrosis [35, 43]. The presence of shiny white structures has an OR 2.5–9.7 for melanoma [23, 43].

Blotches are structureless areas with heavy pigmentation obscuring the visualization of any other dermoscopic structures. An isolated blotch located toward the center of a reticular nevus is considered to be regular and is found in nevi (Fig. 9.2d). A blotch is irregular if it is off center (closer to the periphery of the lesion, Fig. 9.3h) or if multiple blotches are found within a lesion [22]. The pigment corresponds to melanin present throughout all layers of the epidermis with or without dermal involvement [17]. Irregular blotches have an OR 1.88–4.1 for melanoma [23, 24, 29, 30].

Structureless areas are light brown or tan areas that encompass more than 10% of the lesion. Those that are located at the periphery of a lesion are considered irregular (Figs. 9.3i and 9.8), while those with a central location are considered regular. The peripheral tan structureless areas correspond to areas of flattened DEJ with pagetoid spread of melanocytes [17]. Peripheral structureless areas have an OR 2.9 for melanoma [29].

There are numerous terms in dermoscopy that describe vessel morphology and distribution. Short curved linear vessels analogous to a comma are typical of benign dermal nevi. The presence of any other vascular structure in a melanocytic lesion should raise concern for melanoma. **Polymorphous vasculature** or the presence of multiple types of vessels (i.e., dotted, coiled, looped, and serpentine) in one lesion is indicative of malignancy [22], and has an OR 2.0–3.04 for melanoma [23, 29, 30] (Figs. 9.3j, 9.6, and 9.7).

In the clinical setting, the practitioner is required to integrate the clinical context with physical findings in order to formulate a differential diagnosis. Based on the practitioner's impression, management decisions can be discussed with the patient. Incorporating dermoscopy into this equation can appear daunting. In the next section, we walk through several dermoscopic algorithms to successfully integrate dermoscopy into the clinical approach to a lesion.

Diagnostic/Triage Algorithms

With dermoscopy, practitioners can evaluate pigmented and non-pigmented lesions to determine which lesion requires a biopsy [44]. There are several methods for incorporating this into clinical practice. We focus on pattern analysis, two-step algorithm, and triage amalgamated dermoscopy algorithm (TADA).

Pattern Analysis

Pattern analysis, first described by Pehamberger et al. [45], assesses heterogeneity in the structure, color, pattern, and margin of a lesion. While pattern analysis has been shown to have superior diagnostic performance, it draws upon a practitioner's experience [24]. As more clinicians incorporate dermoscopy into their practice [46], algorithms that aid new users in diagnosing and managing a diverse array of skin lesions are needed. In this section, we cover the two-step algorithm, mentioned earlier, and TADA.

The Two-Step Algorithm

The first step of the two-step algorithm differentiates melanocytic from non-melanocytic lesions. A lesion that does not contain melanocytic structures should be evaluated to see if it has any structures indicative of a dermatofibroma, basal cell carcinoma (BCC), squamous cell carcinoma (SCC), seborrheic keratosis (SK), and angioma/angiokeratoma. In order to correctly apply the two-step algorithm, it is important to be able to identify common non-melanocytic lesions, which include dermatofibroma, BCC, SCC, SK, and angioma/angiokeratoma. While outside the scope of this chapter, these non-melanocytic lesions can be reliably diagnosed with the aid of dermoscopy using features specific for these lesions [18, 44, 47]. If the lesion does not fit into any non-melanocytic category, the presence of vascular structures associated with melanocytic structures, such as comma, dot, serpentine, coiled, or polymorphous vessels, indicates that the lesions should be evaluated in the second step. An unclassifiable lesion should be considered melanocytic and analyzed in the second step of the algorithm [24]. The second step uses the presence and/or absence of melanoma-specific features to help clinicians classify melanocytic lesions as benign (melanocytic nevus), suspicious, or malignant (melanoma). Clinicians can then proceed to reassure the patient or monitor/biopsy the lesion (Fig. 9.9).

Several algorithms have been developed to assist dermoscopy users in the second step. The melanoma-specific features can achieve high sensitivity and specificity for the diagnosis of melanoma (range of sensitivity 70.6–82.4% and range of specificity 40.2–59.4%) [23]. Intended as an aid for new users, these algorithms include the ABCD Rule, the 7-point checklist, the Menzies' method, the CASH algorithm, and the "chaos and clues" algorithm [48–52]. In essence, nevi tend to manifest one of the benign patterns (Fig. 9.2) and any lesion with one of the aforementioned melanoma-specific structures should raise concern for melanoma.

Triage Amalgamated Dermoscopy Algorithm (TADA)

TADA is a dermoscopic algorithm that serves as a comprehensive guide to managing pigmented and non-pigmented skin lesions through previously validated dermoscopic criteria (Fig. 9.10) [26, 37, 43, 53–57]. The unique feature of TADA is that it first asks users to identify if the lesion is an unequivocal dermatofibroma, angioma, or SK. If the user is confident that the lesion evaluated can be classified as one of these three benign lesions, it is then excluded from further evaluation and the patient can be reassured. Since these lesions are excluded from further analysis, these lesions must be unequivocal.

In the second step, the user assesses a lesion for architectural disorder [58]. In a study by the International Dermoscopy Society, architectural disorder was the most powerful discriminator for melanoma (OR of 6.6) and had the best interobserver agreement among study participants (intraclass correlation coefficient of 0.43, where 0 corresponds to agreement by chance and 1 is perfect agreement) [23]. However, malignancy can present in an organized manner, as evident with spitzoid, nodular, and amelanotic melanomas (Figs. 9.5 and 9.6) [59]. Therefore, TADA includes additional features found in organized malignant lesions: starburst pattern, blue-black or gray color, shiny white structures, negative network, ulceration/erosion, and/or vessels. The presence of architectural disorder or any of the abovementioned features of an organized malignancy signals the need for a biopsy/excision or a specialist referral.

A pilot study found that dermoscopy novices, including dermatologists and family physicians, with just 1 day of dermoscopy training, achieved 93.3% sensitivity and 74.1% specificity using TADA to evaluate malignant study lesions (melanoma, BCC, SCC) [58]. The study suggested that individuals with limited dermoscopy training and experience can be effective at skin cancer screening, regardless of their medical specialty.

Advantages and Limitations of Dermoscopy

As previously described, dermoscopy improves diagnostic accuracy, allows for digital surveillance leading to the detection of thinner melanomas, and reduces the number of unnecessary biopsies [2, 3, 13, 16]. Dermoscopy also offers additional advantages, such as patient and

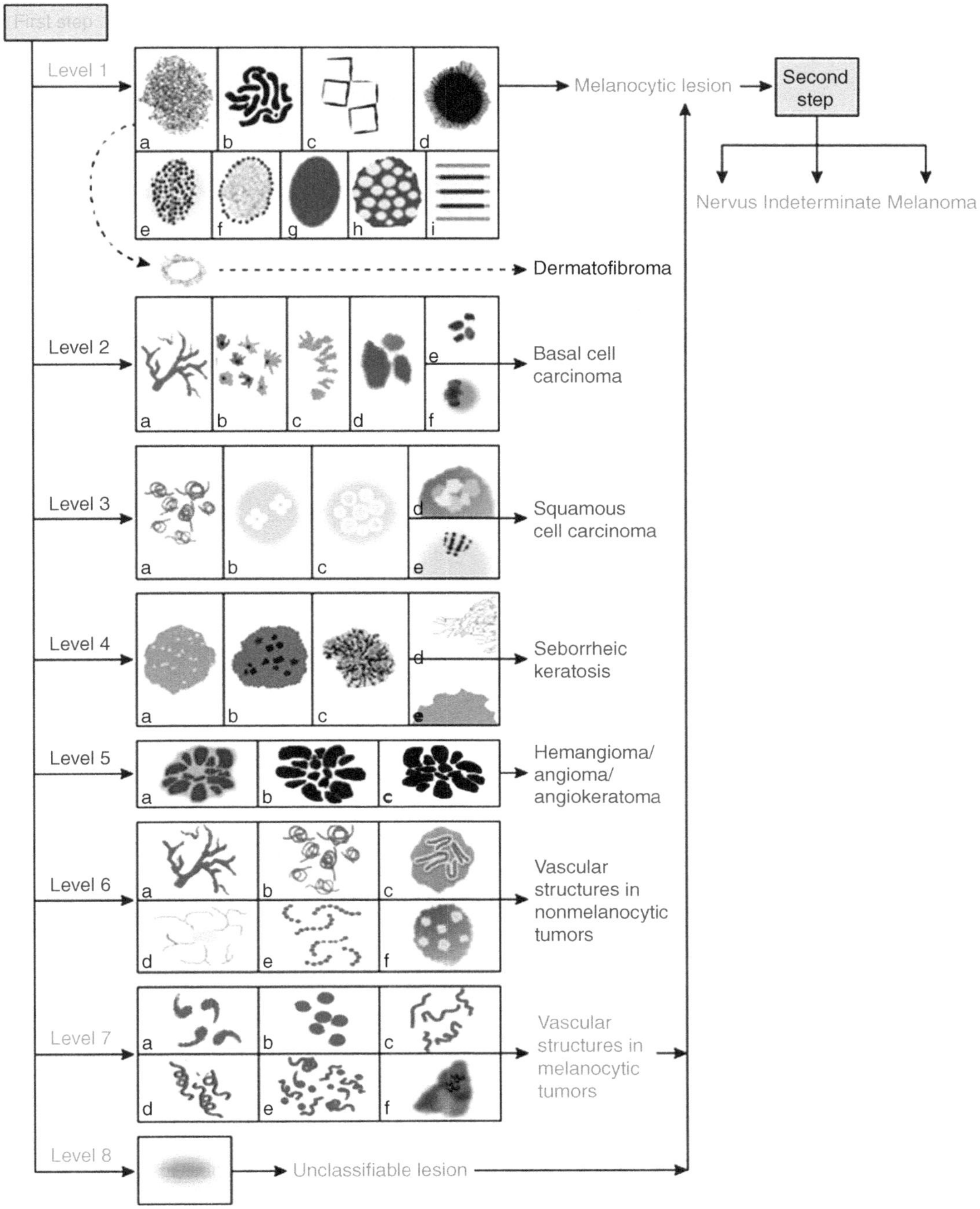

Fig. 9.9 Diagram depicting the two-step algorithm. The first step requires the user to decide whether the lesion is melanocytic. For all practical purposes, the presence of any structure/pattern depicted in level 1 requires the lesion to be evaluated in the second step of the algorithm that is designed to differentiate nevi from melanoma. If the lesion does not have any of the features depicted in level 1 then the lesion is further evaluated to determine if it has any features diagnostic for the most common non-melanocytic lesions encountered in clinical practice (levels 2–6). If, on the other hand, the lesion is determined to have features listed in level 1, level 7, or level 8 then the lesion is considered melanocytic and needs to be evaluated in step 2 of this algorithm. The second step of the algorithm is designed to help identify a lesion as a nevus, melanoma, or indeterminate

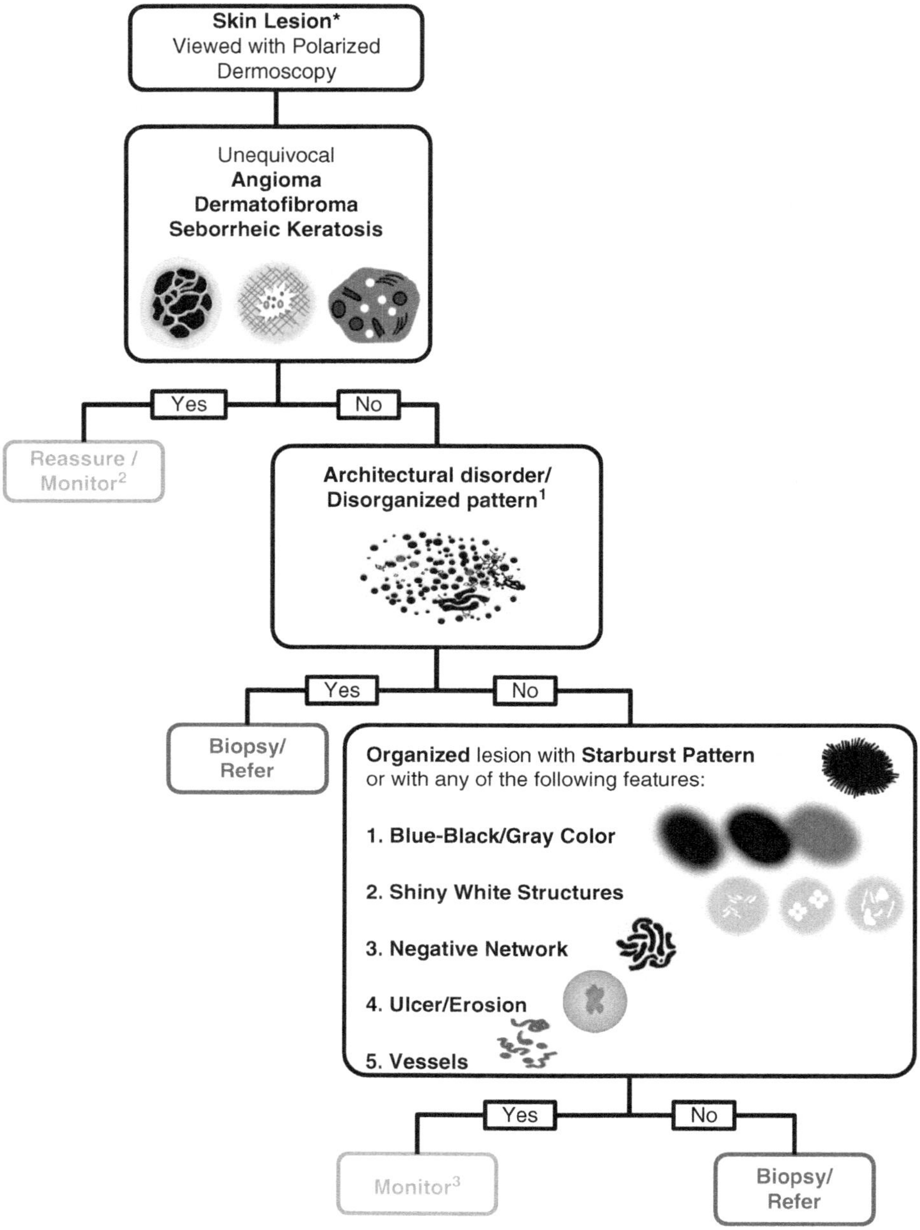

*** This rule does not apply to lesions on glabrous skin (i.e., palms, soles, mucosal surfaces) and nails.**
[1] Colors and structures distributed in an asymmetric/chaotic fashion.
[2] Patient should continue self-monitoring and changes in morphology or symptoms should be brought to attention of their healthcare provider.
[3] Monitoring can include short-term monitoring, long-term monitoring or self-monitoring for change.

Fig. 9.10 Diagram depicting the triage amalgamated dermoscopy algorithm (TADA). This algorithm requires that the lesion be evaluated with polarized dermoscopy. All unequivocal angiomas, dermatofibromas, and seborrheic keratoses can be safely removed from further analysis in the algorithm and the patient can be reassured and, if needed, the lesion can be further monitored. A lesion that is not an unequivocal SK, angioma, or DF is next evaluated for architectural disorder. A lesion with disorder should be biopsied or referred to a specialist. If the lesion is determined to be organized, then it is further evaluated to rule out the slim possibility of a skin cancer presenting itself with a symmetric morphology. Any organized lesion with a starburst pattern, blue-black/gray color, shiny white structure, negative network, ulcer/erosion, or vessel should be biopsied or referred to a specialist. Any lesion that reaches the end of the algorithm with no indication for biopsy or referral can be safely monitored physician reassurance, formation of a more precise differential diagnosis, and enhanced physician confidence in the clinical diagnosis [60]. However, dermoscopy also has its limitations.

Dermoscopy is meant to further inform and add more information to the physical exam and clinical history. Therefore, dermoscopy performed without the appropriate clinical context can lead to lower diagnostic accuracy [61]. Users can rely too heavily on one piece of information (anchoring bias) or use incomplete dermoscopic information to confirm a preexisting diagnostic suspicion (search satisfaction). Furthermore, the misidentification or misinterpretation of structures can lower diagnostic accuracy [62]. Finally, users may not detect early melanomas that lack specific dermoscopic criteria [63]. Therefore, dermoscopy needs to be performed as an adjunct to clinical examination, as relying solely on two-dimensional dermoscopic morphology may miss important information such as texture, consistency, or context of the lesion compared to surrounding lesions. However, despite these limitations, no study has empirically shown that trained dermoscopy users perform worse. This is most likely due to expert integration of patient history and lesional context with the dermoscopy information such as pattern recognition (gestalt) and analytical recognition (dermoscopic criteria) [64].

Conclusion

Dermoscopy offers improved diagnostic accuracy of melanoma. Users can achieve high sensitivity without sacrificing specificity for the diagnosis of melanoma. An improved BMR indicates that for every diagnosed malignancy, fewer benign lesions were unnecessarily removed. In addition, digital dermoscopy allows users to monitor ambiguous lesions for change and diagnose melanomas at an earlier stage. Although dermoscopy has its own learning curve, new users may utilize diagnostic and management algorithms, such as TADA or two-step algorithm to triage lesions for further evaluation and to improve their sensitivity and specificity for discriminating malignant from benign lesions. Finally, with all these improvements, dermoscopy can be a cost-effective screening tool.

Acknowledgments *Funding*: This research was funded in part through the NIH/NCI Cancer Center Support Grant P30 CA008748.

Conflict of interest: The authors have no conflicts of interest to declare.

Permissions: Natalia Jaimes, M.D., has granted us permission to use select schematics throughout this chapter. Natalia Jaimes, M.D., and we retain the copyright to any line drawing included in this submission.

References

1. Carli P, De Giorgi V, Crocetti E, Mannone F, Massi D, Chiarugi A, et al. Improvement of malignant/benign ratio in excised melanocytic lesions in the 'dermoscopy era': a retrospective study 1997–2001. Br J Dermatol. 2004;150(4):687–92. https://doi.org/10.1111/j.0007-0963.2004.05860.x.
2. Vestergaard M, Macaskill P, Holt P, Menzies S. Dermoscopy compared with naked eye examination for the diagnosis of primary melanoma: a meta-analysis of studies performed in a clinical setting. Br J Dermatol. 2008;159(3):669–76. https://doi.org/10.1111/j.1365-2133.2008.08713.x.
3. Salerni G, Teran T, Puig S, Malvehy J, Zalaudek I, Argenziano G, et al. Meta-analysis of digital dermoscopy follow-up of melanocytic skin lesions: a study on behalf of the international Dermoscopy society. J Eur Acad Dermatol Venereol. 2013;27(7):805–14. https://doi.org/10.1111/jdv.12032.
4. Menzies SW, Ingvar C, McCarthy WH. A sensitivity and specificity analysis of the surface microscopy features of invasive melanoma. Melanoma Res. 1996;6(1):55–62. https://doi.org/10.1097/00008390-199602000-00008.
5. Argenziano G, Soyer HP. Dermoscopy of pigmented skin lesions--a valuable tool for early diagnosis of melanoma. Lancet Oncol. 2001;2(7):443–9.
6. Gewirtzman AJ, Saurat JH, Braun RP. An evaluation of dermoscopy fluids and application techniques. Br J Dermatol. 2003;149(1):59–63.
7. Benvenuto-Andrade C, Dusza SW, Agero AL, Scope A, Rajadhyaksha M, Halpern AC, et al. Differences between polarized light dermoscopy and immersion contact dermoscopy for the evaluation of skin lesions. Arch Dermatol. 2007;143(3):329–38. https://doi.org/10.1001/archderm.143.3.329.
8. Wang SQ, Dusza SW, Scope A, Braun RP, Kopf AW, Marghoob AA. Differences in dermoscopic images from nonpolarized dermoscope and polarized dermoscope influence the diagnostic accuracy and confidence level: a pilot study. Dermatol Surg. 2008;34(10):1389–95. https://doi.org/10.1111/j.1524-4725.2008.34293.x.
9. Nehal KS, Oliveria SA, Marghoob AA, Christos PJ, Dusza S, Tromberg JS, et al. Use of and beliefs about baseline photography in the management of patients with pigmented lesions: a survey of dermatology residency programmes in the United States. Melanoma Res. 2002;12(2):161–7.

10. Argenziano G, Puig S, Zalaudek I, Sera F, Corona R, Alsina M, et al. Dermoscopy improves accuracy of primary care physicians to triage lesions suggestive of skin cancer. J Clin Oncol. 2006;24(12):1877–82. https://doi.org/10.1200/JCO.2005.05.0864.
11. Bafounta M, Beauchet A, Aegerter P, Saiag P. Is dermoscopy (epiluminescence microscopy) useful for the diagnosis of melanoma? Results of a meta-analysis using techniques adapted to the evaluation of diagnostic tests. Arch Dermatol. 2001;137(10):1343–50.
12. Kittler H, Pehamberger H, Wolff K, Binder M. Diagnostic accuracy of dermoscopy. Lancet Oncol. 2002;3(3):159–65.
13. Tromme I, Sacré L, Hammouch F, Legrand C, Marot L, Vereecken P, et al. Availability of digital dermoscopy in daily practice dramatically reduces the number of excised melanocytic lesions: results from an observational study. Br J Dermatol. 2012;167(4):778–86. https://doi.org/10.1111/j.1365-2133.2012.11042.x.
14. Argenziano G, Cerroni L, Zalaudek I, Staibano S, Hofmann-Wellenhof R, Arpaia N, et al. Accuracy in melanoma detection: a 10-year multicenter survey. J Am Acad Dermatol. 2012;67(1):54–9. https://doi.org/10.1016/j.jaad.2011.07.019.
15. Tromme I, Legrand C, Devleesschauwer B, Leiter U, Suciu S, Eggermont A, et al. Cost-effectiveness analysis in melanoma detection: a transition model applied to dermoscopy. Eur J Cancer. 2016;67:38–45. https://doi.org/10.1016/j.ejca.2016.07.020.
16. Haenssle H, Hoffmann S, Holzkamp R, Samhaber K, Lockmann A, Fliesser M, et al. Melanoma thickness: the role of patients' characteristics, risk indicators and patterns of diagnosis. J Eur Acad Dermatol Venereol. 2015;29(1):102–8. https://doi.org/10.1111/jdv.12471.
17. Yadav S, Vossaert K, Kopf A, Silverman M, Grin-Jorgensen C. Histopathologic correlates of structures seen on dermoscopy (epiluminescence microscopy). Am J Dermatopathol. 1993;15(4):297–305.
18. Ahnlide I, Zalaudek I, Nilsson F, Bjellerup M, Nielsen K. Preoperative prediction of histopathologic outcome in basal cell carcinoma—flat surface and multiple small erosions predict superficial basal cell carcinoma in lighter skin types. Br J Dermatol. 2016;175(4):751–61. https://doi.org/10.1111/bjd.14499.
19. Sahin MT, Ozturkcan S, Ermertcan AT, Gunes AT. A comparison of dermoscopic features among lentigo senilis/initial seborrheic keratosis, seborrheic keratosis, lentigo maligna and lentigo maligna melanoma on the face. J Dermatol. 2004;31(11):884–9.
20. Pan Y, Chamberlain AJ, Bailey M, Chong AH, Haskett M, Kelly JW. Dermatoscopy aids in the diagnosis of the solitary red scaly patch or plaque-features distinguishing superficial basal cell carcinoma, intraepidermal carcinoma, and psoriasis. J Am Acad Dermatol. 2008;59(2):268–74. https://doi.org/10.1016/j.jaad.2008.05.013.
21. Gonzalez-Alvarez T, Carrera C, Bennassar A, Vilalta A, Rull R, Alos L, et al. Dermoscopy structures as predictors of sentinel lymph node positivity in cutaneous melanoma. Br J Dermatol. 2015;172(5):1269–77. https://doi.org/10.1111/bjd.13552.
22. Kittler H, Marghoob AA, Argenziano G, Carrera C, Curiel-Lewandrowski C, Hofmann-Wellenhof R, et al. Standardization of terminology in dermoscopy/dermatoscopy: results of the third consensus conference of the International Society of Dermoscopy. J Am Acad Dermatol. 2016;74(6):1093–106. https://doi.org/10.1016/j.jaad.2015.12.038.
23. Carrera C, Marchetti MA, Dusza SW, Argenziano G, Braun RP, Halpern AC, et al. Validity and reliability of dermoscopic criteria used to differentiate nevi from melanoma: a web-based International Dermoscopy Society Study. JAMA Dermatol. 2016;152(7):798–806. https://doi.org/10.1001/jamadermatol.2016.0624.
24. Argenziano G, Soyer HP, Chimenti S, Talamini R, Corona R, Sera F, et al. Dermoscopy of pigmented skin lesions: results of a consensus meeting via the internet. J Am Acad Dermatol. 2003;48(5):679–93. https://doi.org/10.1067/mjd.2003.281.
25. Zalaudek I, Docimo G, Argenziano G. Using dermoscopic criteria and patient-related factors for the management of pigmented melanocytic nevi. Arch Dermatol. 2009;145(7):816–26. https://doi.org/10.1001/archdermatol.2009.115.
26. Marghoob AA, Usatine RP, Jaimes N. Dermoscopy for the family physician. Am Fam Physician. 2013;88(7):441–50.
27. Argenziano G, Fabbrocini G, Carli P, De Giorgi V, Delfino M. Epiluminescence microscopy: criteria of cutaneous melanoma progression. J Am Acad Dermatol. 1997;37(1):68–74.
28. Massi D, De Giorgi V, Soyer HP. Histopathologic correlates of dermoscopic criteria. Dermatol Clin. 2001;19(2):259–68. https://doi.org/10.1016/S0733-8635(05)70264-3.
29. Menzies SW, Kreusch J, Byth K, Pizzichetta MA, Marghoob A, Braun R, et al. Dermoscopic evaluation of amelanotic and hypomelanotic melanoma. Arch Dermatol. 2008;144(9):1120–7. https://doi.org/10.1001/archderm.144.9.1120.
30. Haenssle HA, Korpas B, Hansen-Hagge C, Buhl T, Kaune KM, Rosenberger A, et al. Seven-point checklist for dermatoscopy: performance during 10 years of prospective surveillance of patients at increased melanoma risk. J Am Acad Dermatol. 2010;62(5):785–93. https://doi.org/10.1016/j.jaad.2009.08.049.
31. Tschandl P, Rosendahl C, Kittler H. Dermatoscopy of flat pigmented facial lesions. J Eur Acad Dermatol Venereol. 2015;29(1):120–7. https://doi.org/10.1111/jdv.12483.
32. Vanden Daelen A, Ferreira I, Marot L, Tromme I. A digital Dermoscopy follow-up illustration and a histopathologic correlation for angulated lines in Extrafacial Lentigo Maligna. JAMA Dermatol. 2016;152(2):200–3. https://doi.org/10.1001/jamadermatol.2015.4132.
33. Lallas A, Tschandl P, Kyrgidis A, Stolz W, Rabinovitz H, Cameron A, et al. Dermoscopic clues to differenti-

ate facial lentigo maligna from pigmented actinic keratosis. Br J Dermatol. 2016;174(5):1079–85. https://doi.org/10.1111/bjd.14355.
34. Botella-Estrada R, Requena C, Traves V, Nagore E, Guillen C. Chrysalis and negative pigment network in Spitz nevi. Am J Dermatopathol. 2012;34(2):188–91. https://doi.org/10.1097/DAD.0b013e3182222ac1.
35. Pizzichetta MA, Canzonieri V, Soyer PH, Rubegni P, Talamini R, Massone C. Negative pigment network and shiny white streaks: a dermoscopic-pathological correlation study. Am J Dermatopathol. 2014;36(5):433–8. https://doi.org/10.1097/dad.0000000000000019.
36. Bassoli S, Ferrari C, Borsari S, Giusti F, Magnoni C, Pellacani G, et al. Negative pigment network identifies a peculiar melanoma subtype and represents a clue to melanoma diagnosis: a dermoscopic study of 401 melanomas. Acta Derm Venereol. 2013;93(6):650–5. https://doi.org/10.2340/00015555-1588.
37. Pizzichetta MA, Talamini R, Marghoob AA, Soyer HP, Argenziano G, Bono R, et al. Negative pigment network: an additional dermoscopic feature for the diagnosis of melanoma. J Am Acad Dermatol. 2013;68(4):552–9. https://doi.org/10.1016/j.jaad.2012.08.012.
38. Malvehy J. Handbook of dermoscopy. London: Informa Healthcare; 2006.
39. Salopek TG, Kopf AW, Stefanato CM, Vossaert K, Silverman M, Yadav S. Differentiation of atypical moles (dysplastic nevi) from early melanomas by dermoscopy. Dermatol Clin. 2001;19(2):337–45.
40. Marchell R, Marghoob AA, Braun RP, Argenziano G. Dermoscopy of pigmented Spitz and reed nevi: the starburst pattern. Arch Dermatol. 2005;141(8):1060. https://doi.org/10.1001/archderm.141.8.1060.
41. Alon S, Katrin K, Harold SR. Histopathologic tissue correlations of dermoscopic structures. An Atlas of Dermoscopy. 2nd ed. New York: CRC Press; 2012. p. 10–32.
42. Costa J, Ortiz-Ibanez K, Salerni G, Borges V, Carrera C, Puig S, et al. Dermoscopic patterns of melanoma metastases: interobserver consistency and accuracy for metastasis recognition. Br J Dermatol. 2013;169(1):91–9. https://doi.org/10.1111/bjd.12314.
43. Balagula Y, Braun R, Rabinovitz H, Dusza S, Scope A, Liebman T, et al. The significance of crystalline/chrysalis structures in the diagnosis of melanocytic and nonmelanocytic lesions. J Am Acad Dermatol. 2012;67(2):194.e1–8. https://doi.org/10.1016/j.jaad.2011.04.039.
44. Rosendahl C, Tschandl P, Cameron A, Kittler H. Diagnostic accuracy of dermatoscopy for melanocytic and nonmelanocytic pigmented lesions. J Am Acad Dermatol. 2011;64(6):1068–73. https://doi.org/10.1016/j.jaad.2010.03.039.
45. Pehamberger H, Steiner A, Wolff K. In vivo epiluminescence microscopy of pigmented skin lesions. I. Pattern analysis of pigmented skin lesions. J Am Acad Dermatol. 1987;17(4):571–83.
46. Terushkin V, Oliveria SA, Marghoob AA, Halpern AC. Use of and beliefs about total body photography and dermatoscopy among US dermatology training programs: an update. J Am Acad Dermatol. 2010;62(5):794–803. https://doi.org/10.1016/j.jaad.2009.09.008.
47. Soyer HP, Kenet RO, Wolf IH, Kenet BJ, Cerroni L. Clinicopathological correlation of pigmented skin lesions using dermoscopy. Eur J Dermatol. 2000;10(1):22–8.
48. Argenziano G, Fabbrocini G, Carli P, De Giorgi V, Sammarco E, Delfino M. Epiluminescence microscopy for the diagnosis of doubtful melanocytic skin lesions. Comparison of the ABCD rule of dermatoscopy and a new 7-point checklist based on pattern analysis. Arch Dermatol. 1998;134(12):1563–70.
49. Soyer HP, Argenziano G, Zalaudek I, Corona R, Sera F, Talamini R, et al. Three-point checklist of dermoscopy. A new screening method for early detection of melanoma. Dermatology. 2004;208(1):27–31. https://doi.org/10.1159/000075042.
50. Henning JS, Dusza SW, Wang SQ, Marghoob AA, Rabinovitz HS, Polsky D, et al. The CASH (color, architecture, symmetry, and homogeneity) algorithm for dermoscopy. J Am Acad Dermatol. 2007;56(1):45–52. https://doi.org/10.1016/j.jaad.2006.09.003.
51. Rosendahl C, Cameron A, McColl I, Wilkinson D. Dermatoscopy in routine practice—'chaos and clues'. Aust Fam Physician. 2012;41(7):482–7.
52. Stolz W, Riemann A, Cognetta A, Pillet L. ABCD rule of dermoscopy: a new practical method for early recognition of malignant melanoma. Eur J Dermatol. 1994;4:521–7.
53. Marghoob AABR, Malvehy J, editors. Atlas of dermoscopy. 2nd ed. London: Informa Healthcare; 2012.
54. Lallas A, Moscarella E, Longo C, Kyrgidis A, de Mestier Y, Vale G, et al. Likelihood of finding melanoma when removing a Spitzoid-looking lesion in patients aged 12 years or older. J Am Acad Dermatol. 2015;72(1):47–53. https://doi.org/10.1016/j.jaad.2014.09.037.
55. Argenziano G, Longo C, Cameron A, Cavicchini S, Gourhant JY, Lallas A, et al. Blue-black rule: a simple dermoscopic clue to recognize pigmented nodular melanoma. Br J Dermatol. 2011;165(6):1251–5. https://doi.org/10.1111/j.1365-2133.2011.10621.x.
56. Zalaudek I, Kittler H, Hofmann-Wellenhof R, Kreusch J, Longo C, Malvehy J, et al. "White" network in Spitz nevi and early melanomas lacking significant pigmentation. J Am Acad Dermatol. 2013;69(1):56–60. https://doi.org/10.1016/j.jaad.2012.12.974.
57. Altamura D, Menzies SW, Argenziano G, Zalaudek I, Soyer HP, Sera F, et al. Dermatoscopy of basal cell carcinoma: morphologic variability of global and local features and accuracy of diagnosis. J Am Acad Dermatol. 2010;62(1):67–75. https://doi.org/10.1016/j.jaad.2009.05.035.
58. Rogers T, Marino ML, Dusza SW, Bajaj S, Usatine RP, Marchetti MA, et al. A clinical aid for detecting skin cancer: the Triage Amalgamated Dermoscopic Algorithm (TADA). J Am Board Fam Med. 2016;29(6):694–701. https://doi.org/10.3122/jabfm.2016.06.160079.

59. Argenziano G, Zalaudek I, Ferrara G, Johr R, Langford D, Puig S, et al. Dermoscopy features of melanoma incognito: indications for biopsy. J Am Acad Dermatol. 2007;56(3):508–13. https://doi.org/10.1016/j.jaad.2006.10.029.
60. Benvenuto-Andrade C, Marghoob AA. Ten reasons why dermoscopy is beneficial for the evaluation of skin lesions. Expert Rev Dermatol. 2006;1(3):369–74. https://doi.org/10.1586/17469872.1.3.369.
61. Carli P, De Giorgi V, Argenziano G, Palli D, Giannotti B. Pre-operative diagnosis of pigmented skin lesions: in vivo dermoscopy performs better than dermoscopy on photographic images. J Eur Acad Dermatol Venereol. 2002;16(4):339–46.
62. Binder M, Schwarz M, Winkler A, Steiner A, Kaider A, Wolff K, et al. Epiluminescence microscopy. A useful tool for the diagnosis of pigmented skin lesions for formally trained dermatologists. Arch Dermatol. 1995;131(3):286–91.
63. Skvara H, Teban L, Fiebiger M, Binder M, Kittler H. Limitations of dermoscopy in the recognition of melanoma. Arch Dermatol. 2005;141(2):155–60. https://doi.org/10.1001/archderm.141.2.155.
64. Marghoob AA, Scope A. The complexity of diagnosing melanoma. J Invest Dermatol. 2009;129(1):11–3. https://doi.org/10.1038/jid.2008.388.

International Models of Melanoma Management (Australia)

10

Paul Elmslie

The Clinical Management of Skin Cancer

The phrase, "clinical management," refers to the process that occurs once a suspicious lesion is found or identified by a family physician or general practitioner (GP). Typically, once this lesion is identified, the patient is referred to a dermatologist in order to obtain a tissue diagnosis. If it is determined that the lesion is a melanoma, the dermatologist will then conduct an excisional biopsy and send the sample to the pathologist, who will then confirm the lesion's malignancy and the staging if it is a melanoma.

Once the skin cancer is confirmed, the dermatologist then provides the diagnosis to the patient. Depending on the severity of the case, as well as the dermatologist's experience, the patient will likely be either treated within the dermatologist's practice or referred to a surgeon. Another significant factor is the specialist's access to important resources, and this is often determined by where the patient is located. For example, in certain regional areas, there may be only a general surgeon who is available to remove the lesion, as opposed to a surgical oncologist, plastic surgeon, or dermatologist experienced with Mohs micrographic surgery.

While the clinical management of skin cancer and, more specifically, melanoma is essentially the same in every country, there are notable differences in other aspects of care as well. This section focuses specifically on those clinical management differences in Australia, the UK, and the USA.

Australia

In Australia, the clinical management of skin cancer is a combination of primary care, public and private hospitals, and specialists. The federal government's Medicare system provides patients with a rebate for clinical services delivered by GPs and specialists. Some GPs will accept the Medicare payment as full payment; therefore, the services delivered have no out-of-pocket cost for the patient. Specialists will typically charge the patients privately and then the patients can access the Medicare rebate or use their private health insurance. State governments fund public health care and provide free hospital services to local populations. However, patients are not able to select their own specialists, and waiting lists can be quite long.

The private hospital system enables patients to select a specialist and also to have access to private rooms. Approximately one-half of Australians carry private health insurance [1].

P. Elmslie, M.B.A.
HealthCert International, Singapore, Singapore

National Skin Cancer Centres,
Adelaide, SA, Australia
e-mail: paul@healthcert.com

A. I. Riker (ed.), *Melanoma*, https://doi.org/10.1007/978-3-319-78310-9_10

Currently, private health insurance does not cover primary care services, and only covers specialists and private hospital admissions.

Traditional Pathways

A GP is usually the first clinician to identify a suspicious skin lesion, whether it is presented to the GP by the patient as a suspicious lesion or it is the result of a skin check. A GP may have the necessary skills to perform a punch or shave biopsy, so long as the lesion is not located on a cosmetically sensitive area. If the lesion is a suspected melanoma, an excisional biopsy would be recommended, and a GP would also likely be able to complete this task. (The management of melanomas is discussed in more detail in the following section.)

If the lesion is located on a cosmetically sensitive area, the patient can be referred to a GP who subspecializes in skin cancer. In Australia, these GPs are known as skin cancer doctors, and they are able to conduct surgical procedures of a cosmetically sensitive nature. At a lower cost, they provide quicker access to clinical services for patients who do not have private health insurance or cannot afford to pay privately for a dermatologist or plastic surgeon.

There are also two traditional GP referral options for patients with a diagnosed or suspected melanoma [2] (see Fig. 10.1):

1. Referral to a dermatologist, and then to a surgeon if malignancy is confirmed: If a case is severe, the patient will be referred to a surgical oncologist and then potentially to a radiation oncologist if more aggressive treatment is necessary, especially for an advanced melanoma.
   (a) A patient must first receive a referral from a GP to see a dermatologist. The referral lasts 12 months.
   (b) This is usually only an option for those with economic resources because treatment can range from hundreds to thousands of dollars.
2. Referral to a state-funded public hospital system: This, however, presents its own set of challenges because the hospital system is overloaded and patients could have two very different outcomes:
   (a) A patient with a melanoma is treated within 1 month because a melanoma is considered a category 1 case with a target date of 30 days for treatment.
   (b) Non-melanoma cases have a wait list of more than a year, which means the cancer progresses as a patient waits for treatment.

These options are available to those who live in cities. For Australians living in rural areas, the options tend to be more limited. A dermatologist may visit once a month, but he or she only looks at significant cases. Thus, a GP or skin cancer clinic (which is discussed next) tends to do more diagnostic and low-level management cases. There are also regional hospitals with a visiting surgeon who may perform any necessary surgeries.

Skin Cancer Clinics

Skin cancer clinics are a relatively recent development in Australian health care. These clinics began to open in the mid-1990s. They are staffed

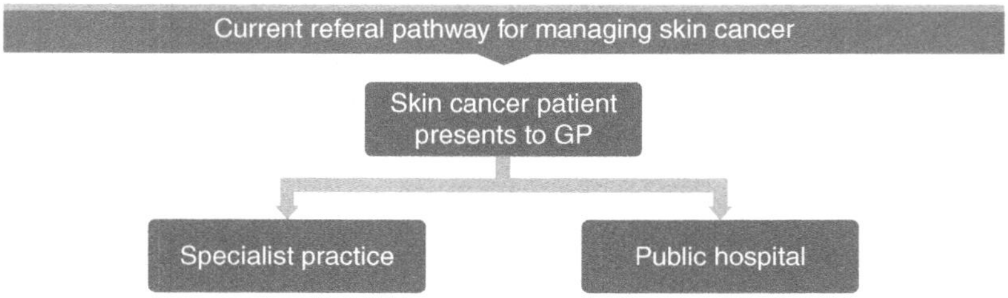

Fig. 10.1 Current referral pathway for managing skin cancer. From "Business Plan for Expansion of the National Skin Cancer Centres for the South Australian Government" (Elmslie 2016, p. 2)

by local GPs with an interest in skin cancer medicine, and they provide lower cost and quicker access to more specialized services. Clinic staff usually manages basal cell and squamous cell carcinomas (BCCs and SCCs) on a daily basis. They also have the skill set to successfully treat early-stage primary melanomas. Anything more significant (stage III, stage IV, etc.) is referred to a specialist or a hospital.

There are now 400 skin cancer clinics in operation across Australia. They are usually small—staffed by two or three doctors—and they are run by the owner/operator in partnership with his colleagues. Approximately 800 GPs work in clinics, out of a GP population of about 28,000. Today, they are considered to be a normal part of skin cancer treatment as well as a standard of care in Australia.

The clinics provide head-to-toe skin exams, on-site biopsies, and on-site treatment for most skin cancers, but patients cannot get any other type of medical services here, including prescriptions. Due to their growing popularity and their success at providing a much-needed service, more generalist GPs are beginning to integrate skin cancer services into their own practices. This is because GPs are becoming frustrated that their patients will see them for normal health concerns but then go to a GP-led skin cancer clinic for their skin cancer concerns.

Challenges in Clinical Management

There are two significant challenges facing the clinical management of skin cancer in Australia.

First, Australia has the highest rate of skin cancer in the world. In fact, every two of three Australians who live to age 70 will get skin cancer [3], and in a population of 23 million more than 750,000 skin cancers are treated every year [4]. Skin cancer is the most costly form of cancer to treat in Australia, with its annual cost to the government of $703 million in 2015 [5]. Approximately 80% of cancers are skin cancers [4].

Second, Australia is a large country with a geographically dispersed population. This makes the delivery of health services challenging, especially in regard to specialist services. Of particular concern to the management of skin cancer is the acute shortage of dermatologists. There are approximately 450 dermatologists to cover the entire population, and while most of these specialists live in the capital cities one-third of Australians live in rural areas. It is not uncommon for a dermatologist to have a 6-month wait list.

Managing Melanoma

Australia's management of melanoma is discussed at length in Section "Efficient/Effective Methods of Diagnosis and Treatment Based on the Australian Model."

United Kingdom

Current clinical management in the UK is part of a single-payer system that is publicly funded. It is unique in that the government funds it in its entirety, regardless of whether it is at a primary care or specialist level. As a result, patients have only the option of being seen at the local hospital for definitive diagnosis and treatment of skin cancer. This does not mean, however, that there are no specialists in private practice. There are a small percentage of specialists who operate within the public sphere. However, this option is typically only available for a wealthy minority who carry private health insurance.

A 2015 study conducted by Public Health England found that the number of melanoma diagnoses for patients living in the most deprived areas, who present either through the 2-week referral or GP referral, is substantially higher than that for those who live in the least deprived areas [6]. The same study found a 2% difference in emergency-room melanoma presentations between those who lived in the most deprived areas versus those living in the least deprived areas [6]. In addition, the 1-year survival rate for melanoma was noticeably lower in patients living in the most deprived areas (95%) versus those living in the least deprived areas (97%) [6].

Overview

When a patient presents to a GP with a suspicious lesion, he is automatically referred to a specialist. This is because of the NICE Guidelines, which effectively prohibit a GP from managing any lesion that is anything more severe than a superficial BCC. Therefore, if a GP finds a suspicious skin lesion, it is always referred into the hospital system.

Depending on the severity of the case, a patient will be seen by a dermatologist, who will make a diagnosis that is confirmed by a histopathologist. Then, the case will be handed over to the hospital surgeons. The severity of the lesion and its cosmetic sensitivity will determine which type of surgeon manages the patient.

Similar to Australia, the UK has also innovated its clinical delivery system to try and deal with the shortage of dermatologists, which is critical considering you are eight times more likely to die of a skin cancer in the UK compared to Australia. This is despite the fact that Australia has eight times the number of cases [7]. In fact, in the last 25 years in the UK, melanoma cases have increased faster than any of the top ten cancers in both men and women [8].

The UK has approximately 600 dermatologists for a population of 60 million people, and many regional or rural areas having little to no dermatology services in the hospitals. The development of the category called a "GP with a Special Interest" (GPwSI), however, has helped provide more dermatology services in the hospital system. These GPwSI in dermatology are required to complete a diploma-level course and undertake continuous professional development and practicing under the supervision of a dermatologist. This allows for the GPwSI to become the frontline of hospital referrals and help filter less significant cases (low-level rashes and infections). (As of this writing, the accreditation for GPwSI in dermatology was under review with the goal of establishing a national accreditation body. Updates are expected in June 2017.)

Challenges in Clinical Management

The UK hospital system divides patients into two groups in terms of waiting times to access dermatology services. Melanoma is considered a "2-week-wait" case. Once a patient is referred, it is recommended he or she be seen within 2 weeks. Many trust hospitals, however, struggle to meet this deadline despite their best efforts. All other skin cancers are placed on an 18-week waiting list. Hospitals also struggle to meet this deadline because of their workload.

Another issue for this system is that many patients with melanomas can be incorrectly referred by the GPs as 18-week-wait cases or as having benign lesions that are referred as suspected melanomas. This is due to low levels of dermoscopy use and training at a primary-care level. Results from a teledermatology study conducted in Hertfordshire, England, confirmed this. Clinical information for 110 patients revealed that 30–50% of 2-week-wait cases were not urgent [9]. This study is discussed in more detail in Section "Teledermatology and Other Educational Projects in the U.K. and its Utility in Clinical Practice."

The UK healthcare system is divided into four separate systems, each called the National Health System. (Northern Ireland's is now officially "Health and Social Care in Northern Ireland," but it is commonly still referred to as NHS.) Each country funds its own system. Though this results in many differences between each system, they are all relatively simple to navigate because general practitioners are responsible for referrals to the local hospitals.

However, like all government-funded health care, the systems are under significant cost pressures and will need to be innovated in the future in order to deal with the aging population and longer life expectancy. Additionally, in the UK, if a drug isn't approved for government funding, you can't access it through the NHS. Therefore, you would have to pay privately for the new and more expensive melanoma drugs available for advanced disease.

Managing Melanoma

In the UK, all melanomas are referred to hospital or specialists for treatment.

USA

The healthcare system in the USA is primarily private, for-profit, and, therefore, very expensive in comparison to almost all other countries. For most people, it is essential to have coverage, especially for substantial, life-threatening situations. It is not unusual for a significant health issue to have costs upwards of $100,000. People can also go bankrupt due to healthcare costs, something you don't see in Australia or the UK. As we have recently witnessed with the introduction of Obamacare in 2010, and the subsequent challenges to it, the US healthcare system is in a constant state of flux, which makes forward planning more difficult for all stakeholders.

The USA also has a Medicare/Medicaid structure to provide healthcare funding for people who meet specific criteria. Medicare is a federally funded program for people over 65 years old or for people with certain disabilities, while Medicaid is a joint state and federally funded program for people with limited income. These programs are similar to the Australian model in that each service has a CPT code associated with it that the medical practice then charges to the government. It also has the challenge that its funding will have to change in the future due to rising costs and government-deficit pressures.

Overview

Family physicians and nurse practitioners that staff primary care clinics do not typically have the skills necessary for diagnosing and treating skin cancers, including melanoma. Therefore, patients with suspected skin cancers are typically referred to a dermatologist, of which there were approximately 13,000-plus in the USA in 2015 [10].

When a patient with a suspicious skin lesion is referred to a dermatologist, a diagnosis is made and confirmed by a histopathologist. Then, the vast majority of cases are sent to a Mohs surgeon—a dermatologist who has undertaken additional training in specific surgical techniques for the treatment of skin cancer. Micrographic surgery is very common in the USA, unlike in the UK or Australia.

Mohs surgery involves the patient having the lesion removed with minimal margins. The lesion is then analyzed with frozen sections to examine the surgical margins and reviewed by the on-site Mohs surgeon for histopathological diagnosis. If the lesion was not completely excised, the Mohs surgeon will remove more tissue along the affected margin. It is especially useful for areas where margin control is important for future patient function or cosmetic purposes.

Challenges in Clinical Management

Skin cancer costs are climbing in the USA at a rate of 126%, compared to a 25% increase in the cost to treat other cancers over the same time period [11]. Treatment costs rose from $3.6 billion in the 5-year period from 2002 to 2006 to $8.1 billion in the 5-year period of 2007–2011 [11].

One reason for such an increase is because Mohs micrographic surgeries (MMS) increased by 700% between 1992 and 2009 [12]. These surgeries normally receive Medicare payments 120–370% more than a standard surgical elliptical excision. This also helps to explain why, during the same period, surgical excisions only increased by 20% [12]. In addition, 1,800 providers billed Medicare for MMS in 2009, a number that increased to 3,209 in 2012 [12]. Approximately one in four skin cancer cases are treated with MMS [12].

These rising costs are increasing awareness and concern over how skin cancers are managed and may lead to future changes, especially because many cases do not need to be managed by the hospital system, which is presently the case. It should be noted, however, that melanomas are a slightly different situation. The vast majority of melanoma cases are managed in the hospital system, and depending on their severity this is as it should be. This will be discussed in more depth in the next section.

Another challenge facing the US management of skin cancer is the evolution of dermatology in the USA. Many dermatologists are moving more toward aesthetic and cosmetic medicine because patients pay cash on the day of their procedure. In contrast, traditional dermatology payments disbursed by an HMO—the private health insurance company—can take 90–120 days to send payments to the provider. As with Australia and the UK, it is a lengthy process to increase the number of dermatologists. Foreseeably, they will also have challenges in providing clinical services due to increased demand and the changing face of dermatology practices.

Managing Melanoma

Over the course of their lifetime, one in five Americans will develop skin cancer (Robinson 2005, cited in [13]). Each year, more than 5.4 million non-melanomas are diagnosed (Rogers 2012, cited in [13]), with more new cases of skin cancer than the combined incidence of breast, prostate, colon, and lung cancer (American Cancer Society, 2017, cited in [13]). The National Cancer Institute estimates that there will be ~87,110 new melanoma cases in the USA in 2017, and of those cases 9730 will result in death (American Cancer Society, 2017, cited in [14]). Though melanoma represents the smallest segment of skin cancer in the USA (less than 5%), it accounts for the most deaths, a rate that has been steadily increasing over the past 40 years (American Cancer Society, 2014, cited in [14]).

Studies have found that even the most experienced dermatopathologists have difficulty distinguishing between benign pigmented lesions and early melanomas. In fact, one study found that, when presented with 140 cases, a panel of dermatopathologists disagreed on 37 of them [15]. Therefore, it is recommended that when a patient presents with a suspicious lesion, it is best to receive a second opinion.

Surgical excision should be the main management tool for melanoma, particularly for cutaneous melanomas that have not spread [14]. Additional treatment is determined by the stage of progression [14]. While stage 0 melanoma requires only excision, stages I through IV could be treated with excision as well as lymph node management, which is first done through lymph node mapping and sentinel lymph node biopsy, as well as one or more of the following (depending on stage): chemotherapy, palliative local therapy, immunotherapy and/or adjuvant therapy, or signal transduction inhibitors [14].

In the USA, there are several different doctors who are trained to treat melanoma. These include dermatologists, medical oncologists, surgical oncologists, and radiation oncologists [16]. Other professionals may be part of the medical team, as well as nurse practitioners and physician assistants [16].

Before beginning treatment, a patient will go through his or her medical history with someone from the medical team [16]. This will include discussing age and health, the stage to which the melanoma has progressed, the likely outcomes of the proposed treatment plan, and the possible side effects from treatment, as well as the patient's feelings toward these side effects [16].

Patients are also advised to get a second opinion, if time allows, or participate in a clinical trial [16].

Efficient/Effective Methods of Diagnosis and Treatment Based on the Australian Model

In Australia, health practitioners have had to innovate due to a number of factors. As previously mentioned, Australia has the highest rate of skin cancer in the world. It also has a population of 23 million people who are spread across a landmass similar in size to the USA. This, coupled with a shortage of specialists who have traditionally been located in major capital cities, has led to long wait lists as well as other challenges.

The traditional model is one where the GP is the first practitioner to whom a patient with a suspected skin cancer or melanoma presents. The GP must then decide whether the patient should be referred to a dermatologist or, if the patient is unable to afford a specialist, whether he or she can be referred to the public hospital. If referred to a dermatologist in private practice, the dermatologist then makes an assessment or final diagnosis of the lesion and determines whether the lesion should be treated in his or her own practice or referred to another specialist.

In the hospital system, the admissions officer is typically the person who makes a determination based on the GP's referral as to how quickly the patient should be seen. The officer determines whether the case should be placed on the category 1 waiting list and seen within 30 days due to a suspected melanoma, or whether the case is category 3, which could put the patient on a wait list of up to 1 year.

Case Study In 2000, a 31-year-old mother of two presented to a primary care practice in Australia with a suspicious lesion of the lip. The GP recognized it as a possible skin cancer but did not have the confidence to make a definitive diagnosis. The patient did not have private health insurance and was therefore unable to afford a dermatologist or surgeon; thus, she was put into the public hospital system. She was unable to be seen in the public hospital for 9 months, and tragically the lesion was an invasive and very aggressive SCC. She died 2 months later.

This case exemplifies the importance of innovation in dealing with skin cancer, particularly in Australia. This woman sought treatment, but due to financial constraints she was unable to access the care that would have saved her life. Her case was the impetus that led to this author's development of a new Australian model of skin cancer treatment.

A New and Better Model

More often than not, the traditional model generally provides good patient outcomes, albeit with long waiting lists and easier access to those who live in major capital cities. The new model, therefore, is not dissimilar to the old model, but it does take into consideration the critical need to provide specialist services outside of the public hospital system to (1) those who may not be able to afford it and (2) those living in rural or regional areas.

Under the new model, GPs are now able to perform 60% of skin cancer diagnoses and treatment. These GPs may practice in their existing primary care practices or in skin cancer clinics. Regardless, they are able to provide a frontline service for diagnosis and treatment and, in many cases, manage low-level melanomas—in situ and level I melanomas—with a high degree of confidence. This is a shift from the situation in many other parts of the world, including the USA and the UK, where primary care physicians do not undertake this type of work. In fact, they would likely refer all suspicious lesions to their specialist colleagues.

Typically, with melanoma, as well as with other aggressive skin cancers such as SCCs, the time from initial diagnosis to treatment is critical due to the fact that some of these cancers can be very aggressive with a high level of morbidity or mortality if left too long without treatment. Therefore, the "ideal model," which is based on the new model in Australia, is designed around providing an optimized service delivery with a focus of trying to minimize the time between initial discovery and diagnosis to definitive treatment.

The Ideal Model

First, a patient would undergo an initial screening—the head-to-toe examination that is required to adequately assess for skin cancer. Because dermatologists do not tend to have enough time to conduct head-to-toe screenings for all of their patients, this is usually done by either a GP or family physician. In the USA, a physician assistant or nurse practitioner might perform the screening. Each of these medical professionals would have training in dermoscopy as well as skills necessary to conduct a skin assessment and diagnose suspicious lesions.

Cytologists are a future potential group of medical professionals who could conduct these screenings. The world of cytology is radically changing and it will soon have a large number of highly skilled people who could quite easily work with dermoscopy to conduct skin cancer screenings.

One of the challenges that must be overcome is the misunderstanding that skin cancers are only a result of sun exposure and therefore only occur on the face, arms, or lower legs. In fact, more than 50% of melanomas are anatomically distributed on the trunk of the body of a male and the trunk and legs of the female. Unless a patient is completely undressed, you may miss 50% of melanomas (see Fig. 10.2).

If a suspicious lesion is found, a biopsy punch or shave or an excisional biopsy must be done. In the ideal model, a family physician, GP, or nurse practitioner with the appropriate training and confidence (particularly when a lesion may be located in a cosmetically sensitive area) can perform the biopsy. Once the biopsy is completed, the biopsied segment would be sent to the dermato- or histopathologist for review and, if it is a melanoma, studied to determine its stage.

Upon reviewing the pathology report, the primary care physician must determine whether to perform a further excision (particularly if it is a melanoma) or refer the patient elsewhere. If the lesion is located in a cosmetically sensitive area or is more advanced, the patient could be referred to a dermatologist or surgeon. However, this would only be possible if the patient has private health insurance or other financial resources. If not, the primary care physician could instead send the patient to a skin cancer clinic, where, for low-level cases, there would be a lower cost and quicker access to services. Many BCC and SCC cases would be referred to these clinics, whereas being referred to a public hospital could lead to up to a year of wait time.

If, however, the patient is referred into the public hospital system, the benefit of having gone through the ideal model is that the patient goes into the hospital already with a known diagnosis.

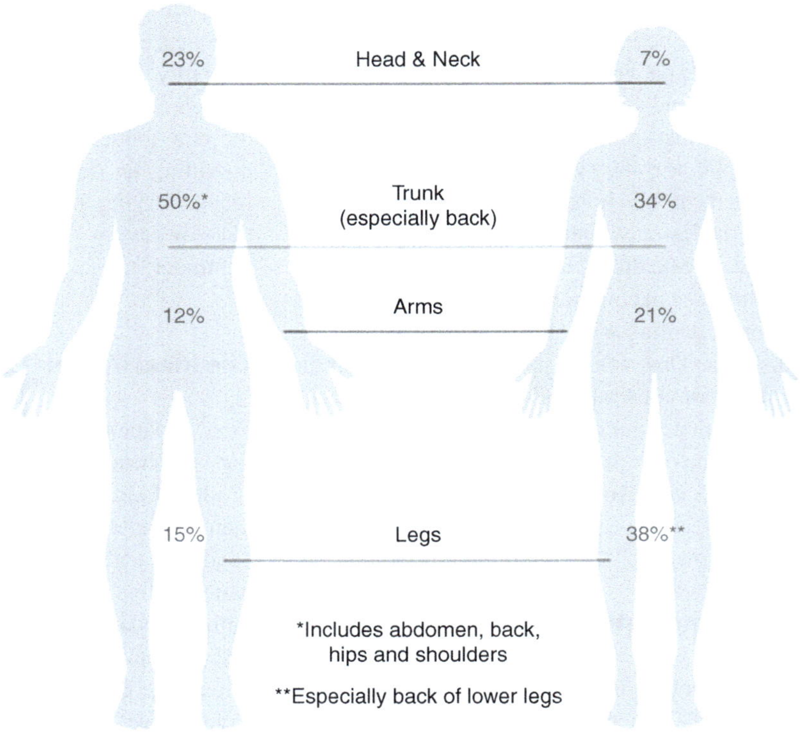

Fig. 10.2 Melanoma distribution from *Skin cancer incidence statistics, December 2015* (Cancer Research UK 2015 [24])

The hospital will know in advance that the patient needs to be seen quickly and would, therefore, provide the appropriate treatment in the required amount of time.

What You Need to Know About Australia and Its Clinicians

The ideal model is capable of providing the shortest timeframe from diagnosis to definitive treatment and, quite probably, at the lowest cost to the government, insurers, and the general public. There is still a lot of work being done, however, by primary care physicians, and this would be an adjustment for many countries. To better understand how this model works, it is important to have a more in-depth understanding of the Australian environment and culture.

Though there are registered and enrolled nurses in Australia, there are effectively no nurse practitioners or physician assistants. Furthermore, though registered and enrolled nurses are permitted to do some skin cancer screenings, the government Medicare system does not reimburse payment for any work that a nurse conducts in the screening or treatment process. As a result, nurses act more as facilitators alongside GPs to enable them to manage and treat more patients each day.

From a primary care perspective, skin cancer is reimbursed quite well. For example, in Medicare, which is the Australian Government-funded rebate system, skin cancer is the most lucrative service a GP can provide. Additionally, the GPs often take a "cowboy approach" to medical practice, meaning that they tend to take on more complex cases and push their clinical limits in comparison to other countries. This is for three reasons. First, as a culture, Australians tend to embrace a certain level of risk.

Second, there is little fear of medical or legal ramifications because it is very rare for doctors in Australia to be sued by a patient. There is an accepted understanding and recognition that doctors will not always get it right and that mistakes are an inevitable part of life. In more than 18 years of building skin cancer clinics, this author (Paul Elmslie) has worked with doctors who have treated thousands upon thousands of patients. I've not ever come across a case where a Medical legal case was brought against any doctor with whom I've worked with. I'm sure this happens occasionally; however, it is exceedingly uncommon compared to the US healthcare system.

Third, when patients have limited options, such as living in a rural or regional area, there is an expectation that the GP can perform the required treatment, to include surgery. Patients simply do not want to travel or will not be able to afford the care provided by a specialist. Regional Australians, by their very nature, are "tough" and would prefer to simply have a lesion cut out by their own doctor and continue on with their lives.

Lessons Learned from the Australian Experience

Due to the severe lack of specialists in Australia, it has become necessary to develop an alternate approach to skin cancer screenings. Skin cancer clinics, which began to form in the late 1990s, are staffed by local GPs who market to their patients that have skin cancer concerns and who don't want to wait several months to see a specialist.

Initially, several issues arose with the development of these clinics. The GPs who staffed them had no more training than their GP colleagues working in nearby primary care practices. As a result, even though these "skin cancer doctors," as they later became known, were only focusing on one element of patient care (which also happened to be the most lucrative), they had no specialized training in skin cancer management.

As a result of this sole focus on skin cancer, patients began to assume that the GPs at the skin cancer clinics were actually dermatologists or other highly trained clinicians. This became problematic because while these clinics were developing across the country, there was no standard of skill developing alongside them.

In 2005, however, discussion began on how to change that, and by 2006 Australia-based HealthCert™, in collaboration with the University of Queensland, developed the world's first certificate through to master's-level university skin cancer program. The aim of this program was to train doctors working in these clinics on a specific skin assessment process.

Standards

The development of a minimum standard for training and care for skin cancer is critical for the success of the ideal model of skin cancer care. GPs should be trained in dermoscopy in particular; otherwise, they will be under-skilled and will ultimately miss potential melanomas. The development of specific standards in Australia remains a challenge, however. As of this writing, there are moves to try and rectify this, but ultimately colleges and the representative bodies of primary care doctors are not keen on the development of too much subspecialization for fear that it will weaken the foundation of general practice.

As a result, the UK model for GPs with special interests will likely become the model taken up in Australia, as it remains one of the best models for skin cancer management in the world.

Opportunities for Citizen Education in the USA Based on the Australian Model

In Australia, an outdoor lifestyle is very much the norm, as the vast majority of the population lives near the coast and therefore spends a lot of time at the beach. Unfortunately, but traditionally, Australians tended to forego sunscreen. As a result, national campaigns to increase awareness of the dangers of sun exposure have become critical.

The main organization fulfilling this purpose in Australia is the Cancer Council. It is a relatively well-funded national organization with its own products, such as sunscreens, and services, such as a public awareness campaign that has been ongoing for more than 20 years. The campaign is well known across the country for its "Sid the Seagull" cartoon mascot, as well as its promotional tune with the phrase, "Slip, Slop, Slap," which encourages you to slip on a shirt, slop on some sunscreen, and slap on a hat. The campaign became so popular that every Australian could sing the jingle. While targeted toward children, it actually educated the wider population about the importance of skin cancer prevention.

Though Sid the Seagull is no longer part of the campaign, his presence sparked a level of public recognition that has only increased over the years. Today, the campaign has evolved to include the words "seek" and "slide" in order to encourage people to also seek shade and slide on sunglasses.

With this campaign, the Cancer Council was able to achieve a high level of public awareness and change community attitudes toward skin cancer. This can be seen on a practical, everyday level. For example, today, in schools across Australia, there is a policy called "no hat, no play." Children are expected to wear a hat to school and are not permitted to play outside unless they are wearing one. There are places, too, where sun structures have been constructed over playgrounds and funded by government and city councils.

There are other organizations in Australia that have made inroads into public awareness. One such organization is Melanoma Patients Australia, which is a support group for people affected by melanoma. In addition to marketing their services to doctors, who in turn provide the information to their patients, they also lead public awareness activities.

The Skin Cancer Institute is a new, global, multidisciplinary organization that focuses solely on skin cancer. Its members include dermatologists, surgeons, histopathologists, primary care GPs, and nurses. The goal of the institute is to optimize limited resources—whether medical or financial, in order to minimize skin cancer's impact.

One core activity on which the Skin Cancer Institute focuses on is building education in nontraditional spaces. For example, it has recently developed programs that train professionals such as hairdressers and masseuses to be able to identify possible malignant skin lesions. This is typically done through the ABCDE rule methodology, so that they can learn how to identify a suspicious skin lesion and communicate this to their clients to seek medical attention.

The Institute is also developing training for medical professionals. The first developed course was for pathologists on the subject of dermoscopy. The program taught pathologists the basic elements of dermoscopy and the characteristics to look for on a surface-based lesion. As photographic images will be incorporated with pathology requests in the future, this skill will be invaluable for pathologists. It will allow them to decide whether more sections will need to be cut for a biopsy if the diagnosis is inconclusive from the existing sections and if the pathologist is concerned about the lesion.

Currently, programs are in development for surgeons and podiatrists, two groups of medical professionals who are not traditionally trained in dermoscopy or skin cancer diagnosis but who are in a position to potentially diagnose suspicious lesions.

Australia's skin cancer clinics, which focus on prevention, diagnosis, and treatment as well as public awareness, are equally important educational tools. The National Skin Cancer Centres, which are a chain of skin cancer clinics, act as low-cost/quick-access referral centers in the local community. Focused on patient education, they produce a series of patient brochures that describe what a suspicious lesion might look like and how to conduct a skin self-examination (see Fig. 10.3).

These centers also lead two important community activities. Due to their focus on patient education, the clinics conduct public presentations on the prevention, self-examination, and early detection of skin cancer. The presentations are given at places such as senior citizen facilities and sporting clubs.

"Information evenings" enable professionals such as GPs, pharmacists, and even hairdressers to assist identifying suspicious skin lesions and then discussing them. This provides an opportunity for people, particularly in nonmedical fields, to learn how to identify possible melanomas. It is important for any professional to whom a person may present with a suspicious lesion to know where to refer him or her, and these "education evenings" provide that.

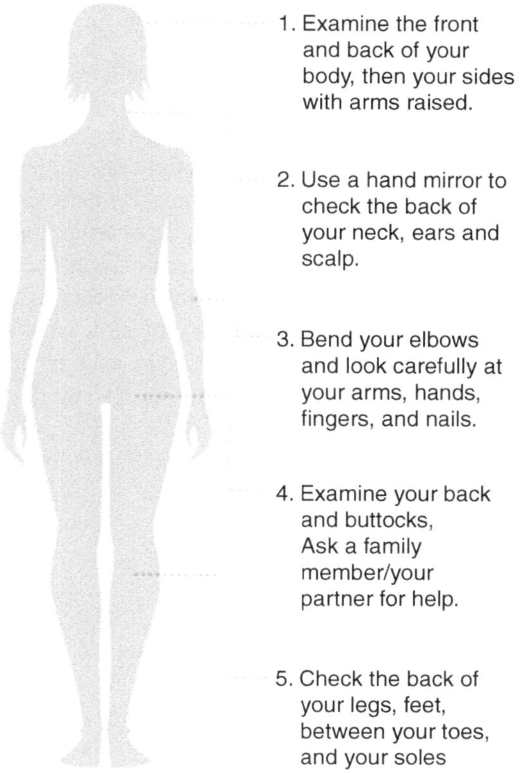

Fig. 10.3 Self-examination from *National Skin Cancer Centre Brochure* ([25] May 2016)

As shown with the Australian model, there are many different opportunities for citizen education in the USA. Organizations such as the American Cancer Society and the American Academy of Dermatologists, as well as smaller private foundations, are excellent educational resources to provide tools similar to those being successfully used across Australia.

Current Educational Efforts in Australia in Skin Cancer Management for Physicians and How These Opportunities Can Be Expanded Internationally

As most of those reading this know, primary care is typically the front line for a patient to enter the healthcare system. The primary care physician determines how the patient is managed and to which medical facility he or she should be referred to.

When dealing with skin cancer patients, however, one of the challenges is that primary care physicians do not have enough training to diagnose a melanoma or successfully assess any lesion that may appear abnormal. Primary care physicians likely did not receive any dermoscopy training, which, even though it has only been introduced more widely in the last 20 years, is an essential skill in the diagnosis of skin cancer. Patients tend to visit their primary care physicians more often than a dermatologist, so training is crucial for a better diagnosis.

When skin cancer clinics began developing across Australia, it was immediately realized that primary care physicians were not adequately trained to diagnose and treat skin cancer. As a result, HealthCert™ developed a course in skin cancer medicine in 2005. Called the Certificate in Primary Care Skin Cancer Medicine, the course was built in collaboration with the University of Queensland through then-Deputy Dean David Wilkinson. With his help, it became a school award course receiving credit into the Master of Medicine (skin cancer) degree at the University's School of Medicine.

Today, the program has developed into nine separate courses in the areas of skin cancer medicine, skin cancer surgery, and dermoscopy. Participants are able to study toward the original professional certificate, an advanced certificate, or a professional diploma. The professional diploma program in general dermatology is of particular importance because many times, a patient will present to his or her primary care physician with what looks like a suspicious lesion, but is really a rash or an infection or some other type of dermatological condition. Doctors who complete the professional diploma training become more educated about the various types of skin problems and can assess them with more confidence.

Professional development is an increasing requirement in many parts of the world. In Australia in particular, it is compulsory in order for doctors to maintain their vocational registration. HealthCert's university-recognized courses instill a high degree of confidence in doctors who want to undertake professional development to better help their patients.

The courses are generally short; they are can be completed online while others are face to face with practical sessions in biopsy and surgical techniques. There is also an online exam. Because the course is specifically designed to give doctors the skills and confidence to manage patients, rather than giving them new qualifications, there is no required specialist licensure. The courses are, however, accredited for CME/CPD. There is also a free course that teaches how to conduct a full head-to-toe skin examination and basic dermoscopy at www.skincancer-training.com.

Sub-specialization is increasing as well, which means doctors are seeing more patients in that particular field. The UK has a successful model of sub-specialization for continuous professional development, and Australia is beginning to follow suit. Additional educational opportunities that have developed include the Master of Medicine at the University of Queensland as well as at the University of Graz in Austria, which also has a Master of Science. Other notable education providers are the Royal Australian College of General Practitioners, Australian College of Rural Remote Medicine, and the Australian College of Dermatologists.

Impact

Education and training should be able to improve a doctor's diagnostic skills in two ways: (1) by identifying lesions that otherwise may have been missed and (2) by reducing the number of unnecessary excisions.

In Australia, there is a ratio of 39 benign excisions to 1 melanoma excision for GPs [17], but additional research shows that with further education this ratio can be reduced to 17–1. As more specific education is obtained in regard to the recognition of skin cancer, the ratio falls even further to 8.5–1 [18]. The ability to reduce the number of unnecessary biopsies will have a profound impact, particularly for a healthcare system that may be under pressure from a funding perspective.

Patient safety is impacted by a doctor's level of skill. A hypothetical situation might be the following: A patient presents with a suspicious lesion, but because his or her clinician is uncertain about what it might be, perhaps because the patient does not have a history of suspicious lesions, it is recommended that the patient does not need to seek further treatment. If the doctor had been trained in dermoscopy, however, and knew specifically how to use and what to look for with a dermatoscope, a better decision could have been made.

Education also reduces waiting times. If a medical professional is able to detect an early-level skin cancer, particularly a melanoma, it can typically be treated within 2–4 weeks. Others that may be in need of more specialist care can be quickly referred. Patient recognition is another area positively affected by training and education. Doctors who complete university-level education are then able to put an award or a certificate on their wall that enables patients to see they have completed professional development classes and have additional skills in a particular area. This is of importance in Australia because some doctors have had no extra training whatsoever, while others have had up to a master's level of additional education. It would be unfair for a patient to believe that these doctors are equally skilled.

Peer recognition is impacted when a doctor has additional training and education. If a general practitioner finds a lesion with which he or she is not comfortable diagnosing or managing, and the patient does not have the insurance and/or wants to wait a year at the local hospital, the GP can then refer the patient to a primary care colleague with more specialized skills. Many doctors now in Australia, once they have obtained a subspecialty skill set, will market themselves to their local GPs for referrals. The National Skin Cancer Centers send referral pads to local GPs to make them aware of the additional skill sets doctors within the centers have developed.

Expanding Internationally

More than 9,500 physicians from 32 countries have completed HealthCert courses at the time of this writing (April 2017). HealthCert is now the largest provider of education for primary care physicians in the world for skin cancer medicine. Three examples of HealthCert's expansion include live presentations in the USA, development of a free online course for the UK's National Health Service (NHS), and an online dermoscopy certificate to diploma course featuring world leading dermatologists/dermoscopists.

Online versions of these courses are becoming more important as HealthCert grows internationally, because distance ought not be an obstacle for additional training and education. The online courses are as effective as those that are live, with the benefit of eliminating the need for travel and time spent outside the office. Practical skills taught in a live environment are still critical. For example, HealthCert uses pork bellies and pig heads as a practice medium to teach doctors how to perform punch and shave biopsies as well as complete deep dermal sutures, elliptical excisions, various flaps, and full-thickness grafts.

International growth can be complicated, however, as different countries have different methods of delivering information to their medical professionals and the potential client may not be the primary care physician. In the USA, for example, the client may not be the family physician or nurse practitioner; it is more likely that the course is sold to a hospital organization of a medical group or health system that does not currently have dermatology services. It also could be a dermatologist who is looking to add this to their skill set for their midlevel providers, such as a nurse practitioner or physician assistant.

In Australia, which is very different from the USA, primary care doctors tend to be sub-contractors who get paid a percentage of the money that they bill for services. As a result, there is an incentive to increase their skills because if they are able to increase the amount they bill, they can take home additional income. In the USA, most doctors are wage employees who work for large groups. As a result, the incentive to upskill is smaller, because even if they do increase their billings, they are unlikely to see any benefits. (It should be noted that rural doctors or doctors with their own practices do not tend to fall into this category.)

In these particular situations, HealthCert must effectively communicate to the people who run the organization the benefits of obtaining these skills for their primary care physicians and other medical professionals, including physician assistants and nurse practitioners. In the UK at this time, medical treatment still falls under one system, the NHS. Doctors are usually employees of the NHS and, therefore, HealthCert would need to encourage the UK Government to help fund education and upskilling courses.

Europe is a very different picture because there are typically no restrictions on the number of training places for dermatologists as there are in other parts of the world like Australia. As a result, there are many, many dermatologists in Europe and little need for primary care physicians to do this work. Therefore, if we were going to expand our education, particularly in dermoscopy education, then dermatologists would be the craft group for us to train in the future.

Canada is similar to Australia in that they both have smaller populations and a small number of specialists. Here, as in Australia, it would be of great benefit for primary care physicians to become more skilled in dermoscopy, low-level diagnosis, and treatment to take some of the heavy load from the specialists. It is important to understand that dermoscopy is the biggest weapon to fight melanoma. It is an essential skill for dermatologists, primary care physicians, and also, arguably, surgeons. Its impact is very well documented, and it is a skill that not only is easy to learn, but can also be learned through very short training courses.

Teledermatology and Other Educational Projects in the UK and Its Utility in Clinical Practice

Teledermatology is a type of telemedicine that enables medical information to be transferred virtually. There are two basic types:

1. *Real time (RT):* An interactive process that requires all participants be present at the same time, even if based in different locations.
2. *Store and forward (S&F):* Participants need not be present at the same time. For example, with teledermatology, healthcare practitioners in remote areas take a digital image of a suspicious skin lesion, which can be done with a low-cost, off-the-shelf digital camera and dermatoscope. The image is forwarded to a specialist for his or her review, who then documents and returns his or her opinion to the remotely located practitioner. This is known as "store and forward" teledermatology.

It is of particular use in areas of the world where health care is not readily available. In Australia especially, because the population is so widely dispersed and dermatologists are primarily located in capital cities, the practice of teledermatology is becoming more useful. Teledermatology has also been used for several years in the UK through various software and models. This section explores several UK-based projects that have shown positive results.

Educational Projects in the UK

For several years, NHS groups in the UK used proprietary teledermatology software through Australia's HealthCert™ to provide patients in rural areas easier access to dermatological services. With the UK's struggle to keep up with hospital caseloads, teledermatology is proving to reduce costs, and provide patients with faster access to care, especially when a severe skin cancer is present.

With the increased use of teledermatology, it is also important to ensure that healthcare professionals have the necessary skill set to successfully incorporate it into their practice. But current dermatology training in medical school is minimal. The average time spent in this specialization is a 2-week period during a student's clinical year. As a result, clinical exposure to common dermatological issues is low. In a 2012 study completed in Edinburgh, UK, the authors advised that additional training be provided, and that e-learning tools in particular would be both cost effective and educationally effective [19].

The following provides a brief overview of several UK projects and studies that have reviewed the effectiveness of teledermatology in modern medical practice.

The Somaliland Project

In 2007, Somaliland's first medical school graduated its inaugural class [20]. But the doctors are located across a large geographical area and their access to medical literature and further training is limited. A teledermatology program between the UK and Somaliland has helped ease these limitations [20]. As part of the program, doctors in Somaliland discuss their clinical cases with UK-based tutors who help them pinpoint areas in need of more attention [20].

Regional Study on the Effect of Teledermatology for All Pigmented Lesions

Since 2004, the Medway Maritime Hospital in Kent, UK, has used a teledermatology service that stores images and patient history [21]. A dermoscopy service was added in 2008 [21]. In this particular study, which included patients from the 2-week-wait clinics, researchers looked at the "effect of teledermoscopy on teledermatology of all pigmented lesions [21]." Approximately 1200 images were reviewed in 2008 and 2009 [21].

As a result of the study, more patients were sent directly to surgery and fewer required a second face-to-face evaluation [21]. In addition, slightly more patients were directly discharged after their pre-dermoscopy teledermatology assessment [21]. According to the participating dermatologists, these findings strengthened their certainty that the use of teledermoscopy leads to improved diagnoses [21].

Hertfordshire Teledermatology Pilot Study

This study aimed to determine the reliability and effectiveness of telediagnosis for patients on the 2-week-referral list [9]. Six GP practices uploaded 110 patients' clinical information as well as three digital images per patient [9]). The study ran alongside the normal 2-week-referral path (Bataille et al.)

Each patient received a telediagnosis by two independent dermatologists, as well as face-to-face consultation and histology if deemed necessary [9]. The two independent dermatologists agreed on 78% of cases [9]. In addition, complete agreement was made in 78% of telediagnoses by one independent dermatologist and the face-to-face consultation, and in 73% of telediagnoses by the other independent dermatologist and face-to-face consultations [9].

The study concluded that between 30 and 50% of all 2-week referrals could be "triaged to other non-urgent pathways" [9]. Though it was recommended that the sample size be increased, the study found that triage of patients in the 2-week-referral pathway could reliably be seen via teledermatology for diagnosis [9].

Choose and Book Software

Choose and Book is a patient referral service software used across the UK. It enables secondary care providers to easily review referrals on a secure network and GPs a pathway to upload patient images and discuss their cases with hospital consultants.

The software has a teledermatology service, but it is often underutilized. In one study, researchers reviewed the use of this service over a 6-month period in the dermatology department of a UK teaching hospital [22]. Sub-services that were observed included data storage, image quality, patient consent and selection, GP training, and even local tariff negotiation [22].

The study concluded that Choose and Book's teledermatology service enables patient's quick access to dermatology consultancy and even reduces the need for secondary referrals in some cases [22].

Teledermatology Service in Kent

A primary care teledermatology service was developed with a group of GPs in Kent to "deliver cost-effective dermatology advice without the necessity of the patients travelling to a secondary care centre" [23]. In the pilot study, conducted between February 2010 and January 2011, two dermatologists with teledermatology experience logged into the KSYOS system each day to review waiting referrals and report daily on cases [23]. Four parameters were consistently observed:

(1) reduced referrals, (2) quality improvement, (3) response time, and (4) learning effect. Over the course of the study, 183 cases were received [23]. The study concluded that the teledermatology service led to an average 9-h response time and that 82% of possible referrals to secondary care were prevented [23]. In addition, GPs found the consultant's reply very helpful in 75% of cases, and helpful in 99% [23].

Future Management of Melanoma

Though there is still debate around the benefits of procedures such as sentinel lymph node biopsy, there are current shifts in treatment that will have a significant impact on the diagnosis and treatment of melanoma.

Training

The belief that every primary care physician and nurse should be trained in dermoscopy is increasing. It is a very simple skill to learn and should be integrated into undergraduate programs, particularly where populations are at higher risk. For example, in Australia, the number of thick melanomas has been decreasing to the point that medical providers are finding more earlier, in situ melanomas. In situ melanomas are not only relatively easy to treat, but they can also be treated at a much lower cost. This means that, when provided with the appropriate training, primary care providers can successfully provide treatment, thus preventing patients from having to go through the substantial physical and financial cost of chemotherapy and radiation.

Screenings

Traditionally, skin cancer screening involves evaluating a person's skin type, family history, personal history, and likely environmental factors, to determine whether a person qualifies as high risk.

The Genome Project, however, is changing this traditional screening process and will enable doctors to know in advance whether a patient has a higher propensity to develop skin cancer in the future, thus immediately making them a candidate for regular screening. This will completely change how the screening of high-risk populations is conducted. Based on this, routine screenings for the general population will ideally become the norm, particularly in areas of the world where melanoma is a high risk. But currently, its cost is still prohibitive in many places.

Teledermatology

At this time, teledermatology is mainly available business-to-business; it is a service used between a primary care doctor and dermatologist. In the future, however, with the continued development of technology, it will increasingly become a direct-to-consumer option. Advancements in teledermatology will enable patients to conduct a self-diagnosis, take clinical and dermatological images of a suspicious lesion, and send them directly to a dermatologist or other skin cancer doctors. In the future, artificial intelligence (AI) will have a profound impact on dermatology service delivery, especially rashes and infections.

Some of these advancements are already in progress. There are now in existence dermatoscopes, made for less than 10 dollars, that can be attached to smartphones with dermatoscope-specific slipcases. In addition, smartphones will likely have high enough resolution to take clinical images clear enough for a medical care provider to evaluate a suspicious lesion.

Digital Full-Body Imaging

The best example of digital full-body imaging at this time is the Canfield Vector WB360, which is currently only available in two research facilities. This tool is composed of a frame with 46 SLR cameras attached to it that can take one image and stitch it together into a 3D body map capable of identifying changes on the body as small as 1 mm.

Using a tool such as this will drastically alter the future management of melanoma. During a skin cancer screening, a patient will get undressed and stand in front of the device, which will then take a photograph and analyze what is new or changing on the patient's body. Then, based on this analysis, the doctor or nurse will discuss with the patient what next step ought to be taken.

Currently, digital full-body imaging is prohibitively expensive, but it is expected that advanced tools such as this will become cheaper and more readily available every 18 months as per Moore's law.

New Immunotherapy Drugs for Melanoma

Drugs such as ipilimumab, nivolumab, and pembrolizumab are capable of treating late-stage melanoma and are specifically for patients for which little can be done because their cancer is so advanced. However, they are relatively new and very expensive, and unfortunately, in some places, the government does not subsidize or reimburse for them. It is reasonable to assume that they will become more readily available and affordable in the future. Based on advancements with these medications, the following question must be asked: Will there eventually be a vaccine for melanoma? The advancements of technology and the changes occurring in how cancer is diagnosed and managed make it reasonably foreseeable that, in the future, patients will not die from skin cancer.

References

1. Australian Bureau of Statistics. Private health insurance. 2013. http://www.abs.gov.au/ausstats/abs@.nsf/lookup/E334D0A98272E4DCCA257B39000F2DCF?opendocument. Accessed 24 Mar 2017.
2. Elmslie P. Business plan for expansion of the national skin cancer centres for the South Australian Government; 2016.
3. Staples, MP, Elwood, M, Burton, RC, Williams, JL, Marks, R, Giles, GG 2006, Non-melanoma skin cancer in Australia: the 2002 national survey and trends since 1985, Med J Aus, 184, 1, pp. 6–10. https://www.mja.com.au/journal/2006/184/1/non-melanoma-skin-cancer-australia-2002-national-survey-and-trends-1985. Accessed 16 May 2017.
4. Cancer Council of Australia. Skin cancer. 2017. http://www.cancer.org.au/about-cancer/types-of-cancer/skin-cancer.html. Accessed 16 May 2017.
5. Fransen M, Karahalios A, Sharma N, English DR, Giles GG, Sinclair RD. Non-melanoma skin cancer in Australia. Med J Aus. 2012;197(10):565–8. https://www.mja.com.au/journal/2012/197/10/non-melanoma-skin-cancer-australia. Accessed 16 May 2017
6. Public Health England. Routes to diagnosis 2015 update: malignant melanoma. 2016. pp. 3–5. Available from Site-Specific Data Briefings 2006–2013 at http://www.ncin.org.uk/publications/routes_to_diagnosis. Accessed 25 May 2017.
7. British Skin Foundation. Skin cancer. n.d. http://www.britishskinfoundation.org.uk/SkinInformation/SkinCancer.aspx. Accessed 25 May 2017.
8. Skin Cancer UK. Skin cancer in the UK: the facts, all-party parliamentary group on skin. n.d. http://www.skcin.org/downloads/SkinCancerUKFacts.pdf. Accessed 25 May 2017.
9. Bataille V, Hargest E, Brown V, Blackwell V, Dawe S, Cooper A, Hamp J. A teledermatology pilot study in Hertfordshire: triage of 2-week-wait referrals: BT-6. Br J Dermatol. 2011;165:137–8.
10. Cegedim. Market profile of U.S. dermatologists one key market insight report. 2015. http://us.imshealth.com/Marketing/GTMN/Market-Profile-of-Dermatologists.pdf. Accessed 16 May 2017.
11. Guy GP, Machlin SR, Ekwueme DU, Yabroff KR. Prevalence and costs of skin cancer treatment in the U.S., 2002–2006 and 2007–2011. Am J Prev Med. 2015;48(2):183–7. https://www.ncbi.nlm.nih.gov/pmc/articles/PMC4603424/. Accessed 16 May 2017
12. Chen JT, Kempton SJ, Rao VK. The economics of skin cancer: an analysis of medicare payment data. Plast Reconstr Surg Glob Open. 2016;4(9):e868. https://www.ncbi.nlm.nih.gov/pmc/articles/PMC5054999/. Accessed 25 May 2017
13. Skin Cancer Foundation. Skin cancer facts & statistics. 2017. http://www.skincancer.org/skin-cancer-information/skin-cancer-facts#melanoma. Accessed 16 May 2017.
14. National Cancer Institute. Melanoma treatment (PDQ®)–health professional version. 2017. https://www.cancer.gov/types/skin/hp/melanoma-treatment-pdq. Accessed 16 May 2017.
15. Corona R, Mele A, Amini M, De Rosa G, Coppola G, Piccardi P, Fucci M, Pasquini P, Faraggiana T. Interobserver variability on the histopathologic diagnosis of cutaneous melanoma and other pigmented skin lesions. J Clin Oncol. 1996;14(4):1218–23. http://ascopubs.org/doi/abs/10.1200/JCO.1996.14.4.1218?url_

ver=Z39.88-2003&rfr_id=ori%3Arid%3Acrossref.org&rfr_dat=cr_pub%3Dpubmed&. Accessed 16 May 2017
16. American Cancer Society. Treating melanoma skin cancer, 2016. https://www.cancer.org/cancer/melanoma-skin-cancer/treating.html. Accessed 23 May 2017.
17. Byrnes P, Ackermann E, Williams ID, Mitchell GK, Askew D. Management of skin cancer in Australia comparison of general practice and skin cancer clinics. Aust Fam Physician. 2007;36(12):1073–5. http://www.racgp.org.au/afp/200712/21114. Accessed 16 May 2017
18. Rosendahl C, Williams G, Eley D, Wilson T, Canning G, Keir J, McColl I, Wilkinson D. The impact of subspecialization and dermatoscopy use on accuracy of melanoma diagnosis among primary care doctors in Australia. J Am Acad Dermatol. 2012;6(5):846–52.
19. Aldridge BR, Maxwell SS, Rees JL. Dermatology undergraduate skin cancer training: a disconnect between recommendations, clinical exposure and competence. BMC Med Educ. 2012;12:27. https://doi.org/10.1186/1472-6920-12-27. Accessed 16 May 2017
20. Ali F, Bowen J, Mahamed J, Finlayson AE. Letter: real-time, intercontinental dermatology teaching of trainee physicians in Somaliland using a dedicated social networking portal. Dermatol Online J. 2011;18(14):16. http://escholarship.org/uc/item/7nt0341d. Accessed 16 May 2017
21. Sheraz A, Halpern SM. Influence of additional dermoscopy images on teledermatology screening of skin lesions. Br J Dermatol. 2011;165:136.
22. Charman CR, Malhomme H, Slocombe G. Teledermatology using choose and book: can it improve your dermatology service? Br J Dermatol. 2011;165:137.
23. Halpern SM, Shall L. Establishment of a primary care-based teledermatology service in Kent. Br J Dermatol. 2011;165(Suppl. 1):135–8.
24. Cancer Research UK. Skin cancer incidence statistics, December 2015. 2015. http://www.cancerresearchuk.org/health-professional/cancer-statistics/statistics-by-cancer-type/skin-cancer/incidence#heading-Four. Accessed 17 May 2017.
25. National Skin Cancer Centre. Brochure; 2016.

Pigmented Lesions: Biopsy Methods and Emerging Non-invasive Imaging Techniques

11

Cindy Wassef, Lea J. Bellomo, and David I. Silverstein

Introduction

Skin cancer incidence continues to increase in the United States, with melanoma accounting for the most deaths. The increase in the number of thin (<1 mm) melanomas diagnosed indicates that a combination of increased diagnostic skills as well as increased awareness may be contributing factors [1, 2]. Given the grave morbidity and mortality associated with thicker lesions, appropriate diagnosis and treatment are imperative. The fundamental step in this cascade is the skin biopsy.

Skin biopsy, however, is not without its controversies. For the majority of cutaneous sites, four major biopsy options exist: shave biopsy, incisional biopsy, scoop or saucerization biopsy, and excisional biopsy. When selecting a biopsy technique, various factors play a role including but not limited to those related directly to the lesion as well as those specific to the patient and the performing physician. In this chapter, our goal is to explore the various biopsy techniques as well as discuss their overall utility and value. We also review special situations and pertinent biopsy techniques. Lastly, while a biopsy still represents the gold standard for tissue diagnosis, we will briefly describe several new and emerging diagnostic non-invasive modalities.

C. Wassef, M.D. · L. J. Bellomo, M.D.
D. I. Silverstein, M.D., F.A.A.D. (✉)
Department of Dermatology, Stony Brook Medicine, Stony Brook, NY, USA
e-mail: cindy.wassef@stonybrookmedicine.edu; lea.bellomo@stonybrookmedicine.edu; david.silverstein@stonybrookmedicine.edu

Evaluation of Pigmented Lesions

Initial clinical history and skin evaluation are always the first steps prior to a biopsy. In most dermatology offices, little equipment exists beyond visual examination and dermoscopy. The most widely used clinical algorithm is the ABCDE criteria. Lesions suspicious for melanoma include those that show asymmetry, border irregularity, variegated or multiple colors, diameter of greater than 6 mm, and evolving or changing lesions. Its utility value in the clinical setting varies. While sensitivity and specificity have been reported to be as high as 90% in some studies, these criteria have fallen short in the detection of a primary melanoma less than 6 mm in diameter and the nodular subtype of melanoma [3].

In conjunction with visual examination, dermoscopy has emerged as an important adjunct for the detection of melanoma. A dermatoscope is a magnifying lens that, in conjunction with a liquid medium and polarized light, can allow direct visualization of features in the epidermis and superficial dermis that are not visible to the naked eye. Its value has been confirmed in multiple studies and meta-analyses that show that adding dermoscopy to the clinical skin exam increased the detection of melanoma compared to

A. I. Riker (ed.), *Melanoma*, https://doi.org/10.1007/978-3-319-78310-9_11

performing only a clinical skin exam [4]. Multiple algorithms have been developed based upon the dermoscopic features identified, with further refinement of various features still in development towards a single unifying algorithm [5].

Equipment, Setup, and Anesthesia

Once the decision is made to biopsy a skin lesion, the next step in performing a satisfactory biopsy is to gather the necessary equipment and local anesthetic and to organize and set up for the procedure. While equipment is dependent upon the type of biopsy being performed, local anesthesia is needed for any biopsy. Minimal equipment is needed to perform skin biopsies and most are readily available in dermatology offices. Personal protective equipment for the physician including non-sterile gloves, goggles, or an eye shield and mask can be used if they are felt to be necessary to protect from any bodily fluid or other materials. Handwashing or use of antiseptic solution is also necessary prior to and after the performance of a biopsy.

Equipment needed usually include a Dermablade™ or a #15 scalpel, a needle holder/driver, tissue forceps, Iris scissors, punch biopsy tool, suture material, and gauze. For hemostasis, there are several options including aluminum chloride, electrocautery, or Monsel's solution. Monsel's solution is iron based and does leave behind residual brown pigment which is both cosmetically displeasing but also can add to difficulties with pathological examination in the event a second biopsy is needed [2]. While biopsy sites are often initially cleaned with 70% alcohol wipes prior to injection with anesthetic, this measure has been shown to be unnecessary and does not decrease the risk of infection. Sanitization of skin is only suggested for a visibly dirty or unclean biopsy site [6].

Lidocaine is the most commonly used anesthetic in dermatologic practice. We typically utilize 1% lidocaine with epinephrine in a 1:100,000 dilution, commonly purchased in this form as single-use vials. Benefits associated with the addition of epinephrine include longer duration of action, vasoconstriction leading to less localized bleeding, and ability to use larger quantities because of decreased systemic diffusion [7]. The full effect of vasoconstriction takes roughly 7–10 min while the duration of action of the anesthetic itself is 1–2 h overall [2]. Lidocaine with epinephrine use is contraindicated in the first trimester of pregnancy and therefore only lidocaine with a maximum volume of 10 mL. Lidocaine with epinephrine is safe to use for digital anesthesia unless the patient has known peripheral vascular disease, connective tissue disease, Raynaud's syndrome, or antiphospholipid syndrome. A single injection of lidocaine with epinephrine into the midline of the phalanx can provide anesthesia for up to 10 h vs. 5 h for lidocaine alone [2, 7, 8]. Patients will often report an "allergy" to lidocaine; however, further investigation may reveal that these perceived allergies are secondary to the sympathetic effects of epinephrine leading to tachycardia and anxiety. A true allergic reaction to lidocaine, an amide anesthetic, should prompt substitution of an ester anesthetic such as procainamide.

Injection of anesthetic is with a small-gauge needle, such as a 30-gauge, ½-in. needle, until a visible wheal is raised of the surrounding area. Anesthetic should be injected adjacent, rather than within the lesion, in order to prevent any disruption of the epidermis or dermis. For larger lesions, a "ring injection" around the perimeter of the lesion can allow for diffusion of the anesthetic more centrally [2]. If the lesion is felt to extend deeper, particularly in certain anatomic sites with a thicker dermis, injection into a deeper plane such as the reticular dermis or superficial adipose tissue may be needed.

There are multiple techniques available to lessen the discomfort associated with the anesthetic injection. Lidocaine 1% with 1:100,000 epinephrine has a known pH of 4.2; thus buffering with 8.4% sodium bicarbonate in a 10:1 ratio has been found to decrease the discomfort of the injection. Buffering lidocaine does not decrease its anesthetic efficacy but does reduce the epinephrine concentration by 25% per week exposed. Warming of the anesthetic solution has also been found to decrease injection pain.

The combination of warming and buffering has been found to produce the greatest benefit in terms of diminishing the pain associated with injection [2, 7]. Needles of a smaller diameter (between 27 and 30 gauge) and slow injection also decrease discomfort. Consequently, a smaller needle also leads to slower injection of anesthetic. Sharper needles lead to less force required to inject into the skin; using a separate needle to draw up anesthetic and then another to inject the patient is a useful way to reduce injection pain. Distraction techniques can range from having the patient look away to tapping at a separate site, having a conversation with the patient, and attempting to gently vibrate the syringe while injecting.

Other anesthetic options seen in many dermatologic practices include topical anesthetics. Topical anesthetics such as EMLA (lidocaine/prilocaine) cream can be used as an adjunct prior to biopsy procedures and local injected anesthetic or as a primary means of numbing. After 2 h under occlusion, EMLA provides anesthesia to a depth of about 5 mm that is deep enough for skin biopsy in areas with a thin-to-moderate dermis [8]. For children, pretreatment with EMLA cream for 45 min under occlusion can ease injection pain, with the full effect seen after 90–120 min. A few other options may include simple application of ice or cryogen to the area [2, 7].

Guidelines for Biopsy

Recommendations on what is regarded as an adequate biopsy for a suspicious skin lesion vary depending on the academic body. The British Academy of Dermatology issued revised guidelines in 2010 indicating that adequate excision of suspicious pigmented lesions should include 2 mm margins of normal skin and a cuff of subcutaneous fat [9]. It advised against performing diagnostic shave biopsies, partial removal of nevi, or routine removal of nevi 5 mm or less. Punch biopsy for lentigo maligna or acral melanoma was deemed acceptable. For subungual melanoma, assurance of the nail matrix in the sample and removal of clinically obvious tumor were advised. These guidelines, however, merely represent recommendations only and should be applied to each patient based upon the clinical situation [9].

The American Academy of Dermatology issued recommendations regarding the biopsy of pigmented lesions in 2011 [10]. For suspicious pigmented skin lesions, narrow excisional biopsy with 1–3 mm margins of normal skin is recommended. Several biopsy techniques are deemed acceptable, such as a standard ellipse, punch biopsy/removal, or a deep-shave biopsy that includes subcutaneous fatty tissue. Under certain circumstances, incisional biopsy may be performed, with clinicopathologic correlation often necessary. For example, suspicious pigmented lesions of the nail bed may be approached with an incisional or excisional biopsy [10]. As previously echoed in the British recommendations, the above recommendations are utilized and applied individually and, in general, will apply to the vast majority of patients.

Biopsy Techniques

Below is a review of the four main biopsy techniques—shave biopsy, scoop or saucerization biopsy, incisional or punch biopsy, and excisional biopsy.

Shave Biopsy

The shave biopsy is the most commonly performed method to evaluate pigmented lesions because of how quickly it can be performed, simplicity of wound care, cosmetic result, and cost-effectiveness [11]. The necessary equipment is shown in Fig. 11.1. Prior to performing the biopsy, it is helpful to finely demarcate the borders of the lesion. A Wood's lamp (365 nm) examination can be helpful in doing so because it enhances (darkens) lesion borders through an increased amount of lesional melanin that causes increased absorption of light compared to the surrounding skin. Once the lesion is clearly defined and marked, the area is then anesthetized

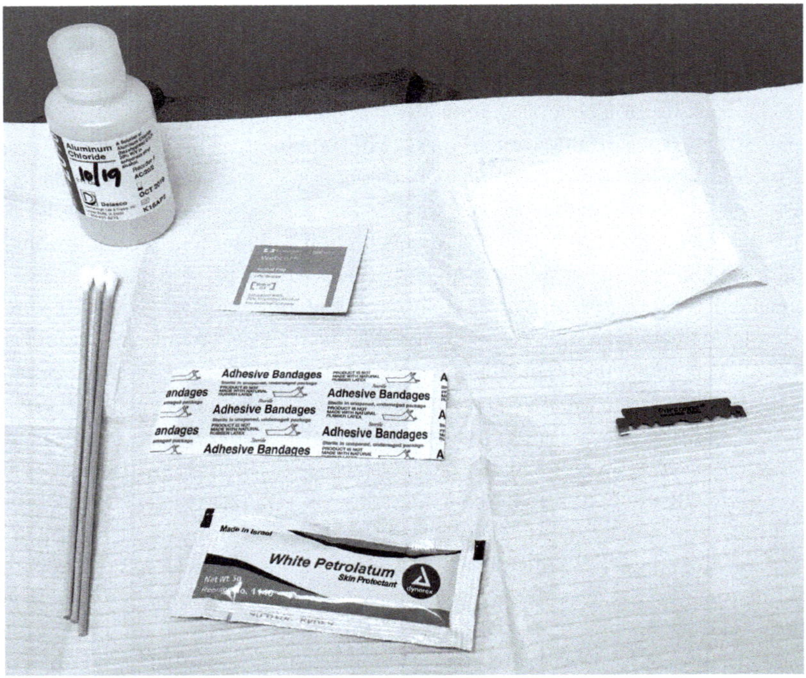

Fig. 11.1 Shave biopsy setup. Shave biopsies require minimal equipment to perform. An alcohol pad is used to sanitize the area. Gillette blade is used for lesion removal with aluminum chloride on a cotton tip applicator for hemostasis. Gauze should be available to apply pressure for bleeding. After bleeding is controlled, white petrolatum and a bandage are used to cover the wound

with lidocaine with epinephrine as previously described. A scalpel (#15 blade) or a flexible razor blade is used to remove the lesion in its entirety if possible, usually with a 1 mm margin of normal surrounding skin. The flexible razor blade allows for alteration of the diameter of the biopsy by curving the blade and alteration of the depth of the biopsy by angling the blade; a greater curvature decreases the diameter of the sample and a deeper angle towards the subcutis increases the depth of the sample [2]. Removing the lesion in its entirety by the aforementioned techniques allows the true depth to be evaluated if need be and it is often recommended that the lesion be re-shaved or completely excised if residual pigment remains.

A disadvantage of this technique is that it can leave a depressed and hypopigmented scar if the biopsy is angled too sharply. Thus, a #15 blade may be a better choice when the skin lesion is flatter and flush with the skin. For this reason, it is ideal for areas of thin skin such as the face and dorsum of the hands. The flexible razor blade is better suited for areas of thick skin such as the back. With experience, however, it is possible to use either blade for biopsy of any skin site with cosmetically acceptable results.

After biopsy, hemostasis is often achieved using aluminum chloride, which deposits small salt plugs into blood vessels. The site is then allowed to heal by secondary intention. Patients are instructed to clean the area with mild soap and keep it moist by coating with Vaseline ointment and covering with a bandage daily until fully healed. The use of antibiotic ointment is not routinely recommended because there is significant risk for allergic contact dermatitis and the overall potential for wound infection is low given the superficial nature of biopsy. Furthermore, recent studies suggest that these antibiotic ointments may select for methicillin-resistant *Staphylococcus aureus* [12]. The use of hydrogen peroxide is also not advised as this may impede the healing process.

Patients should be advised that the biopsy site will look erythematous and inflamed initially and then heal with a yellow fibrinous exudate that is part of the normal healing process. Biopsies on the lower extremities may take up to 1 month or longer to heal completely because of poorer circulation in certain patient populations with peripheral vascular disease, immunosuppression, or diabetes. Given that a shave biopsy is usually selected for small lesions, it tends to provide a generally good cosmetic outcome. The defect created is often circular in shape and shallow so that a significant scar is not evident if the procedure is performed well. Additionally, the scar tends to contract over time, and it is helpful to reassure patients from the outset that the cosmetic defect will likely be smaller than the pigmented lesion with respect to size.

Other benefits of the shave biopsy are the ease of performing the procedure, allowing for an efficient use of office time during a busy day of seeing patients. The shave biopsy is also inexpensive because suture is not needed to close the residual defect. In terms of resident education and training, it is considered an important and standard part of any residency training program in dermatology, with most residents becoming proficient with the shave biopsy early in their training. Other healthcare providers are also capable of performing shave biopsies, an important benefit for patients seeing their primary care physicians. Moreover, in a patient who has many suspicious melanocytic lesions such as that seen in dysplastic nevus syndrome, shave biopsy may be preferable because multiple excisional biopsies can become laborious for both provider and patient. Most providers cannot interrupt their clinic to perform a surgery and must have the patient return for the procedure with significant potential for the patient to be lost to follow-up. The patient may be too fearful to undergo surgery or have scheduling difficulties that may not allow for a return visit in the immediate future. In such cases, shave biopsy may at least allow for immediate diagnostic testing at the time of lesion identification.

A major problem with the shave biopsy technique arises when the procedure is inappropriately selected. For example, larger lesions are more difficult to completely sample and may best be sampled by other means (see later discussion). If a lesion is transected at the base, the true thickness (Breslow's depth) of the lesion cannot be accurately evaluated. Thus, if the lesion returns as a melanoma, where Breslow's depth determines the margins of excision as well as whether to perform a sentinel lymph node biopsy, it is problematic for the surgeon to fully determine this based upon an incomplete Breslow's depth. A recent retrospective study of 139 patients with melanoma showed that 18 patients had a thicker Breslow's depth as determined by excision compared with initial shave biopsy of the lesion. Seven of these patients required additional surgery after the initial wide local excision because of the discrepancy [13].

A more recent study, with a sample size of 600 patients, noted that the initial shave biopsy accurately predicted the lesional depth, translating into the correct surgical treatment strategy in 97% of patients [14]. Thus, when properly performed in the appropriate setting, the shave technique may yield the accurate Breslow's depth in 97% of patients, but it may be incorrect in as much as 10%. The most worrisome scenario could occur if a biopsy is performed too superficially and the pathologist notes that there are atypical features but does not interpret them as a melanoma. Here, it is possible that the deeper portions of the specimen would have resulted in pathologic interpretation as melanoma. Thus, if the pathologist notes that a lesion has significant atypia and it extends to the base of the specimen, it is advisable to have the entirety of the lesion definitively sampled.

Incisional or Punch Biopsy

There are several settings in which an incisional biopsy may be more useful compared to the shave biopsy. For example, as congenital nevi develop, there are often areas within the nevus that become cobblestoned, bleed from irritation, or become darker. An incisional biopsy using a punch biopsy tool is very helpful to sample a certain portion of the larger lesion. Similarly, in a nevus spilus, areas of hyperpigmentation can become darker and may require sampling. Incisional biopsies have been recommended in other circumstances as well, such as extensive or large pigmented lesions with unclear margins, extensive facial lentigo maligna, and pigmented lesions in acral and mucosal areas [15]. The tools and equipment needed to perform a punch biopsy are shown in Fig. 11.2. As with the shave biopsy, the portion of the lesion to be biopsied is clearly marked. A camera is recommended to photograph exactly where in the lesion the biopsy is taken from. Anesthesia is again provided with 1% lidocaine with epinephrine.

The biopsy can be performed using a punch tool, which is placed over the area and rotated in one direction while pressure is applied in a downward direction. The skin lesion should be centered between your fingers and held in the direction of the relaxed skin tension lines so that the punch creates a small ellipse rather than a perfect circle. Depending on the area, the rotation should continue until the hub of the punch is at the surface of the skin. If working in an area of thin skin, the punch should be rotated until the level of the fat is reached. The punch tool is then removed and a tissue forceps is used to gently grasp the specimen without crushing it, and sharp scissors to transect the specimen along the deep fat. For pigmented lesions, the size of the punch should be no smaller than 3 mm so that the pathologist has an adequate specimen for sectioning and processing. A 2 mm punch biopsy would not provide enough tissue for a pathologist to render a diagnosis. Punch biopsies come in many sizes ranging from 1 to 10 mm. Size of punch biopsy is determined by the size of the lesion and whether a whole or only partial sample of the lesion is to be taken. A hemostatic foam or gauze can be used to pack the biopsy site if it is 3 mm. For larger punch sizes, it is recommended to use a simple, interrupted stitch with a nonabsorbable suture to be removed in 5–10 days in the office, depending on the location. If there is concern that the patient cannot return for a suture removal visit, an absorbable suture with cyanoacrylate or other liquid adhesive and Steri-Strips for epidermal re-approximation can be used.

If the lesion is larger than a punch tool, a scalpel with a #15 blade can be used. An ellipse in the direction of skin tension lines is made over the area to be biopsied and removed by cutting down to the layer of the fat. Closure is then performed using dermal and epidermal sutures as needed. Historically, there have been two major issues with incisional biopsy. One is whether putting a defect in the middle of the tumor allows for further spread or seeding of the tumor. This theory has largely been debunked and, if it occurs at all, is not considered clinically relevant [15, 16]. The more important and clinically relevant issue relates to diagnosis and evaluation of the Breslow's depth. Similar to shave biopsies, there

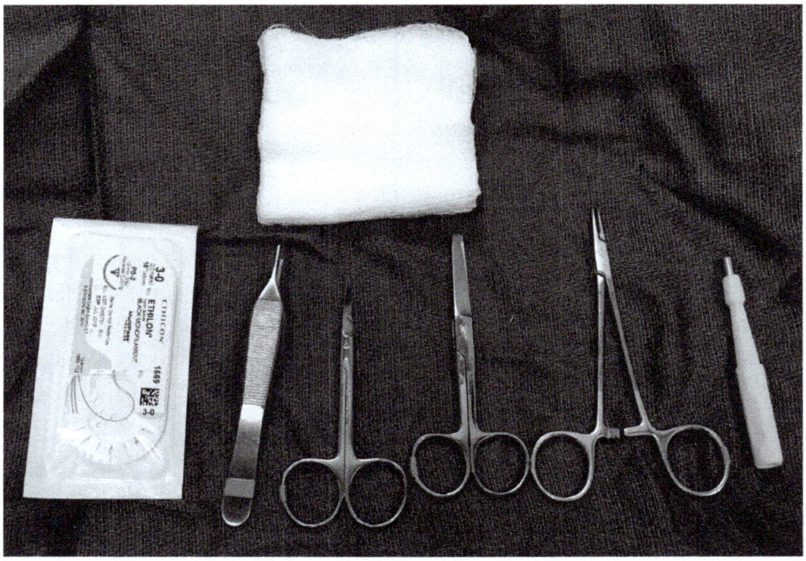

Fig. 11.2 Punch biopsy setup. From left to right, suture, forceps, iris scissors, Mayo dissecting scissors, needle driver, and punch biopsy tool are pictured. The punch biopsy tool is used to sample the specimen with the Adler forceps and Mayo dissecting scissors used for removal. A needle driver and sutures are then used to suture the wound if needed. Gauze should be available to apply pressure for bleeding

is potential for misinterpretation of the true tumor depth with the incisional technique.

Unlike the shave biopsy, which is usually selected with the intent to remove the entire lesion, the incisional biopsy is intended to remove only a portion of the lesion. Some have argued that the most worrisome portion of the lesion, as determined clinically and dermoscopically, should thus be sampled. However, Somach et al. found that there are differences amongst clinicians as to what might represent the most worrisome area of a suspected lentigo maligna lesion [17]. Furthermore, they identified a diagnostic discordance between incisional and excisional biopsy by as much as 40%. Thus, keep in mind that the portion of the lesion most worrisome to a clinician may not correspond to the most histologically aggressive portion of a melanocytic lesion.

Although this observation may be true, once a diagnosis of melanoma is made, most patients subsequently undergo a complete excision with the appropriate surgical margins, with treatment plans modified based upon histopathologic evaluation of the excised specimens. Even though this technique may subject the patient to additional procedures, studies have not documented any negative implications with respect to patient outcome. Pflugfelder et al. retrospectively examined nine such studies, and found no significant difference in patient outcomes when comparing incisional with excisional samples [15]. However, similar to concerns with the shave biopsy, if a lesion is interpreted as melanoma in one region but not another, and the non-melanoma portion of it is sampled, the diagnosis may be missed altogether. Thus, if the pathologist notes that there is atypia with extension to any of the peripheral margins when performing an incisional biopsy, consideration should be given to completely excising the pigmented lesion.

Conversely, a major disadvantage of the incisional biopsy technique is a false-positive result. Evaluation of the symmetry and borders of the lesion is important for the pathologist when interpreting specimens. When an incisional biopsy is performed, the area of interest always extends to the periphery of a sample, thereby making a proper diagnosis difficult to render [18]. For example, histologic melanoma mimickers such as a Spitz nevus or recurrent nevus that can share features of melanoma with regression, for example, may be falsely diagnosed as melanoma when only partially biopsied [19]. In certain situations, an incisional biopsy is an appropriate choice but every effort should be made to provide the pathologist with the entire pigmented lesion when able for the aforementioned reasons.

Excisional Biopsy

Excisional biopsy is considered the gold standard for melanoma diagnosis. It allows the entire lesion to be examined by the dermatopathologist for the margins, Breslow's depth of invasion, and cellular behavior. The excisional biopsy is thus the technique of choice for a pigmented lesion that is suspicious for melanoma. First, the margins of the melanocytic lesion are clearly defined; as mentioned earlier, a Wood's lamp can be helpful to detect subclinical pigmentation. A 2–3 mm margin of excision is performed around the skin lesion, following steps similar to that of other types of biopsies. A scalpel is utilized after local anesthetic has been infiltrated, removing an elliptical area that includes the subcutaneous fat. Once removed, it is important to orient the specimen for the pathologist and provide them with as much information as possible about the lesion, such as anatomic location, description of the lesion, and your preliminary diagnosis. On the extremities, for example, it is preferable to orient excisions vertically, rather than horizontally, to better preserve lymphatic architecture as well as to provide the surgeon the best opportunity to close the residual defect primarily, without requiring placement of a skin graft for wound closure.

Upon the implementation of sentinel lymph node mapping as a sensitive method of examining the first draining lymph nodes in a nodal basin, there was some initial concern as to the effect of performing a biopsy upon the primary site. Several subsequent studies have shown that if there is not significant tissue rearrangement after defect closure, the accuracy of sentinel lymph node biopsy is still quite good, although sentinel lymph node biopsy at the time of wide local excision is preferred [20, 21]. Few studies have attempted to specifically address whether an initial diagnostic excisional biopsy affects the subsequent accuracy of sentinel lymph node biopsy. One study of 60 patients found no difference in lymphatic flow between groups who had previously had diagnostic excisional biopsy for a suspected melanoma [22]. Although no studies directly compare the accuracy of sentinel lymph node biopsy with skin biopsy technique (i.e., shave versus incisional versus excisional), it is generally accepted that narrow excisional biopsy does not alter the subsequent accuracy of a sentinel lymph node biopsy and therefore does not change patient prognosis. If wide local excision does not appreciably alter the accuracy of sentinel lymph node biopsy, it can be assumed that neither should the initial biopsy with narrow margins [23].

Scoop (Saucerization) Biopsy

The scoop biopsy involves utilizing a flexible razor blade that is angled to yield a specimen that extends to the mid-dermis or subcutaneous fat. Thus, it is considered an "excisional biopsy" and may be utilized for lesions that are difficult to remove with an elliptical excision. For example, potential sites include areas where scars may become hypertrophic and spread over time such as the upper back and shoulders or when a patient prefers not to have limitations during the postoperative period. Compared with an elliptical excision that is closed primarily and resulting in a linear scar, saucerization leaves a smaller, rounder scar that may be considered a cosmetically acceptable scar while still providing as much diagnostic tissue as an elliptical excision [11].

Special Situations

Unique situations requiring tailored evaluation include melanonychia, scalp nevi in children, and labial and genital melanotic macules.

Evaluation of Melanonychia

The evaluation of longitudinal melanonychia remains somewhat difficult and will often require performing a biopsy for definitive diagnosis. The most widely accepted biopsy technique is a longitudinal, full-thickness excisional procedure, since a shave biopsy does not always allow adequate evaluation of the true Breslow's depth [24]. Many suggest that before obtaining a biopsy, the nail plate should be viewed "end-on" with dermoscopy because lesions that are present in the dorsal nail plate reflect a melanocytic origin at the proximal nail matrix, whereas lesions present in the ventral nail plate correspond to an origin at the distal nail matrix [25]. Regardless of which biopsy technique is chosen, the procedure is best performed with a digital nerve block using lidocaine and occasionally utilizing a tourniquet (with tourniquet time not exceeding 20 min). There has been much controversy over the years regarding the use of epinephrine in acral areas but it is now generally accepted that it can be used safely in small quantities (not exceeding 3 mL for a single digit) to ensure hemostasis [26].

Shave Biopsy of the Nail Matrix

After achieving adequate anesthesia, tangential incisions are made at the junction of the proximal and lateral nail folds. The skin can be undermined in several ways with sharp dissection along the nail bed plane, with the proximal nail reflected back and thereby exposing the proximal nail plate and underlying matrix. The proximal nail plate is then reflected laterally through the use of an anvil-action nail splitter. This procedure allows full exposure of the proximal nail bed and matrix. The origin of the pigment band is identified and scored with a scalpel blade that is then turned horizontally to shave the specimen. The laterally reflected nail plate is trimmed longitudinally at its lateral free edge and returned to its original position. The proximal nail fold is released and returned to its normal position. The skin is then sutured at each tangential incision [2].

Punch Biopsy of the Nail Matrix

As with the shave biopsy, anesthesia is achieved and proximal nail fold is reflected. The nail plate is left intact because it may serve to help visualize the origin of the pigment. A punch biopsy tool is used to score the overlying plate above the origin of melanonychia and carried down through matrix to bone. Fine-tipped scissors are used to snip the specimen at the level of the periosteum. Given that the underlying nail plate is secure, suturing is not necessary after realigning the proximal nail fold, and a simple pressure dressing may suffice for wound healing [2].

Lateral Longitudinal Excision

A scalpel blade is inserted halfway between the cuticle and distal interphalangeal crease, 1–2 mm medial to the pigmented band. Incision is made through skin and soft tissue to the level of the bone, extending distally through the nail plate and hyponychium, to a level 3–4 mm distal to the digital tip. The blade is then re-inserted proximally at the same starting point and moved laterally, coursing around the entire matrix horn, so that a final elliptical shape is achieved, with a thin margin around the entire pigmented band. Repair is performed by placing a suture that realigns the proximal nail fold to the lateral nail fold, and another at the proximal nail fold and at the hyponychium [2] (Fig. 11.3).

Evaluation of Scalp Nevi in Children

Scalp nevi in children represent a diagnostic challenge because they frequently undergo significant change as the child grows [27]. However, most scalp nevi in children are benign and generally recommendations are conservative observation instead of immediate biopsy. Although nevi in this "special site" are not often associated with problematic clinical behavior, they are more likely to display atypical histologic features, making them somewhat difficult for pathologic evaluation [28, 29]. Thus, if sampling is to be performed, some recommend a full-thickness excisional biopsy with conservative margins in order to provide the dermatopathologist with the most tissue to evaluate [30].

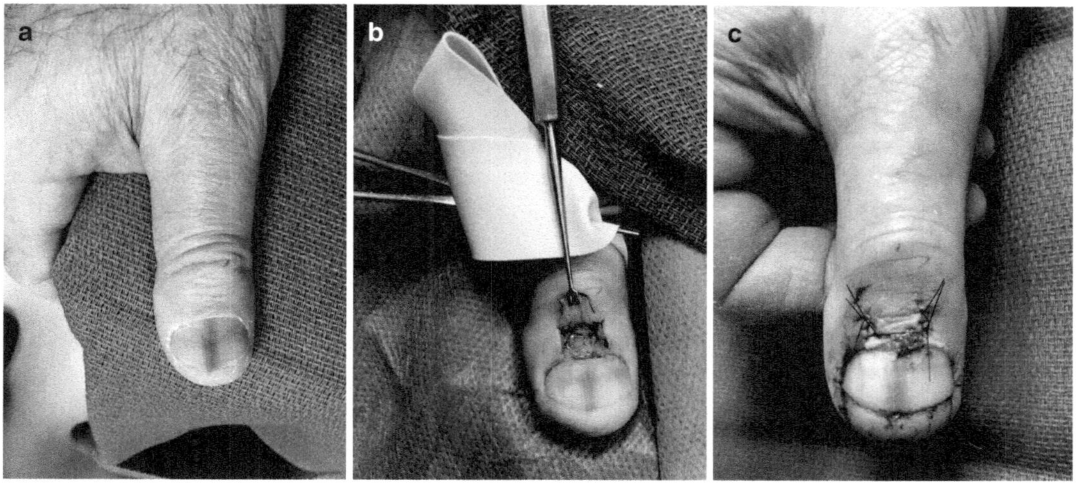

Fig. 11.3 All photos courtesy of Jordan B. Slutsky, MD FAAD. (**a**) Linear melanonychia on right first digit which patient reports has been changing in size in color over the last few years. (**b**) In this photo, the cuticle has been flip backed to reveal the proximal matrix after nerve and local block has been performed. (**c**) After biopsy of the matrix, the cuticular skin is sutured

Labial Melanotic Macules

Melanotic macules on the lips can be due to many causes, including but not limited to sun exposure, medications, physiologic pigmentation, carcinoma, and syndromes such as Laugier-Hunziker or Peutz-Jegher. Biopsy is often indicated and the technique used is dependent upon where on the lip the lesion is located. On the cutaneous lip, a shave biopsy is acceptable if the lesion does not cross the vermilion border. The site can be left to heal by secondary intention and with minimal scarring. On the mucosal lip, a punch biopsy with closure using silk suture (because silk lies down flat and is nonirritating) is preferred. Sutures may be removed at 5 days as the mucosa heals quickly. If the pigmented lesion crosses the vermilion border, a punch biopsy with vertical orientation should be performed. Horizontal orientation may inadvertently cause a noticeable eclabium. Prior to the procedure, the border of the lip should be marked with a gentian violet marking pen so that when the suture is placed to close the defect, the border can be precisely aligned [2].

Genital Melanotic Macules

Genital melanomas are relatively uncommon, with an overall poorer prognosis and earlier tendency towards metastatic spread [31]. For this reason, melanotic macules in the genital region should be monitored closely with serial photography (both clinical and dermatoscopic) to assess for change. If biopsy is required, a punch biopsy using a silk suture for closure is the preferred method. As for oral mucosa biopsies, sutures should be removed at 5 days. Although shave biopsies heal well here, patients often complain of stinging and irritation while wound healing occurs [2].

Non-invasive Options for Pigmented Lesions

Non-invasive diagnostic options are emerging, both as adjuncts to routine biopsy and histopathology, as well as independent diagnostic entities. In this section, we provide an overview of reflectance confocal microscopy, digital multispectral dermoscopy, optical coherence tomography, tape-stripping mRNA, ultrasound, and electrical bioimpedance.

Reflectance Confocal Microscopy

Reflectance confocal microscopy is a method for in vivo imaging of skin and suspicious lesions. It involves the use of lasers to optically section the area of interest into horizontal sections with a depth of 150–200 μm. Black and white images are produced with cellular structures providing different refractive indices (Fig. 11.4). An option to capture vertical images in an indicated location allows for the reconstruction of a three-dimensional area [32].

Its use in dermatology for melanoma and non-melanoma skin cancers has been validated with over 600 indexed articles currently circulating [33]. In one algorithm, two major and four minor criteria were identified for the differentiation of melanoma from nevi. Major criteria included cytologic atypia and non-edged papillae at the basal layer. Minor criteria included round cells in superficial layers spreading upwardly in pagetoid fashion, widespread pagetoid cells, cerebriform clusters in papillary dermis, and nucleated cells within the dermal papillae. Two points were given for the presence of either major criteria and one point was given for the presence of a minor criteria. When this criteria was applied to 102 lesions comprised of primary melanoma, nevi, and Spitz/Reed nevi, a score >5 led to a 96.9% specificity and an 83.8% sensitivity for the diagnosis of melanoma [34].

The challenge now is to transition reflectance confocal microscopy into a typical dermatologic clinical practice. Limitations to its use include, but are not limited to, learning the diagnostic features and algorithms, experience with the tool, and the time needed for imaging and interpretation. Imaging alone can take >10 min, without including the time needed for image interpretation. In addition, image quality can vary greatly

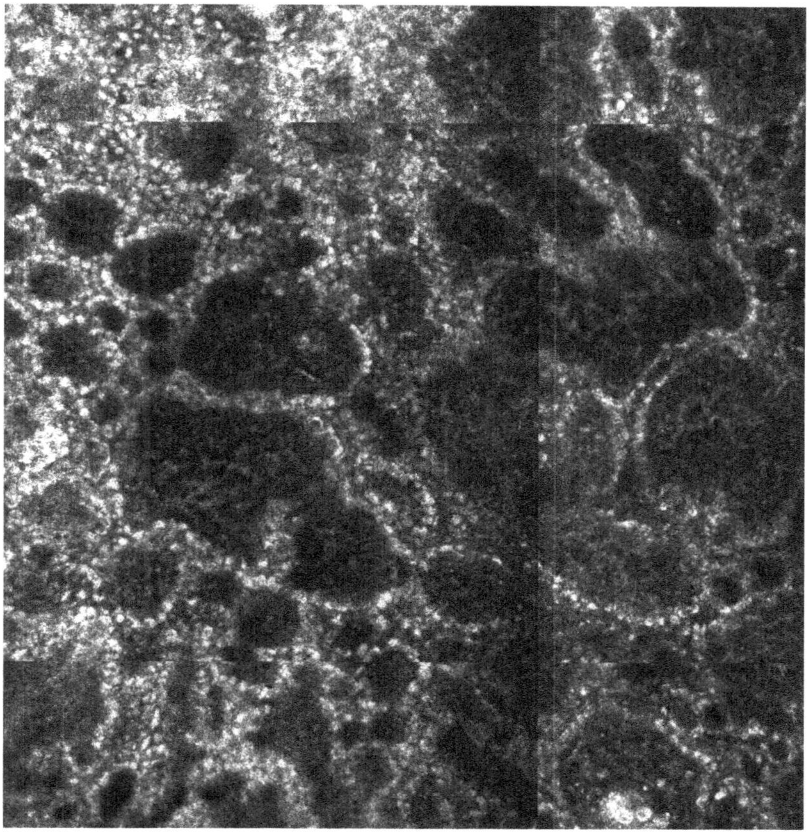

Fig. 11.4 Black and white image generated by reflectance confocal microscopy. This area represents the dermo-epidermal junction with the dermal papillae in horizontal sections versus the traditional bread loaf sections seen with histopathology

depending on the presence of makeup, air bubbles, and movement of the patient or microscope during imaging [32]. Given these challenges, it is evident that reflectance confocal microscopy may not be ideal for every lesion, but rather may benefit more in cosmetically sensitive areas such as the head and neck. It may also be of benefit for the evaluation of lesions in which dermoscopy features are not easily seen, such as with lentigo maligna [33].

In a study of 1279 lesions deemed equivocal on clinical examination, reflectance confocal microscopy was found to be most useful in evaluating both melanoma and non-melanoma skin cancers on the head and neck [33]. This is likely due to the thin epidermis and visualization of deeper structures and sun-damaged skin. This damage results in the atrophy of the epidermis and thinning of the dermo-epidermo junction that allows for adequate confocal imaging and visualization of regression features. Because of its limitation regarding imaging depth, lesions with invasion or microinvasion into the dermis cannot be assessed [35]. Further research is needed to clarify lesional and patient characteristics that can be best imaged with reflectance confocal microscopy.

Digital Multispectral Dermoscopy

Digital multispectral dermoscopy (MelaFind™) is a dermoscope that images pigmented lesions in both the infrared and visible spectra using tailored software. It is indicated for lesions with at least one of the clinical criteria for melanoma. Ten bands of white light are used to illuminate the image followed by multiple imaging with high-quality photos in order to correlate to each spectral band. Images are then conveyed to a computer system for evaluation and compared to a historic imaging database of previously classified lesions.

The database for MelaFind™ contains approximately 9000 biopsied lesions from over 7000 patients. Its intention is to be used as an independent tool to decide whether a biopsy is necessary or not [32, 35, 36].

In a prospective, multicentered, blinded study, 1831 pigmented lesions scheduled for biopsy were imaged prior to their removal. Diagnoses reached by the evaluation of digital multispectral dermoscopy images from multiple blinded pathologists were compared to the gold standard of histopathological diagnosis. Of the 127 biopsied melanomas, a sensitivity of >98% was achieved. In comparison to clinical exam alone, digital multispectral dermoscopy had a specificity that was 9.5% greater than the exam performed by the clinician [36]. There are several disadvantages to the use of this imaging modality. The computer system is extremely sensitive and if every image does not meet parameters, no image is produced. Problems relating to image capture including hair, air bubbles, lack of centering of the lesions, and camera malfunctions also exist [32, 36].

Optical Coherence Tomography

Optical coherence tomography uses infrared light to create cross-sectional microstructural images of tissue. Light from a light source is divided into two paths, one towards the tissue and the other towards a mirror. Light reflected from the tissue sample and that reflected from the mirror are then used to create a false color or grayscale image. Image formation is dependent upon linear structures that include scattering structures, birefringence, and refractive indices. Lesions can be imaged up to a depth of 1 mm [32, 35].

In one study, 92 pigmented lesions previously scheduled for removal and histopathologic evaluation were scheduled for imaging prior to biopsy. No definitive features for benign or malignant lesions were identified to be statistically significant [37]. Features that could be used to differentiate a melanoma from a benign pigmented lesion included unclear demarcation of dermo-epidermal junction, bright horizontal dermal linear structures, vertical dermal icicle-shaped structures, and architectural disarray. However, a few of these features have also been noted in non-melanoma skin cancers. Limitations include no distinct algorithms for the evaluation of pigmented lesions, sensitivity to imaging artifacts, hyperkeratosis, and motion. Images show variation from person to person and variation depending on different sites for the same person. Scar and crust are known to enhance posterior light accentuation [32, 37].

Tape-Stripping mRNA

Tape-stripping mRNA, or epidermal genetic information retrieval, is a technique that uses a special adhesive to noninvasively sample mRNA from the stratum corneum. RNA is then recovered from this adhesive and amplified to evaluate for melanoma-specific genes. Despite the fact that the stratum corneum is made up of non-nucleated cells, mRNA was recovered in this layer and its dispersion is believed to be similar to the dispersion of pigment [32, 38].

In a preliminary study, RNA was harvested from 212 melanoma and nevi via tape stripping. These lesions were later removed for histopathologic diagnosis. A total of 312 genes were identified that differentiate nevi from melanoma. From a data set of 37 melanoma and 37 nevi, a 17-gene classifier set was found that differentiated these lesions with 100% sensitivity and 88% specificity [38]. In a subsequent study, a total of 140 lesions consisting of melanomas, nevi, and other benign entities were sampled via tape stripping and then biopsied for histopathologic diagnosis. Using a previously reported 15-gene classifier set, gene pairs were amplified and rearranged until two genes, CMIP and LINC00518, were found to have a sensitivity of 97.6% and a specificity of 72.7% in the diagnosis of melanoma. With adjustment for a melanoma prevalence of 10%, which is the average seen in clinical practice, a negative predictive value of 99.6% was achieved [39].

Advantages of this technique include no recovery time or healing wound, allowing for the examination of multiple lesions. In the setting of dysplastic nevus syndrome, this could serve as a screening method to determine which lesion within the background of all lesions would warrant a biopsy based upon the presence of various genetic sequences. However, limitations include a lesion size of at least 4 mm as well as loss or inadequate amounts of mRNA. Acral and vulvar skins have also been excluded from studies and their utility for these lesions is unknown [32, 35, 39].

Ultrasound

Ultrasound has been used in dermatology since the 1970s. It is utilized to assist with depth determination of the pigmented lesions. To produce ultrasound images, acoustic energy is released from a transducer and reflected or refracted off of various tissue specimens. The returning waves are processed with images generated by a computer. In comparison to lymph nodes, where optimal frequency for imaging is 7.5–10 Hz, ultrasound transducer for pigmented lesions is optimal at 20 Hz [32]. It has been established that in melanomas thicker than 1 mm ultrasound and histopathology have yielded similar depth measurements. In one study, 28 biopsy-proven melanomas were imaged with ultrasound prior to removal [40]. Ultrasound depth was measured to be within 0.1 mm of measured histopathologic Breslow's depth. Of note, two thin facial melanomas with a Breslow's depth 0.4 mm and 1.0 mm were overestimated by ultrasound, later found to be 1.7 mm and 2.7 mm, respectively. They both displayed dermal elastosis and inflammatory infiltrates that may have contributed to the erroneous measurements [40].

In thinner melanomas (<1 mm), however, overestimations of depth have also been noted. These have been attributed to inflammatory infiltrates confounding depth measurement. Higher frequencies, as high as 100 Hz transducers, have been used to evaluate pigmented lesions with a higher resolution noted; however, this comes at the expense of shorter depth visualization. This could potentially lead to non-visualization of a thicker area in a pigmented lesion. In one study of thin melanomas, 52 lesions of which 6 were melanomas were imaged with a 22 Hz transducer [41]. Lesions were subsequently biopsied and Breslow's depth on histopathology was measured. A manual measurement of depth via ultrasound imaging was also performed. Automated depth measurement from ultrasound imaging was developed via a set of algorithms. Manual measurement was found to overestimate the depth, while the automatic depth measurement underestimated, with the majority of underestimations within <0.1 mm. Ultrasound has the ability to image a lesion up to a depth of 1.5 cm. However, it is difficult to differentiate between a primary melanoma from a dermal metastasis. Image quality is also greatly dependent on operator skill and familiarity with equipment [35].

Electrical Bioimpedance

Electrical bioimpedance measures the current evoked when a voltage source runs through a designated area. Levels of bioimpedance are a function of the structure of not only cells and membranes, but also water content. Sensitivity in the detection of melanoma has been estimated to be 92–100%, with a specificity of 67–80%. When imaging lesions, bioimpedance images are taken from the center of the lesion and from an unaffected area of skin. The entire process is estimated to take ~7 min [32, 35, 42].

Melanoma detection is limited by the high impedance of the stratum corneum. While this does not affect basal cell carcinomas as much because of their location in the epidermis, melanoma is found primary at the dermo-epidermal junction. To rectify this problem, microelectrodes with probes into the stratum corneum have been used as a modified way to detect melanoma using bioimpedance. While technically this does make it an "invasive method," the probes are limited to the stratum corneum only. With this adjustment, nevi were differentiated from a melanoma with a 92% sensitivity and 80% specificity [35, 42, 43].

Conclusion

In conclusion, various techniques exist for the biopsy of pigmented lesions. Lesion characteristics as well as operator comfort are important factors when deciding what techniques to use. With many emerging noninvasive imaging modalities available, the use of these as either independent tools or as adjuncts offers another option particularly when assessing lesions in children or cosmetically sensitive areas. Further research is needed to qualify these modalities as comparable to the gold standard of biopsy before they are used independently.

References

1. Watson M, Geller AC, Tucker MA, Guy GP Jr, Weinstock MA. Melanoma burden and recent trends among non-Hispanic whites aged 15–49 years, United States. Prev Med. 2016;91:294–8.
2. Silverstein D, Mariwalla K. Biopsy of the pigmented lesions. Dermatol Clin. 2012;30(3):435–43.
3. American Academy of Dermatology Ad Hoc Task Force for the ABCDEs of Melanoma, Tsao H, Olazagasti JM, Cordoro KM, Brewer JD, Taylor SC, Bordeaux JS, Chren MM, Sober AJ, Tegeler C, Bhushan R, Begolka WS. Early detection of melanoma: reviewing the ABCDEs. J Am Acad Dermatol. 2015;72(4):717–23.
4. Vestergaard ME, Macaskill P, Holt PE, Menzies SW. Dermoscopy compared with naked eye examination for the diagnosis of primary melanoma: a meta-analysis of studies performed in a clinical setting. Br J Dermatol. 2008;159(3):669–76.
5. Carrera C, Marchetti MA, Dusza SW, Argenziano G, Braun RP, Halpern AC, Jaimes N, Kittler HJ, Malvehy J, Menzies SW, Pellacani G, Puig S, Rabinovitz HS, Scope A, Soyer HP, Stolz W, Hofmann-Wellenhof R, Zalaudek I, Marghoob AA. Validity and reliability of dermoscopic criteria used to differentiate nevi from melanoma: a web-based international dermoscopy society study. JAMA Dermatol. 2016;152(7):798–806.
6. Hutin Y, Hauri A, Chiarello L, Catlin M, Stilwell B, Ghebrehiwet T, Garner J, Injection Safety Best Practices Development Group. Best infection control practices for intradermal, subcutaneous, and intramuscular needle injections. Bull World Health Organ. 2003;81(7):491–500.
7. Strazar AR, Leynes PG, Lalonde DH. Minimizing the pain of local anesthesia injection. Plast Reconstr Surg. 2013;132(3):675–84.
8. Nischal U, Nischal KC, Khopkar U. Techniques of skin biopsy and practical considerations. J Cutan Aesthet Surg. 2008;1(2):107–11.
9. Marsden JR, Newton-Bishop JA, Burrows L, Cook M, Corrie PG, Cox NH, Gore ME, Lorigan P, MacKie R, Nathan P, Peach H, Powell B, Walker C, British Association of Dermatologists Clinical Standards Unit. Revised U.K. guidelines for the management of cutaneous melanoma 2010. Br J Dermatol. 2010;163(2):238–56.
10. Bichakjian CK, Halpern AC, Johnson TM, Foote Hood A, Grichnik JM, Swetter SM, Tsao H, Barbosa VH, Chuang TY, Duvic M, Ho VC, Sober AJ, Beutner KR, Bhushan R, Smith Begolka W, American Academy of Dermatology. Guidelines of care for the management of primary cutaneous melanoma. American Academy of Dermatology. J Am Acad Dermatol. 2011;65(5):1032–47.
11. Shave PH. Punch biopsy for skin lesions. Am Fam Physician. 2011;84(9):995–1002.
12. Suzuki M, Yamada K, Nagao M, Aoki E, Matsumoto M, Hirayama T, Yamamoto H, Hiramatsu R, Ichiyama S, Iinuma Y. Antimicrobial ointments and methicillin-resistant Staphylococcus aureus USA300. Emerg Infect Dis. 2011;17(1):1917–20.
13. Moore P, Hundley J, Hundley J, et al. Does shave biopsy accurately predict the final breslow depth of primary cutaneous melanoma? Am Surg. 2009;75(5):369–73.
14. Zager JS, Hochwald SN, Marzban SS, et al. Shave biopsy is a safe and accurate method for the initial evaluation of melanoma. J Am Coll Surg. 2011;212(4):454–60.
15. Pflugfelder A, Weide B, Eigentler TK, et al. Incisional biopsy and melanoma prognosis: facts and controversies. Clin Dermatol. 2010;28(3):316–8.
16. Sober AJ, Balch CM. Method of biopsy and incidence of positive margins in primary melanoma. Ann Surg Oncol. 2007;14(2):274–5.
17. Somach SC, Taira JW, Pitha JV, et al. Pigmented lesions in actinically damaged skin. Histopathologic comparison of biopsy and excisional specimens. Arch Dermatol. 1996;132(11):1297–302.
18. Elenitsas R, Schuchter LM. The role of the pathologist in the diagnosis of melanoma. Curr Opin Oncol. 1998;10(2):162–9.
19. King R, Hayzen BA, Page RN, et al. Recurrent nevus phenomenon: a clinicopathologic study of 357 cases and histologic comparison with melanoma with regression. Mod Pathol. 2009;22(5):611–7.
20. Gannon CJ, Rousseau DL Jr, Ross MI, et al. Accuracy of lymphatic mapping and sentinel lymph node biopsy after previous wide local excision in patients with primary melanoma. Cancer. 2006;107(11):2647–52.
21. Evans HL, Krag DN, Teates CD, et al. Lymphoscintigraphy and sentinel node biopsy accurately stage melanoma in patients presenting after wide local excision. Ann Surg Oncol. 2003;10(4):416–25.
22. Koller J, Rettenbacher L. The influence of diagnostic biopsies on the sentinel lymph node detection in cutaneous melanoma. Arch Dermatol. 2000;136(9):1176.
23. Morton DL, Thompson JF, Essner R, et al. Validation of the accuracy of intraoperative lymphatic mapping and sentinel lymphadenectomy for early-stage melanoma: a multicenter trial. Multicenter Selective Lymphadenectomy Trial Group. Ann Surg. 1999;230(4):453–63.
24. O'Connor EA, Dzwierzynski W. Longitudinal melonychia: clinical evaluation and biopsy technique. J Hand Surg Am. 2011;36(11):1852–4.

25. Tran KT, Wright NA, Cockerell CJ. Biopsy of the pigmented lesion—when and how. J Am Acad Dermatol. 2008;59(5):852–71.
26. Chowdhry S, Seidenstricker L, Cooney DS, et al. Do not use epinephrine in digital blocks: myth or truth? Part II. A retrospective review of 1111 cases. Plast Reconstr Surg. 2010;126(6):2031–4.
27. Gupta M, Berk DR, Gray C, et al. Morphologic features and natural history of scalp nevi in children. Arch Dermatol. 2010;146(5):506–11.
28. Schaffer J. Update on melanocytic nevi in children. Clin Dermatol. 2015;33(3):368–86.
29. Mason AR, Mohr MR, Koch LH, et al. Nevi of special sites. Clin Lab Med. 2011;31(2):229–42.
30. Fabrizi G, Pagliarello C, Parente P, et al. Atypical nevi of the scalp in adolescents. J Cutan Pathol. 2007;34(5):365–9.
31. Lenane P, Keane CO, Connell BO, Loughlin SO, Powell FC. Genital melanotic macules: clinical, histologic, immunohistochemical, and ultrastructural features. J Am Acad Dermatol. 2000;42(4):640–4.
32. Wassef C, Rao BK. Uses of non-invasive imaging in the diagnosis of skin cancer: an overview of the currently available modalities. Int J Dermatol. 2013;52(12):1481–9.
33. Borsari S, Pampena R, Lallas A, Kyrgidis A, Moscarella E, Benati E, Raucci M, Pellacani G, Zalaudek I, Argenziano G, Longo C. Clinical indications for use of reflectance confocal microscopy for skin cancer diagnosis. JAMA Dermatol. 2016;152(10):1093–8.
34. Pellacani G, Cesinaro AM, Seidenari S. Reflectance-mode confocal microscopy of pigmented skin lesions—improvement in melanoma diagnostic specificity. J Am Acad Dermatol. 2005;53(6):979–85.
35. Rigel DS, Russak J, Friedman R. The evolution of melanoma diagnosis: 25 years beyond the ABCDs. CA Cancer J Clin. 2010;60(5):301–16.
36. Monheit G, Cognetta AB, Ferris L, Rabinovitz H, Gross K, Martini M, Grichnik JM, Mihm M, Prieto VG, Googe P, King R, Toledano A, Kabelev N, Wojton M, Gutkowicz-Krusin D. The performance of MelaFind: a prospective multicenter study. Arch Dermatol. 2011;147(2):188–94.
37. Gambichler T, Regeniter P, Bechara FG, Orlikov A, Vasa R, Moussa G, Stücker M, Altmeyer P, Hoffmann K. Characterization of benign and malignant melanocytic skin lesions using optical coherence tomography in vivo. J Am Acad Dermatol. 2007;57(4):629–37.
38. Wachsman W, Morhenn V, Palmer T, Walls L, Hata T, Zalla J, Scheinberg R, Sofen H, Mraz S, Gross K, Rabinovitz H, Polsky D, Chang S. Noninvasive genomic detection of melanoma. Br J Dermatol. 2011;164(4):797–806.
39. Gerami P, Alsobrook JP 2nd, Palmer TJ, Robin HS. Development of a novel noninvasive adhesive patch test for the evaluation of pigmented lesions of the skin. J Am Acad Dermatol. 2014;71(2):237–44.
40. Machet L, Belot V, Naouri M, Boka M, Mourtada Y, Giraudeau B, Laure B, Perrinaud A, Machet MC, Vaillant L. Preoperative measurement of thickness of cutaneous melanoma using high-resolution 20 MHz ultrasound imaging: a monocenter prospective study and systematic review of the literature. Ultrasound Med Biol. 2009;35(9):1411–20.
41. Andrekute K, Valiukeviciene S, Raisutis R, Linkeviciute G, Makstiene J, R K. Automated estimation of melanocytic skin tumor thickness by ultrasonic radiofrequency data. J Ultrasound Med. 2016;35(5):857–65.
42. Patel JK, Konda S, Perez OA, Amini S, Elgart G, Berman B. Newer technologies/techniques and tools in the diagnosis of melanoma. Eur J Dermatol. 2008;18(6):617–31.
43. Aberg P, Geladi P, Nicander I, Hansson J, Holmgren U, Ollmar S. Non-invasive and microinvasive electrical impedance spectra of skin cancer—a comparison between two techniques. Skin Res Technol. 2005;11(4):281–6.

12 The Pathology of Melanoma

Jane L. Messina and Rahel A. John

Specimen Submission and Evaluation Guidelines

The correct diagnosis of melanoma begins with the submission of an adequate specimen, as well as clinical information that is essential to correlate with the findings. The pathology requisition should include, in addition to the required demographic information such as age and sex, a description of the size of the lesion, its duration, and whether there has been any recent change. If the biopsy is only partially representative of a larger lesion, then it should be clearly stated on the requisition. In practice, there is a wide variety of biopsy techniques employed by those at the forefront of diagnosing melanoma, such as dermatologists, primary care physicians, and surgeons. These include excisional biopsies, shave biopsies, deep scallop shave biopsies, and punch biopsies. All of these techniques have potential pitfalls and can potentially lead to challenges in accurate diagnosis and staging, due to partial sampling and underrepresentation of the lesion. Inadequate sampling of a pigmented lesion may not allow the pathologist to assess all features required to establish the diagnosis of a melanoma from a nevus, including the overall size of the lesion, its circumscription, and its symmetry.

Transection of the base of a lesion may lead to an underestimation of its true depth, leading to inaccurate staging, and therefore decisions about the width of margins and the necessity for regional nodal sampling. Currently, the American Academy of Dermatology recommends excisional biopsy as the preferred method for biopsy of a skin lesion suspicious for melanoma [1–4]. However, excisional biopsies of melanomas are infrequently performed, possibly due to either time constraints in a busy clinic and fairly low sensitivity of the clinical diagnosis for melanoma. The reported rates are as low as 42% for general practitioners and as high as 80% for dermatologists [5]. There is also some concern about the potential for excision resulting in an alteration of the lymphatic drainage and compromise of the sentinel lymph node (SLN) mapping procedure, especially for large primary lesions. Considering the low sensitivity for clinical recognition of melanoma there is also the potential for a morbid excision for a lesion that turns out to be benign [6].

Punch biopsy is still very commonly used in the initial assessment of cutaneous lesions suspicious for melanoma. While they are easy to perform under local anesthesia, biopsies larger than 3 mm require simple suture closure. Punch biopsies are limited in diameter, with 6 mm the largest typically available. Thus, while a punch can

J. L. Messina, M.D. (✉)
Departments of Anatomic Pathology and Cutaneous Oncology, Moffitt Cancer Center, Tampa, FL, USA
e-mail: jane.messina@moffitt.org

R. A. John, M.D.
Department of Pathology, Lutheran General Hospital, Park Ridge, IL, USA
e-mail: bjohn@mdpmail.com

A. I. Riker (ed.), *Melanoma*, https://doi.org/10.1007/978-3-319-78310-9_12

usually provide accurate assessment of dermal depth, their inability to encompass the entire periphery of the lesion puts the dermatopathologist at a disadvantage. This is partly due to an incomplete punch biopsy that hinders the accurate assessment of overall size, circumscription, and symmetry of the lesion. This partial sampling can lead to misdiagnosis, a far more serious error than an inaccurate T-stage. Additionally, in very-large-diameter lesions only partially sampled, there is a potential for inaccurate reporting of depth (if other areas of the pigmented lesion are left in situ and have a thicker Breslow's depth) [1, 7].

Karimipour et al. reported that previous incisional or punch biopsies of melanoma were associated with upstaging in 21% of patients at the time of definitive excision [8]. Proponents of shave biopsy point to its timesaving nature and minimal morbidity, as well as a lack of need for suture placement [2, 9]. Clearly, the ideal shave biopsy should include the full thickness of the melanoma for most accurate staging. Considering the fact that the median tumor depth of melanoma at diagnosis is 0.60 mm [10] this should not be difficult. However, partial biopsies are still seen, likely secondary to the aforementioned low sensitivity of clinical diagnosis. If the shave biopsy measures at least 1 mm in depth, even if the melanoma is greater in thickness, the decision to perform a 2-cm-wide excision and sentinel node biopsy, as recommended by National Comprehensive Cancer Network (NCCN) guidelines, is still not compromised [3, 11]. In a recent large series, melanomas diagnosed by shave biopsy were upstaged in only 3% of subsequent wide excisions [12].

The handling of therapeutic wide excisions varies among institutions, and there have been no prospective or retrospective studies outside of Europe addressing the gross examination protocol for these specimens. While these European studies showed minimal yield from examination of multiple sections, the initial method of diagnosis in these patients is excisional biopsy, which removes nearly all of the primary lesion [13, 14]. In the USA, where shave and punch biopsies are more commonly employed as initial diagnostic methods, there are no studies documenting the positivity rate of subsequent wide excision. There are a wide variety of protocols, and whichever is used it must address the presence and extent of residual tumor and status of as much of the peripheral and deep margin as feasible, in order to facilitate accurate staging. Most centers employ variations of the "bread loaf" method, wherein specimens are serially sectioned and completely submitted after differential inking of margins. However, this is not feasible for excisions larger than 1 cm in diameter by 2 cm in length due to the large number of sections this would produce. Tangential sampling of all or most of the peripheral and deep margins, with enface sectioning of these cuts, as well as submission of serial sections from the residual primary tumor and/or prior biopsy site, is an accepted and valid approach for large excisions.

Evaluation of Primary Melanoma Biopsies

Once properly sampled, the diagnosis of melanoma requires the identification of a constellation of features that distinguish it from its benign nevus counterparts. There is no exact number of features that is required, rather a systematic evaluation of the lesion's growth pattern, cytomorphology, and alterations of the microenvironment such as inflammation and reactive sclerosis. There are fairly characteristic morphologic features that vary by histologic subtype, and these are described below.

Proper evaluation of a biopsy of an atypical pigmented lesion begins with a low-power examination of the architecture of the lesion, assessing the lesion's size and symmetry. If any portion of the biopsy shows incomplete sectioning, cutting of deeper levels is essential to enable evaluation of the entire lesion. If the entire lesion has been sampled, attention should be paid to the border of the lesion. Poor lateral circumscription is a hallmark of melanoma, as evidenced by a trailing edge of solitary, irregularly spaced melanocytes. Next, attention is paid to the junctional component of the lesion.

Within the epidermis, irregularity of size, shape, and spacing of nests (if present) is often seen in melanoma, as well as high cellularity evidenced by confluence of nests. Single cells often predominate, but not always. Suprabasal (defined as above the hypothetical line drawn at the tips of the dermal papillae) nests and single melanocytes are commonly seen. Consumption of the epidermis, defined as the presence of a thinned epidermis overlying expansile junctional nests of melanocytes, was found in 43% of melanomas. This is compared to only 2.5% of severely dysplastic nevi, and absent in mildly dysplastic, congenital, and common nevi [15]. While occasional single melanocytes and even suprabasal melanocytes can be seen in the central, most cellular portions of dysplastic nevi, acral nevi, and nevi with recent actinic exposure, their presence and/or predominance at the edges of a pigmented lesion is suspicious for melanoma [16, 17]. The dermal component of a melanoma is often markedly more cellular than benign counterparts. Any sheetlike growth, with little or no intervening dermis between groups of cells, strongly favors a diagnosis of melanoma.

After the architecture is closely examined, attention should be paid to cytologic features. Malignant melanocytes can range from epithelioid to spindle, and vary in size from small cell variants to large, even ballooned cell types. Often, classic malignant cytologic features such as marked pleomorphism, multinucleation, hyperchromasia, and atypical mitoses are prominent. While 1% of nevi may demonstrate 1–2 superficial mitoses, the presence of mitoses near the base of the lesion is a suspicious finding [18]. More subtle features include lack of maturation of the dermal component, with the presence of pleomorphic melanocytes at the base of the lesion the same size as junctional component—a hallmark of melanoma. Some lesions demonstrate pseudo-maturation, where the overall size of the cell diminishes because of loss of cytoplasm, but the high nuclear/cytoplasmic ratio is maintained [19]. Melanoma typically elicits a distinctive reaction in the dermis, including the presence of an expanded and sclerotic papillary dermis, increased lymphocytic infiltrate, and irregular clumps of melanin-laden macrophages. Elastic fiber staining has been touted to distinguish the distinctive sclerotic peritumoral collagen from the undisturbed stroma of a benign nevus [20].

While the typical melanoma often displays many of the aforementioned features, many lesions only demonstrate a few abnormalities, and thus overlap with benign nevi. Immunohistochemical analysis is often employed to aid in the diagnosis. Melanocyte-specific stains such as Melan-A/Mart-1, Sox10, and MITF can help delineate the size of lesion, cellularity, and presence of pagetoid spread. Melan-A is a cytoplasmic stain that can sometimes give the impression that a lesion is more cellular than it actually is, especially in sun-damaged skin [21]. Therefore, nuclear stains such as Sox10 and MITF are often more helpful in examining biopsies on sun-damaged skin. S-100 has mostly been replaced by Sox10 due to its lack of specificity. One notable pitfall of S-100 is its lack of sensitivity in evaluating lesions of the nail matrix, where 70% of melanoma in situ was negative for S-100 in one study [22]. The monoclonal antibody, HMB-45, is often utilized to identify the gp-100 tumor antigen that is often retained throughout the full thickness of the dermal component in melanoma. It may taper in intensity upon dermal depth in benign nevi, with the exception of blue nevi, deep-penetrating nevi, and some Spitz nevi [23, 24].

Evaluation of proliferation with Ki-67 has both diagnostic and prognostic use. While many melanomas show a proliferation index that overlaps with benign nevi, a proliferation index of >10% is almost always diagnostic of melanoma [25, 26]. Since Ki-67 is expressed in a high percentage of lymphocytes, which can lead to difficulty in interpreting heavily inflamed lesions, combining this marker with Melan-A using two chromogens (MelPro or K-Mart) is quite helpful [27]. Phosphohistone H3 (pHH3) is a marker of cells in mitoses, and can give an accurate assessment of the number of mitoses in a lesion. While there is a significant correlation of pHH3 with manual assessments of mitotic rate, and it can be used to screen for "hot spots" of mitotic activity, it should not replace manual counting of mitoses

[28, 29]. P16 expression is often assessed, since it is lost in up to 63% of melanomas [30] and often retained in benign lesions. While complete loss of expression of p16 was originally thought to indicate homozygous deletion of the CDKN2a gene encoding p16/INK4a and p14ARF (a hallmark of melanoma), it is now known that epigenetic silencing and heterozygous deletion can lead to absence of staining [31]. Therefore, this stain cannot be used as a sole indicator of the malignant potential of a lesion. In the rare lesion with Spitzoid morphology, there are other immunohistochemical stains such as BAP-1 that may also be employed.

Histologic Subtypes of Melanoma

The histologic subtypes of melanoma were first proposed by Clark and Elder in 1986 [32]. These variants show distinctive clinical presentations, clustering in certain ethnic subgroups and geographic locations. While they were originally thought to be distinctive prognostically, it is now known that other histologic features such as tumor depth and presence of ulceration are the major drivers of prognosis in primary melanomas. These subtypes have recently been shown to cluster with certain types of molecular abnormalities, especially with respect to the presence or absence of chronic sun damage [33, 34].

Lentigo maligna melanoma arises in heavily sun-damaged skin, evidenced by abundant solar elastosis and often epidermal atrophy. It is characterized by an in situ growth phase (lentigo maligna) that displays predominantly basally located growth of atypical melanocytes. Pagetoid involvement of the epidermis (so named because of the superficial resemblance of the single epithelioid melanocytes to Paget's disease of the breast) is typically a minor feature, but confluence of single melanocytes is characteristic. There is often a quite prominent adnexal involvement (Fig. 12.1). Occasionally, lesional cells may be quite small and nevoid, but confluent, broad growth is still a feature [35]. The invasive component usually is composed of spindled melanocytes [36], but epithelioid melanocytes may be observed. There is variable cytological atypia, with occasional downward displacement of the dense band of solar elastosis in the background of sun-damaged skin by the tumor nests [37].

Superficial spreading melanoma is characterized by a proliferation of atypical melanocytes, singly and in nests, at all levels within the epidermis (Fig. 12.2). The abundance of pagetoid

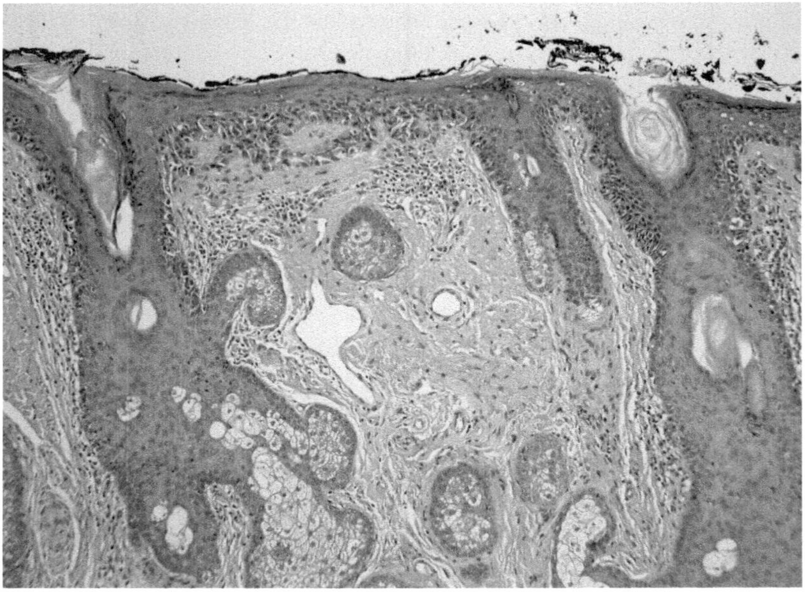

Fig. 12.1 Lentigo maligna (melanoma *in situ* in sun-damaged skin), with marked solar elastosis and growth of confluent melanocytes in a flattened epidermis and extending into adnexal epithelium (×10)

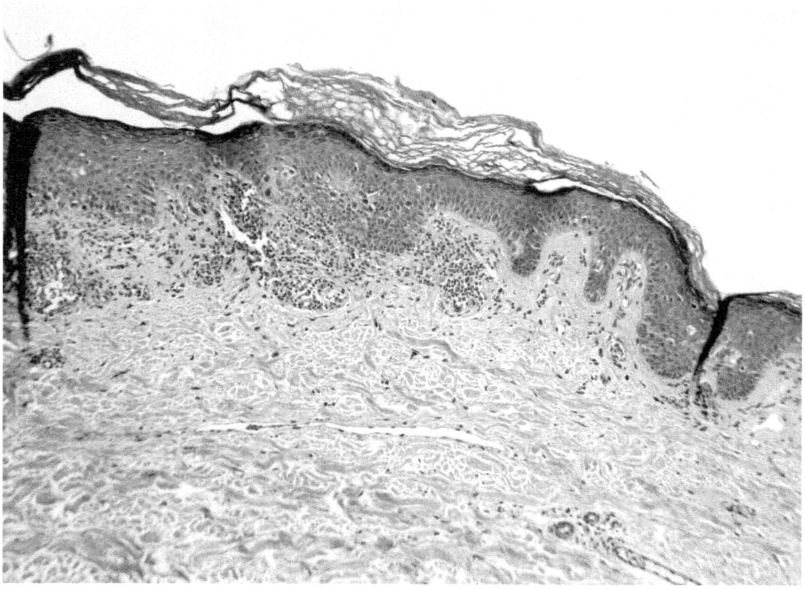

Fig. 12.2 Superficial spreading melanoma, showing confluent nests and single melanocytes with abundant pagetoid spread (×10)

spread has been referred to as "buckshot scatter." The junctional component features poor circumscription, marked variation in nesting, and areas of confluence [38]. Superficial adnexal epithelium may also be involved. Consumption of the epidermis, defined as thinning of the epidermis above and below expansile intraepidermal collections of melanocytes, is present in approximately 40% of cases of malignant melanoma of all types [15]. Consumption is thought to possibly predate cutaneous ulceration, and its presence is helpful in favoring a diagnosis of melanoma over a benign mimicker such as Spitz nevus [39]. Often, the abundant intraepidermal growth of melanocytes in superficial spreading melanoma leads to the formation of clefts from the epidermis, due to lack of adhesive cellular junctions in melanocytes [38]. The infiltrative component of superficial spreading melanoma may be sheetlike or fascicular in growth, and composed of melanocytes with a variety of morphologies, including epithelioid, spindled, and nevoid. There is usually absence of maturation [38].

Nodular melanoma is characterized by entrance in the vertical growth phase early in the development of the lesion, so that there is a minimal junctional component (Fig. 12.3) [40]. The earliest definition of a nodular melanoma specifies that the junctional component should not extend three rete ridges beyond the invasive component [41]. The dermal component may be composed of any morphologic variant of melanoma, including epithelioid and spindle. Nodular melanomas are the variety most commonly ulcerated at presentation [42], and their average thickness at diagnosis is greater than the other subtypes [43]. The NRAS mutation is most frequently found in this variant of melanoma [33].

Acral lentiginous melanoma has a distinctive lentiginous pattern of intraepidermal growth, with single cells predominating over nests. The lentiginous melanocytes often have a perinuclear clear halo, giving a lacunar appearance, or they may have heavily pigmented dendritic processes (Fig. 12.4). Pagetoid spread, however, is usually less prominent than it is in superficial spreading melanoma [44]. Deep extension of in situ growth in adnexal epithelium is often found, with approximately 15% of cases considered amelanotic [45]. The invasive component may consist of epithelioid cells or spindle cells, or it may resemble nevus cells [44]. There may be a desmoplastic stromal response, with the presence of secondary sarcomatous changes, typically osteosarcoma, as a distinctive feature of acral lentiginous melanoma [46].

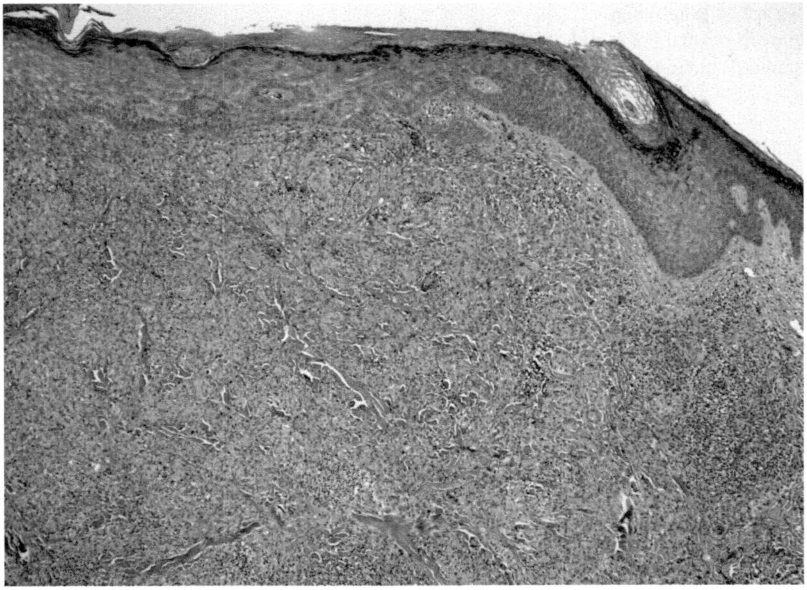

Fig. 12.3 Nodular melanoma, showing invasive dermal component and no extension of melanoma in situ laterally to it (×10)

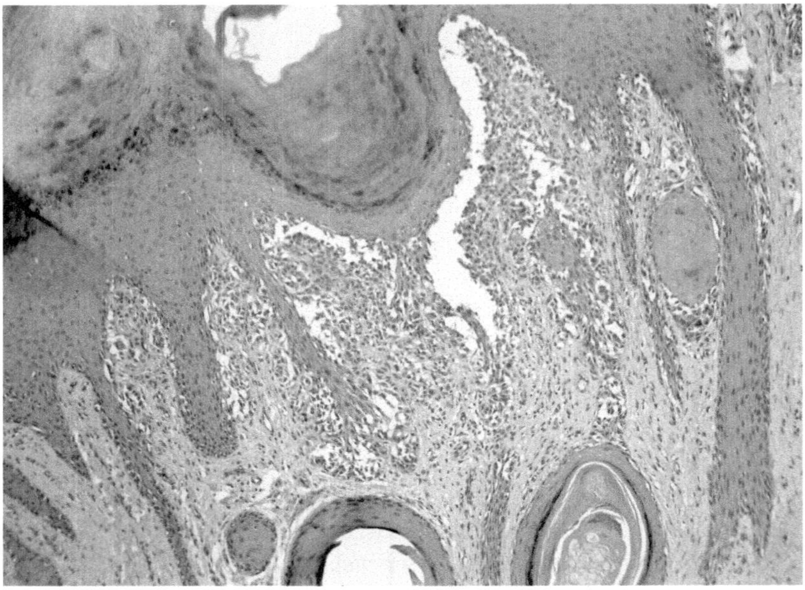

Fig. 12.4 Melanoma on acral skin, showing polyglonal melanocytes with pale cytoplasm and exhibiting separation artifact from dermis due to abundant cellularity (×10)

Desmoplastic melanoma is a distinct subtype of melanoma characterized by a subtle in situ component, and paucicellular dermal growth of spindle cells surrounded by abundant desmoplastic stromal change (Fig. 12.5). The mean Breslow's thickness at presentation is 4 mm [47]. It has been shown that only about 70% of cases demonstrate an in situ component at initial presentation [48]. Desmoplasia is defined as the presence of prominent dermal fibroblasts with abundant production of dermal mucin, mostly hyaluronic acid. These distinct histologic features contribute to the distinct clinical presentation of this lesion, which is often found in sun-damaged skin, rarely pigmented, and often scar-like at presentation [48]. There are two subtypes of desmoplastic melanoma, pure and mixed, with pure desmoplastic melanoma composed of >90% paucicellular dermal spindle cell growth. If >10% of the tumor is cellular, with little intervening stroma between tumor cells, or has an epithelioid morphology, the tumor is classified as mixed [49].

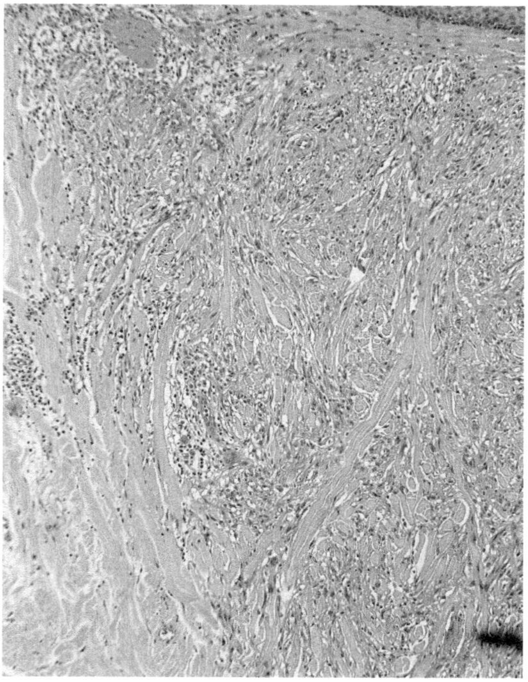

Fig. 12.5 Pure desmoplastic melanoma, showing paucicellular proliferation of slender cells separated by fibromyxoid stroma and infiltrated by lymphocytes (×10)

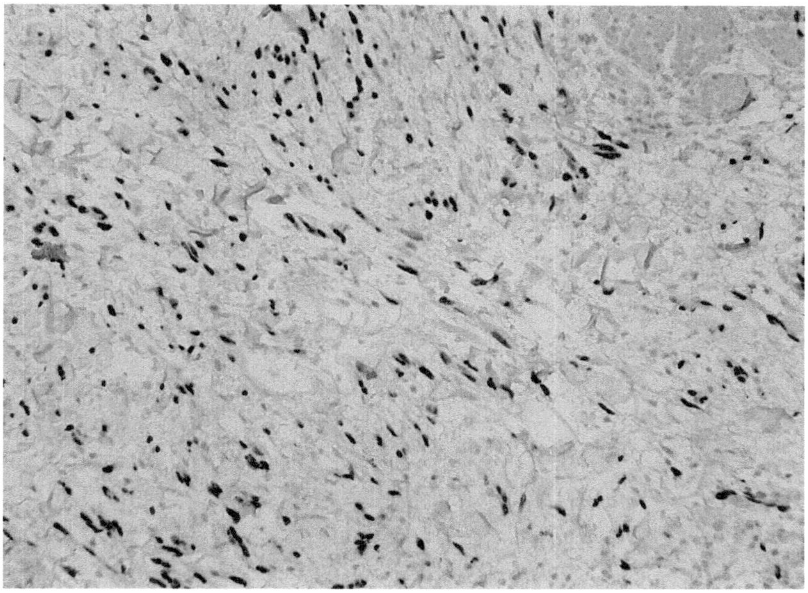

Fig. 12.6 Sox10 staining of desmoplastic melanoma (×20)

This distinction is important, since pure desmoplastic melanoma has a lower rate of sentinel node positivity than mixed and non-desmoplastic melanoma of similar thickness [50]. Both types of desmoplastic melanoma frequently demonstrate perineural invasion and/or small foci of collections of tumor cells resembling nerves, so-called neurotization. Lymphoid follicles are scattered throughout the dermal component of the tumor, giving a distinctive low-power appearance. This subtype of melanoma is distinct immunohistochemically, with desmoplastic melanoma almost always positively staining for S-100 and Sox-10 (Fig. 12.6), but by definition is negative for Melan-A and

HMB-45 [51]. This morphology makes distinction from the malignant peripheral nerve sheath tumors (MPNST) difficult, but a recently described marked, H3K27Me3, is retained in desmoplastic melanoma, lost in 69% of MPNST and in 95% of sporadic MPNST [52]. Delineation of desmoplastic melanoma from spindle cell melanoma (i.e., nodular or superficial spreading melanoma with a spindled dermal component) is often difficult. In contrast to desmoplastic melanoma, spindle cell melanoma is more likely to demonstrate positivity with Melan-A, have a trichrome-negative stroma, and demonstrate more frequent (31 v 5%) BRAF mutation [53].

There are a variety of other unusual subtypes of melanoma that are distinctive on either the basis of histology or the clinical presentation. These include nevoid melanoma (Fig. 12.7), verrucous melanoma, balloon-cell melanoma, animal-type melanoma, signet ring-cell melanoma, Spitzoid melanoma, small-cell melanoma, myxoid melanoma, and melanoma with divergent differentiation such as osteosarcoma and chondrosarcoma [54]. Recognition of these variants is obviously important insofar as the accurate diagnosis and therefore treatment of melanoma are initiated, but these variants do not carry a different prognosis from the common varieties listed above when matched by stage.

The entity "primary dermal melanoma" deserves mention, as the proper staging of a patient who presents with a dermal nodule of melanoma is a common diagnostic dilemma. Not infrequently, although the precise incidence is poorly defined, patients present with a single dermal or subcutaneous nodule of melanoma and the pathologist is unable to identify an epidermal component in order to establish the diagnosis of primary cutaneous melanoma [55]. Whether these represent a primary melanoma arising in the dermis or a metastasis remains a matter of debate. However, available evidence suggests that these dermal or subcutaneous tumors are usually primary melanomas where the epidermal component has regressed or been lost, such as by prior biopsy, trauma (such as repeated scratching), or cryoablation.

Traumatic removal of the epidermal component of a melanoma is quite frequent in areas groomed by shaving, such as the legs in women and face in men. Melanomas located in the dermis and subcutaneous tissues behave more like a thick, primary melanoma or a local recurrence rather than a regional metastasis [56]. Management of these cases benefits greatly from close collaboration with the pathologist as well as a careful history to seek evidence for an initial cutaneous component of the tumor versus a history of a primary melanoma at another site that could have potentially been the source of metastasis. A full metastatic workup may or may not be necessary depending on the level of uncertainty as to whether the lesion represents a primary

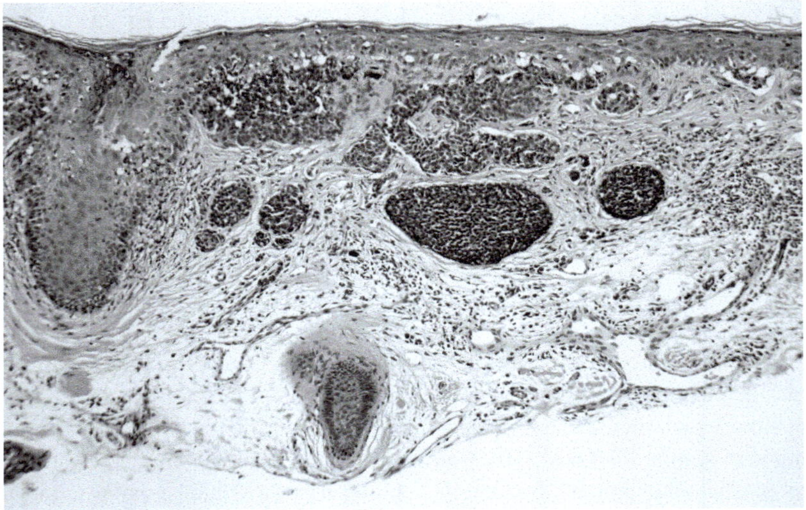

Fig. 12.7 Nevoid melanoma, demonstrating pseudomaturation of dermal component, which remains hyperchromatic and cellular despite diminution in size of cells upon dermal depth (×10)

tumor. For tumors centered in the deep dermis or subcutaneous tissue, a diagnosis of clear cell sarcoma should be entertained, and the specimen referred for analysis for the t(12;22)(q13;q12) translocation. The AJCC staging guidelines for melanoma indicate that for melanomas lacking a primary epidermal component, when an appropriate staging workup does not reveal other sites of metastases, the lesion be managed and staged as a primary melanoma of similar thickness [57]. Oftentimes, the presence of an epidermal component is noted on the wide excision, in retrospect, establishing these lesions as primary cutaneous melanoma.

Molecular Analysis of Diagnostically Challenging Melanocytic Lesions

While a thorough discussion of the benign mimickers of melanoma is beyond the scope of this chapter, a brief discussion of some of the adjunct tests used for diagnostic confirmation may be helpful. Melanocytic neoplasms that demonstrate pathologic overlap with benign lesions, so-called "atypical melanocytic neoplasms" (melanocytic tumors of uncertain malignant potential, superficial atypical melanocytic proliferations of uncertain significance, etc.), are of special interest because of the consequences of both overtreatment (aggressive local and regional surgery) and undertreatment for incorrectly diagnosed lesions. Many of these lesions are diagnostically challenging because of the significant histologic overlap that exists between Spitz nevus and melanoma, cellular blue nevus and melanoma, and nevus and so-called nevoid melanoma. There have been numerous studies documenting the lack of histologic consensus among experts in diagnosing these lesions, as well as the difficulty in predicting their biologic behavior from histology alone [51, 58]. Many of the patients affected by this dilemma are pediatric, with many of their lesions displaying worrisome clinical features [59]. Accordingly, efforts have been made to develop tests to detect basic molecular differences between melanoma and its histologic mimics. One caveat in determining the utility of these tests is that they have been infrequently tested in ambiguous lesions using the gold standard (long-term event-free survival or death from melanoma).

Fluorescence in situ hybridization (FISH) is a commercially available assay to aid in the diagnosis of controversial melanocytic lesions. Melanomas display numerous chromosomal aberrations such as loss of chromosomes 6q, 8p, 9p, and 10q and copy number increases of chromosomes 1q, 6p, 7, 8q, 17q, and 20q, which are not found in nevi. The exception is Spitz nevus, which shows an isolated copy number increase of chromosome 11p in one-fourth of cases, an aberration not found in melanoma [60]. After extensive testing with probes for a number of chromosomal regions, a combination of four probes was demonstrated to have a sensitivity and specificity of 86.7% and 95.4%, respectively, for the diagnosis of melanoma [60].

The first version of the FISH assay employed probes targeting 6p25 (RREB1), centromere 6, 6q23, and 11q13 (CCND1) utilizing formalin-fixed paraffin-embedded tissues [61]. The test has also been used to distinguish intranodal nevi from metastatic melanoma, epithelioid blue nevi from blue nevus-like melanoma, and mitotically active nevi from nevoid melanoma [62–64]. In 2011, an assay employing new probes to 9p21 (CDKN2a), 11q13 (CCND1), 8q24 (MYC), and centromere 9, and maintaining probes for 6p25 (RREB1), was promulgated to increase the sensitivity in evaluating ambiguous Spitzoid neoplasms and to address the issue of false positivity in the setting of polyploidy [65]. This test increased the sensitivity for detection of melanoma to 94% but is still hampered by lack of specificity in evaluation of atypical Spitzoid lesions, as low as 33% [66–69].

In 2012, a commercial test offered by Myriad Genetics became available for use in formalin-fixed biopsies of diagnostically challenging lesions. The myPath test measures mRNA expression of 23 genes by quantitate RT-PCR. A weighting algorithm computes the expression of these genes, which are related to melanocyte differentiation, immune signaling, and others to produce a numerical score between −16 and +11. A negative score supports a benign lesion, while a positive score supports a melanoma malignancy, with a reported sensitivity of 90% and specificity of 91% in unequivocal lesions [70]. A single report testing the utility of this assay in diagnostically challenging lesions has shown that the myPath score agreed with the histologic interpretation of a panel of experts in 64% of cases. This same study showed agreement of FISH result with histologic interpretation in 70% of cases [71].

Comparative genomic hybridization (CGH) is an assay that can detect losses or gains within portions of genomic material and map to their chromosomal regional location. This test uses formalin-fixed, paraffin-embedded (FFPE) tissue and has the advantage of evaluating the whole genome of the entire tissue sample, rather than focusing on specific parts of the genome, such as with FISH. In CGH, the index lesion is compared to normal tissue, with the DNA from both samples allowed to compete for substrate and evaluated based upon the ratio of fluorescence intensity of tumor to normal tissue [72]. A total of 95% of melanomas harbor whole chromosomal gains and/or losses, especially in chromosome 9, followed by chromosome 10, 61, and 8p [73]. In contrast, benign nevi typically show normal CGH, and rarely isolated gains or losses of chromosomal regions in a pattern that does not overlap with melanoma [72]. Spitz nevi can harbor an 11p or 7q gain [61, 72, 74, 75]. One drawback of this test is that it is not widely available, further complicated by issues of difficulties in test cost reimbursement by most major insurance carriers. As such, CGH is mostly employed as part of a comprehensive, expert consultation of a diagnostic lesion at major academic centers.

Recently, mutations in the promoter region of the telomerase reverse transcriptase (TERT) gene, which regulates the activity of telomerase, have been described in melanomas in both adults [76] and children [77]. In a recent study of 56 atypical Spitz tumors and Spitzoid melanomas, the presence of a TERT promotion mutation was the most significant predictor of distant metastatic spread and death. Three of the four patients who died had initially been diagnosed with an atypical Spitzoid lesion [78].

Reporting and Staging of Primary Melanoma

Once a diagnosis of melanoma has been established, examination of the lesion for a variety of pathologic features that are essential for accurate staging is necessary. These features must be accurately measured and recorded to enable the most precise prognostication possible. While the 8th edition of the American Joint Committee on Cancer (AJCC) staging criteria only employs a handful of staging features of primary melanoma, a host of other features have been shown to have prognostic or predictive ability either in univariate or, occasionally, multivariate analysis. Several of these are required by AJCC to be assessed and recorded, though not used for final staging. While one may debate the necessity of evaluating and reporting other non-AJCC-required features, most academic centers continue to report the majority of these, in the spirit of recording this data for possible use in future predictive models.

For the purposes of AJCC staging, tumor depth in millimeters, presence or absence of ulceration, and presence or absence of microsatellite metastases are required to be evaluated and reported in the examination of a primary melanoma biopsy specimen and/or wide local excision. The depth of the tumor measures from the granular layer of the epidermis to the deepest portion of the invasive component. This was first described by Alexander Breslow in 1970 [79], with the Breslow's depth of invasion becoming the most important prognostic feature of a primary melanoma, further defining the T-stage of the lesion. The thickness can only be evaluated accurately in sections cut perpendicular to the epidermis. When the epidermis is absent, the Breslow's depth is measured from the base of the overlying ulcer [42]. Melanoma growing within and continuous with adnexal epithelium is not considered in the measurement of Breslow's depth, unless it is the only focus of invasion [80].

In the newest version of the AJCC staging system, tumor depth is reported to the closest 0.1 mm. While most ocular micrometers have the ability to read to the closest 0.01 mm, the reading would be rounded to the nearest 0.1 mm, rounding down for decimal values ending in 1–4 and rounding up for 5–9 [57]. The 8th edition T1–4 categories continue to be defined by whole-number integers (T1: 0–1.0 mm, T2: >1.0–2.0 mm, T3: >2.0–4.0 mm, T4: >4.0 mm). The T1 category is subdivided as follows: T1a: 0–0.8 mm and T1b: >0.8–1 mm. If tumor thickness cannot be evaluated, the tumor is staged as TX. Melanoma in situ is staged as Tis. Patients with completely regressed melanoma or melanoma of unknown primary are staged as T0.

Tumor ulceration continues to be a part of the T-staging, with its presence upstaging a tumor from T-stage (a) to (b) at any thickness. Ulceration is defined as absence of the full thickness of the epidermis, and is accompanied by reactive change such as fibrin deposition and presence of neutrophils (Fig. 12.8). Mere thinning of the epidermis, presence of scale crust, or narrow, sharp ulceration consistent with traumatic excoriation does not constitute ulceration. In one recent study of 4,661 patients, the 5-year melanoma-specific survival was significantly impacted in patients with an ulcer diameter <5 mm compared to those with an extensively ulcerated (>5 mm) melanoma [81]. Therefore, the 8th edition staging mandates that the maximum extent of ulceration is required to be measured and recorded in millimeters using an ocular micrometer.

While mitotic rate is no longer considered in the staging of a lesion, the AJCC recommends measuring and recording the number of mitoses/mm^2. This is accomplished using the "hot spot" method, wherein the region containing the most mitoses is first identified (Fig. 12.9). Then, after counting mitoses in the initial high-power field, the count is extended to adjacent but nonoverlapping fields until an area 1 mm^2 is counted. The pathologist must know the field diameter of their microscope in order to determine how many high power fields comprise this area, using the formula πr^2. The mitotic rate is recorded as a whole integer. If the invasive component measures <1 mm^2, the number of mitoses found should still be recorded as if they were found in a mm^2. Conversely, if only one mitosis was found in the entire dermal component, then it is recorded as the absolute number. The revisions in recording of tumor depth, ulceration, and mitotic rate will cause some differences in staging of thin melanomas in the revised AJCC staging. For instance, in the 7th edition, a mitotically active lesion measuring 0.70 mm would be recorded as T1b, while in the 8th edition it would be classified as a T1a melanoma. Conversely, a 0.90 mm melanoma with 0 mitoses/mm^2 previously classified as T1a would be T1b in the updated staging system.

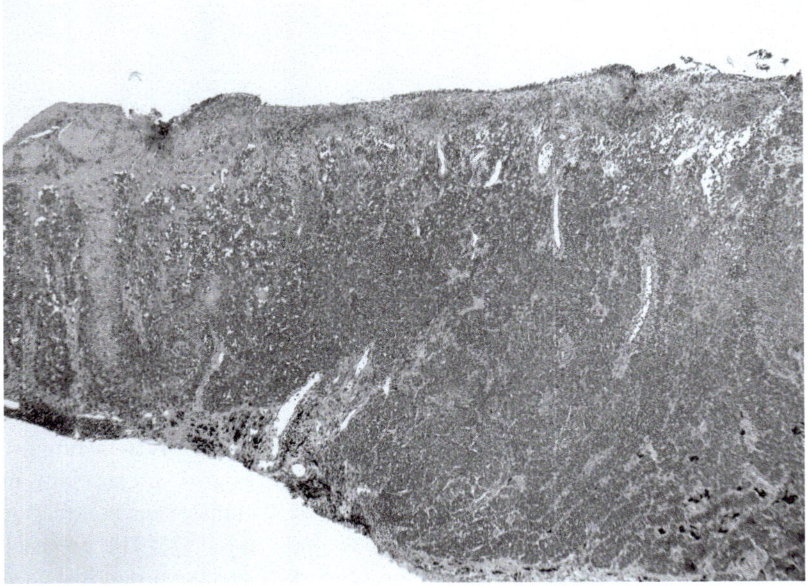

Fig. 12.8 Ulcerated melanoma, demonstrating complete absence of epidermis with surface fibrin deposition and neutrophils

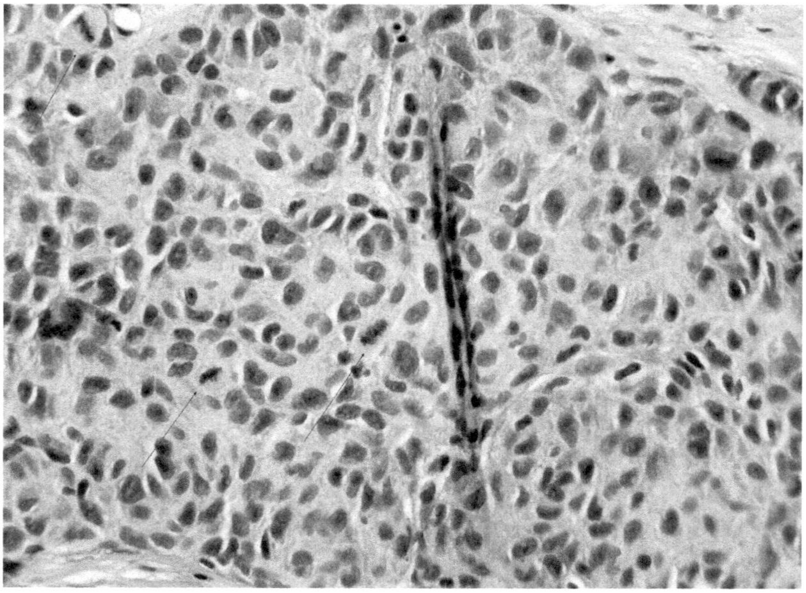

Fig. 12.9 Three mitotic figures in one ×40 field of melanoma, arrows (×40)

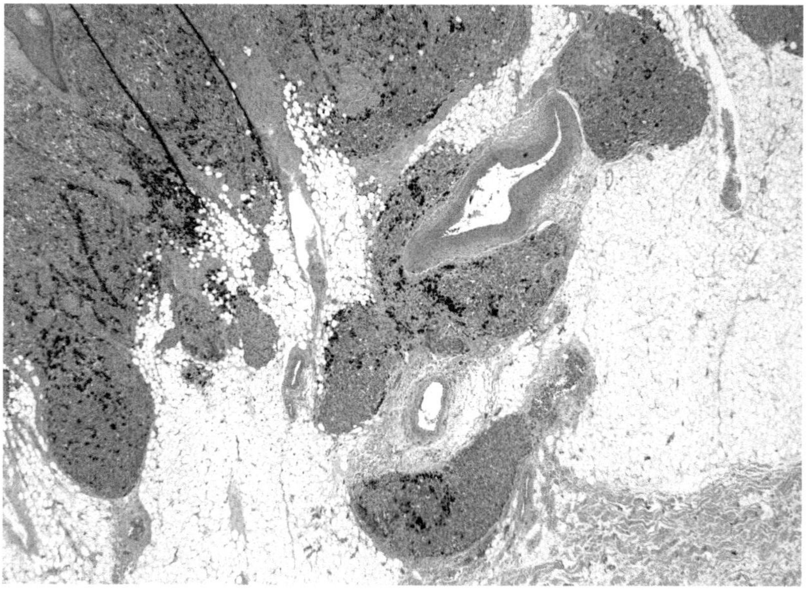

Fig. 12.10 Several subcutaneous nodules of melanoma separate from base of primary consistent with microsatellites (×20)

Microsatellite metastases are defined as microscopic tumor foci within the dermis or subcutaneous fat adjacent to, but discontinuous from, the primary melanoma. Microsatellites must be separated from the primary tumor by normal dermis or fat, not fibrosis or inflammation (Fig. 12.10). These were previously strictly defined as measuring >0.05 mm in size and located at least 0.3 mm from the main primary tumor mass [3]. However, the 8th edition does not delineate a minimum size or distance. Thus, to avoid a potential for "overcall" of microsatellites, it is recommended to examine multiple tissue levels to distinguish these from peri-adnexal extension, especially in tumors with poorly circumscribed interface with the surrounding dermis [57]. The presence of microsatellites is an adverse prognostic factor in primary melanoma.

Patients with microsatellites are classified as Stage III disease, and staged as N1c, N2c, or N3c according to the number of positive regional lymph nodes present [57].

Other non-staging prognostic features required by AJCC to be recorded as a primary tumor characteristic include Clark's level of invasion, tumor-infiltrating lymphocytes, lymphovascular invasion, regression, and neurotropism. The level of invasion, first described by Wallace Clark, is a surrogate for tumor depth, similar to that described by Breslow [82]. Defined as penetration of tumor relative to anatomic landmarks of the dermis, its relative lack of reproducibility is the likely reason for its prognostic significance in univariate, but not most multivariate, analyses [83]. Lymphocytic infiltration of the primary melanoma tumor is a favorable prognostic factor [84], and may predict lower rates of sentinel node positivity [85]. Tumor-infiltrating lymphocytes (TILs) are defined as lymphocytes that surround and extend into nests and individual tumor cells of a melanoma. The tripartite grading scheme most commonly used is absent, non-brisk, and brisk TILs. To classify a tumor as having brisk TILs, the lymphocytes must either infiltrate the entire base of the tumor or diffusely permeate it [57]. Lymphovascular invasion comprises melanoma tumor cell infiltration into either blood vessels or lymphatics. It is recorded as present or absent. A double immunostain for melanoma and lymphatic endothelium has been proposed as a method to augment its recognition, and this phenomenon was demonstrated to be a factor predicting metastasis in patients with clinical stage IB and IIA melanoma [86].

Tumor regression of a melanoma occurs when the host immune response results in destruction of all or a portion of a primary melanoma. Histologically, regression is characterized by the absence of melanoma, associated with superficial dermal fibrosis/sclerosis, accompanied by lymphocytes, melanophages, and epidermal effacement. The mere presence of fibrosis, inflammation, and/or melanophages in the vicinity of viable tumor does not equate to regression, as this requires complete absence of tumor [3]. Regression is scored as present or absent. Regression is often patchy within a tumor, and if regression changes are noted at the margin of excision, re-excision should be considered. The prognostic significance of regression is a matter of debate. While it has been shown to portend a worse prognosis in thin melanomas [87], a systematic review and meta analysis of 14 studies comprising 10,098 patients showed a lower incidence of sentinel node positivity in tumors with regression compared to those without [88]. It is likely that the varied results of these studies stem in part from a lack of a standardized definition or criteria for the diagnosis of regression, as well as poor interobserver reproducibility. Additional prognostic parameters often reported include growth phase (radial or vertical), and presence or absence of a coexisting nevus.

Pathologic Evaluation of Regional Lymph Nodes

Optimal utilization of sentinel node biopsy in the care of melanoma patients requires cooperation between the radiologist, surgeon, and pathologist. Accurate pathologic diagnosis of the sentinel node is central to proper staging, optimal treatment decisions, and precise prognostication of patients with melanoma. Intraoperative handling, gross dissection, and histologic/immunohistochemical (IHC) evaluation techniques are all key components of this process. Although not currently part of routine handling, newer molecular techniques may potentially add to the valuable information gained from evaluating sentinel node specimens.

Standard gross dissection of all types of SLN begins with complete reporting of the anatomic location, SLN number, and if indicated by surgeon the presence or absence of blue dye and radioactivity counts. After proper fixation, any gross lesion, such as pigment or visible tumor, should be described and measured. Unless voluminous, the perinodal fat should not be dissected away, taking care not to disturb the lymph node capsule. If small (<4 mm), the node can be submitted in its entirety, unsectioned. Larger SLN should be serially sectioned at 2–3 mm intervals along the longest axis and completely embedded for histopathologic evaluation [3]. Rapid intraoperative identification of SLN metastases may allow the patient to avoid second surgery and treatment delays. However, frozen section of melanoma SLN has been found to have a low sensitivity, with reported rates ranging from 47 to 59% [89]. While one group found a false-negative rate as low as 5.3% [90], this has not been repeated by others and has not gained widespread acceptance. Thus, due to concerns about tissue exhaustion and cryostat contamination, currently frozen section analysis is not advised in the detection of melanoma [91].

Intraoperative imprint cytology (IIC) gained widespread interest in the early 2000s as a rapid alternative to frozen section that can sample a broader area of tissue with no concerns for tissue usage. After touch imprinting one to several lymph node surfaces to a glass slide, with a variety of staining techniques that have been employed, including Giemsa/Diff-Quik staining, H&E staining, and additional rapid immunohistochemical staining melanoma, IIC has been shown to have a sensitivity of 33–61%, with a negligible false-positive rate. The sensitivity of IIC increases with the tumor stage, as high as 47% in patients with T4 lesions, and rises to 62% when metastases >2 cm in size are present [92]. Thus, it is acceptable to perform IIC in melanoma SLN, and preferable to performing a frozen section, when a metastasis is strongly suspected on gross examination.

Current and past AJCC guidelines recognize two categories of SLN involvement in melanoma: clinically occult micrometastasis and clinically apparent macrometastasis [3]. Micrometastatic melanoma is defined as the presence of morphologically malignant cells positive for at least one IHC marker (S-100, HMB-45, Melan-A/Mart1, Sox10) (Figs. 12.4 and 12.5) and/or melanoma detectable on H&E staining alone [3]. A number of IHC markers have been evaluated for sensitivity and specificity of detection of metastatic melanoma in the SLN. S-100 has the greatest sensitivity (~99%), and Melan-A approaches this in one study (97%) [93]. More recently, Sox10 has been utilized, with sensitivity that is equivalent to S-100, but with added specificity, because unlike S-100 this nuclear stain is negative in nodal dendritic cells and macrophages [94]. S-100 and Melan-A also highlight benign nodal nevi, present in the capsule, trabeculae, and rarely the parenchyma in up to 28% of lymph nodes [95], but these are typically HMB-45 negative [96, 97].

In the 8th edition AJCC schema, the designation of nodal stage of melanoma depends on the number of involved nodes; presence of in-transit, satellite, or microsatellite metastases; and whether tumor was detected by sentinel node staging (a) or clinically (b) [57].

While standardized lymph node examination protocols have been in place in Europe for a number of years, there is no standard protocol mandated in the USA, and several major institutions have developed their own sets of guidelines. The most widely utilized protocol is that of Cochran and colleagues, who advocate cutting ten serial sections from each lymph node section, staining sections 1, 3, 5, and 10 with H&E, 4 with HMB45, and 6 with Mart-1, saving four for possible additional studies [98]. This approach identifies metastatic melanoma in 16–20% of specimens [99]. Numerous studies have demonstrated that extended histopathologic examination of the SLN can improve diagnostic yield.

The current EORTC protocol is modeled after the work by Cook, demonstrating a 34% SLN positivity rate with a protocol that examines six pairs of sections cut at 50 μm intervals, staining 1–6 with H&E and S-100 and level 2 additionally with HMB-45 and pan-melanoma [100]. Spanknebel and colleagues employed a technique of performing S-100, Melan-A, and HMB-45 immunostaining on multiple levels of SLNs step-sectioned 20 times at 50 μm intervals or until the node was exhausted. This identified metastases in 14/39 (35%) of SLN called negative by routine pathologic analysis, for an overall node-positive rate of 61%. The authors concluded that cutting three sections for H&E, S-100, and HMB-45 at three 250 μm intervals had the highest yield, detecting 70% of all nodal micrometastases [101]. While this costly ($1050 in 2005) and time-consuming approach is not practical for routine use, the study highlighted the widespread distribution of tumor cells in SLN, and was one of the first studies to raise the possibility that there may be a SLN tumor burden low enough that may be subclinical and comparative to those patients with node-negative disease [101].

Several studies have suggested that the pattern and burden of SLN tumor involvement may be linked to non-SLN positivity and clinical outcome measures [102, 103]. Starz et al. developed a three-stage schema based on the number of metastases and depth of tumor invasion from the interior of the SLN capsule in mm [104], showing that this schema was predictive of distant metastases and long-term survival. Cochran demonstrated that the two-dimension percentage of involved nodal area could independently predict non-SLN positivity [105]. Dewar demonstrated that a SLN with metastases in the subcapsular region had a lower rate of non-SLN positivity that those with multifocal, extensive, or intraparenchymal disease [106].

The Rotterdam criteria, based on the work by van Akkooi et al., demonstrated that the maximum diameter of the largest metastasis had a significant influence on non-SLN involvement and survival [106]. While none of these criteria have yet been fully validated in a multicenter or prospective study, reporting is recommended. The ongoing European Minitub trial comparing outcome in patients with minimal SLN tumor burden managed by observation versus a complete lymph node dissection (CLND) will likely answer this question.

Pathologic evaluation of the CLND is similarly important for accurate staging. Clearly, this requires submission of at least one section from each grossly identified lymph node. However, there is controversy over the necessity for submission of each lymph node in its entirety, versus a single representative section. Similar to the controversy surrounding optimal methods for evaluation of sentinel nodes, there is debate concerning the necessity for IHC evaluation of non-SLNs [107].

Distant Metastatic Melanoma

Melanoma metastases may be resected as part of the initial diagnostic workup in a patient with a previously undetected or unknown primary, or as a palliative and/or therapeutic excision in a patient with oligometastatic disease. In patients without a prior history of melanoma, a thorough diagnostic workup often includes the IHC markers discussed in Section "Evaluation of Primary Melanoma Biopsies." The most useful markers include a combination of at least one highly sensitive marker such as S-100 or Sox-10, and one highly specific marker such as Melan-A or HMB-45. There are several potential pitfalls to this approach: desmoplastic melanoma may be missed, and tumor of perivascular epithelioid cells (PEComa) and clear-cell sarcoma may have a similar immunoprofile. PEComa is a family of tumors comprising angiomyolipoma, lymphangiomyomatosis, and clear-cell sugar tumor of lung, and most importantly in the differential diagnosis of melanoma PEComa may present as a soft-tissue mass. Soft-tissue and cutaneous PEComa are characterized by nested/fascicular growth of clear cells, often with a perivascular distribution (ref). In one study, all cases expressed at least one melanocytic marker, including HMB-45 (96%), Melan-A (72%), and MiTF (50%) [108]. However, unlike melanoma, they almost always express smooth muscle markers [109].

Clear-cell sarcoma is a tumor of young adults that chiefly arises in the soft tissue of acral locations. It displays compact nests or fascicles of oval cells with clear cytoplasm in a delicate connective tissue framework. S-100 is almost always expressed, as well as HMB-45, Melan-A, and MiTF [110, 111]. There is commonly a translocation of t(12;22)(q13;q12), fusing the EWSR1 gene on chromosome 22 with ATF, a member of the CREB transcription factor family on chromosome 12. This translocation is found in 70% of all cases [112]. As noted previously, desmoplastic melanoma is only positive for Sox-10 and S-100, and thus demonstration of retention of H3K27em3 is required to separate it from MPNST [52].

Finally, the emergence of therapies targeted to specific gene mutations present in melanoma has also changed our evaluation of metastatic melanoma tumors. It is now customary to evaluate metastatic disease at the time of diagnosis for the presence of actionable gene mutations. There are a number of methods employed, such as pyrosequencing, Sanger sequencing of individual genes, or next-generation sequencing, that target a panel of genes. While mutations in BRAF and cKIT are most commonly evaluated [113], there are also therapies and/or therapeutic trials available for patients with mutations of a variety of other genes, including NRAS, MET, EGFR, ALK, ROS1, PIK3CA, mTOR, PTEN, NF1, AKT, and NTRK fusions [114].

In summary, recent knowledge gained from exhaustive mining of clinical and molecular data has revolutionized the ways in which tissue from melanocytic lesions is analyzed and reported. From pathologic microstaging of localized and regionally metastatic disease to submission of tumor tissue for molecular testing to stratify patients for treatment, pathologists and oncologists must be aware of these advances in order to avail their patients of the most relevant treatment options.

References

1. Ng PC, Barzilai DA, Ismail SA, Averitte RL Jr, Gilliam AC. Evaluating invasive cutaneous melanoma: is the initial biopsy representative of the final depth? J Am Acad Dermatol. 2003;48(3):420–4.
2. Riker AI, Glass F, Perez I, Cruse CW, Messina J, Sondak VK. Cutaneous melanoma: methods of biopsy and definitive surgical excision. Dermatol Ther. 2005;18(5):387–93.
3. Balch CM, Gershenwald JE, Soong SJ, Thompson JF, Atkins MB, Byrd DR, Buzaid AC, Cochran AJ, Coit DG, Ding S, Eggermont AM, Flaherty KT, Gimotty PA, Kirkwood JM, McMasters KM, Mihm MC Jr, Morton DL, Ross MI, Sober AJ, Sondak VK. Final version of 2009 AJCC melanoma staging and classification. J Clin Oncol. 2009;27(36):6199–206.
4. Ng JC, Swain S, Dowling JP, Wolfe R, Simpson P, Kelly JW. The impact of partial biopsy on histopathologic diagnosis of cutaneous melanoma: experience of an Australian tertiary referral service. Arch Dermatol. 2010;146(3):234–9.
5. Chen SC, Bravata DM, Weil E, Olkin I. A comparison of dermatologists' and primary care physicians' accuracy in diagnosing melanoma: a systematic review. Arch Dermatol. 2001;137(12):1627–34.
6. Lederman JS, Sober AJ. Does wide excision as the initial diagnostic procedure improve prognosis in patients with cutaneous melanoma? J Dermatol Surg Oncol. 1986;12(7):697–9.
7. Lorusso GD, Sarma DP, Sarwar SF. Punch biopsies of melanoma: a diagnostic peril. Dermatol Online J. 2005;11(1):7.
8. Karimipour DJ, Schwartz JL, Wang TS, Bichakjian CK, Orringer JS, King AL, Huang CC, Johnson TM. Microstaging accuracy after subtotal incisional biopsy of cutaneous melanoma. J Am Acad Dermatol. 2005;52(5):798–802.
9. Roses DF, Ackerman AB, Harris MN, Weinhouse GR, Gumport SL. Assessment of biopsy techniques and histopathologic interpretations of primary cutaneous malignant melanoma. Ann Surg. 1979;189(3):294–7.
10. Criscione VD, Weinstock MA. Melanoma thickness trends in the United States, 1988–2006. J Invest Dermatol. 2010;130(3):793–7.
11. Network, N. C. C. NCCN clinical practice guidelines in oncology for melanoma (Version I.2017); 2016.
12. Zager JS, Hochwald SN, Marzban SS, Francois R, Law KM, Davis AH, Messina JL, Vincek V, Mitchell C, Church A, Copeland EM, Sondak VK, Grobmyer SR. Shave biopsy is a safe and accurate method for the initial evaluation of melanoma. J Am Coll Surg. 2011;212(4):454–60. discussion 460-452
13. Fallowfield ME, Cook MG. Re-excisions of scar in primary cutaneous melanoma: a histopathological study. Br J Dermatol. 1992;126(1):47–51.
14. Martin HM, Birkin AJ, Theaker JM. Malignant melanoma re-excision specimens--how many blocks? Histopathology. 1998;32(4):362–7.
15. Walters RF, Groben PA, Busam K, Millikan RC, Rabinovitz H, Cognetta A, Mihm MC Jr, Prieto VG, Googe PB, King R, Moore DT, Woosley J, Thomas NE. Consumption of the epidermis: a criterion in the differential diagnosis of melanoma and dysplastic nevi that is associated with increasing breslow depth and ulceration. Am J Dermatopathol. 2007;29(6):527–33.
16. Petronic-Rosic V, Shea CR, Krausz T. Pagetoid melanocytosis: when is it significant? Pathology. 2004;36(5):435–44.
17. Huwait H, Hijazi N, Martinka M, Crawford RI. The significance of Melan-A-positive pagetoid melanocytosis in dysplastic nevi. Am J Dermatopathol. 2014;36(4):340–3.
18. Gerami P, Busam K, Cochran A, Cook MG, Duncan LM, Elder DE, Fullen DR, Guitart J, LeBoit PE, Mihm MC Jr, Prieto VG, Rabkin MS, Scolyer RA, Xu X, Yun SJ, Obregon R, Yazdan P, Cooper C, Weitner BB, Rademaker A, Barnhill RL. Histomorphologic assessment and interobserver diagnostic reproducibility of atypical spitzoid melanocytic neoplasms with long-term follow-up. Am J Surg Pathol. 2014;38(7):934–40.
19. Magro CM, Crowson AN, Mihm MC. Unusual variants of malignant melanoma. Mod Pathol. 2006;19(Suppl 2):S41–70.
20. Kamino H, Tam S, Tapia B, Toussaint S. The use of elastin immunostain improves the evaluation of melanomas associated with nevi. J Cutan Pathol. 2009;36(8):845–52.
21. El Shabrawi-Caelen L, Kerl H, Cerroni L. Melan-A: not a helpful marker in distinction between melanoma

in situ on sun-damaged skin and pigmented actinic keratosis. Am J Dermatopathol. 2004;26(5):364–6.
22. Theunis A, Richert B, Sass U, Lateur N, Sales F, Andre J. Immunohistochemical study of 40 cases of longitudinal melanonychia. Am J Dermatopathol. 2011;33(1):27–34.
23. Leleux TM, Prieto VG, Diwan AH. Aberrant expression of HMB-45 in traumatized melanocytic nevi. J Am Acad Dermatol. 2012;67(3):446–50.
24. Uguen A, Talagas M, Costa S, Duigou S, Bouvier S, De Braekeleer M, Marcorelles P. A p16-Ki-67-HMB45 immunohistochemistry scoring system as an ancillary diagnostic tool in the diagnosis of melanoma. Diagn Pathol. 2015;10:195.
25. Li LX, Crotty KA, McCarthy SW, Palmer AA, Kril JJ. A zonal comparison of MIB1-Ki67 immunoreactivity in benign and malignant melanocytic lesions. Am J Dermatopathol. 2000;22(6):489–95.
26. Nasr MR, El-Zammar O. Comparison of pHH3, Ki-67, and survivin immunoreactivity in benign and malignant melanocytic lesions. Am J Dermatopathol. 2008;30(2):117–22.
27. Puri PK, Valdes CL, Burchette JL, Grichnik JM, Turner JW, Selim MA. Accurate identification of proliferative index in melanocytic neoplasms with Melan-A/Ki-67 double stain. J Cutan Pathol. 2010;37(9):1010–2.
28. Tetzlaff MT, Curry JL, Ivan D, Wang WL, Torres-Cabala CA, Bassett RL, Valencia KM, McLemore MS, Ross MI, Prieto VG. Immunodetection of phosphohistone H3 as a surrogate of mitotic figure count and clinical outcome in cutaneous melanoma. Mod Pathol. 2013;26(9):1153–60.
29. Ottmann K, Tronnier M, Mitteldorf C. Detection of mitotic figures in thin melanomas—immunohistochemistry does not replace the careful search for mitotic figures in hematoxylin-eosin stain. J Am Acad Dermatol. 2015;73(4):637–44.
30. Ohta M, Berd D, Shimizu M, Nagai H, Cotticelli MG, Mastrangelo M, Shields JA, Shields CL, Croce CM, Huebner K. Deletion mapping of chromosome region 9p21-p22 surrounding the CDKN2 locus in melanoma. Int J Cancer. 1996;65(6):762–7.
31. Harms PW, Hocker TL, Zhao L, Chan MP, Andea AA, Wang M, Harms KL, Wang ML, Carskadon S, Palanisamy N, Fullen DR. Loss of p16 expression and copy number changes of CDKN2A in a spectrum of spitzoid melanocytic lesions. Hum Pathol. 2016;58:152–60.
32. Clark WH Jr, Elder DE, Van Horn M. The biologic forms of malignant melanoma. Hum Pathol. 1986;17(5):443–50.
33. Curtin JA, Fridlyand J, Kageshita T, Patel HN, Busam KJ, Kutzner H, Cho KH, Aiba S, Brocker EB, LeBoit PE, Pinkel D, Bastian BC. Distinct sets of genetic alterations in melanoma. N Engl J Med. 2005;353(20):2135–47.
34. Bastian BC. The molecular pathology of melanoma: an integrated taxonomy of melanocytic neoplasia. Annu Rev Pathol. 2014;9:239–71.
35. Flotte TJ, Mihm MC Jr. Lentigo maligna and malignant melanoma in situ, lentigo maligna type. Hum Pathol. 1999;30(5):533–6.
36. Penneys NS. Microinvasive lentigo maligna melanoma. J Am Acad Dermatol. 1987;17(4):675–80.
37. Horenstein MG, Norton CL, Evans TN. Displacement of dermal solar elastosis in malignant melanoma. J Cutan Pathol. 2007;34(5):376–80.
38. Price NM, Rywlin AM, Ackerman AB. Histologic criteria for the diagnosis of superficial spreading malignant melanoma: formulated on the basis of proven metastatic lesions. Cancer. 1976;38(6):2434–41.
39. Hantschke M, Bastian BC, LeBoit PE. Consumption of the epidermis: a diagnostic criterion for the differential diagnosis of melanoma and Spitz nevus. Am J Surg Pathol. 2004;28(12):1621–5.
40. Elder DE, Jucovy PM, Tuthill RJ, Clark WH Jr. The classification of malignant melanoma. Am J Dermatopathol. 1980;2(4):315–20.
41. Wanebo HJ, Fortner JG, Woodruff J, MacLean B, Binkowski E. Selection of the optimum surgical treatment of stage I melanoma by depth of microinvasion: use of the combined microstage technique (Clark-Breslow). Ann Surg. 1975;182(3):302–15.
42. Balch CM, Wilkerson JA, Murad TM, Soong SJ, Ingalls AL, Maddox WA. The prognostic significance of ulceration of cutaneous melanoma. Cancer. 1980;45(12):3012–7.
43. Chamberlain AJ, Fritschi L, Giles GG, Dowling JP, Kelly JW. Nodular type and older age as the most significant associations of thick melanoma in Victoria, Australia. Arch Dermatol. 2002;138(5):609–14.
44. Cascinelli N, Zurrida S, Galimberti V, Bartoli C, Bufalino R, Del Prato I, Mascheroni L, Testori A, Clemente C. Acral lentiginous melanoma. A histological type without prognostic significance. J Dermatol Surg Oncol. 1994;20(12):817–22.
45. Phan A, Touzet S, Dalle S, Ronger-Savle S, Balme B, Thomas L. Acral lentiginous melanoma: histopathological prognostic features of 121 cases. Br J Dermatol. 2007;157(2):311–8.
46. Lucas DR, Tazelaar HD, Unni KK, Wold LE, Okada K, Dimarzio DJ Jr, Rolfe B. Osteogenic melanoma. A rare variant of malignant melanoma. Am J Surg Pathol. 1993;17(4):400–9.
47. de Almeida LS, Requena L, Rutten A, Kutzner H, Garbe C, Pestana D, Gomes MM. Desmoplastic malignant melanoma: a clinicopathologic analysis of 113 cases. Am J Dermatopathol. 2008;30(3):207–15.
48. Chen LL, Jaimes N, Barker CA, Busam KJ, Marghoob AA. Desmoplastic melanoma: a review. J Am Acad Dermatol. 2013;68(5):825–33.
49. Busam KJ, Mujumdar U, Hummer AJ, Nobrega J, Hawkins WG, Coit DG, Brady MS. Cutaneous desmoplastic melanoma: reappraisal of morphologic heterogeneity and prognostic factors. Am J Surg Pathol. 2004;28(11):1518–25.
50. Busam KJ. Desmoplastic melanoma. Clin Lab Med. 2011;31(2):321–30.

51. Busam KJ. Desmoplastic Melanoma. Surg Pathol Clin. 2009;2(3):511–20.
52. Prieto-Granada CN, Wiesner T, Messina JL, Jungbluth AA, Chi P, Antonescu CR. Loss of H3K27me3 expression is a highly sensitive marker for sporadic and radiation-induced MPNST. Am J Surg Pathol. 2016;40(4):479–89.
53. Weissinger SE, Keil P, Silvers DN, Klaus BM, Moller P, Horst BA, Lennerz JK. A diagnostic algorithm to distinguish desmoplastic from spindle cell melanoma. Mod Pathol. 2014;27(4):524–34.
54. Mentzel T. Uncommon variants of malignant melanocytic neoplasms. Pathologe. 2007;28(6):445–52.
55. Swetter SM, Ecker PM, Johnson DL, Harvell JD. Primary dermal melanoma: a distinct subtype of melanoma. Arch Dermatol. 2004;140(1):99–103.
56. Cassarino DS, Cabral ES, Kartha RV, Swetter SM. Primary dermal melanoma: distinct immunohistochemical findings and clinical outcome compared with nodular and metastatic melanoma. Arch Dermatol. 2008;144(1):49–56.
57. Gershenwald JE, Scolyer RA, Hess KR, Thompson JF, Long GV, Ross MI, Lazar AJ, Atkins MB, Balch CM, Barnhill R, Bilimoria KY, Brierley JD, Buzaid AC, Byrd DR, Chapman PB, Cochran AJ, Coit DG, Eggermont AM, Elder DE, Faries MB, Flaherty KT, Garbe C, Gardner JM, Gimotty PA, Halpern AC, Haydu LE, Johnson T, Kirkwood JM, Lee AWM, McArthur GA, Mihm MC, Prieto VG, Sober AJ, Wahl RL, Wong SL, Sondak VK. Melanoma of the skin. In: AJCC cancer staging manual. 8th ed. Springer: Switzerland; 2017.
58. Barnhill RL, Argenyi ZB, From L, Glass LF, Maize JC, Mihm MC Jr, Rabkin MS, Ronan SG, White WL, Piepkorn M. Atypical Spitz nevi/tumors: lack of consensus for diagnosis, discrimination from melanoma, and prediction of outcome. Hum Pathol. 1999;30(5):513–20.
59. Tom WL, Hsu JW, Eichenfield LF, Friedlander SF. Pediatric "STUMP" lesions: evaluation and management of difficult atypical Spitzoid lesions in children. J Am Acad Dermatol. 64(3):559–72.
60. Gerami P, Jewell SS, Morrison LE, Blondin B, Schulz J, Ruffalo T, Matushek PT, Legator M, Jacobson K, Dalton SR, Charzan S, Kolaitis NA, Guitart J, Lertsbarapa T, Boone S, LeBoit PE, Bastian BC. Fluorescence in situ hybridization (FISH) as an ancillary diagnostic tool in the diagnosis of melanoma. Am J Surg Pathol. 2009;33(8):1146–56.
61. Scolyer RA, Murali R, McCarthy SW, Thompson JF. Histologically ambiguous ("borderline") primary cutaneous melanocytic tumors: approaches to patient management including the roles of molecular testing and sentinel lymph node biopsy. Arch Pathol Lab Med. 134(12):1770–7.
62. Dalton SR, Gerami P, Kolaitis NA, Charzan S, Werling R, LeBoit PE, Bastian BC. Use of fluorescence in situ hybridization (FISH) to distinguish intranodal nevus from metastatic melanoma. Am J Surg Pathol. 34(2):231–7.
63. Gerami P, Wass A, Mafee M, Fang Y, Pulitzer MP, Busam KJ. Fluorescence in situ hybridization for distinguishing nevoid melanomas from mitotically active nevi. Am J Surg Pathol. 2009;33(12):1783–8.
64. Pouryazdanparast P, Newman M, Mafee M, Haghighat Z, Guitart J, Gerami P. Distinguishing epithelioid blue nevus from blue nevus-like cutaneous melanoma metastasis using fluorescence in situ hybridization. Am J Surg Pathol. 2009;33(9):1396–400.
65. Gerami P, Li G, Pouryazdanparast P, Blondin B, Beilfuss B, Slenk C, Du J, Guitart J, Jewell S, Pestova K. A highly specific and discriminatory FISH assay for distinguishing between benign and malignant melanocytic neoplasms. Am J Surg Pathol. 2012;36(6):808–17.
66. Gaiser T, Kutzner H, Palmedo G, Siegelin MD, Wiesner T, Bruckner T, Hartschuh W, Enk AH, Becker MR. Classifying ambiguous melanocytic lesions with FISH and correlation with clinical long-term follow up. Mod Pathol. 2010;23(3):413–9.
67. Massi D, Cesinaro AM, Tomasini C, Paglierani M, Bettelli S, Dal Maso L, Simi L, Salvianti F, Pinzani P, Orlando C, De Giorgi V, Lukic S, Maiorana A, Santucci M, Canzonieri V. Atypical Spitzoid melanocytic tumors: a morphological, mutational, and FISH analysis. J Am Acad Dermatol. 2011;64(5):919–35.
68. Vergier B, Prochazkova-Carlotti M, de la Fouchardiere A, Cerroni L, Massi D, De Giorgi V, Bailly C, Wesselmann U, Karlseladze A, Avril MF, Jouary T, Merlio JP. Fluorescence in situ hybridization, a diagnostic aid in ambiguous melanocytic tumors: European study of 113 cases. Mod Pathol. 2011;24(5):613–23.
69. Tetzlaff MT, Wang WL, Milless TL, Curry JL, Torres-Cabala CA, McLemore MS, Ivan D, Bassett RL, Prieto VG. Ambiguous melanocytic tumors in a tertiary referral center: the contribution of fluorescence in situ hybridization (FISH) to conventional histopathologic and immunophenotypic analyses. Am J Surg Pathol. 2013;37(12):1783–96.
70. Clarke LE, Warf MB, Flake DD 2nd, Hartman AR, Tahan S, Shea CR, Gerami P, Messina J, Florell SR, Wenstrup RJ, Rushton K, Roundy KM, Rock C, Roa B, Kolquist KA, Gutin A, Billings S, Leachman S. Clinical validation of a gene expression signature that differentiates benign nevi from malignant melanoma. J Cutan Pathol. 2015;42(4):244–52.
71. Minca EC, Al-Rohil RN, Wang M, Harms PW, Ko JS, Collie AM, Kovalyshyn I, Prieto VG, Tetzlaff MT, Billings SD, Andea AA. Comparison between melanoma gene expression score and fluorescence in situ hybridization for the classification of melanocytic lesions. Mod Pathol. 2016;29(8):832–43.
72. Bauer J, Bastian BC. Distinguishing melanocytic nevi from melanoma by DNA copy number changes: comparative genomic hybridization as a research and diagnostic tool. Dermatol Ther. 2006;19(1):40–9.

73. Bastian BC, LeBoit PE, Hamm H, Brocker EB, Pinkel D. Chromosomal gains and losses in primary cutaneous melanomas detected by comparative genomic hybridization. Cancer Res. 1998;58(10):2170–5.
74. Ali L, Helm T, Cheney R, Conroy J, Sait S, Guitart J, Gerami P. Correlating array comparative genomic hybridization findings with histology and outcome in spitzoid melanocytic neoplasms. Int J Clin Exp Pathol. 3(6):593–9.
75. Bastian BC, Olshen AB, LeBoit PE, Pinkel D. Classifying melanocytic tumors based on DNA copy number changes. Am J Pathol. 2003;163(5):1765–70.
76. Horn S, Figl A, Rachakonda PS, Fischer C, Sucker A, Gast A, Kadel S, Moll I, Nagore E, Hemminki K, Schadendorf D, Kumar R. TERT promoter mutations in familial and sporadic melanoma. Science. 2013;339(6122):959–61.
77. Lu C, Zhang J, Nagahawatte P, Easton J, Lee S, Liu Z, Ding L, Wyczalkowski MA, Valentine M, Navid F, Mulder H, Tatevossian RG, Dalton J, Davenport J, Yin Z, Edmonson M, Rusch M, Wu G, Li Y, Parker M, Hedlund E, Shurtleff S, Raimondi S, Bhavin V, Donald Y, Mardis ER, Wilson RK, Evans WE, Ellison DW, Pounds S, Dyer M, Downing JR, Pappo A, Bahrami A. The genomic landscape of childhood and adolescent melanoma. J Invest Dermatol. 2015;135(3):816–23.
78. Lee S, Barnhill RL, Dummer R, Dalton J, Wu J, Pappo A, Bahrami A. TERT promoter mutations are predictive of aggressive clinical behavior in patients with spitzoid melanocytic neoplasms. Sci Rep. 2015;5:11200.
79. Breslow A. Thickness, cross-sectional areas and depth of invasion in the prognosis of cutaneous melanoma. Ann Surg. 1970;172(5):902–8.
80. Scolyer RA, Judge MJ, Evans A, Frishberg DP, Prieto VG, Thompson JF, Trotter MJ, Walsh MY, Walsh NMG, Ellis DW. Data set for pathology reporting of cutaneous invasive melanoma: recommendations from the International Collaboration on Cancer Reporting (ICCR). Am J Surg Pathol. 2013;37(12):1797–814.
81. In 't Hout FE, Haydu LE, Murali R, Bonenkamp JJ, Thompson JF, Scolyer RA. Prognostic importance of the extent of ulceration in patients with clinically localized cutaneous melanoma. Ann Surg. 2012;255(6):1165–70.
82. Clark WH Jr, From L, Bernardino EA, Mihm MC. The histogenesis and biologic behavior of primary human malignant melanomas of the skin. Cancer Res. 1969;29(3):705–27.
83. Buzaid AC, Ross MI, Balch CM, Soong S, McCarthy WH, Tinoco L, Mansfield P, Lee JE, Bedikian A, Eton O, Plager C, Papadopoulos N, Legha SS, Benjamin RS. Critical analysis of the current American Joint Committee on Cancer staging system for cutaneous melanoma and proposal of a new staging system. J Clin Oncol. 1997;15(3):1039–51.
84. Burton AL, Roach BA, Mays MP, Chen AF, Ginter BA, Vierling AM, Scoggins CR, Martin RC, Stromberg AJ, Hagendoorn L, McMasters KM. Prognostic significance of tumor infiltrating lymphocytes in melanoma. Am Surg. 2011;77(2):188–92.
85. Azimi F, Scolyer RA, Rumcheva P, Moncrieff M, Murali R, McCarthy SW, Saw RP, Thompson JF. Tumor-infiltrating lymphocyte grade is an independent predictor of sentinel lymph node status and survival in patients with cutaneous melanoma. J Clin Oncol. 2012;30(21):2678–83.
86. Xu X, Chen L, Guerry D, Dawson PR, Hwang WT, VanBelle P, Elder DE, Zhang PJ, Ming ME, Schuchter L, Gimotty PA. Lymphatic invasion is independently prognostic of metastasis in primary cutaneous melanoma. Clin Cancer Res. 2012;18(1):229–37.
87. Yun SJ, Gimotty PA, Hwang WT, Dawson P, Van Belle P, Elder DE, Elenitsas R, Schuchter L, Zhang PJ, Guerry D, Xu X. High lymphatic vessel density and lymphatic invasion underlie the adverse prognostic effect of radial growth phase regression in melanoma. Am J Surg Pathol. 2011;35(2):235–42.
88. Ribero S, Gualano MR, Osella-Abate S, Scaioli G, Bert F, Sanlorenzo M, Balagna E, Fierro MT, Macripo G, Sapino A, Siliquini R, Quaglino P. Association of Histologic Regression in primary melanoma with sentinel lymph node status: a systematic review and meta-analysis. JAMA Dermatol. 2015;151(12):1301–7.
89. Alkhatib W, Hertzenberg C, Jewell W, Al-Kasspooles MF, Damjanov I, Cohen MS. Utility of frozen-section analysis of sentinel lymph node biopsy specimens for melanoma in surgical decision making. Am J Surg. 2008;196(6):827–32; discussion 832–3
90. Gipponi M, Solari N, Lionetto R, Di Somma C, Villa G, Schenone F, Queirolo P, Cafiero F. The prognostic role of the sentinel lymph node in clinically node-negative patients with cutaneous melanoma: experience of the Genoa group. Eur J Surg Oncol. 2005;31(10):1191–7.
91. Scolyer RA, Thompson JF, McCarthy SW, Gershenwald JE, Ross MI, Cochran AJ. Intraoperative frozen-section evaluation can reduce accuracy of pathologic assessment of sentinel nodes in melanoma patients. J Am Coll Surg. 2005;201(5):821–3; author reply 823–4
92. Badgwell BD, Pierce C, Broadwater JR, Westbrook K, Korourian S, Davis D, Hiatt K, Lee J, Cheung WL, Klimberg VS. Intraoperative sentinel lymph node analysis in melanoma. J Surg Oncol. 2011;103(1):1–5.
93. Karimipour DJ, Lowe L, Su L, Hamilton T, Sondak V, Johnson TM, Fullen D. Standard immunostains for melanoma in sentinel lymph node specimens: which ones are most useful? J Am Acad Dermatol. 2004;50(5):759–64.
94. Jennings C, Kim J. Identification of nodal metastases in melanoma using sox-10. Am J Dermatopathol. 2011;33(5):474–82.

95. Abrahamsen HN, Hamilton-Dutoit SJ, Larsen J, Steiniche T. Sentinel lymph nodes in malignant melanoma: extended histopathologic evaluation improves diagnostic precision. Cancer. 2004;100(8):1683–91.
96. Cochran AJ. The pathologist's role in sentinel lymph node evaluation. Semin Nucl Med. 2000;30(1):11–7.
97. Murray CA, Leong WL, McCready DR, Ghazarian DM. Histopathological patterns of melanoma metastases in sentinel lymph nodes. J Clin Pathol. 2004;57(1):64–7.
98. Morton DL, Wen DR, Wong JH, Economou JS, Cagle LA, Storm FK, Foshag LJ, Cochran AJ. Technical details of intraoperative lymphatic mapping for early stage melanoma. Arch Surg. 1992;127(4):392–9.
99. Morton DL, Cochran AJ, Thompson JF. Authors' response to a letter to the editor re: sentinel node biopsy for early-stage melanoma. Ann Surg. 2007;245(5):828–9.
100. Cook MG, Green MA, Anderson B, Eggermont AM, Ruiter DJ, Spatz A, Kissin MW, Powell BW. The development of optimal pathological assessment of sentinel lymph nodes for melanoma. J Pathol. 2003;200(3):314–9.
101. Spanknebel K, Coit DG, Bieligk SC, Gonen M, Rosai J, Klimstra DS. Characterization of micrometastatic disease in melanoma sentinel lymph nodes by enhanced pathology: recommendations for standardizing pathologic analysis. Am J Surg Pathol. 2005;29(3):305–17.
102. van Akkooi AC, Spatz A, Eggermont AM, Mihm M, Cook MG. Expert opinion in melanoma: the sentinel node; EORTC Melanoma Group recommendations on practical methodology of the measurement of the microanatomic location of metastases and metastatic tumour burden. Eur J Cancer. 2009;45(16):2736–42.
103. van Akkooi AC, Verhoef C, Eggermont AM. Importance of tumor load in the sentinel node in melanoma: clinical dilemmas. Nat Rev Clin Oncol. 2010;7(8):446–54.
104. Starz H, Balda BR, Kramer KU, Buchels H, Wang H. A micromorphometry-based concept for routine classification of sentinel lymph node metastases and its clinical relevance for patients with melanoma. Cancer. 2001;91(11):2110–21.
105. Cochran AJ, Wen DR, Huang RR, Wang HJ, Elashoff R, Morton DL. Prediction of metastatic melanoma in nonsentinel nodes and clinical outcome based on the primary melanoma and the sentinel node. Mod Pathol. 2004;17(7):747–55.
106. Dewar DJ, Newell B, Green MA, Topping AP, Powell BW, Cook MG. The microanatomic location of metastatic melanoma in sentinel lymph nodes predicts nonsentinel lymph node involvement. J Clin Oncol. 2004;22(16):3345–9.
107. Holtkamp LH, Wang S, Wilmott JS, Madore J, Vilain R, Thompson JF, Nieweg OE, Scolyer RA. Detailed pathological examination of completion node dissection specimens and outcome in melanoma patients with minimal (<0.1 mm) sentinel lymph node metastases. Ann Surg Oncol. 2015;22(9):2972–7.
108. Folpe AL, Mentzel T, Lehr HA, Fisher C, Balzer BL, Weiss SW. Perivascular epithelioid cell neoplasms of soft tissue and gynecologic origin: a clinicopathologic study of 26 cases and review of the literature. Am J Surg Pathol. 2005;29(12):1558–75.
109. Goldblum JR, Folpe AL, Weiss SW. Enzinger and Weiss's soft tissue tumors. Philadelphia: Saunders; 2013.
110. Kindblom LG, Lodding P, Angervall L. Clear-cell sarcoma of tendons and aponeuroses. An immunohistochemical and electron microscopic analysis indicating neural crest origin. Virchows Arch A Pathol Anat Histopathol. 1983;401(1):109–28.
111. Swanson PE, Wick MR. Clear cell sarcoma. An immunohistochemical analysis of six cases and comparison with other epithelioid neoplasms of soft tissue. Arch Pathol Lab Med. 1989;113(1):55–60.
112. Langezaal SM, Graadt van Roggen JF, Cleton-Jansen AM, Baelde JJ, Hogendoorn PC. Malignant melanoma is genetically distinct from clear cell sarcoma of tendons and aponeurosis (malignant melanoma of soft parts). Br J Cancer. 2001;84(4):535–8.
113. Jeck WR, Parker J, Carson CC, Shields JM, Sambade MJ, Peters EC, Burd CE, Thomas NE, Chiang DY, Liu W, Eberhard DA, Ollila D, Grilley-Olson J, Moschos S, Neil Hayes D, Sharpless NE. Targeted next generation sequencing identifies clinically actionable mutations in patients with melanoma. Pigment Cell Melanoma Res. 2014;27(4):653–63.
114. National Cancer Institute, N. C. NCI-MATCH Trial (Molecular Analysis for Therapy Choice). 2017. https://www.cancer.gov/about-cancer/treatment/clinical-trials/nci-supported/nci-match. Accessed 30 Apr 2017.

Pediatric Melanoma and Atypical Melanocytic Neoplasms

13

Radhika Sreeraman Kumar, Jane L. Messina, Damon R. Reed, and Vernon K. Sondak

Introduction

Definition and Epidemiology

Pediatric melanoma is a malignant melanocytic lesion in a child from birth to the start of adulthood, variably defined as either age 18 or 21. Pediatric melanoma can be classified by the presence or absence of precursor lesions, age at presentation (see Fig. 13.1), histology, and staging criteria applied to adult melanoma. In children, it is often difficult to establish whether an abnormal melanocytic lesion is unequivocally cancer. Although this difficulty is sometimes due to reticence in diagnosing melanoma in young children, there are a significant number of abnormal melanocytic lesions that are difficult to characterize consistently. We term this broad class as atypical melanocytic neoplasms, and these can be classified based on pathology and metastatic potential [1, 2].

While it is the most common cutaneous malignancy in patients younger than 20 years of age, pediatric melanoma comprises only 0.3–2.0% of all melanomas and 1–3% of pediatric malignancies [3–5]. Melanoma is more prevalent in adolescents than in the younger pediatric population, and was expected to comprise 5% of all cancers diagnosed in this age group in 2017 [6]. Over the past 30 years, the incidence in prepubertal patients has remained stable, while it has been steadily rising in older children by 2.9% per year in the United States. This trend is also mirrored in other parts of the world [7, 8]. Caucasian children account for the majority of new diagnoses; however, the incidence continues to rise in the Hispanic and Native American populations [9]. The rise in melanoma is highest in female adolescents.

R. S. Kumar
Radiation Oncology Services, Riverdale, GA, USA
e-mail: rsreeraman@berkeley.edu

J. L. Messina, M.D.
Departments of Anatomic Pathology and Cutaneous Oncology, Moffitt Cancer Center, Tampa, FL, USA

Departments of Pathology and Cell Biology and Dermatology, University of South Florida Morsani College of Medicine, Tampa, FL, USA
e-mail: jane.messina@moffitt.org

D. R. Reed
Departments of Cutaneous Oncology and Sarcoma Oncology, Moffitt Cancer Center, Tampa, FL, USA

Pediatric Cancer and Blood Disorders Institute, Johns Hopkins All Children's Hospital, St Petersburg, FL, USA
e-mail: damon.reed@moffitt.org

V. K. Sondak (✉)
Department of Cutaneous Oncology, Moffitt Cancer Center, Tampa, FL, USA

Departments of Oncologic Sciences and Surgery, University of South Florida Morsani College of Medicine, Tampa, FL, USA
e-mail: Vernon.sondak@moffitt.org

A. I. Riker (ed.), *Melanoma*, https://doi.org/10.1007/978-3-319-78310-9_13

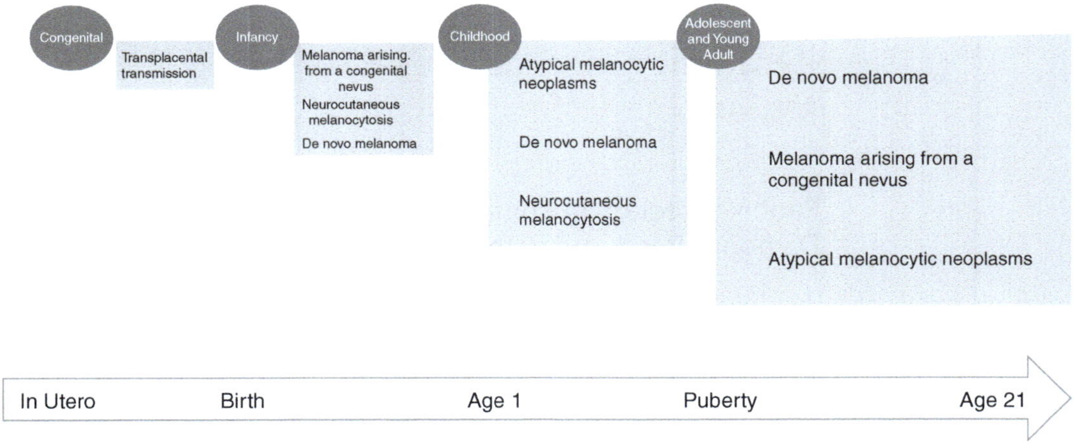

Fig. 13.1 Pediatric melanoma presentations according to age. The width of the textbox is roughly proportional to the incidence of melanoma (and/or atypical melanocytic neoplasms) occurring in each period (adapted from Sreeraman Kumar et al. [101])

Classification and Risk Factors

General Risk Factors

The risk factors for pediatric melanoma are somewhat age dependent. While genetic risk factors and benign precursor lesions are more common in prepubertal patients, the risk factors for adolescents are similar to those of adults: sun exposure, fair skin, and tanning bed use [8, 10].

Congenital/Neonatal Melanoma: In Utero to 1 Year

Congenital and neonatal melanoma is rare, and the incidence has remained steady over the past 30 years [4, 11].

Transplacental Transmission

Although it is extremely rare, melanoma can spread from mother to fetus via transplacental transmission. Available literature includes fewer than 30 cases and is mainly descriptive [12–16]. The factors that have been associated with this rare but devastating event are maternal diagnosis of node-positive disease >3 years prior to pregnancy, development of metastatic melanoma in the mother during the third trimester, primiparity, male fetal gender, birth at greater than 36 weeks gestation, and maternal age less than 30 [14, 17]. Clearly, some of these factors are associated with a patient's ability, desire, and/or willingness to become pregnant after a prior melanoma diagnosis. For example, younger women with no prior children and a long interval since their melanoma diagnosis may be more motivated to become pregnant and accept the risks associated with recurrence of their disease in the pre- or postpartum period.

For transplacental transmission to occur, metastatic melanoma must first lodge in and grow in the maternal side of the placenta, where it can be detected by histopathologic analysis conducted after delivery. In cases with placental metastases, two-thirds of infants were alive 1.5 years after birth, so the finding of melanoma in the placenta does not guarantee that transplacental transmission will occur [15, 17]. In the small number of cases where transmission to the fetus across the placenta has been reported, the diagnosis portends a poor prognosis, and the majority of these newborns ultimately die within the first year of life [15, 16, 18, 19]. Placental metastases have been reported even in mothers with early-stage melanoma, and thus we recommend thorough pathologic examination of the placenta after delivery in all women with a history of invasive melanoma. An evaluation showing no evidence of melanoma can provide the new mother with a strong sense of reassurance that transplacental transmission was unlikely to have occurred.

Proving that neonatal melanoma was transmitted transplacentally and not occurring de novo is possible. Karyotyping analysis or fluorescence in situ hybridization (FISH) can be used when transplacental melanoma transmission is suspected in males (as an XX chromosome in the tumor would confirm maternal origin). Efforts to quantify the copy number of sex chromosomes in genomic DNA purified from a fetal tumor biopsy specimen suspected to be of maternal origin have also been conducted [20].

Melanoma in a Giant Pigmented Nevus

Congenital melanocytic nevi (CMN) are present at, or very shortly after, birth. They are benign melanocytic proliferations and are classified by the size the lesions are projected to attain at adulthood, assuming growth congruent with the growth of the child, because the risk of malignant transformation rises with the size of the nevus. Small CMN are those projected to be less than 1.5 cm in diameter; medium CMN will be between 1.5 and 20 cm; and large CMN will be greater than 20 cm [21]. The definitions of what constitutes a giant (as opposed to a large) CMN vary. Some use body surface area measurements rather than projected adult size [22]. Giant CMN are either G1 (40–60 cm) or G2 (>60 cm), but other features besides nevus size, particularly satellite nevus counts and physical features such as color, surface change, and hypertrichosis, appear to also impact the risk of malignant transformation [23]. Location is also a factor: axial CMN are more likely to develop melanoma than CMN in extremities [24]. Giant CMN are most likely to give rise to pediatric melanoma, although the estimated risk varies. Small and medium CMN have a lifetime risk of 2–5%, but most of the melanomas within these nevi that do occur are diagnosed in adulthood, not in childhood. In contrast, patients with giant CMN are more likely to develop melanoma in adolescence or even early childhood.

A meta-analysis of 432 patients with CMN found that 0.7% developed melanoma, and a more recent, prospective, observational study of patients (median age of 6) noted two pediatric patients who developed melanoma [25, 26]. Although the median age of diagnosis for melanoma arising in CMN is 7 years, the median age of diagnosis for patients with fatal cases is 3 years [27]. The early onset of melanoma in CMN patients is the rationale for surgical removal of these lesions in early childhood. *NRAS* mutations have been seen in congenital nevi, and while the studies are conflicting *BRAF* V600E mutations may be seen in 12–30% of cases [28–30]. One-third of cases of fatal childhood melanoma arising in the setting of congenital nevi also had neurocutaneous melanocytosis [31].

Neurocutaneous Melanoma

Neurocutaneous melanoma is exceptionally rare. It originates in the background of neurocutaneous melanocytosis, which is also termed "congenital melanocytic nevus syndrome." This syndrome involves benign and malignant proliferation of melanocytes in the central nervous system, in conjunction with a giant CMN or with more than three small-to-medium CMN. As many as 4–11% of patients with giant CMN will develop symptomatic neurocutaneous melanocytosis [22, 26, 32]. Presenting symptoms include headache, vomiting, seizures, neuropsychiatric disturbance, or myelopathy, often the result of increasing intracranial pressure. Most patients develop symptoms by age 10 and have intractable seizures and neurocognitive delay [32]. Neurocutaneous melanocytosis is associated with the development of melanoma in 40–60% of cases. Patients may develop melanoma involving the skin, brain, or leptomeninges. Due to the difficulty of resection, risk of leptomeningeal infiltration, and lack of available targeted agents, the prognosis is poor [33, 34]. Genomic studies have indicated that *NRAS* mosaicism and post-zygotic mutations in codon 61 are associated with the onset of neurocutaneous melanocytosis [35]. Recent studies suggest the involvement of activated Wnt signaling as an additional factor leading to the varied natural histories of neurocutaneous melanocytosis. The mitogen-activated protein pathway (MAPK) may play a role, as its inhibition was noted to halt the development of neurocutaneous melanocytosis in animal studies [36]. One clinical case series investigating trametinib (a MEK inhibitor) in patients with neurocutaneous melanoma demonstrated symptomatic improvement, though patients eventually succumbed to the disease [37].

De Novo/Sporadic Melanoma

There are only 14 cases of de novo melanoma in infancy reported to date [38, 39]. Of these, three have succumbed to the disease. There are no known risk factors, and diagnosis is challenging, given some histologic overlap with giant CMN. Comparative genomic hybridization may be helpful to establish the diagnosis [39].

Childhood Melanoma: 1 Year to Puberty

The most relevant biologic cutoff to divide childhood and adolescent melanoma seems to be puberty, when hormone-driven changes in melanocyte physiology occur. Although Tanner stage may be an accurate method of determining postpubertal adolescence, retrospectively ascertaining whether a child has undergone puberty is difficult. Thus, most studies use an arbitrary threshold of age 10 or 12 as a substitute to distinguish between prepubertal and postpubertal cases.

De Novo/Sporadic Melanoma

Most childhood melanomas are not associated with CMN or genetic syndromes. The risk factors for these sporadic cases have not been firmly established. However, such cases are primarily associated with UV radiation exposure, fair skin, and multiple nevi just as in adults [10]. Prepubertal patients, however, are more likely than adolescents to be non-Caucasian. Consequently, the role of UV exposure for these patients remains ambiguous [40].

Arising from Giant CMN and Dysplastic Nevi

Childhood melanomas, like neonatal melanomas, can develop from giant CMN. One-third of childhood melanomas originate from giant CMN or another precursor lesion, including common and dysplastic nevi [21, 22, 24, 33, 40–45].

CMN (Please See "Melanoma in a Giant Pigmented Nevus")

Spitz Nevi

Spitz nevi are benign melanocytic proliferations that present more commonly in the pediatric population. Like melanoma, they can be melanocytic or amelanotic, and can have irregular borders. However, most are less than 1 cm in diameter, and up to 80% spontaneously involute during childhood. Intermediate between benign Spitz nevi and melanoma are the atypical spitzoid tumors (AST). Some of these atypical, but not unequivocally malignant-appearing, lesions have the potential to metastasize (i.e., they are unrecognized melanomas). High-risk factors for recurrence and metastasis include ulceration, asymmetry, and large diameter. All patients with atypical Spitz tumors should be monitored carefully clinically, but particularly those with lesions with the aggressive features mentioned above. Immunohistochemistry (IHC) can be helpful in distinguishing AST from melanoma [46]. A new study revealed differences in miRNA expression levels between the two tumor types, particularly a decrease in the expression of miR-155-5p in spitzoid melanomas [47].

Genetic Syndromes

Germline mutations that result in alterations to cell cycle tumor suppressors and genes involved in DNA damage repair confer sensitivity to DNA damage. These are associated with an increased risk of melanoma in children, adolescents, and adults alike.

Xeroderma Pigmentosum

Xeroderma pigmentosum is an autosomal recessive genetic disorder of nucleotide excision repair. Affected individuals are sensitive to DNA damage by UV radiation. By age 8, they generally develop non-melanoma skin cancer; by age 21, 5–13% of xeroderma pigmentosum patients have been diagnosed with melanoma [45, 48].

Familial Melanoma Syndromes

Familial melanoma syndromes are not particularly well characterized in either the pediatric or the adult populations. However, genomic studies are providing further insight into the mutations leading to multiple and recurrent melanomas. *CDKN2A* is the most common high-risk melanoma susceptibility locus. Mutations in this gene are associated with dysplastic (atypical) nevus syndrome, >100 nevi, nevi of buttocks/feet, multiple primary melanomas, and in some cases an increased risk for pancreatic cancer [49]. These germline mutations are present in <5% of prepubertal melanomas [50, 51]. Rarer familial melanoma syndromes include germline *BAP1*, *BRCA2*, and *MC1R* mutations. However, they are more closely associated with adult rather than pediatric melanoma.

Adolescent and Young Adult Melanoma

Adolescent and young adult melanoma comprises patients from puberty to age 21. The incidence in this cohort of pediatric melanoma continues to rise, largely due to the increasing rate in teenage girls [52]. The risk factors are thought to be similar to that for adults, which include ultraviolet radiation exposure, tanning bed use, fair skin, family history of melanoma, and presence of multiple and atypical nevi [40, 42, 43, 52–55]. Other risk factors include xeroderma pigmentosum and germline mutations involving cell cycle mediators, as for prepubertal melanoma.

Clinical Presentation

General

Pediatric melanoma presents with its own clinical signs and symptoms, which vary by age grouping, as do the epidemiologic factors enumerated above. In adult melanoma, the classic criteria are asymmetry, irregular borders, variation in color, diameter >6 mm, and evolution. However, 60% of prepubertal melanomas and 40% of adolescent melanomas do not exhibit these characteristics [43, 53, 56]. Cordoro et al. noted that 77% of patients younger than 10 years old presented with an amelanotic lesion, with Ferrari et al. noting that 88% of patients had well-circumscribed lesions [53, 57]. Accordingly, the traditional diagnostic criteria have been expanded to include the following new criteria for pediatric melanoma: amelanotic, bump/bleeding, uniform or no color, and de novo/any diameter (see Table 13.1) [3, 57]. While the criteria have not been validated in prospective studies, they nonetheless provide a framework for further evaluation.

Table 13.1 Characteristics of pediatric melanoma compared to the classic adult "ABCDE" criteria

	Classic adult melanoma	Pediatric melanoma
A	Asymmetry	Amelanotic
B	Border irregularity	Bump and bleeding
C	Color variation	Colorless or uniform color
D	Diameter	De novo development/any diameter
E	Evolution	Evolution

This table describes the classic features of adult melanoma and the additional features seen in pediatric melanoma (adapted from Cordoro et al. [57])

Congenital/Neonatal Melanoma

Congenital melanomas associated with maternofetal transmission develop in the background of maternal metastatic melanoma, and as such this potential risk can be of concern to pregnant women with a history of melanoma. Due to the risk of maternofetal melanoma transmission, we recommend the routine submission of the placenta at the time of delivery for pathologic analysis with IHC staining for melanocyte lineage antigens such as S-100 and/or Melan-A. The presence of melanoma cells on the fetal side of the placenta suggests potential maternal-fetal spread, and infants should be carefully monitored during the first year of life and beyond for signs and symptoms of metastatic melanoma. The majority of, if not all, neonatal melanoma cases arising from maternal-fetal transmission are diagnosed within the first year of birth [15, 18].

Infants with melanoma unrelated to transplacental transmission usually have melanoma from a CMN. Neonates have a distinct presentation from older patients in that they are less likely to arise from an atypical junctional proliferation or melanoma in situ. Patients tend to have pink or dark papules within CMN or nodules in the dermal component of CMN. These are difficult to diagnose, given that features typically of concern, such as ulceration, can be found in benign proliferative nodules within CMN [27]. In cases of neurocutaneous melanocytosis, neonatal patients present with symptoms of increased intracranial pressure and other neurologic symptoms.

Childhood Melanoma: Age 1–Puberty

While there is no classic presentation of prepubertal melanoma, they tend to exhibit alternative diagnostic criteria, such as amelanosis, bleeding, nodularity with uniform color, and diameter <6 mm that persist after being monitored for an extended period of time. Prepubertal patients are more likely than adolescents to have extremity or head and neck presentation, nodular rather than superficial lesions, and multiple nevi [3, 4, 40].

Adolescent and Young Adult: Puberty–21

More than 75% of pediatric melanoma patients are diagnosed in adolescence or young adulthood. Similar to prepubertal patients, 40% will present with atypical presentations, such as amelanotic, symmetric papular, or a nodular appearance and "evolution." The most common pre-biopsy diagnosis in this age group is pyogenic granuloma [57]. In contrast to younger children, they are more likely to have superficial spreading, rather than nodular, melanomas and more likely to have a truncal primary site [4].

Initial Clinical and Pathologic Workup

The rarity of pediatric melanoma, along with the plethora of benign nevi in the pediatric population, makes the diagnosis of malignancy difficult. The potential for delay in diagnosis is quite high, with a recent study finding an initial clinical misdiagnosis in 25% of their cohort [58]. Among experienced pathologists, there was significant diagnostic disagreement, with a kappa coefficient of 0.3, indicating a low degree of inter-observer concordance [59].

Given the high rate of misdiagnosis and delay in diagnosis, suspicious melanocytic lesions should be biopsied and evaluated by an experienced dermatopathologist. Often, cutaneous lesions in children are initially diagnosed as warts, and subsequently treated with a variety of topical agents prior to biopsy. The clinical history, including the presence of a precursor lesion, CMN or nevus, demographics, color, size, extent of biopsy (excisional, partial excision/punch, shave), and photograph of the lesion, can all assist the dermatopathologist in the diagnostic process. The importance of collaboration between clinicians and pathologists by sharing clinical information that can assist in the diagnostic evaluation bears emphasis.

We recommend complete excisional biopsy with a narrow margin of normal skin, allowing for complete pathologic evaluation of both the lesion and its relationship to the surrounding epidermis and subcutis. Preserving the specimen with formalin fixation is adequate, even if specialized IHC and/or molecular testing are needed to evaluate the lesion, allowing for the routine handling of pediatric skin biopsies in the clinic [60, 61]. Fluorescence in situ hybridization (FISH), comparative genomic hybridization (CGH), and gene expression analyses are now increasingly being used as additional tests in the diagnostic process [27, 46, 47, 62, 63].

The initial histopathologic evaluation of the biopsy specimen includes commercially available IHC stains. Proliferation is assessed using mitotic count, augmented when necessary with phosphohistone H3 and/or the proliferation marker Ki-67 [64, 65]. The progressive loss of HMB-45 staining with increasing dermal depth demonstrates melanocytic maturation, characteristic of benign lesions, but is often lost in melanoma [66]. Melanoma, in comparison to benign lesions, is more likely to have increased mitotic activity, high-grade atypia, inflammation and mitotic figures deeper in the dermis, histologic asymmetry, and ulceration [27, 59]. However, there still remains significant inter-observer variation in diagnosis with histological evaluation alone.

More recent studies have evaluated gene expression and CGH as methods of distinguishing malignant lesions from those without metastatic potential. Spitzoid lesions are the most common atypical lesions of uncertain potential. Atypical spitzoid tumors or melanoma may demonstrate a loss of p16 expression by homozygous deletion of *p16/CDKN2A*, but benign Spitz nevi rarely express p16 loss [67–69]. Loss of BAP1 expression has been shown in spitzoid-appearing benign and malignant melanocytic proliferations [70]. Recently, tyrosine kinase fusions involving ALK, ROS-1, NTRK-1, BRAF, or RET have been found in up to 40% of lesions with spitzoid histology. However, these have not yet been shown to be indicative of the metastatic potential of these lesions [62]. Isolated *HRAS* mutations and chromosome 11p gain have been identified in benign spitzoid lesions but not in melanoma (see Fig. 13.2a) [46, 71]. Increase in the copy number of *RREB1* (chromosome 6p25), *MYB* (6q23), and *CCND1* (11q13) is associated with lesions with metastatic potential, i.e., melanoma (see Fig. 13.2b) [46]. More recently, microRNA studies have shown potential to distinguish melanoma from benign lesions [72, 73]. A commercially available gene expression signature (myPath™, Myriad Diagnostics) has been shown to have good sensitivity and specificity on histologically unequivocal lesions, but its performance has only been evaluated in one study comparing results of FISH and myPath score in atypical lesions [74]. In this study, FISH was more frequently in agreement with the histologic diagnosis than myPath (70% vs. 64%).

Pathologic Classification

Spectrum of Melanocytic Neoplasia

The spectrum of melanocytic neoplasms in children ranges among congenital and acquired benign lesions, dysplastic nevi, blue nevi, Spitz nevi, pigmented epithelioid melanocytomas, and progress on to melanoma. There are many lesions along this spectrum that do not fit neatly into one diagnostic category, variably termed as borderline tumors, melanocytic tumors of uncertain malignant potential (MELTUMPS), spitzoid tumors of uncertain malignant potential (STUMP), and atypical Spitz tumors. Although observational, retrospective, and prospective studies have sought to evaluate the natural history of these atypical neoplasms [21, 24, 71, 75–81] considerable ambiguity persists and even among expert dermatopathologists diagnostic disagreement occurs [59]. We will refer to these lesions as "atypical melanocytic neoplasms" in this chapter.

Atypical spitzoid neoplasms are the most common atypical melanocytic neoplasms in the pediatric population, and distinguishing the benign ones from those with metastatic potential is challenging. "Spitzoid" refers to lesions with some, but not all, of the features of a typical (benign) Spitz nevus. Histologically, benign Spitz nevi tend to have uniform hyperplasia in the epidermis, maturation in the dermis, eosinophilic cytoplasm, low mitotic activity (less than 2 mm^2), and pale eosinophilic "Kamino bodies." Often, even benign lesions will have some variations. Thus, differentiating between atypical lesions with metastatic potential and those that are unequivocally benign is difficult.

Recent studies have used CGH, FISH, and more recently gene expression profiling to characterize the metastatic potential of atypical melanocytic neoplasms. These techniques are utilized when several (but not all) elements of either melanoma or a benign nevus are present in a case [82].

CGH evaluates gains and losses of segments of chromosomes across the 23 chromosome pairs (46 chromosomes). Melanomas are more likely than benign lesions to have multiple gains or losses in chromosomes. Karyotype alterations in chromosomes 1q, 6p, 6q, 7p, 8p, 8q, 9p, 10p, 11q, and 17q were found in melanoma and absent in Spitz nevi [46]. Bastian et al. reported that 96% of melanomas in their series had chromosomal gains or losses, while only 13% of atypical melanocytic neoplasms had abnormalities. In contrast to most benign nevi, which have normal karyotypes, and melanoma, which rarely exhibits an *HRAS* mutation, 15% of Spitz nevi and 70% of

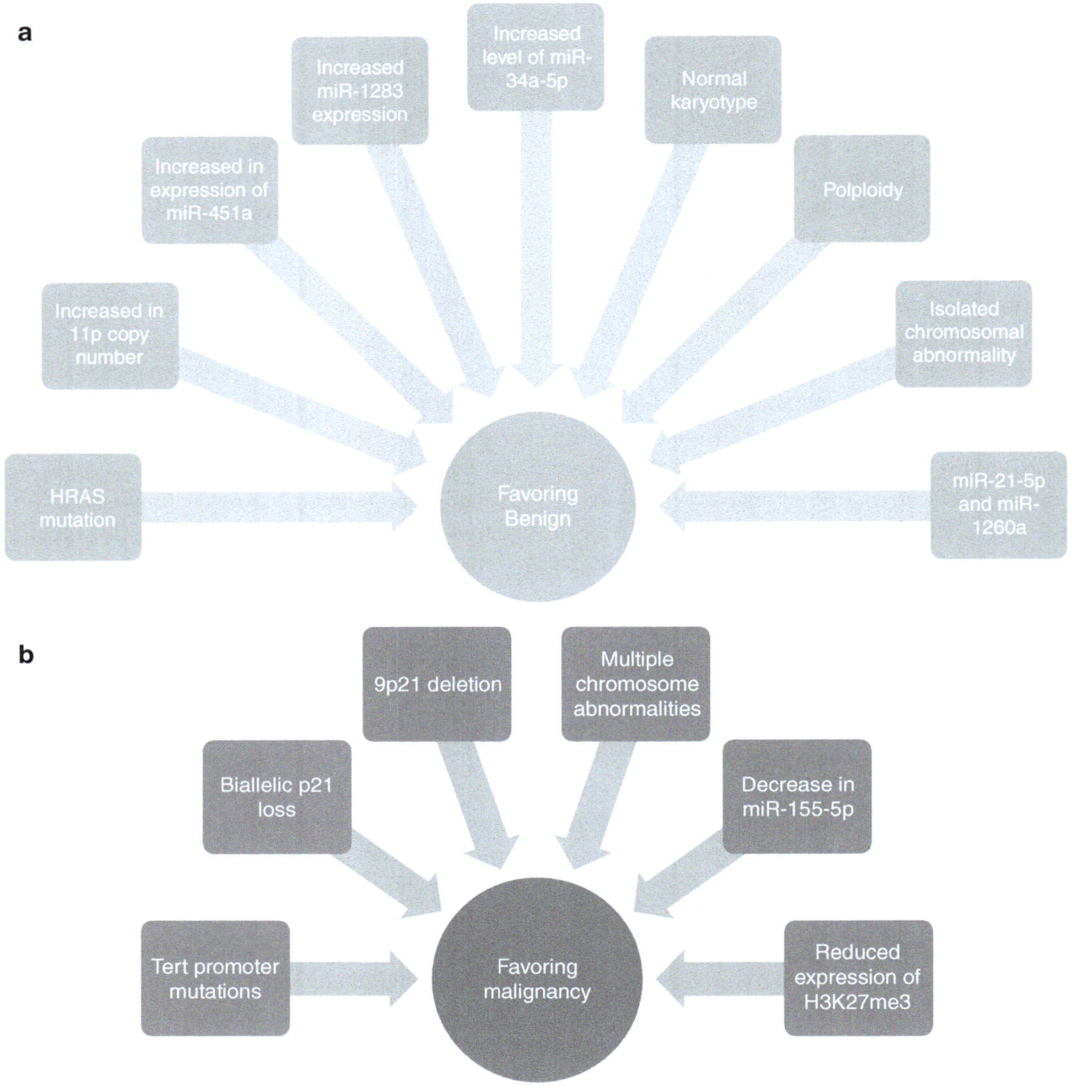

Fig. 13.2 (**a**) Common genetic and chromosomal abnormalities in benign (atypical) pediatric melanocytic neoplasms. (**b**) Common genetic and chromosomal abnormalities in pediatric melanoma

atypical Spitz neoplasms had an increase in the copy number of 11p at the *HRAS* locus [83]. Evaluation of a database of ambiguous melanocytic neoplasms revealed a chromosome 3p21 loss in 6.7% of cases, while loss of *BAP1* was associated with atypical spitzoid melanocytic tumors [84].

Multiple studies have now identified kinase fusions involving ALK, ROS-1, NTRK-1, BRAF, and RET in up to 51% of atypical spitzoid melanocytic tumors [62, 76, 85]. The identification of a fusion protein in a lesion may confer different metastatic potential and clinical evolution depending on the specific fusion. *ALK* mutations were more likely to be found in amelanotic lesions, with *NTRK-1* mutations associated with lesions found to have Kamino bodies and small, arranged nests. Mutations in the *BRAF* gene were more likely to be associated with high-grade atypia, sheets of dysplastic cells, copy number gains, and a predominance of epithelioid cells [86–88]. Lesions with *BRAF* mutations were more likely to be diagnosed as, or develop into, a melanoma. However, the presence of a fusion protein has not yet been definitively shown to be associated with an adverse outcome or recurrence [89].

FISH utilizes nucleic acid probes that bind to portions of chromosomes to detect the presence or absence of known sequences. The first-generation FISH testing utilized probes targeting chromosomes 6p25 (the locus of gene *RREB1*), 6q23 (*MYB*), *Cep6* (the centromere of chromosome 6), and 11q13 (*CCND1*). The results were promising, with a sensitivity of 86.7%, and a specificity of 95.4% in the diagnosis of melanoma compared to benign nevi. The main concern raised was the identification of false-positive test results in tetraploid cases [90]. The next-generation FISH test targeted 6p25, 11q13, 9p21 (*CDKN2A*), and 8q24 (*cMYC*), and it reportedly has greater accuracy with histologically unequivocal melanocytic neoplasms. Nonetheless, in diagnostically challenging spitzoid melanocytic neoplasms, the sensitivity is less than 70%. However, it may be helpful as an adjunct study to assist in diagnosis. Gerami et al. reported that in their series of 64 patients with atypical Spitz tumors analyzed by FISH, 9 of the 11 patients who developed advanced disease or died had deletion of 9p21, which results in loss of *p16/CDKN2A* [77]. A later study of patients with fusion proteins revealed a recurrence in only those with 9p21 loss [89].

There are further studies investigating the role of epigenetics and hypermethylation as biomarkers of melanoma. In a study of patients with melanoma arising from CMN compared to proliferative nodules, there was reduced expression of H3K27me3 in melanomas but not in the (benign) proliferative nodules [91]. Increased telomerase activity, associated with mutations of the *TERT* promoter, was found in 12 of 15 melanomas and 2 of 26 atypical spitzoid tumors [92]. Another study of 54 patients with atypical spitzoid melanocytic neoplasms found *TERT* promoter mutations in the 4 patients who developed disseminated disease, but not in the 52 who remained free of disease [93]. Among adolescents and young adults, TERT promoter methylation with or without a TERT promoter mutation was associated with worse recurrence-free survival [94]. MicroRNA analysis of spitzoid lesions revealed a decrease in miR-155-5p in melanoma, with an increase in miR-451a, miR-1283, miR-34a-5p, miR-21-5p, and miR-1260a in benign lesions [47].

Taken together, each of these new tests could serve as additional diagnostic studies. Furthermore, there may be other clues in an atypical melanocytic lesion that may reveal its metastatic potential, in particular the involvement of regional draining lymph nodes. However, this, too, is contentious. A study of 541 patients with atypical spitzoid lesions noted 303 patients who underwent sentinel lymph node biopsy. Of these, 119 (39%) were found to have positive sentinel lymph nodes, with 97 subsequently undergoing a completion lymph node dissection. This study reported a median follow-up of 59 months, showing that 99% of patients with a positive sentinel lymph node were still alive. While this study suggests that atypical spitzoid lesions may have a higher rate of lymph node involvement than melanomas, the involvement of sentinel lymph nodes in atypical spitzoid neoplasms may not have the same negative prognosis as in patients with unequivocal melanoma [95].

Of unequivocal melanomas, the most common histologic subtype of melanoma in children is the superficial spreading subtype, which comprises from 9 to 62% of cases, depending on the study. Nodular melanomas are more commonly seen in prepubertal cases and comprise between 12 and 34% of cases. The incidence of spitzoid melanomas is thought to between 2 and 17% of pediatric melanomas (see Table 13.2), but this may be over- or underreported, as many studies did not report Spitz type as a distinct category.

Categorization of Pediatric Melanocytic Neoplasia

In addition to the diagnostic challenge of atypical melanocytic neoplasms, the lack of a standard terminology creates confusion between pathologists and clinicians regarding the exact nature of

Table 13.2 Histologic subtypes of pediatric melanoma based on single-institution series

	Superficial spreading (%)	Nodular (%)	Acral lentiginous	Spitzoid	Other/unclassified/ NOS (%)
Paradela et al. [44] (n = 128)	48	34	4%	Not reported separately	14
Livestro et al. [43] (n = 73)	62	12	1%	Not reported separately	25
Aldrink et al. [41] (n = 136)	49	21	4%	2%	24
Han et al. [56] (n = 62)	47	23	0%	4%	26
Cordoro et al. [57] (n = 60)	9	30	0%	13%	48
Brecht et al. [114] (n = 443)	51	15	2%	Not reported separately	32
Dean et al. [5] (n = 78)	38	12	Not reported separately	Not reported separately	50
Freemyer et al. [108] (n = 185)	35	29	2%	17%	17
Total (n = 1165)	46	21	2%	4%	28

a lesion. A recent study noted that the "Spitz" terminology was used by 90% of surveyed pathologists, but treatment recommendations varied widely [96, 97]. The lack of standardization makes it difficult for clinicians to adequately communicate the nature of the lesion, the risk for metastasis and death, as well as the treatment options to patients and their families. To create an objective scale, we adopted a system to classify melanocytic lesions from a spectrum of unequivocally benign to unequivocally malignant. This system is derived from the original 5-point "BiRAD" system for categorizing the results of mammography, and is similar to a proposal for categorizing dysplastic nevi [98, 99]. We have implemented this system in our practice and find it useful in our conversations between pathologist and clinician and the patient/family. It also allows us to better convey evolution of the diagnostic process to patients, wherein an initial uncertain diagnosis can be clarified as additional pathologic analyses are performed or new clinical features emerge [100, 101].

Category 1: Benign

The lesions in this category have histologic features characteristic of an unequivocally benign lesion, and include Spitz nevi, pigmented spindle cell nevi of Reed, blue nevi, deep-penetrating nevi, CMN, proliferative nodule in congenital nevi, benign melanocytic nevi, dysplastic melanocytic nevi, and speckled lentiginous nevi. No additional evaluation is necessary beyond complete excision, as appropriate [102].

Category 2: Atypical Melanocytic Neoplasm, Favor Benign

The atypical melanocytic neoplasms in this category have most, but not all, of the features of one of the unequivocally benign lesions noted above. There are a few nontypical features seen, such as focal areas of proliferation/mitoses, focal increases in cellularity, or focal cellular atypia. Alternatively, we use this category when an incomplete biopsy precludes full evaluation, and a benign diagnosis cannot be rendered with certainty. Thus, these lesions should all be completely excised to assess the areas of the lesion not sampled with the initial biopsy. After complete excision, no further evaluation or management is necessary for category 2 lesions.

Category 3: Atypical Melanocytic Neoplasm, Not Amenable to Further Classification

The lesions in this category have atypical features indicating possible metastatic potential, but no features allowing the pathologist to definitively classify the lesion as likely malignant or likely benign. These have been given names like spitzoid tumors of uncertain malignant potential (STUMP), spitzoid atypical melanocytic proliferation of uncertain significance (SAMPUS), and melanocytic tumor of uncertain malignant potential (MELTUMP). This category also includes other melanocytic lesions for which the potential for recurrence or metastasis is unknown, such as the pigmented epithelioid melanocytoma, atypical cellular blue nevi, and BAP1-deleted melanocytic neoplasms.

CGH, FISH, and microRNA analysis can be helpful in further assessing the benign or malignant nature of these lesions. An atypical spitzoid lesion in category 3 by histopathologic criteria with a single chromosomal aberration in chromosome 11p might be appropriately recategorized as an atypical Spitz nevus, favor benign (category 2). An identical-appearing lesion with multiple FISH and chromosomal abnormalities in a high percentage of cells would be considered concerning for melanoma. This lesion would be more accurately reported as an atypical spitzoid lesion, favoring a spitzoid melanoma (category 4).

Category 3 lesions should always be completely excised. The re-excision specimen should be carefully examined for hints of any residual neoplasm that could allow for a more definitive diagnosis to be made. Furthermore, for patients with lesions in this category, sentinel node biopsy may be offered, with the understanding that the finding of lesional cells in the sentinel node may, or may not, allow for a reclassification as unequivocally malignant (see below).

Category 4: Atypical Melanocytic Neoplasm, Favor Malignant

The lesions in category 4 have a significant number of atypical features worrisome for malignancy, but they lack sufficient features to allow for the definite diagnosis of melanoma. These are lesions that have at least some potential to metastasize or recur, with numerous reports of category 4-type lesions leading to recurrence, metastatic disease, or death (and hence ultimate reclassification into category 5). While there are areas of overlap with this category and category 3, there are enough features to warrant more concern. Such features include Spitz-like neoplasms with high dermal cellularity, deep dermal or subcutaneous extension, high mitotic rate in the deep dermis, asymmetry and/or necrosis, or atypical cellular blue neoplasms that are large, with necrosis and/or increased mitoses $>2/\text{mm}^2$, with clinical features of ulceration and/or bleeding [58, 103, 104].

Category 4 lesions should always be excised to negative margins, and we generally recommend they be treated as an unequivocal melanoma of similar depth. At our institution, we would perform a sentinel lymph node biopsy for lesions 1 mm or thicker in Breslow's depth. CGH and FISH are often helpful and may provide sufficient evidence for the pathologist to render an outright malignant diagnosis (category 5). In contrast to category 3 lesions, lesional cells in the sentinel node, particularly in the parenchyma or growing in an expansile method, should be considered to represent evidence that the lesion is indeed malignant.

Category 5: Melanoma

Category 5 lesions express classic histopathologic features of an unequivocal melanoma. The number of melanomas in the pediatric population that exhibit spitzoid characteristics adds to the difficulty in rendering a diagnosis of unequivocal melanoma. However, when the classic features are present, a dermatopathologist should not hesitate to render this diagnosis simply because of the young age of the patient.

Further Evaluation and Reclassification of Atypical Melanocytic Neoplasms

Treatment decisions made on the initial biopsy specimen, particularly when based on a partial sampling of the lesion, are subject to change as subsequent information becomes available. Physicians, patients, and families must recognize the uncertainty involved with the diagnosis of pediatric melanocytic lesions. As additional studies are performed during the course of workup and diagnosis, a lesion that initially could not be categorized unequivocally as either benign or malignant on initial biopsy may be reclassified into a different diagnostic category. All lesions in category 2, 3, or 4 should be completely excised to negative margins. The re-excision pathology should be evaluated by an experienced dermatopathologist. Further investigation with CGH, FISH, and expression profiling as well as sentinel node biopsy (for category 3 and 4 lesions) should be considered in diagnostically challenging cases; this may lead to a definitive diagnosis. Finally, long-term clinical follow-up can result in reclassification of a benign or an atypical lesion to malignant based on disease progression or metastasis.

Diagnostic and Treatment Paradigms for Pediatric Melanoma and Atypical Melanocytic Neoplasms

Preoperative Staging Workup

For patients diagnosed with unequivocal melanoma at initial biopsy, the next step in evaluation is a thorough physical examination. Of importance are determining the presence of any residual pigmented lesion at the primary site and examination of the regional lymph nodes. If the regional lymph nodes are enlarged or hard to examine, ultrasonography can be helpful. Often, an ultrasound-guided fine-needle aspiration can be performed in order to establish a diagnosis of stage III melanoma prior to resection.

Due to the risks of ionizing radiation in prepubertal children and adolescents [105, 106], CT and PET/CT scans should generally be used preoperatively only for the following indications: patients with clinically positive lymph nodes in whom a biopsy establishes stage III melanoma, and those with clinical signs and symptoms of metastasis. Newer protocols such as PET/MRI reduce exposure to ionizing radiation and may be preferable for evaluation, if available [107]. Patients with atypical lesions (categories 2, 3, or 4) should undergo a thorough evaluation of the regional lymph nodes, including ultrasonography, if necessary. Otherwise, preoperative radiologic imaging is not indicated for patients with these lesions. No routine laboratory tests are needed in pediatric patients with atypical or malignant lesions aside from those required for pre-surgical evaluation.

Given the rarity of pediatric melanoma and the multidisciplinary approach required for treatment, patients should routinely be referred to a specialized center. Freemeyer et al. compared patients treated at an NCI-designated comprehensive cancer center with patients treated at a non-designated center. There was a significant disease-free and overall survival benefit, particular for stage III and stage IV patients, when they underwent their initial surgical evaluation at an NCI-designated comprehensive cancer center [108].

Wide Excision

The primary treatment for localized cutaneous melanomas and for all atypical melanocytic lesions is surgical removal. A complete excision is recommended for all categories of atypical melanocytic neoplasms. For category 4 or 5 lesions (suspected or diagnosed melanoma), wide excision is indicated, even if the initial biopsy had negative margins. Due to the previous exclusion of children from randomized trials evaluating margin width, there is no standard margin of excision for pediatric melanoma. When compared to melanomas of the same thickness in adults, pediatric melanoma appears to have a lower risk of local recurrence [43, 109]. For children younger than 14, we use a 1 cm margin for melanomas regardless of thickness and in all primary sites. We have not seen any local recurrences with this protocol [56, 110]. For older children, we employ the standard adult guidelines for margins of excision: 1 cm for lesions ≤1 mm in thickness at all anatomical sites and for tumors 1–2 mm in thickness in locations where a wider margin would require a skin graft or result in severe deformity, and for tumors on the head and neck or distal extremities; we perform 2 cm margins for most thicker lesions. For category 2 and 3 lesions, we utilize a maximum of a 1 cm margin, regardless of location. The goal of surgery is to achieve a final negative pathologic margin. In the rare cases where residual neoplasm is present at the excision margin, further re-excision is indicated. If re-excision of a category 2 or 3 lesion with less than a 1 cm margin uncovers a category 4 or 5 lesion, further excision is generally recommended.

Indications for Sentinel Lymph Node Biopsy

The role of sentinel lymph node biopsy in pediatric melanoma and atypical melanocytic neoplasms remains controversial. Sentinel lymph node biopsy is a well-tolerated procedure that enables accurate surgical staging, which can guide further treatment decisions. The majority of pediatric melanoma patients have node-negative disease and an excellent prognosis [11, 44, 54, 78, 111–114]. Such patients are at low risk for recurrence and can be followed with routine clinical and dermatologic surveillance. The significance of a negative sentinel node biopsy in reassuring to the patient and family should not be undervalued. In some cases, however, the sentinel lymph node or nodes contain cells identical to the primary tumor. In fact, the incidence of positive sentinel lymph nodes in atypical melanocytic neoplasms appears to be as great as, or greater than, that seen with pediatric melanoma [95]. For both atypical melanocytic neoplasms and pediatric melanoma, the incidence is higher than in adults with melanomas of similar thickness. However, the prognosis of sentinel node-positive pediatric patients is significantly better than for adults [43].

Indications for Sentinel Node Biopsy in Pediatric Melanoma

The argument for sentinel lymph node biopsy as a prognostic tool for pediatric melanoma is based on numerous studies that revealed that recurrence and death are more likely in patients with positive sentinel lymph nodes [1, 11, 114–116]. The risk of late side effects of removing one or two lymph nodes from a nodal basin is relatively low [117]. Over 20% of pediatric patients with clinically negative lymph nodes and a primary melanoma $\geq$1 mm in thickness are found to have positive sentinel lymph nodes. The indications for nodal evaluation in the pediatric population are similar to those for adults. In our practice, we utilize sentinel lymph node biopsies in pediatric patients with melanomas $\geq$1 mm in thickness in the absence of contraindications. We are selective for older children with lesions >0.75 mm in Breslow's thickness with ulceration and/or a mitotic rate $\geq 1/\text{mm}^2$, as in adults [118]. Because very young children rarely present with melanomas less than 1 mm in depth, our knowledge of the value of a sentinel lymph node biopsy is limited in this population, but we would consider it on a case-by-case basis.

Indications for Sentinel Node Biopsy in Pediatric Atypical Melanocytic Neoplasms

Recent articles have argued for a limited role for sentinel lymph node biopsy in the absence of a definite diagnosis of melanoma, as the prognostic significance of a positive sentinel lymph node is unclear [65, 95, 119]. It is clear that lesional cells from benign nevi, like cellular blue nevi and Spitz nevi, can be found in regional lymph nodes, and therefore it is difficult to distinguish metastatic melanoma from benign nevus cells. Even patients with category 1 (unequivocally benign) nevi can have nodal nevi, collections of benign nodal melanocytes. The melanocytic deposits in benign Spitz nevi are similar in appearance to the primary lesion, most commonly subcapsular, and are small in size [120]. In contrast, the nodal melanocytes arising from category 4 atypical melanocytic neoplasms and melanoma are more likely to be present in the parenchyma of the lymph node. The presence of expansile tumor deposits, necrosis, nodal effacement, sheets of malignant cells rather than nest of melanocytes, and involvement of multiple lymph nodes would favor metastasis from a primary lesion that is melanoma. Many cases of atypical melanocytic neoplasms with nodal involvement have features that are between the characteristics of benign nodal melanocytes and unequivocal involvement with melanoma. However, clinical studies have shown few, or even no, recurrences for atypical melanocytic neoplasms with positive sentinel nodes. There are a few small series of atypical melanocytic neoplasms managed with excision alone, showing no evidence of recurrent disease [1, 71, 75, 121]. A systemic review of 541 patients with atypical spitzoid lesions revealed that 39% of patients had nodal involvement, and at almost 5 years of follow-up 99% of patients with positive lymph nodes were alive without disease [95].

In contrast, we have seen multiple cases where patients initially diagnosed with pediatric atypical neoplasms developed recurrent melanoma and have even died, often many years after their initial diagnosis. Even in "unequivocal" pediatric melanoma, many of the recurrences and deaths from disease occur more than 5 years after initial diagnosis [56, 112, 118]. Thus, studies with short or incomplete follow-up must be carefully viewed with this in mind.

The most convincing case in favor of sentinel lymph node biopsy for pediatric atypical neoplasms is the uncertainty associated with the diagnosis. The variation in diagnoses, even among experienced dermatopathologists, is well noted. Cases of documented fatal outcomes were originally deemed as atypical or benign, when examined by experienced dermatopathologists in a blinded fashion [59, 122]. An atypical diagnosis from the initial biopsy may not accurately reflect the malignant nature of the lesion. Although the consequence of atypical cells in the sentinel node is not always clear, the presence of expansile nodules of tumor cells may expose a malignancy that otherwise would have been overlooked. The finding of negative sentinel nodes can reassure the patient and family that despite the uncertainty the patient has been treated appropriately if the diagnosis is indeed melanoma.

Surgical Management of the Sentinel Node-Positive Nodal Basin

The main aspects of managing of the pediatric melanoma patient with a positive sentinel lymph node are largely drawn from the adult literature. The standard of care is completion lymphadenectomy (radical lymph node dissection) after the diagnosis of a positive sentinel node biopsy [123]. In adults, involved non-sentinel nodes are found in only 15–20% of lymphadenectomy patients [124–126]. In the pediatric population, there is limited data on the rates of non-sentinel node involvement, with one study even suggesting that it may be lower than in adults, while another suggests that it is higher than in adults [111, 127].

The rates of lymphedema are lower for pediatric patients undergoing radical lymphadenectomy compared to adults. In our experience, the sensory neuropathy and numbness seen in the adult population after lymphadenectomy are rarely of lasting clinical significance in children. However, the infection risk of a radical lymph node dissection can be a problem, especially for younger patients who are more at risk for lifelong consequences. Conversely, teenagers and young adults may be noncompliant with the close follow-up recommended for node-positive patients not undergoing completion lymphadenectomy. Thus, we recommend a completion lymphadenectomy on a case-by-case basis. For each patient, we consider the extent of tumor involvement in the sentinel nodes, the number of sentinel nodes involved, the location of the positive sentinel node, the age of the child, the findings on the preoperative lymphoscintigraphy and the ability of the patient to be compliant with follow-up. For example, a young child may benefit greatly from even a few years of delay in performing a lymphadenectomy, which can decrease both the acute and late risks. Thus, in this case, we may defer a completion lymphadenectomy for a time in the future. Adolescents and older patients must be evaluated to ensure that they will be compliant with the follow-up schedule, which can last for years as they leave for college, employment, etc. Removing the regional nodes in a timely fashion (after a positive sentinel node biopsy) may be a preferred approach if long-term follow-up cannot be assured.

All patients with positive sentinel lymph nodes for whom completion lymph node dissection is deferred should undergo ultrasound surveillance of the involved nodal basin at least two to three times per year. This should continue over a period of 3–5 years, followed by a decreased frequency of every 6–12 months. They are advised to return promptly to clinic if they develop any signs or symptoms of a recurrence.

Surgical Management of the Clinically Node-Positive Nodal Basin

Sentinel node biopsy can identify occult nodal metastasis and, in some cases, the management of patients with positive sentinel nodes can involve observation. However, the pediatric patient with clinically detected lymph node metastases should routinely undergo a radical lymphadenectomy of the involved nodal basin, unless there is evidence of distant metastatic disease. The same surgical principles used in adults to determine the extent of dissection are also utilized in children. As in adults, the role of pelvic ("deep") node dissection in patients with inguinal node-positive disease is inadequately defined. If the iliac or obturator nodes are deemed suspicious for metastatic disease by pre-surgical radiographic evaluation, the indication for lymphadenectomy is clear. However, deep lymphadenectomy should be considered for patients with numerous, large involved inguinal nodes, even in the absence of radiologic evidence of pelvic lymph node involvement. In adults, studies suggest that including the external iliac and obturator nodes with an inguinofemoral node dissection does not increase long-term morbidity [128, 129]. Our own experience in our practice in adults and children also supports this approach.

Adjuvant Systemic Therapy

Systemic adjuvant therapy is commonly used in the adult population with high-risk disease. Due to the exclusion of children from most previous melanoma trials, as well as the relative rarity of pediatric melanoma, there is limited information regarding adjuvant systemic treatment in the pediatric melanoma population.

Interferon α-2b

The best studied agent in pediatric melanoma is interferon α-2b, which is approved for use in the adjuvant treatment of adult node-positive melanoma [130]. Three single-institution studies have retrospectively evaluated the feasibility of using high-dose interferon α-2b in stage III resected pediatric melanoma [131–133]. Pediatric patients tolerated the treatment well and needed fewer dose adjustments than adult patients. In one study of five stage III patients, two patients required dose modification in the induction phase, while two patients required dose modification in the maintenance phase due to abnormal liver function tests [133]. A prospective study of 15 patients with sentinel node-positive melanoma underwent treatment with high-dose interferon, with 8 initially diagnosed with atypical melanocytic neoplasms and subsequently reclassified as melanoma. All patients enrolled in the study were able to complete the initial induction phase, and only one patient was unable to complete the maintenance phase due to toxicity. Two of 15 patients developed recurrent disease during treatment. One underwent complete resection and one died of metastatic melanoma. A third patient developed metastases after treatment and succumbed to disease [132].

Because subcutaneous injection of interferon α-2b three times a week is inconvenient, particularly in children, the pegylated interferon α-2b (peg-interferon) form may be a better option for children. It can be administered once a week [134–136] and has a more favorable pharmacokinetic profile that is suitable for maintenance therapy [137]. A recent study of a hybrid interferon and peg-interferon regimen in children and adolescents with resected high-risk melanoma confirmed that it was well tolerated. Of 23 patients on the trial, all patients completed induction therapy, 18 patients completed all prescribed therapy, and only 3 patients discontinued treatment due to toxicity. The quality-of-life scores showed an improvement after the intravenous component of the treatment (induction) was delivered [138]. Our preference in children with stage III melanoma, particularly before puberty, has been to utilize this hybrid approach with adjuvant interferon α-2b given IV for 1 month, followed by maintenance peg-interferon weekly for 12 months. However, the development of newer adjuvant therapy regimens in adults has the potential to make all forms of interferon adjuvant therapy obsolete.

Alternative Adjuvant Regimen and Therapeutic Agents Under Evaluation

The side effects and duration of treatment for high-dose interferon have led to the investigation of alternate dosing regimens. SWOG S0008, an intergroup phase III randomized control trial, compared high-dose interferon for 1 year to biochemotherapy given for only 9 weeks (dacarbazine, cisplatin, vinblastine, interleukin-2, interferon, and granulocyte-stimulating factor given every 21 days for three cycles). While the study primarily included adult patients, children aged 10 and older were eligible for enrollment. For all patients enrolled, there was a statistically significant improvement in median recurrence-free survival (4 years for patients receiving biochemotherapy vs. 1.9 years for high-dose interferon) and 5-year recurrence-free survival (48% vs. 39%). Overall survival, however, was not different between the two study arms [139]. Age-specific results were not reported, but this study offers one alternative for postpubertal children unable to commit to a year of adjuvant therapy.

In recent years, there has been an explosion of new agents shown to improve survival in adults with metastatic melanoma, and older regimens like biochemotherapy and even interferon have almost entirely been abandoned. New options for treating unresectable metastatic melanoma may be beneficial in the adjuvant setting in children as they have proven to be in adults. Ipilimumab, a human monoclonal antibody to cytotoxic T-cell lymphocyte antigen 4, has been investigated in the adjuvant setting for stage III melanoma and found to have a significant 5-year recurrence-free survival benefit of 40.8 vs. 30.3% when compared to observation alone. There was an improvement in 5-year metastasis-free survival and overall survival, despite 53.3% of patients discontinuing treatment due to toxicity. However, there were a high number of grade 3 and 4 toxicities with ipilimumab, and 1.1% of patients in the ipilimumab arm died of immune-related adverse events [140]. The optimum dosing is currently being investigated. E1609 (NCT01274338) compares high-dose interferon to two doses of ipilimumab, the high-dose initial investigated in the adjuvant setting, and a lower dose consistent with that approved for use in metastatic disease, and includes children aged 15 and older. This will likely provide the first opportunity to evaluate these newer agents in the adjuvant therapy of melanoma in any portion of the pediatric population.

The use of anti-PD1 antibody therapy has particular promise in the adjuvant setting, given its lower toxicity and greater efficacy compared to ipilimumab [141]. Preliminary results of a randomized trial in adult patients with stage III melanoma show that the anti-PD1 antibody, nivolumab, is less toxic and improves relapse-free survival compared to high-dose ipilimumab [142]. There is no information yet available about the impact of anti-PD1 adjuvant therapy on overall survival, and no anti-PD1 agent has yet been directly compared to adjuvant interferon, although a clinical trial (S1404, NCT02506) has completed accrual. Most recently, randomized trials have shown the potential for targeted therapy with BRAF and MEK inhibitors (specifically dabrafenib and trametinib) as adjuvant [143] and neoadjuvant (preoperative) therapy [144] for adults with stage III melanoma harboring a BRAF V600 mutation. Pediatric oncologists are gaining experience with these drugs in a variety of childhood malignancies [145], and the field of adolescent and young adult oncology has created new collaborations between medical oncologists and pediatric oncologists. Hence it is likely that these promising findings will be applied to selected younger patients with stage III pediatric melanoma. While ideally clinical trials will be conducted in the pediatric population, the promising adult data makes it likely that reports will emerge with BRAF/MEK inhibitor cohorts being reported from larger volume centers.

Metastatic Disease

Systemic Therapy

Pediatric patients with metastatic melanoma should strongly consider enrollment in a clinical trial, as there is little knowledge about this patient population in terms of efficacy and safety profile. Multiple trials in the adult stage IV melanoma population have shown an increase in survival with BRAF inhibitors (such as vemurafenib and dabrafenib), anti-PD1 antibodies (such as pembrolizumab and nivolumab), and the anti-CTLA antibody ipilimumab. Knowledge of the *BRAF* mutational status is an important component on making treatment decisions for stage IV melanoma. *BRAF* mutations are more common in adolescent and young adults with conventional melanoma than the prepubertal cohort and the older adult melanoma population [146]. There are multiple case reports of vemurafenib and other BRAF inhibitors being used in children for various malignancies (brain, thyroid, etc.) with known *BRAF* mutations with good response.

Melanomas in young children, especially those arising in congenital nevi, predominantly lack *BRAF* mutations, and hence cannot be treated with BRAF inhibitors [147]. A recent study evaluated the use of the MEK inhibitor trametinib for four pediatric patients with *NRAS* mutated melanoma of the central nervous system (congenital nevus syndrome/neurocutaneous melanocytosis). There was a transient improvement that lasted 1–9 months, but eventual progression and death in all these patients [37].

A Phase I trial of ipilimumab was conducted for pediatric patients with advanced solid tumors. Of 33 patients, 12 patients had melanoma. Dose-limiting toxicities were noted at 5 and 10 mg/kg. While there were no tumor responses observed, patients who developed immune-related toxicities after receiving ipilimumab had an improved duration in overall survival [148]. Ipilimumab is currently the only FDA-approved agent for treating pediatric melanoma [149].

Other commercially available agents include pembrolizumab, nivolumab, dabrafenib, and cobimetinib. There is little published data regarding the safety and efficacy of any of these agents in children under the age of 16. Recently, there was a case report involving a patient with congenital melanoma with widespread metastatic disease treated with nivolumab. The patient remains alive with stable disease after 1 year of therapy, which was well tolerated [150].

Palliative Radiation

In the pediatric melanoma population, radiation therapy is reserved for the treatment of unresectable disease or the palliation of metastatic disease, particularly brain lesions. Newer radiation techniques such as intensity-modulated radiation therapy (IMRT), proton beam radiation, image guidance, and stereotactic radiation have yielded more conformal treatments and increased sparing of normal tissue. Case reports and retrospective studies of stereotactic and fractionated radiation in the pediatric population suggest that modern techniques can be used safely in the pediatric population [151, 152]. We suggest that radiation be used selectively as an effective method of palliation.

Follow-Up

There are no specific follow-up recommendations available for pediatric melanoma patients. The National Comprehensive Cancer Center Guidelines for melanoma are typically followed. However, recurrences can occur more than 5 years after diagnosis due to the long natural history of pediatric melanoma [56]. Moreover, early detection of recurrence may allow for surgical intervention and/or a more favorable treatment outcome. These patients are also at risk of developing another (second primary) melanoma. Seventeen percent of pediatric melanoma patients in one series had another melanoma diagnosed within 10 years after initial diagnosis and 24% within 20 years after diagnosis [112]. Therefore, even beyond 5 years, these patients should continue to undergo annual examinations.

Prognosis of Pediatric Melanoma Based on Stage of Disease

Stage of disease is the major factor in determining the overall survival in pediatric melanoma, just as in adults, with localized disease having a more favorable prognosis. The prognosis is likely better for pediatric melanoma patients diagnosed prior to puberty versus in adolescence, and for both groups, better than adults of a similar stage [40, 53, 109]. However, age is not included in current staging systems.

Stages I–II: Localized Disease

Early-stage, localized pediatric melanoma portends an excellent prognosis, with multiple series reporting from 90 to 100% overall survival over 10 years for stage I disease, 79 to 100% for stage II disease with a disease-free survival of more than 70%, and 77.4% overall survival at 20 years [11, 40, 112]. Ulceration, increase in tumor thickness, and Clark level and nodular subtype are associated with a higher local recurrence and metastasis rate and a decreased overall survival, as in adult melanoma [114].

Stage III: Regional Metastatic Disease

Metastatic disease to regional lymph nodes is associated with decreased disease-free and overall survival in comparison to early-stage disease. A recent National Cancer Data Base analysis attempted to determine prognosis in prepubertal vs. postpubertal patients. In patients 10 years or younger, the prognosis was equivalent regardless of lymph node involvement, but a positive lymph node was a negative prognostic factor in adolescents. While the study is subject to retrospective bias and potential inclusion of atypical neoplasms, it is consistent with prior data suggesting that prepubertal patients have a more favorable prognosis than adolescents and both do better than adults with similar staged disease [109]. The overall survival for stage III patients at 10 years was 70–77% [11, 40, 153].

Stage IV: Distant Metastatic Disease

As in adults, distant metastasis in the pediatric population portends a poor prognosis, with 40% overall survival at 5 years and 0% at 10 years, as reported in a large registry series [11].

Prognosis of Atypical Melanocytic Neoplasms

Atypical melanocytic neoplasms are diverse in terms of histology, molecular makeup, and perhaps prognosis. The vast majority of patients with atypical melanocytic neoplasms have an excellent prognosis, yet deaths from melanoma have occurred in children whose initial lesion could not, even in retrospect, be definitely characterized as malignant. Recurrent or metastatic disease is more common in atypical melanocytic neoplasms with ulceration, diameter >1 cm, extension into the subcutaneous tissue, and higher numbers of mitoses. Atypical lesions in postpubertal children are associated with increased risk of metastasis compared to younger children, just as with unequivocal melanoma [80]. Recent studies suggest that lesions with 9p21 deletions and *TERT* promoter mutations have increased potential for recurrence and metastasis [77, 89, 92, 93]. The prognostic significance of sentinel lymph node biopsy is controversial (see Section "Indications for Sentinel Node Biopsy in Pediatric Atypical Melanocytic Neoplasms" above).

Future Directions and Challenges

Knowledge of pediatric melanoma, its natural history and epidemiology, is limited by the rarity of the disease, incomplete data about the cases that do occur, and variations in diagnosis and diagnostic terminology. Most studies are from single-institution series with comparatively small patient numbers, although there has been one large registry study published [11]. The plethora of malignant, atypical, and benign nevi continues to be challenging to distinguish, but recent studies further characterizing lesions with metastatic potential are encouraging. Discovering mutations in melanoma and having available agents to target these mutations provide children who otherwise would have had limited available treatments with potential options. However, for pediatric patients with unresectable or metastatic disease, access to clinical trials testing the latest therapeutic agents is limited. This limits our understanding of the safety profile of these medications as well as their efficacy in children. With greater national and international collaboration between institutions, prospective evaluation, clinical trials, and discovery of tumor markers to assess metastatic potential as well as response to treatment, we will be able to further elucidate the appropriate management and to develop age-specific guidelines for pediatric melanoma.

References

1. Mills OL, Marzban S, Zager JS, Sondak VK, Messina JL. Sentinel node biopsy in atypical melanocytic neoplasms in childhood: a single institution experience in 24 patients. J Cutan Pathol. 2012;39(3):331–6.
2. Reed D, Kudchadkar R, Zager JS, Sondak VK, Messina JL. Controversies in the evaluation and management of atypical melanocytic proliferations in children, adolescents, and young adults. J Natl Compr Cancer Netw. 2013;11(6):679–86.
3. LaChance A, Shahriari M, Kerr PE, Grant-Kels JM. Melanoma: kids are not just little people. Clin Dermatol. 2016;34(6):742–8.
4. Austin MT, Xing Y, Hayes-Jordan AA, Lally KP, Cormier JN. Melanoma incidence rises for children and adolescents: an epidemiologic review of pediatric melanoma in the United States. J Pediatr Surg. 2013;48(11):2207–13.
5. Dean PH, Bucevska M, Strahlendorf C, Verchere C. Pediatric melanoma: a 35 year population-based review. Plast Reconstr Surg Glob Open. 2017;5(e1252):e1252.
6. Siegel RL, Miller KD, Jemal A. Cancer statistics, 2017. CA Cancer J Clin. 2017;67(1):7–30.
7. Senerchia AA, Ribeiro KB, Rodriguez-Galindo C. Trends in incidence of primary cutaneous malignancies in children, adolescents, and young adults: a population-based study. Pediatr Blood Cancer. 2014;61(2):211–6.
8. Slade AD, Austin MT. Childhood melanoma: an increasingly important health problem in the USA. Curr Opin Pediatr. 2014;26(3):356–61.
9. Rajput A, Faizi SA, Nir I, Morris KT, Fahy B, Russell J, Wiggins C. Pediatric melanoma in New Mexico American Indians, Hispanics, and non-Hispanic whites, 1981–2009. Am J Surg. 2014;207(3):412–6.
10. Strouse JJ, Fears TR, Tucker MA, Wayne AS. Pediatric melanoma: risk factor and survival analysis of the Surveillance, Epidemiology and End Results database. J Clin Oncol. 2005;23(21):4735–41.
11. Averbook BJ, Lee SJ, Delman KA, Gow KW, Zager JS, Sondak VK, Messina JL, Sabel MS, Pittelkow MR, Ecker PM, Markovic SN, Swetter SM, Leachman SA, Testori A, Curiel-Lewandrowski C, Go RS, Jukic DM, Kirkwood JM. Pediatric melanoma: analysis of an international registry. Cancer. 2013;119(22):4012–9.
12. Perret-Court A, Fernandez C, Monestier S, Millet V, Tasei AM. Placental metastasis of melanoma: a new case and literature review. Ann Pathol. 2010;30(2):143–6.
13. Shuhaila A, Rohaizak M, Phang KS, Mahdy ZA. Maternal melanoma with placental metastasis. Singap Med J. 2008;49(3):e71–2.
14. Anderson JF, Kent S, Machin GA. Maternal malignant melanoma with placental metastasis: a case report with literature review. Pediatr Pathol. 1989;9(1):35–42.
15. Alexander A, Samlowski WE, Grossman D, Bruggers CS, Harris RM, Zone JJ, Noyes RD, Bowen GM, Leachman SA. Metastatic melanoma in pregnancy: risk of transplacental metastases in the infant. J Clin Oncol. 2003;21(11):2179–86.
16. De Carolis S, Garofalo S, Degennaro VA, Zannoni GF, Salvi S, Moresi S, Di Pasquo E, Scambia G. Placental and infant metastasis of maternal melanoma: a new case. J Obstet Gynaecol. 2015;35(4):417–8.
17. Richardson SK, Tannous ZS, Mihm MC Jr. Congenital and infantile melanoma: review of the literature and report of an uncommon variant, pigment-synthesizing melanoma. J Am Acad Dermatol. 2002;47(1):77–90.
18. Trumble ER, Smith RM, Pearl G, Wall J. Transplacental transmission of metastatic melanoma to the posterior fossa. Case report. J Neurosurg. 2005;103(2 Suppl):191–3.
19. Valenzano Menada M, Moioli M, Garaventa A, Nozza P, Foppiano M, Trimarchi N, Fulcheri E. Spontaneous regression of transplacental metastases from maternal melanoma in a newborn: case report and review of the literature. Melanoma Res. 2010;20(6):443–9.
20. Raso A, Mascelli S, Nozza P, Biassoni R, Negri F, Garaventa A, Tarantino V, Garre ML, Cama A, Capra V. Detection of transplacental melanoma metastasis using quantitative PCR. Diagn Mol Pathol. 2010;19(2):78–82.
21. Tannous ZS, Mihm MC Jr, Sober AJ, Duncan LM. Congenital melanocytic nevi: clinical and histopathologic features, risk of melanoma, and clinical management. J Am Acad Dermatol. 2005;52(2):197–203.
22. Alikhan A, Ibrahimi OA, Eisen DB. Congenital melanocytic nevi: where are we now? Part I Clinical presentation, epidemiology, pathogenesis, histology, malignant transformation, and neurocutaneous melanosis. J Am Acad Dermatol. 2012;67(4):495.e1–17.
23. Price HN, O'Haver J, Marghoob A, Badger K, Etchevers H, Krengel S. Practical application of the new classification scheme for congenital melanocytic nevi. Pediatr Dermatol. 2014;32(1):23–7.
24. DeDavid M, Orlow SJ, Provost N, Marghoob AA, Rao BK, Huang CL, Wasti Q, Kopf AW, Bart RS. A study of large congenital melanocytic nevi and associated malignant melanomas: review of cases in the

New York University Registry and the world literature. J Am Acad Dermatol. 1997;36(3 Pt 1):409–16.
25. Krengel S, Hauschild A, Schafer T. Melanoma risk in congenital melanocytic naevi: a systematic review. Br J Dermatol. 2006;155(1):1–8.
26. Wramp ME, Langenbruch A, Augustin M, Zillikens D, Krengel S. Clinical course, treatment modalities, and quality of life in patients with congenital melanocytic nevi—data from the German CMN registry. J Dtsch Dermatol Ges. 2017;15(2):159–67.
27. Wood BA. Paediatric melanoma. Pathology. 2016;48(2):155–65. https://doi.org/10.1016/j.pathol.2015.12.001.
28. Salgado CM, Basu D, Nikiforova M, Bauer BS, Johnson D, Rundell V, Grunwaldt LJ, Reyes-Mugica M. BRAF mutations are also associated with neurocutaneous melanocytosis and large/giant congenital melanocytic nevi. Pediatr Dev Pathol. 2015;18(1):1–9.
29. Phadke PA, Rakheja D, Le LP, Selim MA, Kapur P, Davis A, Mihm MC Jr, Hoang MP. Proliferative nodules arising within congenital melanocytic nevi: a histologic, immunohistochemical, and molecular analyses of 43 cases. Am J Surg Pathol. 2011;35(5):656–69.
30. Charbel C, Fontaine RH, Malouf GG, Picard A, Kadlub N, El-Murr N, How-Kit A, Su X, Coulomb-L'Hermine A, Tost J, Mourah S, Aractingi S, Guegan S. NRAS mutation is the sole recurrent somatic mutation in large congenital melanocytic nevi. J Invest Dermatol. 2014;134(4):1067–74.
31. Neuhold JC, Friesenhahn J, Gerdes N, Krengel S. Case reports of fatal or metastasizing melanoma in children and adolescents: a systemcatic analysis of the literature. Pediatr Dermatol. 2015;32(1):13–22.
32. Jain P, Kannan L, Kumar A, Sigamani E, Suri V, Basheer N, Suri A, Gulati S. Symptomatic neurocutaneous melanosis in a child. JAMA Neurol. 2013;70(4):516.
33. Ruiz-Maldonado R, Tamayo L, Laterza AM, Duran C. Giant pigmented nevi: clinical, histopathologic, and therapeutic considerations. J Pediatr. 1992;120(6):906–11.
34. Kadonaga JN, Frieden IJ. Neurocutaneous melanosis: definition and review of the literature. J Am Acad Dermatol. 1991;24 ((5):747–55.
35. Kinsler VA, Thomas AC, Ishida M, Bulstrode NW, Loughlin S, Hing S, Chalker J, McKenzie K, Abu-Amero S, Slater O, Chanudet E, Palmer R, Morrogh D, Stanier P, Healy E, Sebire NJ, Moore GE. Multiple congenital melanocytic nevi and neurocutaneous melanosis are caused by postzygotic mutations in codon 61 of NRAS. J Invest Dermatol. 2013;133(9):2229–36.
36. Pawlikowski JS, Brock C, Chen SC, Al-Olabi L, Nixon C, McGregor F, Paine S, Chanudet E, Lambie W, Holmes WM, Mullin JM, Richmond A, Wu H, Blyth K, King A, Kinsler VA, Adams PD. Acute inhibition of MEK suppresses congenital melanocytic nevus syndrome in a murine model driven by activated NRAS and Wnt signaling. J Invest Dermatol. 2015;135(8):2093–101.
37. Kinsler VA, O'Hare P, Jacques T, Hargrave D, Slater O. MEK inhibition appears to improve symptom control in primary NRAS-driven CNS melanoma in children. Br J Cancer. 2017;116(8):990–3.
38. Asai J, Takenaka H, Ikada S, Soga F, Kishimoto S. Congenital malignant melanoma: a case report. Br J Dermatol. 2004;151(3):693–7.
39. Su A, Low L, Li X, Zhou S, Mascarenhas L, Barnhill RL. De novo congenital melanoma: analysis of 2 cases with array comparative genomic hybridization. Am J Dermatopathol. 2014;36(11):915–9.
40. Lange JR, Pallis BE, Chang DC, Soong SJ, Balch CM. Melanoma in children and teenagers: an analysis of patients from the National Cancer Database. J Clin Oncol. 2007;25(11):1363–8.
41. Aldrink JH, Selim MA, Diesen DL, Johnson J, Pruitt SK, Tyler DS, Seigler HF. Pediatric melanoma: a single-institution experience of 150 patients. J Pediatr Surg. 2009;44(8):4–21.
42. Downard CD, Rapkin LB, Gow KW. Melanoma in children and adolescents. Surg Oncol. 2007;16(3):215–20.
43. Livestro DP, Kaine EM, Michaelson JS, Mihm MC, Haluska FG, Muzikansky A, Sober AJ, Tanabe KK. Melanoma in the young: differences and similarities with adult melanoma. A case-matched controlled analysis. Cancer. 2007;110(3):614–24.
44. Paradela S, Fonseca E, Pita-Fernandez S, Kantrow SM, Diwan AH, Herzog C, Prieto VG. Prognostic factors for melanoma in children and adolescents: a clinicopathologic, single-center study of 137 patients. Cancer. 2010;116(18):4334–44.
45. Pappo AS. Melanoma in children and adolescents. Eur J Cancer. 2003;39(18):2651–61.
46. Dika E, Ravaioli GM, Fanti PA, Neri I, Patrizi A. Spitz nevi and other spitzoid neoplasms in children: overview of incidence data and diagnostic criteria. Pediatr Dermatol. 2017;34(1):25–32.
47. Latchana N, Regan K, Howard JH, Aldrink JH, Ranalli MA, Peters SB, Zhang X, Gru A, Payne PR, Suarez-Kelly LP, Carson WE 3rd. Global microRNA profiling for diagnostic appraisal of melanocytic Spitz tumors. J Surg Res. 2016;205(2):350–8.
48. Bradford PT, Goldstein AM, Tamura D, Khan SG, Ueda T, Boyle J, Oh KS, Imoto K, Inui H, Moriwaki S, Emmert S, Pike KM, Raziuddin A, Plona TM, DiGiovanna JJ, Tucker MA, Kraemer KH. Cancer and neurologic degeneration in xeroderma pigmentosum: long term follow-up characterises the role of DNA repair. J Med Genet. 2011;48(3):168–76.
49. Bis S, Tsao H. Melanoma genetics: the other side. Clin Dermatol. 2013;31(2):148–55.
50. Berg P, Wennberg AM, Tuominen R, Sander B, Rozell BL, Platz A, Hansson J. Germline CDKN2A mutations are rare in child and adolescent cutaneous melanoma. Melanoma Res. 2004;14(4):251–5.
51. Navid F. Genetic alterations in childhood melanoma. Am Soc Clin Oncol Educ Book. 2012, 2012:589–92.

52. Wong JR, Harris JK, Rodriguez-Galindo C, Johnson KJ. Incidence of childhood and adolescent melanoma in the United States: 1973–2009. Pediatrics. 2013;131(5):846–54.
53. Ferrari A, Bono A, Baldi M, Collini P, Casanova M, Pennacchioli E, Terenziani M, Marcon I, Santinami M, Bartoli C. Does melanoma behave differently in younger children than in adults? A retrospective study of 33 cases of childhood melanoma from a single institution. Pediatrics. 2005;115(3):649–54.
54. Lewis KG. Trends in pediatric melanoma mortality in the United States, 1968 through 2004. Dermatol Surg. 2008;34(2):152–9.
55. Neier M, Pappo A, Navid F. Management of melanomas in children and young adults. J Pediatr Hematol Oncol. 2012;34(Suppl 2):S51–4.
56. Han D, Zager JS, Han G, Marzban SS, Puleo CA, Sarnaik AA, Reed D, Messina JL, Sondak VK. The unique clinical characteristics of melanoma diagnosed in children. Ann Surg Oncol. 2012;19(12):3888–95.
57. Cordoro KM, Gupta D, Frieden IJ, McCalmont T, Kashani-Sabet M. Pediatric melanoma: results of a large cohort study and proposal for modified ABCD detection criteria for children. J Am Acad Dermatol. 2013;68(6):913–25.
58. Mitkov M, Chrest M, Diehl NN, Heckman MG, Tollefson M, Jambusaria-Pahlajani A. Pediatric melanomas often mimic benign skin lesions: a retrospective study. J Am Acad Dermatol. 2016;75(4):706–11.
59. Gerami P, Busam K, Cochran A, Cook MG, Duncan LM, Elder DE, Fullen DR, Guitart J, LeBoit PE, Mihm MC Jr, Prieto VG, Rabkin MS, Scolyer RA, Xu X, Yun SJ, Obregon R, Yazdan P, Cooper C, Weitner BB, Rademaker A, Barnhill RL. Histomorphologic assessment and interobserver diagnostic reproducibility of atypical spitzoid melanocytic neoplasms with long-term follow-up. Am J Surg Pathol. 2014;38(7):934–40.
60. Tang W, David FB, Wilson MM, Barwick BG, Leyland-Jones BR, Bouzyk MM. DNA extraction from formalin-fixed, paraffin-embedded tissue. Cold Spring Harb Protoc. 2009;2009(2):pdb.prot5138.
61. Thirlwell C, Eymard M, Feber A, Teschendorff A, Pearce K, Lechner M, Widschwendter M, Beck S. Genome-wide DNA methylation analysis of archival formalin-fixed paraffin-embedded tissue using the Illumina Infinium HumanMethylation27 BeadChip. Methods. 2010;52(3):248–54.
62. Wiesner T, He J, Yelensky R, Esteve-Puig R, Botton T, Yeh I, Lipson D, Otto G, Brennan K, Murali R, Garrido M, Miller VA, Ross JS, Berger MF, Sparatta A, Palmedo G, Cerroni L, Busam KJ, Kutzner H, Cronin MT, Stephens PJ, Bastian BC. Kinase fusions are frequent in Spitz tumours and spitzoid melanomas. Nat Commun. 2014;5:3116.
63. DeMarchis EH, Swetter SM, Jennings CD, Kim J. Fluorescence in situ hybridization analysis of atypical melanocytic proliferations and melanoma in young patients. Pediatr Dermatol. 2014;31(5):561–9.
64. Nasr MR, El-Zammar O. Comparison of pHH3, Ki-67, and survivin immunoreactivity in benign and malignant melanocytic lesions. Am J Dermatopathol. 2008;30(2):117–22.
65. Casper DJ, Ross KI, Messina JL, Sondak VK, Bodden CN, McCardle TW, Glass LF. Use of anti-phosphohistone H3 immunohistochemistry to determine mitotic rate in thin melanoma. Am J Dermatopathol. 2010;32(7):650–4.
66. McNutt NS, Urmacher C, Hakimian J, Hoss DM, Lugo J. Nevoid malignant melanoma: morphologic patterns and immunohistochemical reactivity. J Cutan Pathol. 1995;22(6):502–17.
67. Conway C, Beswick S, Elliott F, Chang YM, Randerson-Moor J, Harland M, Affleck P, Marsden J, Sanders DS, Boon A, Knowles MA, Bishop DT, Newton-Bishop JA. Deletion at chromosome arm 9p in relation to BRAF/NRAS mutations and prognostic significance for primary melanoma. Genes Chromosomes Cancer. 2010;49(5):425–38.
68. Yazdan P, Cooper C, Sholl LM, Busam K, Rademaker A, Weitner BB, Obregon R, Guitart J, Gerami P. Comparative analysis of atypical spitz tumors with heterozygous versus homozygous 9p21 deletions for clinical outcomes, histomorphology, BRAF mutation, and p16 expression. Am J Surg Pathol. 2014;38(5):638–45.
69. Mason A, Wititsuwannakul J, Klump VR, Lott J, Lazova R. Expression of p16 alone does not differentiate between Spitz nevi and Spitzoid melanoma. J Cutan Pathol. 2012;39(12):1062–74.
70. Wiesner T, Obenauf AC, Murali R, Fried I, Griewank KG, Ulz P, Windpassinger C, Wackernagel W, Loy S, Wolf I, Viale A, Lash AE, Pirun M, Socci ND, Rutten A, Palmedo G, Abramson D, Offit K, Ott A, Becker JC, Cerroni L, Kutzner H, Bastian BC, Speicher MR. Germline mutations in BAP1 predispose to melanocytic tumors. Nat Genet. 2011;43(10):1018–21.
71. McCormack CJ, Conyers RK, Scolyer RA, Kirkwood J, Speakman D, Wong N, Kelly JW, Henderson MA. Atypical Spitzoid neoplasms: a review of potential markers of biological behavior including sentinel node biopsy. Melanoma Res. 2014;24(5):437–47.
72. Grignol V, Fairchild ET, Zimmerer JM, Lesinski GB, Walker MJ, Magro CM, Kacher JE, Karpa VI, Clark J, Nuovo G, Lehman A, Volinia S, Agnese DM, Croce CM, Carson WE 3rd. miR-21 and miR-155 are associated with mitotic activity and lesion depth of borderline melanocytic lesions. Br J Cancer. 2011;105(7):1023–9.
73. Latchana N, Martin del Campo S, Grignol V, Carson M, Clark J, Peters S, Carson III W. Classifications of indeterminate melanomas by microRNA profiling. In: Perspectives in melanoma XVIII, Dublin, Ireland, September 19, 2014.
74. Minca EC, Al-Rohil RN, Wang M, Harms PW, Ko JS, Collie AM, Kovalyshyn I, Prieto VG, Tetzlaff MT, Billings SD, Andea AA. Comparison between melanoma gene expression score and fluorescence

in situ hybridization for the classification of melanocytic lesions. Mod Pathol. 2016;29(8):832–43.
75. Cerrato F, Wallins JS, Webb ML, McCarty ER, Schmidt BA, Labow BI. Outcomes in pediatric atypical Spitz tumors treated without sentinel lymph node biopsy. Pediatr Dermatol. 2012;29(4):448–53.
76. Rand AJ, Flejter WL, Dowling CA, Brooke LM, Boland GM, Kroshinsky D, Rosenblum IR, Herandez-Perez M, Reimann JDR. Atypical ALK-positive Spitz tumors with 9p21 homozygous deletion: report of two cases and review of the literature. J Cutan Pathol. 2018;45(2):136–40.
77. Gerami P, Cooper C, Bajaj S, Wagner A, Fullen D, Busam K, Scolyer RA, Xu X, Elder DE, Abraham RM, Prieto VG, Guitart J, Liu P, Pestova E, Barnhill RL. Outcomes of atypical Spitz tumors with chromosomal copy number aberrations and conventional melanomas in children. Am J Surg Pathol. 2013;37(9):1387–94.
78. Moscarella E, Zalaudek I, Cerroni L, Sperduti I, Catricala C, Smolle J, Hofmann-Wellenhof R, Sgambato A, Pellacani G, Argenziano G. Excised melanocytic lesions in children and adolescents: a 10-year survey. Br J Dermatol. 2012;167(2):368–73.
79. Barnhill RL. The Spitzoid lesion: rethinking Spitz tumors, atypical variants, 'Spitzoid melanoma' and risk assessment. Mod Pathol. 2006;19(Suppl 2):S21–33.
80. Spatz A, Calonje E, Handfield-Jones S, Barnhill RL. Spitz tumors in children: a grading system for risk stratification. Arch Dermatol. 1999;135(3):282–5.
81. Zaal LH, Mooi WJ, Klip H, van der Horst CM. Risk of malignant transformation of congenital melanocytic nevi: a retrospective nationwide study from The Netherlands. Plast Reconstr Surg. 2005;116(7):1902–9.
82. North JP, Garrido MC, Kolaitis NA, LeBoit PE, McCalmont TH, Bastian BC. Fluorescence in situ hybridization as an ancillary tool in the diagnosis of ambiguous melanocytic neoplasms: a review of 804 cases. Am J Surg Pathol. 2014;38(6):824–31.
83. Bastian BC, Olshen AB, LeBoit PE, Pinkel D. Classifying melanocytic tumors based on DNA copy number changes. Am J Pathol. 2003;163(5):1765–70.
84. Yeh I, Mully TW, Wiesner T, Vemula SS, Mirza SA, Sparatta AJ, McCalmont TH, Bastian BC, LeBoit PE. Ambiguous melanocytic tumors with loss of 3p21. Am J Surg Pathol. 2014;38(8):1088–95.
85. Botton T, Yeh I, Bastian BC. Melanoma BRAF fusions (Letter). Clin Cancer Res. 2014;20(24):6631.
86. Amin SM, Haugh AM, Lee CY, Zhang B, Bubley JA, Merkel EA, Verzi AE, Gerami P. A Comparison of morphologic and molecular features of BRAF, ALK, and NTRK1 fusion spitzoid neoplasms. Am J Surg Pathol. 2017;41(4):491–8.
87. Kiuru M, Jungbluth A, Kutzner H, Wiesner T, Busam KJ. Spitz tumors: comparison of histological features in relationship to immunohistochemical staining for ALK and NTRK1. Int J Surg Pathol. 2016;24(3):200–6.
88. Wiesner T, Kutzner H, Cerroni L, Mihm MC Jr, Busam KJ, Murali R. Genomic aberrations in spitzoid melanocytic tumours and their implications for diagnosis, prognosis and therapy. Pathology. 2016;48(2):113–31.
89. Lee CY, Sholl LM, Zhang B, Merkel EA, Amin SM, Guitart J, Gerami P. Atypical Spitzoid neoplasms in childhood: a molecular and outcome study. Am J Dermatopathol. 2017;39(3):181–6.
90. Gerami P, Jewell SS, Morrison LE, Blondin B, Schulz J, Ruffalo T, Matushek P 4th, Legator M, Jacobson K, Dalton SR, Charzan S, Kolaitis NA, Guitart J, Lertsbarapa T, Boone S, LeBoit PE, Bastian BC. Fluorescence in situ hybridization (FISH) as an ancillary diagnostic tool in the diagnosis of melanoma. Am J Surg Pathol. 2009;33(8):1146–56.
91. Busam KJ, Shah KN, Gerami P, Sitzman T, Jungbluth AA, Kinsler V. Reduced H3K27me3 expression is common in nodular melanomas of childhood associated with congenital melanocytic nevi but not in proliferative nodules. Am J Surg Pathol. 2017;41(3):396–404.
92. Bahrami AE, Easton J, Mulder H, Lee S, Barnhill R, Pappo AS. Analysis of TERT promoter mutations in pediatric melanoma. J Clin Oncol. 2014;32(5s Suppl):abstr 9023.
93. Lee S, Barnhill RL, Dummer R, Dalton J, Wu J, Pappo A, Bahrami A. TERT promoter mutations are predictive of aggressive clinical behavior in patients with spitzoid melanocytic neoplasms. Sci Rep. 2015;5:11200.
94. Seynnaeve B, Lee S, Borah S, Park Y, Pappo A, Kirkwood JM, Bahrami A. Genetic and epigenetic alterations of TERT are associated with inferior outcome in adolescent and young adult patients with melanoma. Sci Rep. 2017;7:45704.
95. Lallas A, Kyrgidis A, Ferrara G, Kittler H, Apalla Z, Castagnetti F, Longo C, Moscarella E, Piana S, Zalaudek I, Argenziano G. Atypical Spitz tumours and sentinel lymph node biopsy: a systematic review. Lancet Oncol. 2014;15(4):e178–83.
96. Zhao G, Lee KC, Peacock S, Reisch LM, Knezevich SR, Elder DE, Piepkorn MW, Elmore JG, Barnhill RL. The utilization of spitz-related nomenclature in the histological interpretation of cutaneous melanocytic lesions by practicing pathologists: results from the M-Path study. J Cutan Pathol. 2017;44(1):5–14.
97. Lee KC, Peacock S, Weinstock MA, Zhao GA, Knezevich SR, Elder DE, Barnhill RL, Piepkorn MW, Reisch LM, Carney PA, Onega T, Lott JP, Elmore JG. Variation among pathologists' treatment suggestions for melanocytic lesions: a survey of pathologists. J Am Acad Dermatol. 2017;76(1):121–8.
98. D'Orsi CJ, Bassett LW, Geig SA, Jackson VP, Kopans DB, Linver MN, et al. ACR BI-RADS mammography. In: ACR breast imaging reporting and data system, Breast Imaging Atlas. 4th ed. 2003. p. 193–8.

99. Piepkorn MW, Barnhill RL, Elder DE, Knezevich SR, Carney PA, Reisch LM, Elmore JG. The MPATH-Dx reporting schema for melanocytic proliferations and melanoma. J Am Acad Dermatol. 2014;70(1):131–41.
100. Sondak VK, Messina JL. Unusual presentations of melanoma: melanoma of unknown primary site, melanoma arising in childhood, and melanoma arising in the eye and on mucosal surfaces. Surg Clin North Am. 2014;94(5):1059–73.
101. Sreeraman Kumar R, Messina JL, Reed D, Navid F, Sondak VK. Pediatric melanoma and atypical melanocytic neoplasms. Cancer Treat Res. 2016;167:331–69.
102. Lallas A, Apalla Z, Ioannides D, Lazaridou E, Kyrgidi A, Broganelli P, Alfano R, Zalaudek I, Argenziano G. Update on dermoscopy of Spitz/Reed naevi and management guidelines by the International Dermoscopy Society. Br J Dermatol. 2017;177(3):645–55. https://doi.org/10.1111/bjd.15339.
103. Urso C. A new perspective for Spitz tumors? Am J Dermatopathol. 2005;27(4):364–6.
104. Barnhill RL, Argenyi Z, Berwick M, Duray PH, Erickson L, Guitart J, Horenstein MG, Lowe L, Messina J, Paine S, Piepkorn MW, Prieto V, Rabkin MS, Schmidt B, Selim A, Shea CR, Trotter MJ. Atypical cellular blue nevi (cellular blue nevi with atypical features): lack of consensus for diagnosis and distinction from cellular blue nevi and malignant melanoma ("malignant blue nevus"). Am J Surg Pathol. 2008;32(1):36–44.
105. Miglioretti DL, Johnson E, Williams A, Greenlee RT, Weinmann S, Solberg LI, Feigelson HS, Roblin D, Flynn MJ, Vanneman N, Smith-Bindman R. The use of computed tomography in pediatrics and the associated radiation exposure and estimated cancer risk. JAMA Pediatr. 2013;167(8):700–7.
106. Pearce MS, Salotti JA, Little MP, McHugh K, Lee C, Kim KP, Howe NL, Ronckers CM, Rajaraman P, Sir Craft AW, Parker L, Berrington de Gonzalez A. Radiation exposure from CT scans in childhood and subsequent risk of leukaemia and brain tumours: a retrospective cohort study. Lancet. 2012;380(9840):499–505.
107. Gatidis S, Schmidt H, Gucke B, Bezrukov I, Seitz G, Ebinger M, Reimold M, Pfannenberg CA, Nikolaou K, Schwenzer NF, Schafer JF. Comprehensive oncologic imaging in infants and preschool children with substantially reduced radiation exposure using combined simultaneous (1)(8) F-fluorodeoxyglucose positron emission tomography/magnetic resonance imaging: a direct comparison to (1)(8) F-fluorodeoxyglucose positron emission tomography/computed tomography. Investig Radiol. 2016;51(1):7–14.
108. Freemyer B, Hamilton E, Warneke CL, Ali AM, Herzog C, Hayes-Jordan A, Austin M. Treatment outcomes in pediatric melanoma - Are there benefits to specialized care? J Pediatr Surg. 2016;51(12):2063–7.
109. Lorimer PD, White RL, Walsh K, Han Y, Kirks RC, Symanowski J, Forster MR, Sarantou T, Salo JC, Hill JS. Pediatric and adolescent melanoma: a National Cancer Data Base update. Ann Surg Oncol. 2016;23(12):4058–66.
110. Wong JY, Sondak VK. Unanswered questions about margin recommendations for primary cutaneous melanoma. J Natl Compr Cancer Netw. 2012;10(3):357–65.
111. Howman-Giles R, Shaw HM, Scolyer RA, Murali R, Wilmott J, McCarthy SW, Uren RF, Thompson JF. Sentinel lymph node biopsy in pediatric and adolescent cutaneous melanoma patients. Ann Surg Oncol. 2010;17(1):138–43.
112. Howman-Giles R, Shaw HM, Scolyer RA, Murali R, Wilmott J, McCarthy SW, Uren RF, Thompson JF. Sentinel lymph node biopsy in pediatric and adolescent patients: a proven technique. J Surg Oncol. 2012;104(4):405–19.
113. Stanelle EJ, Busam KJ, Rich BS, Christison-Lagay ER, Dunkel IJ, Marghoob AA, Halpern A, Coit DG, La Quaglia MP. Early-stage non-Spitzoid cutaneous melanoma in patients younger than 22 years of age at diagnosis: long-term follow-up and survival analysis. J Pediatr Surg. 2015;50(6):1019–23.
114. Brecht IB, Garbe C, Gefeller O, Pfahlberg A, Bauer J, Eigentler TK, Offenmueller S, Schneider DT, Leiter U. 443 paediatric cases of malignant melanoma registered with the German Central Malignant Melanoma Registry between 1983 and 2011. Eur J Cancer. 2015;51(7):861–8.
115. Han D, Turner L, Reed D, Messina JL, Sondak VK. The prognostic significance of lymph node metastasis in pediatric melanoma and atypical melanocytic proliferations. Expert Rev Dermatol. 2013b;8(2):103–6.
116. Morton DL, Thompson JF, Cochran AJ, Mozzillo N, Nieweg OE, Roses DF, Hoekstra HJ, Karakousis CP, Puleo CA, Coventry BJ, Kashani-Sabet M, Smithers BM, Paul E, Kraybill WG, McKinnon JG, Wang HJ, Elashoff R, Faries MB. Final trial report of sentinel-node biopsy versus nodal observation in melanoma. N Engl J Med. 2014;370(7):599–609.
117. Palmer PE 3rd, Warneke CL, Hayes-Jordan AA, Herzog CE, Hughes DP, Lally KP, Austin MT. Complications in the surgical treatment of pediatric melanoma. J Pediatr Surg. 2013;48(6):1249–53.
118. Han D, Zager JS, Shyr Y, Chen H, Berry LD, Iyengar S, Djulbegovic M, Weber JL, Marzban SS, Sondak VK, Messina JL, Vetto JT, White RL, Pockaj B, Mozzillo N, Charney KJ, Avisar E, Krouse R, Kashani-Sabet M, Leong SP. Clinicopathologic predictors of sentinel lymph node metastasis in thin melanoma. J Clin Oncol. 2013a;31(35):4387–93.
119. Coit DG, Ernstoff MS, Busam KJ. Is pediatric melanoma always malignant? Cancer. 2013;119(22):3910–3.
120. Harms KL, Lowe L, Fullen DR, Harms PW. Atypical Spitz tumors: a diagnostic challenge. Arch Pathol Lab Med. 2015;139(10):1263–70.

121. Ludgate MW, Fullen DR, Lee J, Lowe L, Bradford C, Geiger J, Schwartz J, Johnson TM. The atypical Spitz tumor of uncertain biologic potential: a series of 67 patients from a single institution. Cancer. 2009;115(3):631–41.
122. Barnhill RL, Argenyi ZB, From L, Glass LF, Maize JC, Mihm MC Jr, Rabkin MS, Ronan SG, White WL, Piepkorn M. Atypical Spitz nevi/tumors: lack of consensus for diagnosis, discrimination from melanoma, and prediction of outcome. Hum Pathol. 1999;30(5):513–20.
123. Wong SL, Balch CM, Hurley P, Agarwala SS, Akhurst TJ, Cochran A, Cormier JN, Gorman M, Kim TY, McMasters KM, Noyes RD, Schuchter LM, Valsecchi ME, Weaver DL, Lyman GH. Sentinel lymph node biopsy for melanoma: American Society of Clinical Oncology and Society of Surgical Oncology joint clinical practice guideline. J Clin Oncol. 2012;30(23):2912–8.
124. Rossi CR, De Salvo GL, Bonandini E, Mocellin S, Foletto M, Pasquali S, Pilati P, Lise M, Nitti D, Rizzo E, Montesco MC. Factors predictive of non-sentinel lymph node involvement and clinical outcome in melanoma patients with metastatic sentinel lymph node. Ann Surg Oncol. 2008;15(4):1202–10.
125. McMasters KM, Wong SL, Edwards MJ, Chao C, Ross MI, Noyes RD, Viar V, Cerrito PB, Reintgen DS. Frequency of nonsentinel lymph node metastasis in melanoma. Ann Surg Oncol. 2002;9(2):137–41.
126. Murali R, Desilva C, Thompson JF, Scolyer RA. Non-Sentinel Node Risk Score (N-SNORE): a scoring system for accurately stratifying risk of non-sentinel node positivity in patients with cutaneous melanoma with positive sentinel lymph nodes. J Clin Oncol. 2010;28(29):4441–9.
127. Urso C, Borgognoni L, Doria M, Tinacci G, Zini E. Non-sentinel lymph node involvement in a patient with an atypical Spitz tumor and a positive sentinel node. Report of a case and review of the literature. J Cutan Pathol. 2009;36(5):586–90.
128. Faries MB, Thompson JF, Cochran A, Elashoff R, Glass EC, Mozzillo N, Nieweg OE, Roses DF, Hoekstra HJ, Karakousis CP, Reintgen DS, Coventry BJ, Wang HJ, Morton DL, Group MC. The impact on morbidity and length of stay of early versus delayed complete lymphadenectomy in melanoma: results of the Multicenter Selective Lymphadenectomy Trial (I). Ann Surg Oncol. 2010;17(12):3324–9.
129. Sarnaik AA, Puleo CA, Zager JS, Sondak VK. Limiting the morbidity of inguinal lymphadenectomy for metastatic melanoma. Cancer Control. 2009;16(3):240–7.
130. Kirkwood JM, Strawderman MH, Ernstoff MS, Smith TJ, Borden EC, Blum RH. Interferon alfa-2b adjuvant therapy of high-risk resected cutaneous melanoma: the Eastern Cooperative Oncology Group Trial EST 1684. J Clin Oncol. 1996;14(1):7–17.
131. Chao MM, Schwartz JL, Wechsler DS, Thornburg CD, Griffith KA, Williams JA. High-risk surgically resected pediatric melanoma and adjuvant interferon therapy. Pediatr Blood Cancer. 2005;44(5):441–8.
132. Navid F, Furman WL, Fleming M, Rao BN, Kovach S, Billups CA, Cain AM, Amonette R, Jenkins JJ, Pappo AS. The feasibility of adjuvant interferon alpha-2b in children with high-risk melanoma. Cancer. 2005;103(4):780–7.
133. Shah NC, Gerstle JT, Stuart M, Winter C, Pappo A. Use of sentinel lymph node biopsy and high-dose interferon in pediatric patients with high-risk melanoma: the Hospital for Sick Children experience. J Pediatr Hematol Oncol. 2006;28(8):496–500.
134. Eggermont AM, Suciu S, Santinami M, Testori A, Kruit WH, Marsden J, Punt CJ, Sales F, Gore M, Mackie R, Kusic Z, Dummer R, Hauschild A, Musat E, Spatz A, Keilholz U, Group EM. Adjuvant therapy with pegylated interferon alfa-2b versus observation alone in resected stage III melanoma: final results of EORTC 18991, a randomised phase III trial. Lancet. 2008;372(9633):117–26.
135. Eggermont AM, Suciu S, Testori A, Kruit WH, Marsden J, Punt CJ, Santinami M, Sales F, Schadendorf D, Patel P, Dummer R, Robert C, Keilholz U, Yver A, Spatz A. Ulceration and stage are predictive of interferon efficacy in melanoma: results of the phase III adjuvant trials EORTC 18952 and EORTC 18991. Eur J Cancer. 2012;48(2):218–25.
136. Herndon TM, Demko SG, Jiang X, He K, Gootenberg JE, Cohen MH, Keegan P, Pazdur R. US Food and Drug Administration approval: peginterferon-alfa-2b for the adjuvant treatment of patients with melanoma. Oncologist. 2012;17(10):1323–8.
137. Daud AI, Xu C, Hwu WJ, Urbas P, Andrews S, Papadopoulos NE, Floren LC, Yver A, Deconti RC, Sondak VK. Pharmacokinetic/pharmacodynamic analysis of adjuvant pegylated interferon alpha-2b in patients with resected high-risk melanoma. Cancer Chemother Pharmacol. 2011;67(3):657–66.
138. Navid F, Herzog CE, Sandoval J, Daryani VM, Stewart CF, Gattuso J, Mandrell B, Phipps S, Chemaitilly W, Sykes A, Davidoff AM, Shulkin BL, Bahrami A, Furman WL, Mao S, Wu J, Schiff D, Rao B, Pappo A. Feasibility of pegylated interferon in children and young adults with resected high-risk melanoma. Pediatr Blood Cancer. 2016;63(7):1207–13.
139. Flaherty LE, Othus M, Atkins MB, Tuthill RJ, Thompson JA, Vetto JT, Haluska FG, Pappo AS, Sosman JA, Redman BG, Moon J, Ribas A, Kirkwood JM, Sondak VK. Southwest Oncology Group S0008: a phase III trial of high-dose interferon alfa-2b versus cisplatin, vinblastine, and dacarbazine, plus interleukin-2 and interferon in patients with high-risk melanoma—an intergroup study of Cancer And Leukemia Group B, Children's Oncology Group, Eastern Cooperative Oncology Group, and Southwest Oncology Group. J Clin Oncol. 2014;32(33):3771–8.
140. Eggermont AM, Chiarion-Sileni V, Grob JJ, Dummer R, Wolchok JD, Schmidt H, Hamid O, Robert C,

Ascierto PA, Richards JM, Lebbe C, Ferraresi V, Smylie M, Weber JS, Maio M, Bastholt L, Mortier L, Thomas L, Tahir S, Hauschild A, Hassel JC, Hodi FS, Taitt C, de Pril V, de Schaetzen G, Suciu S, Testori A. Prolonged survival in stage III melanoma with ipilimumab adjuvant therapy. N Engl J Med. 2016;375(19):1845–55.

141. Robert C, Schachter J, Long GV, Arance A, Grob JJ, Mortier L, Daud A, Carlino MS, McNeil C, Lotem M, Larkin J, Lorigan P, Neyns B, Blank CU, Hamid O, Mateus C, Shapira-Frommer R, Kosh M, Zhou H, Ibrahim N, Ebbinghaus S, Ribas A. Pembrolizumab versus ipilimumab in advanced melanoma. New Eng J Med. 2015;372(26):2521–32.
142. Weber J, Mandala M, Del Vecchio M, Gogas HJ, Arance AM, Cowey CL, Dalle S, Schenker M, Chiarion-Sileni V, Marquez-Rodas I, Grob J, Butler MO, Middleton MR, Maio M, Atkinson V, Queirolo P, Gonzalez R, Kudchadkar RR, Smylie M, Meyer N, Mortier L, Atkins MB, Long GV, Bhatia S, Lebbé C, Rutkowski P, Yokota K, Yamazaki N, Kim TM, de Pril V, Sabater J, Qureshi A, Larkin J, Ascierto PA. Adjuvant nivolumab versus ipilimumab in resected Stage III or IV melanoma. N Engl J Med. 2017;377(19):1824–35.
143. Menzies AM, Haydu LE, Visintin L, Carlino MS, Howle JR, Thompson JF, Kefford RF, Scolyer RA, Long GV. Distinguishing clinicopathologic features of patients with V600E and V600K BRAF-mutant metastatic melanoma. Clin Cancer Res. 2012;18(12):3242–9.
144. Lu C, Zhang J, Nagahawatte P, Easton J, Lee S, Liu Z, Ding L, Wyczalkowski MA, Valentine M, Navid F, Mulder H, Tatevossian RG, Dalton J, Davenport J, Yin Z, Edmonson M, Rusch M, Wu G, Li Y, Parker M, Hedlund E, Shurtleff S, Raimondi S, Bhavin V, Donald Y, Mardis ER, Wilson RK, Evans WE, Ellison DW, Pounds S, Dyer M, Downing JR, Pappo A, Bahrami A. The genomic landscape of childhood and adolescent melanoma. J Invest Dermatol. 2015;135(3):816–23.
145. Merchant MS, Wright M, Baird K, Wexler LH, Rodriguez-Galindo C, Bernstein D, Delbrook C, Lodish M, Bishop R, Wolchok JD, Streicher H, Mackall CL. Phase I clinical trial of ipilimumab in pediatric patients with advanced solid tumors. Clin Cancer Res. 2016;22(6):1364–70.
146. Bristol-Myers Squibb. U.S. Food and Drug Administration expands approval of Yervoy (ipilimumab) to include pediatric patients 12 years and older with unresectable or metastatic melanoma. Bristol-Myers Squibb online press release July 24, 2017. https://news.bms.com/press-release/corporatefinancial-news/us-food-and-drug-administration-expands-approval-yervoy-ipilim
147. Weyand AC, Mody RJ, Rabah RM, Opipari VP. PD-1 inhibition in congenital pigment synthesizing metastatic melanoma. Pediatr Blood Cancer. 2017;65(1):e26702.
148. Stinauer MA, Kavanagh BD, Schefter TE, Gonzalez R, Flaig T, Lewis K, Robinson W, Chidel M, Glode M, Raben D. Stereotactic body radiation therapy for melanoma and renal cell carcinoma: impact of single fraction equivalent dose on local control. Radiat Oncol. 2011;6:34.
149. Weintraub D, Yen CP, Xu Z, Savage J, Williams B, Sheehan J. Gamma knife surgery of pediatric gliomas. J Neurosurg Pediatr. 2012;10(6):471–7.
150. Ferrari A, Bisogno G, Cecchetto G, Santinami M, Maurichi A, Bono A, Vajna De Pava M, Pierani P, Bertolini P, Rossi CR, De Salvo GL. Cutaneous melanoma in children and adolescents: the Italian rare tumors in pediatric age project experience. J Pediatr. 2014;164(2):376–82.e1–2.
151. Georgina V. Long, Axel Hauschild, Mario Santinami, Victoria Atkinson, Mario Mandalà, Vanna Chiarion-Sileni, James Larkin, Marta Nyakas, Caroline Dutriaux, Andrew Haydon, Caroline Robert, Laurent Mortier, Jacob Schachter, Dirk Schadendorf, Thierry Lesimple, Ruth Plummer, Ran Ji, Pingkuan Zhang, Bijoyesh Mookerjee, Jeff Legos, Richard Kefford, Reinhard Dummer, John M. Kirkwood. Adjuvant Dabrafenib plus Trametinib in Stage III -Mutated Melanoma. N Engl J Med. 2017;377(19): 1813–1823.
152. Rodabe N Amaria, Peter A Prieto, Michael T Tetzlaff, Alexandre Reuben, Miles C Andrews, Merrick I Ross, Isabella C Glitza, Janice Cormier, Wen-Jen Hwu, Hussein A Tawbi, Sapna P Patel, Jeffrey E Lee, Jeffrey E Gershenwald, Christine N Spencer, Vancheswaran Gopalakrishnan, Roland Bassett, Lauren Simpson, Rosalind Mouton, Courtney W Hudgens, Li Zhao, Haifeng Zhu, Zachary A Cooper, Khalida Wani, Alexander Lazar, Patrick Hwu, Adi Diab, Michael K Wong, Jennifer L McQuade, Richard Royal, Anthony Lucci, Elizabeth M Burton, Sangeetha Reddy, Padmanee Sharma, James Allison, Phillip A Futreal, Scott E Woodman, Michael A Davies, Jennifer A Wargo. Neoadjuvant plus adjuvant dabrafenib and trametinib versus standard of care in patients with high-risk, surgically resectable melanoma: a single-centre, open-label, randomised, phase 2 trial. The Lancet Oncol. 2018;19(2):181–193.
153. Francisco Bautista, Angelo Paci, Veronique Minard-Colin, Christelle Dufour, Jacques Grill, Ludovic Lacroix, Pascale Varlet, Dominique Valteau-Couanet, Birgit Geoerger. Vemurafenib in pediatric patients with mutated high-grade gliomas. Pediatr Blood Cancer. 2014;61(6):1101–1103.

Melanoma in Pregnancy

14

Joanna L. Walker, Annie Wang,
George Kroumpouzos, and Martin A. Weinstock

Melanocytic Nevi in Pregnancy

Melanocytic nevi should be monitored during pregnancy, and a biopsy performed for significant change or features of malignant melanoma (MM) [1]. Historically, change in BMN pigmentation during pregnancy was once considered to be a normal hormonally driven phenomenon. This hypothesis was derived from other pregnancy-induced pigmentary disorders, such as melasma and *linea nigra,* whereby sex hormone signaling increases pigment production. However, no correlation between sex hormone signaling and pigmentation has been proven with BMN in pregnancy.

Melanocytic nevus enlargement and/or darkening can occur during pregnancy, but the rate of malignant transformation of BMN is not increased according to histologic and clinical data [2]. While the natural course of BMN is not altered by pregnancy, dysplastic nevi (DN) in patients with dysplastic nevus syndrome (DNS) may have an increased risk for malignant change [3].

Evidence for pregnancy's effect on DN comes from Ellis et al., examining 17 females with DNS where nevi were photographed and prospectively followed. The rate of change in nevi increased 3.9-fold in pregnancy compared to the nonpregnant state, with the risk of change in DN found to be 1.6 times higher [3]. One patient in the study developed MM during pregnancy [3]. Altered estrogen receptor (ER) expression in changing DN is a plausible mechanism for elevated rate of change during pregnancy. ERβ expression is higher in DN compared with BMN and expression correlates with the grade of atypia [2]. The ERβ receptor is upregulated in BMN, but not DN during pregnancy, and it appears to have protective antitumoral effects [2]. Interpretation of this data is difficult as ER signaling is complex, the effects of endogenous estrogen binding to ERβ on DN are unknown, and the newly identified G protein-coupled ER (GPER) has not been studied in DN. Further studies are needed to clarify the significance of ER expression in melanocytic lesions and the natural course of DN in pregnancy.

J. L. Walker, M.D. (✉) · M. A. Weinstock, M.D., Ph.D.
Department of Dermatology, The Warren Alpert Medical School of Brown University, Providence, RI, USA

Division of Dermatology, Veterans Affairs Medical Center, Providence, RI, USA
e-mail: Joanna_walker@brown.edu; maw@brown.edu

A. Wang, M.D.
Department of Dermatology, Hawaii Permanente Medical Group, Honolulu, HI, USA

G. Kroumpouzos, M.D., Ph.D.
Department of Dermatology, The Warren Alpert Medical School of Brown University, Providence, RI, USA

Department of Dermatology, Medical School of Jundiai, Sao Paulo, Brazil

Division of Dermatology, Veterans Affairs Medical Center, Providence, RI, USA
e-mail: gk@gkderm.com

A. I. Riker (ed.), *Melanoma*, https://doi.org/10.1007/978-3-319-78310-9_14

Mild histologic changes in melanocytic nevi may occur in pregnancy. A histopathologic review reported a slight increase in atypical histologic features in nevi of pregnant patients, compared with those of non-pregnant controls. The atypical findings were not of a sufficient degree to result in diagnostic confusion in distinguishing between benign nevus and MM [4]. Interestingly, the histologic features were no different compared with male controls [4]. A smaller histologic study by Chan et al. documented more mitotic figures and higher mitotic rates in nevi from pregnant patients compared with non-pregnant controls, supporting a theory of higher "activation" of cells during pregnancy. They also described a distinctive morphologic pattern of clustered epithelioid melanocytes in the superficial dermis that was more common in BMN from pregnant cases (81% vs. 27% of controls) [5] (Fig. 14.1).

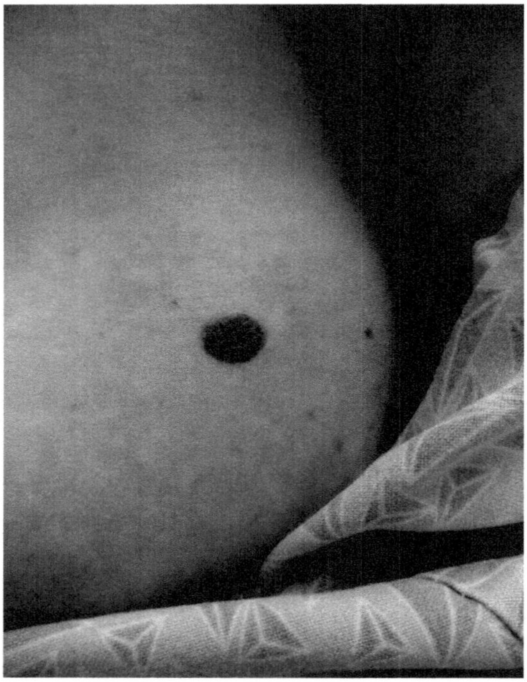

Fig. 14.1 Nevus on the left breast that enlarged, became lighter, and more raised during pregnancy. Pathology showed moderate melanocytic atypia with expansile dermal nest and elevated Ki67 expression (5%) on dermal melanocytes. No atypia or signs of proliferation were present on the residual lesion that was excised 9 months post-partum

Studies evaluating clinical and dermoscopic changes in nevi during pregnancy report either no change [6] or changes in size, pigment network, and/or vascular structures that return to normal within approximately 12 months postpartum [7–9]. Physical stretching of the skin, increased vascularity, and behavioral modifications such as reduced exposure to sunlight are postulated to contribute to pregnancy-associated changes in nevi [9]. BMN on the breasts and abdomen are more likely to change as tissue expands in these regions [7, 10, 11]. Growth in diameter is less common on areas such as the back, occurring in 0–9.5% of BMN between the first and third trimester [12, 13].

Pregnancy-associated dermoscopic changes include lightening or darkening of pigment, reduced thickness and prominence of pigment network, peripheral pigment globules, and increased vascularity (increased dotted or comma-shaped vascular structures) [6–9, 11, 12]. A dermoscopic scoring system for BMN change during pregnancy has documented minimal, but statistically significant, change occurring in ~10–19% of nevi [7, 8, 12] (Table 14.1.).

Traditional dermoscopic criteria for dysplasia such as asymmetry, irregular pigment network, and blue-white veil should not be attributed to physiologic gestational changes [9]. Clinically suspicious lesions should always warrant a biopsy to obtain a pathologic diagnosis, performed in the same manner as a non-pregnant patient. Excision of a dysplastic nevus with severe cytologic atypia may be safely postponed until postpartum. However, there may be certain circumstances whereby an immediate re-excision may be considered [14] (Fig. 14.2).

Table 14.1. Pregnancy-associated dermoscopic changes in melanocytic nevi

Lightened or darkened pigment
Reduced pigment network prominence
Peripheral pigment globules
Increased vascular structures

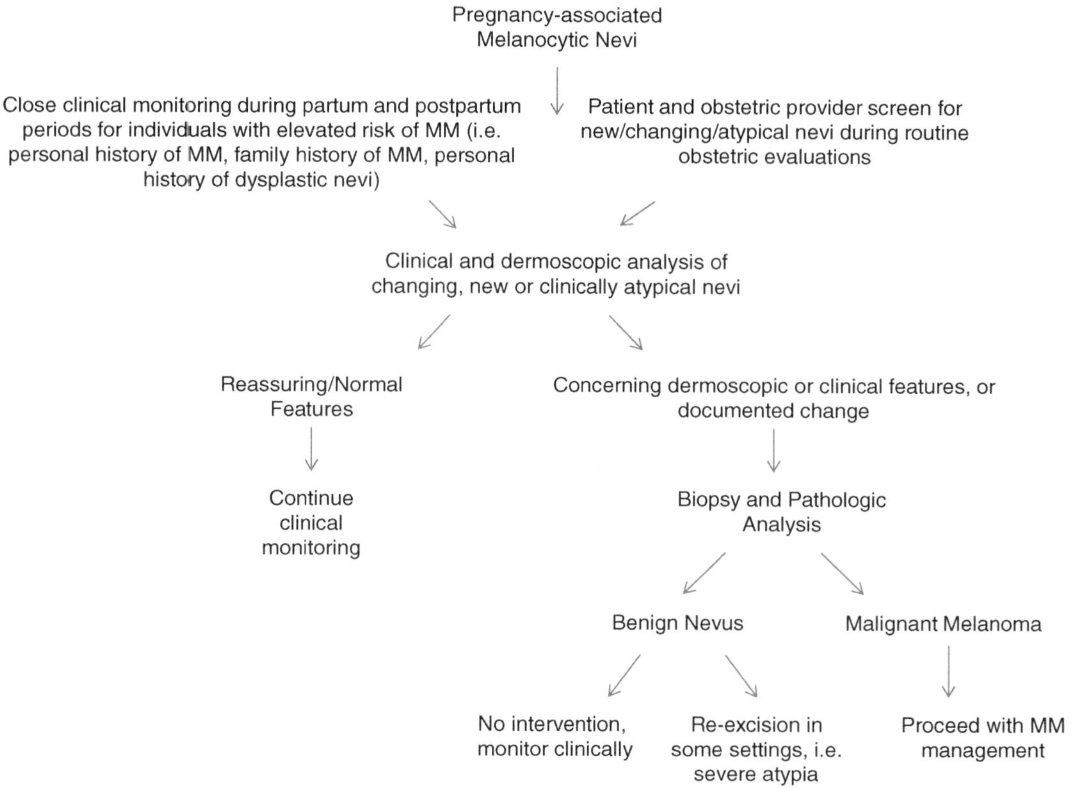

Fig. 14.2 Pregnancy-associated MM

MM in Pregnancy

Introduction

MM is the most common malignancy in pregnancy, accounting for 24–33% of all malignancies diagnosed during pregnancy in Swedish, Norwegian, and Australian population studies [15–18]. One-third of MMs affecting women occur during childbearing age [15, 16] and 3.3–11.8% of cases in this group are associated with pregnancy [18, 19]. Approximately 8% of all MM diagnoses occur during pregnancy [20]. PAMM incidence is rising due to the increasing incidence of MM in younger females and trends in the delay in childbearing [18, 21–23]. The incidence of PAMM in Australia increased from 37.1 to 51.84 per 100,000 maternities between 1994 and 2008, with maternal age accounting for the difference in cases [24].

The conventional definition of pregnancy-associated cancer is a diagnosis occurring during pregnancy through 1-year postpartum. While the definition of PAMM in the literature varies from inclusion of pregnancy only and/or 1–5 years postpartum, the definition of PAMM here includes the diagnosis during pregnancy and up to 1 year after delivery.

Pathophysiology

Pregnancy-induced changes in the immune milieu, hormone levels, metabolic activity, lymphangiogenesis, and fetal cell microchimerism underlie theories for altered tumor and host behavior in PAMM. Evidence of poorer outcome in pregnant mice with MM stimulates efforts to identify potential pathogenic mechanisms [25]. The interplay of various pregnancy-specific changes is complex, with some factors having a seemingly protective role against MM and others associated with increased risk (Table 14.2).

The immune milieu in pregnancy shifts toward a T-helper cell 2 (Th2)-dominant phenotype with increased cellular tolerance and relative immunosuppression. Cancer cells and fetal trophoblast cells survive through biologic mechanisms that promote "immune escape" via natural killer and regulatory T cells [26]. Human leukocyte antigen (HLA)-G expression suppresses immune surveillance via dampened response against tumor antigens and sustains immune tolerance by inducing CD4+ lymphocyte differentiation into regulatory T cells (Tregs). Tregs and trophoblast expression of HLA-G prevent maternal rejection of the semi-allogeneic fetus. In a similar manner, cancer cells alter the local immune response through these pathways to allow tumor progression [27]. In fact, increased Treg cells correlate with a worse outcome in metastatic MM [28]. It is unknown whether the trophoblast alteration in Tregs affects surveillance and response to MM and evidence of suppressed immune response to PAMM is lacking. In fact, increased peri-tumoral lymphocytic infiltrates are seen in PAMM compared with non-PAMM tumors [29]. The prognostic implications of the inflammatory reaction in this setting are unknown.

The effects of sex hormones on the development and outcome of MM are varied and poorly understood. Female gender and multiparity are associated with improved MM survival and MM outcomes in some studies [24, 29–31]. An Australian population-based study reported a 40% decreased risk of PAMM in females with at least three prior pregnancies compared with nulliparous females [24]. However, the association between parity and decreased MM risk has been shown for both male and female genders, suggesting environmental over hormonal or biologic factors [32].

Table 14.2 Potential factors in pathophysiology and outcome in PAMM[a]

Protective	Increased peri-tumoral inflammation
Unclear/mixed effect on outcome	Female hormone levels
	Estrogen receptor expression on tumor cells
	Fetal cell microchimerism
Unfavorable	Increased lymphangiogenesis
	Reduced cellular immunity/ increased tumor tolerance
	Increased metabolic activity

[a]Further research is needed to clarify the role of these factors in PAMM

MM cells have estrogen receptors [33, 34] but it is unclear whether it is a "hormone-responsive" tumor. Some theorize that elevated estrogen levels have a detrimental effect on MM outcome, but recent data suggests that estrogen signaling on tumor cells is more complex than initially thought, and possibly could even have favorable effects. Additionally, treatment of metastatic MM with the antiestrogen drug, tamoxifen, does not seem to affect outcome [35, 36].

Estrogen receptors are expressed differently in PAMM. There is higher expression of G protein-coupled estrogen receptor (GPER) in PAMM compared with non-PAMM (78% vs. 28%) and in most of these cases ERβ is co-expressed [34]. GPER and ERβ co-expression correlates with favorable pathologic prognostic features such as lower Breslow's depth, fewer mitoses, increased peri-tumoral lymphocytic infiltrates, and a decreased risk of metastasis [34]. Loss of ERβ expression promotes tumorigenesis [34, 37].

Pregnancy is well known to represent a state of increased metabolic activity, with some studies showing an increased mitotic activity in tumors associated with pregnancy [5]. However, several studies analyzing mitotic rate and immunohistochemical markers for PAMM tumors do not show increased tumor proliferation rates [29, 38]. Pregnancy-associated plasma protein-A (PAPPA) is a metalloproteinase that influences insulin growth factor and tumor transition from the epidermis to the mesenchyme. The serum levels of PAPPA are increased in pregnancy, suggesting that increased levels can correlate with increased MM cell migration and worse survival, particularly for advanced-stage MM [39].

The most compelling data on pregnancy's role in the pathogenesis of MM relates to recent data on the increased lymphangiogenesis and fetal microchimeric cells. Pregnant mice with MM were shown to have larger tumors, increased metastases, and poorer survival as well as increased lymphatic vessels compared with non-pregnant controls [25, 40, 44]. Increased lymphatic vessel size and lymphatic intra-tumoral area were also documented in MMs from human pregnant individuals, with no increase in blood vessel angiogenesis [25, 40]. Prior studies increased MM tumor lymphangiogenesis with an increased risk for lymph node invasion and a higher hazards ratio of 5.5 of finding a sentinel lymph node with metastatic disease [41, 42]. While the mouse model showing increased lymphangiogenesis is more representative of advanced MM, the potential correlation between poorer outcomes associated with pregnancy requires further exploration.

A study evaluating fetal cell microchimerism (FCM) provided a potential mechanism for MM tumor lymphatic formation unique to pregnancy. FCM is the phenomenon whereby fetal cells enter the maternal circulation, persist, and act as progenitor cells that may differentiate into other cell lines, particularly in the setting of damaged tissue. The role of FCM in cancer is quite complex and in many studies they appear to have a protective effect for the mother [43]. In the case of MM, such cells are found in the majority of tumors in pregnant mice and humans, often expressing endothelial cell markers. In fact, they were found to cluster in the form of vessels in some instances, leading the authors to hypothesize that fetal-derived lymphatic progenitor cells acquired during gestation lead to increased MM-associated lymphatics [44]. Further studies are required to explore these concepts further and evaluate potential clinical impact for these findings.

Outcomes and Prognosis

Maternal Risks

There is insufficient evidence to determine if pregnancy affects MM prognosis and an overall consensus is lacking. Historically, the prevailing view was that PAMM portended worse outcomes based on several case series in the 1950s–1990s [45–48]. Subsequently, some controlled studies have disproven this belief, while others continue to show poorer outcomes in this population. Variability in the definition of PAMM complicates the interpretation of results, as studies include MM cases ranging from diagnosis 1 year prior to pregnancy, and during pregnancy only, to inclusion of diagnosis 2 or more years following pregnancy. Further analysis of several studies has shown a wide variation in applied statistical methods, as well as a lack of other confounding factors such as staging, tumor thickness, and anatomic location. Table 14.3 summarizes research findings on PAMM's influence on prognosis.

Table 14.3 Studies on prognosis of melanoma arising in pregnancy[a]

First author, publication year	Study design and country: pregnant cases (stage)	Findings
Pregnancy has no effect on prognosis		
Jones et al. 2017 [20]	Prospective hospital-based cohort United States 156 cases (stages 0–III) Complete dataset, controlled analyses	No difference in stage, recurrence, disease-free interval, melanoma-specific survival, or overall survival
Johansson et al. 2014 [57] (extension of Lens et al. 2004 [55])	Retrospective population-based cohort Sweden 1019 cases (include pregnancy and 2 years postpartum; 247 during pregnancy) staging data available in 59%, mostly early stage	No difference in MSS or OS between cases and controls (HR 1.05 CI 0.81–1.36) Sub-analysis with non-significant ↓ mortality in pregnant cases (HR 0.79, CI 0.44–1.41)
O'Meara et al. 2005 [56]	Retrospective population-based cohort United States 412 cases; MM diagnosed during or within 1 year of pregnancy (all stages, but survival analysis limited to localized disease)	No difference in stage, tumor thickness, or prognosis (HR for death 0.79, $p = .57$)

(continued)

Table 14.3 (continued)

First author, publication year	Study design and country: pregnant cases (stage)	Findings
Daryanani et al. 2003 [60]	Retrospective clinic-based cohort	Pregnancy does not affect survival
	The Netherlands	Non-significant ↑ tumor thickness in pregnancy
	46 cases (stage I/II)	
Travers et al. 1995 [61]	Retrospective clinic-based cohort	Trend toward better survival in pregnant MM pts ($p = .08$)
	United States	
	45 cases in pregnancy or 1 year postpartum (stage "clinically localized")	↑ thickness in tumors in PAMM
MacKie et al. 1991[b] [92]	Retrospective clinic-based cohort	No effect on DFI or survival after correcting for tumor thickness
	United Kingdom	
	92 cases (stage I/II MM)	
Wong et al. 1989 [62]	Retrospective clinic-based cohort	No differences in tumor location, histologic features, and 5-year survival between groups
	United States	
	66 cases (stage I MM)	
Adverse effect of pregnancy on prognosis		
Kyrgidis et al. 2017 [49]	Meta-analysis	↑ Risk of mortality (HR 1.17 CI 1.03–1.33), ↓ OS
	Pooled data from 14 studies	
		↓ DFS (HR 1.50 CI 1.19–1.90)
Byrom et al. 2015 [51]	Meta-analysis	↑ Risk of melanoma death (HR 1.56 CI 1.23–1.99)
	Pooled data from 4 studies (Lens, Mackie, Stensheim, Moller)	Addition of Tellez study increases HR to 1.64 (53)
		Repeat analysis with exclusion of Moller and other adjustments show HR non-significantly elevated [52]
Tellez et al. 2015 [63]	Retrospective hospital-based cohort	5.1 ↑ odds of death ($p = .03$), 6.7 ↑ odds of metastasis ($p = .01$), 9.2 ↑ odds of local recurrence ($p = .01$)
	United States	Discrepancies in staging, criticism for methods [65, 66]
	41 cases (all stages, mostly stage I/II) during or within 1 year of preg (19 during preg)	
Moller et al. 2013 [58]	Retrospective population-based cohort	↑ risk of death (HR 1.92 CI 1.42–3.01)
	United Kingdom	Study design
	306 cases (all stages) *diagnosis during 1 year postpartum only* (no cases during pregnancy); stage available for 72%	examined the effect of recent childbirth on outcome, did not examine MM during pregnancy
Stensheim et al.2008 [16]	Retrospective population-based cohort	↑ risk of cause-specific death (HR 1.52, CI 1.01–2.31); no longer significant when adjusted for tumor location. No difference in survival
	Norway	
	160 cases (stage not stated; Breslow's depth available for 55%)	
Slingluff et al. 1989 [48] (extension of Reintgen et al. 1985 [70])	Retrospective clinic-based cohort	Thicker MMs ($p = .05$), ↑ metastatic disease ($p = .008$) but no difference in OS between groups (Slingluff)
	United States	
	100 cases (all stages, but 98% with stage I/II)	↓ DFI in pts compared to controls ($p = .04$); no difference in OS (Reintgen)
Trapeznikov et al. 1989 [64]	Russia	↓ 10-year survival in pts compared to controls ($p < .05$)
	102 cases (all stages)	

HR hazard ratio, *DFI* disease-free interval, *DFS* disease-free survival, *MSS* melanoma-specific survival, *OS* overall survival, *MM* malignant melanoma, *pts* patients, *preg* pregnancy, ↑ increased, and ↓ decreased

Table is substantially modified from Tierney E, Krounpouzos G, Rogers G. Skin Tumors. In: Kroumpouzos G, editor. Text Atlas of Obstretric Dermatology. Philadelphia: Lippincott Williams & Wilkins Publishers. 2013; 141–151

[a]Table includes only studies of ≥40 patients

[b]143 completed pregnancy before MM; 85 diagnosed/treated before pregnancy; 68 diagnosed between pregnancies

Recent meta-analyses suggest increased mortality for PAMM, but the results are controversial based on differences in inclusion criteria, methods of statistical analyses, and poor quality of evidence in included studies such as retrospective case–control study design, incomplete data that lacks confounding factors, and inconsistent definition and analysis of outcomes [49–54]. Mortality is increased by 17% and recurrence by 50% in PAMM according to a meta-analysis by Kyrgidis et al. Sensitivity analyses addressed the heterogeneity in case definition, study design, and ability to control for stage and tumor depth, and the effect of PAMM on mortality remained. However, the overall grade for the quality of evidence was too low to have confidence in the estimate according to the author's analysis [49].

A meta-analysis by Byrom et al. showed a 56% increase in the mortality risk for PAMM and a hazards ratio of 1.64 [51, 53]. The study design and analysis were criticized for selection bias and improperly utilized statistical methods that included the pooling of the hazard ratio outcomes. In addition, the study with the greatest weight in the analysis included cases during postpartum only, evaluating the effect of recent childbirth on MM outcome as opposed to the other studies evaluating MM during pregnancy. When the results are recalculated according to alternative definitions and inclusion criteria, the adverse survival outcome is no longer found to be statistically significant [52, 54].

Population-based cohort studies are the highest level of evidence available for PAMM. Most of the available evidence shows no worsened survival for PAMM, but some results are conflicting and pertinent confounding factors, such as staging data, are missing in some of the larger studies [55–58]. In addition to the population-based cohort studies with largely negative results, several single-institution cohort and case–control studies on localized PAMM fail to show that pregnancy has any adverse influence on outcomes [20, 38, 59–62]. Conversely, others demonstrate poorer survival and outcomes for PAMM [63, 64], but again the utilized methods and statistical analyses have been questioned [65, 66]. Increased gravity at diagnosis was associated with worse survival in early-stage PAMM in one study [20]. This finding was not noted in stage III disease, and overall pregnancy did not portend worse outcome or survival in that study [20].

The effect of pregnancy on stage III and IV malignant melanoma is unclear, as controlled studies lack adequate numbers of advanced MMs in pregnancy. Two retrospective case series summarize outcomes for a total of 52 stage III and IV PAMMs, but interpretation is difficult without a comparison group [67, 68]. Theoretically, several behavioral and biologic mechanisms negatively affect late-stage PAMM outcomes. With the advent of effective systemic therapies that lack safety data in pregnancy, there is the risk for substandard and delayed care in late-stage PAMM [48, 56]. Additionally, the mechanisms of increased lymphangiogenesis during pregnancy are more likely to be impactful with invasive tumors.

Delay in diagnosis during pregnancy can cause an increase in postpartum MM diagnoses, i.e., a "rebound effect" in incidence, later stage disease, and poorer outcome [15, 17]. Diagnostic delay likely explains the increased tumor thickness of PAMM compared with controls in some studies [24, 48, 61, 69, 70] and accounts for some trends showing decreased survival in PAMM. Alternatively, increased tumor depth in PAMM could be interpreted as more aggressive disease associated with pregnancy, but the majority of studies do not find pregnancy as an adverse prognostic factor in MM when tumor depth and stage are controlled. In fact, PAMM cases were actually diagnosed at an earlier stage in a study involving patients under close surveillance in a pigmented lesion clinic [38].

Several adverse maternal effects have been reported for pregnancy-associated cancers including increased hospitalizations, cesarean section delivery, sepsis, thromboembolic events, and severe maternal morbidity [17]. However, studies with separate analyses for PAMM indicate that the incidence of thromboembolic events is not increased [71], and the risk of hospitalization is lower in MM compared with that of other pregnancy-associated cancers [72]. Potential

PAMM complications and maternal risks include those relevant to MM treatment, late-stage disease, and emotional stress.

Fetal Risks

While the majority of research focuses on maternal health risks for PAMM, few studies analyze potential adverse fetal effects. The risk for cesarean delivery and planned preterm birth are elevated in pregnancy-associated cancers and PAMM [17]. Prematurity is the most common fetal adverse outcome associated with PAMM, typically iatrogenic, and much more common in advanced-stage MM (occurring in 56% of stage III/IV cases) [67, 68]. Whether MM diagnosis during pregnancy affects infant birth weight is unclear. PAMM was associated with large-for-gestational age (LGA) newborns in one study [17] and lower mean birth weight in another [73], and two population studies showed no influence on birth weight [56, 74].

Adverse fetal effects are more likely to occur from the diagnostic and therapeutic interventions, particularly in stage III and IV MM. A recent report included cases treated with surgery, lymph node biopsy (11 cases), lymph node dissections (10 cases), radiation (3 cases), and chemotherapy (1 case) during pregnancy, showing uneventful adverse newborn outcomes [68]. In a retrospective review of 22 stage III and IV PAMM cases at a single institution, there were no neonatal deformities or severe fetal complications noted, except for one spontaneous abortion occurring after a lymph node dissection in the first trimester [67].

The fetal risk is most clearly defined for advanced-stage MM when there is a substantial risk for placental and fetal metastasis; fortunately, this is a rare occurrence. MM is the most common type of pregnancy-related cancer that also metastasizes to the placenta and fetus. Forty to 58% of all metastatic cancers to the fetus are due to MM [75–77]. One review highlighted that in all cases of fetal metastasis, microscopic evidence of metastatic MM was found in all placentas, and all mothers had visceral metastases (stage IV) [75]. In a separate study, 87 cases of maternal MM were reviewed, of which 17% (15 of 87 patients) had placental involvement, but only 40% of those (6 of the 15 patients) were found to have fetal metastasis [77]. On average, cases of metastatic MM presented in the fetus around 4.5 months post-partum (range: 0 to 20 months). The most common sites of metastasis were the liver and subcutaneous tissues [77].

Management

There are no NCCN guidelines for MM in pregnancy. The current standard of care is to manage melanocytic lesions in pregnant females just as one would in nonpregnant females. Once a histopathologic confirmation of MM is made, staging and prognostication, including evaluation of maternal and fetal risks from diagnostic procedures, surgery and systemic chemotherapy, targeted therapy, and immunotherapy, should be performed. When imaging is required for staging, modalities using ionizing radiation should be avoided whenever possible. Magnetic resonance imaging (MRI) is a diagnostic tool to be used when other nonionizing diagnostic procedures such as ultrasound are deemed inadequate. MRI is safe for both mother and fetus in the second and third trimesters, but its use in the first trimester is typically reserved for clinically imperative cases [78] (Fig. 14.3).

Treatment

The surgical management of MM is the same for pregnant women as it is for nonpregnant women. Biopsies of suspicious lesions should not be delayed. Local anesthesia, with the minimum necessary amount of lidocaine 1% (pregnancy category B), for shave, punch, or excisional biopsy, ensures prompt diagnosis and carries minimal risks to mother and fetus. Subsequent re-excision of MM lesions with appropriate wide margins based on tumor Breslow's depth is recommended for all localized MM and should not be postponed.

In thicker lesions (>0.8 mm Breslow's thickness) and tumor stage ≥T1b, the sentinel lymph

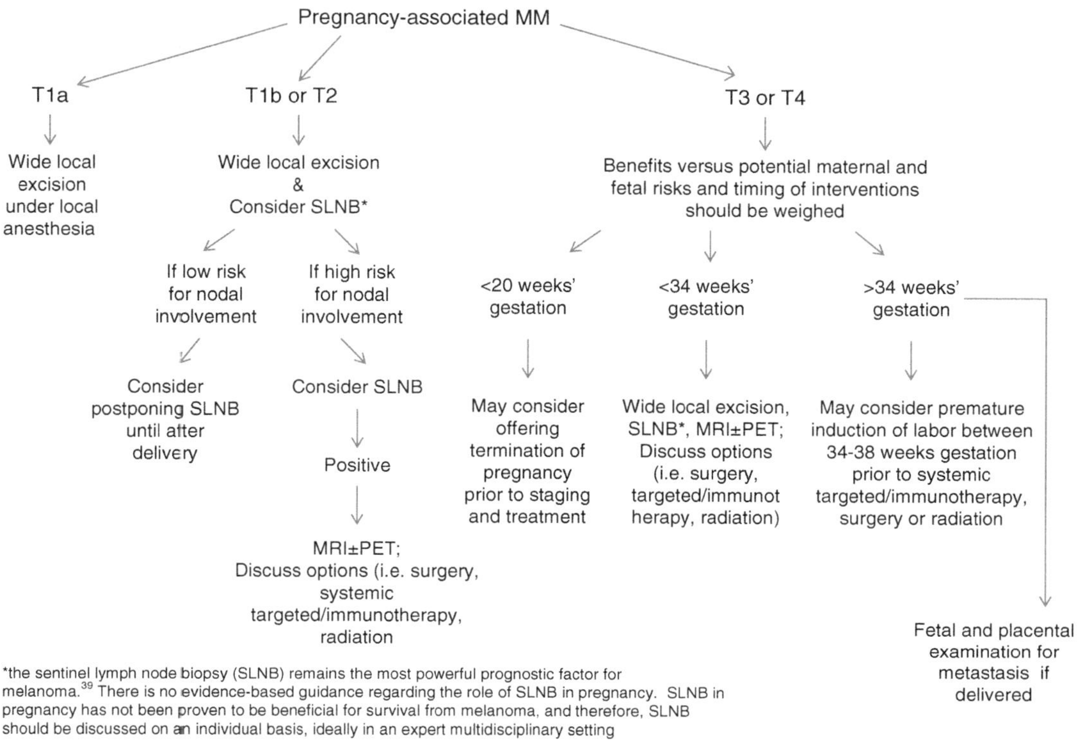

Fig. 14.3 Pregnancy-associated melanocytic nevi

node biopsy (SLNB) is a powerful prognostic test [77], which is useful for staging but has no impact on MM survival. There is no evidence-based guidance regarding the role and timing of SLNB in pregnancy, and therefore SLNB should be discussed on an individual basis, ideally within the confines of a comprehensive cancer center that specializes in the multidisciplinary management of melanoma. Radiopharmaceuticals with a short half-life, such as preoperative intradermal technetium-99 m-sulfur colloid, deliver <5 mGy of radiation and have not been associated with any maternal or fetal adverse effects [79]. The use of radiocolloid alone for SLNB, without blue dye, is recommended to prevent potential complications, such as anaphylactic reactions [14, 80]. Some authors suggest postponing SLNB until after delivery for pregnant patients with a perceived low risk for nodal involvement (stage T1b to T2b) [81]. For patients without advance disease, premature delivery should be avoided [68].

For stage III/IV disease, the benefits versus potential maternal and fetal risks of staging and treatment should be weighed [82]. Indications for complete lymph node or therapeutic lymph node dissection in regional metastatic MM (stage III) are the same as for a nonpregnant patient. If advanced-stage MM is diagnosed in the first trimester, termination of pregnancy may be offered. However, there is no specific guideline for this since it is unknown if pregnancy affects the outcome of MM in the mother [82], and the risk for fetal metastasis is very low.

The need for imaging and systemic therapies that pose fetal risk must also be considered. For the patients needing systemic therapy or radiation, premature induction of delivery at 34 weeks prior to the initiation of therapy can be considered [83]. However, this decision will depend on several factors, including the specific therapy's risk for fetal harm compared with the dangers of delayed treatment of MM.

There is scarce safety data for adjuvant and newer targeted or immunomodulatory therapy (such as interferon-α, BRAF inhibitors, MEK inhibitors, anti-CTLA-4 monoclonal antibodies, or PD1 inhibitors) during pregnancy. One report of vemurafenib use in pregnancy resulted in premature cesarean delivery for fetal distress but, fortunately, did not result in any fetal malformations [84]. Ipilimumab, an anti-CTLA-4 antibody, is known to cross the placenta and has been associated with urogenital tract malformations, miscarriages, stillbirths, premature births, and neonatal death in monkeys [85]. The anti-PD1 antibodies (nivolumab and pembrolizumab) have resulted in fetal loss, but no increase in birth defects in animal studies [86]. There is no safety data in human pregnancy; therefore, the use of such medications should be restricted to experienced practitioners after extensive discussion and evaluation of the potential risks and benefits on a case-by-case basis [87].

Fetal Metastasis

Since melanoma may metastasize to the placenta and the fetus [75–77], gross and microscopic evaluation of the placenta postpartum is recommended. This is performed with immunohistochemical staining for MM antigens in all stage IV metastatic melanoma patients [77]. In neonates without metastases at birth, careful evaluation and monitoring for the next 24 months are recommended, including periodic evaluation at wellness checks with full body examination of the skin. Baseline chest X-ray and liver enzymes, including lactate dehydrogenase, every 6 months, are also advocated by some experts [77].

Counseling

Preconception counseling for women with a history of MM and a desire to conceive can be a difficult discussion for healthcare providers. There are no evidence-based guidelines regarding pregnancy after a diagnosis of MM [87]. Discussion points include patient prognosis and maternal/fetal risks should recurrence occur during pregnancy. If chemotherapy or immunotherapy were used, their potential effects on fertility should be acknowledged. Overall, fertility and pregnancy rates are decreased in cancer survivors.

However, MM may be an exception, as post-cancer pregnancy rates do not appear to be adversely affected in women with a prior MM [88]. Additionally, fetal adverse outcomes such as congenital abnormalities, stillbirth, low birth weight, and preterm birth are not increased for gestations occurring after a diagnosis of MM [73, 74]. There is no evidence to suggest that a post-cancer pregnancy worsens outcomes or prognosis in females with treated MM [16, 30, 89, 90]. Several reviews have failed to show an increase in MM recurrence, or a decrease in survival, associated with pregnancy after a diagnosis of MM. This data is predominantly derived from patients with stage I/II MM and a detrimental effect for those with a higher stage MM diagnosis cannot be ruled out [89–91].

Tumor thickness remains the single most important predictor of recurrence. MacKie et al. documented a <10% 5-year MM recurrence rate in tumors <1.5 mm thickness, as compared with a 30% 5-year mortality risk for tumors 1.5–3.5 mm in Breslow's depth [92]. Tumors thicker than 3.5 mm had >50% mortality [92]. The same authors also showed that 83% of recurrence in stage II occurred within 2 years of the initial treatment [92]. Based on this data, the authors proposed waiting 2 years after surgery before becoming pregnant.

Schwartz et al. supported the 2-year wait for thinner MMs, and also recommended waiting 3–5 years for thicker lesions [14]. In a retrospective review of 22 cases of stage III and IV PAMM, the median time between primary melanoma and regional or distant disease occurring during pregnancy was 16 months, with a range of 0–10 years [67]. In general, however, a waiting period prior to becoming pregnant is not shown to alter outcomes. Recommendations should be made on a case-by-case basis after weighing the risks and benefits of recurrence risk with the age of the patient and eagerness to conceive.

It is worth noting that there is no evidence that oral contraceptives or hormone replacement therapies have any role in the natural history of MM. The decision to use either of the above should be based on a thorough evaluation of health and familial risk factors beyond that of a MM history [93–96].

Conclusions

Controversy remains regarding the effect of pregnancy on MM outcomes, especially for stage III and IV, but it is clear that early diagnosis and treatment are imperative to improve outcomes. This requires countering former assumptions regarding the normalcy of changing pigmented lesions during pregnancy, with prompt biopsy of changing or worrisome lesions. Future studies are necessary to clarify the role of pregnancy in MM prognostication. In general, treatment for PAMM should be according to standard guidelines, but in some cases consideration for fetal and maternal health may individualize the timing and course of staging and therapy.

References

1. Walker JL, Wang AR, Kroumpouzos G, Weinstock MA. Cutaneous tumors in pregnancy. Clin Dermatol. 2016;34(3):359–67.
2. Nading MA, Nanney LB, Boyd AS, Ellis DL. Estrogen receptor beta expression in nevi during pregnancy. Exp Dermatol. 2008;17(6):489–97.
3. Ellis DL. Pregnancy and sex steroid hormone effects on nevi of patients with the dysplastic nevus syndrome. J Am Acad Dermatol. 1991;25(3):467–82.
4. Foucar E, Bentley TJ, Laube DW, Rosai J. A histopathologic evaluation of nevocellular nevi in pregnancy. Arch Dermatol. 1985;121(3):350–4.
5. Chan MP, Chan MM, Tahan SR. Melanocytic nevi in pregnancy: histologic features and Ki-67 proliferation index. J Cutan Pathol. 2010;37(8):843–51.
6. Wyon Y, Synnerstad I, Fredrikson M, Rosdahl I. Spectrophotometric analysis of melanocytic naevi during pregnancy. Acta Derm Venereol. 2007;87(3):231–7.
7. Akturk AS, Bilen N, Bayramgurler D, Demirsoy EO, Erdogan S, Kiran R. Dermoscopy is a suitable method for the observation of the pregnancy-related changes in melanocytic nevi. J Eur Acad Dermatol Venereol. 2007;21(8):1086–90.
8. Rubegni P, Sbano P, Burroni M, Cevenini G, Bocchi C, Severi FM, et al. Melanocytic skin lesions and pregnancy: digital dermoscopy analysis. Skin Res Technol. 2007;13(2):143–7.
9. Zampino MR, Corazza M, Costantino D, Mollica G, Virgili A. Are melanocytic nevi influenced by pregnancy? A dermoscopic evaluation. Dermatol Surg. 2006;32(12):1497–504.
10. Sanchez JL, Figueroa LD, Rodriguez E. Behavior of melanocytic nevi during pregnancy. Am J Dermatopathol. 1984;6(Suppl):89–91.
11. Strumia R. Digital epiluminescence microscopy in nevi during pregnancy. Dermatology. 2002;205(2):186–7.
12. Gunduz K, Koltan S, Sahin MT, EF E. Analysis of melanocytic naevi by dermoscopy during pregnancy. J Eur Acad Dermatol Venereol. 2003;17(3):349–51.
13. Pennoyer JW, Grin CM, Driscoll MS, Dry SM, Walsh SJ, Gelineau JP, et al. Changes in size of melanocytic nevi during pregnancy. J Am Acad Dermatol. 1997;36(3 Pt 1):378–82.
14. Tierney EKG, Tumors RGS. In: Kroumpouzos G, editor. Text atlas of obstretric dermatology. Philadelphia: Lippincott Williams & Wilkins Publishers; 2013. p. 141–51.
15. Andersson TM, Johansson AL, Fredriksson I, Lambe M. Cancer during pregnancy and the postpartum period: a population-based study. Cancer. 2015;121(12):2072–7.
16. Stensheim H, Moller B, van Dijk T, Fossa SD. Cause-specific survival for women diagnosed with cancer during pregnancy or lactation: a registry-based cohort study. J Clin Oncol. 2009;27(1):45–51.
17. Lee YY, Roberts CL, Dobbins T, Stavrou E, Black K, Morris J, et al. Incidence and outcomes of pregnancy-associated cancer in Australia, 1994–2008: a population-based linkage study. BJOG. 2012;119(13):1572–82.
18. Eibye S, Kjaer SK, Mellemkjaer L. Incidence of pregnancy-associated cancer in Denmark, 1977–2006. Obstet Gynecol. 2013;122(3):608–17.
19. Lens M, Rosdahl I, Newton-Bishop J. Cutaneous melanoma during pregnancy: is the controversy over? J Clin Oncol. 2009;27(19):e11–2; author reply e3–4
20. Jones MS, Lee J, Stern SL, Faries MBI. Pregnancy-associated melanoma associated with adverse outcomes? J Am Coll Surg. 2017;225(1):149–58.
21. Peccatori FA, Azim HA Jr, Orecchia R, Hoekstra HJ, Pavlidis N, Kesic V, et al. Cancer, pregnancy and fertility: ESMO clinical practice guidelines for diagnosis, treatment and follow-up. Ann Oncol. 2013;24(Suppl 6):vi160–70.
22. Purdue MP, Freeman LE, Anderson WF, Tucker MA. Recent trends in incidence of cutaneous melanoma among US Caucasian young adults. J Invest Dermatol. 2008;128(12):2905–8.
23. Bleyer WA. Cancer in older adolescents and young adults: epidemiology, diagnosis, treatment, survival, and importance of clinical trials. Med Pediatr Oncol. 2002;38(1):1–10.

24. Bannister-Tyrrell M, Roberts CL, Hasovits C, Nippita T, Ford JB. Incidence and outcomes of pregnancy-associated melanoma in New South Wales 1994–2008. Aust N Z J Obstet Gynaecol. 2015;55(2):116–22.
25. Khosrotehrani K, Nguyen Huu S, Prignon A, Avril MF, Boitier F, Oster M, et al. Pregnancy promotes melanoma metastasis through enhanced lymphangiogenesis. Am J Pathol. 2011;178(4):1870–80.
26. Cristiani CM, Palella E, Sottile R, Tallerico R, Garofalo C, Carbone E. Human NK cell subsets in pregnancy and disease: Toward a new biological complexity. Front Immunol. 2016;7:656.
27. Johansen LL, Lock-Andersen J, Hviid TV. The pathophysiological impact of HLA class Ia and HLA-G expression and regulatory T cells in malignant melanoma: a review. J Immunol Res. 2016;2016:6829283.
28. Baumgartner JM, Gonzalez R, Lewis KD, Robinson WA, Richter DA, Palmer BE, et al. Increased survival from stage IV melanoma associated with fewer regulatory T cells. J Surg Res. 2009;154(1):13–20.
29. Fabian M, Toth V, Somlai B, Harsing J, Kuroli E, Rencz F, et al. Retrospective analysis of clinicopathological characteristics of pregnancy associated melanoma. Pathol Oncol Res. 2015;21(4):1265–71.
30. Vihinen P, Vainio-Kaila M, Talve L, Koskivuo I, Syrjanen K, Pyrhonen S. Previous pregnancy is a favourable prognostic factor in women with localised cutaneous melanoma. Acta Oncol. 2012;51(5):662–8.
31. Roh MR, Eliades P, Gupta S, Tsao H. Cutaneous melanoma in women. Int J Womens Dermatol. 2015;1(1):21–5.
32. Kaae J, Andersen A, Boyd HA, Wohlfahrt J, Melbye M. Reproductive history and cutaneous malignant melanoma: a comparison between women and men. Am J Epidemiol. 2007;165(11):1265–70.
33. Zhou JH, Kim KB, Myers JN, Fox PS, Ning J, Bassett RL, et al. Immunohistochemical expression of hormone receptors in melanoma of pregnant women, nonpregnant women, and men. Am J Dermatopathol. 2014;36(1):74–9.
34. Fabian M, Rencz F, Krenacs T, Brodszky V, Harsing J, Nemeth K, et al. Expression of G protein-coupled estrogen receptor, GPER in melanoma and in pregnancy-associated melanoma. J Eur Acad Dermatol Venereol. 2017;31(9):1453–61.
35. Beguerie JR, Xingzhong J, Valdez RP. Tamoxifen vs. non-tamoxifen treatment for advanced melanoma: a meta-analysis. Int J Dermatol. 2010;49(10):1194–202.
36. Lens MB, Reiman T, Husain AF. Use of tamoxifen in the treatment of malignant melanoma. Cancer. 2003;98(7):1355–61.
37. Bardin A, Boulle N, Lazennec G, Vignon F, Pujol P. Loss of ERbeta expression as a common step in estrogen-dependent tumor progression. Endocr Relat Cancer. 2004;11(3):537–51.
38. Merkel EA, Martini MC, Amin SM, Yelamos O, Lee CY, Sholl LM, et al. A comparative study of proliferative activity and tumor stage of pregnancy-associated melanoma (PAM) and non-PAM in gestational age women. J Am Acad Dermatol. 2016;74(1):88–93.
39. Prithviraj P, Anaka M, McKeown SJ, Permezel M, Walkiewicz M, Cebon J, et al. Pregnancy associated plasma protein-A links pregnancy and melanoma progression by promoting cellular migration and invasion. Oncotarget. 2015;6(18):15953–65.
40. Rodero MP, Prignon A, Avril MF, Boitier F, Aractingi S, Khosrotehrani K. Increase lymphangiogenesis in melanoma during pregnancy: correlation with the prolactin signalling pathway. J Eur Acad Dermatol Venereol. 2013;27(1):e144–5.
41. Dadras SS, Lange-Asschenfeldt B, Velasco P, Nguyen L, Vora A, Muzikansky A, et al. Tumor lymphangiogenesis predicts melanoma metastasis to sentinel lymph nodes. Mod Pathol. 2005;18(9):1232–42.
42. Massi D, Puig S, Franchi A, Malvehy J, Vidal-Sicart S, Gonzalez-Cao M, et al. Tumour lymphangiogenesis is a possible predictor of sentinel lymph node status in cutaneous melanoma: a case-control study. J Clin Pathol. 2006;59(2):166–73.
43. Cirello V, Fugazzola L. Novel insights into the link between fetal cell microchimerism and maternal cancers. J Cancer Res Clin Oncol. 2016;142(8):1697–704.
44. Nguyen Huu S, Oster M, Avril MF, Boitier F, Mortier L, Richard MA, et al. Fetal microchimeric cells participate in tumour angiogenesis in melanomas occurring during pregnancy. Am J Pathol. 2009;174(2):630–7.
45. Conybeare RC. Malignant melanoma and pregnancy: report of 3 cases. Obstet Gynecol. 1964;24:451–4.
46. Riberti C, Marola G, Bertani A. Malignant melanoma: the adverse effect of pregnancy. Br J Plast Surg. 1981;34(3):338–9.
47. Pack GT, Scharnagel IM. The prognosis for malignant melanoma in the pregnant woman. Cancer. 1951;4(2):324–34.
48. Slingluff CL Jr, Reintgen DS, Vollmer RT, Seigler HF. Malignant melanoma arising during pregnancy. A study of 100 patients. Ann Surg. 1990;211(5):552–7. discussion 8-9
49. Kyrgidis A, Lallas A, Moscarella E, Longo C, Alfano R, Argenziano G. Does pregnancy influence melanoma prognosis? A meta-analysis. Melanoma Res. 2017;27(4):289–99.
50. Mendizabal E, De Leon-Luis J, Gomez-Hidalgo NR, Joigneau L, Pintado P, Rincon P, et al. Maternal and perinatal outcomes in pregnancy-associated melanoma. Report of two cases and a systematic literature review. Eur J Obstet Gynecol Reprod Biol. 2017;214:131–9.
51. Byrom L, Olsen C, Knight L, Khosrotehrani K, Green AC. Increased mortality for pregnancy-associated melanoma: systematic review and meta-analysis. J Eur Acad Dermatol Venereol. 2015;29(8):1457–66.
52. Martires KJ, Stein JA, Grant-Kels JM, Driscoll MS. Meta-analysis concerning mortality for pregnancy-associated melanoma. J Eur Acad Dermatol Venereol. 2016;30(10):e107-e8.
53. Khosrotehrani K, Olsen CM, Byrom L, Green AC. Melanoma during pregnancy: level of evidence

and principles of precaution. J Am Acad Dermatol. 2017;76(1):e29–e30.
54. Kyrgidis A, Argenziano G, Moscarella E, Longo C, Alfano R, Lallas A. Increased mortality for pregnancy-associated melanoma: different outcomes pooled together, selection and publication biases. J Eur Acad Dermatol Venereol. 2016;30(9):1618.
55. Lens MB, Rosdahl I, Ahlbom A, Farahmand BY, Synnerstad I, Boeryd B, et al. Effect of pregnancy on survival in women with cutaneous malignant melanoma. J Clin Oncol. 2004;22(21):4369–75.
56. O'Meara AT, Cress R, Xing G, Danielsen B, Smith LH. Malignant melanoma in pregnancy. A population-based evaluation. Cancer. 2005;103(6):1217–26.
57. Johansson AL, Andersson TM, Plym A, Ullenhag GJ, Moller H, Lambe M. Mortality in women with pregnancy-associated malignant melanoma. J Am Acad Dermatol. 2014;71(6):1093–101.
58. Moller H, Purushotham A, Linklater KM, Garmo H, Holmberg L, Lambe M, et al. Recent childbirth is an adverse prognostic factor in breast cancer and melanoma, but not in Hodgkin lymphoma. Eur J Cancer. 2013;49(17):3686–93.
59. Silipo V, De Simone P, Mariani G, Buccini P, Ferrari A, Catricala C. Malignant melanoma and pregnancy. Melanoma Res. 2006;16(6):497–500.
60. Daryanani D, Plukker JT, De Hullu JA, Kuiper H, Nap RE, Hoekstra HJ. Pregnancy and early-stage melanoma. Cancer. 2003;97(9):2248–53.
61. Travers RL, Sober AJ, Berwick M, Mihm MC Jr, Barnhill RL, Duncan LM. Increased thickness of pregnancy-associated melanoma. Br J Dermatol. 1995;132(6):876–83.
62. Wong JH, Sterns EE, Kopald KH, Nizze JA, Morton DL. Prognostic significance of pregnancy in stage I melanoma. Arch Surg. 1989;124(10):1227–30; discussion 30–1
63. Tellez A, Rueda S, Conic RZ, Powers K, Galdyn I, Mesinkovska NA, et al. Risk factors and outcomes of cutaneous melanoma in women less than 50 years of age. J Am Acad Dermatol. 2016;74(4):731–8.
64. Trapeznikov NN, Khasanov Sh R, Iavorskii VV. Melanoma of the skin and pregnancy. Vopr Onkologii. 1987;33(6):40–6.
65. Driscoll MS, Martires K, Bieber AK, Pomeranz MK, Grant-Kels JM, Stein JA. Pregnancy and melanoma. J Am Acad Dermatol. 2016;75(4):669–78.
66. Martires KJ, Pomeranz MK, Stein JA, Grant-Kels JM, Driscoll MS. Pregnancy-associated melanoma (PAMM): is there truly a worse prognosis? Would not sound alarm bells just yet. J Am Acad Dermatol. 2016;75(2):e77.
67. Pages C, Robert C, Thomas L, Maubec E, Sassolas B, Granel-Brocard F, et al. Management and outcome of metastatic melanoma during pregnancy. Br J Dermatol. 2010;162(2):274–81.
68. de Haan J, Lok CA, de Groot CJ, Crijns MB, Van Calsteren K, Dahl Steffensen K, et al. Melanoma during pregnancy: a report of 60 pregnancies complicated by melanoma. Melanoma Res. 2017;27(3):218–23.
69. Miller E, Barnea Y, Gur E, Leshem D, Karin E, Weiss J, et al. Malignant melanoma and pregnancy: Second thoughts. J Plast Reconstr Aesthet Surg. 2010;63(7):1163–8.
70. Reintgen DS, McCarty KS Jr, Vollmer R, Cox E, Seigler HF. Malignant melanoma and pregnancy. Cancer. 1985;55(6):1340–4.
71. Bleau N, Patenaude V, Abenhaim HA. Risk of venous thrombo-embolic events in pregnant patients with cancer. J Matern Fetal Neonatal Med. 2016;29(3):380–4.
72. Lee YY, Roberts CL, Young J, Dobbins T. Using hospital discharge data to identify incident pregnancy-associated cancers: a validation study. BMC Pregnancy Childbirth. 2013;13:37.
73. Langagergaard V. Birth outcome in women with breast cancer, cutaneous malignant melanoma, or Hodgkin's disease: a review. Clin Epidemiol. 2010;3:7–19.
74. Langagergaard V, Puho EH, Lash TL, Norgard B, Sorensen HT. Birth outcome in Danish women with cutaneous malignant melanoma. Melanoma Res. 2007;17(1):31–6.
75. Dildy GA III, Moise KJ, Carpenter RJ Jr, et al. Maternal malignancy metastatic to the products of conception: a review. Obstet Gynecol Surv. 1989;44:5.
76. Eltorky MKV, Osborne P, et al. Placental metastasis from maternal carcinoma: a report of three cases. J Reprod Med. 1995;40:4.
77. Alexander A, Samlowski WE, Grossman D, Bruggers CS, Harris RM, Zone JJ, et al. Metastatic melanoma in pregnancy: risk of transplacental metastases in the infant. J Clin Oncol. 2003;21(11):2179–86.
78. Patenaude Y, Pugash D, Lim K, Morin L, Diagnostic Imaging C, Lim K, et al. The use of magnetic resonance imaging in the obstetric patient. J Obstet Gynaecol Can. 2014;36(4):349–63.
79. Andtbacka RH, Donaldson MR, Bowles TL, Bowen GM, Grossmann K, Khong H, et al. Sentinel lymph node biopsy for melanoma in pregnant women. Ann Surg Oncol. 2013;20(2):689–96.
80. Hu Y, Melmer PD, Slingluff CL Jr. Localization of the sentinel lymph node in melanoma without blue dye. Ann Surg. 2016;263(3):588–92.
81. Broer N, Buonocore S, Goldberg C, Truini C, Faries MB, Narayan D, et al. A proposal for the timing of management of patients with melanoma presenting during pregnancy. J Surg Oncol. 2012;106(1):36–40.
82. Leachman SA, Jackson R, Eliason MJ, Larson AA, Bolognia JL. Management of melanoma during pregnancy. Dermatol Nurs. 2007;19(2):145–52. 61
83. Beyeler M, Hafner J, Beinder E, Fauchere JC, Stoeckli SJ, Fehr M, et al. Special considerations for stage IV melanoma during pregnancy. Arch Dermatol. 2005;141(9):1077–9.
84. Maleka A, Enblad G, Sjors G, Lindqvist A, Ullenhag GJ. Treatment of metastatic malignant melanoma with vemurafenib during pregnancy. J Clin Oncol. 2013;31(11):e192–3.

85. Grunewald S, Jank A. New systemic agents in dermatology with respect to fertility, pregnancy, and lactation. J Dtsch Dermatol Ges. 2015;13:277.
86. Wang SCLY, Piao HL, Hong XW, Zhang D, Xu YY, et al. PD-1 and Tim-3 pathways are associated with regulatory CD8+ T cell function in decidua and maintenance of normal pregnancy. Cell Death Dis. 2015;6:e1738.
87. Ribero S, Longo C, Dika E, Fortes C, Pasquali S, Nagore E, et al. Pregnancy and melanoma: A European-wide survey to assess current management and a critical literature overview. J Eur Acad Dermatol Venereol. 2017;31(1):65–9.
88. Stensheim H, Cvancarova M, Moller B, Fossa SD. Pregnancy after adolescent and adult cancer: a population-based matched cohort study. Int J Cancer. 2011;129(5):1225–36.
89. Byrom L, Olsen CM, Knight L, Khosrotehrani K, Green AC. Does pregnancy after a diagnosis of melanoma affect prognosis? Systematic review and meta-analysis. Dermatol Surg. 2015;41(8):875–82.
90. Brady MS, Noce NS. Pregnancy is not detrimental to the melanoma patient with clinically localized disease. J Clin Aesthet Dermatol. 2010;3(3):22–8.
91. Albersen M, Westerling VI, van Leeuwen PA. The influence of pregnancy on the recurrence of cutaneous malignant melanoma in women. Dermatol Res Pract. 2010;2010
92. MacKie RM, Bufalino R, Morabito A, Sutherland C, Cascinelli N. Lack of effect of pregnancy on outcome of melanoma. For the World Health Organisation Melanoma Programme. Lancet. 1991;337(8742):653–5.
93. Karagas MR, Zens MS, Stukel TA, Swerdlow AJ, Rosso S, Osterlind A, et al. Pregnancy history and incidence of melanoma in women: a pooled analysis. Cancer Causes Control. 2006;17(1):11–9.
94. Naldi LAA, Imberti GL, Giordano L, Gallus S, La Vecchia C. Oncology Study Group of the Italian Group for Epidemiologic Research in Dermatology (GISED). Cutaneous malignant melanoma in women. Phenotypic characteristics, sun exposure, and hormonal factors: a case-control study from Italy. Ann Epidemiol. 2005;15:5.
95. Lea CSHE, Hartge P, et al. Reproductive risk factors for cutaneous melanoma in women: a case-control study. Am J Epidemiol. 2007;165:8.
96. Mackie RM, Bray CA. Hormone replacement therapy after surgery for stage I or II cutaneous melanoma. Br J Cancer. 2004;90:2.

Mucosal Melanoma

15

Lauge Hjorth Mikkelsen and Steffen Heegaard

Introduction

Malignant melanoma in mucosal membranes is an aggressive and extremely rare disease comprising approximately 0.03% of all cancers and 1.3% of all melanomas (Table 15.1) [1, 2]. In recent years, cutaneous melanoma has been studied in detail, but due to its rarity, mucosal melanoma is poorly described in the literature [2–6]. The present literature often relies on retrospective investigations and the level of evidence is generally low. The epidemiology, etiology, pathogenesis, and prognostic factors remain largely unknown, with no established consensus on appropriate guidelines for either diagnosis or treatment [3–6].

Mucosal melanomas can occur in all mucosal membranes in the body, including the conjunctiva [3]. Apart from conjunctival melanoma, most mucosal melanomas appear in occult locations, and symptoms arise in an advanced stage of disease where lymph node involvement or distant metastases are often present [3–5]. Distant metastasis frequently occurs in the lungs, liver, and bones [3, 5]. The treatment of choice is surgery, but unfortunately long-term survival is still quite difficult to achieve [3, 4]. Furthermore, the clinical diagnosis is often delayed due to the fact that many mucosal melanomas are amelanotic and pathologists seem to be relatively unaware of the diagnosis at these uncommon locations [3, 4]. All of these factors make mucosal melanoma management exceedingly challenging, and novel treatment modalities along with detailed clinical and pathological guidelines are needed in order to improve the prognosis and long-term outcome [2–7]. In this chapter, we describe mucosal melanomas as a specific disease entity with special focus on etiology and management. Although a large part of the vulva is considered modified skin and not true mucosa, vulvar melanoma is also discussed in this chapter.

L. H. Mikkelsen, M.D. · S. Heegaard, M.D., D.M.Sc. (✉)
Eye Pathology Section, Department of Pathology and Department of Ophthalmology, Rigshospitalet, University of Copenhagen, Copenhagen, Denmark
e-mail: lauge.hjorth.mikkelsen@regionh.dk; sthe@sund.ku.dk

Epidemiology and Demographics

Conjunctival melanomas along with sinonasal melanomas represent the most frequently occurring mucosal melanomas, each having an incidence of approximately 0.5 per million/year [3, 8–10]. A recent study reported an incidence for sinonasal melanoma of 0.9 per million/year in the Danish population [11]. Anorectal melanomas have an incidence of approximately 0.4 per million/year, while melanoma in the oral cavity and in the vagina has an annual incidence of 0.2 per million/year [3, 7, 9, 12]. Melanoma is the second most common malignant vulvar disease after squamous cell carcinoma, and it appears in approximately 0.2/100,000/year [7]. Smaller series and case studies have reported melanoma

A. I. Riker (ed.), *Melanoma*, https://doi.org/10.1007/978-3-319-78310-9_15

Table 15.1 Mucosal melanoma of various organ systems

Location	Incidence	Gender ratio (M:F)	Median age (years)	Prognosis (5-year survival)
Conjunctiva	0.5 per million/year	1:1	58	86.3%
Respiratory tract				
Sinonasal	0.5 per million/year	1:1	75	30%
Larynx	60 cases reported	4:1	60	<10%
Lung	30 cases reported	1:1	54	<25%
Gastrointestinal				
Oral cavity	0.2 per million/year	2:1	65	12.5%
Esophagus	337 cases reported	2:1	65	37%
Stomach	20 cases reported	1:1	65	0%
Small intestine	18 cases reported	1:1	56	0%
Colon	12 cases reported	1:1	60	21%
Anorectal	0.4 per million/year	1:2	68	20%
Gall bladder	31 cases reported	1:1	50	n/a
Biliary tract	9 cases reported	8:1	45	0.33%
Urological				
Urinary bladder	18 cases reported	1:1	62	<10%
Urethra	160 cases reported	1:2	73	<10%
Genital tract				
Penis	100 cases reported	Only male	75	22.5%
Vulva[a]	2 per million/year	Only female	68	30%
Vagina	0.2 per million/year	Only female	60	17.4%
Cervix	80 cases reported	Only female	55	7.8%

n/a not available [with kind permission from Acta Pathologica, Microbiologica et Immunologica Scandinavica (Mikkelsen et al. APMIS, 2016)]
[a]The vulva is generally considered modified skin

in numerous other mucosal membranes, but clear incidence rates of these sites are not available [3]. While the incidence of cutaneous melanomas is rapidly increasing, the incidence of mucosal melanomas has been considered stable [3, 5, 13, 14]. However, while the incidence of conjunctival melanoma in the Danish population was found to be stable in the period from 1943 to 1997 [15], recent studies from Finland, Sweden, and Denmark have reported an increasing frequency in these countries [14, 16, 17].

Additionally, the incidence of sinonasal melanoma in the Swedish population has also been found to be increasing in the period from 1960 to 2000 [13]. Furthermore, a recent study has shown the incidence of anorectal melanoma to be increasing in the American population [18]. Overall, slightly more women seem to be affected, with the main reason due to women suffering from anorectal melanoma (M:F = 1:2). This is compounded by the relatively high incidence of melanoma in the female genital tract and vulva [3, 18–24]. Mucosal melanoma is mainly a disease of the elderly, and most patients are diagnosed after their sixth decade of life, regardless of the affected organ system [3–5, 14]. A general racial predisposition does not appear to exist [9, 25, 26]. However, conjunctival melanoma and vulvar melanoma occur almost exclusively in Caucasians, and sinonasal melanoma is also more frequent in Caucasians compared to Blacks [8, 27, 28]. Sinonasal melanoma and especially oral melanoma seem to occur more frequently in Asian populations compared to Caucasians [26]. Oral melanoma has been found to represent up to 8% of all melanomas in Japanese people [2].

Etiology and Pathogenesis

Malignant melanomas are tumors caused by a malignant transformation of melanocytes derived from neural crest cells [3, 5, 29]. Melanocytes travel along and together with peripheral nerves and other neural crest-derived cells from the neural crest to their definitive destinations in numerous microenvironments, as well as the mucosal membranes [29]. Melanocytes have been found in most mucosal membranes, but their function in these locations remains unknown [30]. Mucosal melanomas share the neural crest origin with melanotic schwannomas and other pigmented neural crest-derived tumors [29]. Melanomas may potentially share more biological features with other neural crest-derived tumors. Mucosal melanomas most frequently arise *de novo* from a single melanocyte located within a mucosal membrane where a preexisting melanotic lesion is not present [8, 30].

Additionally, melanoma may arise in any preexisting melanocytic lesion [30]. Mucosal melanomas have been reported in preexisting benign melanosis (melanotic macule) of the esophagus, nasal cavity, vulva, vagina, and rectum [30–32]. Regarding anorectal and colon melanomas, the clinician must keep in mind that melanosis coli is not a melanocytic lesion. Mucosal melanocytic nevi have been identified in various mucosal membranes, namely in the oral mucosa; however, there is no evidence of increased risk of malignant transformation in these lesions [30, 33]. An exception is conjunctival melanomas that may potentially arise in a conjunctival nevus in 2–40% of the cases [17, 34, 35]. Vulvar melanomas may be divided into those emerging from the follicular skin and those emerging from the glabrous skin (a broad transition zone consisting of modified skin without hair follicles separating true hairy skin on the labia majora and the true mucosal epithelium in the vagina). Interestingly, a Swedish study showed that melanomas of the glabrous skin were almost exclusively *de novo* melanomas, while melanomas of the hairy skin often developed within a preexisting nevus [36].

In the literature, pure mucosal melanoma in situ is a very rarely reported condition [30]. This may be due to authors reporting the lesion under different names, such as atypical lentigo, atypical pigmented macules, precancerous melanoma, and atypical melanotic hyperplasia [30]. Another plausible explanation may be that these lesions never cause symptoms prior to malignant transformation. Due to the lack of symptoms, most are found accidentally by the dentist or a gynecologist during routine clinical examination. Histologically, mucosal melanoma in situ is defined as an intraepithelial proliferation of cytologically atypical melanocytes [37]. These lesions may be found in several organ systems and the prognosis is favorable after complete surgical removal [38]. A German study found a melanoma in situ component in two-thirds of all cases of sinonasal melanomas [37]. Mucosal melanoma in situ needs further investigation and classification in a universal mucosal melanoma staging manual.

In Caucasian populations, 42–75% of conjunctival melanomas seem to arise in a premalignant lesion, a so-called primary acquired melanosis (PAM), which may be considered a melanoma in situ [8, 17, 39]. PAM is mostly considered a clinical diagnosis and is described as a unilateral, flat, brown lesion with patches of pigmentation confined to the conjunctiva with or without involvement of the eyelid skin or cornea [8, 39]. Histopathologically, PAM is characterized by a neoplastic proliferation of the conjunctival melanocytes and by using specific histological criteria. It can be subdivided into PAM with atypia (PAM+) and without atypia (PAM−). PAM+ has a high risk of progression to melanoma, especially when vertical invasion of the epithelium by the conjunctival melanocytes is observed. Pagetoid spread and epithelioid cytology are also features pointing towards progression of a PAM+ lesion to becoming a melanoma [8, 10, 39, 40]. There is much debate in regard to the grading of PAM because the term "melanosis" has been associated with both benign and premalignant lesions. For this reason, a grading system of premalignant lesions using the more appropriate terms "conjunctival melanocytic intraepithelial neoplasia" (C-MIN) and "hypermelanosis" has been proposed [41].

While sun exposure is a known risk factor for the development of a cutaneous melanoma, no clear risk factors have been identified for mucosal melanomas [3, 5]. Exposure to tobacco and formaldehyde has been proposed to play a role in sinonasal and oral melanoma, but clear evidence is lacking [42, 43]. The presence of *BRAF* mutations along with a UV light signature consisting of multiple cytosine-to-thymine (C > T) transitions in sun-exposed conjunctival melanoma suggests a role of sun exposure in the pathogenesis of these tumors, but further investigations are needed [44].

Molecular Biology and Genetic Features

In recent years, the genetics and molecular features of cutaneous melanoma have been extensively studied with various next-generation sequencing techniques [45]. However, the genomic landscape of mucosal melanomas remains sparsely elucidated. The discovery and application of molecularly based targeted therapies have revolutionized the treatment of melanoma, and this makes the identification of specific molecular targets even more important today and for the future.

Whole-Genome Sequencing

Furney et al. performed whole-genome sequencing and exome sequencing on ten mucosal melanomas from various locations outside of the eye [46]. This study showed that mucosal melanomas carry a relatively low mutational burden. The mucosal melanoma samples harbored an average of 8.193 somatic, single-nucleotide variants (SNVs) [46], while sun-exposed cutaneous melanomas have been found to harbor an average of 84.495 SNVs (i.e., a factor of 10) [47]. The study also revealed a high rate of copy number and structural variants in mucosal melanoma [46, 48]. Other studies have shown that mucosal melanomas have specific patterns of chromosomal aberrations differing from cutaneous melanomas [49, 50]. Overall, these findings suggest mucosal melanomas as a distinct entity driven by distinct molecular pathways [48].

MAPK Pathway: *BRAF, NRAS,* and *KIT*

The Ras-Raf-MEK-ERK (or MAPK) pathway is over-activated in most melanomas (Fig. 15.1) [51]. In cutaneous melanoma, activation of this pathway mainly occurs through mutations leading to activation of the *BRAF*, *NRAS*, or *KIT* genes [51]. *BRAF* mutations are found in about 50% of cutaneous melanoma [45]. Similarly, conjunctival melanomas have about the same overall percentage of 50%, resembling the frequency found in cutaneous melanoma [10, 52, 53]. *BRAF* mutations have been identified as early events in conjunctival melanoma development, and these mutations are highly associated with sun exposure [10]. The conjunctiva is the only mucosal membrane exposed to the sun, and most *BRAF* mutated conjunctival melanomas are confined to the sun-exposed bulbar conjunctiva [10]. This suggests that conjunctival melanomas can be induced by both sun exposure and other factors.

Apart from the conjunctiva, *BRAF* mutations only occur in 10–17% of mucosal melanomas [3, 48, 54]. While frequent in cutaneous melanoma, *NRAS* mutations only seem to be present in 5–14% of mucosal melanomas [48, 49, 54]. An exception is a Swedish study that found *NRAS* mutations in 43% of vaginal melanomas, suggesting a different *NRAS* mutation rate among various locations [55].

While both *BRAF* and *NRAS* mutations are rare in mucosal melanoma, the MAPK pathway seems to be frequently activated by mutations in the *KIT* gene. This gene codes for an upstream tyrosine kinase (c-KIT or CD117) ultimately activating the MAPK pathway [48, 51]. Beadling et al. found *KIT* mutations in 15% of mucosal melanomas [56]. Swedish studies have identified *KIT* mutations in 4% (nasal cavity), 9% (anorectal), and 35% (vulva) of mucosal melanomas, suggesting considerable variation between tumor sites [54, 55]. Curtin et al. found *KIT* mutations and copy number increase in 39% of 102 primary mucosal melanomas of various locations [57]. Santi et al. screened 31 anorectal melanomas and

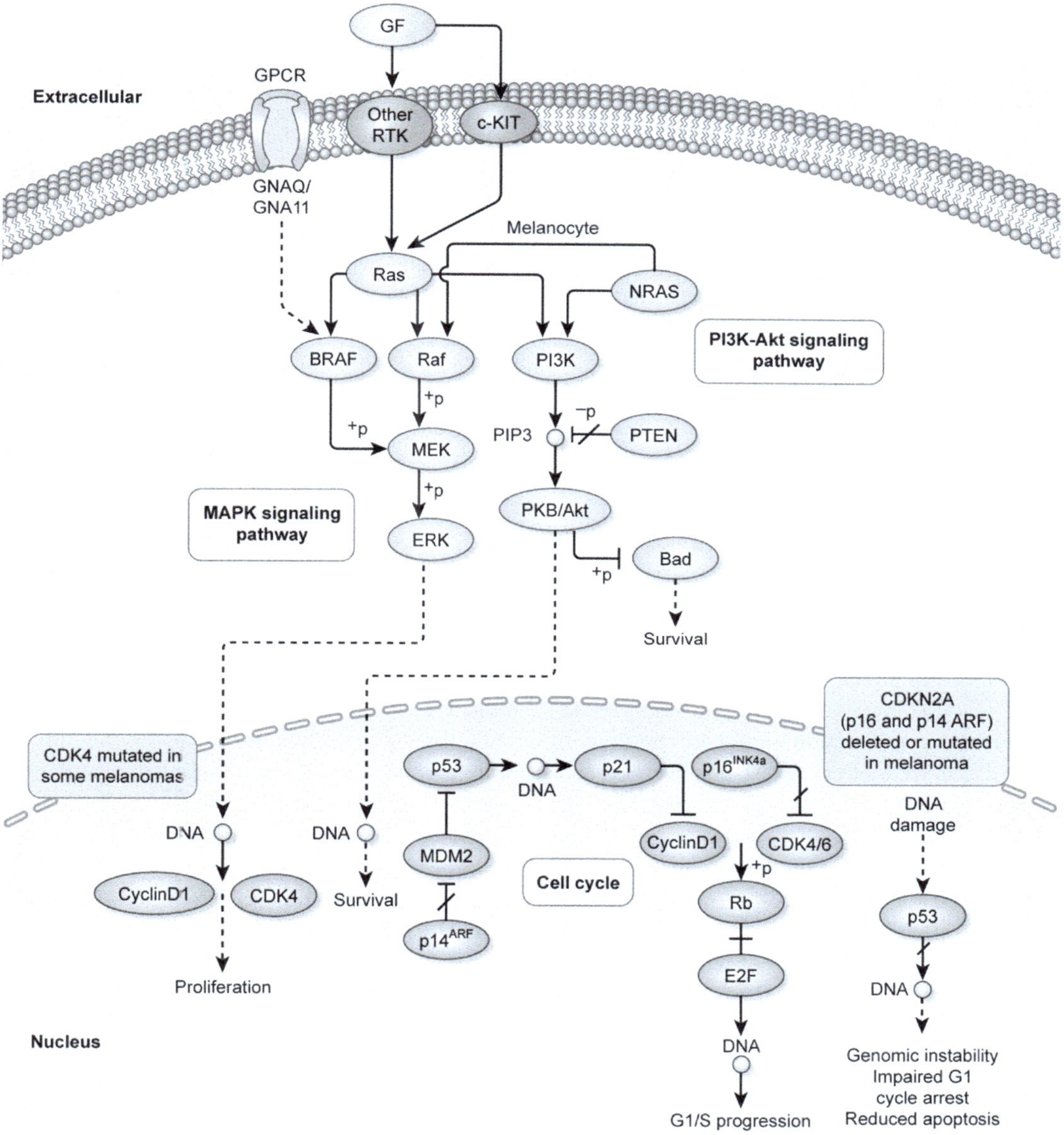

Fig. 15.1 Genetic alterations involved in the development of mucosal melanoma. Mucosal melanoma may develop due to four different mechanisms: activation of the MAPK pathway or the PI3K-Akt pathway, or mutations in the *CDKN2A* or *CDK4* genes. The MAPK pathway may be activated at several levels by mutations in numerous genes, including the *KIT*, *BRAF*, *NRAS*, and *GNAQ/GNA11* genes. Activation of this pathway results in proliferation of the tumor cell. The PI3K-Akt pathway may be activated by mutations in the *NRAS* or the *PTEN* genes resulting in enhanced survival of the tumor cell. Mutations in the *CDK4 or CDKN2A* genes may activate intranuclear pathways allowing the cell to progress into the cell cycle G1/S phase resulting in proliferation. *GF* growth factor, *GPCR* G protein-coupled receptor, *RTK* receptor tyrosine kinase, *P* phosphorylation

found *KIT* mutations in 35.5% [58]. Although there is some variation in the frequency reported by different authors, *KIT* is generally considered more important in mucosal melanoma compared to *NRAS* and *BRAF*.

Other Genetic Features

The PI3K-AKT and CDKN2A pathways have been shown to promote melanomagenesis, and it seems that these pathways are important in the development of mucosal melanoma (Fig. 15.1) [48]. Curtin et al. found a significantly altered expression of *PTEN* (a tumor suppressor that acts as an upstream inhibitor of the PI3K-AKT pathway) in mucosal melanomas compared to other melanoma subtypes [49]. A recent study reported the loss of *PTEN* in 50% of sinonasal melanomas [59]. Total loss of the CDKN2A locus and amplifications of the *CDK4* gene have also been found to be more common in mucosal melanomas compared to other melanoma subtypes [49]. Hsieh et al. found amplification and overexpression of cyclin D1 in 61% of cyclin D1-positive oral melanomas [60]. These findings suggest that the PI3K-AKT and CDKN2A pathways are important in the development of mucosal melanoma, in particular due to the relatively low frequency of identified mutations in genes affecting the MAPK pathway.

Uveal melanomas harbor aberrations of the *GNAQ* or the *GNA11* genes, but these mutations have never been identified in conjunctival melanoma [3]. On the other hand, *NRAS* and *BRAF* mutations are extremely rare in uveal melanoma [3]. *GNAQ/GNA11* mutations are generally not considered to occur in mucosal melanoma, but surprisingly a newer study found *GNAQ/GNA11* mutations in 9.5% (27/284) of mucosal melanomas in Chinese patients [61]. In this study, *GNAQ/GNA11* mutations were associated with a poor prognosis [61]. Targeted treatment for *GNAQ/GNA11* is currently not available [48].

Recent studies have identified *TERT* promoter region mutations in conjunctival melanoma and sinonasal melanomas; however, the role of these aberrations remains unclear [27, 62].

MiRNA Expression

Apart from studies utilizing human melanoma cell lines, the number of studies investigating miRNA in mucosal melanomas is very limited [63]. The largest study identified 25 differentially expressed miRNAs in 37 conjunctival melanomas. In this study, 24 miRNAs were upregulated and 1 was downregulated. Several of the identified miRNAs have previously been found in cutaneous melanoma. The study concluded that there was no difference in the expression of these 25 miRNAs compared to sinonasal melanoma [63]. Additional research is essential in order to identify potential prognostic miRNAs or therapeutic target miRNAs.

Diagnosis

Primary mucosal melanomas are rare conditions, and metastases to the mucosa from other melanomas always have to be excluded [3–5]. Therefore, a detailed clinical history should be obtained focusing on prior cutaneous, ocular, or mucosal melanomas [3]. A clinical full-body examination of the skin with the use of dermoscopy along with a full ophthalmological examination including ophthalmoscopy should always be performed in case of a suspected or confirmed mucosal melanoma [3]. The main differential diagnosis of a pigmented mucosal melanoma is a melanosis or a metastasis from a cutaneous melanoma. Macroscopically, melanomas appear as a flat, macular, or elevated lesion [3, 5]. The tumor may be polypoid, ulcerated, brown to black colored, and/or adherent to underlying tissue [3, 5]. Sinonasal melanomas often present as a polypoid, fleshy, or friable mass [2]. Amelanotic melanomas are frequent in all mucosal locations and may look like most other tumors without any specific tumor characteristics [3]. Most amelanotic vulvar melanomas emerge from glabrous skin [36]. The final diagnosis is made by histopathology [3, 5]. Uveal melanoma with extraocular extension should always be excluded in cases of a conjunctival melanoma [8, 39, 64].

Symptomatology

In general, symptoms of mucosal melanoma present at an advanced tumor stage [3–5]. The symptoms are mostly unspecific and relate to the affected organ system. The hallmark of conjunctival melanomas is the presence of a nodular, elevated tumor of the conjunctiva and only about 60% is pigmented brown or black [8, 14]. Patients with sinonasal melanoma often present with unilateral nasal obstruction, epistaxis, and a mass tumor [65]. In advanced stages, sinonasal melanoma may cause proptosis, diplopia, pain, and facial deformities [9]. Oral melanomas are often asymptomatic [20]. Laryngeal melanomas mainly present with hoarseness due to impingement upon the recurrent laryngeal nerve in some cases [2]. Esophageal melanomas may present with dysphagia and pain, and lower gastrointestinal melanomas may present with bleeding, anemia, bowel obstruction, weight loss, or pain [66, 67]. Urogenital melanomas may present with hematuria, bleeding, discharge, and dysuria [7, 68].

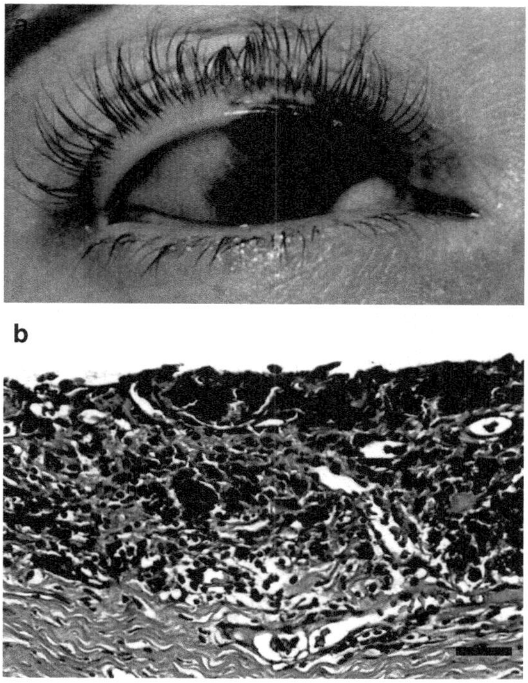

Fig. 15.2 Conjunctival melanoma. (**a**) Clinical photograph showing a conjunctival melanoma involving the upper palpebral conjunctiva. Melanomas at this location are non-UV-exposure induced and may share pathogenic features with mucosal melanomas confined to other sun-shielded mucosal membranes. (**b**) Micrograph of the same conjunctival melanoma. The tumor cells invade the stroma and abundant melanin is present (H&E, bar = 50 μm)

Location

Mucosal melanomas are found in all mucosal membranes, with a tendency for them to appear close to transition zones between the skin and mucosal membranes (Table 15.1) [3]. Studies also show that more melanocytes are found in mucosal membranes closer to the skin (e.g., the oral cavity or rectum) compared to more internal locations, such as the ileum [5]. This may be due to the relatively low number of tight junctions in mucosal membranes compared to the skin, allowing skin melanocytes to travel horizontally from the skin part of the transition zones into the mucosal membrane. Distant metastases from mucosal melanoma are mainly seen in the lung, liver, and non-regional lymph nodes [69]. Most conjunctival melanomas are confined to the sun-exposed limbal zone of the bulbar conjunctiva [8, 14, 34]. Melanomas of the palpebral conjunctiva and caruncle are rare (Fig. 15.2) [8, 14, 34].

Approximately 50% of mucosal melanomas of the head and neck are located in the sinonasal cavity, while about 40% confined to the oral cavity [2–4]. The majority of sinonasal melanomas are located in the anterior part of the inferior turbinates, followed by the septum and the middle turbinates [11, 70]. Melanoma in the paranasal sinuses is rare, with the maxillary sinus being the most commonly affected [11, 70]. Oral melanomas often involve the gingiva and the hard palate, while lesions in the buccal and lip mucosa are very rare [2, 11]. The remaining ~10% of head/neck melanomas are extremely rare and confined to the pharynx, supraglottic larynx, true vocal cords, and lungs [2, 3].

Distal gastrointestinal melanomas represent another large group of mucosal melanomas. The transitional zone is the area surrounding the dentate line that separates the anal skin from the rectal mucosal. It is important to distinguish between melanomas originating from the rectal mucosa (about 40%) and those originating from the abundant melanocytes in the proximal anal canal (about one-third), since the latter have a skin origin and are not classified as pure mucosal melanomas [4]. Other gastrointestinal melanomas are mainly found in the middle or lower esophagus, ileum, ascending colon, and neck of the gall bladder. Most vaginal melanomas are located in the anterior wall within the lower third of the vagina [7]. In about 85% of vulvar melanoma, the tumor originates in the labia minora, clitoris, or inner (glabrous, non-hairy) part of the labia majora [7]. Urethral melanoma is often located in the distal part of the urethra [7]. Bladder melanoma can be found in all parts of the bladder [7]. Penile melanoma is often found on the glans [3].

Radiology and Imaging

Radiological examination is important for accurate tumor staging, surgical planning, and surveillance of patients [69, 71]. The Danish Melanoma Group recommends the use of a computed tomography (CT) scan along with magnetic resonance imaging (MRI) in order to characterize the extent of sinonasal melanomas [72]. The National Comprehensive Cancer Network (NCCN) recommends chest imaging in cases of a biopsy-confirmed mucosal melanoma [73]. A positron emission tomography/computer tomography (PET/CT) fusion scan is recommended to detect potential clinically unsuspected metastatic disease [72, 73]. Apart from mucosal melanomas in the head and neck region, CT and PET/CT are of relatively limited value in the evaluation of local disease [71]. The MRI features of mucosal melanoma depend on the melanin content and the presence or absence of hemorrhage [74]. Melanotic melanomas can be separated from other tumors because they reveal a distinct MRI signal pattern comprised of a hyperintense signal on T1-weighted scans and a hypointense signal on T2-weighted scans [74]. Mucosal melanomas are often seen as a homogenous enhancement pattern on MRI [74]. A combined [^{18}F]fluorodeoxyglucose-PET/CT scan has been shown to be superior to a conventional CT scan in detecting lymph node metastasis and distant metastases in anorectal melanoma [24]. Although the role of this scan is well established in cutaneous melanoma management, its utility still needs further validation in large-scale trials regarding mucosal melanoma [71].

Biopsy

Incisional biopsies are associated with an unfavorable prognosis in conjunctival melanoma and should be avoided [14, 40]. There have not been any studies evaluating the role of incisional biopsies in mucosal melanomas outside the conjunctiva, with a standard tissue biopsy, such as a punch or shave biopsy, currently recommended in order to establish the definitive diagnosis [3, 33]. In mucosal melanoma, the diagnosis must be established on the basis of a full-thickness biopsy of the lesion [75]. In vulvar melanoma, excisional biopsies are the preferred method of tissue diagnosis [75].

Histopathology and Immunohistochemistry

Histopathological examination is recommended in all mucosal melanomas in order to confirm the diagnosis and stage of the tumor [3, 72]. The histological features of mucosal melanoma are similar to those found in cutaneous melanomas, with tumors showing a range from epithelioid to spindle-shaped tumor cells, including mixed types (Fig. 15.3). Amelanotic mucosal melanomas are frequently found and have been reported in up to 45% of cases [43]. The melanoma cells may grow in a sheetlike fashion or in nests [3, 8, 37, 39]. Approximately 75% of conjunctival melanomas are associated with a preexisting PAM with atypia, and 20% are associated with a nevus or PAM without atypia [8, 39]. Invasion of tumor cells from the epithelium into the substantia propria is the hallmark of any mucosal melanoma [39].

Pathologic analysis of suspected lesions includes immunohistochemical staining for

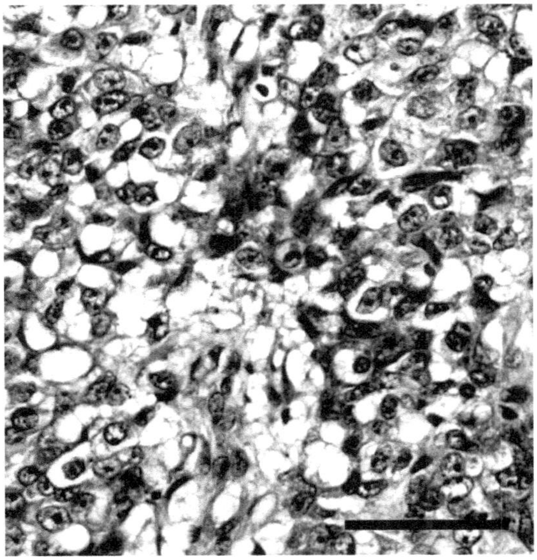

Fig. 15.3 High-power micrograph of a melanoma in the small intestine. Pleomorphic epithelioid tumor cells are seen with large polymorphic nuclei. Mitotic figures are observed (H&E, bar = 50 μm)

S-100, HMB-45, tyrosinase, and Melan-A/Mart-1 [3, 37, 64]. Melan-A with red chromogen may be quite useful in order to separate tumor cells from pigment. A proliferative tumor cell index, such as Ki-67, is highly recommended within the final pathology report. Furthermore, the mutational status regarding *BRAF* and *KIT* genes should be evaluated in order to identify those patients who may be a candidate for select targeted therapy [76].

Staging

There is currently no universal system for the staging of mucosal melanomas [3]. Clark's level is not applicable due to the diverging anatomy and absence of histological landmarks in mucosal membranes compared to skin. The 8th Edition of the American Joint Committee on Cancer (AJCC) tumor-node-metastasis (TNM) classification system suggests a staging system regarding upper respiratory tract melanomas [77]. This classification starts with T3 primary tumors, ignoring smaller T1 and T2 tumors. The AJCC manual suggests both a clinical and pathological staging system for conjunctival melanoma [77]. Apart from the AJCC classification, other systems for head/neck melanoma have been proposed by various authors [65, 78–80].

Tumor thickness seems to be an important prognostic factor in most kinds of melanoma [3, 80, 81]. Ballantyne et al. have suggested a simple three-step staging system that includes stage 1 (localized disease), stage 2 (lymph node involvement), and stage 3 diseases (distant metastases) [79]. Prasad et al. proposed a classification system based upon histological evaluation of tumor invasion that is divided into three distinct tissue compartments, inclusive of melanoma in situ [78]. This system appears to be useful in predicting poor survival for patients with localized, lymph node-negative, and early-stage head/neck melanoma [78]. Another staging system for head/neck melanomas has been proposed by Thompson et al. based on the TNM system. In this system, the presence of distant metastases was the most important factor in predicting patient survival [65]. However, the AJCC classification has been shown to be beneficial in staging sinonasal melanoma [82]. Oral melanomas may be staged according to the AJCC or according to a simple TNM staging system that is combined with a microstaging system of stage 2 tumors, as proposed by Meleti et al. [83].

It has been suggested that the most appropriate staging for anorectal melanoma should allow for some variations of the TNM classification system; however, no true consensus has been agreed upon [24, 84]. The staging for vaginal melanoma primarily utilizes the current AJCC staging system for cutaneous melanoma [85]. Due to the lack of surface keratin and granular layers of the vaginal mucosal membrane, Breslow's thickness should be properly measured from the mucosal surface to the deepest level of invasion within the mucosal membranes [85]. Vulvar melanomas may be staged using the AJCC staging system for cutaneous melanoma [85]. A universal staging algorithm is needed in order to have an accurate method of comparison between tumors of different mucosal origin.

Treatment and Prognosis

The current recommended management of mucosal melanoma is generally based upon physician experience and small cohort studies of treatment, with some difficulty in developing evidence-based treatment guidelines. Although definitive, and often radical, resection has long been the initial treatment of choice, less invasive and morbid procedures have been examined in recent years [6, 22]. There does not appear to be a major difference in survival or clinical outcome between those patients treated with radical surgery and less invasive procedures [3]. A thorough discussion about all possible treatment options with patients and family members is very important, with mutual decision-making based upon the risks and benefits of each treatment modality. The quality of life and associated morbidities of a radical surgery should be discussed in detail before definitive surgery is recommended. The role of lymph node biopsies and/or elective node dissection remains unclear. It is highly advisable to include mucosal melanoma patients in any possible clinical trials utilizing novel, nonoperative therapies, especially those with an advanced tumor stage where surgery may result in significant morbidity and/or disfigurement.

Surgery

Conjunctival Melanoma

Ophthalmologists treat all three melanoma subtypes: uveal melanoma, conjunctival melanoma, and cutaneous melanoma on the eyelids [86]. Conjunctival melanomas represent only 5% of these tumors, and the majority are confined to the sun-exposed bulbar conjunctiva [8, 15]. The treatment of choice is complete surgical resection (*en bloc*) using a no-touch technique with a 3–5 mm surgical margin [17, 34, 87]. To avoid local recurrences, at least one additional treatment modality has to be applied: local brachytherapy, cryotherapy, or local chemotherapy (mitomycin C, interferon alfa-2b, or 5-fluorouracil) [14, 17, 27, 34]. In a large Danish study, patients treated with surgery alone without adjuvant therapy showed an increased risk of both locoregional and distant metastases, with increased risks of melanoma-related and all-cause mortality [14]. Poor prognostic factors include extrabulbar location, increased tumor thickness, nodular appearance, and de novo origin [8, 14, 35]. Local recurrence is very common and is also a poor prognostic sign. Lymphatic spread to regional lymph nodes, as well as to distant sites, such as skin, adrenal glands, brain, and lungs, has been reported [8, 17, 34]. The melanoma-related 10-year mortality rate is approximately 30% [8, 14, 15, 17, 88]. Sentinel lymph node biopsy has been suggested as a safe and feasible procedure in evaluating conjunctival melanoma [89, 90]. However, there is a need for large-scale studies investigating the relationship between a positive sentinel node and ultimate clinical outcome [90].

Mucosal Melanoma of the Sinonasal and Oral Cavity

Melanomas of the mucosal membranes in the head/neck region constitute about 50% of all mucosal melanomas located outside the conjunctiva [2–4]. Surgery remains the gold standard in head/neck mucosal melanoma [2, 3, 72, 73]. The NCCN and the Danish Melanoma Group have produced detailed guidelines regarding head/neck melanoma management [3, 73]. The NCCN treatment guidelines suggest wide surgical resection followed by adjuvant radiotherapy as the treatment of choice regarding AJCC stage T3 and T4aN0 tumors [73]. In addition, the guidelines also suggest some form of neck dissection in cases of a positive lymph node (T3–T4aN1 tumors) [73]. Primary radiotherapy or systemic chemotherapy is recommended for treatment of T4b and T4c tumors [73]. Mutilating procedures are discouraged, and, even with complete resection, recurrence rates of up to 50% are observed. Therefore, some authors advocate considering aggressive adjuvant therapy, regardless of margin status [26, 70].

According to the NCCN guidelines, melanoma of the oral cavity should be managed with wide surgical resection for T3 and T4a tumors [73]. It is suggested that more advanced tumor stages be managed with primary radiotherapy or systemic chemotherapy [73]. The Danish Melanoma Group recommends primary surgery for all head/neck melanomas, concluding that adjuvant radiotherapy or systemic chemotherapy may be beneficial for local control [72]. However, the use of adjuvant therapy has not been associated with improved survival compared to treatment with surgery alone [11, 43]. An *en bloc* resection should be attempted whenever feasible, with intraoperative frozen section analysis performed for margins whenever possible [33, 73].

Approximately 80% of sinonasal melanomas present as a localized disease, with only a few cases identified as having lymph node or distant metastases at the time of diagnosis [2]. However, up to 50% of patients will present with distant metastases during the course of their disease [2]. A Danish study found recurrence in 72% of patients, regardless of treatment [11]. The 3-year overall survival rate for sinonasal melanoma is about 45%, with a 5-year survival rate of ~30% [11, 26, 91]. The 5-year survival rate of oral melanoma is ~15% [3, 33]. Histologically, confirmed negative resection margins seem to be a positive predictor for survival in head and neck melanomas, but unfortunately this can be technically difficult to achieve due to the complex anatomical structures [11, 26, 43, 91]. Advanced age, multiple tumor sites, presence of necrosis, and amelanotic tumor histology have all been shown to negatively impact long-term survival [26, 37, 43].

In recent years, surgeons have favored the use of endoscopic resection in order to reduce post-surgical morbidity [3]. A recent study found a significantly better survival rate in patients who underwent an endoscopically assisted surgery compared to patients who only received open surgery [92]. Endoscopic resection has not been associated with an increased risk of death compared with more radical surgical procedures, such as craniofacial resection [91]. In general, elective lymph node dissection is not routinely performed or recommended in mucosal melanoma of the head and neck [73]. However, due to a high frequency of lymph node spread in oral melanoma, lymph node dissection may be performed [11].

Mucosal Melanoma of the Anus and Rectum

Approximately 25% of these tumors seem to be without evidence of pigmentation, deemed amelanotic [93]. Due to the fact that a high percentage of cutaneous melanoma patients will present with gastrointestinal metastases on autopsy, all patients with gastrointestinal melanomas should be carefully examined for metastatic disease from a regressed cutaneous melanoma [24, 67]. Aside from the above-mentioned radiological imaging modalities, this includes upper endoscopy, colonoscopy, and video endoscopy of the small bowel in order to exclude metastatic disease. Surgery remains the treatment of choice, but unfortunately no guidelines regarding optimal surgical management exist [3, 24]. Historically, anorectal melanoma has been treated with an abdominoperineal resection, but in recent years the less invasive transanal excision has been favored [22]. The choice of surgical intervention is still controversial and agreement on a gold standard of treatment has not been firmly established. Large, retrospective epidemiological studies have not shown a significant difference in overall survival when comparing the different surgical approaches [22, 24].

Due to the associated postoperative morbidity, transanal excision with free margins should be favored, with more radical procedures such as abdominoperineal resection reserved for those patients where less invasive procedures are not feasible [22]. Histologically free surgical margins seem to correlate with improvements in overall survival [22, 94]. Patients without free margins on transanal excision may be reoperated on, either with a second attempt at transanal excision or with salvage/delayed abdominoperineal resection [22]. Wide local excision has not been shown to alter the median survival time [94]. Patients with perirectal lymph node metastases identified on PET/CT may benefit from curative abdominoperineal resection [24]. The prognosis is particularly poor, with a mean survival time of about 20 months, for both anal and rectum melanoma, regardless of the type of surgical intervention chosen [67].

The overall 5-year survival rate is <20% for rectal melanomas and only 10% when lymph node metastases are present [22]. Some studies suggest a longer median survival (27 months) regarding rectal melanomas [93]. The overall prognosis for anal melanomas (10% 5-year survival) seems to be lower than for rectal melanomas [93]. Recurrence is quite frequent and occurs in about 60% of anal and 70% of rectal melanomas [22, 67, 93]. Presence of distant metastases has a particularly poor prognosis with no long-term survivors beyond 5 years [22]. Negative lymph node status at the time of surgery seems to improve the prognosis, suggesting a role of lymph node resection in the management [22, 67]. However, large-scale studies will be needed in order to guide the development of meaningful treatment protocols. Cases of laparoscopic abdominoperineal resection have been reported, with larger studies needed to further evaluate this technique as a valid operative approach [95].

Melanoma of the Vulva

Most vulvar melanomas are actual cutaneous melanomas, mainly located in non-sun-exposed areas. For many years, the standard treatment of vulvar melanoma was a radical vulvectomy, regardless of tumor size, location, thickness, or level of invasion [7]. However, the overall survival does not seem to improve with radical surgery compared to wide local excision and hemi- or partial vulvectomy [7]. It is advisable to excise a vulvar melanoma with a Breslow's thickness of <2.0 mm with clinical margins of at least 1 cm. Vulvar melanoma with a thickness >2.0 mm should be excised with a 2 cm margin of surrounding skin [28].

The role of lymph node dissection in vulvar melanoma remains controversial [96]. Sentinel lymph node mapping of the inguinal nodal basins by an experienced surgeon is technically feasible, and is currently recommended in the management of vulvar melanoma [28]. Lymphadenectomy may be considered in select patients where palpable or clinically suspicious regional adenopathy is identified [28]. Poor prognostic factors are the presence of ulceration, macroscopic amelanosis, advanced age, Breslow's thickness >2.0 mm, and advanced AJCC stage [96, 97]. In recent years, the 5-year overall survival of vulvar melanoma has improved to about 80% for early-stage tumors [85, 96]. However, recurrence rates are close to 60%, and the 5-year survival rate for more advanced tumor stages remaining at about 30% [28, 96].

Mucosal Melanoma of the Vagina

The optimal surgical approach for vaginal melanoma has not been firmly established. It is evident that patients treated surgically have a better prognosis than those treated without surgery [98]. Vaginal melanoma has historically been surgically managed with forms of "radical" surgery, such as a pelvic exenteration. Unfortunately, "radical" surgery in this case is poorly defined, covering a variety of surgical procedures that range from local excision with total hysterectomy, subtotal vaginectomy, vaginectomy without vulvectomy and total vulvectomy, etc. [99]. Radical surgery has not been proven to increase the long-term prognosis compared to more conservative procedures, and in recent years the treatment of choice has been wide local excision of the primary mucosal melanoma with surgical margin of 1–2 cm [100, 101]. Authors suggest at least a 1 cm margin regarding tumors with a Breslow's depth of <2 mm, and a 2 cm margin for melanomas that are >2 mm in thickness [98]. Furthermore, radical procedures are often associated with an increased morbidity and a decreased quality of life due to the complexity of the operation and close anatomical relationship to the surrounding structures.

Recently, a Japanese group attempted to carry out a systematic review of radical procedures for the treatment of vaginal melanoma, examining whether radical surgery improves the short-term survival and locoregional control [99]. This study introduced a scoring system to classify the grade of radicality in various procedures and concluded that vaginal melanoma patients may benefit from more radical procedures [99]. However, total pelvic exenteration does not seem to significantly increase the overall survival [98]. Larger studies on the effect of radical vs. non-radical procedures are thus necessary. Systemic recurrence continues to be a major problem, as high as 80% in some studies (80%), metastasizing to the liver and lungs in many instances [98, 100]. Many will present with disseminated disease at the time of initial diagnosis, with a poor 5-year survival rate of ~20% [7, 98]. The role for sentinel lymph node biopsy or elective lymphadenectomy is unclear and possibly considered with each patient, taking into account the associated risks and morbidity associated with complete [28, 98].

Mucosal Melanoma of Other Rare Sites

Due to the very small number of cases of mucosal melanoma confined to other locations than the above mentioned, it is difficult to define the role of different treatment regimens in these tumors. Radical surgery is the treatment of choice regarding melanomas of the larynx, lung, stomach, small and large intestines, biliary tract, uterine cervix, urethra, penis, and urinary bladder [3, 7, 19, 23, 67, 68, 100, 102–106]. However, the prognosis for these rare tumor sites remains extremely poor (see Table 15.1). Most mucosal melanomas may spread to regional lymph nodes at an early stage, but the prognostic role of these metastases remains unknown [102].

Radiotherapy

In general, mucosal melanomas are not considered to be radiosensitive; thus the role and utility of radiotherapy remain unclear [3, 26, 33, 107]. Definitive radiotherapy of head/neck mucosal melanoma has not been shown to significantly benefit patients with respect to local control or overall survival [26, 43, 92, 107]. This may be due to the fact that most patients treated primarily with radiation suffer from an advanced, inoperable tumor stage or that the patient may not be a surgical candidate [26, 107]. A systematic review of head/neck melanoma management concluded that local control rates ranged from 0 to 61% and that overall 5-year survival rates were as low as 13–18% [26].

Authors have reported total radiation dosages exceeding 50 Gy, with no clear association between total dose and overall survival observed [26, 107]. The NCCN treatment guidelines for advanced head/neck melanoma management recommend radiotherapy for gross disease using a conventional fractionation scheme (2 Gy per fraction to a total postoperative dose of 60–66 Gy, possibly up to 70 Gy) [73]. Few studies have compared the effect of conventional fractionation with that of hypofractionation, and the results have been inconclusive [26]. Primary radiotherapy may be attempted for advanced-stage cervical melanoma primarily for palliation of symptoms [100, 108]. Overall, primary radiotherapy should be considered an option in cases of non-operable mucosal melanoma due to significant tumor spread or medical inoperability [7, 26, 107]. It has not been possible to identify an optimal fractionation scheme, with the radiotherapy regimen determined by a radiation oncologist on a patient-per-patient basis [7, 26, 107]. The ability to tolerate the radiation dosage, proximity of the tumor to surrounding critical structures, and overall performance status must be taken into account in all treatment decisions [107].

Adjuvant radiotherapy has been associated with improved local control in mucosal melanomas. However, it does not seem to affect overall survival or the development of distant metastases, regardless of primary tumor location [11, 26, 92, 98, 109, 110]. Some authors suggest that adjuvant radiotherapy is only indicated in head/neck melanoma with negative surgical margins, nodal metastases, and critical structure involvement (i.e., the dura) [91]. Most authors suggest the use of a total dosage exceeding 50 Gy in the adjuvant setting for head/neck melanoma [26]. The role of radiation therapy in anorectal melanoma remains controversial and relatively unknown. Some authors suggest local excision in combination with hypofractionated radiotherapy as a sphincter-sparing alternative to abdominoperineal resection [109]. Adjuvant radiotherapy in combination with surgery may be beneficial compared to surgery alone in the treatment of anorectal melanoma [24]. A large systematic review of genital melanoma suggests that the use of adjuvant radiotherapy in advanced tumor stages may be beneficial in obtaining locoregional control [24]. Conjunctival melanoma may be treated effectively using a ruthenium^{106}-plaque. The plaque may be used as an adjuvant therapy after surgery [111]. Adjuvant local brachytherapy using a vaginal cesium^{137}-cylinder has also been proposed in vaginal melanoma [7, 101].

Novel Radiotherapy

The role of particle radiotherapy has not yet been firmly established in mucosal melanoma. Due to the poor and inconclusive results of photon radiotherapy regarding survival, particle beam radiotherapy may be a favorable treatment modality of mucosal melanoma in the future. High-dose proton beam therapy has shown some initial promising results in the treatment of head/neck melanoma [112]. A proton beam has the unique physical feature called the Bragg peak, which allows the beam to deposit maximum energy in the tissue at a designated depth [112]. In a Japanese study, 20 patients followed a hypofractionated treatment schedule of 3.5 Gy relative biological effectiveness (RBE) per fraction, administered daily with a total dose of 70 Gy RBE (20 fractions) [112]. In this study, the overall 5-year survival time was 54% and equal to that of surgery [112]. Zenda et al. allocated 32 sinonasal melanoma patients to a hypofractionated scheme administering a total 60 Gy equivalents (GyE) in 15 fractions with a dose fraction of 4 Gy [113]. The 3-year survival in this study was 46% and comparable to conventional photon radiotherapy [113].

Fast neutron radiotherapy is a high linear energy transfer (LET) radiation that has shown to be effective in radioresistant malignancies by generating significant tumor cell death compared to a low LET [26]. Furthermore, the total dose is particularly lower than using photon radiotherapy [26]. Liao et al. reviewed 14 patients treated with fast neutron radiotherapy and found increased locoregional control with a 5-year local control rate of 66% [114]. However, the overall survival was not significantly different, with patients dying due to early distant metastases [114]. Two patients developed serious osteoradionecrosis as an adverse effect [114].

Carbon-ion radiotherapy has both the biological advantage of the high LET from the neutron beam and the same physical properties, and as with proton beam therapy includes the Bragg peak [26]. A Japanese study including 72 head/neck melanoma patients found a 5-year overall locoregional control rate of 84%, with a 5-year survival rate of 39% [115]. Naganawa et al. treated 19 oral mucosal melanoma patients with carbon-ion therapy and found a 5-year local control rate of almost 90% along with an overall survival of 57%, suggesting that carbon-ion radiotherapy is an effective treatment for oral malignant melanoma [116]. A study investigating carbon-ion radiotherapy of gynecological melanoma found a local control rate of 50% and an overall survival equal to surgery, with acceptable adverse effects that were deemed tolerable [117]. These findings suggest that carbon-ion therapy could be a favorable therapy regarding local control in head/neck mucosal melanoma.

Robotic stereotactic body radiotherapy using the CyberKnife® has shown promising results in the treatment of head and neck cancers regarding local control and toxicity [26]. The advantages of the CyberKnife® are the ability to deliver high doses of energy to the tumors and sparing of the adjacent unaffected peripheral tissues and/or organs [26]. Ozyigit et al. reported on four patients with mucosal melanoma treated with the CyberKnife®, two for definitive treatment and two in the adjuvant setting [118]. Three patients demonstrated complete remission and one patient had a partial remission [118].

Chemotherapy

In general, standard chemotherapy and biotherapy have not been shown to be effective in mucosal melanoma. Regimens including various combinations of cisplatin, vinblastine, temozolomide, dacarbazine, interferon-α, or interleukins have been proposed [5–7, 75]. Dacarbazine in combination with interferon-α and interleukin-2 has shown some benefit in head/neck melanoma [9]. Lian et al. found some effect of a regimen combining temozolomide and cisplatin in the postoperative treatment of resected mucosal melanoma [119]. However, the results of these therapies are not so promising regarding mucosal melanoma, with a considerable risk of developing serious toxic effects [6, 75, 100]. The role of chemotherapy used as preoperative or adjuvant therapy remains unclear because of the lack of consistency in the literature. The patient groups are extremely heterogeneous and the regimens are rarely explained in detail [24].

Targeted Therapy

As previously mentioned, a large fraction of mucosal melanomas seems to harbor amplifications of the *KIT* gene. The KIT inhibitor, imatinib, has been shown to be effective in the treatment of cutaneous melanoma [6, 120]. It also appears that such patients with *KIT* amplifications may benefit from imatinib [6, 121]. Patients harboring aberrations in exon 11 (L576P) or exon 13 (K642E) show better response rates compared to patients having *KIT* amplifications or alterations in other regions [4, 6, 28, 120]. It is advisable to rule out *NRAS* mutation before initiating KIT inhibitor treatment, because an underlying *NRAS* mutation may activate the MAPK pathway downstream of the *KIT* mutation [76].

The BRAF inhibitors, dabrafenib and vemurafenib, have revolutionized the treatment of metastatic cutaneous melanoma [6]. Many authors suggest BRAF inhibition as a promising advance in the treatment of mucosal melanoma. However, the rate of *BRAF* mutations in mucosal melanoma is relatively low, limiting this as a potent treatment option for mucosal melanoma [2, 120]. We recommend screening for *BRAF* mutation, and, if the mutation is present, similar treatment regimens utilized for cutaneous melanoma may be applicable. It is notable that most melanomas will develop resistance to single-agent BRAF inhibition, and a combination with a MEK inhibitor has been shown to increase both disease-free and overall survival [122–124].

Immunotherapy

Treatment with ipilimumab, a monoclonal antibody that blocks the cytotoxic T-lymphocyte antigen-4 (CTLA-4) receptor, has been shown to impact the overall survival in the treatment of advanced cutaneous melanoma [6, 120]. No randomized trials exist at present for the treatment of mucosal melanoma, but smaller case studies demonstrate a benefit of this agent in treating mucosal melanoma [4, 6]. One such study showed a 12% response rate along with an overall survival time of 4.3–6.4 months [125].

Another novel treatment option is identification of an antibody that blocks the programmed death-1 (PD-1) receptor on activated T cells, which ultimately leads to an enhanced ability of the T cells to eradicate tumor cells. Two PD-1 antibodies, nivolumab and pembrolizumab, have been approved for the first-line treatment of metastatic melanoma [126–128]. Response rates of up to 32% have been identified in mucosal melanoma, which are comparable to those found in cutaneous melanoma [129]. Thus, it is clear that checkpoint inhibition therapy has become a promising treatment option in mucosal melanoma, with further studies planned for the future. A large, pooled analysis of data for anti-PD-1 therapy in combination with ipilimumab in mucosal melanoma has shown that this combination has a synergistic efficacy when compared to each given alone. However, combination therapy was associated with high rates of grade 3 or 4 adverse effects [127]. Given the fast development of novel agents, these must be studied in large, multicenter studies of mucosal melanoma.

References

1. Chang AE, Karnell LH, Menck HR. The National Cancer Data Base report on cutaneous and noncutaneous melanoma. Cancer. 1998;85:1664–78.
2. Lourenco S, Fernandes J, Hsieh R, Coutinho-Camillo CM, Bologna S, Sangueza M, et al. Head and neck mucosal melanoma: a review. Am J Dermatopathol. 2014;36(7):578–87.
3. Mikkelsen LH, Larsen AC, Buchwald CV, Drzewiecki KT, Prause JU, Heegaard S. Mucosal malignant melanoma—a clinical, oncological, pathological and genetic survey. APMIS. 2016;124(6):475–86.
4. Carvajal RD, Spencer S, Lydiatt W. Mucosal melanoma: a clinically and biologically unique disease entity. J Natl Compr Cancer Netw. 2012;10(3):345–56.
5. Mihajlovic M, Vlajkovic S, Jovanovic P, Stefanovic V. Primary mucosal melanomas: a comprehensive review. Int J Clin Exp Pathol. 2012;5(8):739–53.

6. Spencer KR, Mehnert JM. Mucosal melanoma: epidemiology, biology and treatment. Cancer Treat Res. 2016;167:295–320.
7. Piura B. Management of primary melanoma of the female urogenital tract. Lancet Oncol. 2008;9:973–81.
8. Seregard S. Conjunctival melanoma. Surv Ophthalmol. 1998;42(4):321–50.
9. Gavriel H, McArthur G, Sizeland A. Review: mucosal melanoma of the head and neck. Melanoma Res. 2011;21(4):257–66.
10. Larsen AC, Dahl C, Dahmcke CM, Lade-Keller J, Siersma VD, Toft PB, et al. BRAF mutations in conjunctival melanoma: investigation of incidence, clinicopathological features, prognosis and paired premalignant lesions. Acta Ophthalmol. 2016;94(5):463–70.
11. Lawaetz M, Birch-Johansen F, Friis S, Eriksen JG, Kiss K, Gade S, et al. Primary mucosal melanoma of the head and neck in Denmark, 1982–2012: Demographic and clinical aspects. A retrospective DAHANCA study. Acta Oncol (Stockholm, Sweden). 2016;55(8):1001–8.
12. McLaughlin CC, Wu XC, Jemal A, Martin HJ, Roche LM, Chen VW. Incidence of noncutaneous melanomas in the U.S. Cancer. 2005;103:1000–7.
13. Jangard M, Hansson J, Ragnarsson-Olding B. Primary sinonasal malignant melanoma: a nationwide study of the Swedish population, 1960–2000. Rhinology. 2013;51(1):22–30.
14. Larsen AC, Dahmcke CM, Dahl C, Siersma VD, Toft PB, Coupland SE, et al. Conjunctival melanoma: a retrospective review of presentation, treatment and outcome and investigation of features associated with BRAF mutations. JAMA Ophthalmol. 2015;133(11):1295–303.
15. Isager P, Østerlind A, Engholm G, Lindegaard J, Heegaard S, Overgaard J, et al. Uveal and conjunctival malignant melanoma in Denmark, 1943–97: incidence and validation study. Ophthalmic Epidemiol. 2005;12:223–32.
16. Triay E, Bergman L, Nilsson B, All-Eircsson C, Seregard S. Time trends in the incidence of conjunctival melanoma in Sweden. Br J Ophthalmol. 2009;93:1524–8.
17. Tuomaala S, Eskelin S, Tarkkanen A, Kivelä T. Population-based assessment of clinical characteristics predicting outcome of conjunctival melanoma in whites. Invest Ophthalmol Vis Sci. 2002;43:3399–408.
18. Callahan A, Anderson WF, Patel S, Barnholtz-Sloan JS, Bordeaux JS, Tucker MA, et al. Epidemiology of anorectal melanoma in the United States: 1992 to 2011. Dermatol Surg. 2016;42(1):94–9.
19. Terada T, Saeki N, Toh K, Uwa N, Sagawa K, Mouri T, et al. Primary malignant melanoma of the larynx: a case report and literature review. Auris Nasus Larynx. 2007;34:105–10.
20. Hicks MJ, Flaitz CM. Oral mucosal melanoma: epidemiology and pathobiology. Oral Oncol. 2000;36: 152–69.
21. Sabanathan S, Eng J, Pradhan GN. Primary malignant melanoma of the esophagus. Am J Gastroenterol. 1989;84:1475–81.
22. Iddings DM, Fleisig AJ, Chen SL, Faries MB, Morton DL. Practice patterns and outcomes for anorectal melanoma in the USA, reviewing three decades of treatment: is more extensive surgical resection beneficial in all patients? Ann Surg Oncol. 2010;17:40–4.
23. Oliva E, Quinn TR, Amin MB, Eble JN, Epstein JI, Srigley JR, et al. Primary malignant melanoma of the urethra: a clinicopathologic analysis of 15 cases. Am J Surg Pathol. 2000;24(6):785–96.
24. Falch C, Mueller S, Kirschniak A, Braun M, Koenigsrainer A, Klumpp B. Anorectal malignant melanoma: curative abdominoperineal resection: patient selection with 18F-FDG-PET/CT. World J Surg Oncol. 2016;14(1):185.
25. Neugut AI, Kizelnik-Freilich S, Ackerman C. Black-White differences in risk for cutaneous, ocular, and visceral melanomas. Am J Public Health. 1994;84(11):1828–9.
26. Lazarev S, Gupta V, Hu K, Harrison LB, Bakst R. Mucosal melanoma of the head and neck: a systematic review of the literature. Int J Radiat Oncol Biol Phys. 2014;90(5):1108–18.
27. Sheng X, Li S, Chi Z, Si L, Cui C, Mao L, et al. Prognostic factors for conjunctival melanoma: a study in ethnic Chinese patients. Br J Ophthalmol. 2015;99(25):990–6.
28. Leitao MM Jr. Management of vulvar and vaginal melanomas: current and future strategies. Am Soc Clin Oncol Educ Book. 2014;2014:e277–81.
29. Agarwalla PK, Koch MJ, Mordes DA, Codd PJ, Coumans JV. Pigmented lesions of the nervous system and the neural crest: Lessons from embryology. Neurosurgery. 2015;78(1):142–54.
30. Saida T, Kawachi S, Takata M, Kurita H, Kurashina K, Kageshita T, et al. Histopathological characteristics of malignant melanoma affecting mucous membranes : a unifying concept of histogenesis. Pathology. 2004;36(5):404–13.
31. Righi A, Dimosthenous K. Primary malignant melanoma of the rectum arisinf against a background of rectal melanosis. Int J Surg Pathol. 2008;16(3):335–6.
32. Guzman RP, Wightman R, Ravinsky E, Unruh HW. Primary malignant melanoma of the eosophagus with diffuse melanocytic atypia and melanoma in situ. Am J Clin Pathol. 1984;92:802–4.
33. Meleti M, Mooi WJ, Casparie MK, van der Waal I. Melanocytic nevi of the oral mucosa—no evidence of increased risk for oral malignant melanoma; An analysis of 119 cases. Oral Oncol. 2007;43:976–81.
34. Missotten GS, Keijser S, De Keizer RJ, De Wolff-Rouendaal D. Conjunctival melanoma in the Netherlands: a nationwide study. Invest Ophthalmol Vis Sci. 2005;46:75–82.
35. Shields CL, Markowitz JS, Belinsky I, Schwartzstein H, George NS, Lally SE. Conjunctival melanoma:

outcomes based on tumour origin in 382 consecutive cases. Ophthalmology. 2011;118(2):389–95.
36. Ragnarsson-Olding BK, Kanter-Lewensohn LR, Lagerlöf B, Nilsson BR, Ringborg UK. Malignant melanoma of the vulva in a nationwide , 25-year study of 219 Swedish females clinical observations and histopathologic features. Cancer. 1999;86(7):1273–84.
37. Mochel MC, Duncan LM, Piris A, Kraft S. Primary mucosal melanoma of the sinonasal tract: a clinicopathologic and immunohistochemical study of thirty-two cases. Head Neck Pathol. 2015;9(2):236–43.
38. Sedassari BT, Lascane NA, de Freitas AL, Mautoni MC, Sotto MN, Gallottini MH, et al. In situ melanoma of the gingiva associated with dense inflammation and pigment deposition: a potential diagnostic pitfall in evaluating stromal invasion. Head Neck Pathol. 2016;10(4):547–51.
39. Jacobiec FA, Folberg R, Iwamoto T. Clinicopathologic characteristics of premalignant and malignant melanocytic lesions of the conjunctiva. Ophthalmology. 1989;96(2):147–66.
40. Shields CL, Shields JA, Gündüz K, Cater J, Mercado GV, Gross N, et al. Conjunctival melanoma: risk factors for recurrence, exenteration, metastasis, and death in 150 consecutive patients. Arch Ophthalmol. 2000;118:1497–507.
41. Damato B, Coupland S. Conjunctival melanoma and melanosis: a reappraisal of terminology, classification and staging. Clin Exp Ophthalmol. 2008;36:786–95.
42. Holmstrom M, Lund VJ. Malignant melanomas of the nasal cavity after occupational exposure to formaldehyde. Br J Ind Med. 1991;48(1):9–11.
43. Zhu W, Zou B, Wang S. Clinicopathological features and prognosis of sinonasal mucosal malignant melanoma: a retrospective study of 83 cases in a chinese population. ORL J Otorhinolaryngol Relat Spec. 2016;78(2):94–104.
44. Rivolta C, Royer-Bertrand B, Rimoldi D, Schalenbourg A, Zografos L, Leyvraz S, et al. UV light signature in conjunctival melanoma; not only skin should be protected from solar radiation. J Hum Genet. 2015;61(4):361–2.
45. Zhang T, Dutton-Regester K, Brown KM, Hayward NK. The genomic landscape of cutaneous melanoma. Pigment Cell Melanoma Res. 2016;29(3):266–83.
46. Furney SJ, Turajlic S, Stamp G, Nohadani M, Carlisle A, Thomas JM, et al. Genome sequencing of mucosal melanomas reveals that they are driven by distinct mechanisms from cutaneous melanoma. J Pathol. 2013:230(3):261–9.
47. Berger MF, Hodis E, Heffernan TP, Deribe YL, Lawrence MS, Protopopov A, et al. Melanoma genome sequencing reveals frequent PREX2 mutations. Nature. 2012;485(7399):502–6.
48. Si L, Wang X, Guo J. Genotyping of mucosal melanoma. Chin Clin Oncol. 2014;3(3):34.
49. Curtin JA, Fridlyand J, Kageshita T, Patel HN, Busam KJ, Kutzner H, et al. Distinct sets of genetic alterations in melanoma. N Engl J Med. 2005;353(20):2135–47.
50. Bastian BC, Olshen AB, LeBoit PE, Pinkel D. Classifying melanocytic tumors based on DNA copy number changes. Am J Pathol. 2003;163(5):1765–70.
51. Dahl C, Guldberg P. The genome and epigenome of malignant melanoma. The genome and epigenome of malignant melanoma. Acta Pathol Microbiol Immunol Scand. 2007;115(10):1161–76.
52. Spendlove HE, Damato BE, Humphreys J, Barker KT, Hiscott PS, Houlston RS. BRAF mutations are detectable in conjunctival but not uveal melanomas. Melanoma Res. 2004;14(6):449–52.
53. Lake SL, Jmor F, Dopierala J, Taktak AG, Coupland SE, Damato BE. Multiplex ligation-dependent probe amplification of conjunctival melanoma reveals common BRAF V600E gene mutation and gene copy number changes. Invest Ophthalmol Vis Sci. 2011;52(8):5598–604.
54. Zebary A, Jangard M, Omholt K, Ragnarsson-Olding B, Hansson J. KIT, NRAS and BRAF mutations in sinonasal mucosal melanoma: a study of 56 cases. Br J Cancer. 2013;109(3):559–64.
55. Omholt K, Grafström E, Kanter-Lewensohn L, Hansson J, Ragnarsson-Olding BK. KIT pathway alterations in mucosal melanomas of the vulva and other sites. Clin Cancer Res. 2011;17(12):3933–42.
56. Beadling C, Jacobson-Dunlop E, Hodi FS, Le C, Warrick A, Patterson J, et al. KIT gene mutations and copy number in melanoma subtypes. Clin Cancer Res. 2008;14(21):6821–8.
57. Curtin J, Busam K, Pinkel D, Bastian BC. Somatic activation of KIT in distinct subtypes of melanoma. J Clin Oncol. 2006;24(26):4340–6.
58. Santi R, Simi L, Fucci R, Paglierani M, Pepi M, Pinzani P, et al. KIT genetic alterations in anorectal melanomas. J Clin Pathol. 2015;68(2):130–40.
59. Turri-Zanoni M, Medicina D, Lambardi D, Ungari M, Balzarini P, Rossini C, et al. Sinonasal mucosal melanoma: molecular profile and therapeutic implications from a series of 32 cases. Head Neck. 2013;35(8):1066–77.
60. Hsieh R, Nico MS, Coutinho-camillo CM, Buim ME, Sangueza M, Lourenço SV. The CDKN2A and MAP kinase pathways: molecular roads to primary oral mucosal melanoma. Am J Dermathol Pathol. 2013;35(2):167–75.
61. Sheng X, Kong Y, Li Y, Zhang Q, Si L, Cui C, et al. GNAQ and GNA11 mutations occur in 9.5% of mucosal melanoma and are associated with poor prognosis. Eur J Cancer. 2016;65:156–63.
62. Jangard M, Zebary A, Ragnarsson-Olding B, Hansson J. TERT promoter mutations in sinonasal malignant melanoma: a study of 49 cases. Melanoma Res. 2015;25(3):185–8.
63. Larsen AC, Mikkelsen LH, Borup R, Kiss K, Toft PB, Von Buchwald C, et al. MicroRNA expression profile in conjunctival melanoma. Invest Opthalmol Vis Sci. 2016;57(10):4205.

64. Jacobiec FA, Bhat P, Colby KA. Immunohistochemical studies of conjunctival nevi and melanomas. Arch Ophthalmol. 2010;128(2):174–83.
65. Thompson LD, Wieneke JA, Miettinen M. Sinonasal tract and nasopharyngeal melanomas: a clinicopathologic study of 115 cases with a proposed staging system. Am J Surg Pathol. 2003;27:594–611.
66. Volpin E, Sauvanet A, Couvelard A, Belghiti J. Primary malignant melanoma of the esophagus: a case report and review of the literature. Dis Esophagus. 2002;15:244–9.
67. Cheung MC, Perez EA, Molina MA, Jin X, Gutierrez JC, Franceschi D, et al. Defining the role of surgery for primary gastrointestinal tract melanoma. J Gastrointest Surg. 2008;12:731–8.
68. Pacella M, Gallo F, Gastaldi C, Ambruosi C, Carmignani G. Primary malignant melanoma of the bladder. Int J Urol. 2006;13:635–7.
69. Grozinger G, Mann S, Mehra T, Klumpp B, Grosse U, Nikolaou K, et al. Metastatic patterns and metastatic sites in mucosal melanoma: a retrospective study. Eur Radiol. 2016;26(6):1826–34.
70. Patel SG, Prasad ML, Escrig M, Singh B, Shaha AR, Kraus DH, et al. Primary mucosal malignant melanoma of the head and neck. Head Neck. 2002;24:247–57.
71. O'Regan K, Breen M, Ramaiya N, Jagannathan J, DiPiro PJ, Hodi FS, et al. Metastatic mucosal melanoma: imaging patterns of metastasis and recurrence. Cancer Imaging. 2013;13(4):626–32.
72. Birch-Johansen F, Buchwald CV, Drzewiecki KT. Slimhinde melanomer i hoved-halsregionen [In Danish] Copenhagen2013. www.melanoma.dk
73. Pfister DG, Ang KK, Brizel DM, Burtness B, Cmelak AJ, Colevas AD, et al. Mucosal melanoma of the head and neck. J Natl Compr Cancer Netw. 2012;10(3):320–38.
74. Surabhi VR, Menias CO, Amer AM, Elshikh M, Katabathina VS, Hara AK, et al. Tumors and tumorlike conditions of the anal canal and perianal region: MR imaging findings. Radiographics. 2016;36(5):1339–53.
75. Ferraioli D, Lamblin G, Mathevet P, Hetu J, Berakdar I, Beurrier F, et al. Genital melanoma: prognosis factors and treatment modality. Arch Gynecol Obstet. 2016;294(5):1037–45.
76. Schaefer T, Satzger I, Gutzmer R. Clinics, prognosis and new therapeutic options in patients with mucosal melanoma: a retrospective analysis of 75 patients. Medicine. 2017;96(1):e5753.
77. AJCC Cancer Staging Manual. 8th ed. Springer International Publishing; 2016.
78. Prasad ML, Patel SG, Huvos AG, Shah JP, Busam KJ. Primary mucosal melanoma of the head and neck: a proposal for microstaging localized, Stage I (lymph node-negative) tumors. Cancer. 2004;100(8):1657–64.
79. Ballantyne AJ. Malignant melanoma of the skin of the head and neck. An analysis of 405 cases. Am J Surg. 1970;120(4):425–31.
80. Shah J, Huvos A, Strong E. Mucosal melanomas of the head and neck. Am J Surg. 1977;134:531–5.
81. Chung AF, Woodruff JM, Lewis JL Jr. Malignant melanoma of the vulva: a report of 44 cases. Obstet Gynecol. 1975;45(6):638–46.
82. Gal TJ, Silver N, Huang B. Demographics and treatment trends in sinonasal mucosal melanoma. Laryngoscope. 2011;121(9):2026–33.
83. Meleti M, Leemans CR, Mooi WJ, Vescovi P, van der Waal I. Oral malignant melanoma: a review of the literature. Oral Oncol. 2007;43(2):116–21.
84. Chae WY, Lee JL, Cho DH, Yu CS, Roh J, Kim JC. Preliminary suggestion about staging of anorectal malignant melanoma may be used to predict prognosis. Cancer Res Treat. 2016;48(1):240–9.
85. Seifried S, Haydu LE, Quinn MJ, Scolyer RA, Stretch JR, Thompson JF. Melanoma of the vulva and vagina: principles of staging and their relevance to management based on a clinicopathologic analysis of 85 cases. Ann Surg Oncol. 2015;22(6):1959–66.
86. Damato B, Coupland S. Ocular melanoma. Saudi J Ophthalmol. 2012;26(2):137–44.
87. Damato B, Coupland SE. Management of conjunctival melanoma. Expert Rev Anticancer Ther. 2009;9(9):1227–39.
88. Norregaard JC, Gerner N, Jensen OA, Prause JU. Malignant melanoma of the conjunctiva: occurrence and survival following surgery and radiotherapy in a Danish population. Albrecht Von Graefes Arch Klin Exp Ophthalmol. 1996;234(9):569–72.
89. Pfeiffer ML, Ozgur OK, Myers JN, Peng A, Ning J, Zafereo ME, et al. Sentinel lymph node biopsy for ocular adnexal melanoma. Acta Ophthalmol. 2017;95(4):e323–8.
90. Mendoza PR, Grossniklaus HE. Sentinel lymph node biopsy for eyelid and conjunctival tumors: what is the evidence? Int Ophthalmol Clin. 2015;55(1):123–36.
91. Lombardi D, Bottazzoli M, Turri-Zanoni M, Raffetti E, Villaret AB, Morassi ML, et al. Sinonasal mucosal melanoma: a 12-year experience of 58 cases. Head Neck. 2016;38(Suppl 1):E1737–45.
92. Won TB, Choi KY, Rhee CS, Jin HR, Yi JS, Dhong HJ, et al. Treatment outcomes of sinonasal malignant melanoma: a Korean multicenter study. Int Forum Allergy Rhinol. 2015;5(10):950–9.
93. Bello DM, Smyth E, Perez D, Khan S, Temple LK, Ariyan CE, et al. Anal versus rectal melanoma: does site of origin predict outcome? Dis Colon Rectum. 2013;56(2):150–7.
94. Nilsson PJ, Ragnarsson-Olding BK. Importance of clear resection margins in anorectal malignant melanoma. Br J Surg. 2010;97(1):98–103.
95. Han J, Shi C, Dong X, Wang J, Wen H, Wang B, et al. Laparoscopic abdomino-perineal resection for patients with anorectal malignant melanoma: a report of 4 cases. J Biomed Res. 2016;30(5):436–40.
96. Iacoponi S, Rubio P, Garcia E, Oehler MK, Diez J, Diaz-De la Noval B, et al. Prognostic factors of recurrence and survival in vulvar melanoma: sub-

group analysis of the VULvar CANcer study. Int J Gynecol Cancer. 2016;26(7):1307–12.
97. Ragnarsson-Olding BK. Primary malignant melanoma of the vulva an aggressive tumor for modeling the genesis of non-UV light-associated melanomas. Acta Oncol. 2004;43(5):421–35.
98. Frumovitz M, Etchepareborda M, Sun CC, Soliman PT, Eifel PJ, Levenback CF, et al. Primary malignant melanoma of the vagina. Obstet Gynecol. 2010;116(6):1358–65.
99. Todo Y, Okamoto K, Suzuki Y, Minobe S, Kato H. Radicality of initial surgery for primary malignant melanoma of the vagina. Melanoma Res. 2016;26(2):173–80.
100. Lee JH, Yun J, Seo JW, Bae GE, Lee JW, Kim SW. Primary malignant melanoma of cervix and vagina. Obstet Gynecol Sci. 2016;59(5):415–20.
101. Leitao MM, Cheng X, Hamilton AL, Siddiqui NA, Jurgenliemk-Schulz I, Mahner S, et al. Gynecologic Cancer InterGroup (GCIG) consensus review for vulvovaginal melanomas. Int J Gynecol Cancer. 2014;24(9):117–22.
102. Gao S, Li J, Feng X, Shi S, He J. Characteristics and surgical outcomes for primary malignant melanoma of the esophagus. Sci Rep. 2016;6:23804.
103. Ost D, Joseph C, Sogoloff H, Menezes G. Primary pulmonary melanoma: case report and literature review. Mayo Clin Proc. 1999;74:62–6.
104. Khalid U, Saleem T, Imam AM, Khan MR. Pathogenesis, diagnosis and management of primary melanoma of the colon. World J Surg Oncol. 2011;9:14.
105. Papes D, Altarac S, Arslani N, Rajkovic Z, Antabak A, Cacic M. Melanoma of the glans penis and urethra. Urology. 2014;83(1):6–11.
106. Smith NE, Taube JM, Warczynski TM, Collier KD, Pawlik TM. Primary biliary tract melanoma: report of a case and review of the literature. Int J Surg Case Rep. 2012;3:441–4.
107. Pittaka M, Kardamakis D, Spyropoulou D. Comparison of international guidelines on mucosal melanoma of the head and neck: a comprehensive review of the role of radiation therapy. In vivo (Athens, Greece). 2016;30(3):165–70.
108. Cantuaria G, Angioli R, Nahmias J, Estape R, Penalver M. Primary malignant melanoma of the uterine cervix: case report and review of the literature. Gynecol Oncol. 1999;75:170–4.
109. Kelly P, Zagars GK, Cormier JN, Ross MI, Guadagnolo BA. Sphincter-sparing local excision and hypofractionated radiation therapy for anorectal melanoma: a 20-year experience. Cancer. 2011;117(20):4747–55.
110. Kirschner AN, Kidd EA, Dewees T, Perkins SM. Treatment approach and outcomes of vaginal melanoma. Int J Gynecol Cancer. 2013;23(8):1484–9.
111. Damato B, Coupland SE. An audit of conjunctival melanoma treatment in Liverpool. Eye (Lond). 2009;23(4):801–9.
112. Fuji H, Yoshikawa S, Kasami M, Murayama S, Onitsuka T, Kashiwagi H, et al. High-dose proton beam therapy for sinonasal mucosal malignant melanoma. Radiat Oncol (London, England). 2014;9:162.
113. Zenda S, Akimoto T, Mizumoto M, Hayashi R, Arahira S, Okumura T, et al. Phase II study of proton beam therapy as a nonsurgical approach for mucosal melanoma of the nasal cavity or para-nasal sinuses. Radiother Oncol. 2016;118(2):267–71.
114. Liao JJ, Parvathaneni U, Laramore GE, Thompson JA, Bhatia S, Futran ND, et al. Fast neutron radiotherapy for primary mucosal melanomas of the head and neck. Head Neck. 2014;36(8):1162–7.
115. Yanagi T, Mizoe JE, Hasegawa A, Takagi R, Bessho H, Onda T, et al. Mucosal malignant melanoma of the head and neck treated by carbon ion radiotherapy. Int J Radiat Oncol Biol Phys. 2009;74(1):15–20.
116. Naganawa K, Koto M, Takagi R, Hasegawa A, Ikawa H, Shimozato K, et al. Long-term outcomes after carbon-ion radiotherapy for oral mucosal malignant melanoma. J Radiat Res. 2017;58(4):517–22.
117. Karasawa K, Wakatsuki M, Kato S, Kiyohara H, Kamada T. Clinical trial of carbon ion radiotherapy for gynecological melanoma. J Radiat Res. 2014;55(2):343–50.
118. Ozyigit G, Cengiz M, Yazici G, Yildiz F, Sezen D, Yildiz D, et al. Robotic stereotactic body radiotherapy in the treatment of sinonasal mucosal melanoma: report of four cases. Head Neck. 2013;35(3):E69–73.
119. Lian B, Si L, Cui C, Chi Z, Sheng X, Mao L, et al. Phase II randomized trial comparing high-dose IFN-alpha2b with temozolomide plus cisplatin as systemic adjuvant therapy for resected mucosal melanoma. Clin Cancer Res. 2013;19(16):4488–98.
120. Carvajal RD, Antonescu CR, Wolchok JD, Chapman PB, Roman RA, Teitcher J, et al. KIT as a therapeutic target in metastatic melanoma. JAMA. 2011;305(22):2327–34.
121. Hodi FS, Corless CL, Giobbie-Hurder A, Fletcher JA, Zhu M, Marino-Enriquez A, et al. Imatinib for melanomas harboring mutationally activated or amplified KIT arising on mucosal, acral, and chronically sun-damaged skin. J Clin Oncol. 2013;31(26):3182–90.
122. Larkin J, Ascierto PA, Dreno B, Atkinson V, Liszkay G, Maio M, et al. Combined vemurafenib and cobimetinib in BRAF-mutated melanoma. N Engl J Med. 2014;371(20):1867–76.
123. Long GV, Stroyakovskiy D, Gogas H, Levchenko E, de Braud F, Larkin J, et al. Combined BRAF and MEK inhibition versus BRAF inhibition alone in melanoma. N Engl J Med. 2014;371(20):1877–88.
124. Robert C, Karaszewska B, Schachter J, Rutkowski P, Mackiewicz A, Stroiakovski D, et al. Improved overall survival in melanoma with combined dabrafenib and trametinib. N Engl J Med. 2015;372(1):30–9.
125. Del Vecchio M, Di Guardo L, Ascierto PA, Grimaldi AM, Sileni VC, Pigozzo J, et al. Efficacy and safety of ipilimumab 3mg/kg in patients with pretreated, metastatic, mucosal melanoma. Eur J Cancer. 2014;50(1):121–7.

126. Thierauf J, Veit JA, Lennerz JK, Weissinger SE, Affolter A, Doscher J, et al. Expression of Kallikrein-related peptidase 6 in primary mucosal malignant melanoma of the head and neck. Head Neck Pathol. 2017;11(3):314–20.
127. D'Angelo SP, Larkin J, Sosman JA, Lebbe C, Brady B, Neyns B, et al. Efficacy and safety of nivolumab alone or in combination with ipilimumab in patients with mucosal melanoma: a pooled analysis. J Clin Oncol. 2017;35(2):226–35.
128. Robert C, Schachter J, Long GV, Arance A, Grob JJ, Mortier L, et al. Pembrolizumab versus ipilimumab in advanced melanoma. N Engl J Med. 2015;372(26):2521–32.
129. Shoushtari AN, Munhoz RR, Kuk D, Ott PA, Johnson DB, Tsai KK, et al. The efficacy of anti-PD-1 agents in acral and mucosal melanoma. Cancer. 2016;122(21):3354–62.

Uveal Melanoma

16

Ronald W. Milam Jr. and Anthony B. Daniels

Introduction

The three main types of primary ocular melanoma are eyelid, conjunctival, and uveal melanoma, each fundamentally different from each other. Eyelid and conjunctival melanomas are external to the eye itself, while uveal melanoma refers strictly to intraocular melanomas. Eyelid melanomas can be considered essentially identical to cutaneous melanoma, as they both possess the same pathogenesis, genetic alterations, risk factors, and general principles of metastasis and treatment. The reader is referred to other sections of this book for further detailed discussion on cutaneous melanoma. The conjunctiva is the thin, clear external mucous membrane that covers the front of the eye, extending from the peripheral edge of the cornea (the corneal limbus) over the anterior sclera (termed the bulbar conjunctiva). It then loops back onto the posterior surface of the eyelids (termed the palpebral conjunctiva) (Fig. 16.1). While not identical to cutaneous melanoma, it is important to recognize that conjunctival melanoma has several features reminiscent of its cutaneous counterpart.

It is important to note that, when referring to "ocular melanoma," some sources will group together both conjunctival and uveal melanomas [1]. Occasionally, even periocular cutaneous melanoma is included when some sources discuss "eye melanomas." However, uveal (intraocular) melanoma is unique from both conjunctival and cutaneous melanoma in its clinical and molecular features as well as its risk factors, genetics, pathogenesis, metastatic behavior, and treatment [2–7]. Therefore, it is important to think of uveal melanoma as a separate entity from the other two [8]. This chapter focuses predominantly on primary uveal melanoma, which is 7.5–17.5 times more common than conjunctival melanoma [5, 9–12]. A brief discussion of conjunctival melanoma is found at the end of this chapter.

Basic Ocular Definitions (Fig. 16.1)

- *Uvea*: The pigmented layer of the eye, often referred to as the uveal tract. It is composed of three intraocular structures (choroid, ciliary body, and iris) that are morphologically and functionally distinct but contiguous with one another. Uveal melanoma arises from melanocytes within these three structures.
- *Choroid*: The pigmented vascular layer of the eye that lies between the retina and the sclera. It is the most posterior portion of the uvea.

R. W. Milam, Jr., M.D.
Department of Ophthalmology and Visual Sciences, Vanderbilt University Medical Center, Vanderbilt Eye Institute, Nashville, TN, USA

A. B. Daniels, M.D., M.Sc. (✉)
Department of Ophthalmology and Visual Sciences, Department of Radiation Oncology, Vanderbilt-Ingram Cancer Center, Vanderbilt University Medical Center, Nashville, TN, USA

Program in Cancer Biology, Vanderbilt University, Nashville, TN, USA
e-mail: Anthony.b.daniels@vanderbilt.edu

A. I. Riker (ed.), *Melanoma*, https://doi.org/10.1007/978-3-319-78310-9_16

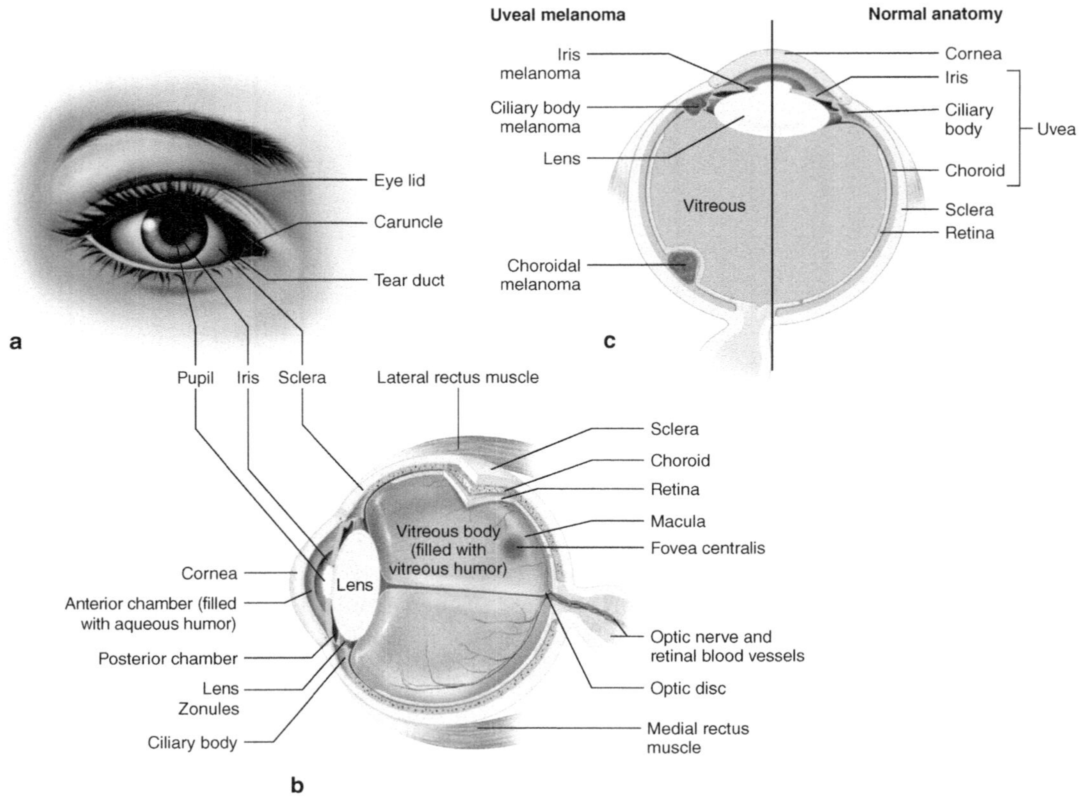

Fig. 16.1 Visual glossary of ocular anatomy. (**a**) External view with ocular surface and adnexal structures. (**b**) Sagittal cross section of the eye displaying intraocular anatomy. (**c**) Simplified cross section of the eye highlighting the normal uveal tract (on the *right*) and highlighting the location of the three locations of uveal melanoma (iris, ciliary body, and choroid) on the *left*

- *Ciliary body*: The pigmented vascular structure of the eye that connects the iris to the choroid. It consists of ciliary muscles (which alter the shape of the lens to allow the eye to focus on near objects) and ciliary processes (which produces the aqueous humor). It is the middle portion of the uvea.
- *Iris*: The thin circular pigmented structure that lies between the cornea and the lens. It has a dynamic aperture in the center that is known as the pupil. Eye color is defined by the color of one's iris. It is the most anterior portion of the uvea.
- *Aqueous humor*: The clear fluid produced by the ciliary body, which is composed primarily of water. It contains oxygen and nutrients that nourish the anterior structures of the eye, including the cornea.

Epidemiology

Uveal melanoma is the most common primary intraocular malignancy in adults [13] and is comprised of melanomas involving the choroid, ciliary body, and iris (Figs. 16.1, 16.2, and 16.3). Uveal melanoma represents 3–5% of all melanomas in the body, and the uvea is the second most common location, after the skin, from which primary melanomas arise [5, 14]. It is estimated that there are approximately 1,500–2,000 new cases of uveal melanoma diagnosed in the United States each year [5, 8], with the choroid accounting for 81–90% of these cases. Melanomas of the ciliary body are the second most common location for uveal melanomas and they comprise 5–8% of cases, while iris melanomas are the least common, representing only

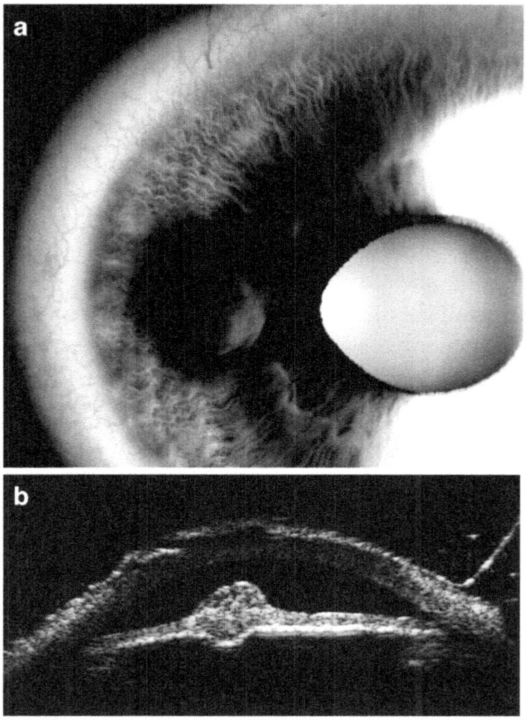

Fig. 16.2 Iris melanoma. (**a**) Anterior segment photographs of a small iris melanoma. (**b**) Ultrasound biomicroscopy (UBM) of the lesion seen in (**a**)

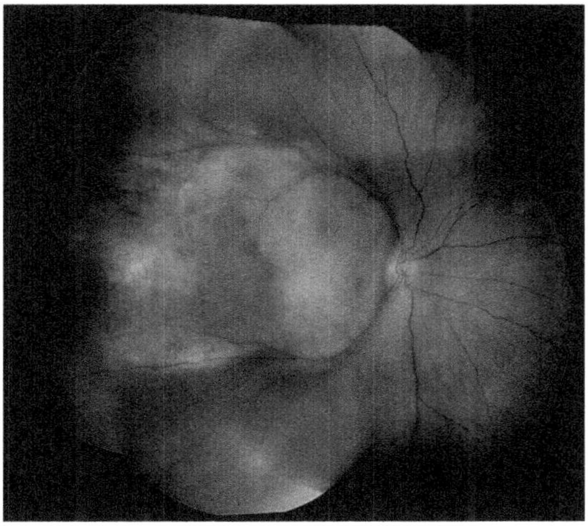

Fig. 16.3 Medium-sized amelanotic melanoma involving the macula and abutting the optic nerve (juxtapapillary)

3–5% of cases [9, 14, 15]. Infrequently, more than one site of the uveal tract may be involved, such as uveal melanomas that are large enough to involve both the iris and ciliary body (termed "iridociliary melanoma") or both the ciliary body and the choroid (termed "ciliochoroidal melanoma").

The annual incidence of uveal melanoma in the United States and Europe is 5–8 cases per million per year. Unlike cutaneous melanoma, where the incidence has been on the rise, the worldwide incidence of uveal melanoma has remained stable over the past several decades [5, 9, 10, 16]. Previously, a geographical trend in incidence change was identified, with the incidence of uveal melanoma observed to increase significantly with an increase in latitude of birth (4.91-fold increase from 20–22 degrees latitude to 47–48 degrees latitude) [17]. However, a further meta-analysis has shown that latitude of birth is not an independent risk factor for development of uveal melanoma. Rather, this trend reflects the genetic predisposition for uveal melanoma of populations living in these higher latitudes, with a higher incidence in countries having larger Scandinavian or Caucasian populations (higher latitude countries) and a lower incidence in East Asia and Africa (lower latitude countries) where there is a lower proportion of Scandinavian or Caucasian populations [5, 10, 18, 19].

Uveal melanoma primarily afflicts older Caucasian adults, with a peak age at diagnosis of 70–79 years, with men and women being equally affected [5]. However, uveal melanoma can occur over a wide age range, with diagnoses being reported anywhere from 6 to 100 years of age [14, 20, 21]. Caucasians represent 97.8% of cases in the United States, with a Caucasian-to-African-American ratio of 196:1 [5]. Population studies estimate the annual incidence of uveal melanoma, based on ethnicity, to be 4351 for Caucasian-non-Hispanics, 1154 for Hispanics, 875 for Asians, and 316 for Africans [22].

Risk Factors for Developing Uveal Melanoma

Several studies and meta-analyses have identified a variety of risk factors that put certain individuals at a higher risk for developing uveal melanoma. These risk factors include presence of light-colored irides, fair skin, cutaneous freckles, increased number of common cutaneous nevi, atypical cutaneous nevi, propensity to sunburn/inability to tan, iris nevi, ocular melanocytosis, dysplastic nevus syndrome, inactivating *BAP1* gene mutation, and welding as an occupation [18, 23–27]. In comparison, similar risk factors have been shown to be important in the development of cutaneous melanoma, including blonde or red hair, fair skin color, light eye color, skin freckling, presence of cutaneous nevi, and sensitivity to sunlight [28]. It has been shown that ultraviolet (UV) light/sunlight exposure is the most significant modifiable risk factor for cutaneous melanoma [29–31]. However, the effect of sunlight on the development of uveal melanoma has not been thoroughly identified as a major risk factor.

There is conflicting data from numerous studies which have investigated the role of UV/sunlight exposure in the development of uveal melanoma. For example, melanoma is more likely to arise within the posterior pole of the eye, where sunlight exposure is thought to be greatest. However, the preponderance of evidence suggests that UV light damage is not causative in the pathogenesis of posterior uveal (choroidal and ciliary body) melanoma [27, 32–34]. This is supported by the fact that the types of deoxyribonucleic acid (DNA) damage typically seen with UV light, such as C-to-T transitions, are not as commonly observed with uveal melanomas [35–39]. Similarly, genes mutated in cutaneous melanomas arising in sun-exposed or chronically sun-damaged skin, such as BRAF and NRAS, are not mutated in uveal melanoma (see Genetics section below) [40–42].

Genetics and Pathogenesis of Uveal Melanoma

Uveal melanoma harbors a relatively limited number of conserved genetic mutations, which are responsible for its oncogenesis and progression to metastatic disease [36–38, 43, 44]. This is in contrast to many other solid tumors, including cutaneous melanoma, which carry a much wider variety of pathogenic and passenger mutations. Chromosomal anomalies associated with uveal melanoma consist primarily of derangements in chromosomes 1, 3, 6, and 8 [45–50]. Further discussion of these chromosomal alterations and their implications for patient prognosis is given in detail later in this chapter. This section reviews the major genes and epigenetic modifications involved in the pathogenesis of uveal melanoma.

It is important to mention that the specific genetic variants underlying the development of uveal melanoma differ completely from those observed with cutaneous melanoma. The most commonly observed high-risk susceptibility genes associated with cutaneous melanoma include *CDKN2A*, *CDK4*, *MITF*, and *MC1R* [51]. Furthermore, cutaneous melanoma is typically driven by mitogen-activated protein kinase (*MAPK*) activating mutations in *BRAF* (40–50% of cases) and *NRAS* (10–25% of cases) or by loss-of-function mutations in the *NF1* gene (14% of cases) [52].

In contrast, uveal melanoma contains a more limited number of conserved mutations found almost exclusively in the *GNAQ*, *GNA11*, *SF3B1*, *EIF1AX*, and *BAP1* genes. Mutations in *GNAQ* and *GNA11* occur early and are found in approximately 83–91% of all primary uveal melanomas and are always mutually exclusive to one another [38, 43]. Mutations in *SF3B1*, *EIF1AX*, and *BAP1* are present, in addition to the early *GNAQ/GNA11* mutations. As with *GNAQ/GNA11*, mutations in *SF3B1*, *EIF1AX*, and *BAP1* are all also mutually exclusive from each other [37, 43, 53].

Uveal melanomas arise from uveal melanocytes. The timing of the major genetic mutational events that lead to melanocytic malignant transformation is largely predictable. Progression from uveal melanocyte to nevus is characterized by specific mutations in either *GNAQ* or *GNA11*, followed by a mutation in either *SF3B1* or *EIF1AX*. In turn, this causes a transformation from nevus to a "low-metastatic-risk" uveal melanoma. Alternatively, after the initial *GNAQ/GNA11* mutation, a uveal nevus may transform into a "high-metastatic-risk" uveal melanoma by acquiring a subsequent independent pathogenic derangement in the *BAP1* gene (Fig. 16.4).

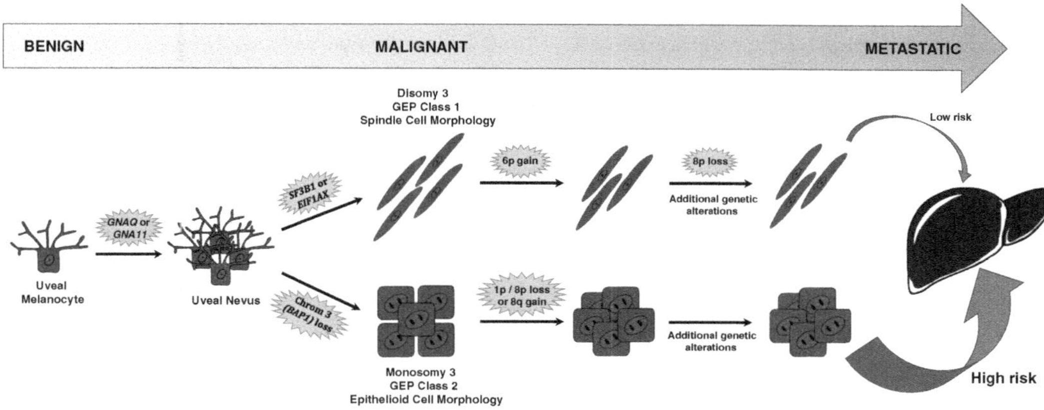

Fig. 16.4 Genetic pathway of uveal melanoma. The first step in the genetic development of a uveal melanoma starts with a uveal melanocyte acquiring a mutation in either *GNAQ* or *GNA11*, creating a uveal nevus. During melanomagenesis, the nevus then progresses along on one of the two mutually exclusive pathways. Some tumors will develop chromosome 3 loss (monosomy 3) with loss of *BAP1*, leading to a melanoma with high metastatic risk and Class 2 gene expression profile (GEP). Alternatively, tumors may instead acquire a mutation in either *SF3B1* or *EIF1AX*, leading to a melanoma with low metastatic risk and Class 1 GEP. After the initial genetic bifurcation, tumors may then acquire subsequent genetic derangements in chromosomes 1, 6, and 8, which are themselves independent modifiers of metastatic risk and patient mortality. Adapted with permission of Wiley

GNAQ and GNA11 Gene Mutations

GNAQ/11 each encodes for G protein-related alpha subunits of a larger cellular protein complex. Mutations in these genes are somatically acquired and almost exclusively occur within the GTPase catalytic domain at codon 209 in exon 5 [36, 38, 43]. Inactivating mutations at this site prevent hydrolysis of GTP, subsequently locking the mutated protein in its activated configuration and resulting in constitutive activation of many downstream pathways such as MEK/ERK. This causes YAP hypo-phosphorylation and nuclear localization, resulting in transcriptional activation of numerous cell cycle genes [36, 37, 54, 55]. Mutations in *GNAQ/11* lead to precursor uveal nevi, but alone are not sufficient to lead to melanoma. *GNAQ/11* mutations have been observed in nevi and melanomas at all stages of malignant progression, independent of other well-known oncogenic mutations. As such, *GNAQ/11* mutations represent the earliest genetic event in the pathogenesis from uveal melanocyte to melanoma [56].

BAP1 Gene Mutations

BRCA-1-associated protein-1 *(BAP1)* is located on chromosome 3p21. *BAP1* functions as a tumor-suppressor gene, and therefore requires functional loss of both copies of the gene in order to cause malignant transformation of a cell (i.e., a single functional copy of *BAP1* is adequate to maintain normal cellular function). The BAP1 protein is linked to many critical intracellular processes required for maintaining normal cellular function. Although its exact role in the oncogenesis of uveal melanoma remains unclear, it is certain that maintaining at least one functional copy of *BAP1* is critical for normal cellular growth, chromatin regulation, and DNA damage repair. Furthermore, it has been shown that reduction in BAP1 activity can result in regression of cellular differentiation of uveal melanoma cells, which is likely the underlying oncogenic driving force in cells with *BAP1* mutations [57].

There are two ways in which uveal melanocytes may develop total functional loss of *BAP1* (i.e., functional loss of both copies of *BAP1*). First, patients may carry a single mutant *BAP1* gene and then acquire a subsequent loss of the other, wild-type, *BAP1* gene via an inactivating mutation or total chromosome 3p21 loss, resulting in complete loss of cellular BAP1 function. Second, a uveal melanocyte may exhibit loss of *BAP1* heterozygosity by one parent cell, incorrectly contributing two mutant *BAP1* genes to a daughter cell during mitosis, creating isodisomy (also known as uniparental disomy). By this mechanism, a melanocyte may acquire two copies of inactivated *BAP1* genes, and therefore exhibit complete loss of *BAP1* function [58]. Both genetic mutations and histone deacetylase enzymes have been shown to play a role in the inactivation of *BAP1*, with inactivating mutations observed in up to 84% of uveal melanomas that metastasize [59]. Genetic prognostication and metastatic disease are discussed later in this chapter.

SF3B1 Gene Mutations

The splicing factor 3B subunit 1 (*SF3B1*) gene encodes for a subunit of the splicing factor component of a larger intracellular spliceosome complex. This complex functions to splice precursor messenger ribonucleic acid (mRNA) into mature transcription products. The wild-type *SF3B1* gene product anchors the precursor mRNA onto the spliceosome complex, facilitating correct mRNA splicing. Mutations of the *SF3B1* gene can result in critical mRNA splicing errors that may result in downstream protein product dysfunction, cell cycle derangements, and ultimately melanomagenesis [60–62].

EIF1AX Gene Mutations

The eukaryotic translation initiation factor 1A, X-linked (*EIF1AX*) gene encodes for a protein involved in the translation of other intracellular proteins. Its exact mechanism of oncogenesis in uveal melanoma is not well understood at present. Mutations in the *EIF1AX* gene have been reported in up to 24% of primary uveal melanomas [63, 64].

Rb, p53, and PTEN Gene Mutations

In uveal melanomas, mutations in the retinoblastoma (*Rb*), phosphatase and tensin homolog (*PTEN*), and *p53* tumor-suppressor genes are exceedingly rare. However, most uveal melanomas exhibit some degree of inhibition of the Rb and p53 pathways, even in the presence of wild-type *Rb* and *p53* genes. This apparent loss of Rb and p53 activity is due to the overexpression of cyclin D1 and MDM2, respectively. Reduced Rb and p53 activity allows for disinhibited progression through the cell cycle and further malignant transformation [65–67].

The loss of *PTEN* activity has also been reported in a subset of uveal melanomas and is thought to result in increased downstream activity of PI3K/AKT signaling, which in turn activates many other downstream targets that lead to cellular proliferation [68]. In one study, up to 11% of uveal melanomas were found to have mutations in *PTEN*. Furthermore, there are other small studies suggesting that reduced patient survival may be associated with uveal melanomas containing *PTEN* mutations [68–73].

Epigenetics in Uveal Melanoma

Epigenetics is the study of mitotically inherited cellular influences that alter genetic function, but are not caused by direct DNA nucleotide alterations. Over the past two decades, it has become more apparent that these epigenetic factors play an important role in the modification of chromatin, resulting in dynamic alterations in the expression of DNA. It is now known that epigenetics plays an important role in the development of numerous pathologies and cancers, with several epigenetic mechanisms centrally involved in the malignant transformation and progression of melanoma.

The most notable epigenetic factors include DNA methylation and alterations of histones through acetylation or methylation. Collectively, this has been termed the "epigenome," and a "histone code" has been theorized. The histone code can be modified significantly by major regulators of transcription, such as polycomb group (PcG) proteins and histone-modifying enzymes (HMEs) such as histone acetyltransferases (HATs) or histone deacetylases (HDACs) [74].

Recently, Herlihy and colleagues showed that reduced expression levels of HMEs and PcG proteins were associated with uveal melanoma harboring monosomy 3, with the gene expression profile (GEP) Class 2 [75], both of which are characteristics associated with increased metastatic risk. Currently, the role of epigenetics in the pathogenesis and treatment of uveal melanoma is still in its infancy. However, there have been some small studies elucidating potential future directions for utilizing epigenetic modification in the treatment of uveal melanoma [75, 76].

Summary of Genetic Pathogenesis of Uveal Melanoma

In summary, it is well known that the genetic pathway for uveal melanoma bifurcates at an early stage in its pathogenesis. The initial genetic alteration involves an early mutation in either GNAQ or GNA11. Mutations in GNAQ/11 result in the development of a uveal nevus, but a mutation in either of these genes alone is not fully sufficient for a uveal melanocyte to complete malignant transformation [36, 43, 53, 77]. After this initial mutation in either GNAQ or GNA11, the cell acquires another separate pathogenic mutation in either *SF3B1 or EIF1AX* (leading to melanoma with a lower metastatic risk) or *BAP1* (leading to melanoma with a high metastatic risk). Each of these mutations is mutually exclusive to the others [63], and this bifurcation results in two mutually exclusive and genetically distinct uveal melanoma subtypes (Fig. 16.4) [36, 45, 78].

Evaluation and Diagnosis of Primary Uveal Melanoma

Uveal melanoma arises from uveal melanocytes, and may either develop from a long-standing choroidal nevus or arise de novo, without progressing from a precursor nevus. However, there is no data documenting the proportion of melanomas that arise from nevus vs. de novo. In fact, the overwhelming majority of published literature only reports rates of growth and transformation of uveal nevi into melanomas, with only two case reports documenting truly de novo choroidal melanomagenesis [79, 80]. Additionally, it is reasonable to assume that some larger reports of nevi progression may actually include melanoma variants that arose de novo but were initially misclassified. Consequently, it is difficult to establish an accurate incidence of malignant transformation from nevus vs. incidence of de novo melanomagenesis. Given the lack of documentation of uveal melanomas arising de novo, experts believe that the overwhelming majority of melanomas evolve along a continuum between benign uveal nevus and melanoma, analogous to cutaneous nevi and melanoma [81, 82].

Diagnosis of Primary Uveal Melanoma

The diagnosis of uveal melanoma is determined by the clinical judgment of the evaluating ophthalmologist, and is based on patient presentation with a detailed physical examination using biomicroscopy and ophthalmoscopy. Adjuvant diagnostic imaging techniques may be used as well to look for the presence of high-risk features, suggesting uveal melanoma over a benign nevus. Studies have shown that the rarity of uveal melanoma may play a role in the correct diagnosis (i.e., differentiating a melanoma from a nevus) being missed by comprehensive ophthalmologists who may only observe this disease a few times during their career. In fact, it is estimated that a comprehensive ophthalmologist practicing in the United States will see one new case of uveal melanoma per decade of practice [20, 83]. Consequently, given uveal melanoma's high rate of metastasis and mortality [84–87], along with its evolution along a continuum from benign to malignant, careful ophthalmologic examination by a trained and experienced clinician remains critical.

Differential Diagnosis of Uveal Melanomas

There are numerous other benign and malignant neoplasms of the retina, the outer lying retina pigment epithelium (RPE) and choroid, all of which can mimic the appearance of ciliary body or choroidal melanoma on physical exam. The differential diagnosis of a solitary, pigmented lesion includes uveal melanoma, choroidal nevus, melanocytoma, congenital hypertrophy of the RPE (CHRPE), hemorrhage in the subretinal or suprachoroidal space, and metastatic cutaneous melanoma. The differential diagnosis of a solitary amelanotic lesion includes amelanotic uveal melanoma, choroidal hemangioma, metastatic choroidal tumors, solitary choroidal granuloma (from sarcoidosis or tuberculosis), posterior scleritis, and prominent vortex ampulla [88]. The differential diagnosis of pigmented melanocytic iris lesions includes iris nevus, iris melanoma, primary iris cyst, essential iris atrophy, iris foreign body, peripheral anterior synechiae, iris metastasis, leiomyoma, melanocytoma, and other rare entities [89].

Delays in Early Diagnosis of Primary Uveal Melanoma

Despite the high mortality rate associated with metastatic disease, studies have not conclusively shown that early diagnosis and treatment of primary uveal melanoma have an impact upon improving a patient's survival. However, there are numerous studies demonstrating that early diagnosis prevents disease-related morbidity by reducing the rate of enucleation (removal of the entire eye) and increasing the rate of eye-sparing treatment with radiotherapy. Enucleation rates for delayed diagnoses are 44–52%, compared to the 17–29% for cases without diagnostic delays [20, 87, 90]. Several reports show that diagnostic delays result from an initial misdiagnosis in 23–42% of cases. Diagnostic delays are associated with a significant delay in the onset of treatment, with an average time to treatment of 6.6 months for cases with diagnostic delays compared to 4.2 weeks for cases without delays [20, 90]. Cited reasons include tumors located in areas difficult to observe on exam (such as in the anterior choroid or ciliary body), the presence of media opacities (such as cataracts) that may obstruct the view, and the presence of other ocular pathologies that may incorrectly explain visual symptoms which are actually caused by the melanoma [83, 90].

Patient Presentation

Large, prospective studies have shown that 69–72% of patients with uveal melanoma present symptomatically. The most common presenting symptom is blurry vision, occurring in 37.8% of symptomatic patients, followed by photopsias (flashes of lights) in 8.6%, floaters in 7.0%, visual field loss in 6.1%, visible tumor in 3.1%, and pain in 2.4%. Larger tumors are more likely to present with some of these symptoms due to secondary effects from the tumor, such as associated serous retinal detachment which may cause reduced vision, visual field deficits, and photopsias [20, 90]. On the other hand, 28–31% of patients present completely asymptomatic and are diagnosed on routine ophthalmic screening exams. Rarely, a long-standing blind eye or an eye with a very dense cataract may harbor an occult uveal melanoma. Therefore, eye care providers must routinely and thoroughly evaluate eyes with a poor view to the posterior pole (e.g., due to dense cataracts, diseased corneas, or phthisis bulbi) with ocular ultrasonography, in order to monitor for the development of an occult tumor [91].

Clinical Features of Ciliary Body and Choroidal Melanomas

Melanomas of the ciliary body and choroid typically present as a solitary, elevated, pigmented, or amelanotic lesion. Ciliary body and choroidal melanomas are typically dome shaped (Figs. 16.2 and 16.5) with 60% of choroidal melanomas being located within 3 mm of the optic disc or fovea. There may be clumps of overlying orange pigment, due to collection of lipofuscin associated with the melanoma (Fig. 16.6). In some cases, serous fluid may leak from the tumor and

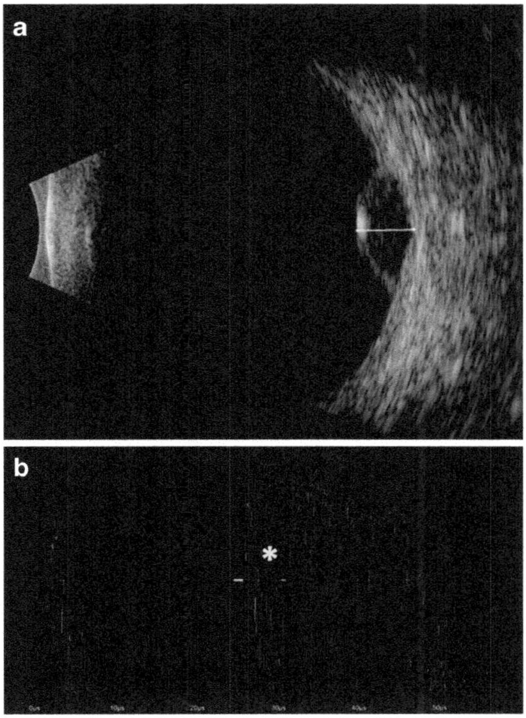

Fig. 16.5 Choroidal melanoma ultrasonography. (**a**) B-scan ultrasonography of choroidal melanoma, demonstrating the characteristic dome shape, and acoustic hollowness. (**b**) The corresponding A-scan ultrasonography of the same melanoma, displaying low-medium internal reflectivity (*yellow asterisk*) with vascular spikes

collect underneath the retina, causing an associated serous retinal detachment or subretinal hemorrhage (Fig. 16.6).

Large ciliary body and choroidal melanomas are often easy for the trained ophthalmologist to diagnose on physical exam, based on the presence of high-risk clinical features that distinguish them from smaller benign nevi. However, the distinction between small- and medium-sized nevi versus melanomas can be difficult, with adjuvant imaging modalities quite useful as an aid in making the correct diagnosis. Such imaging modalities include fundus photography, ophthalmic ultrasonography, ultrasound biomicroscopy (UBM), optical coherence tomography (OCT), fundus autofluorescence (FAF), fluorescein angiography (FA), indocyanine green (ICG), and magnetic resonance imaging (MRI).

Anterior Segment and Fundus Photography

Anterior segment and fundus photography employ the use of a specialized camera attached to a biomicroscope with a light source. This camera is used to capture high-resolution photographs of the anterior segment (iris, cornea, conjunctiva, and sclera) and fundus (the back of the inside of the eye) (Figs. 16.2, 16.3, 16.6, and 16.8). Fundus photography is mainly used for monitoring and documenting any change in the pigmentation and borders uveal nevi, melanomas, and other suspicious lesions requiring monitoring for growth. Fundus photography allows for lesions to be documented and compared over time. Any documented change or growth of a nevus may represent malignant transformation, necessitating treatment.

Ophthalmic Ultrasonography

Ophthalmic ultrasonography (USG) is the single most valuable diagnostic tool available to the experienced clinician to aid in diagnosis, monitoring, and documenting growth for uveal melanoma. Serial USG measurements are used to monitor for any change in tumor dimensions over time, with an increasing basal diameter or apical height highly suggestive of malignant transformation and growth [8, 92, 93]. Additionally, USG is indispensable for accurately evaluating lesions through retinal detachments and dense media opacities that would otherwise obstruct the examiner's direct view of the lesion in question. Clinicians utilize both B-scan and A-scan USG to accurately evaluate lesions suspicious for the diagnosis of melanoma (Figs. 16.5 and 16.7).

Traditional USG B-scans use a 10 MHz transducer that provides a resolution of 300–400 μm, and is used to reliably define the tumor extent, shape, and dimensional measurements. Typical features of choroidal and ciliary body melanomas on B-scan USG include a dome or mushroom shape, apical height >3 mm, choroidal excavation, acoustic hollowness, and posterior shadowing

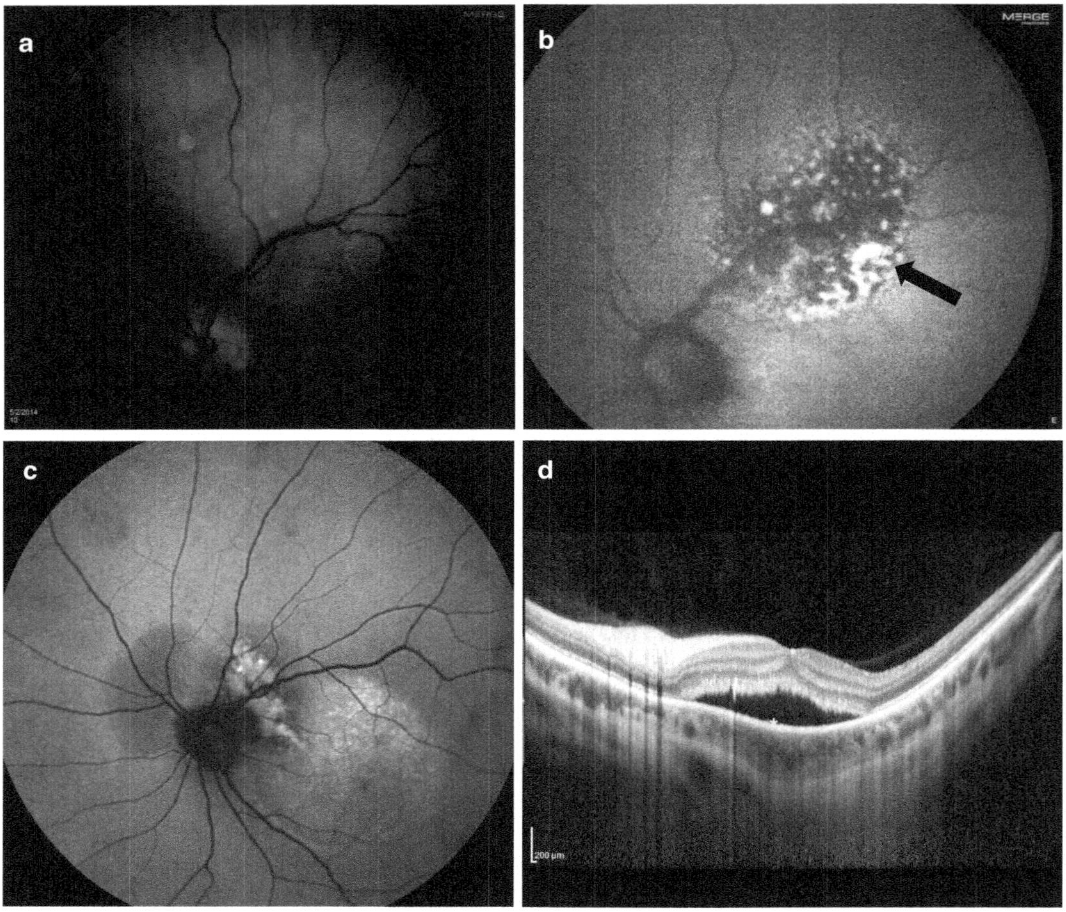

Fig. 16.6 (**a**) Color fundus photography of a choroidal melanoma with several high-risk features, including the presence of orange pigment (*arrow*) and juxtapapillary location abutting the optic nerve head. (**b**) Fundus autofluorescence of the choroidal melanoma displayed in (**a**), demonstrating hyper-autofluorescence (*arrow*) corresponding to the orange pigment seen on the fundus photograph. (**c**) Another fundus autofluorescence of a different choroidal melanoma, also displaying some hyper-autofluorescence of orange pigment and subtle subretinal fluid. (**d**) Spectral domain optical coherence tomography (OCT) of the choroidal melanoma displayed in (**c**). This OCT highlights the presence of subretinal fluid (*asterisk*)

(Figs. 16.5 and 16.7) [94]. Mushroom shape on USG (Fig. 16.7) is nearly pathognomonic for choroidal melanoma [95], which occurs as a result of melanoma extension through Bruch's membrane (the innermost layer separating the choroid from the retina). Another concerning feature on USG is the presence of an apical height >3 mm, as these lesions are very likely to be melanoma [8, 93]. In addition to B-scan USG, there are characteristic features on A-scan that are highly suggestive of the diagnosis of uveal melanoma. The classic acoustic features of uveal melanoma seen on A-scan USG include homogenous, low-to-medium internal reflectivity, solid consistency with no "after movement," and echographic signs of vascularity, such as fast vertical flickering A-scan spikes (Fig. 16.5) [96].

Ultrasound Biomicroscopy

Ultrasound biomicroscopy (UBM) is a separate ultrasonography technique that is used primarily to evaluate the anterior segment of the eye,

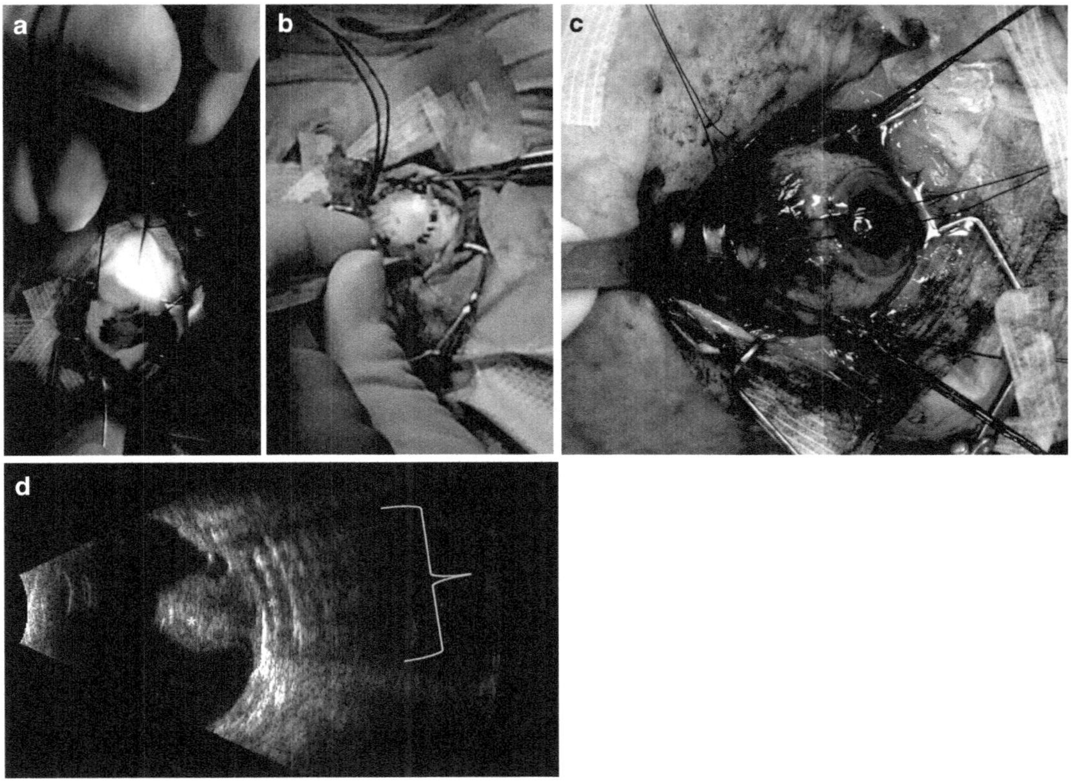

Fig. 16.7 Radioactive brachytherapy plaque placement. (**a**) Traction sutures have been placed around the superior and inferior rectus muscles and the eye has been rotated. The lateral rectus muscle has been disinserted to allow better access to the underlying tumor. A light is shined into the eye in this photo, transilluminating the melanoma on the surface of the overlying sclera. (**b**) This transillumination shadow is then marked to delineate the borders of the tumor. The radioactive plaque is sewn to the sclera to cover the previously marked tumor borders. (**c**) The gold plaque shell can be seen on the left side of the eye. (**d**) Intraoperative ultrasound showing a mushroom-shaped choroidal melanoma (*yellow asterisk*) and the correctly placed brachytherapy plaque (*green asterisk*) with acoustic shadowing posterior (*green bracket*) to the plaque

including the iris, ciliary body, anterior chamber, and cornea. Compared to conventional ophthalmic A-scan and B-scan ultrasonography, UBM uses a higher frequency transducer (35–100 MHz) to capture anterior segment images with a higher resolution approaching 20–60 μm [97]. While standard B-scan ultrasonography of the eye is useful for evaluation of posterior choroidal melanomas, UBM's higher resolution is better for imaging smaller uveal melanomas of the ciliary body and iris. UBM improves on the axial and lateral resolution of conventional B-scan imaging by a factor of ten, and its imaging penetrates up to 4 mm, which is sufficient to image most ciliary body and iris melanomas [98]. Due to its superior resolution and penetration over USG, UBM demonstrates superior accuracy in acquiring dimensional measurements and localization of uveal melanomas involving the ciliary body and peripheral iris (Fig. 16.2) [99].

Fundus Autofluorescence

Fundus autofluorescence (FAF) is a noninvasive retinal imaging modality that provides a density map of lipofuscin, the predominant fluorophore in the retinal pigment epithelium (RPE). Fluorophores are naturally occurring molecules that absorb light of a particular wavelength, and then emit (autofluoresce) light of a distinctly separate wavelength. Classically, FAF utilizes blue light to excite the lipofuscin, and then collects the subsequent fluorescent emissions to form a brightness map that reflects the distribution of lipofuscin located in the RPE. The RPE is the pigmented, outermost layer of cells that lines the retina, serving multiple functions to support and nourish the retina photoreceptors. In clinical practice, FAF is used as a reliable noninvasive method to estimate the viability of the RPE [100].

For choroidal melanomas, FAF is used to assess the health of the overlying RPE, which may demonstrate characteristics that differentiate choroidal nevus from melanoma [101]. FAF features associated with choroidal nevus include overlying hypo-autofluorescence (56% of cases), homogenous hyper-autofluorescence (25% of cases), or iso-autofluorescence (19% of cases). Hypo-autofluorescence on FAF is a sign that is suggestive of chronic RPE atrophy associated with the underlying lesion. Signs of chronicity are more likely to represent a benign nevus over melanoma. Such chronic changes indicate that a particular lesion has been present for an extended time period that is long enough for these changes to manifest. Therefore, chronic changes are indirect signs of slow or minimal growth, which is the major characteristic of a nevus.

Contrasting FAF of nevi, choroidal melanomas are more likely to demonstrate distinct hyper-autofluorescence that corresponds directly to intrinsic lipofuscin deposition (seen as orange pigmentary deposits on physical exam) (Fig. 16.6). While the absence of this FAF feature does not rule out the diagnosis of melanoma, its presence suggests malignancy. Thus, the diagnostic utility of FAF in uveal melanoma is most beneficial for potentially highlighting subtle lipofuscin aggregates (orange pigmentation) of uveal melanomas that may be missed on the clinical exam alone [101–103]. Some researchers have demonstrated quantification of FAF images using imaging software to quantify the amount of autofluorescence and differentiate between clinically benign and malignant choroidal melanocytic lesions [104].

Optical Coherence Tomography

Optical coherence tomography (OCT) is both a noncontact and noninvasive ophthalmic imaging technique commonly used in ophthalmology. It is utilized to quickly and accurately visualize in vivo cross-sectional images of ocular tissues in a wide variety of diseases. Modern OCTs are capable of producing high-definition images with a resolution of up to 5 μm. This technique uses the interference patterns of laser light that is shined onto, and reflected from, the ocular tissue to create high-definition cross-sectional images of the cornea, iris, ciliary body, retina, and choroid. OCT is not regularly employed as a diagnostic tool for uveal melanomas, as it has shown limited use for evaluating lesions >3 mm in thickness or lesions with heavy pigmentation [105, 106]. However, when utilized, OCT is primarily used to confirm the presence of subtle subretinal fluid associated with uveal melanoma and which may be missed on clinical exam alone (Fig. 16.6). Other less common roles of OCT for uveal melanoma include obtaining dimensional measurements of small tumors and differentiating congenital hypertrophy of the retina pigment epithelium (CHRPE) from choroidal melanoma.

Fluorescein Angiography

Fluorescein angiography (FA) is a relatively more invasive chorioretinal vascular imaging technique that involves injecting a fluorescent dye into the patient's bloodstream. While the dye circulates through the retinal and choroidal vasculature in the back of the eye, serial fundus images are captured. FA is not routinely used to evaluate or monitor uveal nevi/melanomas, as it has limited ability to distinguish between the two and there is no pathognomonic FA characteristic for either of these lesions. However, it is important to note that FA can demonstrate a "dual-circulation" pattern in up to 61% of choroidal melanomas, which is a sign of secondary choroidal vascularization in tumors that have broken through Bruch's membrane beneath the RPE [107].

Indocyanine Green Angiography

Indocyanine green angiography (ICGA) is an ophthalmic imaging technique that is used to evaluate the choroidal vasculature, but has a limited role for evaluating uveal melanomas. ICGA is similar to FA, in that it involves the injection of a dye into the patient's bloodstream, with subsequent serial imaging of the ocular fundus while the dye circulates through the choroidal blood vessels. However, ICGA is better for imaging the choroid, utilizing near-infrared light, which penetrates the RPE to activate the indocyanine green dye in the choroidal vessels. These features allow for ICGA to evaluate the integrity of the choroidal vascular system.

While ICGA may demonstrate hypocyanescence of uveal melanomas, this finding is not reliably characteristic and its role in the diagnosis, evaluation, and monitoring of uveal melanoma remains rare and limited. ICGA may be most useful in distinguishing choroidal melanoma from choroidal hemangiomas if this distinction is not apparent to the clinician on physical exam, as the choroidal vessel patterns differ between these two entities [108]. There are previous studies suggesting that ICGA may be capable of detecting prognostically significant microvasculature patterns (such as closed vascular loops that are only seen on histopathological biopsy evaluations) [109, 110]. However, these studies have not been validated and this imaging modality continues to have limited utility in the evaluation of uveal melanoma.

Computed Tomography and Magnetic Resonance Imaging

Computed tomography (CT) and magnetic resonance imaging (MRI) are rarely used for the evaluation of primary uveal melanomas. Uveal melanomas may be seen as hyperdense on CT imaging and may demonstrate mild-to-moderate enhancement with contrast dye. With MRI, they appear hyper-intense on T1-weighted images and hypo-intense on T2-weighted images [88]. While large melanomas can be seen on both imaging modalities, with MRI able to demonstrate extrascleral extension in rare cases of larger tumors [111], the role of CT and MRI for primary uveal melanomas remains limited. The principal role of CT and MRI in uveal melanoma is for monitoring the development of systemic metastatic spread of the disease, rather than for imaging the primary tumor itself. In usual practice, CT and MRI of the orbit are only used when treatments such as stereotactic radiosurgery are being planned (see treatment section below), or if optic nerve invasion is suspected.

Monitoring Uveal Melanoma Over Time

Imaging modalities are not only useful for aiding in the correct diagnosis on initial evaluation, but also invaluable for serially following suspicious lesions that may not have the typical features of melanoma. Of the previously mentioned modalities, B-scan ultrasonography and fundus photography are the most useful and most regularly utilized methods for monitoring growth and change in appearance over time. Any documentation of rapid growth would be indicative of malignancy and therefore indicate urgent treatment. The appearance of new subretinal fluid is likewise worrisome for malignant transformation.

Clinical Features of Iris Melanomas

Iris melanomas may be well circumscribed (90%) (Fig. 16.2) or diffuse (10%) and are much less common than ciliary body or choroidal melanoma. Due to their anterior and more visible location in the front of the eye, iris melanomas are diagnosed an average of 10–20 years earlier than their ciliary body and choroidal counterparts [88, 112]. In most cases, iris melanomas are noticed due to a change in iris color (iris heterochromia) or pupil distortions (corectopia). Iris melanomas are most commonly located in the inferior quadrant of the iris (45% of cases) and may be associated with pupillary border abnormalities, secondary glaucoma, ectropion uveae (posterior iris pulled forward through the pupillary margin), hyphema (bleeding in the anterior chamber), and extraocular extension [88, 112–114]. Evaluation of iris melanoma includes exam with the slit lamp, gonioscopy (evaluation of the anterior chamber angle and trabecular meshwork), photos, and UBM. Occasionally, anterior segment OCT can be helpful, but in general UBM is superior to OCT in assessing iris melanomas. This is because UBM penetrates deeper into the tumor, allowing better characterization of the posterior border of the iris tumor and therefore more accurate measurements compared to OCT [115].

Lesion Characteristics Associated with High Risk for Malignancy, Growth, and Metastasis

In addition to differentiating uveal melanocytic lesions (nevi and melanomas) from other entities on the differential diagnosis, the ophthalmologist is often called upon to determine if a uveal melanocytic lesion is benign (nevus) or malignant (melanoma). At the extremes, when lesions are either very small or very large, the diagnosis of nevus or melanoma (respectively) is straightforward. However, it can be difficult to differentiate a small melanoma from a large or an atypical nevus. In this indeterminate range, there are certain ophthalmoscopic and imaging features that are associated with subsequent growth, serving as indicators that a particular lesion represents a small melanoma rather than a nevus.

Analogous to the ABCDEs of cutaneous melanoma, ophthalmologists look for specific clinical features that portend a higher risk of malignancy and active growth. These high-risk clinical features are remembered by the mnemonic, "To Find Small Ocular Melanomas Using Helpful Hints" (TFSOMUHH) [92, 116–118]. These features are used to distinguish benign uveal nevi from small melanomas and include

- T—Tumor **T**hickness >2 mm
- F—Subretinal **F**luid
- S—**S**ymptoms
- O—**O**range pigment
- M—**M**argin of tumor within 3 mm of the optic disc
- UH—**U**ltrasound **H**ollowness
- H—*Absence* of **H**alo

Although not included in the mnemonic, the *absence* of yellow drusen deposits (a sign of chronicity) is also a risk factor for growth.

The median hazards ratio for lesions with 1–2 of the above features is 3; for 3–4 features is 5; for 5–6 features is 9; and for all 7 features is 21 [92, 116–118]. It is important to note that *the presence of three or more of the above features conveys a >50% risk of active growth* (i.e., melanoma).

Small uveal melanomas are defined as 3 mm or less in diameter, with this cutoff chosen based upon calculations of tumor doubling time and the associated likelihood of metastatic conversion. Despite the classification as "small," these tumors still portend a very real risk for metastasis and mortality for the patient. For example, it has been theorized that the average size of uveal melanoma at the time of metastasis is 3 mm in basal diameter and 1.5 mm in thickness (a small melanoma) [119, 120]. Furthermore, it is estimated that micrometastatic seeds have already developed approximately 5 years prior to the initial diagnosis or treatment of the primary melanoma [119]. On the other hand, small nevi have a <1% chance for malignant transformation and pose minimal risk for vision loss or death [121]. Thus, it is imperative for the ophthalmologist to scrutinize each choroidal nevus for the presence of any high-risk features that may suggest a diagnosis of uveal melanoma over nevus [81].

Clinical features that are more consistent with a benign choroidal nevus include the presence of drusen (yellow subretinal deposits of lipids and proteins), RPE changes, and presence of a hypopigmented halo surrounding the lesion (Fig. 16.8). These features represent secondary signs of chronicity. When drusen, a halo, or RPE changes are associated with a melanocytic lesion less than

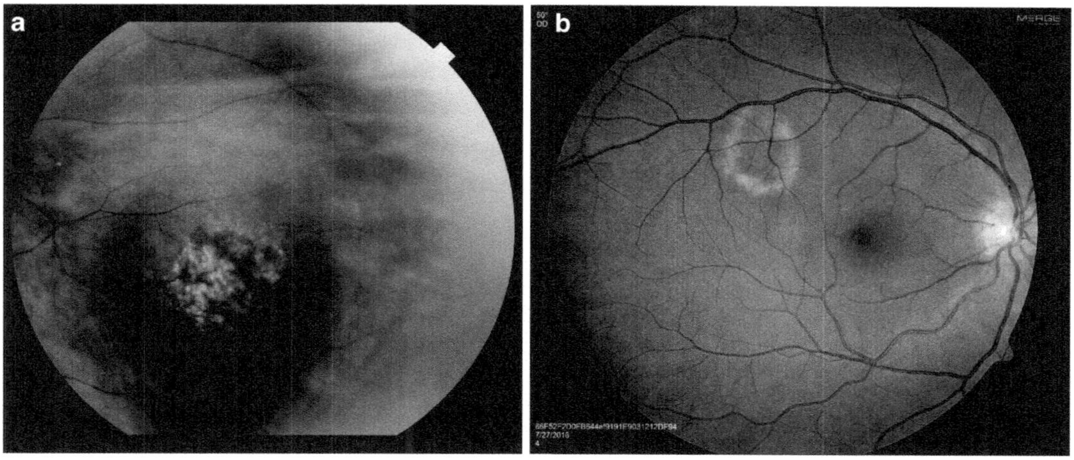

Fig. 16.8 Benign choroidal nevi. (**a**) Benign nevus with overlying yellow drusen and lack of other high-risk malignant features. (**b**) Benign choroidal nevus of the superior macula with a reassuring halo, suggesting a diagnosis of nevus rather than melanoma

3 mm in thickness, it can generally be assumed that the lesion has been present for years without significant growth, strongly supporting a diagnosis of benign nevus. However, nevus malignant transformation is still possible in the future. Therefore, these lesions must be monitored over time for any changes in appearance, presence of any TFSOMUHH features, or any documented growth in dimensions [92, 116–118].

It is important to remember that the *sine qua non* of uveal melanoma malignant transformation is increasing basal diameter or apical height observed over serial measurements. It is recommended, and considered the standard of practice, to follow patients with uveal nevi regularly, typically reexamining small nevi every 6 months initially, followed annually afterwards if the lesion remains stable. Monitoring must be performed by a qualified eye care provider for life [31]. The authors have treated patients who experienced obvious evidence of tumor growth and malignant transformation of uveal melanocytic lesions that had previously been stable over the course of >26 years of observation (including photographic evidence of stability going back several decades). Thus, it must be impressed upon patients the importance of continued monitoring even of those lesions that have been stable for a long time.

Clinical and Histopathologic Characteristics Associated with an Increased Risk of Metastasis

Uveal melanoma location, size, histopathology, and genetics have all been shown to impact risk for metastasis and patient survival [87]. Tumor location and size are readily evaluated in the outpatient clinical setting with tumor histopathology and genetic evaluation both requiring surgical biopsy in the operating room. In this section, we discuss how tumor size, location, and histopathology relate to patient prognosis. The genetics of uveal melanoma and how it relates to prognosis will be discussed later in this chapter.

Tumor Location

Ciliary body involvement of uveal melanoma is a clinical feature associated with a poorer prognosis when compared to iris or choroidal location. Relative to iris and choroid locations, ciliary body involvement has been associated with accelerated growth and an increased risk for development of metastasis within the first 3 years after diagnosis. However, the risk for metastasis after 3 years diminishes to that equal of tumors without ciliary body involvement [49, 122–124].

It is thought that contraction of the ciliary body muscles leads to increased mechanical progression of tumor cells through the adjacent ciliary blood vessels. However, anterior tumors (i.e., tumors involving the ciliary body) typically are not discovered until they are large enough to become symptomatic. It is plausible that ciliary body location may be a surrogate for late disease presentation, explaining the observed increased metastatic risk [87, 123].

On the other hand, iris melanomas have a much lower rate of metastasis when compared to their choroidal and ciliary body counterparts [124]. As previously discussed, these tumors are often easily visible to the naked eye, and are picked up early both by physicians and by patients themselves. Thus, this earlier detection may be at least partly responsible for the lower rate of metastasis [124].

Tumor Size

When ophthalmologists discuss uveal melanomas, they describe them in terms of relative sizes, such as small, medium, and large. As defined by the Collaborative Ocular Melanoma Study (COMS) [118, 125–128], these sizes are standardized, and convey increasingly higher risk for metastasis and mortality with increasing size.

- Small uveal melanomas: <3 mm height, <10 mm diameter
- Medium uveal melanomas: 3–8 mm height, <16 mm diameter
- Large uveal melanomas: >8 mm height or >15 mm diameter

Increasing basal diameter and thickness are risk factors associated with increased metastasis and mortality, even after treatment with enucleation [129, 130]. As tumor thickness increases, so does the 3-, 5-, and 10-year mortality rate [93]. Since this is true even among eyes that underwent enucleation, this observation obviates the question as to whether metastasis occurred in the setting of unsuccessful local therapy, given that enucleation always achieves local tumor control (except in cases of extraocular extension of tumor at presentation).

High-Metastatic-Risk Histopathologic Features of Uveal Melanoma

There are three main histopathologic features associated with a poorer prognosis for patients with uveal melanoma: higher proportion of epithelioid cells, higher mitotic activity, and presence of closed vascular loops. Uveal melanomas arise from uveal melanocytes and are comprised of two major cell types, spindle-shaped cells and epithelioid cells (or a mixture of both spindle and epithelioid cells). On histopathologic evaluation, an increasing proportion of epithelioid-type cells is associated with a progressively worse prognosis [124]. This proportion is calculated by counting the number of epithelioid cells per high-power field [87], with the 10-year mortality of 5× higher in patients with >0.5 epithelioid cells per high-power field [123].

High mitotic activity is another histopathological feature associated with higher rates of metastasis and mortality for patients with uveal melanoma. Mitotic activity is measured by the number of mitotic cells seen per high-power field. In a study of 217 uveal melanomas, McLean and colleagues found that mitotic activity was a prognostic feature that is independent of tumor size. McLean's group also found that the 6-year mortality rate was 3.6-fold higher with uveal melanoma demonstrating high mitotic activity compared to those with low activity [131].

The third major high-risk histopathologic feature of uveal melanoma is the presence of closed vascular loops. These loops represent the intrinsic dual-vascular circulation of uveal melanomas. The presence of these closed vascular loops has been shown to correlate with a markedly reduced overall patient survival from 90 to 50%, even after treatment [109].

It is important to note that all three of the preceding findings can only be readily discerned if the eye is enucleated, whereas the vast majority of eyes are treated with globe-conserving therapies.

Fine-Needle Aspiration Biopsy of Uveal Melanoma

Uveal melanoma biopsies are performed using fine-needle aspiration (FNA), as excisional biopsy is often not possible without blinding the patient or removing the eye completely. While endoresection has been reported either as primary therapy or in conjunction with radiotherapy, it is not currently standard-of-care treatment for posterior (ciliary body or choroidal) uveal melanoma. It should be stressed that FNA biopsies require a skilled and experienced vitreoretinal or ocular oncology specialist in collaboration with an experienced cytopathologist. The major role of FNA biopsy of uveal melanomas is for prognostication, and is rarely required for the purpose of making the correct diagnosis.

As previously discussed, the diagnosis of uveal melanoma is ultimately a clinical one, based upon the physical examination and clinical judgment of as-experienced ophthalmologist. In fact, the COMS reported a >99% diagnostic accuracy for patients who had the typical high-risk features of uveal melanoma [118, 132, 133]. Furthermore, FNA biopsy is of limited utility in differentiating melanoma from a nevus, as even melanoma cells can have benign-appearing nuclear morphology [134, 135]. Even in the hands of very experienced ocular cytopathologists, FNA biopsies may not be able to unequivocally differentiate benign nevus from melanoma [135, 136]. However, there may be rare situations in which the diagnosis is uncertain and diagnostic biopsies may be helpful, such as with amelanotic lesions without typical melanoma features, within eyes that have media opacity (such as vitreous hemorrhage) or in differentiating between a primary choroidal melanoma versus a metastasis [134, 136, 137]. Studies have shown that diagnostic biopsy with FNA can be safely used to assist in the diagnosis of iris melanoma in small suspicious melanocytic lesions. In 100 consecutive biopsies with FNA, Shields et al. demonstrated that an adequate sample could be obtained with minimal complications in 99% of cases [138].

Biopsy with FNA plays a much more significant role in prognostication. While FNA is rarely performed for diagnostic purposes, it is very commonly performed to obtain genetic material to aid with patient metastatic stratification and prognosis. Prognostic biopsies are useful for assessing high-risk genetic features and obtaining a specific gene expression profile (GEP) on uveal melanoma [139–141]. Uveal melanoma genetics and its relation to tumor behavior and prognosis are discussed in further detail later in this chapter.

Staging of Uveal Melanomas

During the evaluation of uveal melanoma, the ophthalmologist may use clinical features to stage the tumor and provide prognostic data for patients. However, molecular analysis of the tumor has largely surpassed and replaced the prognostication based upon clinical features alone. In general, staging is performed using the COMS staging criteria, which divides tumors into small, medium, and large categories (see previous section on Clinical and Histopathology Characteristics Associated with Metastatic Uveal Melanoma). Additionally, as with cutaneous melanomas, the American Joint Commission on Cancer (AJCC) has specific staging criteria for uveal melanoma as well [142].

AJCC Staging of Uveal Melanomas

The AJCC uses clinical (rather than genetic) characteristics to classify ciliary body and choroidal melanomas on a T1 through T4 grading scale, based on tumor basal diameter, thickness, involvement of ciliary body, and degree of extraocular extension [142–145]. For iris melanoma, the AJCC staging includes specific criteria based on tumor size, location, clock hours of iris involvement, extension into the ciliary body or choroid, features of secondary glaucoma, and extraocular extension [142, 145]. Shields et al. conducted a retrospective review of 7731 patients with posterior uveal melanoma and found that patients had a twofold increase in risk for both metastasis and death with each increase in AJCC classification from T1 through T4 [143]. While the AJCC system has been shown to be predictive, the COMS classification system is more widely used.

Systemic Evaluation

The overall long-term metastatic rate for primary uveal melanoma is ~50%, with a 15-year mortality rate that is similar at about 50% [85, 86, 146]. Thus, the systemic evaluation of uveal melanoma is directed primarily at detecting metastatic disease. Unlike cutaneous melanoma, metastatic spread of uveal melanoma is hematogenous, involving the liver in more than 90% of cases, with the second most common site of metastasis being the lungs [5, 16, 125–127, 130, 147]. Central nervous system (CNS) metastasis from uveal melanoma is extraordinarily rare, to the point that the brain is not even included in standard staging imaging. Systemic evaluation for metastatic disease includes measuring serum transaminases (AST, ALT, and GGT) to evaluate for hepatocyte structural compromise that may result from liver metastases, as well as liver ultrasonography, CT, or MRI [148]. Chest plain-film radiographs (CXR) have a poor sensitivity and are rarely able to demonstrate lung metastases without liver involvement seen first [148].

Monitoring for metastatic spread is highly individualized and based on a patient's metastatic risk. Patients with GEP Class 1B or Class 2 uveal melanomas (i.e., tumors with relatively higher metastatic risk) are generally monitored every 6 months with multiphasic contrasted CT of the abdomen, with or without CT imaging of the chest. Patients with GEP Class 1A tumors are typically monitored less frequently with CT imaging, or are monitored at the same 6-month interval but without radiation-based imaging modalities (such as with liver ultrasonography).

This is primarily due to the desire to balance the benefit of surveillance imaging with the risk of additional repeat radiation exposure in the setting of lower risk GEP Class 1A uveal melanomas [87]. There is some data on the use of serum monoclonal antibody screening with melanoma-associated antigen (MAA). However, there are no studies that definitively support the clinical utility of serum MAA in detecting subclinical metastases [149].

Treatment of Primary Uveal Melanoma

Historically, all uveal melanomas were treated by removing the entire eye (a procedure called enucleation). Enucleation was performed in order to remove the tumor *in toto* in an attempt to prevent metastatic spread and death. This traditional treatment paradigm was challenged in the 1970s by Zimmerman et al., who theorized that surgical enucleation may actually worsen prognosis by physically promoting liberation of tumor cells and hematogenous dissemination during the act of enucleating the eye. Thus, the "Zimmerman hypothesis" was born, emphasizing the concern that traditional enucleation may increase rates of metastasis [150, 151].

Inspired by Zimmerman's provocative challenge to the traditional standard of treatment, the multicenter COMS investigational group was formed, and ultimately disproved Zimmerman's theory [125, 130, 147, 152]. Furthermore, the COMS showed that enucleation of the eye had no benefit over conservative eye-preserving radiotherapy in relation to metastatic rate and mortality for small- and medium-sized melanomas. In fact, radiotherapy maintained the same metastatic and mortality rate as enucleation for these tumors while adding the benefit of significantly reduced morbidity and preservation of vision over enucleation [118, 125–128, 130, 147].

As a result of the COMS, the treatment paradigm has shifted from enucleation to preservation of both the eye and maintained vision through the use of focal radiotherapy whenever possible. Today, radioactive plaque brachytherapy is the most commonly used treatment for COMS small- and medium-size tumors. Enucleation is now reserved for COMS large-size tumors not amenable to radiotherapy, where radiotherapy would lead to excessive ocular and adnexal morbidity and significant vision loss. Furthermore, enucleation is also reserved as a secondary treatment for tumors that recur following initial treatment with radiotherapy, or for eyes that have become blind and painful from neovascular glaucoma or other complications after radiotherapy [2, 4, 5, 87].

Treatment of Ciliary Body and Choroidal Melanomas

Radioactive Plaque Brachytherapy

Radioactive plaque brachytherapy remains the most commonly used treatment for ciliary body and choroidal melanomas <10 mm in apical height [2, 4, 5]. The prefix "brachy" is derived from the Greek word meaning "short range." Therefore, the moniker "brachytherapy" refers to the short distance between the source of radiation and the target treatment tissue. Brachytherapy for uveal melanoma consists of placing radioactive isotopes (most commonly iodine-125 (^{125}I), ruthenium-106 (^{106}Ru), and palladium-103 (^{103}Pd)) [4, 153] that release ionizing X-ray radiation that is then absorbed by the nearby tissues, breaking DNA bonds and leading to tumor cell death. Presently, in the United States, the most common radioactive brachytherapy plaques for uveal melanoma use ^{125}I, while ^{106}Ru is popular in Europe [154].

Radioactive plaque brachytherapy is performed in the operating room with the patient under general anesthesia (Fig. 16.7). An incision is created in the conjunctiva (called a peritomy) that overlies the ciliary body or choroidal melanoma. The eye is then rotated and a light is shined into the eye through the pupil. This creates transillumination of the sclera from the light inside the eye, with the tumor casting a shadow on the sclera. This shadow is then marked on the scleral surface, delineating the borders of the tumor. In some small or lightly pigmented tumors, the borders may be better delineated using binocular indirect ophthalmoscopy with scleral indentation and marking by the surgeon.

Once the tumor's base is outlined on the scleral surface, a clear-centered plaque is centered over the marked borders, to ensure that the actual radioactive plaque will fit appropriately and adequately. This plaque has the same dimensions and the same eyelet positions as the radioactive plaque, and appropriate eyelet locations are marked on the scleral surface. Sutures are pre-placed at these eyelet markings. A nonradioactive "dummy" plaque is then temporarily sutured into position using these pre-placed eyelet sutures. Intraoperative ultrasonography can be used to ensure that the plaque is centered and completely covers the intended treatment area of the tumor. The dummy plaque is then removed and replaced by the radioactive plaque and intraoperative ultrasonography is again used to ensure appropriate plaque placement with adequate tumor coverage (Fig. 16.7).

The use of intraoperative ultrasonography has been shown to improve plaque placement rates and to reduce treatment failure rates from geographic miss to near 0% [4, 155]. Furthermore, the use of a nonradioactive "dummy" plaque for the initial tumor localization reduces the overall radiation exposure to the surgeon, as any adjustments to plaque location can be made with the nonradioactive "dummy" plaque [156]. Most radioactive brachytherapy plaques are designed to emit focal low levels of radiation at a rate of 0.6–1.2 Gy/h over a period of 5–7 days [153]. A team-based approach is key for the successful treatment and dose planning for the patient. The most appropriate dose rate should be based on the detailed evaluation and collaboration of both the ocular oncologist and radiation oncologist [157]. Plaque brachytherapy is best suited for the treatment of COMS small- to medium-sized melanomas, but can lead to scleral melt and necrosis when used for thicker tumors. This is because of the higher radiation dose exposed to the scleral bed of larger melanomas. Other radiation modalities should be considered for larger tumors [3, 4].

The advantage of treating with plaque brachytherapy is that the plaques can be made in a variety of shapes and sizes to fit varying tumors and tumor locations, such as notched plaques used for tumors adjacent to the optic nerve. The therapeutic advantage of plaque brachytherapy is that the radiation dose distribution follows an inverse square law with the radiation dose dropping off exponentially with increasing distance from the plaque. This means that ocular and adnexal structures farther away from the melanoma will receive exponentially less radiation than the target melanoma. Another therapeutic advantage is that the gold plaque shell shields the orbit and adjacent ocular tissue from unwanted exposure to radiation [4, 158].

Charged Particle Therapy

Particle beam radiation therapy (PBT) is an effective treatment option for primary uveal melanomas, and is sometimes referred to as external beam particle therapy (EBPT). Both protons and charged helium ions have been used in the treatment for uveal melanoma, with proton beam being the most widely studied and widely used charged particle [159–165]. The biologic effect of protons and helium ions does not significantly differ from that of the X-rays emitted with radioactive brachytherapy. Similar to brachytherapy, charged particles interact with the planetary electrons of target tissues, causing electron excitation and ionization of atoms within the tumor. Additionally, protons interact with atomic nuclei, dislodging other heavy particles that then go on to incite additional therapeutic damage to adjacent tumor cells. The ultimate target is tumor DNA molecules, leading to DNA damage and strand break, followed by mitotic crisis and apoptosis.

Proton beam radiotherapy is more useful than traditional external beam radiotherapy for uveal melanomas, requiring more precise localization of radiation to the target area. This is especially true with tumors located adjacent to critical structures that require sparing of radiation. Proton beam therapy takes advantage of a phenomenon known as the Bragg peak effect, which allows for high-radiation dose deposition within the targeted melanoma, followed by abruptly diminishing dosages directly behind the tumor, limiting unwanted radiation to posterior tissues such as the brain. Therefore, PBT is a useful alternative to brachytherapy for treating tumors that would otherwise be difficult to treat with plaques, such as melanomas abutting or surrounding the optic nerve [154, 158, 166].

Prior to irradiation with charged particles, the patient is taken to the operating room where the globe is transilluminated and the tumor borders are marked on the scleral surface. Next, nonferromagnetic tantalum clips are sewn to the sclera over the surface markings, delineating the borders of the base of the tumor. This serves to outline the base of the tumor and localize the target treatment zone. Next, the patient is taken to the cyclotron (the source of the charged particles) and the beam is aimed at the patient's eye in line with the tumor. For most uveal melanomas, the patient is typically given 50–70 cobalt gray equivalents (CGE) divided into five fractions [4, 167].

The major limitation of charged particle therapy with proton beam is the cost associated with creating centers with cyclotrons capable of delivering this treatment. As a result, these treatment centers are rare and the patient cost for this therapy can be prohibitive. Proton therapy has not been widely adopted because of these reasons and because there is a lack of evidence to demonstrate an advantage of PBT over more cost-effective treatments such as plaque brachytherapy for uveal melanoma [4].

External Beam Radiotherapy

External beam radiotherapy (EBRT) refers to the use of an external source to create photons of ionizing X-rays or gamma rays that are then focused and directed at the target tissue. The external source for EBRT is most often a linear accelerator. For the treatment of uveal melanoma, the main form of EBRT in use today is stereotactic radiosurgery (SRS), which is a technique that most often refers to high-precision, gamma-based or X-ray-based photon therapy. SRS occurs with the patient inside a CT scanner and utilizes 3-dimensional tumor localization, with radiation beams cross-firing from multiple directions precisely onto the targeted tumor. The high degree of precision allows for the delivery of very high doses of radiation to the tumor with minimal collateral damage to noninvolved adjacent ocular tissues.

Traditionally, EBRT is performed by first immobilizing (paralyzing) the treatment eye with retrobulbar anesthesia. Sometimes the eye is further immobilized by placing horizontal rectus muscle stay sutures to firmly position the eye in a specific orientation. Alternatively, a fixation point target can be provided, with patients instructed to maintain fixation on this target, thus "immobilizing" their own eye. A stereotactic frame is then applied to the patient's head and MRI or CT imaging is utilized with the head frame to precisely localize the tumor within the eye. The head frame also serves to immobilize the patient's head.

While the patient's head and eye are adequately immobilized, radiation is then precisely delivered to the tumor, either as a single dose or with fractionation. SRS is useful for patients with large melanomas who do not want enucleation, although it has been used for small- medium-sized melanomas as well [168]. It can also be useful for posterior uveal melanoma or melanomas that are adjacent to the optic nerve, similar to the advantage of charged particle irradiation. Thus, SRS may be capable of treating certain tumors for which brachytherapy treatment may not be possible, or in which brachytherapy may give too large a dose to the scleral bed [4]. Studies have shown that gamma-based SRS does not compromise survival when compared to enucleation [169]. However, there is no proven survival benefit to any one radiotherapy technique over the others [170–173].

Transpupillary Thermotherapy

Transpupillary thermotherapy (TTT) is a noninvasive treatment modality that utilizes infrared diode laser light at a wavelength of 810 nm, shined through a dilated pupil onto the choroidal melanoma. As the laser light is absorbed by the pigmented tumor cells, the temperature of the tumor increases to 45–60°F, causing thermal obliteration of the tumor's vascular supply and subsequent tumor necrosis [174]. TTT is limited to the treatment of only COMS small-sized choroidal melanomas, as TTT only penetrates to a maximum depth of 4 mm [174]. TTT is most efficacious when used with heavily pigmented small tumors, as the absorption of the diode laser increases with increasing pigmentation. Conversely, TTT is not a good choice for treatment of medium- to large-sized tumors or amelanotic tumors. However, for small heavily pigmented choroidal tumors, TTT has the benefit of causing immediate tumor necrosis with less damage to surrounding normal ocular tissues compared to methods of radiotherapy [174]. However, TTT alone has fallen out of favor as a primary treatment for uveal melanoma. The majority of the time, TTT is used as an adjuvant to consolidate treatment at the tumor edges following radiotherapy.

Treatment of Primary Iris Melanomas

Small (<3 mm basal diameter) iris melanocytic lesions suspicious for nevus vs. melanoma in an otherwise asymptomatic patient can be monitored for growth with periodic slit lamp exams and photography. However, once there is documented growth, these lesions are presumed to be melanoma and require urgent treatment with either radioactive plaque brachytherapy or PBT. Surgical excision may be utilized in very select cases. Enucleation is rarely used for iris melanomas and is reserved for special cases of large diffuse iris melanomas in eyes with poor vision potential or in cases with recurrence of melanoma [33, 88].

Radiotherapy for Iris Melanomas

Radioactive plaque brachytherapy and PBT are the current preferred treatment modalities for iris melanomas. These modalities provide the greatest relative benefit over surgical excision in tumors with extensive tumor seeding and in non-resectable iris tumors. Both plaque brachytherapy and PBT have been shown to achieve local control in 92% of cases [175–177]. For a detailed discussion on plaque brachytherapy and PBT see the section above on the treatment of ciliary body and choroidal melanomas.

Surgical Excision of Iris Melanomas

While surgical excision of choroidal melanomas is generally not possible without blinding or enucleating the eye, there is a limited role for the excision of melanomas localized to the iris. For these tumors, surgical excision involves removal of the entire tumor by removing the part of the iris (partial iridectomy) housing the tumor. If the iris melanoma also involves the anterior chamber angle, then the surgeon must remove a portion of the trabecular meshwork as well (iridotrabeculectomy). For iris melanomas with ciliary body extension, a portion of the iris and ciliary body must be removed at the time of tumor excision (iridocyclectomy) [88, 112]. Because these are large and invasive procedures that sometimes are associated with high ocular morbidity, radiotherapy has now become the primary treatment modality in most cases.

Control Rates for Treatment of Primary Uveal Melanoma

Radioactive Plaque Brachytherapy

Local control rates for radioactive plaque brachytherapy are excellent, with rates that approach 90–95% [160, 178, 179]. The Mayo Clinic has published data on its control rates and complication rates with the use of ^{125}I plaque brachytherapy, demonstrating a favorable recurrence rate of 8% and a posttreatment enucleation rate of 8%. It also demonstrated that 22% of patients maintained a visual acuity of better than 20/40 after brachytherapy [180].

Charged Particle Therapy

Proton beam therapy has shown similarly favorable results as brachytherapy, with recurrence rates of 2–4% and secondary enucleation rates of 7–11%. Additionally, up to 44% of patients treated with PBT have been shown to maintain visual acuity of better than 20/40 [159, 164, 172, 181–183]. The Curie Institute-Orsay Proton Therapy Center has published its data from more than 20 years of experience treating uveal melanomas with PBT. It has shown a 5-year survival rate of 99%, a 5-year metastatic-free survival rate of 81%, and a 5-year overall survival rate of 79% [159]. There are other smaller studies that have demonstrated similar results, confirming that PBT does not compromise patient survival when compared to enucleation [184, 185].

External Beam Radiotherapy

Study results for the control rates of EBRT have also been similar to those of brachytherapy and PBT. EBRT has demonstrated a 5-year uveal melanoma control rate of 94% and a secondary enucleation rate of 2.4–14%, with 14–33% of patients maintaining a visual acuity of better than 20/200 [168, 171, 186–188]. Other smaller studies have corroborated these results [169, 189–191].

Transpupillary Thermotherapy

Recurrence of choroidal melanoma after treatment with TTT ranges from 9 to 12%, with a direct correlation between tumor recurrence and number of high-risk features present (i.e., features predictive of tumor growth—TFSOMUHH) [174, 192]. Therefore, TTT is less preferable for tumors having multiple high-risk characteristics of the TFSOMUHH. TTT is best used as an adjuvant treatment to enhance local control after plaque brachytherapy. There is no difference in visual acuity outcomes with adjuvant TTT compared to brachytherapy alone [193].

Side Effects and Complications of Treatment

Radiotherapy and Charged Particle Therapy

The acute side effects of all radiotherapy modalities, including radioactive plaque brachytherapy, charged particle therapy, and various forms of EBRT, result in acute local intraocular inflammation and irritation of the conjunctiva and sclera. Acute inflammation is short-lived and less concerning than the long-term side effects. The most significant side effects from radiation therapy are typically delayed and increase over time after treatment. The most common delayed side effects include radiation-induced retinopathy, choroidopathy, optic neuropathy, retinal neovascularization, intraretinal microangiopathy, chorioretinal atrophy, vitreous hemorrhage, cataract formation, iris neovascularization, and neovascular glaucoma, and symptomatic dry eyes (keratoconjunctivitis sicca). Less common side effects of radiotherapy include retinal detachment and scleral melt [165, 178, 179, 194, 195]. Development of secondary malignancy after treatment with radiotherapy is extremely rare with all these modalities. This is due to the sparing of unnecessary radiation exposure to the surrounding healthy ocular and adnexal tissues. The most common cause of vision loss after radiotherapy for uveal melanoma is radiation retinopathy and optic neuropathy, which both progressively worsen over time after treatment. The most common side effect necessitating enucleation after radiotherapy is neovascular glaucoma [154, 159].

Transpupillary Thermotherapy

Although it is the least invasive treatment modality, TTT is not without its own unique side effects and complications. The most common side effects of TTT include development of vitreoretinal traction (44% of cases), branch retinal vein occlusion (26–41% of cases), branch retinal artery occlusion (12% of cases), cystoid macular edema (9–23% of cases), epiretinal membrane (23% of cases), and vitreous hemorrhage (10% of cases). Other rare long-term complications include retinal neovascularization, chorioretinal scarring, retinal detachment, optic nerve atrophy, optic disc edema, and cataract formation [174, 192]. In addition, since TTT destroys the overlying retina, treatment of macular or juxtapapillary tumors can lead to immediate vision loss.

Prognostic Characteristics and Genetic Testing

Because metastatic disease carries a very high risk of mortality for patients with primary uveal melanoma [130], there has been a significant amount of effort directed towards elucidating the clinicopathologic features that are most closely associated with the overall risk of metastasis. As previously discussed, clinicopathologic characteristics were traditionally used to classify uveal melanomas into high- and low-risk categories for development of metastatic disease and death. However, chromosomal analysis and genetic testing have proven to be much more reliable prognostic tools and are the mainstay of prognostic classification at the present time.

Chromosomal Abnormalities

Uveal melanoma is associated with several genetic and epigenetic derangements that are tightly linked to the risk for metastasis and patient mortality. Chromosomal anomalies that provide prognostic value for patients with uveal melanoma include derangements of chromosomes 1, 3, 6, and 8 [45–47]. A gain in chromosome 6p is associated with a relatively good prognosis compared to other chromosomal derangements. The chromosomal anomalies shown to be strongly linked to poorer prognosis (increased mortality from uveal melanoma) include loss of chromosome 3, loss of chromosome 1p, and gain of chromosome 8q. Complete or partial loss of chromosome 3 is the most significant prognostic alteration in uveal melanoma, with monosomy 3 being highly associated with a significantly increased risk for metastatic disease and decreased patient survival [45, 47, 139, 140, 196, 197].

The presence of chromosome 3 loss or 8q gain each correlates with high-risk clinicopathologic features, including increasing tumor basal diameter, ciliary body involvement, presence of epithelioid cell type, high mitotic index, and closed vascular loops [198]. The presence of either chromosome 1p loss or 8q gain in combination with loss of chromosome 3 has an additive effect on the risk of metastasis and death. Specifically, a large study by Damato et al. demonstrated that the 10-year disease-specific mortality for uveal melanomas was 0% for melanomas without chromosome 3 loss, 55% for melanomas having chromosome 3 loss without 8q gain, and 71% for melanomas with concurrent chromosome 3 loss and 8q gain [198].

These chromosomal derangements were initially discovered using standard karyotyping methods [47] and have been validated by other genetic studies, including gene expression profiling (GEP) and multiplex ligation-dependent probe amplification (MLPA), among others. GEP and MLPA are quick and inexpensive commercially available tests that have become the gold standard of prognostication for uveal melanoma, used to reliably and accurately stratify patients into groups of low and high risk for metastasis and death [45, 140, 198].

Gene Expression Profiling

Gene expression profiling (GEP) is a technique that allows for the measurement of the activity of thousands of genes at once, allowing the clinician to discern the global transcriptome of the sample tissue. GEP can be used for rapid detection of the up- or downregulation of select genes. It can be performed even on a very tiny amount of tumor tissue obtained via FNA biopsies. Once the tumor sample is obtained, mRNA is then converted to cDNA and subsequently hybridized to gene chips. Microarray analysis is then performed using these gene chips to quantify the relative upregulation or downregulation of specific genes. For uveal melanomas, tissue samples are typically obtained by FNA biopsy at the time of radioactive brachytherapy plaque placement or immediately after enucleation of the eye [44].

GEP for uveal melanoma was first introduced by Harbour et al. in 2004 and has since been shown to accurately and reliably classify uveal melanomas into two distinct classes (Class 1 and Class 2) with tremendous prognostic utility in accurately predicting metastatic risk and patient mortality [139, 199]. The current technique for GEP of uveal melanoma has evolved into a 15-gene PCR-based assay that reliably segregates tumors into relatively good and poor prognostic classes. The present GEP assay quantifies the expression patterns of 12 class-discriminating genes and 3 control genes. This assay has been validated in a large multicenter prospective clinical trial, correctly classifying uveal melanomas in 97.2% of cases [199]. GEP testing is presently commercially available, providing the treating physician with accurate prognostic information regarding the patient's risk for metastasis and mortality [63, 140].

GEP Class 1 tumors have a low metastatic risk and are associated with gains in chromosome 6p and 8q. These tumor cells closely resemble normal uveal melanocytes or low-grade uveal melanomas and are further subdivided into GEP Class 1A and Class 1B, with Class 1A carrying a 0–2% 5-year metastatic risk and Class 2B carrying a 21% 5-year risk for metastasis. GEP Class 2B tumors also carry an additional increased risk of developing late metastases [63, 78, 139, 200].

GEP Class 2 uveal melanomas resemble primitive stem cells and represent higher grade uveal melanomas. They have more aneuploidy and are most often associated with the loss of chromosome 3, chromosome 1p, and chromosome 8p. These tumors are strongly associated with inactivating mutations of *BAP1*, located on chromosome 3p21. GEP Class 2 melanomas are considered to be very-high-risk tumors, carrying a 72% 5-year risk for metastasis [63, 200].

A limitation of GEP is the potential for limited classification accuracy in small uveal melanomas, which may have genetic heterogeneity within the tumor itself. Augsburger et al. demonstrated a discordance of GEP classification in 11.3% of tumors when biopsy sampling was performed at different sites within a single tumor. They also showed a correlation between tumor height and degree of GEP discordance. Thicker tumors tended to show less discordance, compared to a higher level of intratumoral heterogeneity in thinner tumors. This study demonstrated the risk of prognostic misclassification if GEP is performed on a single-site FNA biopsy. Augsburger et al. suggested considering GEP testing on two separate biopsy sites to reduce this risk [201].

Preferentially Expressed Antigen in Melanoma

To further increase the prognostic accuracy of GEP, a genome-wide analysis was performed, to identify other biomarkers that were altered in patients with uveal melanoma. In this effort, Field et al. discovered that mRNA expression of the cancer-testis antigen, preferentially expressed antigen in melanoma (PRAME), was a biomarker for metastasis of uveal melanoma, independent of either GEP Class 1 or GEP Class 2 profiles [202]. The mechanism by which PRAME expression relates to uveal melanoma progression to metastatic disease is not fully understood. PRAME testing for uveal melanoma is commercially available in conjunction with standard GEP testing.

Multiplex Ligation-Dependent Probe Amplification

Multiplex ligation-dependent probe amplification (MLPA) was first described in 2002 by Schouten et al. as a novel technique with the ability to detect relative quantities of up to 40 different DNA sequences within a single test [203]. With this technique, uveal melanoma DNA is obtained from FNA biopsy, denatured, and then mixed with DNA probes that target specific select genes on chromosomes 1p, 3, 6, and 8. The probes then hybridize to the target DNA sequence, and are amplified using PCR. Lastly, the amplified selected sequences are separated and identified by electrophoresis. The separated products are then quantified to determine the relative expression of each gene product [203, 204].

In 2007, Coupland and colleagues at the Liverpool Ocular Oncology Centre created a novel technique for assessing known chromosomal derangements in uveal melanomas. Coupland's group replaced traditional FISH testing for uveal melanoma with an MLPA reaction that targeted 38 loci across chromosomes 1p, 3, 6, and 8 [45, 204]. Using this novel technique, their group was able to show that MLPA can detect gain or loss of a much larger number of multiple chromosome segments (as many as 50 targets) in one single reaction, and with higher resolution than traditional FISH [203, 204]. Unlike GEP, which is marketed as a stand-alone assay for uveal melanoma prognostication, MLPA is intended to be used in conjunction with other uveal melanoma clinical and clinicopathologic features to provide prognostic utility. In this way, MLPA has been shown to provide similar prognostic accuracy as GEP. MLPA is also presently commercially available [198].

Use of Clinicopathologic Features with Genetic Tests

As previously mentioned, clinicopathologic features alone were traditionally used to stratify patients into high and low risk for metastatic disease and disease-related death. Recently, however, modern genetic and molecular testing techniques (such as GEP and MLPA) have proven to be far superior to clinicopathologic features alone in predicting metastasis and mortality [45, 140, 198, 202, 204, 205]. Still, there is data supporting the role of clinicopathologic features in conjunction with MLPA to improve prognostic accuracy and reliability, and therefore there is a nomogram for predicting metastasis which includes both MLPA and clinical tumor characteristics. In addition, there is recent evidence to suggest that there may be utility in combining tumor characteristics such as largest basal diameter with GEP results to improve prognostic accuracy [141, 198].

Uveal Melanoma Metastases

Unlike metastatic spread of melanomas of the skin, conjunctiva, and eyelids, which is primarily lymphatic, metastatic spread of primary uveal melanoma is hematogenous with a strong predilection for the liver. Once metastatic disease develops, it is uniformly fatal, with a 1-year survival rate of 13% and a 5-year survival rate approaching 0% (mean survival is ~6 months) [16, 206–209]. The most common sites for metastasis are the liver (91%), lung (26%), bone (18%), skin (12%), and lymph nodes (11%). Uveal melanoma does not metastasize to the brain, except for the rare, late-stage presentation of direct extension of the primary to the brain via the optic nerve, or perhaps in very rare patients with widespread metastatic disease [86, 126]. Thus, the presence of brain melanoma metastases from an unknown primary source should not routinely necessitate a dilated ophthalmologic examination to rule out uveal melanoma. Furthermore, patients with a history of primary uveal melanoma who later develop brain melanoma metastases should be evaluated for a second primary melanoma outside the eye that might be the origin of the brain metastasis.

As previously discussed, the overall long-term rate of metastasis for primary uveal melanoma is ~50%, and results in a 15-year mortality rate that approaches 40–50% [85, 86, 146]. Despite significant advances in the treatment of primary uveal melanoma with good local tumor control rates, the 5-year survival rate remains 72–84% [5, 206, 208, 210]. This observed reduced 5-year survival is largely the result of the high rate of metastasis, even despite successful treatment of the primary. For example, although rates of local ocular tumor control exceed 90% with radiotherapy, approximately half of these treated patients will develop metastases extending out to decades following the initial diagnosis [16, 208, 211]. This trend is observed even in patients who receive early treatment with enucleation (complete removal of the eye and tumor) and is presumably due to the presence of previously disseminated micrometastatic disease at the time of treatment for the primary intraocular tumor [87, 212].

Uveal melanoma is a disease that affects primarily older aged individuals who, because of their advanced age, likely have other numerous systemic comorbidities (such as pulmonary and cardiovascular disease) that also carry their own mortality risk for this age group. However, 20 years after treatment of primary uveal melanoma, even in this advanced-age cohort, the number one cause of death is related to uveal melanoma metastatic disease [213]. This evidence, along with the observation of metastatic disease decades after enucleation, suggests that micrometastatic seeds spread to the liver early in the life of the primary tumor and then lie dormant for decades before overt active metastatic disease develops [120, 212, 214]. In fact, these dormant micrometastases have been directly observed in the livers of patients with a history of uveal melanoma and who have died of an unrelated event [212, 215]. Survival after diagnosis of metastatic disease is generally 2–9 months [143]. Even though the majority of metastases develop within the first 5 years after initial diagnosis, metastatic disease remains the most common overall cause of death in uveal melanoma patients for up to 20 years after the initial diagnosis has been made [127, 213].

Treatment of Metastatic Uveal Melanoma

Presently, there is no good data to demonstrate any significant benefit from adjuvant chemotherapy, immunotherapy, radiotherapy, or surgical therapy in reducing the rate of development of metastatic disease [3, 216–221]. Treatment of metastatic disease has been explored with numerous and diverse treatment modalities, including systemic chemotherapy, immunotherapy, hepatic arterial chemotherapy, hepatic artery chemoembolization, regional immunotherapy, and surgical metastasectomy. To date, results of these treatment modalities have shown only modest metastatic tumor response and limited survival benefit [3, 126, 145, 209, 216–220, 222–231].

Given that the majority of patients with metastatic disease present with diffuse liver involvement, surgical resection is generally not a viable treatment. Surgical resection may be considered only in very select cases where patients present with only a few, localized, and easily accessible hepatic lesions. Survival results from focal resection still remain modest at best [3]. It is important to note that although MEK, BRAF, and KIT inhibitors have been transformative for the treatment of cutaneous melanoma, these treatments do not appear to be nearly as effective for the treatment of either primary or metastatic uveal melanoma [36, 37, 43, 53, 232]. Similarly, while immunotherapy appears transformative for the field of metastatic cutaneous melanoma, most metastatic uveal melanomas do not appear to respond to these treatments [221, 233–240].

Surveillance for Development of Metastatic Disease

Although radiographically or clinically apparent metastases are only found in 3% of patients with uveal melanoma at the time of diagnosis [241, 242], everyone agrees that all patients with a new diagnosis of uveal melanoma should undergo systemic staging with imaging [243–245]. This generally consists of CT, MRI, or PET-CT imaging of the chest and abdomen. Due to the very low incidence of CNS metastases from uveal melanoma, the CNS is generally not imaged [241, 243–245]. Beyond this, there is controversy surrounding the role and utility of subsequent surveillance imaging for metastases. While everyone agrees that the risk of developing subsequent metastases is high, there is a difference of opinions regarding the utility of potentially identifying metastases earlier through surveillance imaging when there are no effective treatments for those metastases.

While there is evidence that surveillance imaging leads to prolonged survival following the identification of metastases, this is felt to largely represent lead-time bias, while actual patient survival is not extended [246]. In general, most ocular oncologists do recommend systemic surveillance imaging for metastases, because there are many clinical trials into which patients without end-stage disease could enroll, and because a certain small fraction of patients will respond to one or another class of currently available treatments. This surveillance imaging generally consists of CT or MRI imaging of the liver, with or without CT imaging of the chest [243, 244, 247]. Abdominal ultrasound, in experienced hands, has been shown to be an effective screening modality for the liver, in nonobese patients, and has the benefit of avoiding additional radiation exposure to the patient [248]. Any additional benefit of liver function tests in patients undergoing an imaging-based screening regimen is unclear [148]. As treatments for metastatic uveal melanoma improve, the importance of surveillance imaging will increase.

Association with Systemic Disease

Uveal melanoma is largely an isolated and independent disease for the overwhelming majority of patients. In contrast to cutaneous melanoma, uveal melanoma presents with a positive family history of uveal melanoma only 1.6% of the time [249–251]. However, there are a few other notable diseases and syndromes that are known to be associated with an increased risk for uveal melanoma. These include *BAP1* cancer syndrome, dysplastic nevus syndrome, xeroderma pigmentosum, and oculodermal melanocytosis (Nevus of Ota) [250, 252–254]. The *BAP1* cancer syndrome is associated with an increased risk for development of numerous malignancies, including uveal melanoma, cutaneous melanoma, cutaneous basal cell carcinoma, malignant mesothelioma, clear cell renal cell cancer, abnormal skin lesions termed "melanocytic BAP1-mutated atypical intradermal tumors" (MBAITs), breast cancer, cholangiocarcinoma, non-small-cell lung adenocarcinoma, meningioma, and neuroendocrine carcinoma [253].

Thus, a patient with cutaneous melanoma without any of these other *BAP1*-associated malignancies is unlikely to have any significant difference from the general population regarding the risk for developing uveal melanoma. Therefore, ophthalmic uveal melanoma screening examinations are not typically warranted for patients with simple, isolated cutaneous melanoma in the absence of a cancer syndrome. Even patients with a family history of cutaneous melanoma do not have an increased risk for uveal melanoma unless the cutaneous melanoma is associated with a cancer predisposition syndrome like *BAP1* cancer syndrome, dysplastic nevus syndrome, or xeroderma pigmentosum

[250, 253–255]. Alternatively, patients with uveal melanoma have an 11% increased risk for developing other secondary malignancies such as renal cell carcinoma or cutaneous melanoma. This increased risk is thought to be attributable to germline *BAP1* mutations [256].

Conjunctival Melanoma

The conjunctiva is the thin, clear mucous membrane that is external to the eye and covers the front portions of the sclera, extending from the peripheral edge of the cornea to the eyelid fornix and then looping back onto the posterior surface of the eyelids (Fig. 16.1). Conjunctival melanomas may arise from a conjunctival nevus, primary acquired melanosis (PAM) of the conjunctiva, or de novo [257]. Conjunctival melanomas are rare and have an incidence of 0.2–0.5 per million Caucasians [12]. In fact, uveal melanoma is 7.5 to 17.5 times more common than conjunctival melanoma [5, 9–12]. However, conjunctival melanoma represents 52–53% of all malignant conjunctival tumors [258, 259].

As previously mentioned, it is important to understand that conjunctival melanoma is not intraocular, and is therefore quite different from uveal melanoma. In fact, conjunctival melanoma has many more characteristics and features in common with cutaneous melanoma, including genetics, sun exposure as a risk factor, treatment approach, and propensity for lymphatic spread [6, 13, 28, 260–263]. For example, like cutaneous melanoma, the incidence of conjunctival melanoma in the United States has doubled over the past 50 years from 0.27 to 0.54 per million. Like cutaneous melanoma, this rise is thought to be attributable to increasing UV light exposure [11, 12]. Staging for cutaneous melanoma is via the TNM staging criteria similar to cutaneous melanoma [142].

Treatment of Conjunctival Melanomas

While treatment for primary uveal melanoma is primarily with radiotherapy, conjunctival melanoma is largely a surgical disease, much like its cutaneous counterpart [2–6]. In the past, conjunctival melanomas were treated with extreme measures, such as exenteration (complete removal of the eyeball along with the surrounding orbital fat, extraocular muscles, nerves, and eyelids), because these tumors were thought to be extremely invasive [264]. However, in 1996, Norregaard et al. demonstrated that there was no significant difference in tumor recurrence or patient survival between aggressive exenteration and conservative surgical excision [261]. The results from Norregaard's study dramatically changed the treatment paradigm and conservative treatment is now the mainstay for most conjunctival melanomas [260].

Today, techniques for limited (but complete) excision of the visible tumor with a wide local margin have been widely published. Adjuvant topical chemotherapy with mitomycin C eye drops is commonly used. Excisional biopsy of the melanoma is performed in the operating room with wide surgical margins, employing a no-touch technique, in which the tumor itself is never touched with the surgical instruments, to prevent spread to uninvolved tissues. Alcohol may be used to assist in removing any corneal epithelium that may be involved. Next, a double-freeze-thaw cryotherapy technique is applied to the edges of the limbus and conjunctiva that were excised. Recurrence is then monitored with serial examinations and photography, and periodic surveillance map biopsies of the conjunctiva may be performed if there is concern for recurrence [260, 265].

Recurrence Rates for Conjunctival Melanoma

Despite optimal surgical treatment with acceptable negative surgical margins and negative repeat map biopsies, the prognosis is highly variable and somewhat unpredictable, with significant rates of recurrence and metastases [266]. Recent published recurrence rates are 26% at 5 years, 51% at 10 years, and 65% at 15 years. Metastases are seen in up to 26% of patients at 10 years after treatment. Similar to cutaneous melanoma, the most frequent sites of metastasis for conjunctival melanoma are the regional lymph nodes, with subsequent progression to the brain, liver, and lung. Death from metastatic conjunctival melanoma has been reported to be 13% at 8 years after the initial diagnosis [267].

Areas of Future Study

Over the past several decades, our understanding of the genetics, pathophysiology, risk factors, and prognostic features of uveal melanoma has greatly improved. We understand how uveal melanomas develop from a melanocyte to a benign nevus to a malignant melanoma. Our treatment paradigm has shifted from complete removal of the eye (enucleation) to eye- and vision-sparing treatment with radiotherapy [4]. However, despite excellent local treatment control rates, our ability to prevent or treat metastases is very poor. Once metastases develop, there are currently no good treatment options and patient mortality is nearly 100% at 5 years [207–209].

Furthermore, with the development of genetic prognostication for uveal melanoma, we are now equipped to accurately predict which patients will develop metastatic disease. We also understand that micrometastatic spread to the liver happens very early in the primary disease state, with long periods of micrometastatic dormancy. However, we do not understand how these undetectable micrometastases stay dormant, nor why they ultimately may reactivate, causing overt metastatic disease. Further studies are needed to fully elucidate the pathophysiology of this process and to develop therapies to prevent this reactivation or treat the metastatic tumors once they form.

A potential novel treatment modality on the horizon may utilize epigenetic regulation of genes to treat both primary and metastatic uveal melanoma. The term epigenetics refers to mitotically inherited factors that alter genetic expression but are not caused by direct changes in the primary DNA sequence [268]. Over the past two decades, it has been shown that epigenetics plays an important role in a multitude of diseases and cancers. Epigenetic mechanisms are responsible for producing dynamic modifications of chromatin structure, resulting in relatively more or less compaction of DNA. Ultimately, epigenetic mechanisms produce fluent alterations in gene expression. Relatively recently, the mechanisms underlying a number of epigenetic alterations have been elucidated, including DNA methylation and histone modification through acetylation or methylation. As a result of these discoveries, the terms "epigenome" and "histone code" have been coined [269].

Recent studies have demonstrated strong evidence that aberrant histone modifications play a critical role in the oncogenesis of several malignancies, and prognostic outcomes have been associated with changes in the global cellular patterns of histone modifications in these malignancies [270–273]. It has been shown that the histone code can be altered by modifications to major regulators of transcription, such as the polycomb group (PcG) of proteins and histone-modifying enzymes (HMEs) such as histone acetyltransferases (HATs) or histone deacetylases (HDACs) [74, 274].

In 2015, Herlihy et al. showed that monosomy 3 and GEP Class 2 uveal melanomas are associated with reduced expression levels of several HMEs and PcG proteins [75]. Furthermore, Landreville et al. have shown that histone deacetylase (HDAC) inhibitors can reverse uveal melanoma cellular morphology into a more differentiated state and inhibit growth of these malignant cells in vivo [75, 76]. Future treatments for primary and metastatic uveal melanoma may therefore focus on harnessing the epigenetic regulation of the aberrant genes associated with this disease. Although initial results are intriguing, more studies are needed to better explore and validate these strategies as potential future treatment options.

References

1. Howlader N, Noone A, Krapcho M, Miller D, Bishop K, Kosary C, et al. Cancer Statistics Review, 1975–2014—SEER Statistics, National Cancer Institute. SEER Cancer Statistics Review, 1975–2014. 2016. http://seer.cancer.gov/csr/1975_2014/
2. Shields JA, Shields CL. Management of posterior uveal melanoma. In: Intraocular tumors: a textbook and Atlas. Philadelphia: WB Saunders; 1992. p. 171–205.

3. Weis E, Salopek TG, McKinnon JG, Larocque MP, Temple-Oberle C, Cheng T, et al. Management of uveal melanoma: a consensus-based provincial clinical practice guideline. Curr Oncol. 2016;23(1):e57–64.
4. Milam RW, Batson SA, Breazzano MP, Ayala-Peacock DN, Daniels AB. Modern and novel radiotherapy approaches for the treatment of uveal melanoma. Int Ophthalmol Clin [Internet]. 2017;57(1):11–27.
5. Singh AD, Turell ME, Topham AK. Uveal melanoma: trends in incidence, treatment, and survival. Ophthalmology. 2011;118(9):1881–5.
6. Bichakjian CK, Halpern AC, Johnson TM, Foote Hood A, Grichnik JM, Swetter SM, et al. Guidelines of care for the management of primary cutaneous melanoma. J Am Acad Dermatol. 2011;65(5):1032–47.
7. Tsao H, Atkins MB, Sober AJ. Management of cutaneous melanoma. N Engl J Med [Internet]. 2004;351(10):998–1012. http://www.nejm.org/doi/full/10.1056/NEJMra041245
8. Chattopadhyay C, Kim DW, Gombos DS, Oba J, Qin Y, Williams MD, et al. Uveal melanoma: from diagnosis to treatment and the science in between. Cancer [Internet]. 2016;122(15):2299–12. http://onlinelibrary.wiley.com/doi/10.1002/cncr.29727/abstract;jsessionid=58601C38771BB3963A9DD2C1864E3DB2.f02t01
9. Singh AD, Topham A. Incidence of uveal melanoma in the United States: 1973–1997. Ophthalmology. 2003;110(5):956–61.
10. Virgili G, Gatta G, Ciccolallo L, Capocaccia R, Biggeri A, Crocetti E, et al. Incidence of uveal melanoma in Europe. Ophthalmology. 2007;114(12):2309–15.
11. Tuomaala S, Kivelä T. Correspondence regarding Conjunctival melanoma: is it increasing in the United States? Am J Ophthalmol [Internet]. 2003 [cited 2017 Aug 18];136(6):1189–90; author reply 1190.
12. Yu GP, Hu DN, McCormick S, Finger PT. Conjunctival melanoma: is it increasing in the United States? Am J Ophthalmol. 2003;135(6):800–6.
13. Chang AE, Karnell LH, Menck HR. The National Cancer Data Base report on cutaneous and noncutaneous melanoma: a summary of 84,836 cases from the past decade. The American College of Surgeons Commission on Cancer and the American Cancer Society. Cancer. 1998;83(8):1664–78.
14. McLaughlin CC, Wu XC, Jemal A, Martin HJ, Roche LM, Chen VW. Incidence of noncutaneous melanomas in the U.S. Cancer. 2005;103(5):1000–7.
15. Damato B. Progress in the management of patients with uveal melanoma. The 2012 Ashton Lecture. Eye [Internet]. 2012;26(9):1157–72.
16. Cerbone L, Van Ginderdeuren R, Van den Oord J, Fieuws S, Spileers W, Van Eenoo L, et al. Clinical presentation, pathological features and natural course of metastatic uveal melanoma, an orphan and commonly fatal disease. Oncology. 2014;86(3):185–9.
17. Yu G-P, Hu D-N, McCormick SA. Latitude and incidence of ocular melanoma. Photochem Photobiol [Internet]. 2006 [cited 2017 Oct 3];82(6):1621. http://www.ncbi.nlm.nih.gov/pubmed/16922607
18. Nayman T, Bostan C, Logan P, Burnier MN. Uveal melanoma risk factors: a systematic review of meta-analyses. Curr Eye Res [Internet]. 2017 [cited 2017 Aug 19];42(8):1085–93. http://www.ncbi.nlm.nih.gov/pubmed/28494168
19. Yu G-P, Hu D-N, McCormick SA. Latitude and incidence of ocular melanoma. Photochem Photobiol. 2006;82(6):1621.
20. Damato EM, Damato BE. Detection and time to treatment of uveal melanoma in the United Kingdom: an evaluation of 2384 patients. Ophthalmology. 2012;119(8):1582–9.
21. Andreoli MT, Mieler WF, Leiderman YI. Epidemiological trends in uveal melanoma. Br J Ophthalmol [Internet]. 2015;99(11):1550–3. http://www.ncbi.nlm.nih.gov/pubmed/25904122
22. Kivela T. The epidemiological challenge of the most frequent eye cancer: retinoblastoma, an issue of birth and death. Br J Ophthalmol [Internet]. 2009 Sep 1 [cited 2017 Oct 3];93(9):1129–31. http://www.ncbi.nlm.nih.gov/pubmed/19704035
23. Weis E, Shah CP, Lajous M, Shields JA, Shields CL. The association of cutaneous and iris nevi with uveal melanoma: a meta-analysis. Ophthalmology. 2009;116(3):536–43.
24. Shields CL, Kaliki S, Livesey M, Walker B, Garoon R, Bucci M, et al. Association of ocular and oculodermal melanocytosis with the rate of uveal melanoma metastasis: analysis of 7872 consecutive eyes. JAMA Ophthalmol [Internet]. 2013;131(8):993–1003. http://www.ncbi.nlm.nih.gov/pubmed/23681424
25. Harbour JW, Onken MD, Roberson ED, Duan S, Cao L, Worley LA, et al. Frequent mutation of BAP1 in metastasizing uveal melanomas. Science. 2010;330(6009):1410–3.
26. Gallagher RP, Elwood JM, Rootman J, Spinelli JJ, Hill GB, Threlfall WJ, et al. Risk factors for ocular melanoma: Western Canada Melanoma Study. J Natl Cancer Inst. 1985;74(4):775–8.
27. Shah CP, Weis E, Lajous M, Shields JA, Shields CL. Intermittent and chronic ultraviolet light exposure and uveal melanoma: a meta-analysis. Ophthalmology. 2005;112(9):1599–607.
28. Holman HDAJ, Armstrong BK. Pigmentary traits, ethnic origin, benign nevi, and family history as risk factors for cutaneous malignant melanoma. J Natl Cancer Inst. 1984;72(2):257–66.
29. Mark Elwood J, Jopson J. Melanoma and sun exposure: an overview of published studies. Int J Cancer. 1997;73(2):198–203.
30. Whiteman DC, Stickley M, Watt P, Hughes MC, Davis MB, Green AC. Anatomic site, sun exposure, and risk of cutaneous melanoma. J Clin Oncol. 2006;24(19):3172–7.

31. Shields CL. The hunt for the secrets of uveal melanoma. Clin Exp Ophthalmol. 2008;36:277–80.
32. Tucker MA, Shields JA, Hartge P, Augsburger J, Hoover RN, Fraumeni Jr JF. Sunlight exposure as risk factor for intraocular malignant melanoma. N Engl J Med [Internet]. 1985;313(13):789–92. http://www.ncbi.nlm.nih.gov/pubmed/4033707
33. Kaliki S, Shields C. Uveal melanoma: relatively rare but deadly cancer. Eye [Internet]. 2016 [cited 2017 Aug 28];31:241–57. http://www.nature.com.proxy.library.vanderbilt.edu/eye/journal/v31/n2/pdf/eye2016275a.pdf
34. Schmidt-Pokrzywniak A, Jöckel K-H, Bornfeld N, Sauerwein W, Stang A. Positive interaction between light iris color and ultraviolet radiation in relation to the risk of uveal melanoma: a case-control study. Ophthalmology [Internet]. 2009 Feb [cited 2017 Oct 3];116(2):340–8. http://linkinghub.elsevier.com/retrieve/pii/S0161642008010063
35. Brash DE, Rudolph JA, Simon JA, Lin A, McKenna GJ, Baden HP, et al. A role for sunlight in skin cancer: UV-induced p53 mutations in squamous cell carcinoma. Proc Natl Acad Sci [Internet]. 1991;88(22):10124–8. http://www.pnas.org/cgi/doi/10.1073/pnas.88.22.10124
36. Onken MD, Worley LA, Long MD, Duan S, Council ML, Bowcock AM, et al. Oncogenic mutations in GNAQ occur early in uveal melanoma. Invest Ophthalmol Vis Sci. 2008;49(12):5230–4.
37. Van Raamsdonk CD, Bezrookove V, Green G, Bauer J, Gaugler L, O'Brien JM, et al. Frequent somatic mutations of GNAQ in uveal melanoma and blue naevi. Nature. 2009;457(7229):599–602.
38. Van Raamsdonk CD, Griewank KG, Crosby MB, Garrido MC, Vemula S, Wiesner T, et al. Mutations in GNA11 in uveal melanoma. N Engl J Med. 2010;363(23):2191–9.
39. De Lange MJ, Razzaq L, Versluis M, Verlinde S, Dogrusöz M, Böhringer S, et al. Distribution of GNAQ and GNA11 mutation signatures in uveal melanoma points to a light dependent mutation mechanism. PLoS One. 2015;10(9):e0138002.
40. Cruz F, Rubin BP, Wilson D, Town A, Schroeder A, Haley A, et al. Absence of BRAF and NRAS mutations in uveal melanoma. Cancer Res. 2003;63(18):5761–6.
41. Rimoldi D, Salvi S, Liénard D, Lejeune FJ, Speiser D, Zografos L, et al. Lack of BRAF mutations in uveal melanoma. Cancer Res. 2003;63(18):5712–5.
42. Davies H, Bignell GR, Cox C, Stephens P, Edkins S, Clegg S, et al. Mutations of the BRAF gene in human cancer. Nature. 2002;417(6892):949–54.
43. Daniels AB, Lee JE, MacConaill LE, Palescandolo E, Van Hummelen P, Adams SM, et al. High throughput mass spectrometry-based mutation profiling of primary uveal melanoma. Invest Ophthalmol Vis Sci. 2012;53(11):6991–6.
44. Milam RW, Daniels AB. Genetics of uveal melanoma. In: eLS: encyclopedia of life sciences. Hoboken: John Wiley and Sons Ltd, 2018.
45. Coupland SE, Lake SL, Zeschnigk M, Damato BE. Molecular pathology of uveal melanoma. Eye (Lond). 2013;27(2):230–42.
46. Maat W, Ly LV, Jordanova ES, de Wolff-Rouendaal D, Schalij-Delfos NE, Jager MJ. Monosomy of chromosome 3 and an inflammatory phenotype occur together in uveal melanoma. Invest Ophthalmol Vis Sci. 2008;49(2):505–10.
47. Prescher G, Bornfeld N, Horsthemke B, Becher R. Chromosomal aberrations defining uveal melanoma of poor prognosis. Lancet (London, England). 1992;339(8794):691–2.
48. Prescher G, Bornfeld N, Hirche H, Horsthemke B, Jockel KH, Becher R. Prognostic implications of monosomy 3 in uveal melanoma. Lancet (London, England). 1996;347(9010):1222–5.
49. Damato B, Duke C, Coupland SE, Hiscott P, Smith PA, Campbell I, et al. Cytogenetics of uveal melanoma: a 7-year clinical experience. Ophthalmology. 2007;114(10):1925–31.
50. Cassoux N, Rodrigues MJ, Plancher C, Asselain B, Levy-Gabriel C, Rouic LL-L, et al. Genome-wide profiling is a clinically relevant and affordable prognostic test in posterior uveal melanoma. Br J Ophthalmol. 2014;98(6):769–74.
51. Delaunay J, Martin L, Bressac-de Paillerets B, Duru G, Ingster O, Thomas L. Improvement of genetic testing for cutaneous melanoma in countries with low to moderate incidence. JAMA Dermatol [Internet]. 2017 [cited 2017 Oct 3]; http://www.ncbi.nlm.nih.gov/pubmed/28903138
52. Cancer Genome Atlas Network. Genomic classification of cutaneous melanoma. Cell [Internet]. 2015;161(7):1681–96. http://linkinghub.elsevier.com/retrieve/pii/S0092867415006340
53. Daniels AB, Abramson DH. c-KIT in uveal melanoma: big fish or red herring? Arch Ophthalmol (Chicago, Ill 1960). 2009;127(5):695–7.
54. Feng X, Degese MS, Iglesias-Bartolome R, Vaque JP, Molinolo AA, Rodrigues M, et al. Hippo-independent activation of YAP by the GNAQ uveal melanoma oncogene through a trio-regulated rho GTPase signaling circuitry. Cancer Cell. 2014;25(6):831–45.
55. Yu FX, Luo J, Mo JS, Liu G, Kim YC, Meng Z, et al. Mutant Gq/11 promote uveal melanoma tumorigenesis by activating YAP. Cancer Cell. 2014;25(6):822–30.
56. Bauer J, Kilic E, Vaarwater J, Bastian BC, Garbe C, de Klein A. Oncogenic GNAQ mutations are not correlated with disease-free survival in uveal melanoma. Br J Cancer. 2009;101(5):813–5.
57. Matatall KA, Agapova OA, Onken MD, Worley LA, Bowcock AM, Harbour JW. BAP1 deficiency causes loss of melanocytic cell identity in uveal melanoma. BMC Cancer. 2013;13:371.
58. White VA, McNeil BK, Horsman DE. Acquired homozygosity (isodisomy) of chromosome 3 in uveal melanoma. Cancer Genet Cytogenet. 1998;102(1):40–5.

59. van Essen TH, van Pelt SI, Versluis M, Bronkhorst IH, van Duinen SG, Marinkovic M, et al. Prognostic parameters in uveal melanoma and their association with BAP1 expression. Br J Ophthalmol. 2014;98(12):1738–43.
60. Yavuzyigitoglu S, Koopmans AE, Verdijk RM, Vaarwater J, Eussen B, van Bodegom A, et al. Uveal melanomas with SF3B1 mutations: a distinct subclass associated with late-onset metastases. Ophthalmology. 2016;123(5):1118–28.
61. Bonnal S, Vigevani L, Valcarcel J. The spliceosome as a target of novel antitumour drugs. Nat Rev Discov. 2012;11(11):847–59.
62. Maciejewski JP, Padgett RA. Defects in spliceosomal machinery: a new pathway of leukaemogenesis. Br J Haematol. 2012;158(2):165–73.
63. Field MG, Harbour JW. Recent developments in prognostic and predictive testing in uveal melanoma. Curr Opin Ophthalmol. 2014;25(3):234–9.
64. Martin M, Masshofer L, Temming P, Rahmann S, Metz C, Bornfeld N, et al. Exome sequencing identifies recurrent somatic mutations in EIF1AX and SF3B1 in uveal melanoma with disomy 3. Nat Genet. 2013;45(8):933–6.
65. Coupland SE, Anastassiou G, Stang A, Schilling H, Anagnostopoulos I, Bornfeld N, et al. The prognostic value of cyclin D1, p53, and MDM2 protein expression in uveal melanoma. J Pathol. 2000;191(2):120–6.
66. Brantley MA Jr, Harbour JW. Inactivation of retinoblastoma protein in uveal melanoma by phosphorylation of sites in the COOH-terminal region. Cancer Res. 2000;60(16):4320–3.
67. Brantley MA Jr, Harbour JW. Deregulation of the Rb and p53 pathways in uveal melanoma. Am J Pathol. 2000;157(6):1795–801.
68. Abdel-Rahman MH, Yang Y, Zhou XP, Craig EL, Davidorf FH, Eng C. High frequency of submicroscopic hemizygous deletion is a major mechanism of loss of expression of PTEN in uveal melanoma. J Clin Oncol. 2006;24(2):288–95.
69. Ehlers JP, Worley L, Onken MD, Harbour JW. Integrative genomic analysis of aneuploidy in uveal melanoma. Clin Cancer Res. 2008;14(1):115–22.
70. Stambolic V, Suzuki A, de la Pompa JL, Brothers GM, Mirtsos C, Sasaki T, et al. Negative regulation of PKB/Akt-dependent cell survival by the tumor suppressor PTEN. Cell. 1998;95(1):29–39.
71. Li J, Yen C, Liaw D, Podsypanina K, Bose S, Wang SI, et al. PTEN, a putative protein tyrosine phosphatase gene mutated in human brain, breast, and prostate cancer. Science. 1997;275(5308):1943–7.
72. Maehama T, Dixon JE. The tumor suppressor, PTEN/MMAC1, dephosphorylates the lipid second messenger, phosphatidylinositol 3,4,5-trisphosphate. J Biol Chem. 1998;273(22):13375–8.
73. Chang F, Lee JT, Navolanic PM, Steelman LS, Shelton JG, Blalock WL, et al. Involvement of PI3K/Akt pathway in cell cycle progression, apoptosis, and neoplastic transformation: a target for cancer chemotherapy. Leukemia. 2003;17(3):590–603.
74. Thiagalingam S, Cheng KH, Lee HJ, Mineva N, Thiagalingam A, Ponte JF. Histone deacetylases: unique players in shaping the epigenetic histone code. Ann N Y Acad Sci. 2003;983:84–100.
75. Herlihy N, Dogrusoz M, van Essen TH, Harbour JW, van der Velden PA, van Eggermond MC, et al. Skewed expression of the genes encoding epigenetic modifiers in high-risk uveal melanoma. Invest Ophthalmol Vis Sci. 2015;56(3):1447–58.
76. Landreville S, Agapova OA, Matatall KA, Kneass ZT, Onken MD, Lee RS, et al. Histone deacetylase inhibitors induce growth arrest and differentiation in uveal melanoma. Clin Cancer Res. 2012;18(2):408–16.
77. Field MG, Harbour JW. GNAQ/11 mutations in uveal melanoma: is YAP the key to targeted therapy? Cancer Cell. 2014;25(6):714–5.
78. Onken MD, Ehlers JP, Worley LA, Makita J, Yokota Y, Harbour JW. Functional gene expression analysis uncovers phenotypic switch in aggressive uveal melanomas. Cancer Res. 2006;66(9):4602–9.
79. Sahel JA, Pesavento R, Frederick AR, Albert DM. Melanoma arising de novo over a 16-month period. Arch Ophthalmol (Chicago, Ill 1960) [Internet]. 1988;106(3):381–5. http://www.ncbi.nlm.nih.gov/pubmed/3278703
80. Aleksidze N, Medina CA, Singh AD. De novo evolution of a small choroidal melanoma. Ocul Oncol Pathol [Internet]. 2015 [cited 2017 Dec 2];1(2):83–7. http://www.ncbi.nlm.nih.gov/pubmed/27231689
81. Shields CL, Furuta M, Mashayekhi A, Berman EL, Zahler JD, Hoberman DM, et al. Clinical spectrum of choroidal nevi based on age at presentation in 3422 consecutive eyes. Ophthalmology. 2008;115(3):546–552.e2.
82. Shields CL, Kaliki S, Furuta M, Mashayekhi A, Shields JA. Clinical spectrum and prognosis of uveal melanoma based on age at presentation in 8,033 cases. Retina. 2012;32:1363–72.
83. Bove R, Char DH. Nondiagnosed uveal melanomas. Ophthalmology. 2004;111(3):554–7.
84. Scotto J, Fraumeni JF Jr, Lee JA. Melanomas of the eye and other noncutaneous sites: epidemiologic aspects. J Natl Cancer Inst. 1976;56(3):489–91.
85. Augsburger JJ, Schneider S, Freire J, Brady LW. Survival following enucleation versus plaque radiotherapy in statistically matched subgroups of patients with choroidal melanomas: results in patients treated between 1980 and 1987. Graefes Arch Clin Exp Ophthalmol. 1999;237(7):558–67.
86. Kapoor A, Beniwal V, Beniwal S, Mathur H, Kumar HS. Management of uveal tract melanoma: a comprehensive review. J Egypt Natl Canc Inst. 2016;28(2):65–72.
87. Nichols EE, Richmond A, Daniels AB. Tumor characteristics, genetics, management, and the risk of metastasis in uveal melanoma. Semin Ophthalmol. 2016;31(4):304–9.

88. Shields JA, Shields CL. Intraocular tumors: an atlas and textbook. 3rd ed. Philadelphia: Lippincott Williams & Wilkins; 2015. 608 p.
89. Shields JA, Sanborn GE, Augsburger JJ. The differential diagnosis of malignant melanoma of the iris. A clinical study of 200 patients. Ophthalmology [Internet]. 1983 [cited 2017 Dec 5];90(6):716–20. http://www.ncbi.nlm.nih.gov/pubmed/6888862
90. Ah-Fat FG, Damato BE. Delays in the diagnosis of uveal melanoma and effect on treatment. Eye (Lond). 1998;12(Pt 5):781–2.
91. Eagle Jr RC, Grossniklaus HE, Syed N, Hogan RN, Lloyd WC, Folberg R, et al. Inadvertent evisceration of eyes containing uveal melanoma. Arch Ophthalmol [Internet]. 2009;127(2):141–5.
92. Shields CL. Choroidal nevus transformation into melanoma. Arch Ophthalmol. 2009;127(8):981–7.
93. Shields CL, Furuta M, Thangappan A, Nagori S, Mashayekhi A, Lally DR, et al. Metastasis of uveal melanoma millimeter-by-millimeter in 8033 consecutive eyes. Arch Ophthalmol (Chicago, Ill 1960) [Internet]. 2009;127(8):989–98. http://www.ncbi.nlm.nih.gov/pubmed/19667335
94. Fuller DG, Snyder WB, Hutton WL, Vaiser A. Ultrasonographic features of choroidal malignant melanomas. Arch Ophthalmol (Chicago, Ill 1960) [Internet]. 1979 [cited 2017 Oct 3];97(8):1465–72. http://www.ncbi.nlm.nih.gov/pubmed/464871
95. Bedi DG, Gombos DS, Ng CS, Singh S. Sonography of the eye. Am J Roentgenol. 2006;187(4):1061–72.
96. Ossoinig KC. Standardized echography: basic principles, clinical applications, and results. Int Ophthalmol Clin [Internet]. 1979 [cited 2017 Oct 3];19(4):127–210. http://www.ncbi.nlm.nih.gov/pubmed/395120
97. Pavlin CJ, McWhae JA, McGowan HD, Foster FS. Ultrasound biomicroscopy of anterior segment tumors. Ophthalmology [Internet]. 1992 [cited 2017 Oct 3];99(8):1220–8. http://www.ncbi.nlm.nih.gov/pubmed/1513574
98. Pavlin CJ, McWhae JA, McGowan HD, Foster FS. Ultrasound biomicroscopy of anterior segment tumors. Ophthalmology. 1992;99(8):1220–8.
99. Conway RM, Chew T, Golchet P, Desai K, Lin S, O'Brien J. Ultrasound biomicroscopy: role in diagnosis and management in 130 consecutive patients evaluated for anterior segment tumours. Br J Ophthalmol [Internet]. 2005 [cited 2017 Oct 3];89(8):950–5. http://www.ncbi.nlm.nih.gov/pubmed/16024841
100. Yung M, Klufas MA, Sarraf D. Clinical applications of fundus autofluorescence in retinal disease. Int J Retin Vitr [Internet]. 2016 [cited 2017 Oct 18];2(1):12. http://journalretinavitreous.biomedcentral.com/articles/10.1186/s40942-016-0035-x
101. Shields CL, Pirondini C, Bianciotto C, Materin MA, Harmon SA, Shields JA. Autofluorescence of choroidal nevus in 64 cases. Retina [Internet]. 2008;28(8):1035–43. http://www.ncbi.nlm.nih.gov/pubmed/18779708
102. Almeida A, Kaliki S, Shields CL. Autofluorescence of intraocular tumours. Curr Opin Ophthalmol [Internet]. 2013;24(3):222–32. http://www.ncbi.nlm.nih.gov/pubmed/23429597
103. Lavinsky D, Belfort RN, Navajas E, Torres V, Martins MC, Belfort R. Fundus autofluorescence of choroidal nevus and melanoma. Br J Ophthalmol [Internet]. 2007;91(10):1299–302. http://www.pubmedcentral.nih.gov/articlerender.fcgi?artid=2000998&tool=pmcentrez&rendertype=abstract
104. Albertus DL, Schachar IH, Zahid S, Elner VM, Demirci H, Jayasundera T. Autofluorescence quantification of benign and malignant choroidal nevomelanocytic tumors. JAMA Ophthalmol [Internet]. 2013;131(8):1004–8. http://www.ncbi.nlm.nih.gov/pubmed/23787920
105. Espinoza G, Rosenblatt B, Harbour JW. Optical coherence tomography in the evaluation of retinal changes associated with suspicious choroidal melanocytic tumors. Am J Ophthalmol. 2004;137:90–5.
106. Shields CL, Mashayekhi A, Materin MA, Luo CK, Marr BP, Demirci H, et al. Optical coherence tomography of choroidal nevus in 120 patients. Retina. 2005;25:243–52.
107. Augsburger JJ, Golden MI, Shields JA. Fluorescein angiography of choroidal malignant melanomas with retinal invasion. Retina [Internet]. 1984 [cited 2017 Oct 18];4(4):232–41. http://www.ncbi.nlm.nih.gov/pubmed/6531518
108. Shields CL, Shields JA, De Potter P. Patterns of indocyanine green videoangiography of choroidal tumours. Br J Ophthalmol [Internet]. 1995 [cited 2017 Oct 19];79(3):237–45. http://www.ncbi.nlm.nih.gov/pubmed/7703202
109. Folberg R, Rummelt V, Parys-Van Ginderdeuren R, Hwang T, Woolson RF, Pe'er J, et al. The prognostic value of tumor blood vessel morphology in primary uveal melanoma. Ophthalmology [Internet]. 1993;100(9):1389–98. https://doi.org/10.1016/S0161-6420(93)31470-3
110. Mueller AJ, Bartsch D-U, Folberg R, Mehaffey MG, Boldt HC, Meyer M, et al. Imaging the microvasculature of choroidal melanomas with confocal indocyanine green scanning laser ophthalmoscopy. Arch Ophthalmol [Internet]. 1998;116(1):31–9. http://www.ncbi.nlm.nih.gov/pubmed/9445206
111. Tartaglione T, Pagliara MM, Sciandra M, Caputo CG, Calandrelli R, Fabrizi G, et al. Uveal melanoma: evaluation of extrascleral extension using thin-section MR of the eye with surface coils. Radiol Med [Internet]. 2014 [cited 2017 Oct 19];119(10):775–83. http://www.ncbi.nlm.nih.gov/pubmed/24469990
112. Henderson E, Margo CE. Iris melanoma. Arch Pathol Lab Med [Internet]. 2008;132(2):268–72. http://www.ncbi.nlm.nih.gov/pubmed/18251588
113. Shields CL, Shields JA, Shields MB, Augsburger JJ. Prevalence and mechanisms of secondary intraocular pressure elevation in eyes with intraocular tumors. Ophthalmology [Internet].

1987;94(7):839–46. http://www.ncbi.nlm.nih.gov/pubmed/3658352
114. Shields CL, Kaliki S, Shah SU, Luo W, Furuta M, Shields JA. Iris melanoma: features and prognosis in 317 children and adults. J AAPOS. 2012;16(1):10–6.
115. Bianciotto C, Shields CL, Guzman JM, Romanelli-Gobbi M, Mazzuca D, Green WR, et al. Assessment of anterior segment tumors with ultrasound biomicroscopy versus anterior segment optical coherence tomography in 200 cases. Ophthalmology. 2011;118(7):1297–302.
116. Shields CL, Shields JA, Kiratli H, De Potter P, Cater JR. Risk factors for growth and metastasis of small choroidal melanocytic lesions. Trans Am Ophthalmol Soc. 1995;93:259.
117. Shields CL, Cater J, Shields JA Singh AD, Santos MC, Carvalho C Combination of clinical factors predictive of growth of small choroidal melanocytic tumors. Arch Ophthalmol [Internet]. 2000;118(3):360–4. http://www.ncbi.nlm.nih.gov/pubmed/10721958
118. Factors predictive of growth and treatment of small choroidal melanoma: COMS Report No. 5. The Collaborative Ocular Melanoma Study Group. Arch Ophthalmol [Internet]. 1997;115(12):1537–44. http://www.ncbi.nlm.nih.gov/pubmed/9400787
119. Eskelin S, Pyrhönen S, Summanen P, Hahka-Kemppinen M, Kivelä T. Tumor doubling times in metastatic malignant melanoma of the uvea: Tumor progression before and after treatment. Ophthalmology. 2000;107(8):1443–9.
120. Eskelin S, Kivel T, References F. Uveal melanoma: implications of tumor doubling time. author's reply. Ophthalmology [Internet]. 2001 [cited 2017 Aug 26];108(5):830–1. http://www.aaojournal.org/article/S0161-6420(00)00608-4/pdf
121. Chien JL, Sioufi K, Surakiatchanukul T, Shields JA, Shields CL. Choroidal nevus: a review of prevalence, features, genetics, risks, and outcomes. Curr Opin Ophthalmol. 2017;28(3):228–37.
122. Scholes AG, Damato BE, Nunn J, Hiscott P, Grierson I, Field JK. Monosomy 3 in uveal melanoma: correlation with clinical and histologic predictors of survival. Invest Ophthalmol Vis Sci. 2003;44(3):1008–11.
123. Seddon JM, Albert DM, Lavin PT, Robinson N. A prognostic factor study of disease-free interval and survival following enucleation for uveal melanoma. Arch Ophthalmol [Internet]. 1983;101(12):1894–9. http://www.ncbi.nlm.nih.gov/pubmed/6651594
124. Singh AD, Shields CL, Shields JA. Prognostic factors in uveal melanoma. Melanoma Res. 2001;11(3):255–63.
125. Diener-West M, Earle JD, Fine SL, Hawkins BS, Moy CS, Reynolds SM, et al. The COMS randomized trial of iodine 125 brachytherapy for choroidal melanoma, III: initial mortality findings. COMS Report No. 18. Arch Ophthalmol (Chicago, Ill 1960). 2001;119(7):969–82.
126. Mortality in patients with small choroidal melanoma. COMS report no. 4. The Collaborative Ocular Melanoma Study Group. Arch Ophthalmol (Chicago, Ill 1960) [Internet]. 1997;115(7):886–93. http://www.ncbi.nlm.nih.gov/pubmed/9230829
127. Group COMS. The COMS randomized trial of iodine 125 brachytherapy for choroidal melanoma: V. Twelve-year mortality rates and prognostic factors: COMS report No. 28. Arch Ophthalmol (Chicago, Ill 1960). 2006;124(12):1684–93.
128. Margo CE. The Collaborative Ocular Melanoma Study: an overview. Cancer Control. 2004;11(5):304–9.
129. Diener-West M, Hawkins BS, Markowitz JA, Schachat AP. A review of mortality from choroidal melanoma. II. A meta-analysis of 5-year mortality rates following enucleation, 1966 through 1988. Arch Ophthalmol. 1992;110(2):245–50.
130. Hawkins BS, Group COMS. The Collaborative Ocular Melanoma Study (COMS) randomized trial of pre-enucleation radiation of large choroidal melanoma: IV. Ten-year mortality findings and prognostic factors. COMS report number 24. Am J Ophthalmol. 2004;138(6):936–51.
131. McLean MJ, Foster WD, Zimmerman LE. Prognostic factors in small malignant melanomas of choroid and ciliary body. Arch Ophthalmol [Internet]. 1977;95(1):48–58.
132. Shields CL, Sioufi K, Alset AE, Boal NS, Casey MG, Knapp AN, et al. Clinical features differentiating benign from malignant conjunctival tumors in children. JAMA Ophthalmol [Internet]. 2017;135(3):215–24. http://archopht.jamanetwork.com/article.aspx?doi=10.1001/jamaophthalmol.2016.5544
133. Vine A, Sneed S, Elner V, Wolter R, Willis J, Itani K, et al. Accuracy of diagnosis of choroidal melanomas in the Collaborative Ocular Melanoma Study. COMS report no. 1. Arch Ophthalmol. 1990;108(9):1268–73.
134. Biscotti CV, Singh AD. Uveal metastases. In: Monographs in clinical cytology [Internet]. 2011 [cited 2017 Dec 5]. p. 17–30. http://www.ncbi.nlm.nih.gov/pubmed/22024581
135. Eide N, Walaas L. Fine-needle aspiration biopsy and other biopsies in suspected intraocular malignant disease: a review. Acta Ophthalmol [Internet]. 2009 [cited 2017 Dec 5];87(6):588–601. http://www.ncbi.nlm.nih.gov/pubmed/19719804
136. Singh AD, Biscotti CV. Fine needle aspiration biopsy of ophthalmic tumors. Saudi J Ophthalmol Off J Saudi Ophthalmol Soc [Internet]. 2012 [cited 2017 Dec 5];26(2):117–23. http://www.ncbi.nlm.nih.gov/pubmed/23960981
137. Augsburger JJ, Shields JA, Folberg R, Lang W, O'Hara BJ Claricci JD. Fine needle aspiration biopsy in the diagnosis of intraocular cancer. Cytologic-histologic correlations. Ophthalmology [Internet]. 1985 [cited 2017 Dec 5];92(1):39–49. http://www.ncbi.nlm.nih.gov/pubmed/3974994

138. Shields CL, Manquez ME, Ehya H, Mashayekhi A, Danzig CJ, Shields JA. Fine-needle aspiration biopsy of iris tumors in 100 consecutive cases: technique complications. Ophthalmology. 2006;113(11):2080–6.
139. Onken MD, Worley LA, Ehlers JP, Harbour JW. Gene expression profiling in uveal melanoma reveals two molecular classes and predicts metastatic death. Cancer Res. 2004;64(20):7205–9.
140. Harbour JW, Chen R. The decisionDx-UM gene expression profile test provides risk stratification and individualized patient care in uveal melanoma. PLoS Curr. 2013;5. doi:https://doi.org/10.1371/currents.eogt.af8ba80fc776c8f1ce8f5dc485d4a618.
141. Walter SD, Chao DL, Feuer W, Schiffman J, Char DH, Harbour JW. Prognostic implications of tumor diameter in association with gene expression profile for uveal melanoma. JAMA Ophthalmol. 2016;134(7):734–40.
142. Edge S, Byrd DR, Compton CC, Fritz AG, Greene FL, Trotti A. In: AJCC cancer staging manual [Internet]. 7th ed. New York: Springer; 2010. p. 547–59. http://www.springer.com/it/book/9780387884400#aboutBook
143. Shields CL, Kaliki S, Furuta M, Fulco E, Alarcon C, Shields JA. American Joint Committee on Cancer classification of posterior uveal melanoma (tumor size category) predicts prognosis in 7731 patients. Ophthalmology. 2013;120(10):2066–71.
144. Kujala E, Damato B, Coupland SE, Desjardins L, Bechrakis NE, Grange JD, et al. Staging of ciliary body and choroidal melanomas based on anatomic extent. J Clin Oncol. 2013;31(22):2825–31.
145. Malignant melanoma of the uvea staging form. In: AJCC cancer staging manual. 7th ed. New York City: Springer; 2010. p. 555.
146. Faulkner-Jones BE, Foster WJ, Harbour JW, Smith ME, Davila RM. Fine needle aspiration biopsy with adjunct immunohistochemistry in intraocular tumor management. Acta Cytol. 2005;49(3):297–308.
147. Earle JD. Results from the Collaborative Ocular Melanoma Study (COMS) of enucleation versus preoperative radiation therapy in the management of large ocular melanomas. Int J Radiat Oncol Biol Phys. 1999;43(5):1168–9.
148. Hicks C, Foss AJ, Hungerford JL. Predictive power of screening tests for metastasis in uveal melanoma. Eye. 1998;12:945–8.
149. Wang MX, Shields JA, Donoso LA. Subclinical metastasis of uveal melanoma. Int Ophthalmol Clin [Internet]. 1993 [cited 2017 Aug 27]:33(3):119–27. http://www.ncbi.nlm.nih.gov/pubmed/8407176
150. Zimmerman L, McLean I. Changing concepts concerning the malignancy of ocular tumors. Arch Ophthalmol. 1975;78:487–94.
151. Zimmerman LE, McLean IW, Foster WD. Does enucleation of the eye containing a malignant melanoma prevent or accelerate the dissemination of tumour cells. Br J Ophthalmol. 1978;62(6):420–5.
152. Earle J, Kline RW, Robertson DM. Selection of iodine 125 for the Collaborative Ocular Melanoma Study. Arch Ophthalmol (Chicago, Ill 1960). 1987;105(6):763–4.
153. Marwaha G, Macklis R, Singh AD, Wilkinson A. Brachytherapy. Dev Ophthalmol. 2013;52:29–35.
154. Cox J, Ang K. Radiation oncology: rational, technique, results. 9th ed. Philadelphia: Mosby Elsevier; 2010.
155. Chang MY, Kamrava M, Demanes DJ, Leu M, Agazaryan N, Lamb J, et al. Intraoperative ultrasonography-guided positioning of iodine 125 plaque brachytherapy in the treatment of choroidal melanoma. Ophthalmology. 2012;119(5):1073–7.
156. Classic KL, Furutani KM, Stafford SL, Pulido JS. Radiation dose to the surgeon during plaque brachytherapy. Retina. 2012;32(9):1900–5.
157. Nag S, Quivey JM, Earle JD, Followill D, Fontanesi J, Finger PT, et al. The American Brachytherapy Society recommendations for brachytherapy of uveal melanomas. Int J Radiat Oncol Biol Phys. 2003;56(2):544–55.
158. Finger PT. Radiation therapy for choroidal melanoma. Surv Ophthalmol. 1997;42(3):215–32.
159. Dendale R, Rouic LL-L, Noel G, Feuvret L, Levy C, Delacroix S, et al. Proton beam radiotherapy for uveal melanoma: results of Curie Institut-Orsay proton therapy center (ICPO). Int J Radiat Oncol Biol Phys. 2006;65(3):780–7.
160. Wilson MW, Hungerford JL. Comparison of episcleral plaque and proton beam radiation therapy for the treatment of choroidal melanoma. Ophthalmology. 1999;106(8):1579–87.
161. Char DH, Kroll SM, Castro J. Ten-year follow-up of helium ion therapy for uveal melanoma. Am J Ophthalmol. 1998;125(1):81–9.
162. Gragoudas ES, Lane AM. Uveal melanoma: proton beam irradiation. Ophthalmol Clin North Am. 2005;18(1):111–8. ix
163. Vavvas D, Kim I, Lane AM, Chaglassian A, Mukai S, Gragoudas E. Posterior uveal melanoma in young patients treated with proton beam therapy. Retina. 2010;30(8):1267–71.
164. Young LH, Gragoudas ES. Macular uveal melanoma treated with proton beam irradiation. 10-year follow-up observation with histopathologic correlation. Retina. 1994;14(1):43–6.
165. Gragoudas E, Li W, Goitein M, Lane AM, Munzenrider JE, Egan KM. Evidence-based estimates of outcome in patients irradiated for intraocular melanoma. Arch Ophthalmol (Chicago, Ill 1960). 2002;120(12):1665–71.
166. Mourtada F, Koch N, Newhauser W. 106Ru/106Rh plaque and proton radiotherapy for ocular melanoma: a comparative dosimetric study. Radiat Prot Dosimetry. 2005;116(1–4 Pt 2):454–60.
167. Gragoudas ES, Lane AM, Regan S, Li W, Judge HE, Munzenrider JE, et al. A randomized controlled trial of varying radiation doses in the treatment of cho-

roidal melanoma. Arch Ophthalmol (Chicago, Ill 1960). 2000;118(6):773–8.
168. Fakiris AJ, Lo SS, Henderson MA, Witt TC, Worth RM, Danis RP, et al. Gamma-knife-based stereotactic radiosurgery for uveal melanoma. Stereotact Funct Neurosurg. 2007;85(2–3):106–12.
169. Cohen VM, Carter MJ, Kemeny A, Radatz M, Rennie IG. Metastasis-free survival following treatment for uveal melanoma with either stereotactic radiosurgery or enucleation. Acta Ophthalmol Scand. 2003;81(4):383–8.
170. Abrams MJ, Gagne NL, Melhus CS, Mignano JE. Brachytherapy vs. external beam radiotherapy for choroidal melanoma: Survival and patterns-of-care analyses. Brachytherapy. 2016;15(2): 216–23.
171. Sikuade MJ, Salvi S, Rundle PA, Errington DG, Kacperek A, Rennie IG. Outcomes of treatment with stereotactic radiosurgery or proton beam therapy for choroidal melanoma. Eye (Lond). 2015;29(9):1194–8.
172. Damato B, Kacperek A, Chopra M, Campbell IR, Errington RD. Proton beam radiotherapy of choroidal melanoma: the Liverpool-Clatterbridge experience. Int J Radiat Oncol Biol Phys. 2005;62(5):1405–11.
173. Weber DC, Bogner J, Verwey J, Georg D, Dieckmann K, Escude L, et al. Proton beam radiotherapy versus fractionated stereotactic radiotherapy for uveal melanomas: a comparative study. Int J Radiat Oncol Biol Phys. 2005;63(2):373–84.
174. Shields CL, Shields JA, Perez N, Singh AD, Cater J. Primary transpupillary thermotherapy for small choroidal melanoma in 256 consecutive cases: outcomes and limitations. Ophthalmology. 2002 Feb;109(2):225–34.
175. Rahmi A, Mammar H, Thariat J, Angellier G, Herault J, Chauvel P, et al. Proton beam therapy for presumed and confirmed iris melanomas: a review of 36 cases. Graefes Arch Clin Exp Ophthalmol. 2014;252(9):1515–21.
176. Shields CL, Shah SU, Bianciotto CG, Emrich J, Komarnicky L, Shields JA. Iris melanoma management with iodine-125 plaque radiotherapy in 144 patients: impact of melanoma-related glaucoma on outcomes. Ophthalmology. 2013;120(1):55–61.
177. Demirci H, Shields CL, Shields JA, Eagle RC, Honavar SG. Diffuse iris melanoma: a report of 25 cases. Ophthalmology. 2002;109(8):1553–60.
178. Melia BM, Abramson DH, Albert DM, Boldt HC, Earle JD, Hanson WF, et al. Collaborative ocular melanoma study (COMS) randomized trial of I-125 brachytherapy for medium choroidal melanoma. I. Visual acuity after 3 years COMS report no. 16. Ophthalmology. 2001;108(2):348–66.
179. Finger PT, Berson A, Szechter A. Palladium-103 plaque radiotherapy for choroidal melanoma: results of a 7-year study. Ophthalmology. 1999;106(3):606–13.
180. Jensen AW, Petersen IA, Kline RW, Stafford SL, Schomberg PJ, Robertson DM. Radiation complications and tumor control after 125I plaque brachytherapy for ocular melanoma. Int J Radiat Oncol Biol Phys. 2005;63(1):101–8.
181. Gragoudas ES, Egan KM, Seddon JM, Walsh SM, Munzenrider JE. Intraocular recurrence of uveal melanoma after proton beam irradiation. Ophthalmology. 1992;99(5):760–6.
182. Munzenrider JE. Uveal melanomas. Conservation treatment. Hematol Oncol Clin North Am. 2001;15(2):389–402.
183. Egger E, Schalenbourg A, Zografos L, Bercher L, Boehringer T, Chamot L, et al. Maximizing local tumor control and survival after proton beam radiotherapy of uveal melanoma. Int J Radiat Oncol Biol Phys. 2001;51(1):138–47.
184. Seddon JM, Gragoudas ES, Albert DM, Hsieh CC, Polivogianis L, Friedenberg GR. Comparison of survival rates for patients with uveal melanoma after treatment with proton beam irradiation or enucleation. Am J Ophthalmol. 1985;99(3):282–90.
185. Seddon JM, Gragoudas ES, Egan KM, Glynn RJ, Howard S, Fante RG, et al. Relative survival rates after alternative therapies for uveal melanoma. Ophthalmology. 1990;97(6):769–77.
186. Dinca EB, Yianni J, Rowe J, Radatz MW, Preotiuc-Pietro D, Rundle P, et al. Survival and complications following gamma knife radiosurgery or enucleation for ocular melanoma: a 20-year experience. Acta Neurochir. 2012;154(4):605–10.
187. Wackernagel W, Holl E, Tarmann L, Avian A, Schneider MR, Kapp K, et al. Visual acuity after Gamma-Knife radiosurgery of choroidal melanomas. Br J Ophthalmol. 2013;97(2):153–8.
188. Wackernagel W, Holl E, Tarmann L, Mayer C, Avian A, Schneider M, et al. Local tumour control and eye preservation after gamma-knife radiosurgery of choroidal melanomas. Br J Ophthalmol. 2014;98(2):218–23.
189. Mueller AJ, Talies S, Schaller UC, Horstmann G, Wowra B, Kampik A. Stereotactic radiosurgery of large uveal melanomas with the gamma-knife. Ophthalmology. 2000;107(7):1381–8.
190. Rennie I, Forster D, Kemeny A, Walton L, Kunkler I. The use of single fraction Leksell stereotactic radiosurgery in the treatment of uveal melanoma. Acta Ophthalmol Scand. 1996;74(6):558–62.
191. Zehetmayer M, Kitz K, Menapace R, Ertl A, Heinzl H, Ruhswurm I, et al. Local tumor control and morbidity after one to three fractions of stereotactic external beam irradiation for uveal melanoma. Radiother Oncol. 2000;55(2):135–44.
192. Mashayekhi A, Shields CL, Rishi P, Atalay HT, Pellegrini M, McLaughlin JP, et al. Primary transpupillary thermotherapy for choroidal melanoma in 391 cases: Importance of risk factors in tumor control. Ophthalmology. 2015;122(3):600–9.
193. Harbour JW, Meredith TA, Thompson PA, Gordon ME. Transpupillary thermotherapy versus plaque radiotherapy for suspected choroidal melanomas. Ophthalmology. 2003;110(11):2207–14.

194. Finger PT, Berson A, Ng T, Szechter A. Palladium-103 plaque radiotherapy for choroidal melanoma: an 11-year study. Int J Radiat Oncol Biol Phys. 2002;54(5):1438–45.
195. Lommatzsch PK, Werschnik C, Schuster E. Long-term follow-up of Ru-106/Rh-106 brachytherapy for posterior uveal melanoma. Graefes Arch Clin Exp Ophthalmol. 2000;238(2):129–37.
196. Mensink HW, Vaarwater J, Kilic E, Naus NC, Mooy N, Luyten G, et al. Chromosome 3 intratumor heterogeneity in uveal melanoma. Invest Ophthalmol Vis Sci. 2009;50(2):500–4.
197. Shields CL, Ganguly A, Bianciotto CG, Turaka K, Tavallali A, Shields JA. Prognosis of uveal melanoma in 500 cases using genetic testing of fine-needle aspiration biopsy specimens. Ophthalmology. 2011;118(2):396–401.
198. Damato B, Dopierala JA, Coupland SE. Genotypic profiling of 452 choroidal melanomas with multiplex ligation-dependent probe amplification. Clin Cancer Res. 2010;16(24):6083–92.
199. Onken MD, Worley LA, Char DH, Augsburger JJ, Correa ZM, Nudleman E, et al. Collaborative Ocular Oncology Group report number 1: prospective validation of a multi-gene prognostic assay in uveal melanoma. Ophthalmology. 2012;119(8):1596–603.
200. Chang SH, Worley LA, Onken MD, Harbour JW. Prognostic biomarkers in uveal melanoma: evidence for a stem cell-like phenotype associated with metastasis. Melanoma Res. 2008;18(3):191–200.
201. Augsburger JJ, Correa ZM, Augsburger BD. Frequency and implications of discordant gene expression profile class in posterior uveal melanomas sampled by fine needle aspiration biopsy. Am J Ophthalmol. 2015;159(2):248–56.
202. Field MG, Decatur CL, Kurtenbach S, Gezgin G, van der Velden PA, Jager MJ, et al. PRAME as an independent biomarker for metastasis in uveal melanoma. Clin Cancer Res. 2016;22(5):1234–42.
203. Schouten JP, McElgunn CJ, Waaijer R, Zwijnenburg D, Diepvens F, Pals G. Relative quantification of 40 nucleic acid sequences by multiplex ligation-dependent probe amplification. Nucleic Acids Res. 2002;30(12):e57.
204. Damato B, Dopierala J, Klaasen A, van Dijk M, Sibbring J, Coupland SE. Multiplex ligation-dependent probe amplification of uveal melanoma: correlation with metastatic death. Invest Ophthalmol Vis Sci. 2009;50(7):3048–55.
205. Schopper VJ, Correa ZM. Clinical application of genetic testing for posterior uveal melanoma. Int J Retin Vitr. 2016;2:4. eCollection 2016
206. Singh AD, Topham A. Survival rates with uveal melanoma in the United States: 1973–1997. Ophthalmology. 2003;110(5):962–5.
207. Yonekawa Y, Kim IK. Epidemiology and management of uveal melanoma. Hematol Oncol Clin North Am. 2012;26(6):1169–84.
208. Kujala E, Makitie T, Kivela T. Very long-term prognosis of patients with malignant uveal melanoma. Invest Ophthalmol Vis Sci. 2003;44(11):4651–9.
209. Bishop KD, Olszewski AJ. Epidemiology and survival outcomes of ocular and mucosal melanomas: a population-based analysis. Int J Cancer. 2014;134(12):2961–71.
210. Burr JM, Mitry E, Rachet B, Coleman MP. Survival from uveal melanoma in England and Wales 1986 to 2001. Ophthalmic Epidemiol. 2007;14(1):3–8.
211. Virgili G, Gatta G, Ciccolallo L, Capocaccia R, Biggeri A, Crocetti E, et al. Survival in patients with uveal melanoma in Europe. Arch Ophthalmol (Chicago, Ill 1960). 2008;126(10):1413–8.
212. Grossniklaus HE. Progression of ocular melanoma metastasis to the liver: the 2012 Zimmerman lecture. JAMA Ophthalmol [Internet]. 2013;131(4):462–9. http://www.ncbi.nlm.nih.gov/pubmed/23392528
213. Lane AM, Kim IK, Gragoudas ES. Long-term risk of melanoma-related mortality for patients with uveal melanoma treated with proton beam therapy. JAMA Ophthalmol. 2015;133(7):792–6.
214. Singh AD, Rennie IG, Kivela T, Seregard S, Grossniklaus H. The Zimmerman-McLean-Foster hypothesis: 25 years later. Br J Ophthalmol [Internet]. 2004 [cited 2017 Dec 5];88(7):962–7. http://www.ncbi.nlm.nih.gov/pubmed/15205248
215. Borthwick NJ, Thombs J, Polak M, Gabriel FG, Hungerford JL, Damato B, et al. The biology of micrometastases from uveal melanoma. J Clin Pathol [Internet]. 2011 [cited 2017 Dec 8];64(8):666–71. http://www.ncbi.nlm.nih.gov/pubmed/21593344
216. Mahipal A, Tijani L, Chan K, Laudadio M, Mastrangelo MJ, Sato T. A pilot study of sunitinib malate in patients with metastatic uveal melanoma. Melanoma Res. 2012;22(6):440–6.
217. Huppert PE, Fierlbeck G, Pereira P, Schanz S, Duda SH, Wietholtz H, et al. Transarterial chemoembolization of liver metastases in patients with uveal melanoma. Eur J Radiol. 2010;74(3):e38–44.
218. Schmittel A, Schuster R, Bechrakis NE, Siehl JM, Foerster MH, Thiel E, et al. A two-cohort phase II clinical trial of gemcitabine plus treosulfan in patients with metastatic uveal melanoma. Melanoma Res. 2005;15(5):447–51.
219. Agarwala SS, Panikkar R, Kirkwood JM. Phase I/II randomized trial of intrahepatic arterial infusion chemotherapy with cisplatin and chemoembolization with cisplatin and polyvinyl sponge in patients with ocular melanoma metastatic to the liver. Melanoma Res. 2004;14(3):217–22.
220. Kivela T, Suciu S, Hansson J, Kruit WH, Vuoristo MS, Kloke O, et al. Bleomycin, vincristine, lomustine and dacarbazine (BOLD) in combination with recombinant interferon alpha-2b for metastatic uveal melanoma. Eur J Cancer. 2003;39(8):1115–20.
221. Breazzano MP, Milam RW, Batson SA, Johnson DB, Daniels AB. Immunotherapy for Uveal Melanoma. Int Ophthalmol Clin. 2017;57(1):29–39.

222. Bhatia S, Moon J, Margolin KA, Weber JS, Lao CD, Othus M, et al. Phase II trial of sorafenib in combination with carboplatin and paclitaxel in patients with metastatic uveal melanoma: SWOG S0512. PLoS One. 2012;7(11):e48787.
223. Homsi J, Bedikian AY, Papadopoulos NE, Kim KB, Hwu WJ, Mahoney SL, et al. Phase 2 open-label study of weekly docosahexaenoic acid-paclitaxel in patients with metastatic uveal melanoma. Melanoma Res. 2010;20(6):507–10.
224. Fiorentini G, Aliberti C, Del Conte A, Tilli M, Rossi S, Ballardini P, et al. Intra-arterial hepatic chemoembolization (TACE) of liver metastases from ocular melanoma with slow-release irinotecan-eluting beads. Early results of a phase II clinical study. In Vivo. 2009;23(1):131–7.
225. O'Neill PA, Butt M, Eswar CV, Gillis P, Marshall E. A prospective single arm phase II study of dacarbazine and treosulfan as first-line therapy in metastatic uveal melanoma. Melanoma Res. 2006;16(3):245–8.
226. Schmittel A, Schmidt-Hieber M, Martus P, Bechrakis NE, Schuster R, Siehl JM, et al. A randomized phase II trial of gemcitabine plus treosulfan versus treosulfan alone in patients with metastatic uveal melanoma. Ann Oncol. 2006;17(12):1826–9.
227. Patel K, Sullivan K, Berd D, Mastrangelo MJ, Shields CL, Shields JA, et al. Chemoembolization of the hepatic artery with BCNU for metastatic uveal melanoma: results of a phase II study. Melanoma Res. 2005;15(4):297–304.
228. Schmidt-Hieber M, Schmittel A, Thiel E, Keilholz U. A phase II study of bendamustine chemotherapy as second-line treatment in metastatic uveal melanoma. Melanoma Res. 2004;14(6):439–42.
229. Alexander HR Jr, Libutti SK, Pingpank JF, Steinberg SM, Bartlett DL, Helsabeck C, et al. Hyperthermic isolated hepatic perfusion using melphalan for patients with ocular melanoma metastatic to liver. Clin Cancer Res. 2003;9(17):6343–9.
230. Alexander HR, Libutti SK, Bartlett DL, Puhlmann M, Fraker DL, Bachenheimer LC. A phase I-II study of isolated hepatic perfusion using melphalan with or without tumor necrosis factor for patients with ocular melanoma metastatic to liver. Clin Cancer Res. 2000;6(8):3062–70.
231. Pyrhonen S, Hahka-Kemppinen M, Muhonen T, Nikkanen V, Eskelin S, Summanen P, et al. Chemoimmunotherapy with bleomycin, vincristine, lomustine, dacarbazine (BOLD), and human leukocyte interferon for metastatic uveal melanoma. Cancer. 2002;95(11):2366–72.
232. Eroglu Z, Smalley KSM, Sondak VK. Improving patient outcomes to targeted therapies in melanoma. Expert Rev Anticancer Ther [Internet]. 2016;16(6):633–41. http://www.ncbi.nlm.nih.gov/pubmed/27137746
233. Maio M, Danielli R, Chiarion-Sileni V, Pigozzo J, Parmiani G, Ridolfi R, et al. Efficacy and safety of ipilimumab in patients with pre-treated, uveal melanoma. Ann Oncol. 2013;24(11):2911–5.
234. Luke JJ, Callahan MK, Postow MA, Romano E, Ramaiya N, Bluth M, et al. Clinical activity of ipilimumab for metastatic uveal melanoma: a retrospective review of the Dana-Farber Cancer Institute, Massachusetts General Hospital, Memorial Sloan-Kettering Cancer Center, and University Hospital of Lausanne experience. Cancer. 2013;119(20):3687–95.
235. Buder K, Gesierich A, Gelbrich G, Goebeler M. Systemic treatment of metastatic uveal melanoma: review of literature and future perspectives. Cancer Med. 2013;2(5):674–86.
236. Moser JC, Pulido JS, Dronca RS, McWilliams RR, Markovic SN, Mansfield AS. The Mayo Clinic experience with the use of kinase inhibitors, ipilimumab, bevacizumab, and local therapies in the treatment of metastatic uveal melanoma. Melanoma Res. 2015;25(1):59–63.
237. Page DB, Postow MA, Callahan MK, Wolchok JD. Checkpoint modulation in melanoma: an update on ipilimumab and future directions. Curr Oncol Rep. 2013;15(5):500–8.
238. Topalian SL, Hodi FS, Brahmer JR, Gettinger SN, Smith DC, McDermott DF, et al. Safety, activity, and immune correlates of anti-PD-1 antibody in cancer. N Engl J Med. 2012;366(26):2443–54.
239. Wolchok JD, Kluger H, Callahan MK, Postow MA, Rizvi NA, Lesokhin AM, et al. Nivolumab plus ipilimumab in advanced melanoma. N Engl J Med. 2013;369(2):122–33.
240. Algazi AP, Tsai KK, Shoushtari AN, Munhoz RR, Eroglu Z, Piulats JM, et al. Clinical outcomes in metastatic uveal melanoma treated with PD-1 and PD-L1 antibodies. Cancer [Internet]. 2016 [cited 2017 Dec 8];122(21):3344–53. http://doi.wiley.com/10.1002/cncr.30258
241. Finger PT, Kurli M, Reddy S, Tena LB, Pavlick a C. Whole body PET/CT for initial staging of choroidal melanoma. Br J Ophthalmol. 2005;89(10):1270–4.
242. Freton A, Chin KJ, Raut R, Tena LB, Kivelä T, Finger PT. Initial PET/CT staging for choroidal melanoma: AJCC correlation and second nonocular primaries in 333 patients. Eur J Ophthalmol [Internet]. 2012 [cited 2017 Dec 8];22(2):236–43. http://www.ncbi.nlm.nih.gov/pubmed/21959680
243. Diener-West M, Reynolds SM, Agugliaro DJ, Caldwell R, Cumming K, Earle JD, et al. Screening for metastasis from choroidal melanoma: The Collaborative Ocular Melanoma Study group report 23. J Clin Oncol. 2004;22(12):2438–44.
244. Eskelin S, Pyrhönen S, Summanen P, Prause JU, Kivelä T. Screening for metastatic malignant melanoma of the uvea revisited. Cancer. 1999;85(5):1151–9.
245. Kuan a K, Jackson FI, Hanson J. Multimodality detection of metastatic melanoma. J R Soc Med. 1988;81(10):579–82.

246. Marshall E, Romaniuk C, Ghaneh P, Wong H, McKay M, Chopra M, et al. MRI in the detection of hepatic metastases from high-risk uveal melanoma: a prospective study in 188 patients. Br J Ophthalmol [Internet]. 2013 [cited 2017 Dec 8];97(2):159–63. http://www.ncbi.nlm.nih.gov/pubmed/23159448
247. Semelka RC, Martin DR, Balci C, Lance T. Focal liver lesions: comparison of dual-phase CT and multisequence multiplanar MR imaging including dynamic gadolinium enhancement. J Magn Reson Imaging. 2001;13(3):397–401.
248. Choudhary MM, Gupta A, Bena J, Emch T, Singh AD. Hepatic ultrasonography for surveillance in patients with uveal melanoma. JAMA Ophthalmol [Internet]. 2016 [cited 2017 Dec 8];134(2):174. http://www.ncbi.nlm.nih.gov/pubmed/26633182
249. Gupta MP, Lane AM, DeAngelis MM, Mayne K, Crabtree M, Gragoudas ES, et al. Clinical characteristics of uveal melanoma in patients with germline BAP1 mutations. JAMA Ophthalmol. 2015;133(8):881–7.
250. Rai K, Pilarski R, Boru G, Rehman M, Saqr AH, Massengill JB, et al. Germline BAP1 alterations in familial uveal melanoma. Genes Chromosomes Cancer. 2017;56(2):168–74.
251. Njauw C-NJ, Kim I, Piris A, Gabree M, Taylor M, Lane AM, et al. Germline BAP1 inactivation is preferentially associated with metastatic ocular melanoma and cutaneous-ocular melanoma families. In: Dadras SS, editor. PLoS One [Internet]. 2012 [cited 2017 Dec 8];7(4):e35295. http://www.ncbi.nlm.nih.gov/pubmed/22545102
252. Rai K, Pilarski R, Cebulla CM, Abdel-Rahman MH. Comprehensive review of BAP1 tumor predisposition syndrome with report of two new cases. Clin Genet. 2016;89(3):285–94.
253. Pilarski R, Rai K, Cebulla C, Abdel-Rahman M. BAP1 tumor predisposition syndrome. In: Pagon RA, Adam MP, Ardinger HH, Wallace SE, Amemiya A, Bean LJH, et al., editors. Seattle (WA): University of Washington, Seattle. GeneReviews is a registered trademark of the University of Washington, Seattle. All rights reserved; 1993. (GeneReviews(R)).
254. Hammer H, Oláh J, Tóth-Molnár E. Dysplastic nevi are a risk factor for uveal melanoma. Eur J Ophthalmol [Internet]. 1996 [cited 2017 Aug 19];6(4):472–4. http://www.ncbi.nlm.nih.gov/pubmed/8997595
255. Abdel-Rahman MH, Rai K, Pilarski R, Davidorf FH, Cebulla CM. Germline BAP1 mutations misreported as somatic based on tumor-only testing. Fam Cancer. 2016;15(2):327–30.
256. Laíns I, Bartosch C, Mondim V, Healy B, Kim IK, Husain D, et al. Second primary neoplasms in patients with uveal melanoma: a SEER database analysis. Am J Ophthalmol. 2016;165:54–64.
257. Shields JA, Shields CL. Eyelid, conjunctival, and orbital tumors: an atlas and textbook. 3rd ed. Philadelphia: Lippincott Wolters Kluwers; 2016. 806 p
258. Shields CL, Demirci H, Karatza E, Shields JA. Clinical survey of 1643 melanocytic and nonmelanocytic conjunctival tumors. Ophthalmology. 2004;111:1747–54.
259. Shields CL, Alset AE, Boal NS, Casey MG, Knapp AN, Sugarman JA, et al. Conjunctival Tumors in 5002 Cases. Comparative Analysis of Benign Versus Malignant Counterparts. The 2016 James D. Allen Lecture. Am J Ophthalmol. 2017;173:106–33.
260. Ciralsky J, Colby K. Conjunctival melanomas: can the cancer stem cell hypothesis be applied? Semin Ophthalmol [Internet]. 2009 [cited 2017 Oct 26];24(3):161–5. http://www.tandfonline.com/doi/full/10.1080/08820530902802351
261. Norregaard JC, Gerner N, Jensen OA, Prause JU. Malignant melanoma of the conjunctiva: occurrence and survival following surgery and radiotherapy in a Danish population. Graefes Arch Clin Exp Ophthalmol [Internet]. 1996 [cited 2017 Oct 26];234(9):569–72. http://www.ncbi.nlm.nih.gov/pubmed/8880155
262. Shields CL, Chien JL, Surakiatchanukul T, Sioufi K, Lally SE, Shields JA. Conjunctival tumors:review of clinical features, risks, biomarkers, and outcomes—the 2017 J. Donald M. Gass lecture. Asia-Pacific J Ophthalmol [Internet]. 2017 [cited 2017 Aug 18];6(2):109–20. http://www.ncbi.nlm.nih.gov/pubmed/28399347
263. Katsambas A, Nicolaidou E. Cutaneous malignant melanoma and sun exposure. Recent developments in epidemiology. Arch Dermatol [Internet]. 1996;132(4):444–50. http://www.ncbi.nlm.nih.gov/pubmed/8629849
264. Foster CS, Azar DT, Dohlman CH. Smolin and Thoft's the cornea: scientific foundations and clinical practice. Philadelphia: Lippincott Williams and Wilkins. 1339 p
265. Poothullil AM, Colby KA. Topical medical therapies for ocular surface tumors. Semin Ophthalmol. 2006;21:161–9.
266. Sugiura M, Colby KA, Mihm MC, Zembowicz A. Low-risk and high-risk histologic features in conjunctival primary acquired melanosis with atypia: Clinicopathologic analysis of 29 cases. Am J Surg Pathol. 2007;31(2):185–92.
267. Shields CL. Conjunctival melanoma: risk factors for recurrence, exenteration, metastasis, and death in 150 consecutive patients. Trans Am Ophthalmol Soc. 2000;98:471–92.
268. Jaenisch R, Bird A. Epigenetic regulation of gene expression: how the genome integrates intrinsic and environmental signals. Nat Genet. 2003;33(Suppl):245–54.
269. Wang Y, Fischle W, Cheung W, Jacobs S, Khorasanizadeh S, Allis CD. Beyond the double helix: writing and reading the histone code. Novartis Found Symp. 2004;259:3–21-169.
270. Barlesi F, Giaccone G, Gallegos-Ruiz MI, Loundou A, Span SW, Lefesvre P, et al. Global histone modi-

fications predict prognosis of resected non small-cell lung cancer. J Clin Oncol. 2007;25(28):4358–64.
271. Park YS, Jin MY, Kim YJ, Yook JH, Kim BS, Jang SJ. The global histone modification pattern correlates with cancer recurrence and overall survival in gastric adenocarcinoma. Ann Surg Oncol. 2008;15(7):1968–76.
272. Seligson DB, Horvath S, Shi T, Yu H, Tze S, Grunstein M, et al. Global histone modification patterns predict risk of prostate cancer recurrence. Nature. 2005;435(7046):1262–6.
273. Song JS, Kim YS, Kim DK, Park SI, Jang SJ. Global histone modification pattern associated with recurrence and disease-free survival in non-small cell lung cancer patients. Pathol Int. 2012;62(3):182–90.
274. Jenuwein T, Allis CD. Translating the histone code. Science. 2001;293(5532):1074–80.

Current Surgical Management of Primary Cutaneous Melanoma

17

Adam I. Riker, Marco Antonio Rajo, Stephen L. Lambert, and Jonathan S. Lam

Abbreviations

CLND	Complete lymph node dissection
ELND	Elective lymph node dissection
NCCN	National Comprehensive Care Network
PET	Positron emission tomography
SLN	Sentinel lymph node(s)
SLNB	Sentinel lymph node biopsy

A Brief History of the Surgical Treatment for Melanoma

The first reported case of a patient described as having melanoma appears within the medical writings of Hippocrates around 460 B.C. Several mummies have been recently discovered from this era, and paleopathologists have noted the presence of diffuse metastases in the bones of the skull and extremities, many with rounded melanotic masses in the skin [1]. John Hunter, of St George's Hospital in London, England, was the first physician who successfully surgically removed a recurrent melanoma of the lower jaw in 1787. The specimen is still preserved as Hunter's specimen #219 at the Hunterian Museum of the Royal College of Surgeons in London [2]. It was Renee Laennec, more famous for his invention of the stethoscope, who first described melanoma as the "cancer noire," or the black cancer, later coining the term "melanosis" in 1812 [3].

In 1820, William Norris described the first case of melanoma in the English literature. When he incised through the original tumor, he said, "I found the texture to be heterogeneous; it was of a reddish and whitish brown tint throughout, not very unlike the internal structure of a nutmeg" [4]. Norris later published the first comprehensive study of melanoma, titled "eight cases of melanosis with pathological and therapeutic remarks" [5]. This manuscript is the first observational analysis of a group of patients with melanoma, accurately describing many of the epidemiological, clinical, and pathological features of patients with melanoma, of which many of his observations remain true to the present day. In 1837, Isaac Parish, a 26-year-old surgeon, published the first case of melanoma in North America, and after a treatment of purgatives, leeches, and poultice of ground elm, his patient quickly fell victim to her disease [6].

Samuel Cooper, a British surgeon, recognized in 1840, that metastatic melanomas were untreatable and he stated, "the only chance for benefit

A. I. Riker, M.D., F.A.C.S. (✉) · M. A. Rajo, M.D.
J. S. Lam, M.D.
Section of Surgical Oncology, Department of Surgery, School of Medicine, Louisiana State University, New Orleans, LA, USA
e-mail: ariker@lsuhsc.edu; mrajoa@lsuhsc.edu; jlam1@lsuhsc.edu

S. L. Lambert, M.D.
Department of Family Medicine, Health Science Center, Louisiana State University, New Orleans, LA, USA
e-mail: slamb3@lsuhsc.edu

A. I. Riker (ed.), *Melanoma*, https://doi.org/10.1007/978-3-319-78310-9_17

depends upon the early removal of the disease…" [7], an observation that has held true until recent times. In 1858, Oliver Pemberton published his observations on a collection of 60 cases of cutaneous and ocular melanoma, by far the largest series of patients with melanoma to date, noting the postmortem findings in 33 cases [8]. He was also one of the first surgeons to note the futility of many treatments for advanced disease and was a strong advocate of surgical management of melanoma with wide excision of the primary and extensive resection and removal of the draining lymph node basins.

The concept of the surgical management of melanoma was not uniformly accepted, shunned by many in favor of traditional local therapies with salves and other medicinal treatments passed down from previous generations. However, excision of the primary lesion with wide margins was slowly gaining favor with a small group of surgeons. In 1892, the London surgeon Herbert Snow advocated that melanoma be treated by excision and he noted that: "it is essential to remove, whenever possible, those lymph glands which first receive the infective protoplasm" [9]. In 1903, Frederick Eve described a case series of 45 patients with melanoma treated at the London Hospital, remarking that 80% of the melanoma cases had originated from pigmented moles on the skin [10]. He strongly expressed his views on the surgical management of melanoma, stating in his lecture, "The treatment of melanoma can be given in a few words, free excision or amputation, in accordance with the position and extent of disease…The removal of the nearest chain of lymphatic glands, whether palpably involved or not, should never be omitted; for it may be taken as a matter of certainty that in the great majority of cases they are infected."

In 1905, the Scottish physician William Handley analyzed the lymphatic spread of a melanoma originating from a woman's leg [11]. In 1907, he gave the Hunterian Lecture entitled "Melanotic growths in relation to their operative treatment," in which he strongly supports the views of Frederick Eve, advocating wide excision of the primary melanoma in combination with elective regional lymph node dissection or possibly amputation in selected cases [11]. In this manuscript, he accurately notes that the "permeation of the lymphatics is the principle agent in this local centrifugal spread" of melanoma, recommending a circular incision of about one inch from the edge of the tumor, and another two inches into the subcutaneous fat. This article is of great historical significance, as the recommendations of Handley became the basis for the surgical management of melanoma for the next 50 years.

Until the 1960s, invasive melanoma was considered a high-risk disease that required an extensive local excision for all tumors. In 1969, Wallace H. Clark, Jr., a pathologist at the Massachusetts General Hospital, described a classification system of melanoma based on the extent of tumor invasion relative to the anatomic layers of the skin and related the depth of penetration to overall patient survival [12]. In 1970, Alexander Breslow added a second method of measurement, based upon the true vertical thickness of the tumor, measured in millimeters [13]. This system was found to be a more accurate and reproducible method of measurement, providing an excellent correlation with overall 5-year survival. Comparison of the two systems and other histologic parameters revealed that the tumor thickness, measured in millimeters, was a better predictor of metastasis and overall survival compared to the Clark's level of tumor invasion [14].

In 1978, the pioneering surgeon Donald Morton published the first report of the use of cutaneous lymphoscintigraphy to determine the direction of regional lymphatic drainage in 32 patients with primary malignant melanoma of the trunk [15]. In 1990, at the Society of Surgical Oncology meeting, Morton introduced the use of lymphatic mapping to determine the sentinel lymph node and described the technique of obtaining a sentinel-node biopsy which created a minimally invasive way to stage the tumor status of all nodes in the regional basin [16]. His paper on intraoperative lymphatic mapping for early stage melanoma was initially rejected by several journals until its publication in the *Archives of Surgery* in 1992 [17]. He later developed and published the first landmark trial on sentinel-node biopsy versus nodal observation in melanoma, the MSLT I trial [18].

It is important to recognize the important contributions of past physicians and surgeons, learning from their experiences in the clinical management of patients with melanoma. It is clear that we must continue down the pathways of our predecessors and strive to improve the quality of surgical care for all melanoma patients. Though the basic tenets for the surgical management of primary melanoma and regional nodes have been forged from previous trials, many questions still remain as to the optimal management of patients with later stage disease. As new research continues to surface, physicians, surgeons, and researchers alike continue to develop novel treatment strategies for those patients with advanced disease, many of which do not require the scalpel.

Obtaining the Diagnosis

It is imperative that the diagnosis of cutaneous melanoma be made as early as possible, as this directly correlates with long-term outcome. For decades, physicians have utilized the clinical examination of the skin as the primary screening modality for detecting melanoma. Yet, the ability of the clinician to accurately identify those lesions that are melanoma is highly variable in most cases, making the correct diagnosis in only about 65% of all cases [19–24]. The accuracy rate of detection can be improved by 10–20% with the addition of other imaging tools, such as epiluminescence microscopy and sequential full body photography [25, 26]. However, no matter what observational threshold is being followed, many lesions that are deemed suspicious for melanoma will ultimately undergo a biopsy to obtain a definitive diagnosis. Obtaining a tissue sample by means of whatever method of biopsy, followed by histological examination of the tissue is still considered the "gold standard" for accurately making the diagnosis of primary cutaneous melanoma.

The majority of clinical management guidelines recommend that a pigmented lesion or mole that is deemed suspicious undergo an excisional biopsy as the preferred method of biopsy, obtaining a margin of normal skin of 1–2 mm [19–21]. The depth of the biopsy should encompass the subcutaneous fat, with complete removal of the lesion for a complete and unencumbered histologic examination that will include an accurate Breslow's depth of invasion and other prognostic features [27–29]. The definitive surgical procedure of the primary melanoma should be deferred until the final histologic diagnosis has been made, even for suspected thinner melanomas such as melanoma-in-situ [30–32]. It is imperative for the clinician to be cognizant of cosmetically sensitive areas when performing a biopsy, as this will dictate the type of biopsy performed and the necessity for possibly specialty surgical consultation. Definitive excision of such areas must be deferred until the final diagnosis has been completed, as often the pathological diagnosis yields a benign result that does not require any further surgical intervention [33, 34].

If a punch biopsy is performed, one should obtain the sample from the thickest portion of the lesion, avoiding areas of crusting, ulceration, or necrosis that may grossly underestimate the overall thickness of the tumor. Although the preferred method of biopsy is the excisional biopsy, others will perform a deep shave, or saucerization, of a lesion suspected of being melanoma. This is usually done with either a scalpel or a single-edged razor blade held in a semi-curved position [19]. A saucerization is essentially a modified shave biopsy that samples the deeper dermis, and is achieved by pinching the skin around the lesion while curving the razor blade [35].

One potential drawback of either method is that there remains the possibility of transecting the base of the lesion, thus resulting in a deep margin that is involved with melanoma. This is problematic in that the true Breslow's thickness is not known, creating a diagnostic dilemma for the surgeon in terms of the decision-making for the appropriate surgical margins and whether the draining lymph node basin needs to be evaluated. A second consideration is that biopsy site from a shave biopsy heals by secondary intention, resulting in an inferior cosmetic outcome compared to other techniques.

The main benefit of a punch biopsy is that the specimen can be accurately measured for true depth of invasion. The defect is closed primarily with 1 or 2 interrupted sutures that results in a superior cosmetic outcome compared to a shave biopsy that heals by secondary intention. The primary limitation of the punch biopsy is that for larger lesions (>6 mm), the largest available punch biopsy will be unable to adequately remove the entire lesion, thereby inadequately sampling the adjacent normal skin and histologic architecture. The architectural pattern of the entire specimen, in combination with other cytological features, is of particular importance when diagnosing melanoma [36].

Additionally, there are several other important features that require special attention in order to obtain an accurate diagnosis of melanoma, such as the presence of asymmetry, the lack of circumscription, and the presence (or absence) of scattered atypical melanocytes throughout the epidermis and adnexal epithelium. Such features may not be present if a small punch biopsy is performed and the type of biopsy must be taken into account by the dermatopathologist [35]. In cases of inadequate sampling, it may be necessary to completely remove the lesion with an excisional biopsy in order to confirm the diagnosis of a suspected melanoma.

Once a diagnosis of melanoma had been obtained, staging is essential for prognosis and effective treatment. In 2016, the 8th edition of the American Joint Committee on Cancer (AJCC) staging system for cutaneous melanoma was revised and updated, based on the primary tumor (T), regional lymph node involvement (N), and distant metastatic spread (M) [37].

Surgical Margins of Excision

The surgical management of cutaneous melanoma must always begin with the proper identification and treatment of the primary lesion. With early diagnosis, over 90% of all early stage primary melanomas can be cured by surgical excision alone [38, 39]. The majority of thin primary lesions can be locally excised and closed primarily, generally accomplished with a fusiform excision. Thus, it is important to recognize that achieving negative surgical margins with the appropriate margins of excision will result in the lowest possible local recurrence rates.

The standard operative approach in the past usually included a 3–5 cm margin of normal skin measured from the outer edge of the melanoma in all directions, with most patients requiring a split-thickness skin graft to cover the resulting defect. This extensive surgical procedure resulted in a prolonged hospital stay and associated perioperative complications such as wound infection and skin graft necrosis. Fortunately, as the extent of surgical resection and margins was questioned, several prospective, randomized trials have been performed to address this issue. The first trial that this question, the Intergroup Melanoma Trial, focused on the efficacy of 2-cm vs. 4-cm margins for primary melanomas between 1 and 4 mm in Breslow's thickness [40]. The results of this trial clearly showed an insignificant difference between the local recurrence rate between the two groups, 0.8% in the group who received 2-cm margins and 1.7% for those who had received 4-cm excision margins. Of importance, only 11% of the patients in the 2-cm excision group (compared to 46% in the 4-cm excision group) required a skin graft.

In this trial's 10-year follow-up, no significant differences in the local recurrence rate, disease-free or overall survival was seen [41]. This trial clearly demonstrated that a 2-cm margin of excision is both safe and effective compared to a 4-cm margin for primary melanomas between 1 and 4 mm, with a significant decrease in the need for skin grafting. In a recent prospective, multicenter randomized trial of 936 patients by the Swedish Melanoma Study group, patients were randomly allocated to receive either a 2-cm resection margin or a 4-cm resection margin. The 5-year overall survival of both groups was 65% (p = 0.64) and no significant difference was found, further clarifying that 2-cm resection margins is sufficient [42]. There have been two other trials that have examined 2-cm vs. 5-cm margins for intermediate thickness primary melanomas <2 mm in Breslow's thickness, with both studies showing no difference in local recurrence rates or overall survival [43, 44].

Several randomized trials have established that the overall thickness of the primary melanoma dramatically influences the likelihood of a local recurrence [45]. The World Health Organization (WHO) Melanoma Group study was a prospective, randomized trial comparing patients with primary melanomas ≤2 mm in Breslow's thickness to either 1-cm versus 3-cm surgical margins [46]. There were no local recurrences seen among patients with primary melanomas <1 mm, regardless of what margin was taken. There were four local recurrences seen in patients with primary melanomas between 1 and 2 mm, all occurring within the group that had received 1-cm margins. However, there were no statistically significant differences noted in either group in terms of disease-free and overall survival. This trial has been updated with 15-year follow-up, and again there were no differences noted in disease-free or overall survival [47]. This study provides a clear demonstration that a surgical excision margin of 1 cm is safe and provides excellent local control for melanomas <1 mm in Breslow's thickness.

For primary melanomas with a tumor thickness between 1 and 2 mm, current NCCN guidelines suggest that the margin of excision can be between 1 and 2 cm depending on the anatomic circumstances. If possible, a 2 cm margin of excision should be performed whenever feasible; however, a 1 cm margin is acceptable if placement of a skin graft or an excessively high amount of skin tension will result from taking a larger 2 cm margin. In a review of 576 patients with a melanoma between a 1 and 2 mm in thickness, a comparison between 1 cm vs. 2 cm margins showed no significant difference in overall survival at 8.3 years of follow-up, but the 1 cm margin group did have a local recurrence of 3.6% compared to 0.9% in the 2 cm group [48]. In 2016, Doepker et al. published a retrospective study that compared the use of a 1- or 2-cm resection margin for 965 patients with a 1–2 mm melanoma and reported that using a margin of 1 cm did not increase the risk of local recurrence or disease-specific survival, but the 5-year overall survival for a 1-cm margin was 61.9% vs. 71.2% for a 2-cm margin ($p = 0.004$) [49]. Further data is needed in order to elucidate whether there is a survival benefit for a 2-cm surgical margin vs. a 1-cm margin.

Thomas et al. prospectively examined the excision margins in a defined "high-risk group" of patients with primary melanoma, considered >2 mm in Breslow's thickness in this study [50]. All patients were randomized to either 1-cm or 3-cm margins of excision and they found that a 1-cm margin of excision for melanomas of at least 2 mm in Breslow's thickness was associated with a significantly greater risk of combined (local and regional) recurrence when compared to a 3-cm margin. It is important to note that this high-risk group included *all* primary lesions >2 mm in thickness (median tumor thickness was 3 mm), and therefore the results and conclusions of this trial cannot be directly applied to those patients with only thick (>4 mm) primary lesions. Regardless, this is an important trial because it is the first time that a randomized trial examining surgical margins of excision has demonstrated a significant increase in combined locoregional recurrence with a narrower 1-cm margin. However, there was no statistically significant difference noted in the death rate from melanoma associated with a narrow (1 cm or less) margin of excision for thicker melanomas.

The appropriate surgical margins for a thick primary melanoma (>4 mm) have also been addressed in both retrospective and prospective analyses. The first study was a multi-institutional retrospective review of surgical margins and associated prognostic factors in 278 patients with a thick primary melanoma [51]. This study revealed no significant difference in the local recurrence rate, disease-free or overall survival if margins larger than 2 cm were taken. There does not appear to be any clear advantage (or disadvantage) to removing the deep muscular fascia as part of the definitive excision of the primary melanoma. Several studies have addressed this issue and it does not appear that there is any significant difference in recurrence rates, locally or distant, when the fascia was either left in place or removed as part of the definitive surgery [52, 53].

Truncal and Extremity Melanoma

The surgical management of truncal and extremity melanoma is fairly straightforward, with the basic tenets of surgical therapy to remove the primary melanoma with the appropriate surgical margins. However, certain situations and anatomic locations may alter the surgeon's approach to management, such as melanomas located along the forearm, leg and digits. In particular, a melanoma >2 mm in Breslow's thickness on the forearm will require a 2 cm circumferential excisional margin with a resultant defect of at least 4 × 4 cm. Due to the anatomic limitations of skin mobility in such areas, it is often necessary to utilize a split-thickness skin graft (STSG) for adequate coverage, often taken from the anterolateral aspect of the thigh. Other possible donor sites may include a full-thickness skin graft from the lower quadrant of the abdomen with primary closure of this defect, thereby sparing the patient the increased pain and discomfort associated with a STSG from the thigh.

The majority of primary melanomas located on the back can be treated with the appropriate excision margin followed by skin edge approximation and primary closure. The skin on the back is generally thicker with more laxity compared to other areas of the body, with the resulting defect successfully closed primarily without the need of skin grafting. In order to minimize the amount of tension along the mid-portion of the defect, attention should be given to the orientation of the surgical excision related to the optimal lines of skin tension in order to minimize the need for extensive undermining of the surrounding skin edges. Occasionally, the surgeon may encounter an undue amount of skin tension and this situation is best treated with the placement of a STSG or possibly one of several plastic reconstructive options such as a rotational, advancement or rhomboid skin flap.

Head and Neck Melanoma

The use of SLNB for head and neck melanomas has been recently reviewed in depth and it has been shown to be a safe and valuable tool for experienced surgeons in order to achieve valuable staging information to help guide treatment [54]. Special attention should be paid to the patient with a primary melanoma of the head and neck due to the added anatomic complexity posed within this region. Although the established guidelines are generally followed whenever possible, a melanoma arising within aesthetic areas of the face will often require a compromise in such margins. Every attempt is made at obtaining the appropriate surgical margin and concomitantly achieving the best cosmetic outcome with the lowest possible chance of local recurrence. It is imperative that a thorough discussion of the planned excision be made with the patient, outlining the operative plan and any associated reconstruction being performed. The risks, benefits, and expected cosmetic outcomes should be carefully discussed with the patient, specifically addressing unrealistic expectations of any surgical procedure.

The surgical treatment of the primary tumor of the head and neck includes planning the complete excision of the primary melanoma as well as the reconstructive procedures simultaneously [55]. Some surgeons prefer to stage the excision, waiting for the final pathology prior to performing a definitive reconstruction of the residual defect. In any case, the surgeon should be cognizant of the unique anatomy of the face, considering the relaxed skin tension lines and functional aesthetic. Special consideration should be given to primary melanoma excisions that involve overlying lymph node-bearing areas, such as the parotid gland and neck. A preauricular vertical incision followed by the development of an anterior cervicofacial flap is able to adequately expose the parotid gland or periauricular and upper neck lymph nodes. In the neck, an upper-neck transverse incision or a mid-neck posterior vertical incision provides optimal exposure to the appropriate cervical lymph node basin.

The method of reconstruction of the primary melanoma excision site depends upon several factors such as the location and size of the defect, the functional and aesthetic requirements, and the overall medical condition of the patient. There are numerous possible reconstructive options such as the utility of a STSG, local vascularized and regional tissue flaps as well as myocutaneous flaps. The most common surgical excision of a primary scalp melanoma involves the removal of the appropriate skin margins and underlying subcutaneous fat down to the galea. The underlying periosteum is well vascularized and provides a good base for the proper healing of a STSG. For smaller and even intermediate size scalp excisions, local rotational may be suitable in lieu of skin grafting. In rare cases, extensive surgical excision of the primary melanoma with a large residual defect may require a free flap for adequate wound closure, usually from sites such as the anteriolateral thigh, latissimus or radial forearm muscle.

Small excisions of the cheek can usually be closed within the exaggerated "smile lines" on the face. For larger defects involving the medial portion of the cheek, an inferiorly based cervicofacial rotation advancement flap may provide the optimal aesthetic result. For upper lip defects that are lateral to, and above, the vermillion border, we commonly utilize a cheek advancement flap for optimal cosmetic results. Defects along the medial, central upper lip, and philtrum are best treated by an Abbé lip switch flap for lower lip defects, local rotation flaps are often utilized, bearing in mind that if the defect is a result of a complete excision of the lip, muscle, and mucosa, then one of several lip advancement techniques can be employed. The Karapandzic flap, a rotational, musculomucosal circumoral flap, is an excellent reconstructive choice for lip excisions that have removed between one-third and two-thirds of the lower lip. It allows for muscular continuity and maintains oral competence. Defects that affect the oral commissures are best served with a local rotational flap, such as the Estlander lateral lip-switch flap. If the entire lower lip must be excised, utilization of a radial forearm free flap with palmaris longus sling may be necessary as part of the reconstructive process.

Subungual Melanoma

Subungual melanoma is a type of malignant skin melanoma most commonly diagnosed as an acral lentiginous subtype on histology. This subgroup is more prevalent in darker-skinned individuals, occurring mainly on the palms, soles, and subungual regions. For this reason, such melanomas are often found at a more advanced stage. A subungal melanoma will typically present as a linear brown or black discoloration of the nail known as melanonychia. While melanonychia can be caused by other benign causes, the presence of color variegation, size, ulceration, and extension beyond the nail plate warrant a full-thickness biopsy.

The current standard of care for the surgical treatment of a subungal melanoma remains amputation of the digit one joint space proximal to the subungal melanoma. The appropriate surgical margins should still be measured intraoperatively, with special attention to any evidence of proximal spread beyond the nail bed. Despite the gold standard of digit amputation (with or without a concomitant SLNB), recent literature has suggested that a less aggressive approach may be as beneficial [56–59].

Current Surgical Guidelines and Recommendations

The evolution and collection of data from well-designed clinical trials has allowed us to develop a set of surgical guidelines that are safe, well tolerated, and associated with acceptable locoregional recurrence rates. Strategies that rely on lesser margins of excision, including approaches that rely solely on the pathologist's report of a tumor-free biopsy site margin, offer little savings of morbidity yet risk higher rates of local recurrence. Even patients with thin melanomas (≤1 mm in thickness) deserve an appropriate surgical margin, as recurrence does occur even in this group and is often a harbinger of very poor prognosis and outcome.

National Comprehensive Cancer Network (NCCN) Treatment Guidelines

The National Comprehensive Cancer Network (NCCN) was started in 1995 with the goal of developing a comprehensive set of diagnostic, treatment, and supportive care guidelines for all cancer patients [60]. The NCCN guidelines have become an essential tool to provide comprehensive, evidence-based care of cancer patients. With the rapid increase in knowledge of melanoma driver pathways and immunobiology, a record number of new treatments have been approved in the last few years. These treatment guidelines are constantly updated as new data and information from clinical trials is published, resulting in an effective tool for treatment of cancer patients based upon expert opinion of evidence-based medicine [60].

For a melanoma in-situ [stage 0], we recommend a 5-mm margin of excision. For a primary melanoma that is ≤0.75 mm in Breslow's thickness, the recommendations are to perform a wide local excision with a 1-cm margin. For a stage IA melanoma between 0.76 and 1.0 mm in Breslow's thickness, a further discussion is had as to the risks and benefits of concomitant SLNB. For a stage IB or II melanoma that is greater than 1 mm in Breslow's thickness, a wide local excision with 1–2 cm margins should be performed, with concomitant SLNB. For truncal or proximal extremity melanoma with a Breslow's thickness >2 mm, wide local excision with 2-cm margins should be performed (Table 17.1). In the head and neck region, distal extremities, or other cosmetically sensitive areas, a surgical excision margin of at least 1 cm should be attempted for a primary melanoma with Breslow's thickness >1 mm. If a stage III melanoma is encountered, complete nodal dissection should follow positive SLNB. If nodes are clinically positive, FNA or an alternate form of node biopsy should be obtained prior to excision of the primary tumor. If there is suspicion for clinical, satellite, or in-transit metastasis, biopsy should also be obtained prior to excision of the primary melanoma. Complete surgical excision should still be considered in stage IV disease if the patient is a favorable candidate. For unresectable disease, consideration should be given to a clinical trial or to palliative care in certain situations.

Table 17.1 Recommendations for excision margins of primary cutaneous melanoma

Location	Tumor thickness	Margins
Trunk/proximal extremity	Melanoma in-situ	0.5 cm
	≤1 mm	1 cm
	1–2 mm	1–2 cm
	>2–4 mm	2 cm
	>4 mm	2 cm
Head/neck, distal extremity (or cosmetically sensitive area)	≤1 mm	1 cm
	≤1 mm	At least 1 cm

References

1. Urteaga OB, Pack GT. On the antiquity of melanoma. Cancer. 1967;19:607–10.
2. Home Sir Everhard. Observations on cancer. London. 48 (1805).
3. Laennec RTH. Sur les melanoses. Bull Fac Med Paris. 1812;1:2.
4. Norris W. Case of fungoid disease. Edinburgh Med Surg J. 1820;16:562.
5. Norris W. Eight cases of melanosis with pathological and therapeutical remarks on that disease. London: Longman, Brown, Green, Longman and Roberts; 1857.
6. Parrish I. Case of melanosis. Am J Med Sci. 1837;20:266.
7. Cooper S. The first lines of the theory and practice of surgery. London: Longman; 1840.
8. Pemberton O. Observations on the history, pathology and treatment of cancerous diseases. London: Churchill J; 1858.
9. Snow H. Melanotic cancerous disease. Lancet. 1892;2:872–4.
10. Eve F. Lecture on melanoma. Practitioner. 1903;70:165.
11. Handley WS. The pathology of melanotic growths in relation to their operative treatment (II). Lancet. 1907;1:996–1001.
12. Clark WH Jr, From L, Bernardino EA, Mihm MC Jr. The histogenesis and biologic behavior of primary human malignant melanomas of the skin. Cancer Res. 1969;29:705–27.
13. Breslow A. Thickness, cross-sectional areas and depth of invasion in the prognosis of cutaneous melanoma. Ann Surg. 1970;172:902–8.
14. Breslow A, Cascinelli N, van der Esch EP, Morabito A. Stage I melanoma of the limbs: assessment of prognosis by levels of invasion and maximum thickness. Tumori. 1978;64:273–8.
15. Fee HJ, Robinson DS, Sample WF, et al. The determination of lymph shed by colloidal gold scanning patients with malignant melanoma: a preliminary study. Surgery. 1987;84:626–32.
16. Morton D, Cagle L, Wong J, et al. Intraoperative lymphatic mapping and selective lymphadenectomy: technical details of a new procedure for clinical stage I melanoma. Presented at the Annual Meeting of

the Society of Surgical Oncology; Washington, DC. 1990.
17. Morton DL, Wen DR, Wong JH, et al. Technical details of intraoperative lymphatic mapping for early stage melanoma. Arch Surg. 1992;127:392–9.
18. Morton DL, Thompson JF, Cochran AJ, et al. Sentinel-node biopsy or nodal observation in melanoma. N Engl J Med. 2006;355(13):1307–17.
19. Salopek TG, Slade J, Marghoob AA, et al. Management of cutaneous malignant melanoma by dermatologists of the American Academy of Dermatology. I. Survey of biopsy practices of pigmented lesions suspected as melanoma. J Am Acad Dermatol. 1995;33:441–50.
20. Kanzler MH, Mraz-Gernhard S. Primary cutaneous malignant melanoma and its precursor lesions: diagnostic and therapeutic overview. J Am Acad Dermatol. 2001;54:260–76.
21. Thomas L, Tranchard P, Berard F, Secchi T, Colin C, Moulin G. Semiological value of ABCD criteria in the diagnosis of cutaneous pigmented tumors. Dermatology. 1998;197:11–7.
22. Weinstock MA. Early detection of melanoma. JAMA. 2000;284:886–9.
23. Nachbar F, Soltz W, Merkle T, et al. The ABCD rule of dermatoscopy. High prospective value in the diagnosis of doubtful melanocytic skin lesions. J Am Acad Dermatol. 1994;30:551–9.
24. McGovern TW, Litaker MS. Clinical predictors of malignant pigmented lesions. A comparison of the Glasgow seven-point checklist and the American Cancer Society's ABCD of pigmented lesions. J Dermatol Surg Oncol. 1992;18:22–6.
25. Argenziano G, Soyer H. Dermoscopy of pigmented skin lesions—a valuable toll for early diagnosis of melanoma. Lancet Oncol. 2001;2:443–9.
26. Argenziano G, Fabbrocini G, Carli P, DeGiogi V, Sammarco E, Delfino M. Epiluminescence microscopy for the diagnosis of doubtful melanocytic skin lesions. Comparison of the ABCD rule of dermatoscopy and a new 7-point checklist based on pattern analysis. Arch Dermatol. 1998;134:1563–70.
27. Breslow A. Prognostic factors in the treatment of cutaneous melanoma. J Cutan Pathol. 1979;6:208–12.
28. Clark WH Jr, Elder DE, Guerry DT, et al. Model predicting survival instage I melanoma based on tumor progression. J Natl Cancer Inst. 1989;81:1893–904.
29. Farmer ER. Why a skin biopsy? Arch Dermatol. 2000;136:779–80.
30. Herlyn M, Ferrone S, Ronai Z, Finerty J, Pelroy R, Mohla S. Melanoma biology and progression. Cancer Res. 2001;61:4642–3.
31. Johnson TM, Sondak VK. Melanoma margins: the importance and need for more evidence-based trials. N Engl J Med. 2004;350:757–66.
32. Landthaler M, Braun-Falco O, Leitl A, Konz B, Holzel D. Excisional biopsy as the first therapeutic procedure versus primary wide local excision of malignant melanoma. Cancer. 1989;64:1612–6.
33. Levi F, Randimbison L, LaVecchia C, Te VC, Frandeschi S. Prognostic factors for cutaneous malignant melanoma in Vaud, Switzerland. Int J Cancer. 1998;78:315–9.
34. Macy-Roberts E, Ackerman AB. A critique of techniques for biopsy of clinically suspected malignant melanomas. Am J Dermatopathol. 1982;4:391–8.
35. Riker AI, Glass F, Perez I, Cruse CW, Messina J, Sondak VK. Cutaneous melanoma: methods of biopsy and definitive surgical excision. Dermatol Ther. 2005;18:387–93.
36. Roses D. Biopsy technique for suspected melanoma. Pigment Cell. 1985;7:8–17.
37. Amin MB, Edge S, Greene F, et al., editors. AJCC cancer staging manual. 8th ed. New York: Springer; 2016. p. 563–85.
38. Balch CM, Buzaid AC, Soong SJ, et al. Final version of the American Joint Committee on Cancer staging system for cutaneous melanoma. Cancer. 2001;88:3635–48.
39. Balch CM, Soong SJ, Gershenwald JE, et al. Prognostic factors analysis of 17,600 melanoma patients. Validation of the American Joint Committee on Cancer melanoma staging system. J Clin Oncol. 2001;19:3622–34.
40. Balch CM, Urist MM, Karakousis CP, et al. Efficacy of 2-cm surgical margins for intermediate thickness melanomas (1–4 mm). Results of a multi-institutional randomized surgical trial. Ann Surg. 1993;218(3):262–7.
41. Balch CM, Soong SJ, Ross MI, et al. Long term results of a prospective trial comparing 2 cm vs. 4 cm excision margins for 740 patients with 1–4 mm melanomas. Ann Surg Oncol. 2001;8:101–8.
42. Gillgren P, Drzewiecki KT, Niin M, et al. 2-cm versus 4-cm surgical excision margins for primary cutaneous melanoma thicker than 2mm: a randomised, multicenter trial. Lancet. 2011;378:1635–42.
43. Khayat D, Rixe O, Martin G, et al. Surgical margins in cutaneous melanoma (2 cm versus 5 cm for lesions measuring less than 2.1 mm thick). Cancer. 2003;97:1941–6.
44. Cohn-Cedermark G, Rutqvist LE, Andersson R, et al. Long term results of a randomized study by the Swedish Melanoma Study Group on 2 cm versus 5 cm resection margins for patients with cutaneous melanoma with a thickness of 0.8 to 2.0 mm. Cancer. 2000;89:1495–501.
45. Tanabe KK, Reintgen DS, Balch CM. Local recurrences and their management. In: Balch CM, Houghton AN, Sober AJ, Soong SJ, editors. Cutaneous melanoma. 4th ed. St. Louis, MI: Quality Medical Publishing; 2003. p. 263–73.
46. Veronesi U, Cascinelli N, Adamus J, et al. Thin stage I primary cutaneous malignant melanoma: comparison of excision with margins of 1 or 3 cm. N Engl J Med. 1988;322:1159–62.
47. Santinarni M, Maurici A, Patuzzo R, et al. Impact of clinical trials on the treatment of melanoma. Surg Oncol Clin N Am. 2001;10:935–47.
48. Hudson LE, Maithel SK, Carlson GW, et al. 1 or 2 cm margins of excision for T2 melanomas: do

they impact recurrence or survival? Ann Surg Oncol. 2013;20:346–51.
49. Doepker MP, Thompson ZJ, Fisher KJ, Yamamoto M, Nethers KW, Harb JN, Applebaum MA, Gonzalez RJ, Sarnaik AA, Messina JL, et al. Is a wider margin (2cm vs. 1 cm) for a 1.01-2.0 mm melanoma necessary? Ann Surg Oncol. 2016;23(7):2336–42.
50. Thomas JM, Newton-Bishop J, A'Hern R, et al. Excision margins in high-risk malignant melanoma. N Engl J Med. 2004;350:757–66.
51. Heaton KM, Sussman JJ, Gershenwald JE, et al. Surgical margins and prognostic factors in patients with thick (>4 mm) primary melanoma. Ann Surg Oncol. 1998;5:322–8.
52. Kenady DE, Brown BW, McBride CM. Excision of underlying fascia with a primary malignant melanoma: effect on recurrence and survival rates. Surgery. 1982;92(4):615–8.
53. Sondergaard K, Schou G. Therapeutic and clinicopathological factors in the survival of 1,469 patients with primary cutaneous malignant melanoma in clinical stage I. A multivariate regression analysis. Virchows Arch A Pathol Anat Histopathol. 1985;408(2-3):249–58.
54. Corsten M, Johnson-Obaseki S. Sentinal lymph node biopsy in head and neck melanoma: a review. J Patient-Centered Res Rev. 2014;1(1):27–32.
55. Cruse CW, Wells KE, Reintgen DS. Treatment of the primary in malignant melanoma of the skin. Ann Plast Surg. 1992;28:22–5.
56. Cochran AM, Buchanan PJ, Bueno RA Jr, et al. Subungual melanoma: a review of current treatment. Plast Reconstr Surg. 2014;134(2):259–73.
57. Haddock NT, Wilson SC, Shapiro RL, et al. Wide local en bloc excision of subungual melanoma in situ. Ann Plast Surg. 2014;73(6):640–4.
58. Nakamura Y, Ohara K, Kishi A, et al. Effects of non-amputative wide local excision on the local control and prognosis of in situ and invasive subungual melanoma. J Dermatol. 2015;42(9):861–6.
59. Anda-Juarez MC, Martinez-Velasco MA, Fonte-Avalos V, et al. Conservative surgical management of in situ subungual melanoma: long-term follow-up. An Bras Dermatol. 2016;91(6):846–8.
60. NCCN Clinical Practice Guidelines in Oncology (NCCN Guidelines): Melanoma, version 1.2017. National Comprehensive Cancer Network, Fort Washington, PA. 2016. www.NCCN.org

Mohs Surgery for Melanoma In Situ

18

Joy Kunishige and John Zitelli

Background and Epidemiology

Melanoma in situ (MIS) is a proliferation of malignant melanocytes within the epidermis, without invasion into the dermis. Typically, pigmented macules display the features of melanoma such as variegated color, asymmetry, and irregular border. However, presentation can be varied with some presenting similar to normal freckles or nevi, but distinguished by growth or change. The histologic features include a predominance of individual melanocytes over nests, confluent growth along the epidermis, and pagetoid spread of individual melanocytes into upper layers of the epidermis.

There are four subtypes of MIS: lentigo maligna, superficial spreading, acral lentiginous, and mucosal. Perhaps 75% of MIS can be further classified as lentigo maligna subtype, which has a confusing history. In 1890, it was described as "Hutchinson's melanotic freckle" [1]. Its slow growth led to the hypothesis that it was infectious in etiology. In 1912, Dubreuilh characterized the lesion as precancerous [2]. Some postulated there were two types of lentigo maligna, one that was benign photodamage and one that was malignant [3]. It is still misconstrued by some as a premalignant lesion [4].

Today, lentigo maligna is well established as a subtype of MIS on sun-exposed skin. As such, it occurs in older patients, with peak onset in the seventh and eighth decades of life. Histologically, it contains atypical melanocytes along the basal layer of the epidermis in solitary units or small nests and solar elastosis (abnormal elastin accumulation from excessive sun exposure). Extension of cytologic atypia down follicles and other adnexal structures is common. Though characterized by slow growth, sometimes taking years to diagnose, it is a malignant tumor.

Amelanotic extension is frequently described as an expected feature of lentigo maligna, but it is present in all MIS and invasive melanoma. At least 62% of melanomas contain an area of amelanotic or subclinical extension [5]. Amelanotic extension can be foreshadowed by the loss of freckling, but it is more commonly invisible to the eye. Due to the inability to visualize the border or margin of an MIS or melanoma, standard excision must be performed with an additional safety margin of normal-appearing skin. Discussion of excision guidelines follows.

Aside from subclinical extension, the presence of occult invasive components must be considered. Numerous studies have found that 5–67% of biopsy-proven MIS are later upgraded to invasive melanoma [3, 6–15]. The frequency with which MIS is upgraded depends upon the

J. Kunishige, M.D. (✉)
Department of Plastic Surgery, Zitelli & Brodland Skin Cancer Center, University of Pittsburgh Medical Center, Pittsburgh, PA, USA

J. Zitelli, M.D.
Departments of ENT and Plastic Surgery, Zitelli & Brodland Skin Cancer Center, University of Pittsburgh Medical Center, Pittsburgh, PA, USA

A. I. Riker (ed.), *Melanoma*, https://doi.org/10.1007/978-3-319-78310-9_18

size of the lesion and how thoroughly one examines the specimen. Of note, the invasive area may be 5–10 mm away from the clinically evident lesion [16].

The single-most powerful risk factor for the development of a MIS and melanoma is long-term cumulative UV radiation. Risk factors include fair skin, history of sunburns, tanning bed use, atypical nevi, family history, and immune suppression. Smoking does not appear to be a risk factor [17].

MIS represents 40% of all melanomas diagnosed in the United States and the incidence is rising [18]. Some debate exists as to whether this is due to a true increase versus overdiagnosis. In part, it reflects more biopsies and better histologic criteria such that diagnosis occurs earlier and more accurately. However, studies conclude that increased screening and biopsy alone cannot account for the dramatic increase in incidence [19, 20]. Over 60,000 people in the United States are diagnosed with MIS each year.

Treatment

Given the initial belief that MIS, or at least lentigo maligna, was a premalignant process, plus the frequency with which it occurs, it is not surprising that many treatments have been attempted. Radiation is second-line treatment for patients who are not surgical candidates. It is associated with a 7% recurrence rate and delayed recurrences occurring around 4 years [21]. Topical imiquimod is an inferior option associated with clinical response, but with hidden histologic persistence in at least 25% [22]. Development of invasive disease with satellite metastases has also been reported [23].

MIS is a malignant skin cancer, with an associated risk for becoming a primary, invasive melanoma. Once invasive, it has the same prognosis as other melanomas. It is important to remove the entire lesion for three reasons. First, many MIS are actually invasive. Second, if it is not invasive now, it can be in the future. Twenty-three percent of MIS recur as an invasive melanoma, with a mean Breslow's depth of 0.9 mm [24]. Third, treatment of recurrent lesions is more difficult. Recurrent tumors can track stealthily along scars and be multifocal, lowering cure rates.

The goal of excision is to remove the entire primary lesion. Because it is not possible to visualize the edge of a melanoma with the naked eye, a safety margin must be excised. Guidelines for surgical margins refer to additional tissue that should be excised beyond the visible tumor edge. The guidelines only apply in instances where one is using visual inspection to determine the tumor edge, and they do not apply if instead one uses a microscope to determine the tumor boundary. It is important to understand that the guidelines are recommendations for the clinical surgical margin measured on the patient during excision, and do not refer to histologic margins that may later appear on pathology reports.

Excision guidelines have changed over the past decade to reflect the current best evidence. In 1992, a consensus conference recommended 5 mm excision margins for MIS [25]. This was based on expert opinion at the time, not on high-level studies. Since then, multiple studies have shown that a 5 mm excision margin is inadequate (Table 18.1). A margin of 5 mm will only clear 23–86% of all MIS lesions [3, 8, 9, 12, 26, 27, 29–38].

To determine the surgical margin required to completely excise 97% of MIS, Kunishige et al. prospectively collected data on the treatment of 1,120 MIS lesions. In order to obtain a 97% clearance rate, a 9 mm margin of excision was required [26]. A closer look at this patient population suggested that some lesions on the head and neck actually required a 1.2 cm margin (Author's Unpublished Data). Others have also reported that a 1–1.5 cm margin is necessary [8, 12, 27, 32, 35]. The surgical margin necessary for MIS mirroring that of invasive melanoma makes sense for two reasons: First, studies have not found a correlation between Breslow's depth and the amount of subclinical extension. Second, up to 67% of MIS are actually invasive [3, 6–15].

Clinicians who treat MIS inherently understand that 5 mm margins are not adequate. However, because of the dogma that lentigo

Table 18.1 Melanoma in situ clearance rate with 5 or 6 mm is low

Study	No. of MIS lesions	Follow-up time (month)	Clearance rate with 5- or 6-mm margins
Biernet et al. [29]	76	33	0%
Clayton et al. [30]	81	22	23%
Albertini et al. [31]	42	Unknown	24% if 5 mm
			41% if 6 mm
Moyer et al. [32]	232	101	41%
Agarwal-Antal et al. [33]	92	48	42%
Zalla et al. [12]	46	16	50%
Felton et al. [27]	343	29	65%
Malhotra et al. [50]	109	32	69%
deVries et al. [34]	100	60	~69%
Huilgol et al. [8]	125	38	70%
Hilari et al. [35]	62	Unknown	73.5% if primary
			30.8% if recurrent
Bricca et al. [36]	331	58	84%
Bub et al. [9]	55	57	85%
Kunishige et al. [26]	1120	56	86%
Cohen [3]	45	58	Unknown
Bene et al. [37]	167	63	Unknown

maligna subtype has wide extensions, many question the need for a wider resection margin for other subtypes of MIS. A comparison of 1506 lentigo malignas to 849 other subtypes of MIS found no difference in margin requirements based upon subtype. Both LM and other MIS on the trunk and extremities achieved a 97% clearance with 1 cm margins. Both LM and other MIS on the head and neck achieved 97% clearance with 1.2 cm margins (Author's Unpublished Data).

Indeed, 1 or 1.2 cm margins are not always doable or desirable. In these cases, Mohs surgery should be considered. The Mohs technique is described below, noting that any technique that enables visualization of the entire peripheral margin can be used, such as staged excision or "slow Mohs," and the square technique. The more one sees, the more one can be confident the margin is clear, and thus reduce recurrence rates. In contrast, wide local excision specimens are processed by "breadloaf" technique (Fig. 18.1). The excised ellipse is cut vertically from skin to adipose. A few cross sections are viewed under the microscope. In total, less than 1% of the peripheral margin is examined [39]. Thus, residual MIS is unlikely to be detected and is often missed [40]. If there is 5 mm between each vertical cross section, then there will be a < 20% chance of finding residual tumor. This explains the exasperating tendency of MIS to recur, even when the final pathology report declares "clear" margins: recurrence rate for standard excision of MIS with a 5-mm margin is 8–20% [11, 41, 42].

Mohs surgery for melanoma is safe, effective, and validated (Table 18.2) [3, 7–9, 26–30, 32–34, 37, 40, 43–48, 50–52]. It consistently boasts low recurrence rates that approach zero. It is also associated with improved cure rates for tumors that are recurrent or located on the head and neck [27, 28, 32, 36, 37, 51].

Procedure

Mohs Technique

The biopsy scar and any residual pigment, plus 3 mm of normal-appearing skin, is excised down to the superficial adipose tissue. This debulking specimen is evaluated by routine breadloaf processing (vertical sections) to determine if there is an upgrade in Breslow's

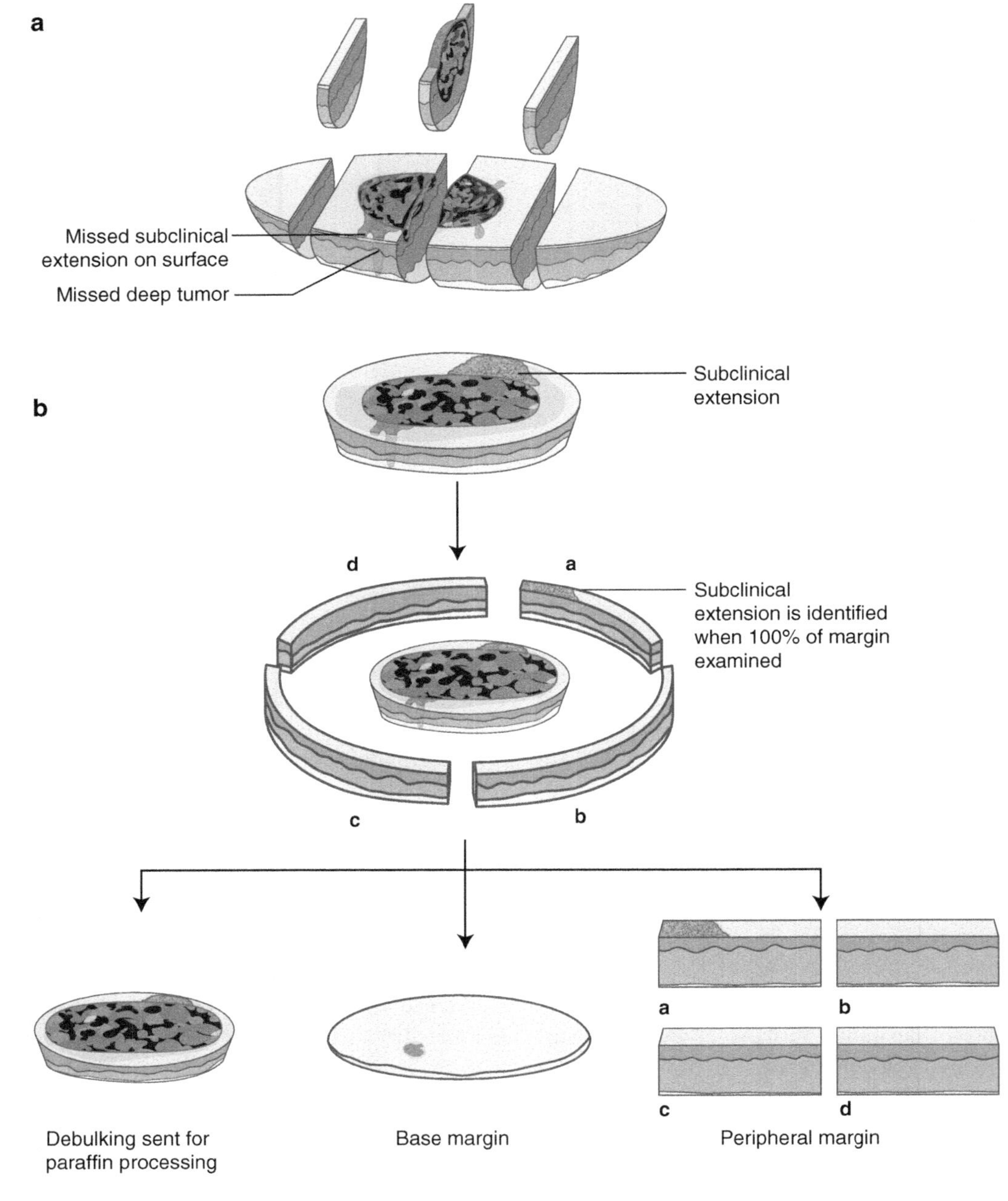

Fig. 18.1 Breadloaf technique enables visualization of less than 1% of the peripheral and deep margin, which is indicated in blue (**a**). Mohs micrographic surgery employs beveled excision and relaxing techniques to flatten the specimen, so that 100% of the peripheral and deep margin can be examined in one plane (**b**)

thickness. This can be done via permanent sections or frozen sections. Immediately after debulking, an additional 3 mm margin is taken laterally and excised as a single piece down to the deep adipose for frozen-section examination by Mohs technique. The peripheral tissue is cut into 1–2 cm strips, then stained with various colors to facilitate orientation and

Table 18.2 Low recurrence rates associated with Mohs technique

Study	# of MIS	Procedure	Follow-up (month)	Recurrence
Bienert et al. [29]	76	Mohs	33	0%
Agarwal-Antal et al. [33]	92	Mohs	48	0%
Johnson et al. [40]	35	SE	Unknown	0%
Jejurikar et al. [43]	42	SE	31	0%
Mahoney et al. [7]	11	SE	4.7	0%
Moller et al. [44]	49	SE	14	0%
Kunishige et al. [26]	2335	Mohs	56	0.3%
Felton et al. [27]	343	Mohs	29	0.3%
Etzkorn et al. [28]	436	Mohs	34	0.5%
Anderson et al. [45]	150	SE	<60	0.7%
Clayton et al. [30]	77	Mohs	22	1%
Bosbous et al. [46]	49	SE	26	1.7%
Bene et al. [37]	116	Mohs	63	1.8%
Nasrati et al. [47]	277	Mohs	103	1.8%
Hou et al. [48]	407	Mohs	95	1.9%
Huilgol et al. [8]	125	Modified SE	38	2%
Moyer et al. [32]	834	SE	10	2%
Cohen et al. [3]	26	Mohs and SE	58	2.2%
Hill et al. [49]	38	Modified SE	25	2.6%
Bub et al. [9]	55	Modified SE	57	3.6%
Malhotra et al. [50]	109	Modified SE	32	3.7%
deVries et al. [34]	100	SE	60	4%
Walling et al. [51]	50	Modified SE	95	6%
Lee et al. [52]	31	Modified SE	42	9.6%
Total	5863	Mohs or SE	45 (mean)	2% (mean)

SE staged excision, *Modified SE* vertical sections were used and entire margin not examined

localization. Frozen sections with and without MART-1 immunostain are reviewed (Fig. 18.2). Any remaining tumor is marked on a map representing the surgical wound. Additional 3 mm margins are excised in exact areas where residual tumor is noted.

Positive margins are defined as those containing at least one of the following: (1) nests of at least 3 atypical melanocytes, (2) melanocytes above the dermoepidermal junction, and (3) nonuniform crowding of cells along the basement membrane. Other histologic findings raising suspicion include: (1) extension of atypical, crowded melanocytes far down adnexal structures, (2) nonuniform distribution of pigment, (3) excessive number of melanophages, and (4) brisk inflammatory response. Increased melanocyte density and mild to moderate confluence alone are typical of melanocytic hyperplasia in sun-damaged skin, and should not be interpreted as melanoma [54, 55]. Using these criteria, the interpretation of frozen sections is comparable to that of paraffin sections [56].

Some Mohs centers utilize additional or alternate immunostains. MITF is a nuclear stain and therefore will only stain melanocytes, whereas MART-1 stains an antigen found on the surface of melanocytes that can sometimes be found in keratinocytes and pseudonests. Though MITF is more specific, the nuclear stain creates faint and tiny dots. MART-1 is sensitive and brightly positive. The rapid 1-hour protocol makes it the most practical and efficient method for Mohs surgeons to judge the presence or absence of melanoma at the margin [54, 57].

The evaluation of melanoma by frozen section requires meticulous lab processing. The immunostain must be applied exactly and without contact with agents that can bind the immunostain and render it useless. Most importantly, the sections of tissue must be very thin. Thicker sections result in viewing a stack of cells, which results in

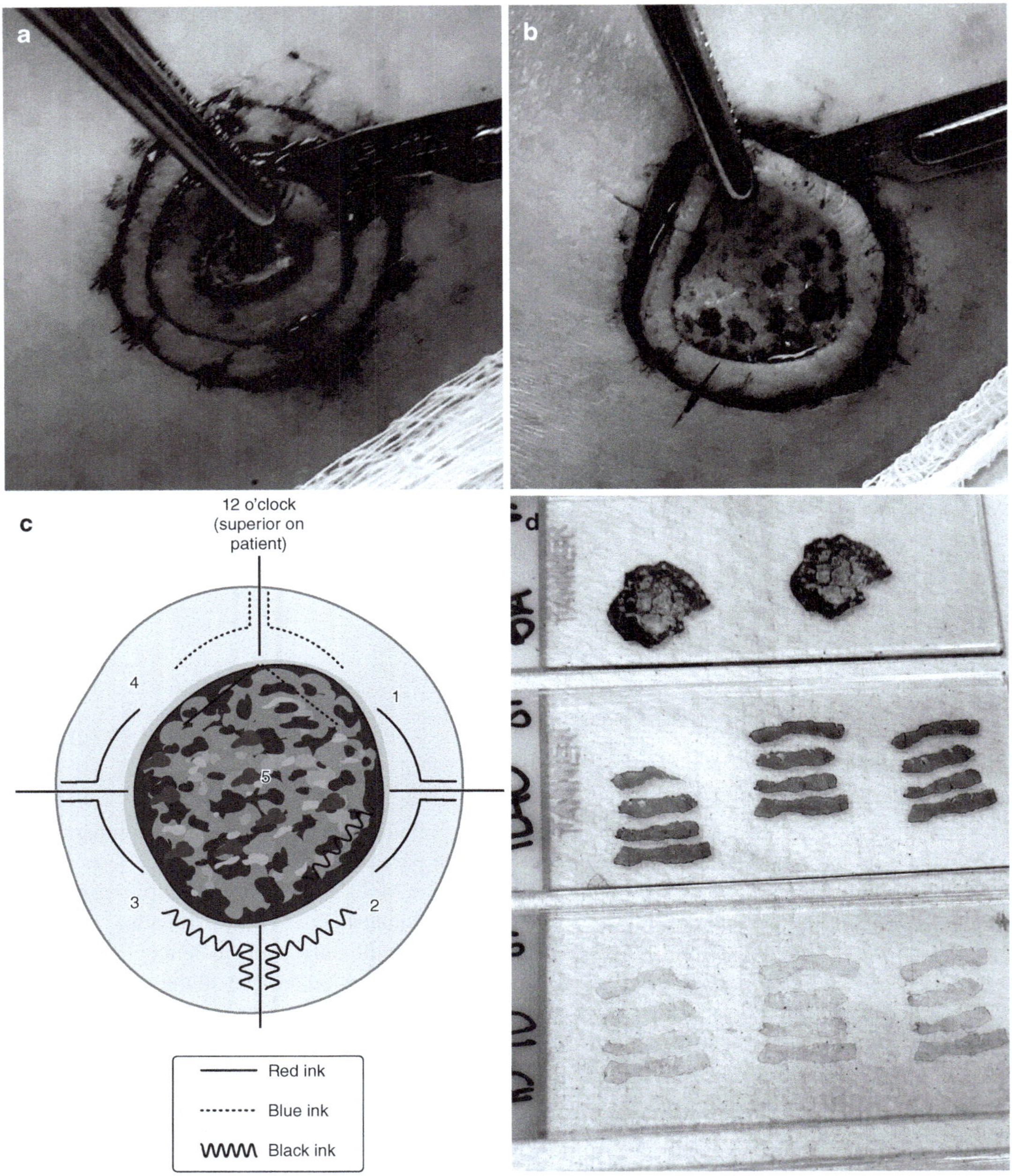

Fig. 18.2 Mohs technique for melanoma. First, the visible tumor is excised and examined with vertical sections (breadloaf technique) to confirm Breslow's thickness (**a**). Next, a peripheral and deep margin of normal-appearing skin is excised down to deep adipose (**b**). The peripheral margin is separated into thin strips to enable en face examination. All sections are inked and mapped (**c**). Frozen sections with and without MART-1 immunostain are reviewed (**d**). Any residual tumor at the margin is mapped then excised

increased stain and false positives. Tangential sections will also cause false positives, because the diagonal stack of melanocytes in the basal layer looks like pagetoid spread. When thin sections with crisp staining cannot be obtained, specimens can be sent out for formalin-fixed permanent sections. Staged excision (slow Mohs) and the square technique are two procedures that utilize permanent sections to visualize the entire peripheral margin.

Staged Excision and Square Procedure

Often called "slow Mohs," staged excision mimics the procedure above, except all tissue is sent out for formalin-fixed permanent processing instead of frozen sections. After excising the central tumor to deep adipose, the first perimeter of tissue is taken. A map is drawn and sent out with the tissue. The resulting wound is dressed with petrolatum ointment and a bandage, and the patient returns in 2–3 days. If additional tissue is needed, this is excised and the patient returns in another 2–3 days. This continues until a tumor-free plane is reached. Then, the patient returns for reconstruction of the defect.

A variant of staged excision is the "square procedure." Here, the desired surgical margin is outlined with geometric angled corners of the lines, such as a square or rectangle. Geometric configuration may facilitate tissue processing. A double-bladed hair transplant scalpel is used to remove a 2–4 mm wide strip of tissue around the tumor. This circumferential band is sent out for permanent section margin evaluation. Additional stages are performed as necessary. Once a tumor-free peripheral plane has been reached, the remaining central "island" of tissue is excised to deep adipose and sent out. With melanoma in situ, it is reasonable to assume the deep margin will be clear and to repair the wound. Of course, if the deep margin proves to contain invasive tumor transected at the base, then additional excision will be necessary [43].

With either of these procedures, the surgeon and pathologist must work together to ensure the entire peripheral margin is evaluated. The circumference of the excision should be embedded *en face*. Modified staged excision refers to the use of vertical, radial, or breadloaf sections to examine part, or all, of the peripheral margin. This will result in higher recurrence rates (Table 18.2).

Clinical Scenarios

Patient referred for lentigo maligna on the right nasal sidewall. This was excised with 6 mm margin. The peripheral and deep margins were examined by standard Mohs technique. No additional stages were needed. The final defect measured 2 cm and was able to be repaired with a local flap (Fig. 18.3). Note that margins narrower than 6 mm may be attempted, with the understanding that there will be a higher probability that additional stages will be needed. The authors routinely use narrower margins of 2 or 3 mm when working near the eye or nasal tip, or when it would allow for simpler reconstruction options.

Patient presented with multiply recurrent MIS on the left cheek. The areas of tumor were delineated via the Mohs procedure, with sparing of some scarred tissue on the lower lid. The wound was repaired with linear repair and graft (Fig. 18.4).

Patient referred for recurrent desmoplastic melanoma arising in an old forehead flap, with the desire to avoid total rhinectomy. He presented with an 8 mm nodule with surrounding induration. The tumor was excised using Mohs technique in four stages. This resulted in a hemi-rhinectomy. The patient returned to his country with plans to pursue reconstruction after one year. If delayed repair is desired to enable monitoring for recurrence, then a skin graft can be applied to prevent wound contraction (Fig. 18.5). Patients may be referred to specialists for reconstruction, or rarely, for additional excision should the tumor invade the skull or nerve foramina.

Controversies and Future Areas of Research

There is no question that complete histologic margin control results in higher cure rates. Looking is better than not looking. However, controversy exists on how to look. Some feel permanent sections are superior to frozen sections for melanoma interpretation. Indeed, frozen sec-

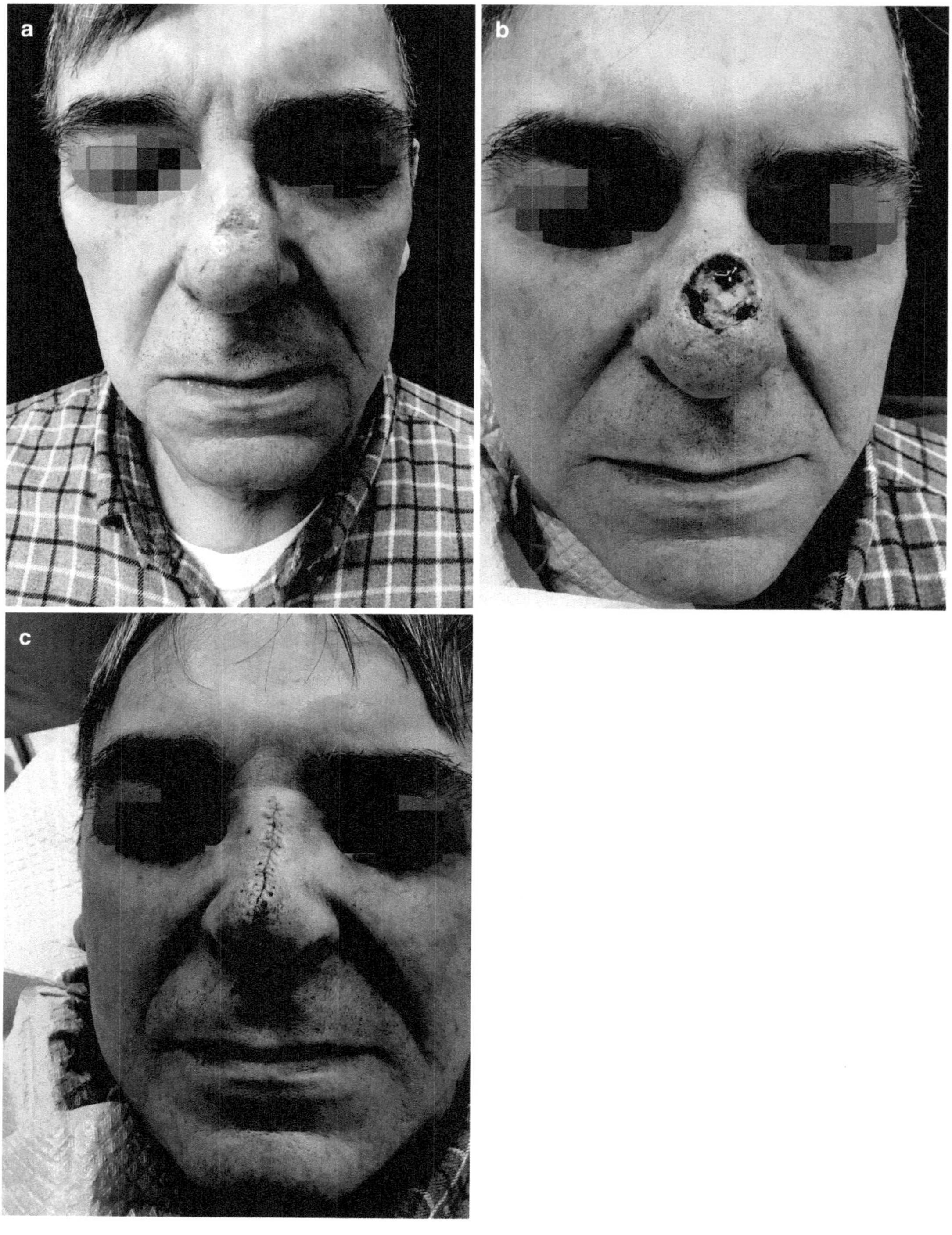

Fig. 18.3 Mohs technique simultaneously offers guaranteed clear margins (**a**, **b**) and tissue conservation enabling repair with local flap (**c**)

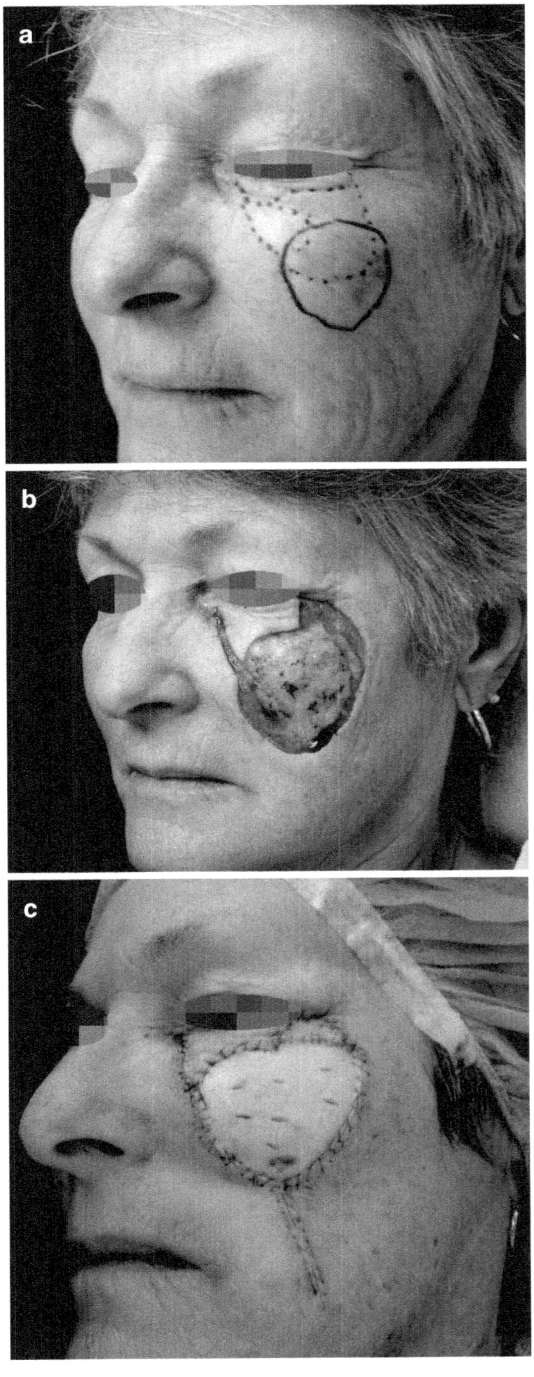

Fig. 18.4 Multiply recurrent melanoma excised with Mohs technique (**a**, **b**), then linear repair and graft (**c**). Checking 100% of the peripheral and deep margin enables the surgeon to excise less tissue than with wide local excision

tions for melanoma are technically difficult. Without an experienced technician and reliably thin sections, the stain will always appear positive, and overcalling will occur. More stages will seem required and large defects will result. The fact that most melanomas can be excised with one stage, in combination with recurrence rates of 0–2%, prove that frozen section analysis is a valid technique.

One study comparing interpretation of frozen section to that of permanent sections found no difference [56]. Another study suggested frozen sections with immunostains may actually be superior to permanent sections: staged excision with permanent sections resulted in a wider margin of resection compared to that of Mohs surgery. The average margin excised was 9.3 mm compared to 6.8 mm for Mohs surgery [26, 32]. This raises the possibility that it is more difficult to distinguish actinic-induced melanocyte proliferation from true malignancy on permanent sections than on frozen sections with MART-1 immunostain. In summary, true Mohs surgery with 100% margin examination, excision and histologic evaluation performed by the same individual, and use of immunostains will yield the lowest recurrence of any method (Table 18.2). However, if thin frozen sections with immunostain cannot reliably be achieved, then staged excision with *en face* processing and permanent sections are a good alternative.

Randomized data may never be available to support Mohs for invasive melanoma. A study by Mayo et al. reported that Mohs surgery and wide local excision had similar recurrence rates [48]. However, the two treatment arms were not randomized. Larger and recurrent lesions, as well as those on the head and neck, were referred for Mohs surgery [48]. A truly randomized study is unlikely, because it is frequently impossible to excise the full 1 cm needed on the head and neck.

Accordingly, the six prospective, randomized, controlled trials behind the guidelines for melanoma excision excluded MIS and virtually

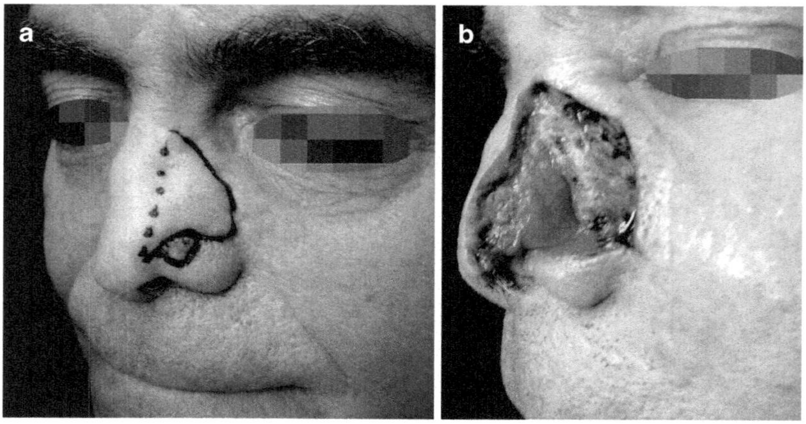

Fig. 18.5 Multiply recurrent desmoplastic melanoma excised, then patient referred to Plastic Surgery for repair (**a**, **b**). This can be done immediately post-operatively or 1–2 weeks later. If delayed repair is desired to enable monitoring for recurrence, then a skin graft can be applied to prevent wound contraction. Repair can be done with confidence that the margin is clear

excluded the head and neck location. Only 16 of 4231 randomized melanomas were on the head and neck [58–63]. Non-randomized studies of head and neck MIS and melanoma suggest that a 1 cm is inadequate for some lesions, clearing as few as 50% [27, 32, 64]. More telling, guideline margins were unable to be executed on 33% of head and neck melanomas [61].

An area of huge impact would be to increase the specificity of melanoma diagnosis. The separation of biologically important MIS from severely atypical photodamage has plagued dermatopathologists for decades, and the answer may lie in gene expression. Gene expression profiling tests already look at a battery of genes within excised melanoma tissue and accurately predict recurrence [65]. And, fluorescence in situ hybridization (FISH) analysis is frequently used to distinguish between benign Spitz nevi and malignant melanoma [66].

Another area of controversy in melanoma management is sentinel lymph node biopsy. The discussion of this is not relevant to a chapter on melanoma in situ. However, there are instances where a MIS is excised, and more thorough examination of the excised tissue results in an upgrade of Breslow's thickness whereby consideration of sentinel lymph node biopsy is warranted. In these cases, sentinel lymph node biopsy can still be performed after repair [67]. However, if this remains a concern of the multidisciplinary team, then frozen sections can be used on the debulking specimen to evaluate for the true Breslow's thickness. An upgrade in thickness would then be determined prior to starting repair, with final repair delayed until after sentinel lymph node biopsy [28].

Finally, the cost of Mohs surgery versus wide local excision is a valid concern. The cost of Mohs surgery (which includes cost of slide preparation and examination) is actually less than the cost of wide local excision plus permanent section evaluation. In a study of 406 tumors that cleared, on average, in 1.6 stages, Mohs surgery cost $805 per tumor compared to $1026 for standard excision with permanent margins [68]. Repair costs are also reduced, because Mohs typically results in smaller wounds that do not need repair or can be closed in a linear fashion. The cost of excision with positive margins and recurrent tumors should also be considered. Knowing that the margin is truly negative before embarking on a complicated reconstruction is invaluable.

Acknowledgement Funding: None

The authors have no conflicts of interest to declare.

References

1. Hutchinson J. Notes on the cancerous process and on new growths in general. Arch Surg (London). 1890;2:83–6.
2. Dubreuilh MW. Lentigo malin des viellards. Ann Dermatol Syphil (Paris). 1894;5:1092–9.
3. Cohen LM. Lentigo maligna and lentigo maligna melanoma. J Am Acad Dermatol. 1997;36:913.
4. Connolly KL, Busam KJ, Nehal KS. Optimizing outcomes for cutaneous head and neck melanoma. JAMA Dermatol. 2017;153(3):267–8.
5. Lawrence CM, Rahim R, Charlton F, Husain A. Prospective study of formalin-fixed mohs surgery and haematoxylin and eosin stains with control contralateral biopsies for lentigo maligna: 5-year follow-up results. Br J Derm. 2014;171:298–303.
6. Dawn ME, Dawn AG, Miller SJ. Mohs surgery for the treatment of MIS: a review. Dermatol Surg. 2007;33:395–402.
7. Mahoney MH, Joseph M, Temple CL. The perimeter technique for lentigo maligna: an alternative to Mohs micrographic surgery. J Surg Oncol. 2005;91(2):120–5.
8. Huilgol SC, Selva D, Chen C, Hill DC, James CL, et al. Surgical margins for lentigo maligna and lentigo maligna melanoma: the technique of mapped serial excision. Arch Dermatol. 2004;140:1087–92.
9. Bub J, Berg D, Slee A, Odland P. Management of lentigo maligna and lentigo maligna melanoma with staged excision. Arch Dermatol. 2004;140:552–8.
10. Megahed M, Schon M, Selimovic D, Schon MP. Reliability of diagnosis of melanoma in situ. Lancet. 2002;359:1921–2.
11. Osborne JE, Hutchinson PEA. follow-up study to investigate the efficacy of initial treatment of lentigo maligna with surgical excision. Br J Plast Surg. 2002;55:611–5.
12. Zalla MJ, Lim KK, Dicaudo DJ, Gagnot MM. Mohs micrographic excision of melanoma using immunostains. Dermatol Surg. 2000;26:771–84.
13. Somach SC, Taira JW, Pitha JV, Everett MA. Pigmented lesions in actinically damaged skin: histopathologic comparison of biopsy and excision specimens. Arch Dermatol. 1996;132:1297–302.
14. Weedon D. A reappraisal of melanoma in situ. J Dermatol Surg Oncol. 1982;8:774–5.
15. Wayte DM, Helwig EB. Melanotic freckle of Hutchinson. Cancer. 1968;21:893–911.
16. Gardner KH, Hill DE, Wright AC, Brewer JD, Arpey CJ. Upstaging from melanoma in situ to invasive melanoma on the head and neck after complete surgical resection. Dermatol Surg. 2015;41:1122–5.
17. Kessides MC, Wheless L, Hoffman-Bolton J, Clipp S, Alani RM, et al. Cigarette smoking and malignant melanoma: a case-control study. J Am Acad Dermatol. 2011;64(1):84–90.
18. Crissione VD, Weinstock MA. Melanoma thickness trends in the United States, 1988–2006. J Invest Dermatol. 2010;130(3):793–7.
19. Linos E, Swetter SM, Cockburn MG, Colditz GA, Clarke CA. Increasing burden of melanoma in the United States. J Invest Dermatol. 2009;129:1666–74.
20. Chen ST, Geller AC, Tsao H. Update on the epidemiology of melanoma. Curr Dermatol Rep. 2013;2:24–34.
21. Farshad A, Burg G, Pannizzon R. A retrospective study of 150 patients with lentigo maligna and lentigo maligna melanoma and the efficacy of radiotherapy using Grenz or soft X-rays. Br J Dermatol. 2002;146(6):1042.
22. Cotter MA, McKenna JK, Bowen GM. Treatment of lentigo maligna with imiquimod before staged excision. Dermatol Surg. 2008;34:147–51.
23. Fisher GH, Lang PG. Treatment of melanoma in situ on sun-damaged skin with topical 5% imiquimod cream complicated by the development of invasive disease. Arch Dermatol. 2003;139:945–7.
24. DeBloom JRII, Zitelli JA, Brodland DG. Invasive growth potential of residual melanoma and MIS. Dermatol Surg. 2010;36:1251–7.
25. Diagnosis and treatment of early melanoma. NIH Consensus Statement. 1991;20:1–26.
26. Kunishige JH, Brodland DG, Zitelli JA. Surgical margins for melanoma in situ. Dermatol Surg. 2011;66(3):438–44.
27. Felton S, Taylor RS, Srivastava D. Excision margins for melanoma in situ on the head and neck. Dermatol Surg. 2016;42:327–34.
28. Etzkorn JR, Sobanko JF, Elenitsas R, Newman JG, Goldbach H, et al. Low recurrence rates for in situ and invasivemelanomas using Mohs micrographic surgery with melanoma antigen recognized by T cells 1 (MART-1) immunostaining: tissue processing methodology to optimize pathologic staging and margin assessment. Dermatol Surg. 2015;72(5):840–50.
29. Bienert TN, Trotter MJ, Arlette JP. Treatment of cutaneous melanoma of the face by Mohs micrographic surgery. J Cutan Med Surg. 2003;7:25–30.
30. Clayton BD, Leshin B, Hitchcock MG, Marks M, White WL. Utility of rush paraffin-embedded tangential sections in the management of cutaneous neoplasms. Dermatol Surg. 2000;26:671–8.
31. Albertini JG, Elston DM, Libow LF, Smith SB, Farley MF. Mohs micrographic surgery for melanoma: a case series, a comparative study of immunostains, an informative case report, and a unique mapping technique. Dermatol Surg. 2002;28:656–65.
32. Moyer JS, Rudy S, Boonstra PS, Kraft C, Chinn SB, et al. Efficacy of staged excision with permanent section margin control for cutaneous head and neck melanoma. JAMA Dermatol. 2017;153(3):282–8.
33. Agarwal-Antal N, Bowen GM, Gerwels JW. Histologic evaluation of lentigo maligna with permanent sections: implications regarding current guidelines. J Am Acad Dermatol. 2002;47:743–8.
34. deVries K, Greveling K, Prens LM, Munte K, Koljenovic S, et al. Recurrence rate of lentigo maligna after micrographically controlled staged surgical excision. Br J Dermatol. 2016;174(3):588–93.
35. Hilari H, Llorca D, Traves V, Villanueva A, Serra-Guillen C, et al. Conventional surgery compared with

slow Mohs microscopic surgery in the treatment of lentigo maligna: a retrospective study of 62 cases. Actas Dermosifiliogr. 2012;103:614–23.
36. Bricca GM, Brodland DG, Ren D, Zitelli JA. Cutaneous head and neck melanoma treated with Mohs micrographic surgery. J Am Acad Dermatol. 2005;52:92–100.
37. Bene NI, Healy C, Coldiron BM. Mohs micrographic surgery is accurate 95.1% of the time for melanoma in situ: a prospective study of 167 cases. Dermatol Surg. 2008;34:660–4.
38. Abide JM, Nahai F, Bennett RG. The meaning of surgical margins. Plast Reconstr Surg. 1984;73:492–7.
39. Kimyai-Asadi A, Katz T, Goldberg LH, Ayala GB, Wang SQ, et al. Margin involvement after the excision of melanoma in situ: the need for complete en face examination of the surgical margins. Dermatol Surg. 2007;33:1434–9.
40. Johnson TM, Headington JT, Baker SR, Lowe L. Usefulness of the staged excision for lentigo maligna and lentigo maligna melanoma: the “square” procedure. J Am Acad Dermatol. 1997;37(5 pt 1):758–64.
41. Pitman GH, Kopf AW, Bart RS, Casson PR. Treatment of lentigo maligna and lentigo maligna melanoma. J Dermatol Surg Oncol. 1979;5:727–37.
42. Coleman WP III, Davis RS, Reed RJ, Krementz ET. Treatment of lentigo maligna and lentigo maligna melanoma. J Dermatol Surg Oncol. 1980;6:476–9.
43. Jejurikar SS, Borschel G, Johnson TM, Lowe L, Brown DL. Immediate, optimal reconstruction of facial lentigo maligna and melanoma following total peripheral margin control. Plast Reconstr Surg. 2007;120(5):1249–55.
44. Moller MG, Pappas-Politis E, Zager JS, Santiago LA, Yu D, et al. Surgical management of melanoma in situ using a staged marginal and central excision technique. Ann Surg Oncol. 2009;16(6):1526–36.
45. Anderson KW, Baker SR, Lowe L, Su L, Johnson TM. Treatment of head and neck melanoma, lentigo maligna subtype: a practical surgical technique. Arch Facial Plast Surg. 2001;3(3):202–6.
46. Bosbous MW, Dzwierzynski WW, Neuburg M. Staged excision of lentigo maligna and lentigo maligna melanoma: a 10-year experience. Plast Reconstr Surg. 2009;124(6):1947–55.
47. Nasrati A, Berliner JG, Goel S, McGuire J, Morhenn V, et al. Outcomes of melanoma ins itu treated with Mohs micrographic surgery compared with wide local excision. JAMA Dermatol. 2017;153(5):436–41. https://doi.org/10.1001/jamadermatol.2016.6138.
48. Hou JL, Reed KB, Knudson RM, Mirzoyev SA, Lohse CM, et al. Five-year outcomes of wide excision and Mohs micrographic surgery for primary lentigo maligna in an academic practice cohort. Dermatol Surg. 2015;41(2):211–8.
49. Hill DC, Gramp AA. Surgical treatment of lentigo maligna and lentigo maligna melanoma. Australas J Dermatol. 1999;40(1):25–30.
50. Malhotra R, Chen C, Huilgol SC, Hill DC, Selva D. Mapped serial excision for periocular lentigo maligna and lentigo maligna melanoma. Opthalmology. 2003;110(10):2011–8.
51. Walling HW, Scupham RK, Bean AK, Ceilley RI. Staged excision versus Mohs micrographic surgery for lentigo maligna and lentigo maligna melanoma. J Am Acad Dermatol. 2007;57(4):659–64.
52. Lee MR, Ryman WJ. Treatment of lentigo maligna with total circumferential margin control using vertical and horizontal permanent sections: a retrospective study. Australas J Dermatol. 2008;49(4):196–201.
53. Valentin-Nogueras SM, Brodland DG, Zitelli JA, Gonzalez-Sepulveda L, Nazario CM. Mohs micrographic surgery using MART-1 immunostain in the treatment of invasive melanoma and melanoma in situ. Dermatol Surg. 2016;42(6):733–44.
54. Bricca GM, Brodland DG, Zitelli JA. Immunostaining melanoma frozen sections: the one hour protocol. Dermatol Surg. 2004;30:403–8.
55. Hendi A, Brodland DG, Zitelli JA. Melanocytes in long-stnading sun-exposed skin: quantitative analysis using the MART-1 immunostain. Arch Dermatol. 2006;142(7):871–6.
56. Zitelli JA, Moy RL, Abell E. The reliability of frozen sections in the evaluation of surgical margins for melanoma. J Am Acad Dermatol. 1991;24:102–6.
57. Sroa N, Campbell S, Ravitskiy L. Immunohistochemistry in Mohs micrographic surgery: a review of the literature. J Clin Aesthet Dermatol. 2009;2(7):37–42.
58. Veronesi U, et al. Narrow excision (1-cm margin). Arch Surg. 1991;126:431–41.
59. Cohn-Cedermark G, et al. Long term results of a RCT by Swedish Melanoma Study Group on 2 versus 5-cm. Cancer. 2000;89:495–501.
60. Balch CM, et al. Long-term results of 2cm vs. 4cm margins for 740 patients with 1-4mm melanoma. Ann Surg Oncol. 2001;8:101–8.
61. Khayat D, et al. Surgical margins in melanoma 2cm versus 5cm for lesions less than 2.1mm. Cancer. 2003;97:1941–6.
62. Gillgren P, et al. 2 versus 4cm surgical excision margins for melanoma thicker than 2mm. Lancet. 2011;378:1635–42.
63. Hayes et al. Wide versus narrow excision margins for high-risk melanoma: longterm follow up. Lancet Once. 2016;17:184–92.
64. Mangold AR, Skinner R, Dueck AC, Sekulic A, Pockaj BA. Risk factors predicting positive margins at primary wide local excision of cutaneous melanoma. Dermatol Surg. 2016;42:646–52.
65. Gerami P, Cook RW, Wilkinson J, Russell MC, Dhillon N, et al. Development of a prognostic genetic signature to predict the metastatic risk associated with cutaneous melanoma. Clin Cancer Res. 2015;21(1):175–83.
66. Gerami P, Scolyer RA, Xu X, Elder DE, Abraham RM, et al. Risk assessment for atypical spitzoid melanocytic neoplasms using FISH to identify chromo-

somal copy number aberrations. Am J Surg Pathol. 2013;37(5):676–8.

67. Gannon CJ, Rousseau DL, Ross MI, Johnson MM, Lee JE, et al. Accuracy of lymphatic mapping and sentinel lymph node biopsy after previous wide local excision in patients with primary melanoma. Cancer. 2006;107(11):2647–52.

68. Ravitskiy L, Brodland DG, Zitelli JA. Cost analysis: Mohs micrographic surgery. Dermatol Surg. 2012;38(4):585–94.

Surgical Management of Head and Neck Melanoma

19

Joseph Zenga, Kevin Emerick, and Shaun Desai

Introduction

Cutaneous malignancy represents the most common group of cancers in the United States, with an estimated incidence as high as four million cases per year and an economic burden that exceeds $3 billion annually [1]. Basal cell carcinoma constitutes the majority of these cases, with cutaneous squamous cell carcinoma comprising ~15%, while melanoma and other uncommon skin malignancies comprise about 5% [2]. Although melanoma accounts for only a small fraction of diagnosed skin cancer, it represents the vast majority of skin cancer-related mortality, with an estimated 9,730 deaths in 2017. The social and economic weight of melanoma mortality is vast, as well, with years of potential life lost and billions lost in productivity. On average in the United States, melanoma mortality shortens life expectancy by over 20 years and over $400,000 is lost in foregone earnings [3].

J. Zenga, M.D. · K. Emerick, M.D.
Department of Otolaryngology—Head and Neck Surgery, Massachusetts Eye and Ear Infirmary, Harvard Medical School, Boston, MA, USA
e-mail: joseph_zenga@meei.harvard.edu; kevin_emerick@meei.harvard.edu

S. Desai, M.D. (✉)
Division of Facial Plastic and Reconstructive Surgery, Department of Otolaryngology—Head and Neck Surgery, Johns Hopkins University School of Medicine, Bethesda, MD, USA
e-mail: sdesai27@jhmi.edu

Importantly, much of the work done in understanding melanoma treatment and outcomes, particularly large randomized trials, includes mainly trunk and extremity disease. The head and neck, however, presents specific anatomic constraints, unique reconstructive challenges, and variable lymphatic drainage. Therefore, pooled data must be interpreted with caution, due to the context of potential differences in clinical behavior and draining lymphatics between the trunk, extremities, and head and neck. This chapter examines the current evidence behind standard treatment recommendations and their applicability to the specific management of head and neck cutaneous melanoma. The risk factors, prognosis, and treatment of mucosal melanoma and specific nonmelanoma head and neck skin cancers are highlighted as well [4].

Head and Neck Cutaneous Melanoma

Primary Site

Margins

There have been six, randomized, controlled trials that have compared narrow (1 or 2 cm) to wide (3–5 cm) margins for cutaneous melanoma [5–10]. These studies included patients with varying melanoma Breslow's thickness (<2 mm [6–8], >2 mm [5, 10], or a range from 1 to 4-mm [9]), and none found a difference in local control

A. I. Riker (ed.), *Melanoma*, https://doi.org/10.1007/978-3-319-78310-9_19

between those undergoing narrow (1–2 cm) versus wide (3–5 cm) margin resections. One study, however, reported an increased locoregional recurrence in patients with 1-cm versus 3-cm margins, primarily due to a higher nodal relapse, which translated into a decreased melanoma-specific survival in the narrow margin group [11].

It should be noted that <1% of patients included in these trials were found to have a primary melanoma of the head or neck, with the majority of patients having a trunk or extremity melanoma. The reasons for this are primarily related to the anatomic constraints of the face, where removing a primary lesion with wider margins is impractical and cosmetically deforming. Extensive resection of aesthetic facial structures such as the eyelid, nasal, or lip skin is avoided, due to the lack of compelling data suggesting any survival benefit for a wider resection beyond 2-cm.

How, then, can the results of these randomized trials be applied to the management of head and neck melanoma? There has not been a randomized trial that has directly compared 1-cm to 2-cm margins, with both margins considered reasonable for a primary melanoma of the head and neck. Currently, the MelmarT Melanoma trial is underway in Australia, in order to address the question of 1- versus 2-cm margins in patients with a Breslow's thickness of >1 mm [12]. Furthermore, conclusions from meta-analyses vary on the adequacy of 1-cm margins [13–16]. Given the heterogeneity and limitations of available data, current NCCN guidelines recommend a 1-cm margin for lesions <1 mm in Breslow's depth, 1–2-cm margins for a primary melanoma 1–2-mm thick, and 2-cm margins for those greater than 2 mm [17].

When critical aesthetic features limit the ability to achieve guideline margins, recurrence and survival outcomes are mixed. Recently, several large series have shown that even for thin melanomas, excision margins of <1 cm may increase the risk of local recurrence [18]. Conversely, recent retrospective reviews of margin width for head and neck melanoma have failed to show differences in recurrence or survival for narrower excision margins aimed to preserve critical elements of facial form and function [19, 20]. Ultimately, further studies are needed to definitively determine the critical margins specific to the head and neck region, and until such trials are completed, the NCCN guidelines should be followed whenever possible [17]. If a margin has to be compromised in one area, such as adjacent to the eyelid, the remaining areas should still be removed with the recommended margins as outlined in the NCCN treatment guidelines.

Immediate Versus Delayed Reconstruction

The accuracy of frozen section analysis in evaluating intraoperative margins for melanoma has been historically unreliable, demonstrating high false-negative rates [21]. Although emerging techniques such as rapid immunostaining may provide some promise, permanent section analysis is the mainstay of recommended treatment for margin analysis for an invasive primary melanoma [17, 22, 23]. Thus, the timing of reconstruction is determined by the likelihood of obtaining a negative margin, combined with wound care concerns and complexity of the reconstruction. In an effort to limit the size of the wound and decreased wound care concerns, some groups advocate for the use of a "window" technique, which is a staged, marginal excision of the tumor borders, followed by a delayed central excision with reconstruction once the margins are deemed negative on final pathology [24]. Nonetheless, with this technique, the deep margin is not assessed until the definitive resection. In large series, positive final margins are found in up to 12% of patients, further associated with adverse prognostic factors such as ulceration, T4-staging, and desmoplastic subtype [25–27]. Conversely, a recent review of 637 patients with head and neck melanoma could not associate any tumor or treatment characteristics with positive margins [27]. Furthermore, outcomes for patients who do recur locally vary considerably in the literature, with a single randomized trial reporting a 5-year overall survival of only 9% in patients with locally recurrent melanoma [9]. When the recurrence is located within the prior surgical scar itself, however, melanoma-specific survival after subsequent wide local resection has been reported as >90% [28]. These differences may be related to the true definition of what represents a local recurrence. It is important to distinguish an adjacent in-transit metastasis, which predicts a high risk of distant metastasis, from a true recurrence of the primary tumor within the scar. For these reasons, immediate reconstruction of defects after resection of a head and neck melanoma should be limited to low-risk lesions or closure techniques that can be more reliably re-resected, such as primary closure or skin grafting. Defects requiring complex wound reconstruction with a local or regional flap associated with a critical area, such as the eyelid, are best reconstructed in a staged fashion.

Regional Nodes

Staging the Clinically Negative Neck

Elective Neck Dissection

Four randomized trials, which included primarily trunk and extremity melanoma, have been performed to compare elective lymph node dissection (ELND) to observation with delayed therapeutic lymph node dissection (TLND) if gross regional disease developed [29–32]. These trials found no significant survival differences between groups, with this outcome due, at least in part, to several unique features of the disease process. Lymphatic drainage basins from cutaneous sites, particularly for head and neck melanoma, are not uniformly predictable, with detailed pathological analysis simply not practical to perform on a large number of excised nodes [33]. ELND may miss the highest echelon, or sentinel, draining nodes and pathological analysis may overlook micrometastases when examining the larger total number of lymph nodes identified within a complete neck dissection. Based on these considerations, ELND is not considered as a standard treatment option according to current NCCN practice guidelines [17].

Sentinel Node Biopsy

Randomized evidence. Given the lack of clear benefit for an immediate ELND, combined with the finding that regional nodal involvement is a critical prognostic factor, sentinel lymph node biopsy (SLNB) was adopted in order to accurately stage the regional nodal basin, without the added morbidity associated with a complete lymph node dissection. The highest level of evidence for the use of SLNB in the regional staging of melanoma came from the Multicenter Selective Lymphadenectomy Trial (MSLT-I) [34]. This trial randomized patients after wide local excision to either observation alone or SLNB. In patients with intermediate thickness melanoma (1 to 4-mm) 10-year melanoma-specific survival was improved in patients with a positive SLNB who underwent a complete neck dissection compared with patients who had a regional recurrence after nodal observation only (56% vs. 41%) [34]. Patients with thick melanoma (>4-mm) did not demonstrate a significant improvement melanoma-specific survival, but regional staging with SLNB in these patients is nonetheless recommended as it provides valuable prognostic information and is important for defining prognosis, risk-stratification, and entry into clinical trials [17]. MSLT-I excluded patients with thin melanoma (<1-mm) and the decision to offer a SLNB in those patients is based largely on retrospective evidence [35]. In these cases, the patient and clinician must balance the risk of occult regional disease with the risks and cost of SLNB. Current guidelines recommend SLNB in a thin melanoma, 0.75 to 1 mm, with high-risk features (ulceration, angiolymphatic invasion, Clark's level 4, or mitosis >1/mm^2) [17].

Application to the head and neck. An important consideration when interpreting the results of randomized data is their applicability to head and neck primary sites. MSLT-I did not report the number of patients included with head and neck melanoma, but only stratified primary site by extremity (45%) compared with other sites (55%). In multivariable analysis, head and neck melanoma was not an independent predictor of recurrence or death in patients undergoing

SLNB. However, the authors did not report the false-negative rate (number of patients who recurred after negative SLNB compared with all true positives) nor survival difference between the observation and SLNB groups for head and neck primary sites [34]. Recent non-randomized data, however, have demonstrated accuracy and reliability for performing a SLNB for the head and neck. A large, prospective study of 353 patients with head and neck melanoma identified a sentinel node in 99.7% of cases and reported a false-negative rate of 14.8% [36]. This compares favorably to the false-negative rate of 20.3% reported in the long-term follow-up of MSLT-I [34]. Additionally, the safety of head and neck SLNB, including preservation of the facial nerve in the parotid basin, has been demonstrated in multiple reports [37, 38].

Completion Neck Dissection

Randomized evidence. In a recently published follow-up trial to MSLT-I, authors of the MSLT-II trial randomized patients with a positive SLNB to either completion lymph node dissection (CLND) or nodal observation with serial imaging by ultrasound [39]. Although 3-year disease-free survival was higher in patients undergoing CLND (68% vs. 63%) based largely on regional control, the 3-year melanoma-specific survival was the same (86% for both groups). This is in contrast to the findings of MSLT-I, that demonstrated an improvement in melanoma-specific survival for patients with a positive SLNB, compared to those who were observed and later recurred. This suggesting that the survival benefit is likely limited to excision and staging of the sentinel nodes only. Further, the rate of lymphedema was significantly higher in patients who underwent CLND (24% vs. 6%). Taken together, these data suggest that although CLND provides prognostic information on the status of non-sentinel nodes and may increase regional control, it does so at the cost of increased morbidity and does not appear to improve overall survival.

Application to the head and neck. In MSLT-II, only 14% of patients included in the study had a head and neck primary site, which may limit the broad generalization of the study's findings to this patient population. Interestingly, the hazard ratio for melanoma-related death was twice as high in patients undergoing nodal observation as compared to CLND in patients with head and neck melanoma. Although this difference did not reach statistical significance, the study was not powered to detect survival differences for head and neck melanoma specifically. Retrospective reports examining the impact of CLND in head and neck melanoma have suggested a potential survival benefit in some patient subgroups [40]. Furthermore, only 11.5% of patients in MLST-II had non-sentinel nodal disease, and it remains unclear if those patients may benefit from accurate staging of non-sentinel nodes for intensification of adjuvant therapy and early entry into clinical trials.

Management of Clinically Positive Nodal Disease

Neck Dissection

The available data on the extent of surgical removal of lymph nodes from the various head and neck regions is limited. The goal of completion lymphadenectomy is to remove known disease and all the regional nodes at risk, while maintaining acceptable associated morbidity. The extent of completion lymphadenectomy for primary head and neck melanoma was not specifically addressed in MLST-II [39]. In a survey of 193 surgeons from 25 countries, the recommended extent of CLND after a positive neck SLNB was selective in 62%, comprehensive in 25%, and super-selective in 3% [41].

Despite this controversy, the potential lymphatic drainage of head and neck cutaneous malignancies is relatively well established. In general, a coronal plan drawn through the external auditory canals separates primary head and neck cutaneous sites that, anterior to this line, drain to the anterior nodal basins (level I-V, preauricular, parotid, submental), and posterior to this line drain to the posterior nodal basins (levels II-V, post-auricular, and suboccipital) [42]. Similarly, the extent of neck dissections should be tailored to address potential drainage sites. Multiple single-institution, retrospective studies have found no difference in regional recurrence or survival in patients undergoing selective as compared to modified radical or radical neck dissection for the treatment of gross regional disease. Critical neurovascular structures (i.e., internal jugular vein and spinal accessory nerve) should be preserved whenever possible [43–46].

Nonetheless, the distribution of regional metastases in head and neck melanoma is not entirely predictable. Some authors have found that up to 25% of patients may have metastases outside of clinically predicted zones and argue for more comprehensive dissection in therapeutic cases [33, 47]. Ultimately, the extent of dissection must balance the likelihood of addressing occult regional disease, the unclear impact of more comprehensive dissection on survival, and the increased risks associated with a more extensive operation.

Parotidectomy

Patients with clinical involvement of the parotid may have up to a 40% risk of occult neck disease and should undergo a neck dissection in addition to a parotidectomy [48]. The extent of neck dissection will depend upon the primary site as discussed above. Involvement of parotid nodes is most commonly associated with primary melanoma of the face, anterior scalp, and ear [47]. Patients with clinical nodal involvement of the superficial parotid lobe may also have deep lobe metastases in over 10% of cases [49]. Those undergoing total parotidectomy in cases of clinical nodal disease in the superficial lobe may have decreased parotid bed recurrence as compared with superficial parotidectomy alone [50]. However, total parotidectomy carries a significantly higher risk of facial nerve injury and cosmetic contour deformity, compared to superficial alone, and must be carefully considered and thoroughly discussed with the patient when deciding upon the extent of parotidectomy.

Adjuvant Radiotherapy

A large, randomized trial examined the effects of adjuvant radiation to the regional nodal basin after surgical resection for cutaneous melanoma [51]. Trial patients were found to have a high risk of regional relapse, which included involvement of at least one parotid, two cervical or axillary, or three inguinal nodes, cervical nodes >3-cm, or the presence of extracapsular nodal extension. Although regional recurrence was significantly lower in patients undergoing adjuvant radiotherapy (21% vs. 36%), radiation-related toxicities were common, and survival outcomes and quality-of-life were similar.

Nonetheless, as the inclusion criteria in this trial were specific and only a quarter of patients were treated for disease in the head and neck, broad application to all parotid and cervical disease is somewhat limited. Several authors have advocated adjuvant radiotherapy in certain subgroups, such as those with extracapsular extension [52, 53]. Although adjuvant radiotherapy to the involved regional nodal basin may decrease nodal relapse, it does not appear to provide an improvement in long-term survival or in the quality-of-life.

Adjuvant Systemic Therapy

Approved Agents

Currently, interferon and ipilimumab are two systemic agents that can be utilized for the adjuvant treatment of stage III, resected melanoma. Although both have demonstrated improvements in recurrence-free survival in randomized trials, as with other large, prospective studies in melanoma, they mainly involve trunk and extremity disease and the application to specific sites of the head and neck remains unclear.

Adjuvant interferon has been the subject of a large number of randomized trials with variable study designs and inclusion criteria. A recent meta-analysis reviewed 17 randomized trials and reported a 17% improvement in disease-free survival and a 9% improvement for overall survival with adjuvant interferon in stage II and III disease [54]. Given the significant heterogeneity between trials, however, patient subgroups which benefit most from therapy are uncertain.

Adjuvant ipilimumab, a monoclonal anti-cytotoxic T-lymphocyte antigen 4 (CTLA-4) antibody, was investigated in the EORTC 18071 clinical trial [55], a randomized trial examining patients with resected stage III disease. Three-year recurrence-free survival was significantly higher in the ipilimumab group (47% vs. 35%). Adverse events were significant, leading to discontinuation of treatment in over 50% and associated with rare, ipilimumab-related fatalities. In a recent trial update, however, overall health-related quality-of-life was found to be similar between ipilimumab and placebo groups [56].

Clinical Trials

Several phase III clinical trials are currently underway, investigating the effects of novel systemic agents in the adjuvant setting after surgical resection. These include immunomodulators, checkpoint inhibitors, targeted therapies, and melanoma vaccines [57–63]. The currently approved agents are being further explored in two trials, one comparing two different doses of ipilimumab with high-dose interferon for stage III-IV disease, with a second study examining the effect of adjuvant pegylated interferon in patients with ulcerated, early stage tumors [57, 58]. Programmed death-1 (PD-1) inhibitors are being investigated in several trials as well. CheckMate 238 compares adjuvant nivolumab to ipilimumab in stage III-IV disease [59], while Keynote-054 compares adjuvant pembrolizumab to a placebo-control in stage III melanoma [60]. Several inhibitors targeting the BRAF and MEK, signaling components of the mitogen-activated protein kinase (MAPK) pathway, are also being studied. BRAF-activating mutations are found in approximately two-thirds of cutaneous melanoma, and MEK is a kinase that is found downstream to the BRAF gene in the MAPK pathway. There are currently two, phase III trials underway targeting this pathway in the adjuvant setting. One evaluates the effects of BRAF-inhibitor vemurafenib in stage II-III disease and the other investigates therapy with the BRAF-inhibitor dabrafenib in combination with the MEK-inhibitor trametinib in stage III disease [61, 62]. Finally, the effects of a melanoma vaccine are being studied. CSF470, a mixture of irradiated melanoma cells from formulated into a vaccine, will be compared to adjuvant interferon in stage II-III disease [63].

Head and Neck Mucosal Melanoma

Overview

Head and neck mucosal melanoma (HNMM) is an aggressive disease with current 5-year survival outcomes below 30% [64]. This is reflected by AJCC staging for which the earliest disease is categorized as T3 and stage III [65]. Almost three-quarters of head and neck mucosal melanoma is of sinonasal in origin. The oral cavity is the second most prevalent location, occurring in >15% of cases. The remainder occurs in other upper aerodigestive tract subsites and occurs only rarely.. Patients with HNMM most commonly present in the sixth or seventh decades without a clear gender predilection. Mucosal melanoma is an uncommon diagnosis, representing less than 1% of all malignant melanoma, with an incidence in the United States of approximately 20–30 cases per million/year [66, 67]. The etiology and risk factors for developing mucosal melanoma are uncertain. Unlike cutaneous melanoma, pathogenesis is not driven by ultraviolet photodamage, and genetic alterations in mucosal and cutaneous melanoma are distinctly different [68]. In addition, there is not a clear relationship between risk factors for other oral malignancies, including tobacco and alcohol use, with development of head and neck mucosal melanoma. Although a direct link is not certain, patients who develop oral or sinonasal mucosal melanoma may have a long history of mucosal melanosis [69, 70].

Management

Given its rarity, few prospective trials have been performed investigating management paradigms in mucosal melanoma, and treatment recommendations rely mainly on smaller single-institution, retrospective trials. When feasible, surgical resection remains the current mainstay of treatment [65]. However, involvement of surgical constraints such as skull base or orbital invasion may lead to unacceptable morbidity in the face of poor overall oncologic prognosis. Although historically, definitive radiotherapy resulted in inferior outcomes to primary surgery-based paradigms, newer radiotherapy techniques, including proton and neutron radiation, have shown promise in the definitive nonsurgical management of mucosal melanoma [71–73]. At this time, however, these treatment paradigms remain experimental and confined to institutions with availability and experience using these techniques, particularly in patients with unresectable disease or those unwilling to undergo operative management.

Primary Site

When performing primary surgery, the necessary extent of resection and width of surgical margins remain unclear. Positive margins have been associated with a worse survival in several reports and efforts should be made to achieve a negative margin of resection [74, 75]. Nonetheless, even surgery with microscopically negative margins may still result in local recurrence in over 40% of patients. Radical surgery to achieve a wide margin of resection may not provide significant benefit while increasing morbidity [76]. Multiple reports have shown equivalent rates of recurrence and survival in patients with sinonasal melanoma undergoing endoscopic surgery, as compared to open transfacial resection [77, 78].

Regional Nodes

Optimal management of the neck remains controversial as well. Although neck dissection is the most common practice for clinically evident regional metastasis, the benefit of elective treatment for the clinically negative lymph node regions is uncertain [65]. Patients with sinonasal melanoma rarely demonstrate regional metastases and prophylactic neck dissection does not appear warranted [79, 80]. However, those with oral mucosal melanoma are at higher risk for regional dissemination, with both rates of occult disease found in elective neck dissections and for regional recurrence in untreated necks >30% in some reports [69, 81]. Although the elective treatment of the neck in oral mucosal melanoma should be considered, its impact on recurrence and survival remain unclear [69, 81, 82]. Due to the limited data available to provide clear guidance, it is important that these treatment decisions are made in a multidisciplinary setting.

Adjuvant Radiotherapy

Adjuvant radiotherapy in the postoperative setting may improve locoregional control [83–85]. There is no clear consensus on the exact indications for adjuvant radiotherapy, although most authors support its use in patients at high risk of recurrence including larger tumors, nodal metastases, close or positive margins, or recurrent disease [84]. Treatment with postoperative radiotherapy appears to be most efficacious when given at higher doses [85]. Adjuvant radiation therapy does not appear to provide an improvement in overall survival [86]. Distant metastatic rates remain high in head and neck mucosal melanoma despite improvements in locoregional control seen with adjuvant radiotherapy [87]. In a review from the National Cancer Database of almost 700 patients with sinonasal melanoma, the 5-year survival was 25% in both patients undergoing surgery alone and surgery with adjuvant radiotherapy [80].

Systemic Therapy

In general, systemic therapies that are indicated for cutaneous melanoma are also recommended for mucosal melanoma in current treatment guidelines [65]. Recently, a single, randomized trial of 189 patients with mucosal melanoma underwent complete surgical resection combined with adjuvant temolozomide and cisplatin. This showed a decrease in locoregional recurrence and improvement in overall survival compared to either observation alone or adjuvant high-dose interferon [88]. For patients with characteristic genetic alterations, some targeted therapies have shown promise. Although targeted BRAF inhibitors, such as vemurafenib, have been shown to be effective in rare cases, unlike cutaneous melanoma, >90% of mucosal melanoma is BRAF wild-type [68, 89]. Mutations in the c-KIT gene have been identified more frequently in mucosal melanoma, with systemic c-KIT inhibitors demonstrating efficacy in recent studies [90]. In a phase II trial, including 13 patients with metastatic mucosal melanoma treated with the c-KIT inhibitor, imatinib, 2 patients had a durable response at 1 year, including 1 complete response [91]. In addition to targeted inhibitors, immunomodulators used in the management of cutaneous melanoma have shown promise in early clinical trials of mucosal melanoma. Rare, long-term durable complete responses have been reported with both ipilimumab, and the PD-1 inhibitor, nivolumab [92, 93].

Special Considerations for Non-melanoma Head and Neck Cutaneous Malignancies

Basal Cell Carcinoma

Basal cell carcinoma (BCC) represents the most common type of cancer, with an incidence of greater than 3 million cases yearly in the United States alone [1]. BCC of the head and neck has a greater risk of recurrence than other sites, particularly in the mask area of the face (nasal, lips, periorbital), chin, mandible, and periauricular areas. Other high-risk features include recurrent tumors, immunosuppression, prior radiotherapy, perineural invasion, and an aggressive histopathological subtype including morpheaform and basosquamous carcinoma [94]. Unlike melanoma, the metastatic potential of BCC is very low, with a distant metastatic rate of <0.1%. Surgical resection is the most common treatment, with Mohs Micrographic Surgery (MMS) a frequently utilized approach for high-risk cases [95]. Long-term results were recently reported of a randomized trial comparing standard excision (SE) to MMS in high-risk BCC of the face, demonstrating a significantly higher 10-year recurrence rate for SE [96]. Definitive radiotherapy may be used for patients who are not surgical candidates; however, in a randomized comparison, radiotherapy resulted in higher recurrence rates, worse cosmetic outcomes, and more treatment-related complications [94, 97, 98].

Adjuvant radiotherapy is recommended for patients with extensive perineural invasion and those whose margins cannot be surgically cleared [99]. For patients with locally advanced or metastatic BCC not amenable to further surgery or radiotherapy, an important class of systemic therapy has recently been developed, targeting the Hedgehog signaling pathway. Both vismodegib and sonidegib are approved Hedgehog pathway inhibitors, which have shown high objective response rates with a subset of patients experiencing a durable response [100, 101]. A phase II clinical trial is underway evaluating the effects of a systemic PD-1 inhibitor (REGN2810) in patients with unresectable or metastatic BCC that is unresponsive to Hedgehog pathway inhibitors [102]. These systemic options are particularly important in the head and neck, where tumors may encroach upon highly sensitive functional or cosmetic areas, providing the possibility of a neoadjuvant, organ-sparing, approach.

Squamous Cell Carcinoma

The majority of cutaneous squamous cell carcinoma (cSCC) has similar risk factors and management to BCC. However, there is a subset of high-risk cSCC that has a higher incidence in the head and neck. These tumors are at high-risk of local recurrence, regional spread (including clinical perineural spread, lymph nodes, and dermal metastasis), as well as distant metastasis. Even when the regional basin is clinically negative, occult regional metastatic disease may be present in over 15% of patients with high-risk cSCC [103]. Current treatment guidelines recommend consideration of SLNB in high-risk cases, although survival benefits are uncertain [104]. Clinical nodal involvement is associated with significantly worse disease-free and overall survival and these patients are managed with surgery and adjuvant radiotherapy [105, 106]. In cases of locally advanced disease not amenable to surgery or further radiotherapy, recommendations for systemic therapy are guided by evidence for mucosal head and neck squamous cell carcinoma, including cisplatin and cetuximab-based regimens [107]. Two, phase II clinical trials are currently underway investigating the outcomes of systemic PD-1 inhibitors (REGN2810 and pembrolizumab) in patients with unresectable or metastatic cSCC, with completion of both studies estimated for 2019 [108, 109].

Merkel Cell Carcinoma

Merkel cell carcinoma (MCC) is an aggressive malignancy with both high locoregional recurrence and distant metastatic potential. It is most commonly found on the head and neck, and like other skin malignancies, ultraviolet exposure is a major risk factor. Unlike other skin cancers, however, development of MCC has been associated with a virus. Present in ~80% of cases, the Merkel Cell Polyomavirus (MCV) has been implicated in oncogenesis and found to clonally integrate into the DNA of MCC samples [110]. The prognostic importance of MCV and the exact pathogenesis of malignant transformation remain uncertain.

Primary surgical resection with 1–2-cm margins is the preferred initial treatment, with SLNB indicated for all cases in which disease is clinically confined to the primary site [111]. Although sentinel node status appears to be an important prognosticator and possibly associated with improved survival in some reports, the value of SLNB remains somewhat controversial given the limitations of the available retrospective data [112–115]. The role for SLNB may be limited because the risk of occult metastasis is so high, well over 50%. Therefore, regional lymph node treatment is often considered, regardless of SLNB status. Adjuvant radiation therapy appears to improve both local and regional disease control as well as overall survival, although the exact indications for radiotherapy are limited by lack of large prospective trials [116–118]. The role of adjuvant systemic therapy in the management of MCC remains unclear, although it may impart benefit in a subset of high-risk patients, such as those with positive surgical margins [116, 119]. However, because the risk of distant metastasis is so high, there is a continued interest in identifying systemic treatments. There are several ongoing phase II trials investigating innovative systemic approaches to advanced and metastatic MCC including adoptive immunotherapy, CTLA-4 inhibitors (ipilimumab), PD-1 inhibitors (nivolumab), PD-L1 inhibitors (avelumab), mTOR inhibitors (MLN0128), and an IL-15 superagonist (ALT-803) [120–123].

Conclusion

Cutaneous malignancies are the most common group of cancers worldwide, afflicting millions of patients annually. Basal and squamous cell carcinomas remain the most common. Although the majority of these have an excellent prognosis, a subset of high-risk tumors is associated with increased recurrence and metastases. Head and neck melanoma, however, leads the majority of skin cancer-related deaths and is associated with an enormous social and economic burden. Although the management of melanoma has been rigorously studied in multiple prospective, randomized trials and large retrospective reviews, the intricacies of treating head and neck melanoma have not been fully investigated. Clinical decisions often must rely on the extrapolation of the clinical data derived from pooled reports and retrospective studies that include only a small number of head and neck primary melanomas. To fully understand the optimal management of melanoma, future prospective trials need to focus on head and neck disease, including appropriate margins, the value of completion neck dissection and the added benefit of radiotherapy. Trials with novel systemic agents are currently underway in an attempt to optimize the adjuvant treatment of head and neck melanoma.

Acknowledgement No financial disclosures or conflicts of interest.

References

1. Wu X, Elkin EE, Marghoob AA. Burden of basal cell carcinoma in USA. Future Oncol. 2015;11(22):2967–74.
2. Mydlarz WK, Weber RS, Kupferman ME. Cutaneous malignancy of the head and neck. Surg Oncol Clin N Am. 2015;24(3):593–613.

3. Ekwueme DU, Guy GP, Li C, Rim SH, Parelkar P, Chen SC. The health burden and economic costs of cutaneous melanoma mortality by race/ethnicity-United States, 2000 to 2006. J Am Acad Dermatol. 2011;65(5 Suppl 1):S133–43.
4. Zenga J, Nussenbaum B, Cornelius LA, Linette GP, Desai SC. Management controversies in head and neck melanoma: a systematic review. JAMA Facial Plast Surg. 2017;19(1):53–62.
5. Gillgren P, Drzewiecki KT, Niin M, et al. 2-cm versus 4-cm surgical excision margins for primary cutaneous melanoma thicker than 2 mm: a randomised, multicentre trial. Lancet. 2011;378(9803):1635–42.
6. Veronesi U, Cascinelli N, Adamus J, et al. Thin stage I primary cutaneous malignant melanoma. Comparison of excision with margins of 1 or 3 cm. N Engl J Med. 1988;318(18):1159–62.
7. Cohn-Cedermark G, Rutqvist LE, Andersson R, et al. Long term results of a randomized study by the Swedish Melanoma Study Group on 2-cm versus 5-cm resection margins for patients with cutaneous melanoma with a tumor thickness of 0.8–2.0 mm. Cancer. 2000;89(7):1495–501.
8. Khayat D, Rixe O, Martin G, et al. Surgical margins in cutaneous melanoma (2 cm versus 5 cm for lesions measuring less than 2.1-mm thick). Cancer. 2003;97(8):1941–6.
9. Balch CM, Soong SJ, Smith T, et al. Long-term results of a prospective surgical trial comparing 2 cm vs. 4 cm excision margins for 740 patients with 1-4 mm melanomas. Ann Surg Oncol. 2001;8(2):101–8.
10. Thomas JM, Newton-Bishop J, A'Hern R, et al. Excision margins in high-risk malignant melanoma. N Engl J Med. 2004;350(8):757–66.
11. Hayes AJ, Maynard L, Coombes G, et al. Wide versus narrow excision margins for high-risk, primary cutaneous melanomas: long-term follow-up of survival in a randomised trial. Lancet Oncol. 2016; 17(2):184–92.
12. Group AaNZMT. MelmarT melanoma margins trial investigating 1 cm v 2 cm wide excision margins for primary cutaneous melanoma. https://clinicaltrials.gov/ct2/show/NCT02385214?term=melmarT&rank=1. Accessed 14 Nov 2015.
13. Sladden MJ, Balch C, Barzilai DA, et al. Surgical excision margins for primary cutaneous melanoma. Cochrane Database Syst Rev. 2009;4:CD004835.
14. Haigh PI, DiFronzo LA, McCready DR. Optimal excision margins for primary cutaneous melanoma: a systematic review and meta-analysis. Can J Surg. 2003;46(6):419–26.
15. Mocellin S, Pasquali S, Nitti D. The impact of surgery on survival of patients with cutaneous melanoma: revisiting the role of primary tumor excision margins. Ann Surg. 2011;253(2):238–43.
16. Lens MB, Dawes M, Goodacre T, Bishop JA. Excision margins in the treatment of primary cutaneous melanoma: a systematic review of randomized controlled trials comparing narrow vs wide excision. Arch Surg. 2002;137(10):1101–5.
17. Melanoma NPM. NCCN clinical practice guidelines in oncology: melanoma. 2017; http://www.nccn.org/professionals/physician_gls/pdf/melanoma.pdf
18. Ross MI, Balch CM. Excision margins of melanoma make a difference: new data support an old paradigm. Ann Surg Oncol. 2016;23(4):1053–6.
19. Rawlani R, Rawlani V, Qureshi HA, Kim JY, Wayne JD. Reducing margins of wide local excision in head and neck melanoma for function and cosmesis: 5-year local recurrence-free survival. J Surg Oncol. 2015;111(7):795–9.
20. Teng J, Halbert T, McMurry TL, Levine PA, Christophel JJ. Histopathologic margin distance in survival in resection of cutaneous melanoma of the head and neck. Laryngoscope. 2015;125(8):1856–60.
21. Prieto VG, Argenyi ZB, Barnhill RL, et al. Are en face frozen sections accurate for diagnosing margin status in melanocytic lesions? Am J Clin Pathol. 2003;120(2):203–8.
22. Chin-Lenn L, Murynka T, McKinnon JG, Arlette JP. Comparison of outcomes for malignant melanoma of the face treated using Mohs micrographic surgery and wide local excision. Dermatol Surg. 2013;39(11):1637–45.
23. Etzkorn JR, Sobanko JF, Elenitsas R, et al. Low recurrence rates for in situ and invasive melanomas using Mohs micrographic surgery with melanoma antigen recognized by T cells 1 (MART-1) immunostaining: tissue processing methodology to optimize pathologic staging and margin assessment. J Am Acad Dermatol. 2015;72(5):840–50.
24. Möller MG, Pappas-Politis E, Zager JS, et al. Surgical management of melanoma-in-situ using a staged marginal and central excision technique. Ann Surg Oncol. 2009;16(6):1526–36.
25. Parrett BM, Kashani-Sabet M, Leong SP, Buncke N, Singer MI. The safety of and indications for immediate reconstruction of head and neck melanoma defects: our early experience. Ann Plast Surg. 2014;72(Suppl 1):S35–7.
26. Sullivan SR, Scott JR, Cole JK, et al. Head and neck malignant melanoma: margin status and immediate reconstruction. Ann Plast Surg. 2009;62(2):144–8.
27. Christophel JJ, Johnson AK, McMurry TL, Park SS, Levine PA. Predicting positive margins in resection of cutaneous melanoma of the head and neck. Laryngoscope. 2013;123(3):683–8.
28. Brown CD, Zitelli JA. The prognosis and treatment of true local cutaneous recurrent malignant melanoma. Dermatol Surg. 1995;21(4):285–90.
29. Veronesi U, Adamus J, Bandiera DC, et al. Delayed regional lymph node dissection in stage I melanoma of the skin of the lower extremities. Cancer. 1982;49(11):2420–30.
30. Sim FH, Taylor WF, Pritchard DJ, Soule EH. Lymphadenectomy in the management of stage I malignant melanoma: a prospective randomized study. Mayo Clin Proc. 1986;61(9):697–705.
31. Cascinelli N, Morabito A, Santinami M, MacKie RM, Belli F. Immediate or delayed dissection of regional

nodes in patients with melanoma of the trunk: a randomised trial. WHO Melanoma Programme. Lancet. 1998;351(9105):793–6.
32. Balch CM, Soong S, Ross MI, et al. Long-term results of a multi-institutional randomized trial comparing prognostic factors and surgical results for intermediate thickness melanomas (1.0 to 4.0 mm). Intergroup Melanoma Surgical Trial. Ann Surg Oncol. 2000;7(2):87–97.
33. Klop WM, Veenstra HJ, Vermeeren L, Nieweg OE, Balm AJ, Lohuis PJ. Assessment of lymphatic drainage patterns and implications for the extent of neck dissection in head and neck melanoma patients. J Surg Oncol. 2011;103(8):756–60.
34. Morton DL, Thompson JF, Cochran AJ, et al. Final trial report of sentinel-node biopsy versus nodal observation in melanoma. N Engl J Med. 2014;370(7):599–609.
35. Andtbacka RH, Gershenwald JE. Role of sentinel lymph node biopsy in patients with thin melanoma. J Natl Compr Canc Netw. 2009;7(3):308–17.
36. Erman AB, Collar RM, Griffith KA, et al. Sentinel lymph node biopsy is accurate and prognostic in head and neck melanoma. Cancer. 2012;118(4):1040–7.
37. Picon AI, Coit DG, Shaha AR, et al. Sentinel lymph node biopsy for cutaneous head and neck melanoma: mapping the parotid gland. Ann Surg Oncol. 2016;23(Suppl 5):9001–9.
38. Schmalbach CE, Nussenbaum B, Rees RS, Schwartz J, Johnson TM, Bradford CR. Reliability of sentinel lymph node mapping with biopsy for head and neck cutaneous melanoma. Arch Otolaryngol Head Neck Surg. 2003;129(1):61–5.
39. Faries MB, Thompson JF, Cochran AJ, et al. Completion dissection or observation for sentinel-node metastasis in melanoma. N Engl J Med. 2017; 376(23):2211–22.
40. Fritsch VA, Cunningham JE, Lentsch EJ. Completion lymph node dissection based on risk of nonsentinel metastasis in cutaneous melanoma of the head and neck. Otolaryngol Head Neck Surg. 2016;154(1): 94–103.
41. Pasquali S, Spillane AJ, de Wilt JH, et al. Surgeons' opinions on lymphadenectomy in melanoma patients with positive sentinel nodes: a worldwide web-based survey. Ann Surg Oncol. 2012;19(13):4322–9.
42. Reynolds HM, Smith NP, Uren RF, Thompson JF, Dunbar PR. Three-dimensional visualization of skin lymphatic drainage patterns of the head and neck. Head Neck. 2009;31(10):1316–25.
43. Van de Vrie W, Eggermont AM, Van Putten WL, Wiggers T. Therapeutic lymphadenectomy in melanomas of the head and neck. Head Neck. 1993; 15(5):377–81.
44. O'Brien CJ, Petersen-Schaefer K, Ruark D, Coates AS, Menzie SJ, Harrison RI. Radical, modified, and selective neck dissection for cutaneous malignant melanoma. Head Neck. 1995;17(3):232–41.
45. Geltzeiler M, Monroe M, Givi B, Vetto J, Andersen P, Gross N. Regional control of head and neck melanoma with selective neck dissection. JAMA Otolaryngol Head Neck Surg. 2014;140(11):1014–8.
46. Supriya M, Narasimhan V, Henderson MA, Sizeland A. Managing regional metastasis in patients with cutaneous head and neck melanoma—is selective neck dissection appropriate? Am J Otolaryngol. 2014;35(5):610–6.
47. Shah JP, Kraus DH, Dubner S, Sarkar S. Patterns of regional lymph node metastases from cutaneous melanomas of the head and neck. Am J Surg. 1991;162(4):320–3.
48. Suton P, Lukšić I, Müller D, Virag M. Lymphatic drainage patterns of head and neck cutaneous melanoma: does primary melanoma site correlate with anatomic distribution of pathologically involved lymph nodes? Int J Oral Maxillofac Surg. 2012;41(4):413–20.
49. Thom JJ, Moore EJ, Price DL, Kasperbauer JL, Starkman SJ, Olsen KD. The role of total parotidectomy for metastatic cutaneous squamous cell carcinoma and malignant melanoma. JAMA Otolaryngol Head Neck Surg. 2014;140(6):548–54.
50. Wertz AP, Durham AB, Malloy KM, Johnson TM, Bradford CR, McLean SA. Total versus superficial parotidectomy for stage III melanoma. Head Neck. 2017;39(8):1665–70.
51. Henderson MA, Burmeister BH, Ainslie J, et al. Adjuvant lymph-node field radiotherapy versus observation only in patients with melanoma at high risk of further lymph-node field relapse after lymphadenectomy (ANZMTG 01.02/TROG 02.01): 6-year follow-up of a phase 3, randomised controlled trial. Lancet Oncol. 2015;16(9):1049–60.
52. Shen P, Wanek LA, Morton DL. Is adjuvant radiotherapy necessary after positive lymph node dissection in head and neck melanomas? Ann Surg Oncol. 2000;7(8):554–9; discussion 560–1
53. Ballo MT, Bonnen MD, Garden AS, et al. Adjuvant irradiation for cervical lymph node metastases from melanoma. Cancer. 2003;97(7):1789–96.
54. Mocellin S, Lens MB, Pasquali S, Pilati P, Chiarion SV. Interferon alpha for the adjuvant treatment of cutaneous melanoma. Cochrane Database Syst Rev. 2013;6:CD008955.
55. Eggermont AM, Chiarion-Sileni V, Grob JJ, et al. Adjuvant ipilimumab versus placebo after complete resection of high-risk stage III melanoma (EORTC 18071): a randomised, double-blind, phase 3 trial. Lancet Oncol. 2015;16(5):522–30.
56. Coens C, Suciu S, Chiarion-Sileni V, et al. Health-related quality of life with adjuvant ipilimumab versus placebo after complete resection of high-risk stage III melanoma (EORTC 18071): secondary outcomes of a multinational, randomised, double-blind, phase 3 trial. Lancet Oncol. 2017;18(3):393–403.
57. Tarhini A. Ipilimumab or high-dose interferon alfa-2b in treating patients with high-risk stage III-IV melanoma that has been removed by surgery. https://clinicaltrials.gov/ct2/show/NCT01274338?term=NCT01274338&rank=1. Accessed 12 Nov 2015.

58. Testori A. Adjuvant PEG intron in ulcerated melanoma. https://www.clinicaltrials.gov/ct2/show/NCT01502696?term=NCT01502696&rank=1. Accessed 12 Nov 2015.
59. Squibb B-M. Efficacy study of nivolumab compared to ipilimumab in prevention of recurrence of melanoma after complete resection of Stage IIIb/c or Stage IV melanoma (CheckMate 238). https://clinicaltrials.gov/ct2/show/NCT02388906?term=NCT02388906&rank=1. Accessed 13 Nov 2015.
60. Corp. MSD. Study of pembrolizumab (MK-3475) versus placebo after complete resection of high-risk stage III melanoma (MK-3475-054/KEYNOTE-054). https://clinicaltrials.gov/ct2/show/NCT02362594?term=NCT02362594&rank=1. Accessed 13 Nov 2015.
61. GlaxoSmithKline. A study of the BRAF inhibitor dabrafenib in combination with the MEK inhibitor trametinib in the adjuvant treatment of high-risk BRAF V600 mutation-positive melanoma after surgical resection. (COMBI-AD). https://www.clinicaltrials.gov/ct2/show/NCT01682083?term=NCT01682083&rank=1. Accessed 14 Nov 2015.
62. Roche H-L. BRIM8: a study of vemurafenib adjuvant therapy in patients with resected cutaneous BRAF mutant melanoma. https://clinicaltrials.gov/ct2/show/NCT01667419. Accessed 14 Nov 2015.
63. Mordoh J. Phase II/III clinical study CSF470 plus BCG plus GM-CSF vs IFN alpha 2b in stage IIB, IIC and III melanoma patients. https://clinicaltrials.gov/ct2/show/NCT01729663?term=melanoma+AND+adjuvant&phase=23&rank=6. Accessed 14 Nov 2015.
64. Schmidt MQ, David J, Yoshida EJ, et al. Predictors of survival in head and neck mucosal melanoma. Oral Oncol. 2017;73:36–42.
65. Members NP. NCCN Clinical practice guidelines in oncology: head and neck cancer. 2017. http://www.nccn.org/professionals/physician_gls/pdf/head-and-neck.pdf. Accessed 28 Aug 2017.
66. Marcus DM, Marcus RP, Prabhu RS, et al. Rising incidence of mucosal melanoma of the head and neck in the United States. J Skin Cancer. 2012;2012:231693.
67. Chang AE, Karnell LH, Menck HR. The National Cancer Data Base report on cutaneous and noncutaneous melanoma: a summary of 84,836 cases from the past decade. The American College of Surgeons Commission on Cancer and the American Cancer Society. Cancer. 1998;83(8):1664–78.
68. Greaves WO, Verma S, Patel KP, et al. Frequency and spectrum of BRAF mutations in a retrospective, single-institution study of 1112 cases of melanoma. J Mol Diagn. 2013;15(2):220–6.
69. Wu Y, Zhong Y, Li C, Song H, Guo W, Ren G. Neck dissection for oral mucosal melanoma: caution of nodular lesion. Oral Oncol. 2014;50(4):319–24.
70. Yao WC, Emerick KS, Kraft S, Holbrook EH. Nasal mucosal melanosis may act as a harbinger of melanoma: a case report. Allergy Rhinol (Providence). 2016;7(3):164–7.
71. Fuji H, Yoshikawa S, Kasami M, et al. High-dose proton beam therapy for sinonasal mucosal malignant melanoma. Radiat Oncol. 2014;9:162.
72. Liao JJ, Parvathaneni U, Laramore GE, et al. Fast neutron radiotherapy for primary mucosal melanomas of the head and neck. Head Neck. 2014;36(8):1162–7.
73. Gal TJ, Silver N, Huang B. Demographics and treatment trends in sinonasal mucosal melanoma. Laryngoscope. 2011;121(9):2026–33.
74. Shuman AG, Light E, Olsen SH, et al. Mucosal melanoma of the head and neck: predictors of prognosis. Arch Otolaryngol Head Neck Surg. 2011;137(4):331–7.
75. Heppt MV, Roesch A, Weide B, et al. Prognostic factors and treatment outcomes in 444 patients with mucosal melanoma. Eur J Cancer. 2017;81:36–44.
76. Lawaetz M, Birch-Johansen F, Friis S, et al. Primary mucosal melanoma of the head and neck in Denmark, 1982–2012: Demographic and clinical aspects. A retrospective DAHANCA study. Acta Oncol. 2016;55(8):1001–8.
77. Swegal W, Koyfman S, Scharpf J, et al. Endoscopic and open surgical approaches to locally advanced sinonasal melanoma: comparing the therapeutic benefits. JAMA Otolaryngol Head Neck Surg. 2014;140(9):840–5.
78. Cao W, Guan B, Yu A, et al. Treatment and outcomes of endoscopic surgery and traditional open resection in sinonasal mucosal melanoma. Acta Otolaryngol. 2017;137(8):862–7.
79. Plavc G, But-Hadžić J, Aničin A, Lanišnik B, Didanović V, Strojan P. Mucosal melanoma of the head and neck: a population-based study from Slovenia, 1985–2013. Radiat Oncol. 2016;11(1):137.
80. Konuthula N, Khan MN, Parasher A, et al. The presentation and outcomes of mucosal melanoma in 695 patients. Int Forum Allergy Rhinol. 2017;7(1):99–105.
81. Yang X, Ren GX, Zhang CP, et al. Neck dissection and post-operative chemotherapy with dimethyl triazeno imidazole carboxamide and cisplatin protocol are useful for oral mucosal melanoma. BMC Cancer. 2010;10:623.
82. Sun CZ, Chen YF, Jiang YE, Hu ZD, Yang AK, Song M. Treatment and prognosis of oral mucosal melanoma. Oral Oncol. 2012;48(7):647–52.
83. Wushou A, Hou J, Zhao YJ, Miao XC. Postoperative adjuvant radiotherapy improves loco-regional recurrence of head and neck mucosal melanoma. J Craniomaxillofac Surg. 2015;43(4):553–8.
84. Krengli M, Jereczek-Fossa BA, Kaanders JH, Masini L, Beldì D, Orecchia R. What is the role of radiotherapy in the treatment of mucosal melanoma of the head and neck? Crit Rev Oncol Hematol. 2008;65(2):121–8.
85. Moreno MA, Roberts DB, Kupferman ME, et al. Mucosal melanoma of the nose and paranasal sinuses, a contemporary experience from the M. D. Anderson Cancer Center. Cancer. 2010;116(9):2215–23.

86. Jarrom D, Paleri V, Kerawala C, et al. Mucosal melanoma of the upper airways tract mucosal melanoma: a systematic review with meta-analyses of treatment. Head Neck. 2017;39(4):819–25.
87. Temam S, Mamelle G, Marandas P, et al. Postoperative radiotherapy for primary mucosal melanoma of the head and neck. Cancer. 2005;103(2):313–9.
88. Lian B, Si L, Cui C, et al. Phase II randomized trial comparing high-dose IFN-α2b with temozolomide plus cisplatin as systemic adjuvant therapy for resected mucosal melanoma. Clin Cancer Res. 2013;19(16):4488–98.
89. Schaefer T, Satzger I, Gutzmer R. Clinics, prognosis and new therapeutic options in patients with mucosal melanoma: a retrospective analysis of 75 patients. Medicine (Baltimore). 2017;96(1):e5753.
90. Kim KB, Alrwas A. Treatment of KIT-mutated metastatic mucosal melanoma. Chin Clin Oncol. 2014;3(3):35.
91. Carvajal RD, Antonescu CR, Wolchok JD, et al. KIT as a therapeutic target in metastatic melanoma. JAMA. 2011;305(22):2327–34.
92. Postow MA, Luke JJ, Bluth MJ, et al. Ipilimumab for patients with advanced mucosal melanoma. Oncologist. 2013;18(6):726–32.
93. Ascierto PA, Vanella V, Grimaldi AM, et al. Complete response to nivolumab monotherapy in a treatment-naive, BRAF wild-type patient with advanced mucosal melanoma and elevated lactate dehydrogenase: a case report from a phase III trial. Cancer Immunol Immunother. 2016;65(11):1395–400.
94. Members NP. NCCN Clinical practice guidelines in oncology: basal cell skin cancer. 2017. https://www.nccn.org/professionals/physician_gls/pdf/nmsc.pdf. Accessed 2 Sept 2017.
95. Bath-Hextall FJ, Perkins W, Bong J, Williams HC. Interventions for basal cell carcinoma of the skin. Cochrane Database Syst Rev. 2007;1:CD003412.
96. van Loo E, Mosterd K, Krekels GA, et al. Surgical excision versus Mohs' micrographic surgery for basal cell carcinoma of the face: a randomised clinical trial with 10 year follow-up. Eur J Cancer. 2014; 50(17):3011–20.
97. Avril MF, Auperin A, Margulis A, et al. Basal cell carcinoma of the face: surgery or radiotherapy? Results of a randomized study. Br J Cancer. 1997;76(1):100–6.
98. Petit JY, Avril MF, Margulis A, et al. Evaluation of cosmetic results of a randomized trial comparing surgery and radiotherapy in the treatment of basal cell carcinoma of the face. Plast Reconstr Surg. 2000;105(7):2544–51.
99. Jackson JE, Dickie GJ, Wiltshire KL, et al. Radiotherapy for perineural invasion in cutaneous head and neck carcinomas: toward a risk-adapted treatment approach. Head Neck. 2009;31(5): 604–10.
100. Sekulic A, Migden MR, Basset-Seguin N, et al. Long-term safety and efficacy of vismodegib in patients with advanced basal cell carcinoma: final update of the pivotal ERIVANCE BCC study. BMC Cancer. 2017;17(1):332.
101. Lear JT, Migden MR, Lewis KD, et al. Long-term efficacy and safety of sonidegib in patients with locally advanced and metastatic basal cell carcinoma: 30-month analysis of the randomized phase 2 BOLT study. J Eur Acad Dermatol Venereol. 2018;32(3):372–81.
102. Pharmaceuticals R. NCT03132636: PD-1 in patients with advanced basal cell carcinoma who experienced progression of disease on hedgehog pathway inhibitor therapy, or were intolerant of prior hedgehog pathway inhibitor therapy. https://clinicaltrials.gov/ct2/show/NCT03132636. Accessed 3 Sept 2017.
103. Durham AB, Lowe L, Malloy KM, et al. Sentinel lymph node biopsy for cutaneous squamous cell carcinoma on the head and neck. JAMA Otolaryngol Head Neck Surg. 2016;142(12):1171–6.
104. Martinez JC, Cook JL. High-risk cutaneous squamous cell carcinoma without palpable lymphadenopathy: is there a therapeutic role for elective neck dissection? Dermatol Surg. 2007;33(4):410–20.
105. Audet N, Palme CE, Gullane PJ, et al. Cutaneous metastatic squamous cell carcinoma to the parotid gland: analysis and outcome. Head Neck. 2004; 26(8):727–32.
106. Moore BA, Weber RS, Prieto V, et al. Lymph node metastases from cutaneous squamous cell carcinoma of the head and neck. Laryngoscope. 2005; 115(9):1561–7.
107. Members NP. NCCN Clinical practice guidelines in oncology: squamous cell skin cancer 2017. https://www.nccn.org/professionals/physician_gls/pdf/squamous.pdf. Accessed 2 Sept 2017.
108. Pharmaceuticals R. NCT02760498: study of REGN2810 in patients with advanced cutaneous squamous cell carcinoma. https://clinicaltrials.gov/ct2/show/NCT02760498. Accessed 2 Sept 2017.
109. Kudchadkar R. NCT02964559: Pembrolizumab in patients with locally advanced or metastatic skin cancer. https://clinicaltrials.gov/ct2/show/NCT02964559. Accessed 3 Sept 2017.
110. Samimi M, Gardair C, Nicol JT, Arnold F, Touzé A, Coursaget P. Merkel cell polyomavirus in merkel cell carcinoma: clinical and therapeutic perspectives. Semin Oncol. 2015;42(2):347–58.
111. Members NP. NCCN clinical practice guidelines in oncology: merkel cell carcinoma. 2017; https://www.nccn.org/professionals/physician_gls/pdf/mcc.pdf. Accessed 3 Sept 2017.
112. Kachare SD, Wong JH, Vohra NA, Zervos EE, Fitzgerald TL. Sentinel lymph node biopsy is associated with improved survival in Merkel cell carcinoma. Ann Surg Oncol. 2014;21(5):1624–30.
113. Thompson JF, Hruby G. The role of sentinel lymph node biopsy in patients with merkel cell carcinoma: uncertainty prevails. Ann Surg Oncol. 2014; 21(5):1517–9.
114. Fritsch VA, Camp ER, Lentsch EJ. Sentinel lymph node status in Merkel cell carcinoma of the head

and neck: not a predictor of survival. Head Neck. 2014;36(4):571–9.

115. Sadeghi R, Adinehpoor Z, Maleki M, Fallahi B, Giovanella L, Treglia G. Prognostic significance of sentinel lymph node mapping in Merkel cell carcinoma: systematic review and meta-analysis of prognostic studies. Biomed Res Int. 2014;2014:489536.
116. Bhatia S, Storer BE, Iyer JG, et al. Adjuvant radiation therapy and chemotherapy in Merkel cell carcinoma: survival analyses of 6908 cases from the National Cancer Data Base. J Natl Cancer Inst. 2016;108(9)
117. Lewis KG, Weinstock MA, Weaver AL, Otley CC. Adjuvant local irradiation for Merkel cell carcinoma. Arch Dermatol. 2006;142(6):693–700.
118. Jouary T, Leyral C, Dreno B, et al. Adjuvant prophylactic regional radiotherapy versus observation in stage I Merkel cell carcinoma: a multicentric prospective randomized study. Ann Oncol. 2012;23(4):1074–80.
119. Chen MM, Roman SA, Sosa JA, Judson BL. The role of adjuvant therapy in the management of head and neck merkel cell carcinoma: an analysis of 4815 patients. JAMA Otolaryngol Head Neck Surg. 2015;141(2):137–41.
120. Chapuis A. NCT02584829: localized radiation therapy or recombinant interferon beta and avelumab with or without cellular adoptive immunotherapy in treating patients with metastatic merkel cell carcinoma. https://clinicaltrials.gov/ct2/show/NCT02584829. Accessed 3 Sept 2017.
121. Rabinowits G. NCT02514824: MLN0128 in recurrent/metastatic merkel cell carcinoma. https://clinicaltrials.gov/ct2/show/NCT02514824. Accessed 3 Sept 2017.
122. Niethammer A. NCT02465957: QUILT-3.009: study of aNK infusions in combination with ALT-803 in patients with stage III (IIIB) or stage (IV) merkel cell carcinoma. https://clinicaltrials.gov/ct2/show/NCT02465957. Accessed 3 Sept 2017.
123. Kim S. NCT03071406: randomized study of nivolumab+Ipilimumab+/− SBRT for metastatic merkel cell carcinoma. https://clinicaltrials.gov/ct2/show/NCT03071406. Accessed 3 Sept 2017.

Management of Melanoma Locoregional Recurrence

20

Clara R. Farley and Keith A. Delman

Abbreviations

BCG	Bacilli Calmette-Guérin
CTLA-4	Cytotoxic T lymphocyte-associated antigen 4
DPCP	Diphencyprone
GM-CSF	Granuloctye-macrophage colony stimulating factor
HILP	Hyperthermic isolated limb perfusion
ILI	Isolated limb infusion
NCCN	National Comprehensive Cancer Network
PD-1	programmed cell death 1
SLNB	Sentinel lymph node biopsy

Introduction

The incidence of melanoma continues to rise, with up to 25% of patients ultimately developing recurrent disease locally or in regional lymph nodes [1, 2]. Locoregional recurrence is defined as recurrence locally at the site of the primary lesion, regionally in the draining lymph node basin, and/or anywhere in between, but excludes distant metastatic disease. It can represent a true recurrence following adequate excision or "persistent" disease due to inadequate excision [2]. Locoregional recurrence can also occur as in-transit metastases, which is defined as cutaneous or subcutaneous recurrence proximal to the primary lesion site and distal to the regional lymph node basin [3]. Historically, local recurrence was distinguished from in-transit metastases by the distance from the site of the primary lesion. A local recurrence is defined as occurring within 2 cm of the initial lesion and in-transit metastases >2 cm from the primary lesion. However, this distinction does not appear to have any significant bearing upon the overall prognosis [4].

Overall rates of local recurrence range from 2 to 3%, but the risk of local recurrence has been shown to increase as the thickness of the primary lesion increases as well as in the setting of ulceration [2, 5, 6]. Similarly, risk factors for in-transit recurrence include increasing depth or mitotic rate, ulceration of the primary lesion and a positive sentinel lymph node biopsy (SLNB) [7–9]. As these risk factors tend to overlap, it is no surprise that patients with in-transit disease are also at a significant risk of further locoregional and distant recurrence [10].

Though the paradigm for the management of patients with melanoma is in a state of considerable flux, surgical resection is the mainstay of therapy for locoregional recurrence and still offers the best chance for long-term cure. For those with unresectable disease, there are several additional treatment modalities to consider. Regional therapy options include hyperthermic isolated limb

C. R. Farley, M.D. (✉) · K. A. Delman, M.D., F.A.C.S.
Department of Surgical Oncology, Emory University Hospital, Atlanta, GA, USA
e-mail: crfarle@emory.edu; kdelman@emory.edu

A. I. Riker (ed.), *Melanoma*, https://doi.org/10.1007/978-3-319-78310-9_20

perfusion (HILP) or isolated limb infusion (ILI), topical therapies, intralesional injection therapies, laser ablation, radiation therapy, and systemic therapy. Systemic therapy and immunotherapy can also be considered in those with unresectable, locoregional disease and widely metastatic disease.

Surgical Therapy

Local and In-Transit Recurrence

Surgical resection carries the best chance of long-term survival for local and regional recurrent disease. This is not a function of the efficacy of surgery, but rather the biology of the disease. It is possible that future treatment modalities may be shown to be as effective as surgical extirpation, but at present, surgical resection of recurrent disease remains a very effective and rapid treatment modality, generally associated with limited complications. For those with biopsy-proven locoregional disease, National Comprehensive Cancer Network (NCCN) guidelines recommend that patients undergo staging with cross-sectional imaging to evaluate for distant metastatic disease prior to surgical intervention. If the workup reveals no evidence of extraregional disease, the surgeon should proceed with complete excision with the goal to obtain microscopically negative margins, as no studies have addressed the potential benefit of taking additional margins in this setting [11].

Many authorities advocate consideration for SLNB in resectable in-transit disease, even in the setting of prior SLNB or lymph node dissection, as it may guide further regional therapy and provide prognostic value [12–14]. Others are more cautious in their approach to treatment in the setting of stage IIIB or greater disease, as the prognosis and treatment of these patients is largely driven by the recurrence itself.

Regional Nodal Recurrence

Completion lymphadenectomy offers the best potentially curative treatment option for patients with recurrent disease confined to the regional lymph node basin. Once regional nodal recurrence is confirmed on biopsy, patients should undergo subsequent workup with radiographic imaging to rule out distant disease [11]. Complete lymph node dissection is indicated for those patients who do not have evidence of systemic disease. For recurrent disease within the inguinal nodal basin, most authors recommend that patients undergo an inguinofemoral, iliac, and obturator pelvic lymph node dissection [15]. Recurrence within the axilla requires formal dissection of nodal levels I, II, and III, while recurrence within the cervical lymph node basin should prompt a modified radical neck dissection of at least levels II, III, IV, and V [16–19]. If disease in the neck is located in the parotid gland, or levels I or VI, then dissection of these regions should be included in the definitive operation.

When used in conjunction with complete lymph node dissection, adjuvant radiation therapy may improve locoregional control and has demonstrated reductions in regional recurrence rates following lymphadenectomy in the neck, axilla, or groin [20–22]. Importantly, radiation therapy has not been shown to improve overall survival, despite some observed benefit in regional control. However, it is has been shown to increase the frequency of postoperative lymphedema following axillary and groin dissections with no impact upon disease-free or overall survival [23].

Palliative Resection

Metastatic disease in melanoma is often widespread, and while curative surgery may be unattainable, palliative surgery may offer an additional surgical option for such patients, many of which have significant and identifiable symptoms due to bulky disease [24, 25]. Palliative resections must be accomplished with minimal morbidity, a limited hospital stay and adequately address a specific symptom. The success of palliative surgery largely rests on the frank and honest preoperative discussion of the goals and expectations among the patient and their family with the surgeon. While palliative surgery does not provide long-term survival benefits in the majority of patients undergoing resection, several studies demonstrate that, in select patients, surgery can be an effective and safe palliative treatment option that can provide symptomatic relief in as high as 77–100% of patients [18, 26, 27].

Regional Therapy

Hyperthermic Isolated Limb Perfusion

When a patient is found to have unresectable locoregional recurrence or in-transit metastases of the extremities, additional therapies should be explored. Undoubtedly, in this era of remarkable progress with systemic therapeutic options, the role of regional therapy is undergoing a dramatic change. Despite these changes, regional therapy remains a tool in the armamentarium of the clinician managing patients with melanoma and can always be considered for patients with unresectable disease limited to an extremity.

HILP is a regional therapy that delivers high-dose chemotherapy to the affected limb [28]. The procedure requires dissection, isolation, and cannulation of the major artery and vein of the limb followed by application of a proximally placed tourniquet to isolate the limb [29]. High concentrations of chemotherapy, typically the alkylating agent melphalan, are then delivered regionally without entering the systemic circulation for 60–90 min. An oxygenated extracorporeal circuit is used to maintain normal oxygenation and acid-base balance during infusion [29]. If indicated, therapeutic regional lymphadenectomy can be performed at the same time as the vessels are already exposed for the procedure.

While most systemic toxicities are avoided with its use, HILP can be associated with significant morbidity. Patients can develop mild skin and soft tissue effects to severe vascular complications, compartment syndrome or limb loss. Lymphedema is the most common complication following HILP and carries an even higher risk in those who undergo concurrent lymph node dissection [29–31]. Complete response rates greater than 50%, with overall response rates of 80%, have been reported. Those with a complete response have demonstrated durable long-term results and improved overall survival [30, 32–34].

Isolated Limb Infusion

ILI was first proposed in the 1990s as a simpler, less invasive alternative to HILP [35]. Vascular access to the artery and vein is obtained percutaneously and under fluoroscopic guidance, 5- or 6-French arterial and venous catheters are positioned in the vessels of the limb to be treated [33]. A proximal tourniquet is then placed to isolate the affected limb from the systemic circulation. An extracorporeal circuit is connected to the catheters for circulation of the chemotherapy. Unlike HILP, supplemental oxygen is not provided. ILI is typically performed for 30 min, creating a hypoxic and acidotic environment in the extremity, which increases the efficacy of melphalan [36].

Overall response rates range from 43 to 88%, with reported complete response rates of 30–41% [30, 33, 36, 37]. ILI is associated with a much lower risk of severe limb-threatening complications and systemic toxicities than HILP and offers additional benefits such as shorter operative time, a minimally invasive approach and the ability to easily repeat the procedure for subsequent recurrences [30, 33, 38]. Disadvantages of ILI, compared to HILP, include its ability to treat less overall area of the affected extremity, lower clinical response rates and shorter durability of response [29]. There are currently no prospective comparisons of HILP versus ILI, but a complete response to either modality is associated with improved overall survival [30, 38, 39].

In 2009, a treatment algorithm for patients with recurrent disease to the lower-extremity was proposed and provides a guide for selecting appropriate regional therapy [38]. For patients with unresectable lower-extremity recurrence and concurrent pelvic lymph node disease, the algorithm advocates for HILP as first line therapy to allow for a completion lymphadenectomy at the time of the procedure. For those patients with unresectable, in-transit metastases localized to an extremity, the algorithm advocates for ILI regional therapy. If a patient fails to respond to ILI, HILP can then be used as salvage therapy [14].

Repeat HILP and ILI are both safe and efficacious options for patients with progressive disease following regional therapy. In this setting, complete response rates of 25–45% have been reported, but it is important to note that the risk of toxicities does increase [37, 40, 41]. While post-therapy surveillance scans have not been proven effective at predicting response to regional therapy, they have been shown to detect subclinical distant disease or regional nodal disease outside the treatment field that was still amenable to resection in 47% of patients [42].

Topical Therapy

While topical therapy is generally considered for areas where surgical options are limited (classically periorbital) and for less invasive disease like melanoma in situ, clinicians will consider its use in some patients with regional disease. This is a particular consideration in those patients with cutaneous metastases on the trunk or scalp as these areas are not amenable to regional perfusion options. The two most notable topical therapies for in-transit melanoma metastases are Diphencyprone (DPCP) and Imiquimod. DPCP is a topical immunotherapy agent that is thought to upregulate the T_H17 lymphocyte pathway [43, 44]. It is important to note that the United States Food and Drug Administration (FDA) has not approved any topical therapy for the treatment of melanoma or melanoma in situ. The data for use of these agents comes from studies performed in either Europe or Australia.

Several small series have shown encouraging partial and complete response rates for patients undergoing weekly topical application of DPCP, either alone or in combination with other agents [45, 46]. These findings are specific to patients with extensive, superficial in-transit melanoma metastases that are not amenable to other therapies. Imiquimod is a topically applied immunomodulator that works as a toll-like receptor agonist [43]. Activation of toll-like receptor 7 induces cytokine secretion leading to downstream activation of effector cells and T_H1 lymphocytes [47, 48]. Several small series have reported regression rates of 50–90% for superficial lesions when imiquimod is used once or twice daily over the course of several months [49, 50].

Intralesional Therapy

Intralesional therapy involves the direct injection of a therapeutic agent into the melanoma lesion. It is most commonly used for unresectable intradermal and subcutaneous recurrent or in-transit lesions. The agents are delivered directly into the lesion, allowing for a much higher concentration to be used with a smaller risk of systemic toxicity. This approach can also induce a systemic immune response against melanoma antigens found within the lesion, thereby inducing regression of other lesions [43, 52].

The first description of intralesional immunotherapy was reported by Morton et al. and used bacilli Calmette-Guérin (BCG) [52]. They reported regression rates of 90% for intradermal lesions into which BCG was injected, along with 17% for regional lesions into which BCG was not injected. More recent data has demonstrated complete regression in 56% of patients when BCG is used in combination with imiquimod. This provided a durable response in 33% of patients when combined with surgical resection of solitary resistant lesions [53]. Rose Bengal (PV-10) is a chemoablative agent that is also used as an intralesional injection and has shown to be directly cytotoxic to melanoma cells. It also stimulates the immune response, as demonstrated by regression rates of 40% in regional lesions into which rose Bengal was not injected [54].

Intralesional immunotherapy has also emerged as a promising regional therapy. Intralesional administration of IL-2 has been explored for in-transit metastatic melanoma and offers the ability to deliver greater local concentrations than standard systemic treatment can safely reach. Small series have demonstrated clinical response in 80–90% of lesions into which IL-2 had been injected, but response rates in untreated regional lesions were less impressive than with BCG therapies [51, 55, 56]. When combined with topical agents such as imiquimod, the use of injected IL-2 has demonstrated significant regression in deeper subcutaneous lesions less responsive to imiquimod alone [57]. Additional cytokines, including interferon-α and interferon-β, have been investigated, but the benefit is controversial as the data on survival outcomes has been largely inconsistent and treatment is associated with significant toxicities [58, 59].

Another promising intralesional immunotherapy is granuloctye-macrophage colony stimulating factor (GM-CSF), originally used as an intralesional immunotherapeutic. More recently, the gene coding for GM-CSF has been inserted in the genome of a modified Herpes virus and used as an intralesional vaccination. The modified virus selectively replicates in tumor cells and secretes GM-CSF [60, 61] locally while replicating and lysing the host cell. Patients exhibiting a response to the vaccine have demonstrated increased dendritic activity locally and decreased numbers of regulatory T cells in lesions into which the virus had been injected [61]. They also demonstrated increased antigen-specific T cells both locally and systemically. Results from Phase I and II trials testing the vaccine were encouraging, prompting a Phase III clinical study called Oncovex (GM-CSF) Pivotal Trial in Melanoma (OPTIM). This trial examined 436 patients with Stage IIIB, IIIC, or IV melanoma and demonstrated an overall response rate of 26.4% for the viral construct versus 5.7% for GM-CSF alone [62, 63]. These results generated considerable enthusiasm and resulted in the FDA approval of this agent as the first oncolytic virus for use in melanoma patients with injectable but unresectable lesions [64].

Laser Therapy

Laser therapy for multifocal, superficial in-transit disease is a minimally morbid, well-tolerated treatment for patients with unresectable lesions. Phototherapy with a pulsed dye laser is a treatment option for visible, superficial intradermal lesions, particularly when lesions are located on the head, neck, or trunk, as these sites are not amenable to other regional therapies such as limb infusion [51]. The laser works by inducing a local inflammatory response and directly lysing tumor cells. It can be combined with topical agents or other modalities in order to achieve local control of micrometastatic disease or for palliation [65]. Carbon dioxide laser ablation is another therapeutic option and may allow treatment of more deeply extending lesions, although wound healing becomes a concern when a larger volume of disease is targeted [66].

Electrochemotherapy

Electrochemotherapy combines high-intensity electrical pulses with the intravenous or intralesional delivery of low-dose cytotoxic drugs [67]. The electrical pulses disrupt cell membrane integrity and cause a local vasoconstriction, increasing the intracellular delivery and local efficacy of the chemotherapeutic agent. Overall response rates of 50–90% have been demonstrated in several published series [67]. Additionally, electrochemotherapy has been shown to be effective in a local control setting for unresectable cutaneous lesions and for the palliative treatment of painful or bleeding lesions. Indications for therapy include proximal lesions of the extremities or lesions on the head, neck, or trunk, while renal failure or allergies to the agents are the primary contraindications [43]. Electrochemotherapy offers many advantages as it has a minimal side effect profile, can be performed under local anesthesia, spares surrounding uninvolved tissue, and can be used in the setting of prior radiation therapy [31].

Radiation Therapy

As noted previously, radiation therapy can be used as an adjuvant for high-risk nodal disease but it can also be used as a palliative option for unresectable nodal, satellite or in-transit disease. The efficacy is greatest in the adjuvant setting for microscopic residual disease, following removal of gross disease or following resection of in-transit metastases with clear margins [51]. There is evidence to suggest that some patients with locoregional recurrence who are unable to undergo resection or regional chemotherapy might achieve improved locoregional control and possibly even improved survival with radiation therapy [68, 69]. For recurrent lesions of the head and neck, where other treatment modalities are unavailable, radiation therapy may be a good option, though with growing options in systemic and injectable therapy, it has fallen out of favor in most circumstances [70].

Due to retrospective and case-series data, widespread adoption of hypofractionation, or high dose per fraction radiation therapy, has been utilized recently [71, 72]. This schedule delivers 30 Gy in five fractions, as opposed to a more standard fractionation of 2 Gy per daily fraction in 3 weeks or more [73]. However, a randomized trial by Burmeister et al. demonstrated improved locoregional control with adjuvant radiation therapy using conventional standard fractionation. This has generated renewed interest in this approach [21].

Systemic Therapy (Immunotherapy and Targeted Agents)

The treatment of metastatic melanoma changed dramatically in 2010, when immunotherapy emerged as a promising treatment option for advanced disease. Ipilimumab, a human monoclonal antibody that inhibits cytotoxic T lymphocyte-associated antigen 4 (CTLA-4), was evaluated in a phase III clinical trial for unresectable stage III and IV melanoma and found to significantly improve overall survival compared to glycoprotein 100 vaccine alone [74]. Since the initial results showing the agent's efficacy in stage IV patients, ipilimumab has also been approved for use as adjuvant therapy for patients with resected disease [75].

Following the success of CTLA-4 blockade, Vemurafenib, a potent inhibitor of mutated BRAF, was shown to have an overall survival rate of 84% at 6 months in patients with metastatic melanoma and a BRAF V600E mutation [76]. Based on these results, vemurafenib was approved for use in metastatic melanoma. The rapid change in the landscape of melanoma therapeutics continued as two subsequent agents, dabrafenib (BRAF inhibitor) and trametinib (MEK inhibitor) were approved for unresectable, metastatic melanoma shortly thereafter. Since these early results, immunotherapeutic options have expanded rapidly with accelerated research agendas driven largely by these successes leading to the evaluation and approval of other checkpoint inhibitors.

Perhaps one of the most dramatic changes in therapeutic options for systemic therapy came in 2014, when pembrolizumab and nivolumab, both highly selective monoclonal antibodies to programmed cell death 1 (PD-1), were approved by the FDA [77]. Both drugs have shown improved antitumor activity and an impressive safety profile. A phase III trial demonstrated that pembrolizumab significantly prolonged progression-free survival (47.3% vs. 26.5%) and 1-year survival rate (74.1% vs. 58.2%) compared to ipilimumab [78]. Furthermore, because of the complementary and non-redundant mechanisms of CTLA-4 and PD-1, combination therapy has been investigated, demonstrating longer progression-free survival (11.5 vs. 6.9 vs. 2.9 months) and higher overall response rates (57.6 vs. 43.7 vs. 19%) when compared to nivolumab or ipilimumab alone [79].

Additional novel immunotherapeutics are currently being investigated and will continue to redefine our treatment strategies for advanced, unresectable melanoma. However, the impressive efficacy of these agents and their relatively mild side effect profile have impacted the algorithm for patients even with disease limited to a limb who previously would have only been considered for regional infusional therapy. Moreover, these successes have prompted investigation into the use of these agents in a neoadjuvant setting. Importantly, for the surgeon, having effective systemic therapy should prompt consideration of a more aggressive approach to therapy, particularly in patients who respond well to systemic treatment, but remain with residual disease. Undoubtedly, the future of the management of patients with locoregional disease will continue to evolve, and will likely include a combination of multiple therapeutic approaches.

References

1. Siegel RL, Miller KD, Jemal A. Cancer statistics, 2017. CA Cancer J Clin. 2017;67:7–30. https://doi.org/10.3322/caac.21387.
2. Karakousis CP, Balch CM, Urist MM, et al. Local recurrence in malignant melanoma: long-term results of the multiinstitutional randomized surgical trial. Ann Surg Oncol. 1996;3(5):446–52.
3. Karakousis CP, Choe KJ, Holyoke ED. Biologic behavior and treatment of intransit metastasis of melanoma. Surg Gynecol Obstet. 1980;150(1):29–32.
4. Singletary SE, Tucker SL, Boddie Jr AW. Multivariate analysis of prognostic factors in regional cutaneous metastases of extremity melanoma. Cancer. 1988; 61(7):1437–40.
5. Francken AB, Accortt NA, Shaw HM, et al. Prognosis and determinants of outcome following locoregional or distant recurrence in patients with cutaneous melanoma. Ann Surg Oncol. 2008;15(5): 1476–84.
6. Balch CM, Soong SJ, Gershenwald JE, et al. Prognostic factors analysis of 17,600 melanoma patients: validation of the American Joint Committee on Cancer melanoma staging system. J Clin Oncol. 2001;19(16):3622–34.
7. Stucky CC, Gray RJ, Dueck AC, et al. Risk factors associated with local and in-transit recurrence of cutaneous melanoma. Am J Surg. 2010;200(6):770–4; discussion 744–5
8. Pawlik TM, Ross MI, Johnson MM, et al. Predictors and natural history of in-transit melanoma after sentinel lymphadenectomy. Ann Surg Oncol. 2005; 12(8):587–96.
9. Kesmodel SB, Karakousis GC, Botbyl JD, et al. Mitotic rate as a predictor of sentinel lymph node positivity in patients with thin melanomas. Ann Surg Oncol. 2005;12(6):449–58.
10. Dong XD, Tyler D, Johnson JL, et al. Analysis of prognosis and disease progression after local recurrence of melanoma. Cancer. 2000;88(5):1063–71.
11. Coit DG, Andtbacka R, Bichakjian CK, et al. Melanoma. J Natl Compr Cancer Netw. 2009;7(3): 250–75.
12. Yao KA, Hsueh EC, Essner R, et al. Is sentinel lymph node mapping indicated for isolated local and in-transit recurrent melanoma? Ann Surg. 2003;238(5):743–7.
13. Coventry BJ, Chatterton B, Whitehead F, et al. Sentinel lymph node dissection and lymphatic mapping for local subcutaneous recurrence in melanoma treatment: longer-term follow-up results. Ann Surg Oncol. 2004;11(3 Suppl):203S–7S.
14. Beasley GM, Tyler DS. Treatment of in-transit melanoma: an opportunity to discover critical knowledge. Oncology (Williston Park). 2011;25(14):1351–2, 1355
15. Badgwell B, Xing Y, Gershenwald JE, et al. Pelvic lymph node dissection is beneficial in subsets of patients with node-positive melanoma. Ann Surg Oncol. 2007;14(10):2867–75.
16. Love TP, Delman KA. Management of regional lymph node basins in melanoma. Ochsner J. 2010;10(2): 99–107.
17. Davis PG, Serpell JW, Kelly JW, Paul E. Axillary lymph node dissection for malignant melanoma. ANZ J Surg. 2011;81(6):462–6.
18. Shada AL, Walters DM, Tierney SN, Slingluff CL Jr. Surgical resection for bulky or recurrent axillary metastatic melanoma. J Surg Oncol. 2012;105(1):21–5.
19. Sawh-Martinez R, Salameh B, Colebunders B, et al. Level I sparing radical neck dissections for cutaneous melanoma in the lymphoscintigram era. Ann Plast Surg. 2012;69(4):422–4.
20. Khan N, Khan MK, Almasan A, et al. The evolving role of radiation therapy in the management of malignant melanoma. Int J Radiat Oncol Biol Phys. 2011;80(3):645–54.
21. Burmeister BH, Henderson MA, Ainslie J, et al. Adjuvant radiotherapy versus observation alone for patients at risk of lymph-node field relapse after therapeutic lymphadenectomy for melanoma: a randomised trial. Lancet Oncol. 2012;13(6):589–97.
22. Agrawal S, Kane JM 3rd, Guadagnolo BA, et al. The benefits of adjuvant radiation therapy after therapeutic lymphadenectomy for clinically advanced, high-risk, lymph node-metastatic melanoma. Cancer. 2009; 115(24):5836–44.
23. Guadagnolo BA, Zagars GK. Adjuvant radiation therapy for high-risk nodal metastases from cutaneous melanoma. Lancet Oncol. 2009;10(4):409–16.
24. Wong SL, Coit DG. Role of surgery in patients with stage IV melanoma. Curr Opin Oncol. 2004;16(2): 155–60. Review
25. Ollila DW. Complete metastasectomy in patients with stage IV metastatic melanoma. Lancet Oncol. 2006; 7(11):919–24. Review
26. Allen PJ, Coit DG. The surgical management of metastatic melanoma. Ann Surg Oncol. 2002;9(8):762–70. Review
27. Wornom IL 3rd, Smith JW, Soong SJ, McElvein R, Urist MM, Balch CM. Surgery as palliative treatment

for distant metastases of melanoma. Ann Surg. 1986;204(2):181–5.
28. Creech O Jr, Krementz ET, Ryan RF, Winblad JN. Chemotherapy of cancer: regional perfusion utilizing an extracorporeal circuit. Ann Surg. 1958;148(4):616–32.
29. Testori A, Verhoef C, Kroon HM, et al. Treatment of melanoma metastases in a limb by isolated limb perfusion and isolated limb infusion. J Surg Oncol. 2011;104(4):397–404.
30. Raymond AK, Beasley GM, Broadwater G, et al. Current trends in regional therapy for melanoma: lessons learned from 225 regional chemotherapy treatments between 1995 and 2010 at a single institution. J Am Coll Surg. 2011;213(2):306–16.
31. Gimbel MI, Delman KA, Zager JS. Therapy for unresectable recurrent and in-transit extremity melanoma. Cancer Control. 2008;15(3):225–32.
32. Alexander Jr HR, Fraker DL, Bartlett DL, et al. Analysis of factors influencing outcome in patients with in-transit malignant melanoma undergoing isolated limb perfusion using modern treatment parameters. J Clin Oncol. 2010;28(1):114–8.
33. Beasley GM, Petersen RP, Yoo J, et al. Isolated limb infusion for in-transit malignant melanoma of the extremity: a well-tolerated but less effective alternative to hyperthermic isolated limb perfusion. Ann Surg Oncol. 2008;15(8):2195–205.
34. Rossi CR, Pasquali S, Mocellin S, et al. Long-term results of melphalan-based isolated limb perfusion with or without low-dose TNF for in-transit melanoma metastases. Ann Surg Oncol. 2010;17(11):3000–7.
35. Thompson JF, Kam PC, Waugh RC, Harman CR. Isolated limb infusion with cytotoxic agents: a simple alternative to isolated limb perfusion. Semin Surg Oncol. 1998;14(3):238–47.
36. Kroon HM, Moncrieff M, Kam PC, Thompson JF. Outcomes following isolated limb infusion for melanoma. A 14-year experience. Ann Surg Oncol. 2008; 15(11):3003–13.
37. Wong J, Chen YA, Fisher KJ, Zager JS. Isolated limb infusion in a series of over 100 infusions: a single-center experience. Ann Surg Oncol. 2013; 20(4):1121–7.
38. Beasley GM, Caudle A, Petersen RP, et al. A multi-institutional experience of isolated limb infusion: defining response and toxicity in the US. J Am Coll Surg. 2009;208(5):706–15; discussion 715–7
39. Sharma K, Beasley G, Turley R, et al. Patterns of recurrence following complete response to regional chemotherapy for in-transit melanoma. Ann Surg Oncol. 2012;19(8):2563–71.
40. Chai CY, Deneve JL, Beasley GM, et al. A multi-institutional experience of repeat regional chemotherapy for recurrent melanoma of extremities. Ann Surg Oncol. 2012;19(5):1637–43.
41. Kroon HM, Lin DY, Kam PC, Thompson JF. Efficacy of repeat isolated limb infusion with melphalan and actinomycin D for recurrent melanoma. Cancer. 2009;115(9):1932–40.
42. Beasley GM, Parsons C, Broadwater G, et al. A multicenter prospective evaluation of the clinical utility of F-18 FDG-PET/CT in patients with AJCC stage IIIB or IIIC extremity melanoma. Ann Surg. 2012;256(2):350–6.
43. Testori A, Faries MB, Thompson JF, et al. Local and intralesional therapy of in-transit melanoma metastases. J Surg Oncol. 2011;104(4):391–6.
44. Martiniuk F, Damian DL, Thompson JF, et al. TH17 is involved in the remarkable regression of metastatic malignant melanoma to topical diphencyprone. J Drugs Dermatol. 2010;9(11):1368–72.
45. Damian DL, Thompson JF. Treatment of extensive cutaneous metastatic melanoma with topical diphencyprone. J Am Acad Dermatol. 2007;56(5):869–71.
46. Damian DL, Shannon KF, Saw RP, Thompson JF. Topical diphencyprone immunotherapy for cutaneous metastatic melanoma. Australas J Dermatol. 2009;50(4):266–71.
47. Hemmi H, Kaisho T, Takeuchi O, et al. Small antiviral compounds activate immune cells via the TLR7 MyD88-dependent signaling pathway. Nat Immunol. 2002;3(2):196–200.
48. Wagner TL, Ahonen CL, Couture AM, et al. Modulation of TH1 and TH2 cytokine production with the immune response modifiers, R-848 and imiquimod. Cell Immunol. 1999;191(1):10–9.
49. Berman B, Poochareon VN, Villa AM. Novel dermatologic uses of the immune response modifier imiquimod 5% cream. Skin Therapy Lett. 2002;7(9):1–6.
50. Florin V, Desmedt E, Vercambre-Darras S, Mortier L. Topical treatment of cutaneous metastases of malignant melanoma using combined imiquimod and 5-fluorouracil. Investig New Drugs. 2012;30(4): 1641–5.
51. Grotz TE, Mansfield AS, Kottschade LA, et al. In-transit melanoma: an individualized approach. Oncology (Williston Park). 2011;25(14):1340–8.
52. Morton D, Eilber FR, Malmgren RA, Wood WC. Immunological factors which influence response to immunotherapy in malignant melanoma. Surgery. 1970;68(1):158–63; discussion 163–4
53. Kidner TB, Morton DL, Lee DJ, et al. Combined intralesional bacille Calmette-Guérin (BCG) and topical imiquimod for in-transit melanoma. J Immunother. 2012;35(9):716–20.
54. Thompson JF, Hersey P, Wachter E. Chemoablation of metastatic melanoma using intralesional rose Bengal. Melanoma Res. 2008;18(6):405–11.
55. Boyd KU, Wehrli BM, Temple CL. Intra-lesional interleukin-2 for the treatment of in-transit melanoma. J Surg Oncol. 2011;104(7):711–7.
56. Radny P, Caroli UM, Bauer J, et al. Phase II trial of intralesional therapy with interleukin-2 in soft-tissue melanoma metastases. Br J Cancer. 2003;89(9):1620–6.
57. Green DS, Bodman-Smith MD, Dalgleish AG, Fischer MD. Phase I/II study of topical imiquimod and intralesional interleukin-2 in the treatment of accessible metastases in malignant melanoma. Br J Dermatol. 2007;156(2):337–45.

58. von Wussow P, Block B, Hartmann F, Deicher H. Intralesional interferon-alpha therapy in advanced malignant melanoma. Cancer. 1988;61(6):1071–4.
59. Fujimura T, Okuyama R, Ohtani T, et al. Perilesional treatment of metastatic melanoma with interferon-beta. Clin Exp Dermatol. 2009;34(7):793–9.
60. Ridolfi L, Ridolfi R. Preliminary experiences of intralesional immunotherapy in cutaneous metastatic melanoma. Hepato-Gastroenterology. 2002;49(44):335–9.
61. Kaufman HL, Kim DW, DeRaffele G, et al. Local and distant immunity induced by intralesional vaccination with an oncolytic herpes virus encoding GM-CSF in patients with stage IIIc and IV melanoma. Ann Surg Oncol. 2010;17(3):718–30.
62. Kaufman HL, Bines SD. OPTIM trial: a phase III trial of an oncolytic herpes virus encoding GM-CSF for unresectable stage III or IV melanoma. Future Oncol. 2010;6(6):941–9.
63. Andtbacka R, Kaufman HL, Collicho F, et al. Talimogene laherparepvec improves durable response rate in patients with advanced melanoma. J Clin Oncol. 2015;33(25):2780–8.
64. Pol J, Kroemer G, Galluzzi L. First oncolytic virus approved for melanoma immunotherapy. Oncoimmunology. 2015;5(1):e1115641.
65. Kottschade LA, Weenig RH, Otley CC, et al. The use of pulsed dye laser in the treatment of melanoma metastatic to the skin: a Mayo Clinic case series. J Am Acad Dermatol. 2010;62(6):e22–5.
66. Gibson SC, Byrne DS, McKay AJ. Ten-year experience of carbon dioxide laser ablation as treatment for cutaneous recurrence of malignant melanoma. Br J Surg. 2004;91(7):893–5.
67. Testori A, Intelisano A, Verrecchia F, et al. Alternatives for the treatment of local advanced disease: electrochemotherapy, limb perfusion, limb infusion, intralesional IL2. What is the role? Dermatol Ther. 2012;25(5):443–51.
68. Olivier KR, Schild SE, Morris CG, et al. A higher radiotherapy dose is associated with more durable palliation and longer survival in patients with metastatic melanoma. Cancer. 2007;110(8):1791–5.
69. Barker CA, Lee NY. Radiation therapy for cutaneous melanoma. Dermatol Clin. 2012;30(3):525–33.
70. Seegenschmiedt MH, Keilholz L, Altendorf-Hofmann A, et al. Palliative radiotherapy for recurrent and metastatic malignant melanoma: prognostic factors for tumor response and long-term outcome: a 20-year experience. Int J Radiat Oncol Biol Phys. 1999; 44(3):607–18.
71. Stevens G, Thompson JF, Firth I, et al. Locally advanced melanoma: results of postoperative hypofractionated radiation therapy. Cancer. 2000;88(1): 88–94.
72. Stevens G, McKay MJ. Dispelling the myths surrounding radiotherapy for treatment of cutaneous melanoma. Lancet Oncol. 2006;7(7):575–83.
73. Rao NG, Yu HH, Trotti A 3rd, Sondak VK. The role of radiation therapy in the management of cutaneous melanoma. Surg Oncol Clin N Am. 2011;20(1):115–31.
74. Hodi FS, O'Day SJ, McDermott DF, et al. Improved survival with ipilimumab in patients with metastatic melanoma. N Engl J Med. 2010;363:711–23.
75. Eggermont AM, Chiarion-Sileni V, Grob JJ, et al. Adjuvant ipilimumab versus placebo after complete resection of high-risk stage III melanoma (EORTC 18071): a randomised, double-blind, phase 3 trial. Lancet Oncol. 2015;16(5):522–3.
76. Chapman PB, Hauschild A, Robert C, et al. Improved survival with vemurafenib in melanoma with BRAF V600E mutation. N Engl J Med. 2011;364:2507–16.
77. Zhu Z, Liu W, Gotlieb V. The rapidly evolving therapies for advanced melanoma—towards immunotherapy, molecular targeted therapy, and beyond. Crit Rev Oncol Hematol. 2016;99:91–9. https://doi.org/10.1016/j.critrevonc.2015.12.002.
78. Robert C, Schachter J, Long GV, Arance A, Grob JJ, Mortier L, Daud A, Carlino MS, McNeil C, Lotem M, Larkin J, Lorigan P, Neyns B, Blank CU, Hamid O, Mateus C, Shapira-Frommer R, Kosh M, Zhou H, Ibrahim N, Ebbinghaus S, Ribas A, KEYNOTE-006 investigators. Pembrolizumab versus ipilimumab in advanced melanoma. N Engl J Med. 2015;372(26): 2521–32. https://doi.org/10.1056/NEJMoa1503093.
79. Larkin J, Hodi FS, Wolchok JD. Combined nivolumab and ipilimumab or monotherapy in untreated melanoma. N Engl J Med. 2015;373(13):1270–1. https://doi.org/10.1056/NEJMc1509660.

Reconstructive Options for Head and Neck Melanoma

21

Ian R. Wisecarver, Charles L. Dupin, and Julian D'Achille

A Brief Introduction

The risk of developing melanoma is skyrocketing. Some data suggests an increase in incidence of 5% per year, faster than any other cancer in the United States [1, 2]. For a bit of perspective, the risk of developing cutaneous melanoma in 1935 was 1 person in 1,500, whereas the risk in 2012 was 1 in 30 [2, 3]. While melanoma accounts for a relatively small portion of skin cancers, roughly 4%, the number of deaths caused by melanoma is disproportionately high, 75% [2]. Head and neck lesions comprise up to 25% of cutaneous melanoma, with 60–90% of these occurring on the face [1, 4, 5]. Scalp, lip, and external ear presentations are much less common [5]. Head and neck melanomas also have a higher local recurrence rate (9–13%) than do melanomas of the trunk or extremities [5, 6]. Melanoma of the face is two times higher in males and significantly more likely to occur in people with lightly colored eyes and a fair complexion [2, 4].

I. R. Wisecarver, B.S.
Louisiana State University Health Sciences Center, New Orleans, LA, USA
e-mail: iwisec@lsuhsc.edu

C. L. Dupin, M.D. (✉) · J. D'Achille, M.D., M.P.H.
Division of Plastic and Reconstructive Surgery, Department of Surgery, Louisiana State University Health Sciences Center, New Orleans, LA, USA
e-mail: cdupin@lsuhsc.edu; jdachi@lsuhsc.edu

Early detection of head and neck melanoma is of the utmost importance and may be the single easiest way to improve patient outcomes. In 1985, the ABCDE method of clinically identifying melanoma was proposed: Asymmetry, irregular Borders, Color variation within the lesion, Diameter ≥6 mm, and Evolution of the lesion over time [7]. An experienced clinician using three of the ABCDE criteria has a sensitivity of 66% and a specificity of 81% [8]. However, histopathologic analysis remains the gold standard and excisional or punch biopsy should be performed on suspicious lesions. Five-year survival rates vary drastically with small changes in Breslow thickness (BT) and reiterate the benefits of early detection: lesions with BT of <1 mm are associated with a 5-year survival rate greater than 94%, while a BT of ≥4 mm carries a 5-year survival rate of <50% [8].

Because most head and neck melanomas occur on the face and ears, even the removal of smaller lesions can be quite disfiguring. The potential for disfigurement, combined with highly variable and complex routes of lymphatic drainage, presents reconstructive surgeons with a difficult choice—how can we balance satisfactory aesthetic and functional results with sufficient oncologic resections? [1]. Unsurprisingly, consensus recommendations for best practice treatment is embroiled in controversy—some parties advocate for aggressive treatment with large margins and others for more conservative treatment to decrease unnecessary tissue loss. The current National Comprehensive

A. I. Riker (ed.), *Melanoma*, https://doi.org/10.1007/978-3-319-78310-9_21

Cancer Network (NCCN) guidelines for wide local excision of melanoma are: 0.5 cm margins for melanoma in situ, 1.0 cm margins for BT of ≤1.0 mm, 1–2 cm margins for BT of 1.01–2.0 mm, and 2 cm margins for BT of ≥2.01 mm [6]. To date, six randomized controlled trials (RCT) have been conducted to evaluate the effectiveness of wide (3–5 cm) vs. narrow (1–2 cm) margins in preventing head and neck melanoma recurrence [9]. No significant difference in local recurrence or overall survival was found between narrow versus wide margins [9]. However, no RCTs have been conducted to directly compare 1 cm vs. 2 cm margins. More conservative criteria (0.5 cm margins for BT <1.0 mm, 0.5–1.0 cm margins for BT of 1.01–2.0 mm, and 1.0 cm margins for BT of >2.0 mm) have been used for resection of melanomatous lesions near critical structures, such as the ear or eyelids, and did not result in a statistical difference in local recurrence rates [6].

Facial reconstruction is often a daunting process. The complex, delicate anatomy of this region demands a depth of understanding and preoperative planning that is uncommon elsewhere on the body. To further complicate matters, there is no one method of reconstruction that is perfectly suited to every geographic region of the face. Identical defects of the eyelid and lip have different functional and aesthetic consequences and may require very different approaches to reconstruction. Most defects of the head and neck may be addressed via primary closure, skin grafting, or local tissue rearrangement. Primary closure may be appropriate for smaller defects. Larger defects closed primarily may place tension on nearby structures and scars may contract over time, distorting the face. Full-thickness skin grafts are suited to defects with underlying collagenous support and sufficient soft tissue to accept a graft. When used inappropriately, however, skin grafts have poor long-term aesthetic results secondary to contracture or color mismatch [10]. Local free-tissue transfer is the workhorse of facial reconstruction and can be accomplished in single- or multi-staged procedures. Free-tissue transfer is ideal for larger defects as it provides stable coverage for extensive defects but without optimal color match and tissue bulk, resulting in acceptable long-term aesthetic and functional results [9].

Melanoma of the head and neck is a potentially devastating disease with an increasing incidence in our society. Early detection, adequate resection, and proper reconstruction are essential to achieve good outcomes for these patients. We hope the following chapters will serve as a general reference for the indications for and methods of reconstruction of head and neck defects secondary to melanoma extirpation.

References

1. Stadelmann W, McMasters K, Digenis A, Reintgen D. Cutaneous melanoma of the head and neck: advances in evaluation and treatment. Plast Reconstr Surg. 2000;105(6):2105–26.
2. Harris C, Bailey J, Blanchaert R. Surgical management of cutaneous melanoma of the head and neck. Oral Maxillofac Surg Clin North Am. 2005;17(2): 191–204.
3. Levine S, Shapiro R. Surgical treatment of malignant melanoma: practical guidelines. Dermatol Clin. 2012;30(3):487–501.
4. Cheriyan J, Wernberg J, Urquhart A. Head and neck melanoma. Surg Clin N Am. 2014;94(5):1091–113.
5. Bricca GM, Brodland DG, Ren D, Zitelli JA. Cutaneous head and neck melanoma treated with Mohs micrographic surgery. J Am Acad Dermatol. 2005;52(1): 92–100.
6. Rawlani R, Rawlani V, Qureshi HA, Kim JY, Wayne JD. Reducing margins of wide local excision in head and neck melanoma for function and cosmesis: 5-year local recurrence-free survival. J Surg Oncol. 2015; 111(7):795–9.
7. Rigel DS, Friedman RJ, Kopf AW, Polsky D. ABCDE—an evolving concept in early detection of melanoma. Arch Dermatol. 2005;141(8):1023–4.
8. Moyer JS. The increasing incidence of melanoma: it may be more than a freckle. JAMA Facial Plast Surg. 2017;19(1):62–3.
9. Zenga J, Nussenbaum B, Cornelius LA, Linette GP, Desai SC. Management controversies in head and neck melanoma: a systematic review. JAMA Facial Plast Surg. 2017;19(1):53–62.
10. Jose RM, Kisku W, Pradhan A, Prinsloo D. Management of complex melanomas of head and neck region. J Plast Reconstr Aesthet Surg. 2010;63(4):573–7.

Reconstruction Options for Ear and Nose Melanoma

22

Charles L. Dupin, Julian D'Achille, and Ian R. Wisecarver

Reconstruction of the Ear: Introduction

The ear is composed of hyaline cartilage and skin. It has subunits which include: the scaphae, the helix, the antihelix, the concha, the lobule, and the tragus (see Fig. 22.1). The skin on the anterior surface is thinner and more tightly adherent than that on the posterior surface. The ear, as a whole, has a robust vascular supply coupled with ample lymphatic drainage. This abundant blood supply makes the tissue of the ear resistant to necrosis, which, in turn, allows surgical manipulation that would be difficult elsewhere in the body.

The lymphatic drainage system of the ear is extensive, with several potential routes of lymphatic spread. In the case of melanoma, the excision of the primary lesion is often performed with a sentinel node harvest, located within the preauricular region, superficial parotid, or the submandibular region. The sentinel nodes may also be located within the five nodal levels of the neck or in the posterior auricular sulcus.

A primary melanoma is infrequently found on the ear. However, when it is encountered on the auricle, it carries a less favorable prognosis than in most other regions [1]. The National Comprehensive Cancer Network (NCCN) standard melanoma resection guidelines dictate that a primary melanoma of the ear should be treated according to the same guidelines as melanoma found in other locations. Thin melanoma requires a 1 cm margin, but a thicker melanoma requires a 2 cm resection margin.

In accordance with these resection guidelines, patients whom undergo resection will normally have a resultant defect roughly 2.5–4.5 cm size. However, some authors have suggested less aggressive margins to conserve precious auricular tissue. Bricca et al. [2] examined surgical margins for the head and neck melanomas in 652 patients, recommending the following surgical margins:

1. 9 mm for MIS and Breslow's depth of 1.01 mm.
2. 12 mm for Breslow's depth 1.01–2.00 mm, 2.01–4.00 mm.
3. At least 12 mm for a Breslow's depth of >4.00 mm.

C. L. Dupin, M.D. (✉) · J. D'Achille, M.D., M.P.H.
Division of Plastic and Reconstructive Surgery, Department of Surgery, Louisiana State University Health Sciences Center, New Orleans, LA, USA
e-mail: cdupin@lsuhsc.edu; jdachi@lsuhsc.edu

I. R. Wisecarver, B.S.
Louisiana State University Health Sciences Center, New Orleans, LA, USA
e-mail: iwisec@lsuhsc.edu

A. I. Riker (ed.), *Melanoma*, https://doi.org/10.1007/978-3-319-78310-9_22

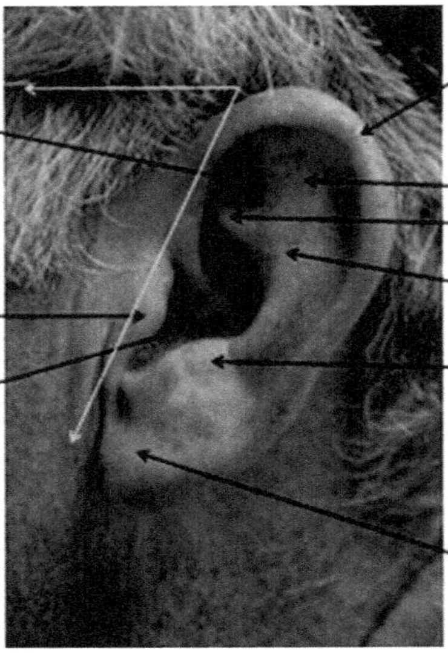

Fig. 22.1 External anatomy of the ear. Note the angle of the anterior ear relative to horizontal

These recommendations were based on evaluation of negative margins achieved with MOH Micrographic Surgery. Unfortunately, there were no cases involving the external ear and thus may not apply to this clinical situation.

A large series of melanomas of the external ear was reported by Jahn et al. [3]. They reported no reduction in survival with reduced margins although the risk of local recurrence was higher. They recommended against removing auricular cartilage unless it made reconstruction simpler. Specifically they did not clarify the issue of the perichondrium. There are other recommendations that minimal excision should include the underlying perichondrium, rendering other means of reconstruction necessary [4].

There have been other recent, limited studies which indicate that the recurrence rate is not increased when using more conservative, smaller resection margins [5, 6]. The tight adherence of the skin on the anterior surface makes it somewhat difficult to remove without exposing, and potentially damaging, underlying cartilage and perichondrium. This presents a challenge for reconstruction because damaged or exposed cartilage will not support a skin graft. Additionally, both anterior and posterior surfaces may require resection if the lesion involves the helical rim. Excision of the skin on the posterior surface is much easier as the skin is not very adherent to the perichondrium.

Skin grafts are a useful and versatile tool for reconstructing defects of the external ear. However, they are only appropriate if the underlying perichondrium, which can support a skin graft, is left intact. This is particularly true of the posterior surface of the ear where the skin is less adherent. On the anterior surface, if the perichondrium is preserved (not just the cartilage), full thickness skin grafts are appropriate. The simple plan to wait a week after excision will usually clarify if the perichondrium is present and graftable as granulation tissue will rapidly cover the perichondrium.

In some portions of the ear, such as the concha, the reconstruction can be simplified by removing underlying exposed but nonessential cartilage. This allows placement of a graft which will benefit from nourishment provided by the opposing side of the ear, where the skin and soft tissue are intact. This method is particularly useful in the concha, where the cartilage can be removed without severely deforming the contour of the ear.

The following algorithm may be helpful when evaluating reconstruction methods for a given defect of the ear (Fig. 22.2).

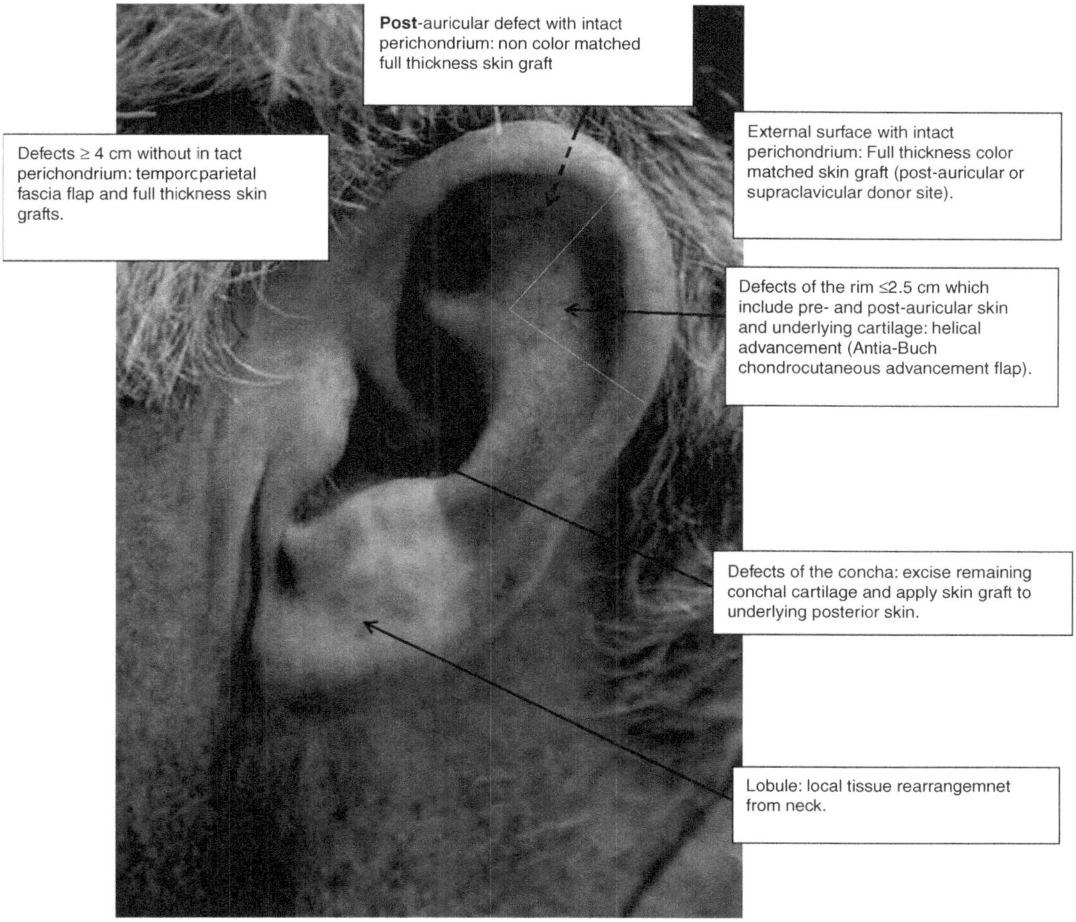

Fig. 22.2 Algorithm for reconstructing defects of the ear

Defects of the Anterior Ear with Intact Perichondrium

As described above, defects of the anterior ear in which intact perichondrium is exposed can be closed with Full-Thickness Skin Grafts (FTSG). These skin grafts will be supported appropriately by the underlying perichondrium and will have good overall graft viability. The postauricular area often serves as the optimal donor site by providing a graft with similar texture and color-match to the skin of the anterior ear (see Fig. 22.3). Following harvest of grafts up to 4 cm wide, the donor site can be closed primarily.

Defects of the Ear with Denuded, Nonessential Cartilage: (Concha Bowl)

Defects which do not have intact perichondrium covering exposed cartilage will not support a skin graft. As such, the exposed cartilage may be excised to expose the inner surface of the posterior skin. The exposed inner surface of the posterior skin provides the requisite blood supply to allow proper take of a FTSG. Again, the post-auricular skin provides optimal texture and color-match when choosing a donor site for FTSG's to repair defects of the anterior auricle (see Fig. 22.4).

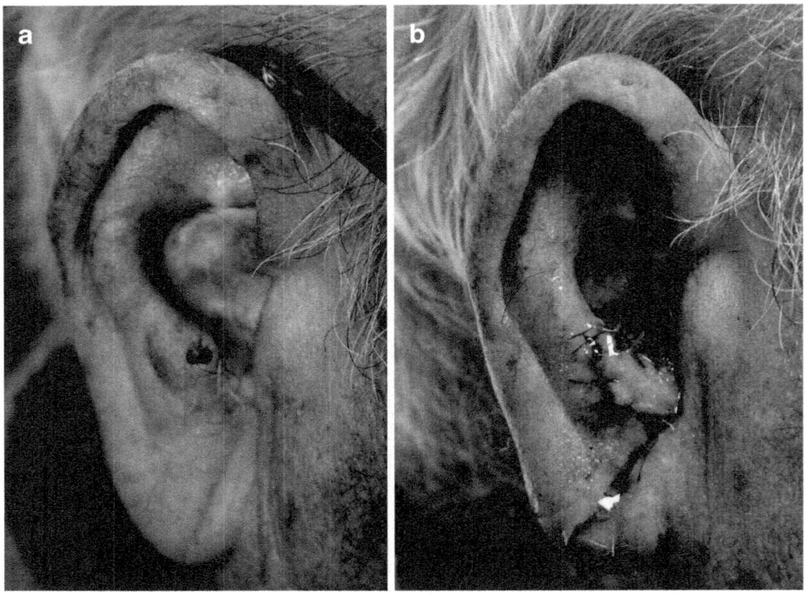

Fig. 22.3 (**a**) Small lesion of the anti-helix to be excised and a color-match graft place on the perichondrium. (**b**) Graft at 1 week with excellent vascular ingrowth

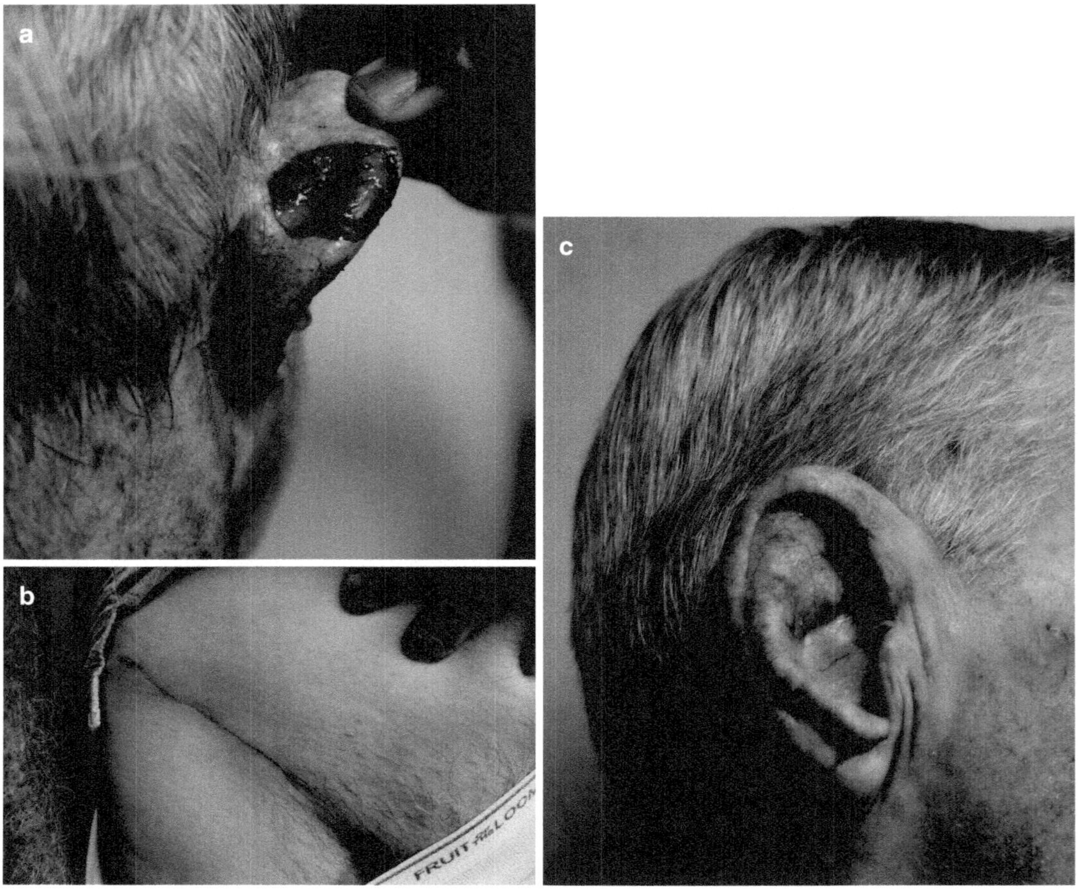

Fig. 22.4 (**a**) 2.5 cm, full thickness defect of the posterior ear with intact perichondrium. The perichondrium at 1 week has excellent granulation present. This will allow appropriate take of an FTSG. (**b**) Healed inguinal-crease donor site of FTSG. (**c**) Final appearance at 4 weeks

Defects of the Posterior Surface of the Ear

Defects of the Scapha, Anti-helix on the Anterior Surface, ≤2 cm in Diameter, with Intact, Essential, Denuded Cartilage

In this scenario, resection of the exposed cartilage will cause unacceptable deformity. It is possible to retain the essential cartilage and achieve appropriate coverage using an auricular flap, which is derived from the pre- or postauricular area and is based either superiorly or posteriorly. A small window through the auricle can be created by excising a small amount of intervening cartilage, allowing the flap to be carried through. In this manner, a posterior-based flap can provide coverage for the anterior auricle.

Unfortunately, this method requires a second stage of reconstruction because the flap will have to be taken down in a separate procedure. However, the post-auricular flap will restore the contour of the ear without decreasing its size and causing subsequent asymmetry with the other ear. It is possible to design a flap 2–3 cm in width and still close most of the post-auricular donor site defect by primary intention. If the donor site cannot be closed primarily, coverage can be achieved with skin grafting (see Fig. 22.5).

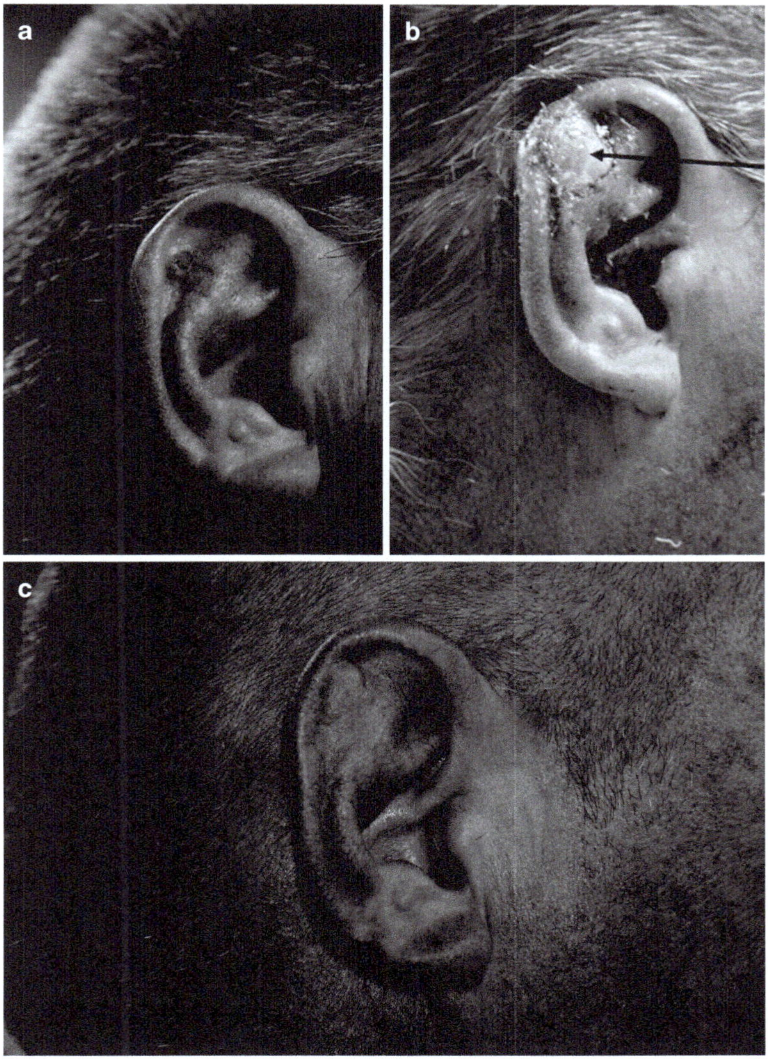

Fig. 22.5 (**a**) Lentigo maligna melanoma of the left ear. This lesion was excised with a 5 mm margin. (**b**) Reconstruction via post-auricular skin flap carried through a window created in the antihelix cartilage. (**c**) Final result after flap release

If more tissue is needed for adequate coverage, two auricular flaps may be implemented simultaneously. One derived from the pre-auricular sulcus and based inferiorly, and the other derived from the post-auricular area and based superiorly. The post-auricular flap will need to be carried through a window created in the intervening cartilage, as described above, to allow coverage of the anterior defect (see Fig. 22.6).

Defects of the Posterior Ear, 2–4 cm in Diameter, with Intact Perichondrium

Such defects can be repaired with a FTSG. If the defect is completely posterior, postoperative patient comfort will take precedence over color-matching and a noncolor-matched donor site will suffice (see Fig. 22.4).

Defects of the Helix ≤2.5 cm in Diameter with Denuded or Absent Cartilage Following Wedge Resection

Wedge resections are often implemented to remove lesions of the middle-upper helix that require excision of both pre-auricular and post-auricular skin. The reconstructive technique of choice, the Antia-Buch helical advancement flap, involves simultaneous V-Y advancement of superior and inferior helical skin flaps and continues to be a reliable method [7, 8].

Incisions following the junction of the antihelix and the helix are made along the anterior surface of the auricle to create superior and inferior helical flaps, which are composed of cartilage and anterior skin. The underlying cartilage is then incised with care being taken not to injure the opposing post-auricular skin, which serves as the blood supply for both helical flaps. The post-auricular skin can be undermined medially to allow further advancement of the superior and inferior helical flaps. When the superior and inferior flaps are advanced towards the middle of the would-be helix, some "cupping" of the helix may develop. Excising a small wedge of scaphal or helical cartilage relieves the cupping and allows for a more natural helical rim shape. The reconstructive process may be streamlined by removing the underlying cartilage and moving the remaining superior and inferior helix together. The final result of the Antia-Buch procedure is a smaller, but adequately shaped, ear (see Fig. 22.7).

Defects of the Lobule

There are a number of procedures for reconstructing the lobule. The most common method for reconstruction of the lobule is the implementation of locoregional flaps, which provide satisfactory substitutes for the missing anterior and posterior skin. A cartilage graft is not required as the lobule is not rigid; however, the flap should be made larger than the original lobule to allow for initial contracture. If necessary, a revision of the flap may be performed to achieve optimal shape.

Large Defects with Denuded or Resected Cartilage

Wide local excision (≥2 cm margins) is the currently accepted surgical resection margins for a melanoma with a Breslow's thickness >1 mm. The resultant defects can be quite large and repair via local tissue rearrangement, such as the Antia-Buch procedure, is often impractical. If the necessary resection is 4–5 cm, the challenge to reconstructing a realistic ear is daunting. If the entire ear is removed, the challenge is that much greater. The most common pathways for reconstruction of large defects of the ear are to rebuild the ear using locoregional flaps and grafts in tandem, if necessary, with costal cartilage grafts or Osseo-integrated implants for definitive coverage [9, 10] (see Fig. 22.8).

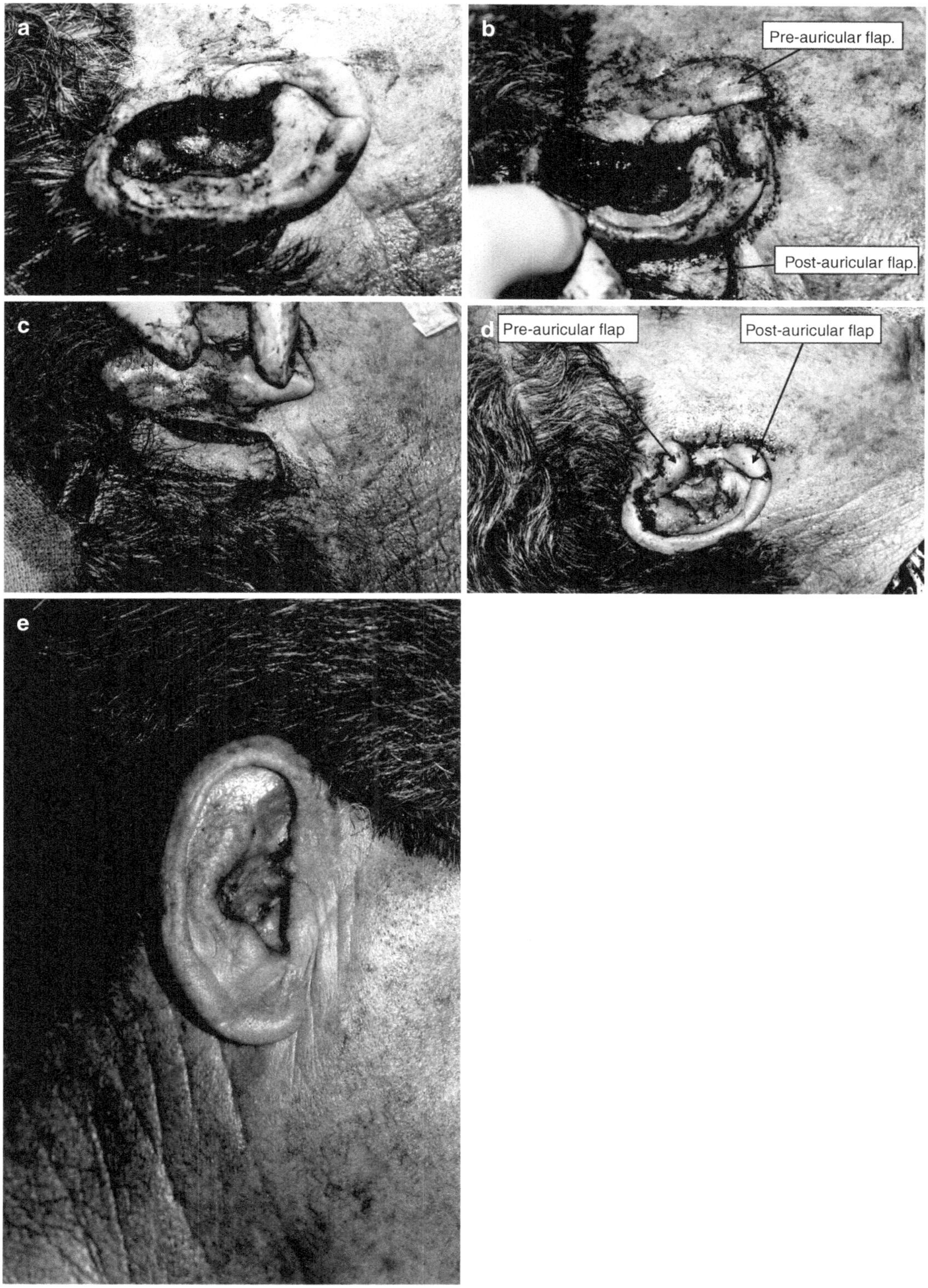

Fig. 22.6 (**a**) Defect of the anterior ear with denuded cartilage—perichondrium is not intact, thus FTSG would not have good take. (**b**) Pre-auricular and post-auricular flaps elevated simultaneously. The posterior flap will enter through a window created in the cartilage. (**c**) Post-auricular flap. (**d**) Flaps inset. (**e**) Final result after release of flaps

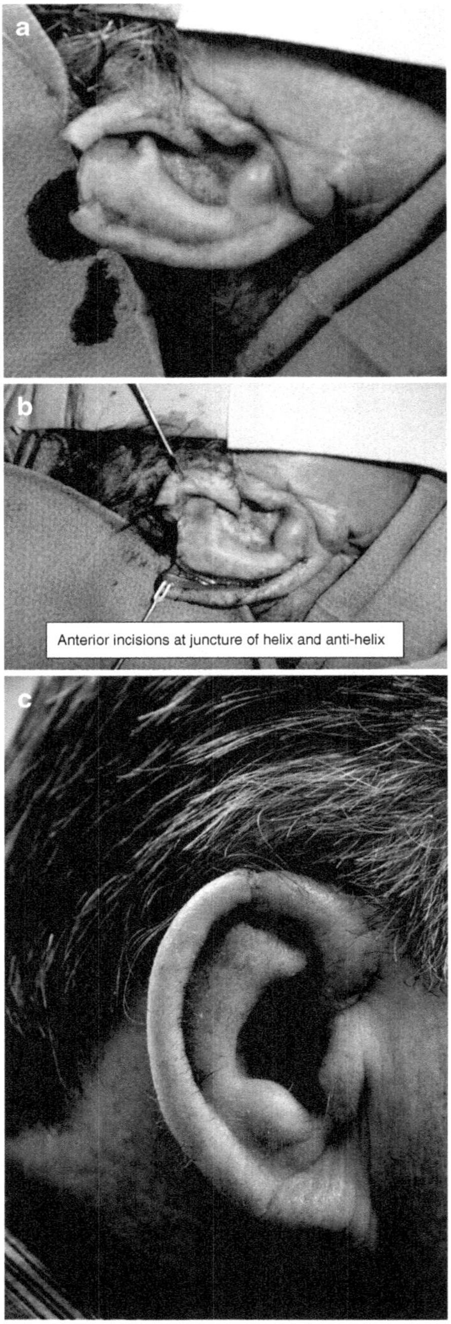

Fig. 22.7 (**a**) Composite, wedge resection of a mid-helix lesion. The resultant defect was approximately 2 cm. The reconstructive method of choice for a defect such as this is Antia-Buch helical advancement. (**b**) Superior and inferior helix flaps, based on the posterior auricular skin, will be advanced simultaneously into the defect. Note: A wedge of scaphal cartilage has been removed to prevent cupping of the reconstructed ear. (**c**) Final result

Defects of the Scapha and Antihelix, 3–4 cm in Diameter with Denuded Cartilage

Reconstructing such a large defect of the scapha and antihelix requires tissue from regional donor sites. The most commonly implemented locoregional flap is the temporoparietal fascial (TPF) flap. The temporoparietal fascia is thin and highly vascular. This fascial plain lies beneath the temporal subcutaneous fat and the underlying deep temporal fascia while covering the temporalis fascia. In approximately 85% of the population, the temporoparietal fascia derives its blood supply from branches of the superficial temporal vessels. TPF flaps are thin and pliable, as such, they can be satisfactorily contoured to cartilaginous defects with complex shapes while still supporting a skin graft. Full thickness grafts are preferred for final closure because they are less likely to contract and subsequently distort the ear (see Fig. 22.9).

Defects of the Helix 4 cm in Diameter

Large defects of the helix reconstructed with TPF flaps and full thickness or split thickness skin grafts harvested from the scalp experience the best outcomes [11–18]. The temporoparietal flap (TPF), however, must have a rigid support framework to provide a realistic post-reconstruction appearance. If underlying cartilage is still present, it may be possible to cover it with a TPF flap. If there is no native cartilage remaining after resection, there are two methods for creating a replacement support. The first is a carved cartilage graft, harvested from the sixth, seventh, and eighth ribs. This method, popularized by Brent, was initially employed in microtia [19–23]. When this method of support is performed correctly, the final result of reconstruction can be highly exacting. However, the process of carving the cartilage graft, achieving appropriate coverage via TPF and FTSG, and stabilizing the ear can be challenging. Additionally, harvesting the rib can result in some deformity of the chest wall.

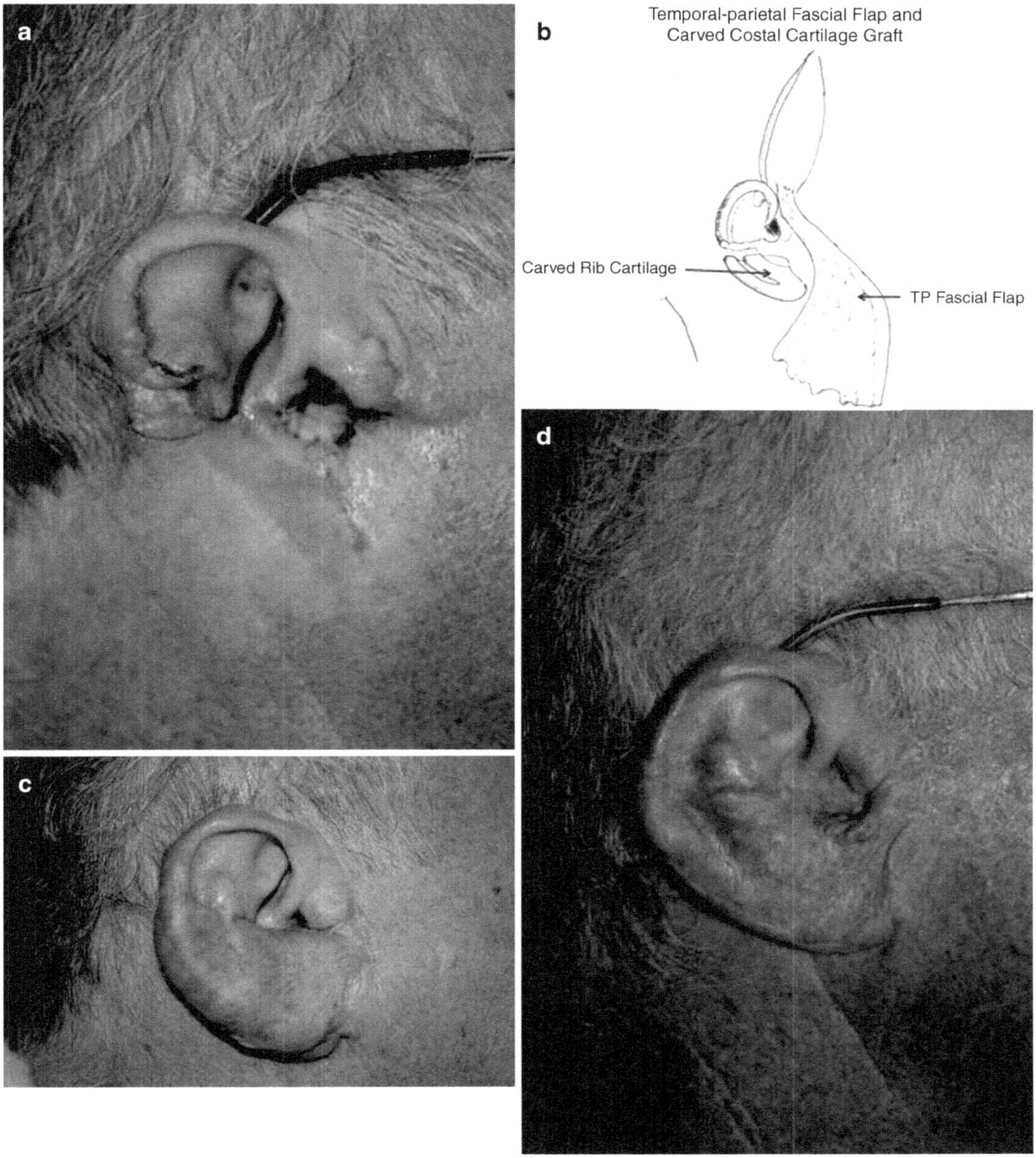

Fig. 22.8 (**a**) This patient presented with a defect comprising the lower half of his ear. The defect will be reconstructed using a costal cartilage graft, temporoparietal fascia flap, and FTSG. (**b**) Diagram of the TFP and Costal Cartilage Graft reconstruction plan. (**c**) Early postoperative appearance. Note the residual edema under the full thickness graft, it will take months to resolve completely. (**d**) Final appearance at 6 months

The second method is the use of a prosthetic framework, such as Silicone and Medpore® materials. Although the use of prosthetic material does not create chest wall deformities, they are more prone to chronic problems such as infection, seroma, and implant extrusion. Prosthetics are also more susceptible to trauma than autologous frameworks. Excellent results have been published in the literature, and it is the authors' opinion that prosthetic frameworks are a suitable alternative to rib-harvest [22–28].

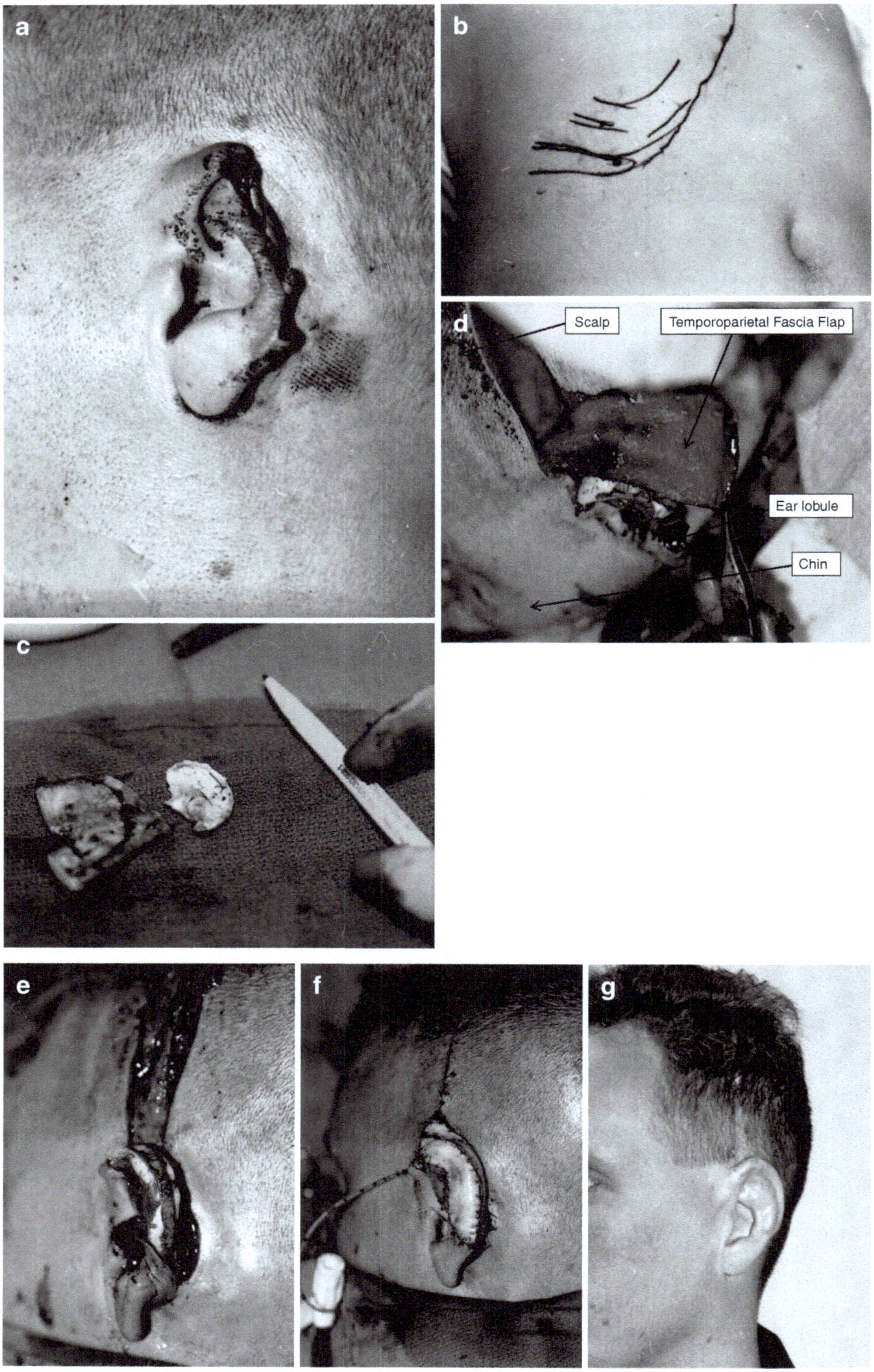

Fig. 22.9 (**a**) Patient with resection involving ≥40% of the posterior ear, including the scapha and helix. (**b**) Costal cartilage (outlined in blue ink) will be harvested to provide a cartilaginous framework for helix reconstruction using TPF flap and FTSG. (**c**) Costal cartilage graft which will be shaped to match the defect template on the right. (**d**) Elevating the TPF flap. (**e**) Costal cartilage graft in place. The TPF flap will be inset over the cartilage graft and then covered with a FTSG. (**f**) TPF flap covered with color-matched FTSG harvested from the supraclavicular area. (**g**) Final result

Reconstruction of the Nose: Introduction

The nose is a central feature of the face which comprises multiple aesthetic subunits. This structural complexity can prove challenging during reconstruction (see Fig. 22.10). Incisions placed in subunit borders tend to form less visible scars because they will be hidden within plane changes. It is also very important to preserve symmetry between paired structures because the human eye can detect even the slightest asymmetry [29, 30]. Many cutaneous malignancies involving the nose often require excision of additional underlying tissue, including bone, cartilage, and, occasionally, the inner lining of the nose. As a rule, resection of melanoma and lentigo maligna requires excision of the skin and subcutaneous tissue; however, special consideration should be given to the amount of tissue excised when these lesions occur on the nose.

Relative to each aesthetic subunit, nasal skin varies in thickness and degree of adherence to underlying tissue. Skin over the dorsum is thick, loose, and non-adherent to an underlying layer of mimetic muscle. The dorsum plane is curvilinear and has a subtle juncture with the tip. The nasal sidewalls are anatomically similar to the dorsum but are flatter, more shadowed, and less prominent.

The skin over the nasal tip and columella is thin and adherent to the underlying cartilage, which makes it difficult to achieve simple closure without subsequent distortion. The nasal tip and columella have underlying, firm, paired lower lateral cartilages which frequently can be seen. The soft tissue triangle has no cartilaginous support and the thin skin is adherent to underlying vestibular skin.

The skin over the alae is tightly bound to underlying fibrocartilage, which, in turn, is adherent to underlying vestibular skin. The rigid skin of the sill is adherent to and covers the feet of the medial crura of the underlying tip cartilage [29].

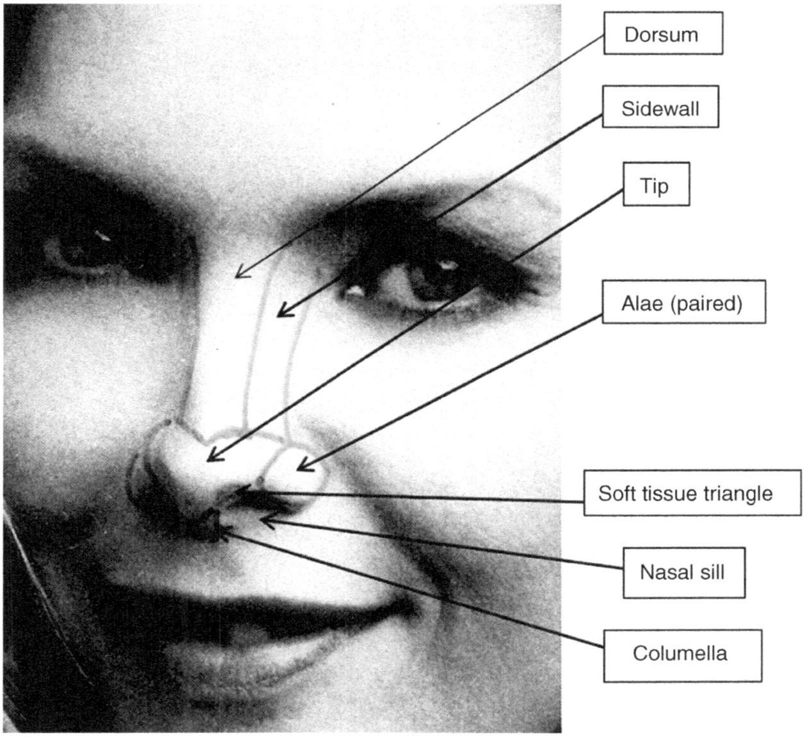

Fig. 22.10 Aesthetic subunits of the nose—the green lines indicate borders between subunits

Optimum Repair by Subunit

Nasal Dorsum

Due to the relatively simple architecture and the loose skin, small lesions may be excised and the defect closed along minimal skin tension lines (MSTL). Defects larger than 10 mm are difficult to close satisfactorily without generating excess wound tension and creating long "dog-ears."

The nasal dorsum can be repaired via full thickness skin graft (FTSG), provided a donor site is available that is appropriately color-matched. A FTSG derived from the forehead, postauricular area, neck, and supraclavicular area produces good, color-matched final results in nasal reconstruction (see Fig. 22.11). Specifically, the "widow's peak" area of the forehead has excellent color-match and thickness. A FTSG from this region can be harvested up to 2 cm in width with minimal donor site distortion. Although melanoma resection involves excision of the skin and subcutaneous tissue above the cartilage, there is often adequate residual soft tissue remaining over the cartilage and bone to properly support a graft and allow for good graft viability [31].

If a defect of the dorsum encroaches on the nasal tip, a *dorsal nasal flap* may be the optimal reconstructive approach. The vascular supply to this flap is derived from terminal branches of the contralateral angular artery. The flap should be elevated with underlying soft tissue intact to ensure its viability [32] (see Fig. 22.12).

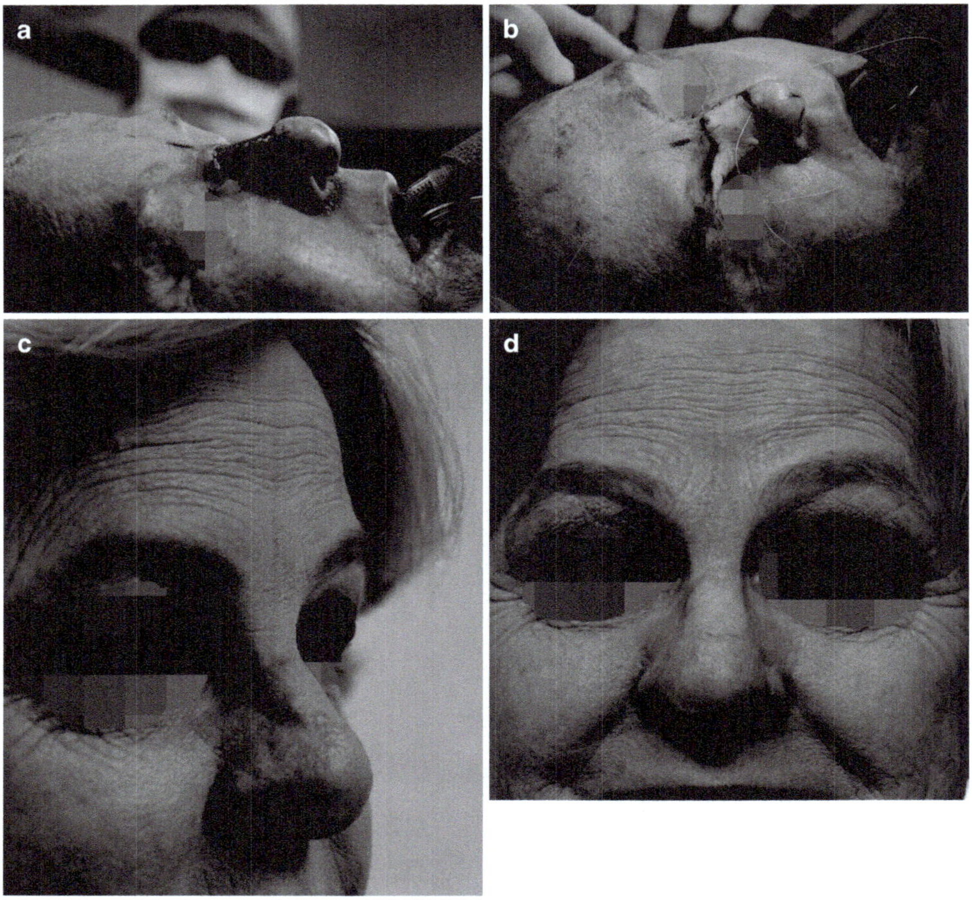

Fig. 22.11 (**a**) Full thickness excision of the nasal dorsum and sidewall. (**b**) Full thickness supraclavicular skin graft sewn in place. (**c**) Post-operative appearance at 1 month. (**d**) Post-operative appearance at 6 months

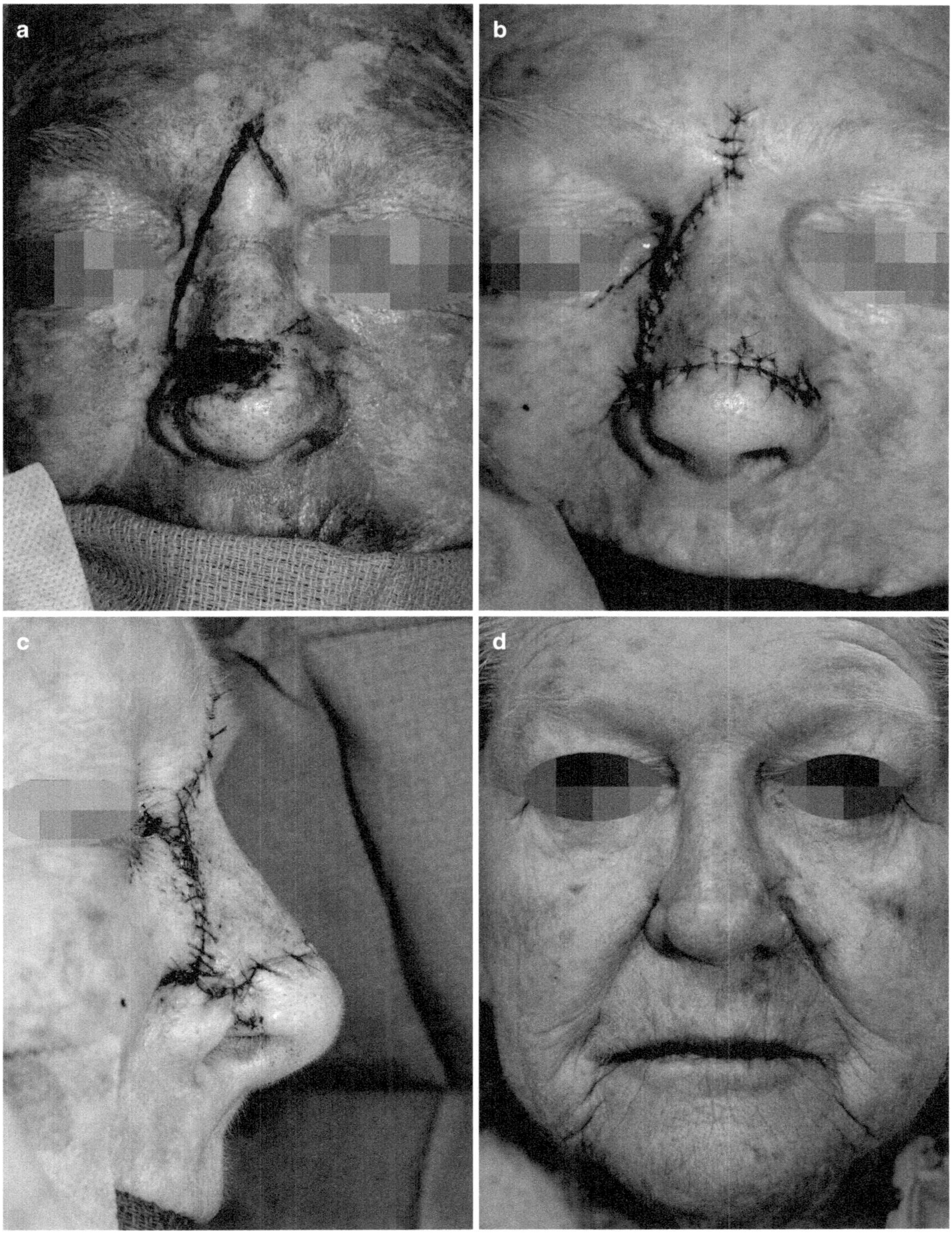

Fig. 22.12 (**a**) Full thickness excision of a lesion involving the supra-tip dorsum. Blue ink outlines the flap, which may easily be advanced to cover the defect. The donor area can be closed with V-Y advancement. (**b**) After elevation and inset frontal view. (**c**) After dorsal nasal flap advancement and inset. (**d**, **e**) Post-operative appearance at 3 months

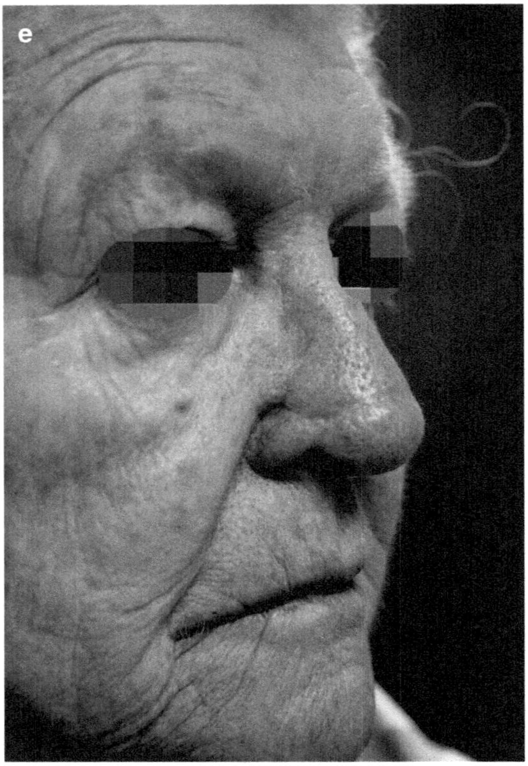

Fig. 22.12 (continued)

Nasal Sidewall

The nasal sidewalls can also be reconstructed with FTSG as long as there is soft tissue covering underlying bone and cartilage [31]. Smaller defects may be closed with local tissue rearrangement, such as the rhomboid flap. When viewing the face, under normal circumstances, the nasal sidewalls are largely in shadow. Thus, scar formation in this subunit is somewhat masked, providing a measure of forgiveness to the reconstructive surgeon [30]. Lesions which are too complex for full thickness grafting may be addressed with local tissue rearrangement, such as the "cocked-hat flap" (see Fig. 22.13).

Nasal Tip

Defects of the tip of the nose, certainly those over 4 mm, are difficult to close primarily. Additionally, the prominence of the nasal tip suggests that scar formation be kept to a minimum. If resection of a lesion requires excising ≥40% of the nasal tip, a better outcome will likely be achieved by removing the remaining skin and reconstructing the entire aesthetic unit [29, 30]. Many techniques have been proposed for reconstruction of the nasal tip; from the author's perspective, the most efficient and relevant are described below.

Skin Grafting

Melanoma excision, as a rule, does not expose the entire underlying cartilage, a FTSG derived from the forehead often provides satisfactory results. Forehead skin is a perfect color-match for nasal tip skin and its ample dermal thickness assures the graft will not appear depressed at final result [31]. Forehead FTSGs should be removed from the "widow's peak" area so as not to preclude the use of a paramedian forehead flap in the future. Grafts larger than 2 cm can be harvested but the donor site should be closed with a "ying-yang" tissue rearrangement to avoid excess tension.

The deep surface of the graft should have a trace of underlying fat. The harvested graft must then be affixed to the nasal tip. Circumferential and quilting sutures, which pass through underlying cartilage, are used to anchor it firmly in place [31]. To prevent desiccation, the graft must be covered with antibiotic ointment two times a day during the first postoperative. These grafts are very reliable; however, the reconstructive surgeon must counsel all patients not to manipulate postoperative graft crusting and to have patience with healing process (see Figs. 22.14 and 22.15).

Bilobed and Rhomboid Flaps

If the underlying soft tissue has been completely removed and bare, or the incised cartilage alone comprises the wound bed, there is not sufficient tissue present to allow for viability of a FTSG. In this case, a flap must be used to cover the exposed cartilage. The bilobed flap provides well-vascularized tissue and has been recommended for coverage of exposed, underlying structures such as described above [33, 34]. This method of local tissue rearrangement relies heavily on successful intraoperative design, the efficacy of which is critical for achieving satisfactory coverage (see Fig. 22.16).

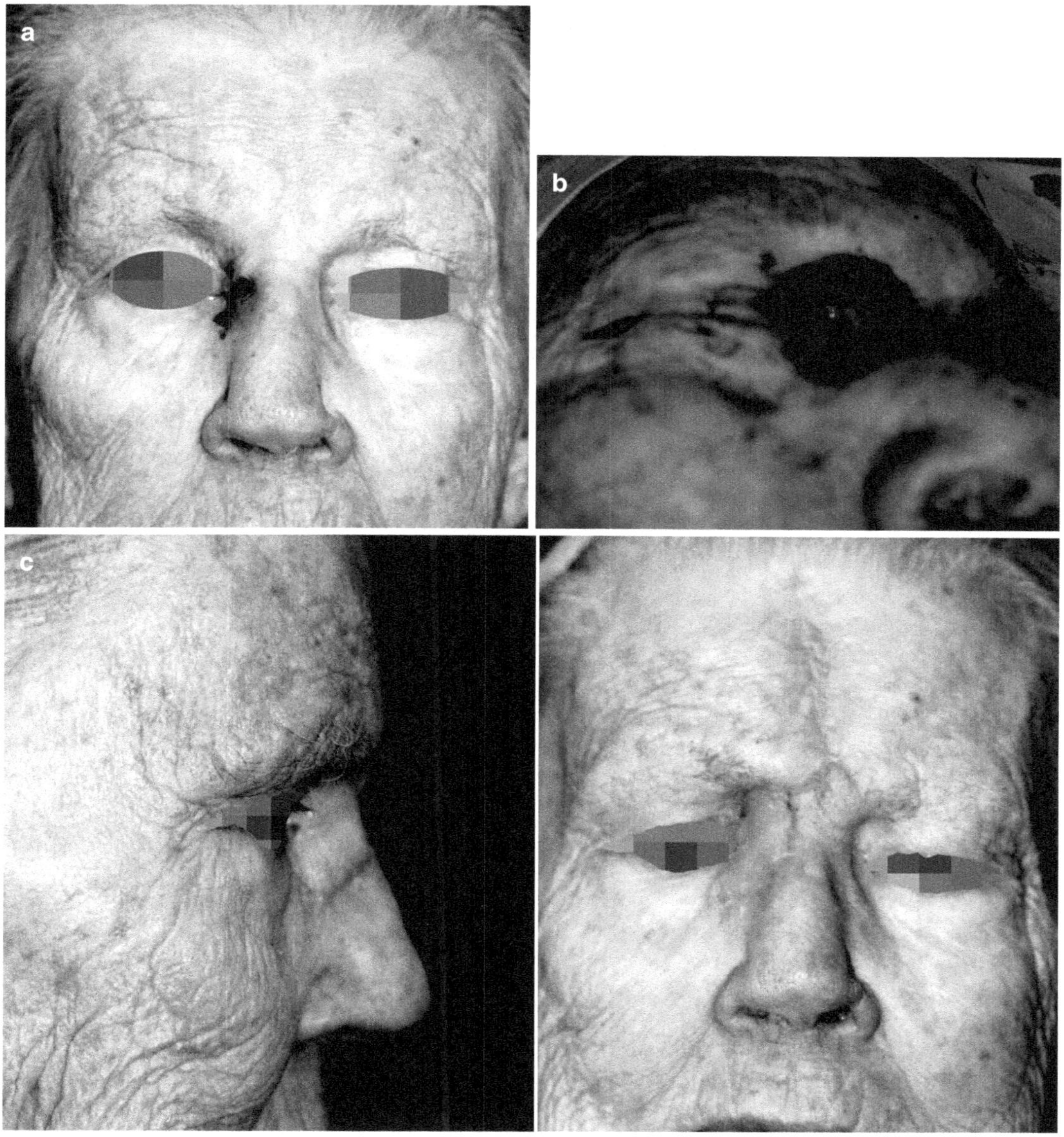

Fig. 22.13 (**a**) Lesion of the nasal sidewall and medial canthal region. (**b**) Nasal sidewall and medial canthal defect. (**c**) Post-operative appearance at 1 month

Unfortunately, there are two significant drawbacks to using the bilobed flap for closure of nasal tip defects. Defects ≥1.5 cm may place tension on the underlying cartilaginous support, resulting in deformity of the tip. The flap also creates a significant amount of scarring at the donor site, which may be difficult to camouflage. Relative to the loose skin of the elderly, this is especially true in young patients with taut skin. Despite these drawbacks, the bilobed flap is an effective tool for the repair of nasal tip defects (see Fig. 22.17).

If the defect involves the tip-alae-sidewall area (i.e., the soft tissue triangle), where there is no native cartilage providing support, the flap may undergo contracture and distort the nasal tip and nostril rim. A cartilage graft, most commonly harvested from the auricle, should be implemented to support the bilobed flap and reduce the likelihood of long-term contracture [35] (see Fig. 22.18).

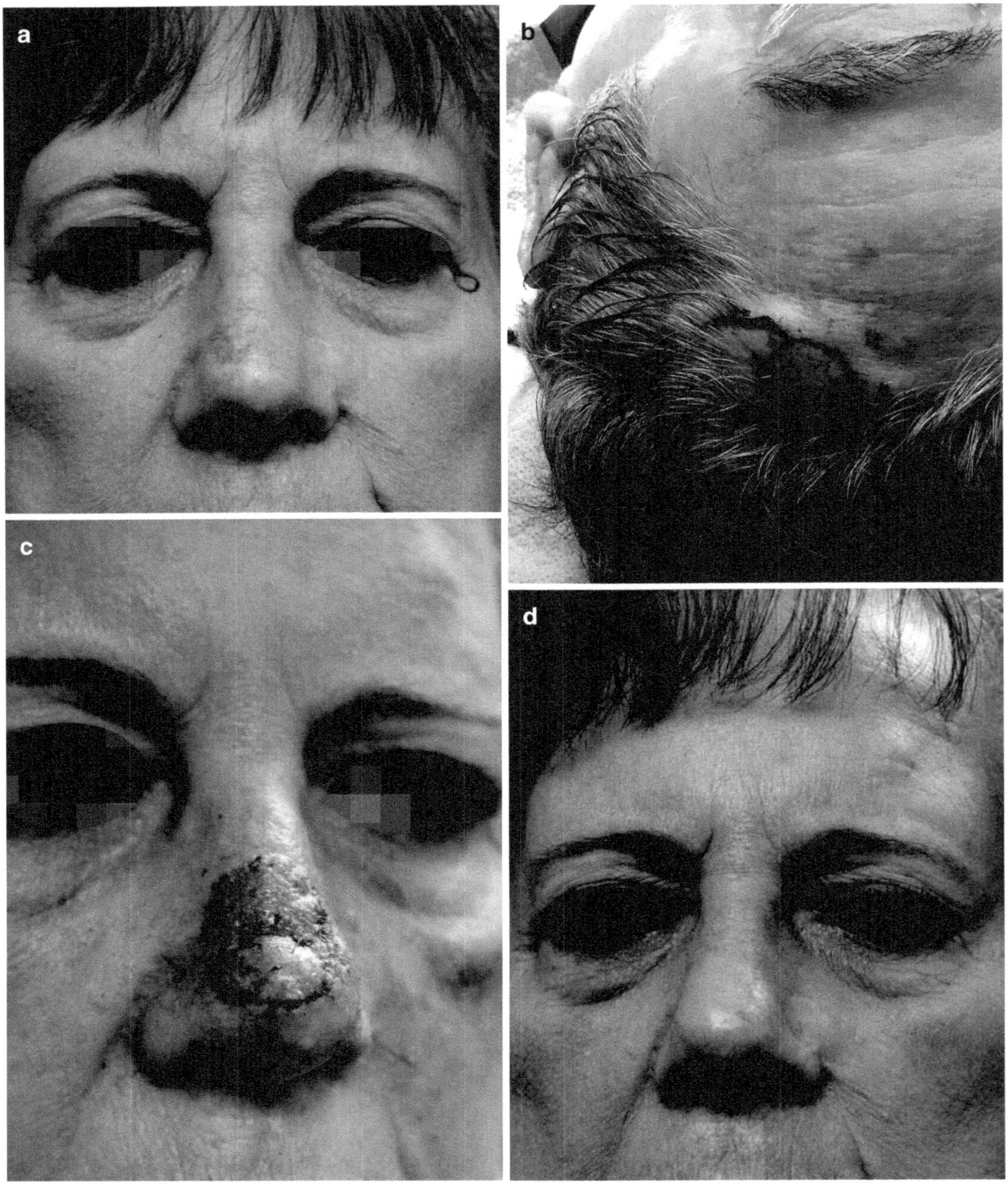

Fig. 22.14 (**a**) Lentigo maligna of the right nasal tip. (**b**) Closure of widow's peak donor site with ying-yang local tissue rearrangement. (**c**) FTSG at 1 week, secured with quilting sutures. (**d**) Final result at 6 months

Another flap that is well suited to the repair of partial nasal tip defects is the rhomboid flap. This form of local tissue rearrangement is especially adept at closing defects of the sidewall and tip junction. This flap, much like the bilobed flap, must be carefully designed such that the tension generated by closure does not distort the donor area. However, we have not found the rhomboid flap suitable for repair of isolated nasal tip defects (see Fig. 23.3 in Chap. 23).

Fig. 22.15 Another patient who underwent FTSG, harvested from the forehead, for repair of a nasal tip defect. Pictured at 2 months post-op

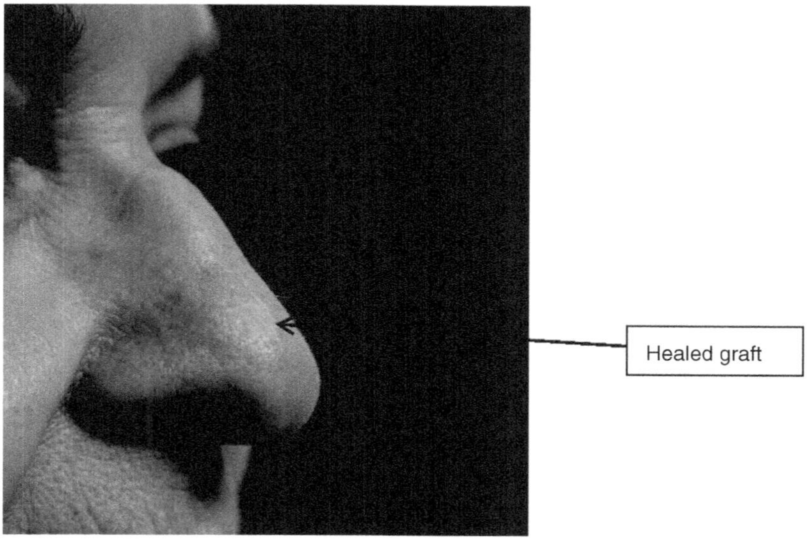

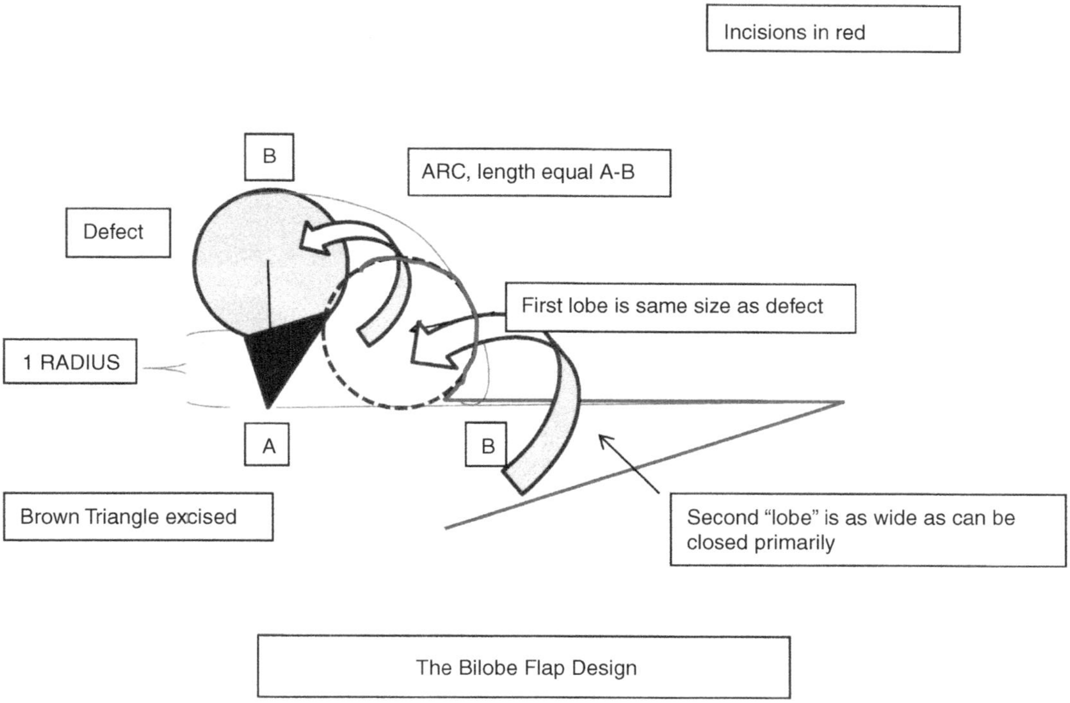

Fig. 22.16 The Bilcbe Flap Design

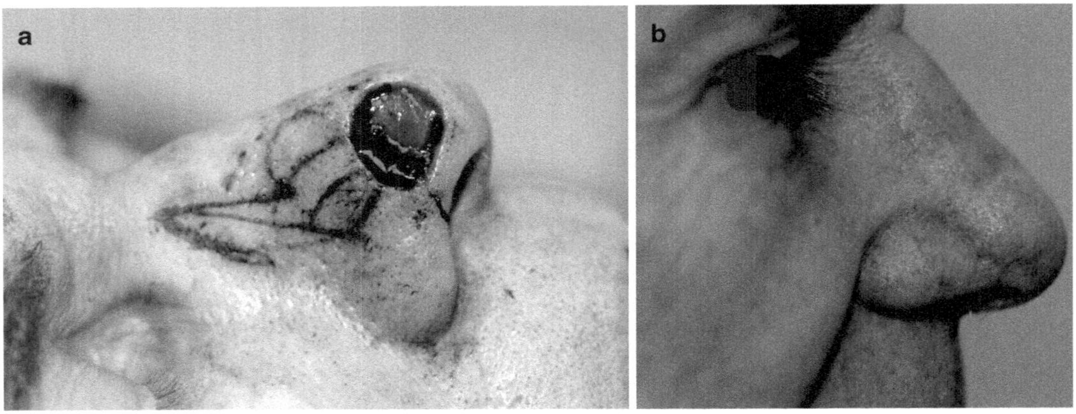

Fig. 22.17 (**a**) Nasal tip defect and bilobed flap design (blue ink). Note that the donor site is parallel to the long axis of the nose. (**b**) Post-operative appearance at 6 months after repair with bilobed flap

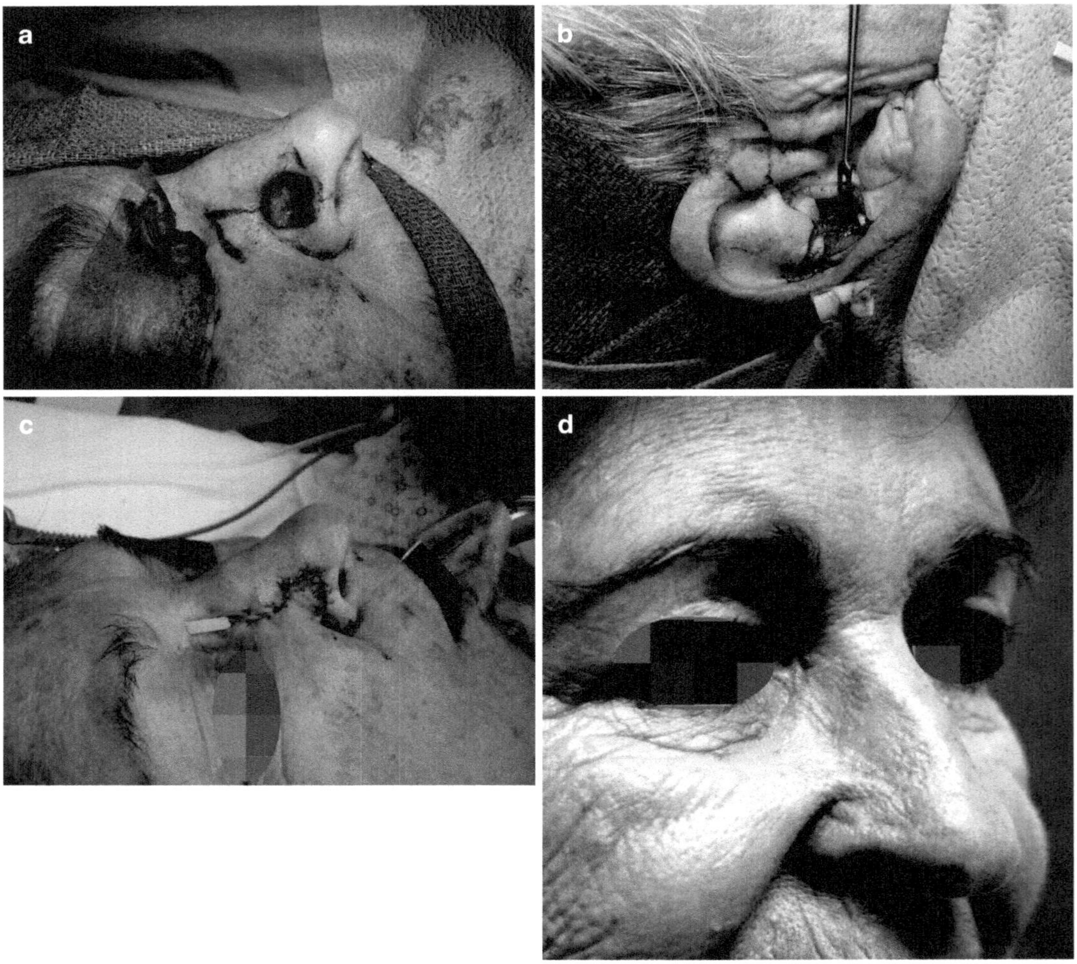

Fig. 22.18 (**a**) Even though only skin was resected from the soft tissue triangle, support must be provided to ensure the rim will not be distorted by wound contracture. (**b**) Auricular cartilage comparable in shape to the defect is harvested and placed in the defect prior to flap inset. (**c**) Bilobed flap rotated into position and inset over the graft. (**d**) Final result at 6 months

Paramedian Forehead Flap

The paramedian forehead flap is the gold standard for tip resurfacing when most, or all, of the tip is resected and when a forehead-derived FTSG is not possible [36, 37]. The paramedian forehead flap is extremely reliable when designed properly. Decisions concerning where to inset the base of the flap on the nasal dorsum is surgeon-dependent and determines the pattern of scar formation. Flaps inset in the supra-tip area result in a scar at the junction of the supra-tip and dorsum. If the remaining dorsal skin is removed, and the flap is inset in the glabella, visible scars of the nasal sidewalls will result (see Fig. 22.19).

The supra-trochlear artery provides the primary blood supply for paramedian forehead flaps. A handheld ultrasound Doppler device may be utilized to help locate the artery, which frequently lies beneath the medial brow hair. It is important that the pedicle width at the brow not exceed 1.5 cm in width. If the pedicle is too wide, it will create tension when rotated down to the nose. The part of the flap which is to cover the defect is drawn on the forehead using a template of the tip defect. If the paramedian forehead flap is chosen for reconstruction, consider resecting the entire tip subunit to avoid placing scars outside the subunit border [36, 37]. The flap should be harvested with margins slightly larger than the template because the templates are inexact and do not account for flap thickness.

The flap is elevated above the pericranium and includes the frontalis muscle and fascia. The flap length requirements can be determined by tethering the proximal end of the template to the brow. If an increase in length is required, the flap elevation may be continued through the brow hair. Ideally, hair-bearing skin is not carried down to the tip defect. However, if it is not possible to avoid harvesting hair-bearing skin of the scalp, the patient can undergo laser treatments for hair removal at a later date.

Reconstruction with a paramedian forehead flap is generally completed in three stages. During Stage I, the flap is elevated and the donor site is partially closed. Full closure of the donor site is usually not possible at this stage; however, if the pericranium is intact, the donor site defect will heal very well by wound contracture. The distal part of the flap can be partially thinned during Stage I in non-smokers.

Stage II is planned for the third post-operative week. At that time, the flap is re-elevated to allow resection of the frontalis muscle and much of the subcutaneous fat. Successful Stage II thinning results in an appropriate thickness match to nasal tip skin. After contouring the flap to match native tissue, quilting sutures are used to secure the flap to underlying cartilage and prevent hematoma formation.

The third, and final, stage entails detaching the paramedian forehead flap from the forehead. Stage III is normally executed 4 weeks after Stage II. However, patients that smoke may require additional post-operative recovery time prior to detachment. Healing and resolution of edema occur more rapidly as the flap remains attached to the forehead for longer periods of time. When the flap is finally released, the proximal portion of the flap can be thinned a final time prior to inset via quilting sutures. The entire flap is not returned to the forehead, rather the brow is realigned and small triangle is set back into the donor site defect.

Nasal Alae

Defects involving the alar rim are somewhat complex because the rim is so sharply demarcated and there is no native cartilage to provide support. For this reason, simple FTSG are not appropriate for reconstruction of the nasal alae because they do not receive adequate support and are likely to undergo contracture and distortion of the rim. Rim reconstruction, much like soft tissue triangle reconstruction, requires harvesting and placing a cartilaginous graft in the defect to prevent wound contracture [35]. There are a variety of approaches to alar reconstruction, the most notable of which are described below.

Composite Graft

A composite graft from the ear can restore the contour of ala defects ≤12 mm in width. The graft is normally harvested from the anterior helix, which can be closed without subsequent deformity [38]. If <40% of the alae has been resected, and the vestibular lining is intact, a composite graft may be used for definitive coverage [38]. If >40% of the alae has been resected, the whole alae should be reconstructed simulta-

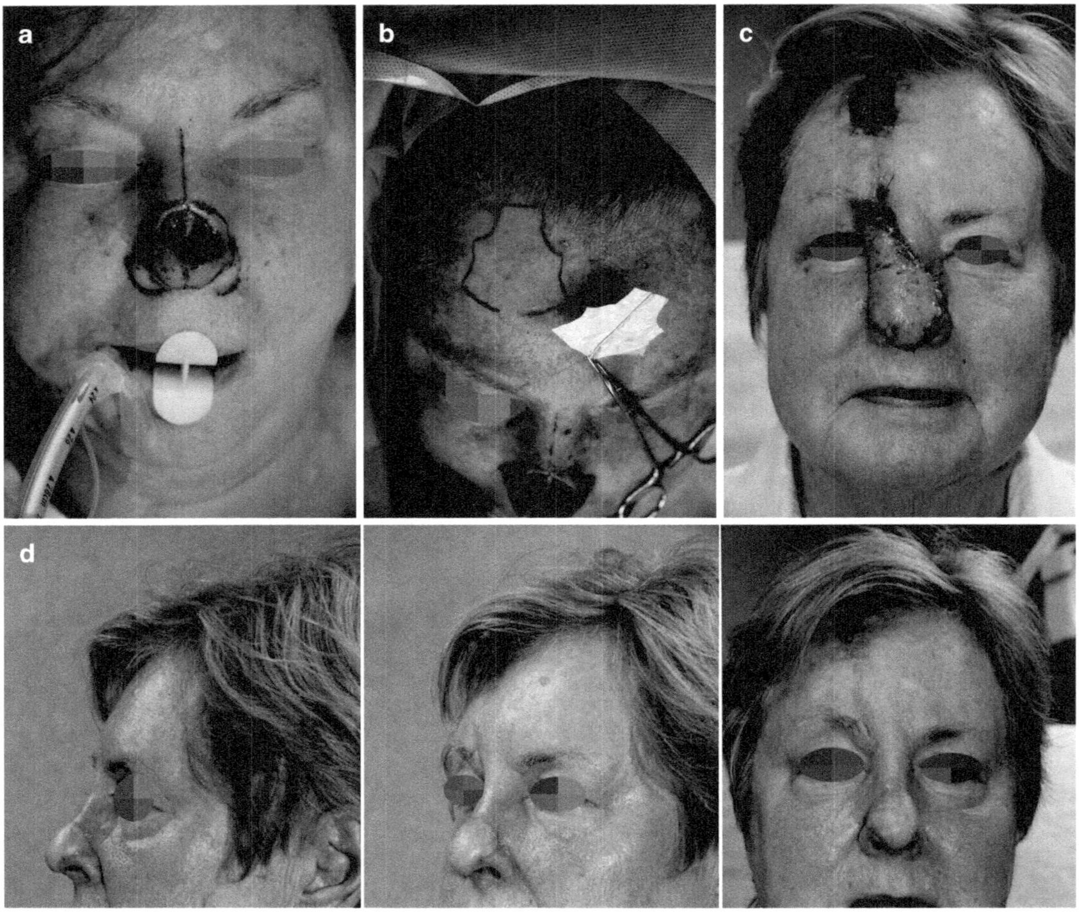

Fig. 22.19 (**a**) Defect of the nasal tip with exposed cartilage. In this patient, the remainder of the nasal tip skin will be excised so the flap may form a uniform, non-scarred surface for the tip at final result. The incision, indicated by blue ink, will be placed in the border between the alae and nasal tip subunits. It proceeds inferiorly along the columella such that the scar will form below the curve of the nasal tip. (**b**) Paramedian forehead flap template (Stage I). Note the marking suture running along the right brow line to the base of the template. (**c**) Flap in place, prior to thinning (Stage II), at 3 weeks post-op. Note the superior portion of the donor site healing by wound contracture. (**d**) Appearance at 4 months after detachment, thinning, and inset (Stage III) of the paramedian forehead flap

neously. Unfortunately, composite grafts larger than 1 cm have poorly predictable take and flap reconstruction is often required. The composite cartilage graft is sutured to the defect and covered with ointment to prevent desiccation. It is critical to be patient and leave the graft alone so it may become a viable composite graft. These grafts frequently appear inviable; however, once they have been placed in the defect, they must be left unmolested (see Fig. 22.20).

Nasolabial Flap

Nasolabial flaps are especially useful in the treatment of elderly patients. Lax tissue in the anterior cheek permits a flap of up to 2 cm in width to be harvested. The blood supply of the nasolabial flap is derived from perforating peri-labial vessels. These vessels are approximately 1–1.5 cm from the lateral alae, which must be left intact to protect the flap's vascular support. It is worth mentioning again that a cartilage graft is required to prevent contracture, even if there was no native cartilage in the subunit prior to resection. To optimize the final aesthetic result of the alar reconstruction, the flap should be lifted at 2 weeks for thinning and contouring. After thinning, the flap is placed back on the incorporated cartilage graft via bolster sutures [39] (see Fig. 22.21).

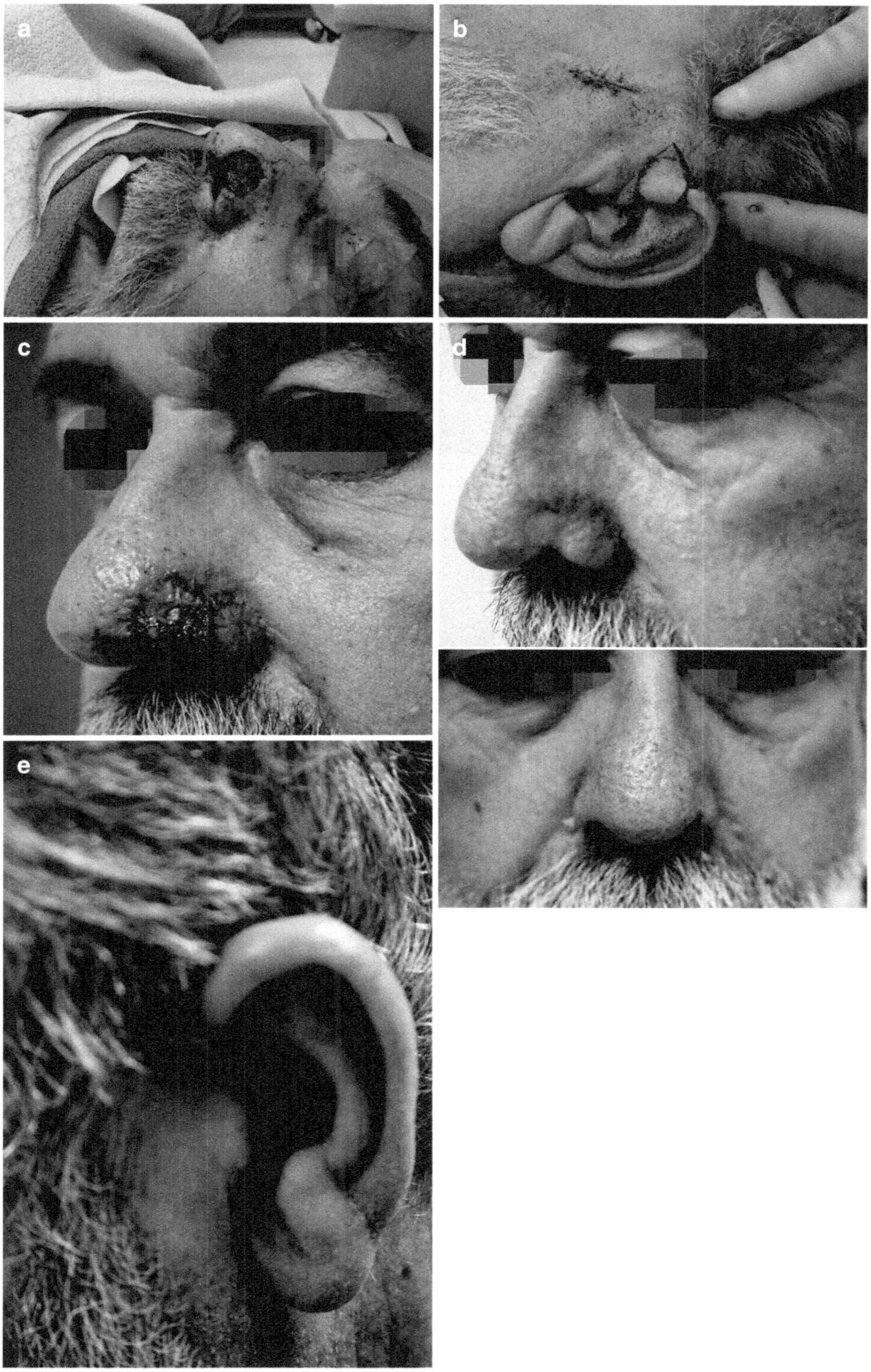

Fig. 22.20 (**a**) Defect involving the rim and alae. The underlying vestibular skin is intact, but there is insufficient support to prevent contracture. (**b**) The composite graft includes anterior skin, underlying cartilage, and posterior skin. The donor site is closed by primary intention. (**c**) Appearance of the composite graft at 1 week post-op. (**d**) Appearance of the composite graft at 3 months post-op. (**e**) Donor site at 3 months post-op

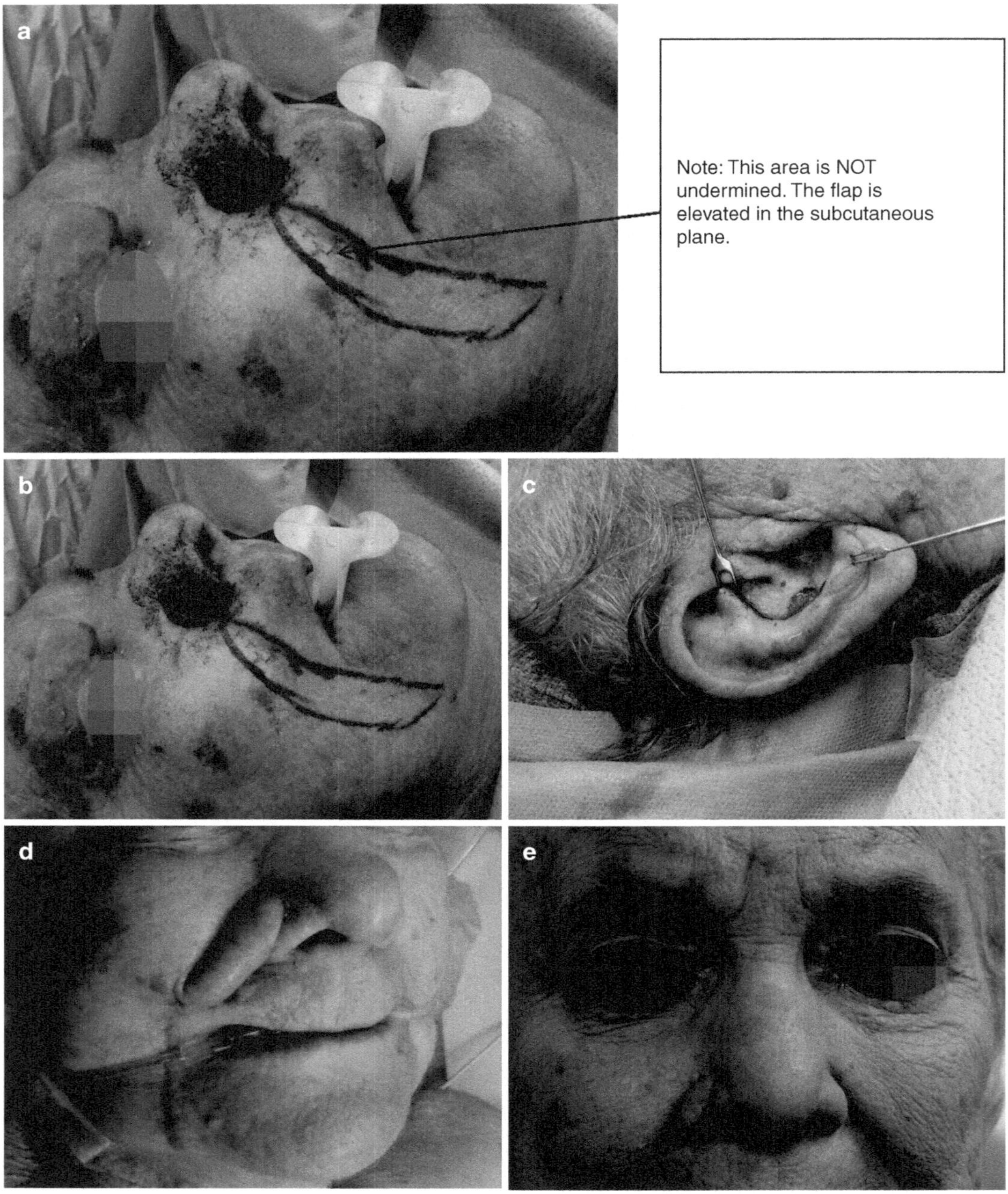

Fig. 22.21 (**a**) Defect of the right nasal ala. The nasolabial flap design is represented in blue ink. A cartilage graft must be placed prior to flap inset. (**b**) A template of the defect is used to determine the size of the auricular cartilage graft. (**c**) Harvesting the auricular cartilage graft. (**d**) Flap inset, prior to thinning at 3 weeks post-op. (**e**) Postoperative appearance at 4 months

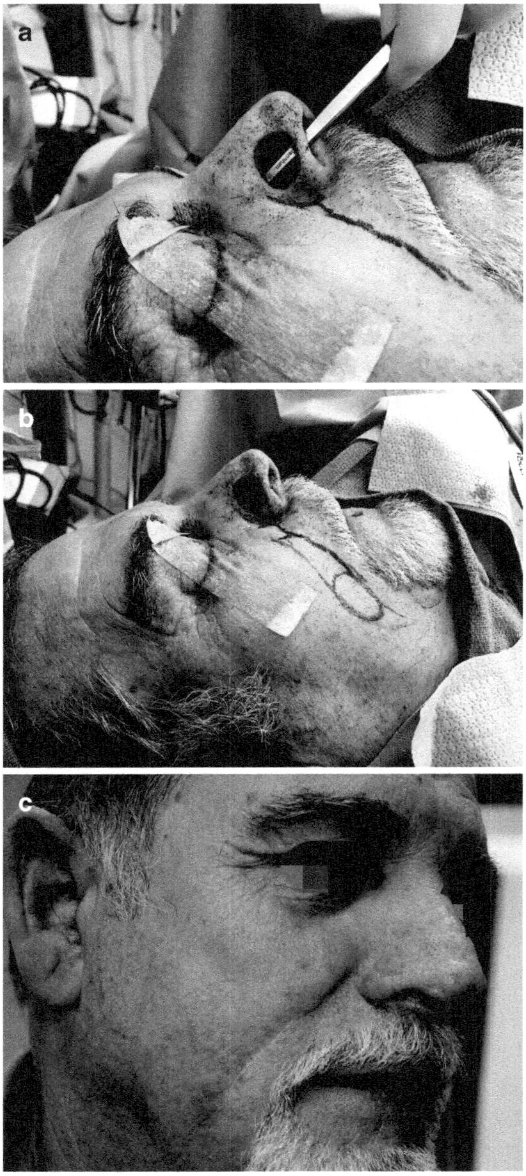

Fig. 22.22 (**a**) The malignancy required transmural resection. (**b**) The nasolabial flap design is represented in blue ink. (**c**) Final result

Nasolabial flaps can also be used for full thickness defects of the alae, as is the case of the patient presented in Fig. 22.22. This patient declined a paramedian forehead flap because of the requisite time commitment of a three-stage reconstructive process and the post-operative appearance associated with Stages I and II (prior to thinning and takedown). His alar defect was reconstructed using a nasolabial flap with a composite graft attached to the undersurface of the flap (see Fig. 22.22).

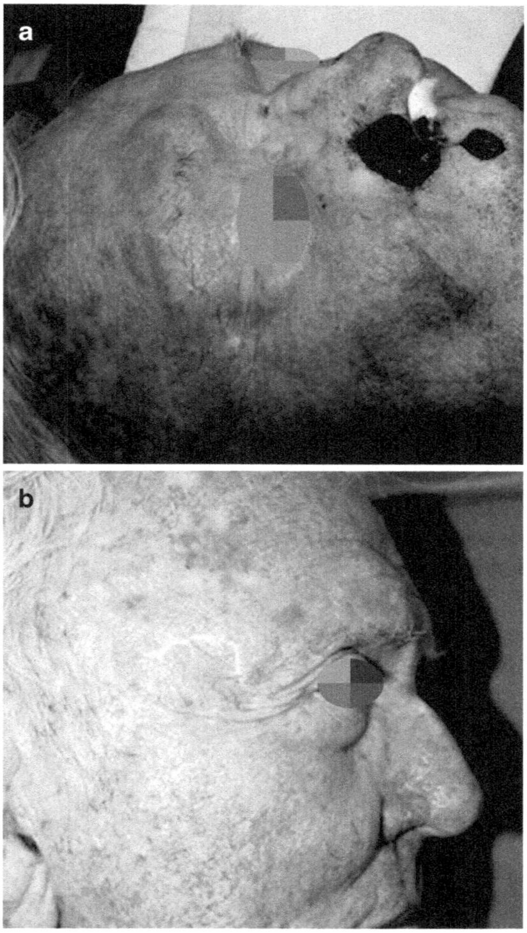

Fig. 22.23 (**a**) Right alar defect with in intact lining. An unsupported FTSG would undergo contracture and deform the ala. (**b**) Appearance of a composite graft reconstruction of the right ala at 4 months

Composite Grafts

Composite grafts are an acceptable, proven method for reconstructing defects of the nasal alae. Composite grafting may be preferable to nasolabial flap harvest, in some patients, because the reconstruction is accomplished in one stage and the surgeon does not create a secondary nasolabial defect at the would-be donor site. The final aesthetic result is generally favorable, depending largely on ability to properly color-match the graft, for appropriately selected patients (see Fig. 22.23).

Paramedian Forehead Flap

If the alar defect is full thickness, the paramedian forehead flap is an option for definitive coverage. Again, an unsupported flap or graft will undergo contracture and deform the ala. For this reason, an auricular cartilage graft to provide structural support must be harvested and inset in the defect prior to flap inset. The first step, however, is to reconstruct the nasal lining using a flap is derived from the nasal membrane. Then, and only then, can the cartilage graft be inset in the defect and the paramedian forehead flap inset on the cartilage graft (see Fig. 22.24).

Columella

Defects of the columella are relatively rare. If they are isolated defects of ≤1 cm, a composite graft, similar to those used in reconstruction of alar rim defects, may be used. If they accompany a defect of the nasal tip, an extension of the paramedian forehead flap may suffice. In columella defects of the elderly, it is possible to utilize two nasolabial flaps for definitive reconstruction. This method first requires the alae to be elevated out of the defect. Next, the nasolabial flaps are turned inward to form the sill and are brought together at the mid-

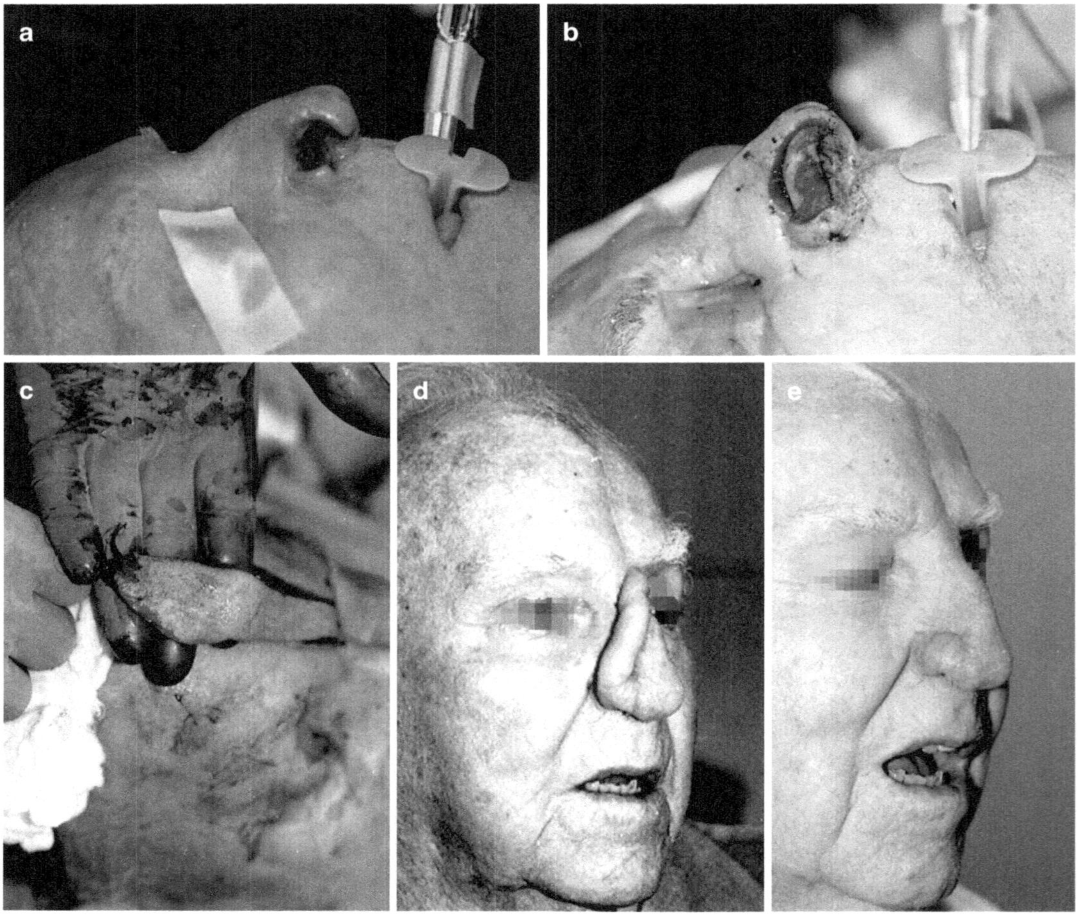

Fig. 22.24 (**a**) Patient with a full thickness defect of the right ala. (**b**) Lining flap and auricular cartilage graft have been inset to provide an appropriate nasal lining and structural support for the paramedian forehead flap. (**c**) Elevation of the paramedian forehead flap. (**d**) Immediately prior to Stage III—proximal flap release and distal flap thinning and inset. (**e**) Post-operative appearance after Stage III. (**f**) Post-operative appearance at 6 months

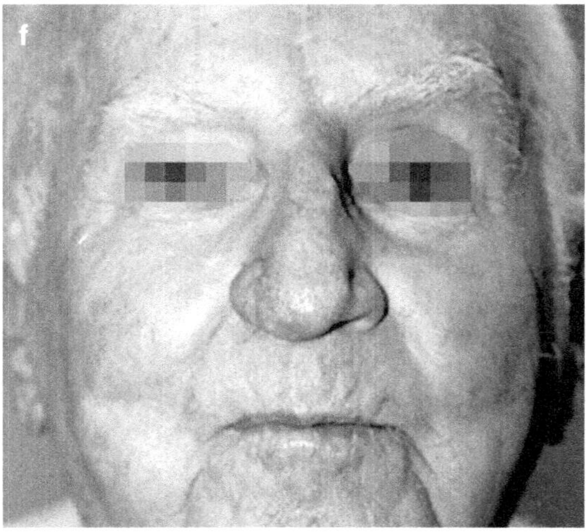

Fig. 22.24 (continued)

line, like "praying hands," to form the columella. The alae are replaced and the flaps contoured during a second procedure at a later date.

Conclusion

Nasal reconstruction is both challenging and rewarding. Sizeable nasal defects are devastating to patients, but oncologic resections must not be compromised. Fortunately, reliable techniques exist to help restore a virtually normal physical appearance. With time, practice, and judicious patient selection, we believe these techniques offer outstanding aesthetic results to patients with significant deformity secondary to resection of malignant nasal lesions.

References

1. Soong S-J, Weiss HL. Predicting outcome in patients with localized melanoma (Ch. 3). In: Balch CM, Houghton AN, Sober AJ, Soong S-J, editors. Cutaneous melanoma. 3rd ed. St Louis: Quality Med Pub; 1998. p. 55.
2. Bricca G, et al. Cutaneous head and neck melanoma treated with Mohs micrographic surgery. J Am Acad Dermatol. 2005;32(1):2099.
3. Jahn H, Breuninger C, et al. Melanoma of the ear: prognostic factors and surgical strategies. Br J Dermatol. 2006;154(2):310–8.
4. Byers RM, et al. Malignant melanoma of the external ear: review of 102 cases. Am J Surg. 1980;140:518.
5. Rawlani R, Rawlani V, Qureshi HA, Kim JY, Wayne JD. Reducing margins of wide local excision in head and neck melanoma for function and cosmesis: 5-year local recurrence-free survival. J Surg Oncol. 2015;111(7):795–9.
6. Zenga J, Nussenbaum B, Cornelius LA, Linette GP, Desai SC. Management controversies in head and neck melanoma: a systematic review. JAMA Facial Plast Surg. 2017;19(1):53–62.
7. Fata JJ. Composite chondrocutaneous advancement flap: a technique for the reconstruction of marginal defects of the ear. Plast Reconstr Surg. 1997;99:1172–5.
8. Bialostocki A, Tan ST. Modified Antia-Buch repair for full thickness upper pole auricular defects. Plast Reconstr Surg. 1999;103:1476–9.
9. Thorne CH, Brecht LE, Bradley JP, Levine JP, Hammerschlag P, Longaker MT. Auricular reconstruction: indications for autogenous and prosthetic techniques. Plast Reconstr Surg. 2001;107:1241–12526.
10. Brent B. The acquired auricular deformity: a systematic approach to its analysis and reconstruction. Plast Reconstr Surg. 1977;59:475–85.
11. Brent B, Byrd HS. Secondary ear reconstruction with cartilage grafts covered by axial, random, and free flaps of temporoparietal fascia. Plast Reconstr Surg. 1983;72:141–52.
12. Brent B, Upton J, Acland RD, Shaw WW, Finseth FJ, Rogers C, Pearl RM, Hentz VR. Experience with the temporoparietal fascial free flap. Plast Reconstr Surg. 1985;76:177–88.
13. Nakai H. Reconstruction of microtia with a contour-accentuated framework and supplemental coverage. Plast Reconstr Surg. 1986;78:604–9.
14. Rose EH, Norris MS. The versatile temporoparietal fascial flap: adaptability to a variety of composite defects. Plast Reconstr Surg. 1990;85:224–32.
15. Tegtmeier RE, Gooding RA. The use of a fascial flap in ear reconstruction. Plast Reconstr Surg. 1977;60:406–11.
16. Park C, Lew D-H, Yoo W-M. An analysis of 123 temporoparietal fascial flaps: anatomic and clinical considerations in total auricular reconstruction. Plast Reconstr Surg. 1999;104:1295–306.
17. Helling ER, Okoro S, Kim G II, Wang PT. Endoscope assisted temporoparietal fascia harvest for auricular reconstruction. Plast Reconstr Surg. 2008;121:1598–605.
18. Nagata S. Secondary reconstruction for unfavorable microtia results utilizing temporoparietal and innominate fascia flaps. Plast Reconstr Surg. 1994;94:254–65.
19. Brent B. Microtia repair with rib cartilage grafts: a review of personal experience with 1000 cases. Clin Plast Surg. 2002;29:257–71.
20. Uppal RS, Sabbagh W, Chana J, Gault DT. Donor-site morbidity after autologous costal cartilage harvest in ear reconstruction and approaches to reducing donor-site contour deformity. Plast Reconstr Surg. 2008;121:1949–55.

21. Thomson HG, Kim TY, Ein SH. Residual problems in chest donor sites after microtia reconstruction: a long-term study. Plast Reconstr Surg. 1995;95:961–8.
22. Fukuda O, Yamada A. Reconstruction of the microticear with autogenous cartilage. Clin Plast Surg. 1978;5:351–66.
23. Kawanabe Y, Nagata S. A new method of costal cartilage harvest for total auricular reconstructionPart I. Avoidance and prevention of intraoperative and postoperative complications and problems. Plast Reconstr Surg. 2006;117:2011–8.
24. Ohmori S, Matsumoto K, Nakai H. Follow-up study on reconstruction of microtia with a silicone framework. Plast Reconstr Surg. 1974;53:555–62.
25. Wellisz T. Clinical experience with the Medpor porous polyethylene implant. Aesthet Plast Surg. 1993;17:339–44.
26. Reinisch J. Microtia reconstruction using a polyethylene implant: An 8-year surgical experience. Presented at the 78th Annual Meeting of the American Association of Plastic Surgeons, Colorado Springs, CO, May 5, 1999.
27. Romo T III, Reitzen SD. Aesthetic microtia reconstruction with Medpor. Facial Plast Surg. 2008;24:120–8.
28. Yang SL, Zheng JH, Ding Z, Liu QY, Mao GY, Ji YP. Combined fascial flap and expanded skin flap for enveloping Medpor framework in microtia reconstruction. Aesthet Plast Surg. 2008;33:518–22.
29. Burget GC, Menick FJ. Subunit principle in nasal reconstruction. Plastic Reconstr Surg. 1985;76(2):239–47.
30. Menick FJ. Artistry in facial surgery: aesthetic perceptions and the subunit principle. In: Furnas D, editor. Clinics in plastic surgery, vol. 14. Philadelphia: WB Saunders; 1987. p. 723.
31. Weathers WM, Bhadkamkar M, Wolfswinkel EM, Thornton JF. Full-thickness skin grafting in nasal reconstruction. Semin Plast Surg. 2013;27(2):90–5.
32. Marchac D, Toth B. The axial frontonasal flap revisited. Plast Reconstr Surg. 1985;76(5):686–94.
33. McGregor JC, Soutar DS. A critical assessment of the bilobed flap. Br J Plast Surg. 1981;34(2):197–205.
34. Zitelli JA. The bilobed flap for nasal reconstruction. Arch Dermatol. 1989;125(7):957–9.
35. Burget GC, Menik FJ. Nasal reconstruction: seeking a fourth dimension. Plast Reconstr Surg. 1986;78(2):145–57.
36. Menick FJ. The aesthetic use of the forehead for nasal reconstruction—the paramedian forehead flaps. In: Tobin G, editor. Clinics in plastic surgery. Philadelphia: WB Saunders; 1990. p. 607.
37. Menick FJ. Ten-year experience in nasal reconstruction with the three-stage forehead flap. Plast Reconstr Surg. 2002;109(6):1839–55.
38. Maves M, Yessenow R. The use of composite auricular grafts in nasal reconstruction. J Dermatol Surg Oncol. 1988;114(9):994–9.
39. Herbert DC. A subcutaneous pedicle cheek flap for reconstruction of ala defects. Br J Plast Surg. 1978;31(2):79–92.

Reconstruction Options for Lip, Cheek, Forehead, and Scalp Melanoma

23

Charles L. Dupin, Julian D'Achille, Ian R. Wisecarver, and Taylor Smith

Compared to the cheek and forehead, melanoma of the upper or lower lip is an infrequent presentation [1]. Resection of an upper or lower lip melanoma using standard resection criteria (0.5 cm margins for melanoma in situ, 1.0 cm margins for Breslow's thickness (BT) of ≤1.0 mm, 1–2 cm margins for BT of 1.01–2.0 mm, and 2 cm margins for BT of ≥2.01 mm) is a daunting task [2]. Following this criteria, excision of a 1.5 mm thick melanoma of the lip requires removal of a 4 cm section of tissue, compromising most of the skin of the lip.

Fortunately, there is published data that seems to indicate that the margins can be reduced without jeopardizing either recurrence rates or survival outcomes. This data suggests that a thin melanoma can be excised with a 0.5 cm margin and thicker melanomas can be excised with a 1 cm margin [2, 3]. The ability to spare even small amounts of tissue greatly reduces the challenge of reconstruction.

The lips are a central feature of the face. The upper lip is a much more complex structure the lower lip. The disparity in anatomic complexity between the upper and lower lips translates well to aesthetic complexity with the lower lip consisting of a single aesthetic subunit while the upper lip comprises multiple subunits (see Fig. 23.1).

Upper lip defects secondary to a melanoma resection are more complicated to reconstruct because of these well-defined features. However, as the face ages, these features become much less defined. Thus, this manner of reconstruction is less difficult to accomplish in elderly patients. The majority of melanoma resections involve only skin and subcutaneous tissue, with wound reconstruction simplified with the need to replace the defect with healthy tissue. However, lesions involving either the vermillion or vermillion cutaneous junction require replacement of both vermillion and skin during reconstruction or resection via pentagonal excision.

Simple Excision

Up to 25% of the lower lip can undergo full-thickness excision with subsequent layered repair and suffer little functional or aesthetic impairment [4]. In the elderly, up to 30 percent of the lower lip can be excised [4, 5]. If additional lip must be resected, tissue will need to be recruited into the defect; however, the initial 25% does not need to

C. L. Dupin, M.D. (✉) · J. D'Achille, M.D., M.P.H.
Division of Plastic and Reconstructive Surgery, Department of Surgery, Louisiana State University Health Sciences Center, New Orleans, LA, USA
e-mail: cdupin@lsuhsc.edu; jdachi@lsuhsc.edu

I. R. Wisecarver, B.S. · T. Smith, B.S.
Louisiana State University Health Sciences Center, New Orleans, LA, USA
e-mail: iwisec@lsuhsc.edu; tsmi21@lsuhsc.edu

A. I. Riker (ed.), *Melanoma*, https://doi.org/10.1007/978-3-319-78310-9_23

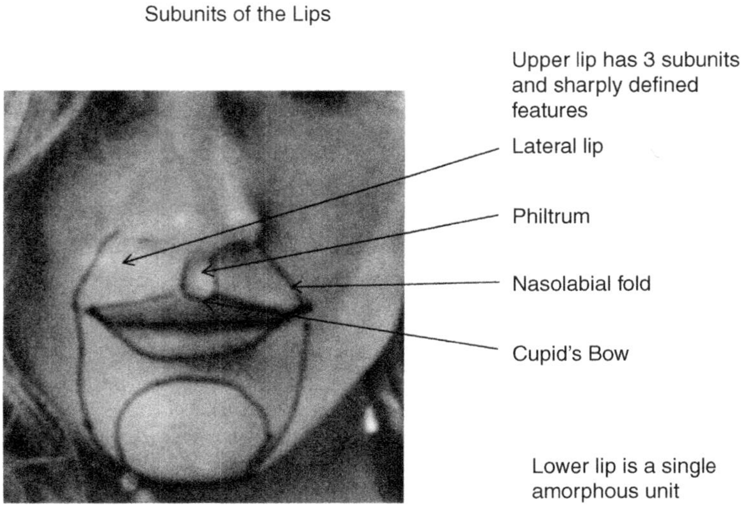

Fig. 23.1 Sub-units of the upper and lower lip

be replaced. Thus, if 50% of the lip is missing, sufficient tissue will be required to replace 25%, rather than the full 50%. If 75% of the lip is missing, the amount of tissue required for appropriate closure will approximate 50% of the normal lip.

Pentagonal Excision

The normal lower lip, in middle-aged adults, is a little over 6 cm in length on average. Lesions requiring resection of ≤1.5 cm of tissue, especially lesions near the vermillion-cutaneous border, may be resected via pentagonal excision [6]. The goal of pentagonal excision is to strategically control the location of maximum tension during closure, so the scar is advanced superiorly and vectors of tension are positioned to avoid notching the lower lip. This technique of resection may seem aggressive, but the manner of closure is such that skin grafts and flap reconstruction are not necessary and good aesthetic results are achieved (see Fig. 23.2).

Pentagonal excision is appropriate for resection of both upper and lower lip lesions [6] (see Fig. 23.3). The result is good closure with little evident distortion, especially if the defect is in the lateral part of the upper lip. Young patients undergoing excision of an upper lip lesion are the exception and may experience some distortion of the lip. For this reason, young patients may be candidates for V-Y advancement rather than a full-thickness pentagonal excision, alternatively, tissue may be moved from the lower lip into the defect.

Vermilionectomy

If the lesion involves the vermillion only, and not the cutaneous part of the lip, the involved vermillion is excised. "Wet" vermillion serves as the tissue replacement substrate and is advanced to the defect from an incision placed in the alveolar mucosal junction. The donor site defect can be closed with a V-Y advancement (see Figs. 23.4 and 23.5).

Skin Grafting

Small defects involving the upper or lower cutaneous lip can be skin grafted [5]. Full-thickness, color-matched skin must be used. The grafts may be taken from the postauricular area or from the forehead (as for the nasal tip). The grafts should be secured with both peripheral and quilting sutures to prevent movement. Even when using

Fig. 23.2 Pentagonal excision. Top: Closing the pentagonal incision places maximum tension at the lower third (red arrow) and creates a vector of force which is directed superiorly (blue arrow). Pressure directed towards the free edge helps prevent notching. Bottom: Closing the wedge incision (red arrow) places maximal tension at the free border and forces the tissue inferior which may lead to notching

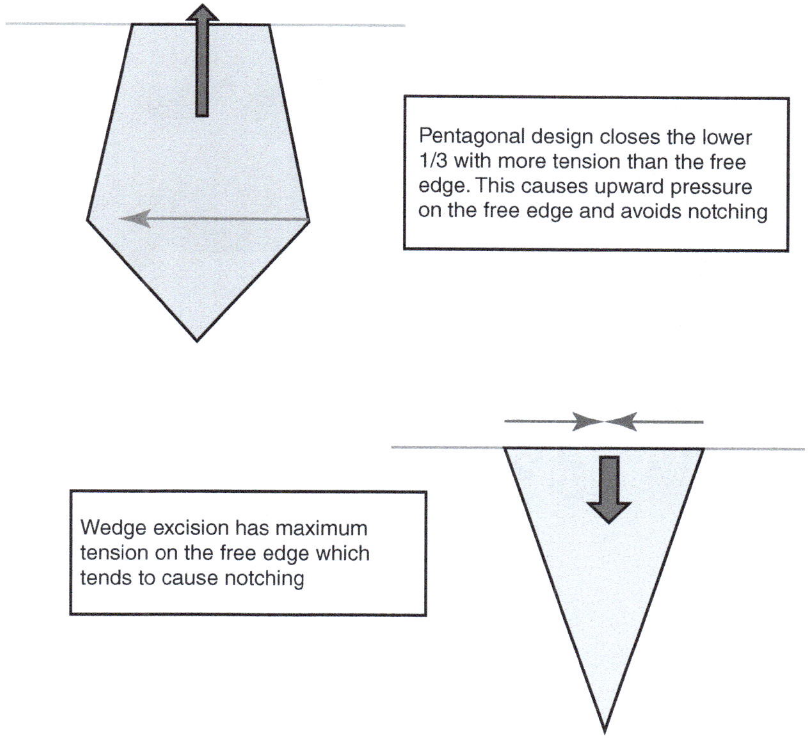

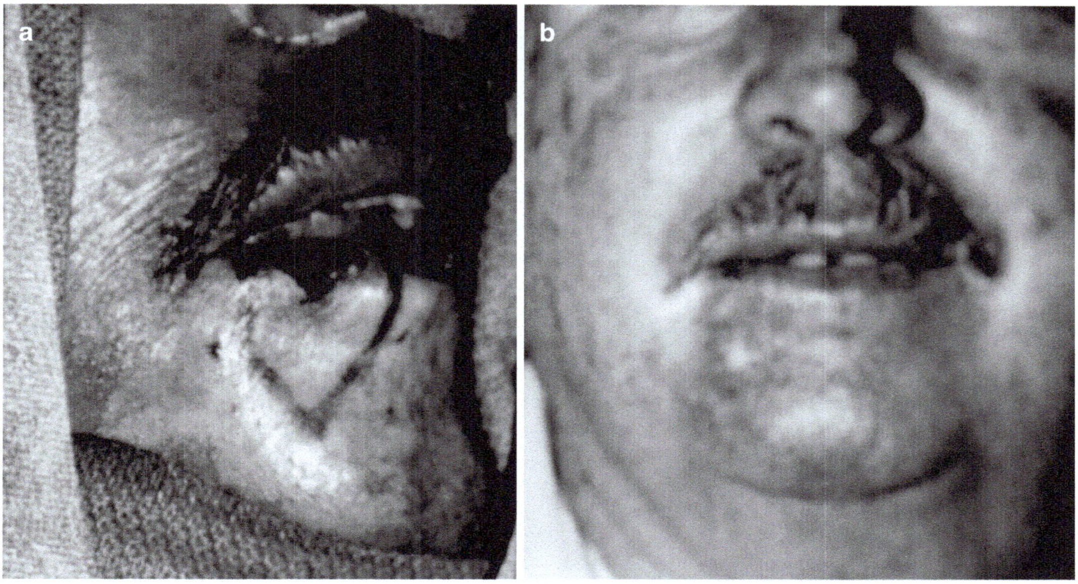

Fig. 23.3 Pentagonal excision of a 1.5 cm defect of the lower lip

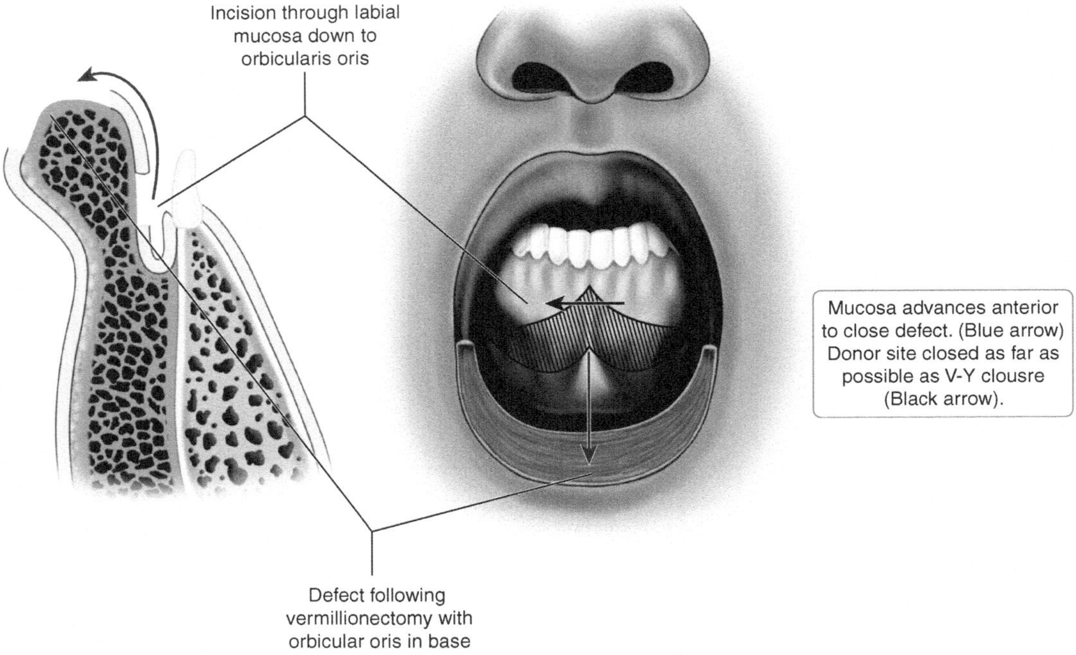

Fig. 23.4 Vermilionectomy

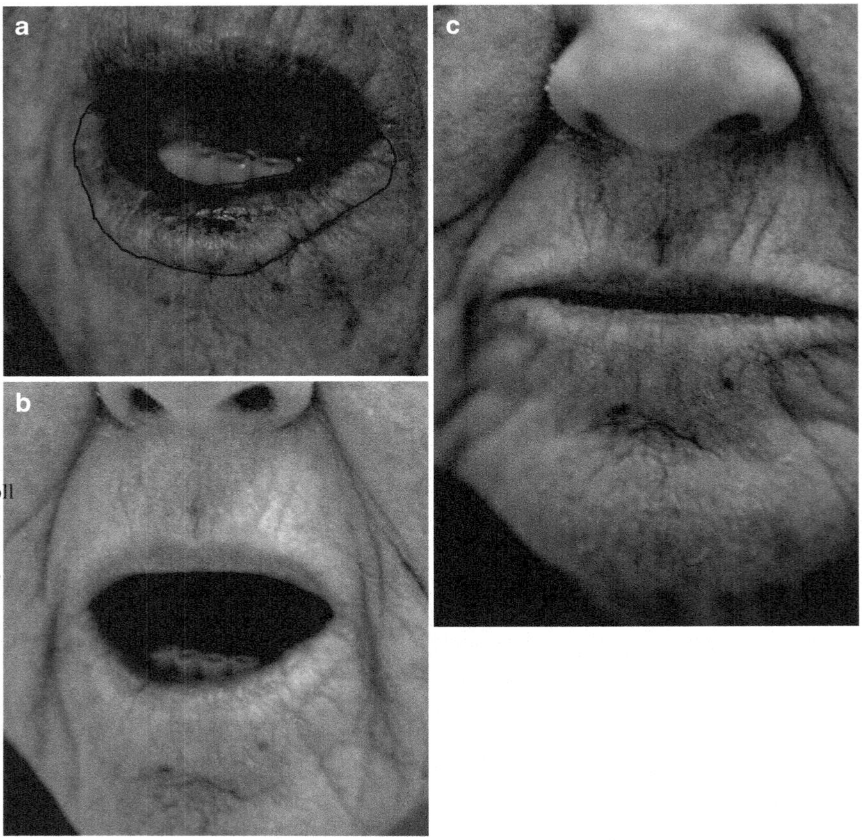

Fig. 23.5 (**a**) Patient requiring lower lip excision of the vermillion and white roll of the lower lip. The blue line represents the tissue to be excised. (**b**, **c**) Postoperative appearance after vermilionectomy. The defect was closed via V-Y advancement as described above

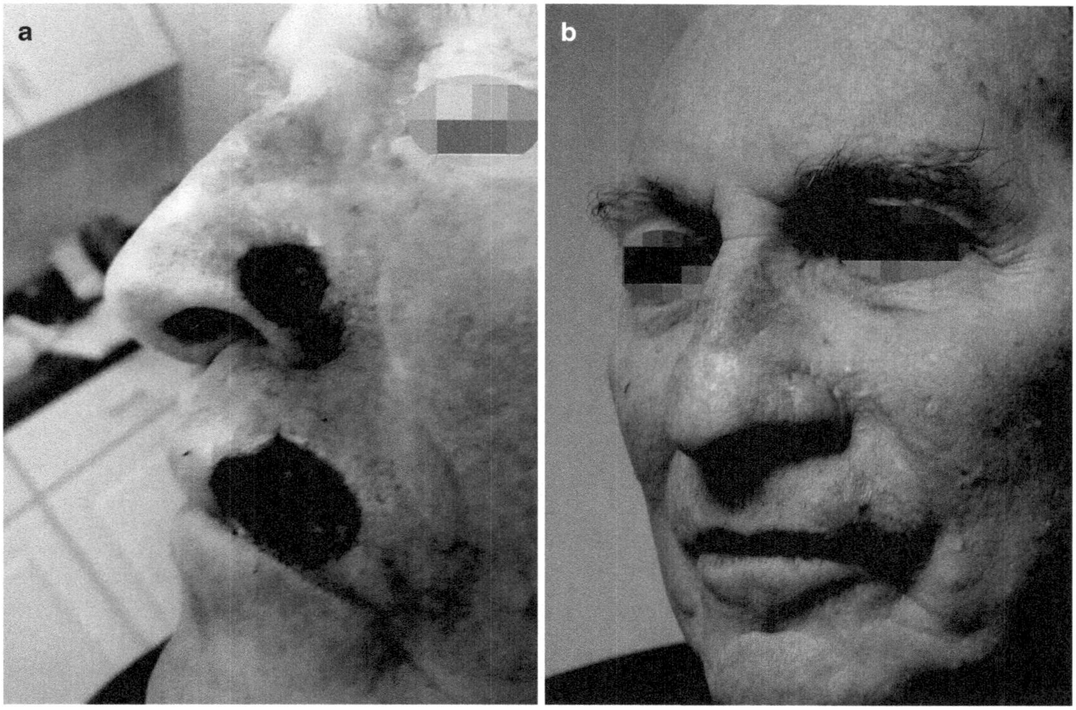

Fig. 23.6 (a) Smaller neoplasm of the left cutaneous lip. Can be treated with excision and full-thickness skin grafting. (b) Patient at 4 weeks post-operative. The small amount of graft contracture will pull the vermillion into place

full-thickness skin grafts for coverage of lip defects, some contracture may be expected because there is no solid structure supporting the graft [7] (see Fig. 23.6).

V-Y Advancement Flaps

If the defect diameter is 1.5–2 cm and involves only the skin, white roll, or vermillion, V-Y advancement flaps can be used to close the defect [8]. V-Y advancement flaps used for oral reconstruction are based on the robust vasculature that supplies the orbicularis oris musculature [8]. Incisions are made through the overlying skin and epimysium of the orbicularis muscle to obtain maximal tissue laxity and allow flap advancement. If the wound includes the vermillion, an opposing V-Y advancement flap can be raised from the oral mucosa in the same manner (see Fig. 23.7).

Mesial Cheek Advancement Techniques

Lesions of the upper and lower lip >2 cm in diameter require transfer of skin from the adjacent area. For upper lip reconstruction, this can be accomplished by removing a crescent of skin at the alar margin and advancing skin from the mesial cheek (see Fig. 23.8). The nasolabial fold is undermined prior to cheek advancement and reconstitutes itself with time. The lower lip can be reconstructed in a similar manner (see Figs. 23.8 and 23.9).

Simple Excision with Mesial Cheek Advancement

In elderly patients, the central features are much less sharply defined. Central upper lip defects of the elderly can be treated via simple resection

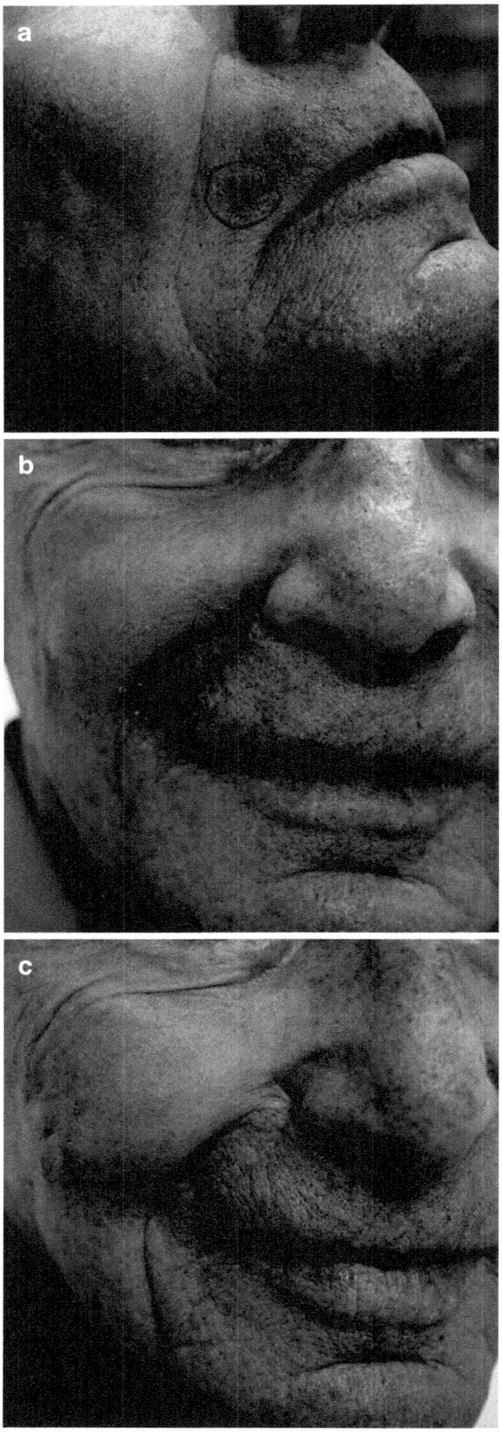

Fig. 23.7 (**a**) Lateral upper lip lesion requiring a 1.5 cm excision. (**b**) Early post-operative appearance. The defect was closed via V-Y advancement. (**c**) Appearance at 2 months

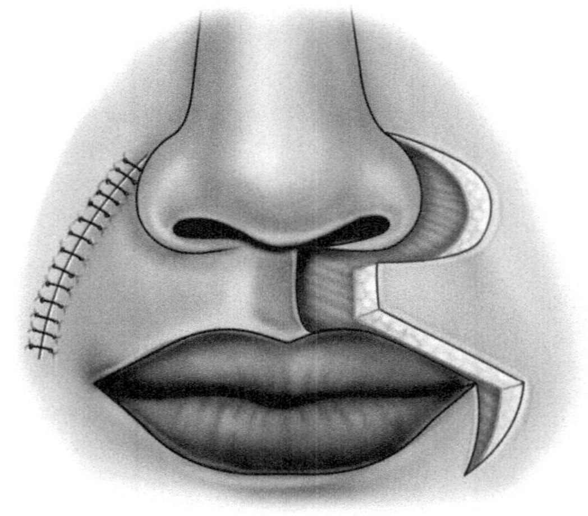

Fig. 23.8 Mesial cheek advancement flap for upper lip reconstruction. Note the crescentic excision lateral to the nasal alae. The optional labial-mental fold excision facilitates more extensive tissue advancement

and subsequent closure with mesial cheek advancement, which provide acceptable aesthetic results (see Fig. 23.10).

Abbe Flap with Mesial Cheek Advancement

Reconstruction of central, upper lip defects in younger patients can be quite challenging. During youth, the philtral ridges are sharp and the recess above "Cupid's Bow" (See Fig. 23.1) is deeper. There is a "pout" of vermillion located centrally beneath the Cupid's bow. In a young patient, excision of this unit without a subsequent, formal reconstructive procedure will inevitably result in significant deformity.

The central aesthetic unit of the upper lip (philtrum) can be reconstructed as a separate subunit using an Abbe flap derived from the lower lip [9]. The Abbe flap contains muscle, mucosa, and skin and derives its blood supply from the inferior labial artery and vein [5, 9]. It can be transferred to the upper lip to replace the philtrum, some recipient site muscle and mucosa must be discarded to create space for the flap.

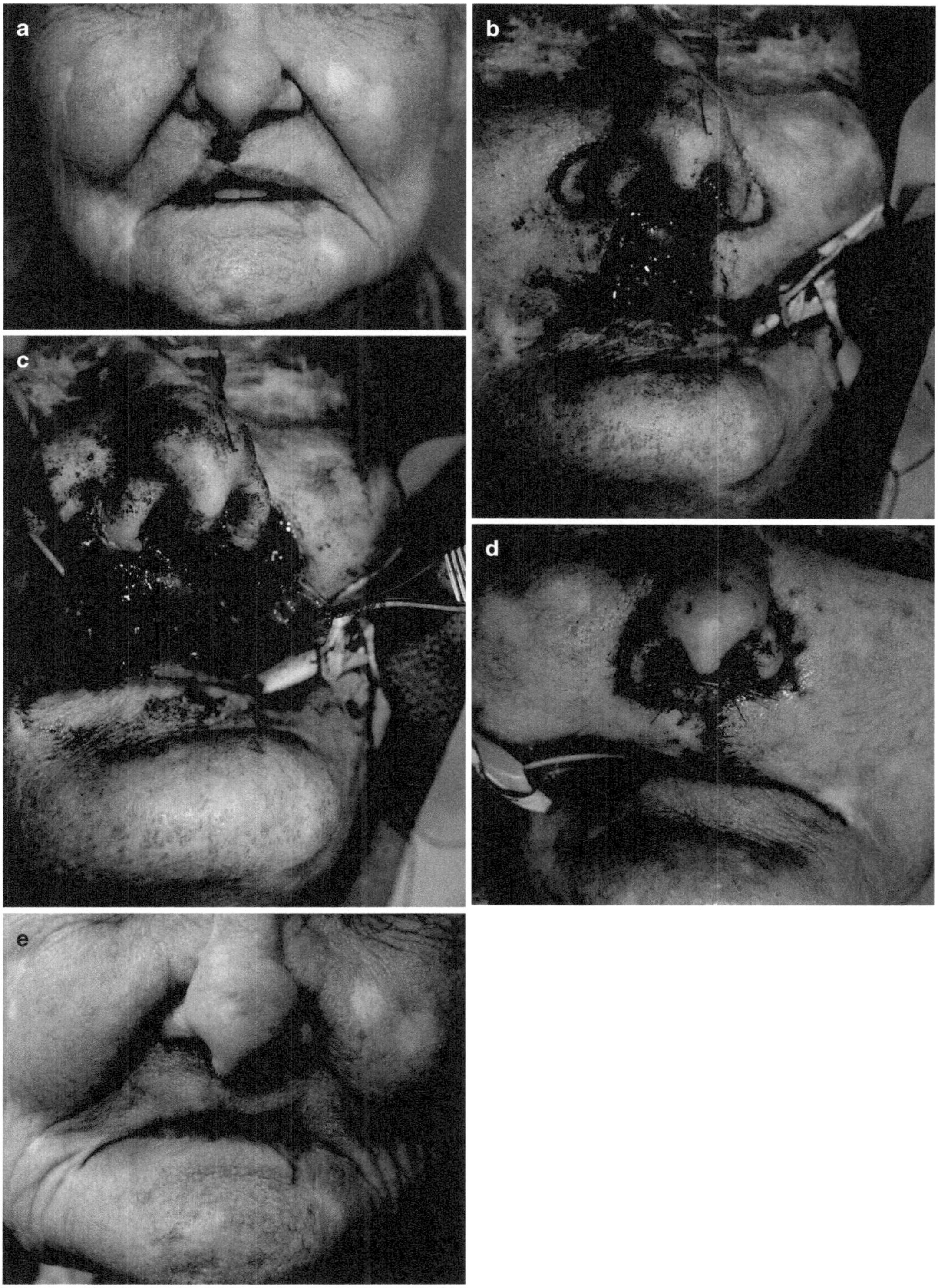

Fig. 23.9 (**a**) Patient with a thin melanoma involving the central upper lip. (**b**) An outline of the mesial cheek advancement flap. (**c**) Flaps elevated and advanced. (**d**) Immediate post-operative result. (**e**) Final result

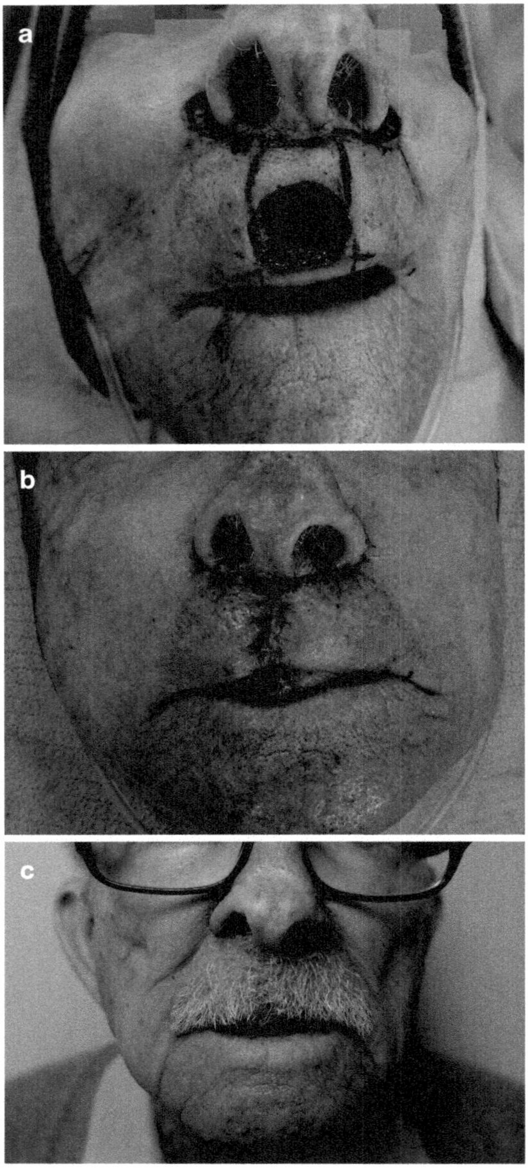

Fig. 23.10 (**a**) Central upper lip defect in an elderly patient. Note the mesial cheek advancement skin markings. (**b**) Mesial cheek advancement—immediate postoperative result. (**c**) Final result

The patient portrayed in Fig. 23.11 had a thin melanoma which involved the philtrum. She underwent complete excision of the philtral skin and part of the left lateral segment. An Abbe flap was performed to reconstruct the philtrum and the lateral segment was reconstructed using an advancement flap from the mesial cheek.

The medial cheek advancement flap can also be used to resurface the lower lip as well if only skin is deficient (see Fig. 23.12).

Webster Modification of the Bernard-Burrow Procedure

Lower lip lesions requiring excision in excess of 2 cm necessitate tissue advancement from the lower cheek. These advancements may be unilateral or bilateral. This technique, known as the Webster modification of the Bernard-Burrow procedure, advances skin, muscle, and mucosa to allow closure of defects comprising up to one-half of the lip [9, 10]. It can also be employed to advance only the skin and subcutaneous tissue, if that is what the situation requires.

Lower cheek advancement is permitted by bilateral excision of a 2 cm triangle of tissue (skin only) lateral to the nasolabial fold. A second set of bilateral triangles, containing only skin, are removed from the lateral chin. The commissure can be incised up to 1 cm in order to release the lip, but no further. If the incision is too wide, the juncture of the mimetic muscles will be destroyed and the lip will not function. Reconstruction of the vermillion component requires an intraoral incision and wet vermillion V-Y advancement, as described above. The wet vermillion is then used to resurface the labial part of the flap. The incision does not extend into the muscle layer, but the muscle layer may be advanced into the defect if necessary. However, muscle advancement should not be required in reconstruction of defects secondary to melanoma resection and only the skin should be advanced. The Webster modification of the Bernard-Borrow procedure may be employed to reconstruct virtually the entire lip (see Fig. 23.13).

Defects of the Cheek

The cheek comprises a large portion of the facial aesthetic unit. Its inferior border is at the neck, the superior border at the scalp, the lateral border at the ear, and the medial border at the nose and

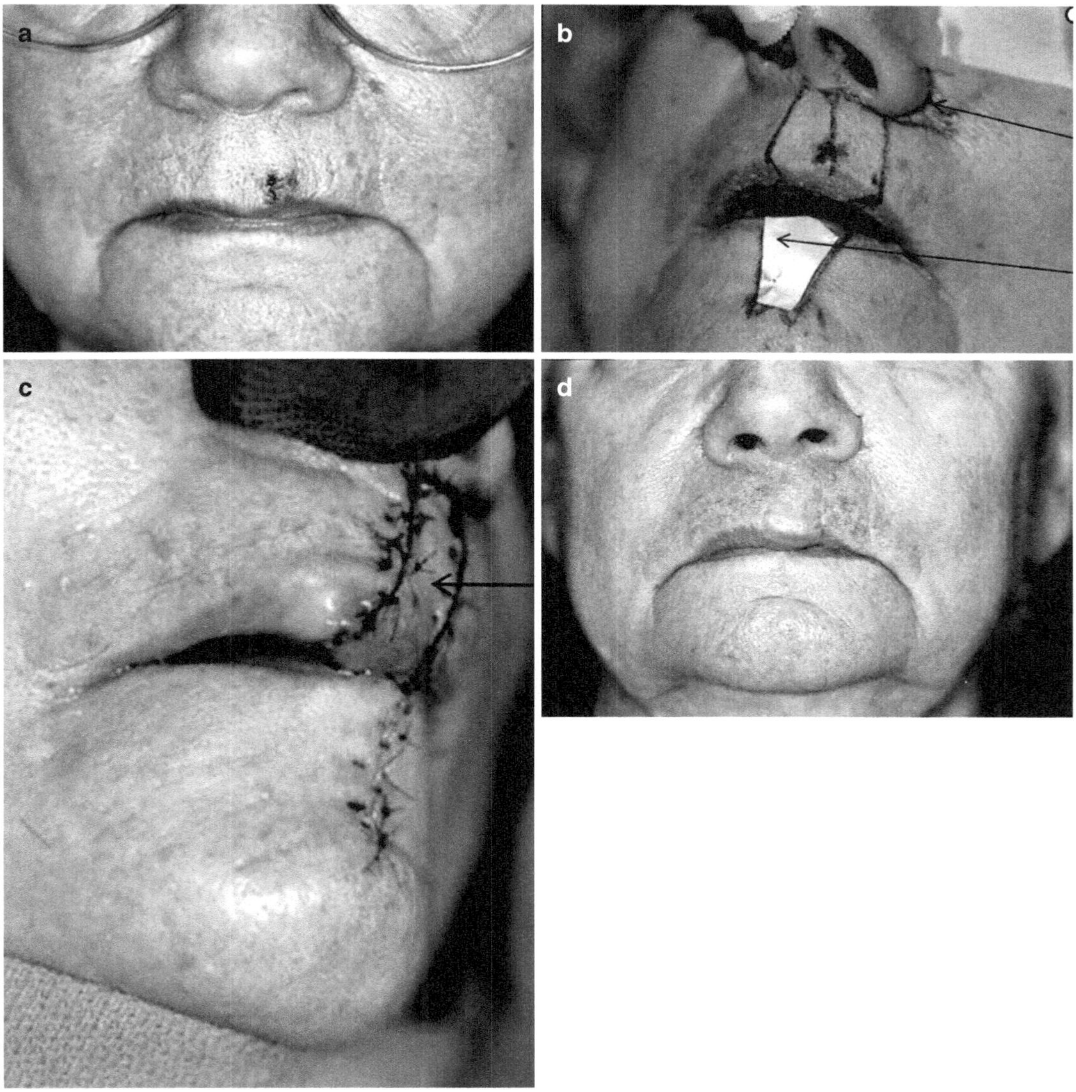

Fig. 23.11 (**a**) Malignant melanoma with a Breslow's thickness of 1.0 mm. (**b**) (Upper arrow) Mesial cheek advancement will be performed to resurface the lateral lip. Note the crescentic excision in the para-alar region. (Lower arrow) Abbe flap template representing the tissue which will be used for philtral reconstruction. (**c**) (Arrow) Abbe flap in place, based on the left inferior labial artery. The donor vessels should be encased in a protective muscular cuff and no attempt should be made to skeletonize them. (**d**) Final result at 3 months with no revisions. We may have improved her aesthetic outcome by advancing more of the cheek flap and anchoring it to the anterior nasal spine

lips [11]. The cheek also has established minimal skin tension lines (MSTL). These lines, seen in the elderly as "wrinkle lines," are the result of movement in the underlying mimetic muscles. Scars aligned with MSTL are favorable.

For the purpose of reconstruction, the cheek can be divided into three general areas. The first area is that which is seen in the mirror and in normal face-to-face contact. In this area, scars are evident to both patient and viewer. The second area is less perceptible, because it is largely in shadow when viewed from the front. The third is the pre-auricular area (see Fig. 23.14).

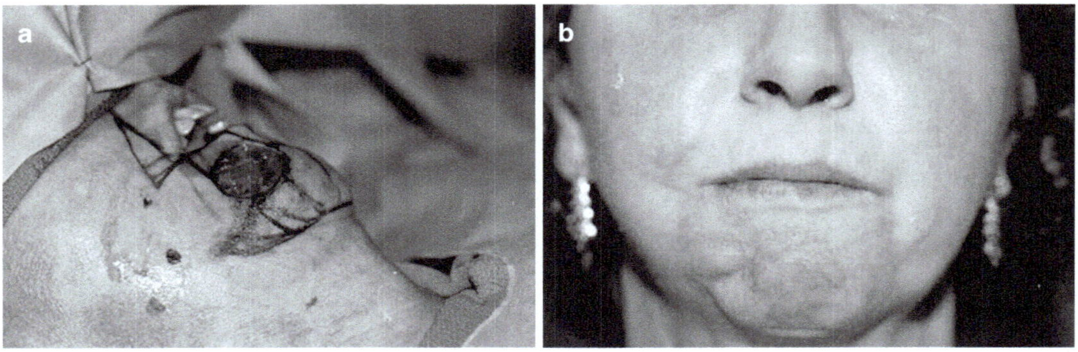

Fig. 23.12 (**a**) Defect of the lower lip with markings for cheek flap. (**b**) Result after 6 months, no revisions

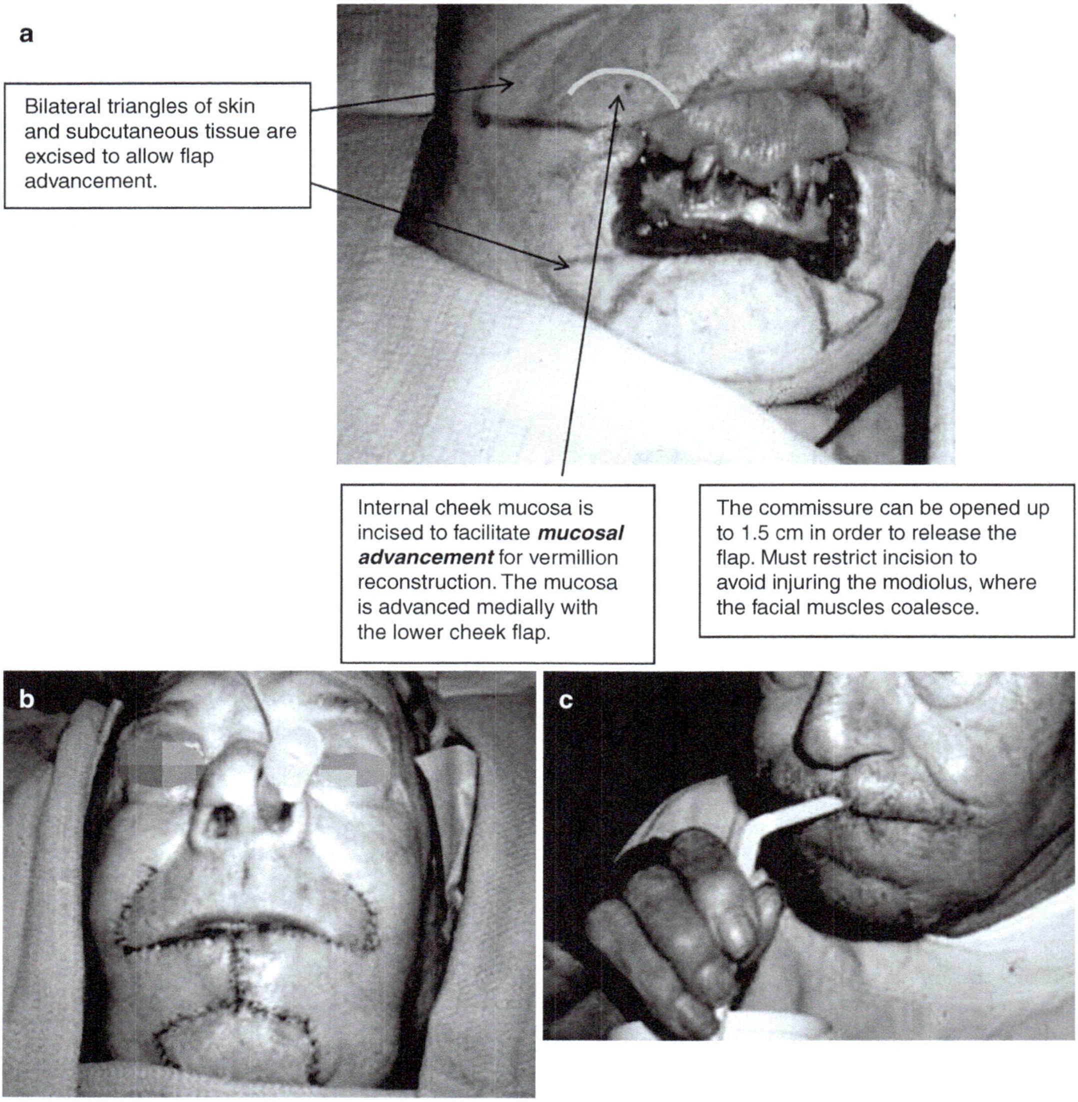

Fig. 23.13 (**a**) Webster modification of the Bernard-Burrow Procedure. (**b**) Immediate post-operative appearance. (**c**) Final result

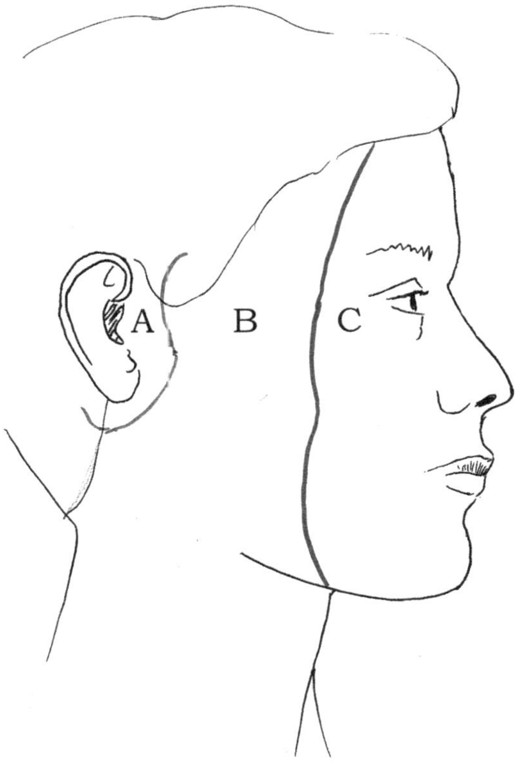

Fig. 23.14 Three aesthetic zones of the cheek. (**a**) Preauricular zone: excisions can be closed with a "facelift" advancement of the cheek into the defect. (**b**) Lateral cheek: Too far anterior to be closed with "facelift" advancement, but lateral enough so it cannot be seen in the mirror. (**c**) Area which can be seen in the mirror and in face-to-face contact

Melanoma excisions, as a rule, remove all of the skin and some subcutaneous tissue while sparing deeper structures. The goal of reconstruction is to repair the defect in such a way that scarring is minimal, less obvious, and may be covered by makeup.

The area most favorable for avoiding visible scars is the immediate preauricular area and anterior to the temporal hairline. Lesions up to 2 cm in diameter may be closed by undermining and advancing the cheek into the defect. Here, laxity of the facial skin allows wound closure in the border between the ear and the face, much like a facelift scar. Scars placed in borders between aesthetic units tend to disappear over time.

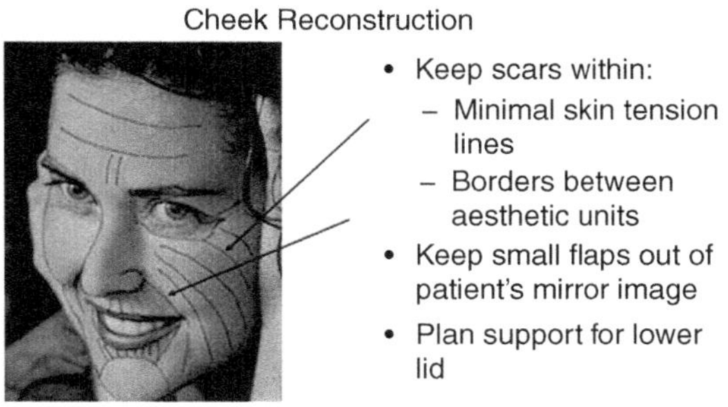

Fig. 23.15 Principles of cheek reconstruction

The second zone, or lateral cheek, is suitable for local tissue rearrangement. Significant laxity in the jowls, cheek skin, and temporal skin allows tissue to be "borrowed" to fill the defect. It is important to avoid deformity in the donor area and to place as many of the scars as possible within the minimal skin tension lines (MSTL). It is also important to avoid deformity of the eyelids when the defect is adjacent to the eye.

There are a number of validated approaches to help minimize deformity and scar formation following excision of cheek lesions. The most notable of which is to place incisions, and therefore scars, in the MSTL. These tension lines, most appreciable in the aging face, are the result of force vectors created by the underlying facial muscles. Incisions along these lines heal very favorably with a good aesthetic result [11]. Scars placed in the borders of subunits are hidden by normal plane changes between aesthetic units. Whenever possible, care must be given to minimize formation of complex scars (such as those which arise from local tissue rearrangement) in the mesial cheek, where they are seen daily in the mirror (see Fig. 23.15).

Defects of the Lateral Cheek

Defects of the lateral cheek which are too far mesial for preauricular incision are frequently closed with local tissue rearrangement. The most useful method of local tissue rearrangement is the rhomboid flap [12]. The rhomboid flap transposes skin from an adjacent area, which has significant tissue laxity, into the defect. One advantage of this

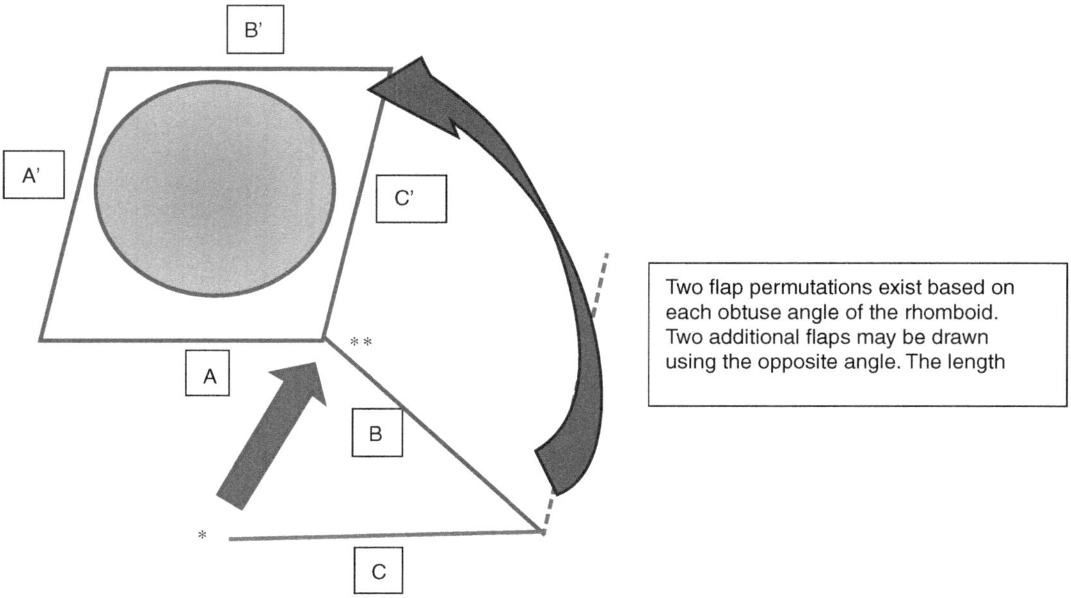

Fig. 23.16 Rhomboid Flap—permutation 1: The flap is incised and elevated with approximately 3 mm of subcutaneous fat. Next, it is rotated into the defect so that **A** meets **A′**, **B** meets **B′**, and **C** meets **C′**. The resulting tension is along the red arrow. This pattern allows the tension to be placed in a manner which prevents donor site deformity. Permutation 2 would be the use of the opposite flap. The choice of flaps is based on the vector of the tension shown in the red arrow. The tension should be placed to avoid deformity in the donor site

method is predictable tension at closure, which can be useful in orienting the flap such that surrounding structures are not deformed (see Fig. 23.16).

The rhomboid flap is especially useful for reconstruction of defects around the orbit and within the lateral cheek zone. First, a pattern, as shown in Fig. 23.16, is drawn on a sterile card to create a template of the potential flap. The template is then positioned about the defect until a favorable vector of tension which utilizes optimum laxity is determined (represented by the red arrow in Fig. 23.16). In the periorbital region, the tension vector should be oriented in a manner which avoids placing downward tension on the eyelid, to prevent ectropion (see Fig. 23.17a–c).

Defects of the Mesial Cheek

Defects of the mesial cheek are readily seen in the mirror. As such, flaps which produce complex scars should be avoided in this area. If placed in the borders between aesthetic units or in MSTL, the cheek rotation-advancement flap can repair large defects of the mesial cheek with favorable scarring [13, 14]. The blood supply can be derived from either the anterior or posterior cheek (see Fig. 23.19).

The proximity of the lids to mesial cheek defects requires that great care be taken to avoid placing downward tension on the lower lid (see Fig. 23.18). A common precaution to prevent ectropion involves affixing flap fascia to the orbital rim via permanent sutures or sutures with bone screw anchors.

The cheek rotation-advancement flap can be raised over very large areas. In nonsmokers, these flaps are reliable even when carried down to the clavicle. Below the zygomatic arch, the superficial fascia may be included to maximize reliability [15] (see Fig. 23.19).

If the defect is in the mesial cheek, the first incision is placed in the nasolabial fold and the second is placed in the MSTL and continues into the preauricular area. The length of incision and

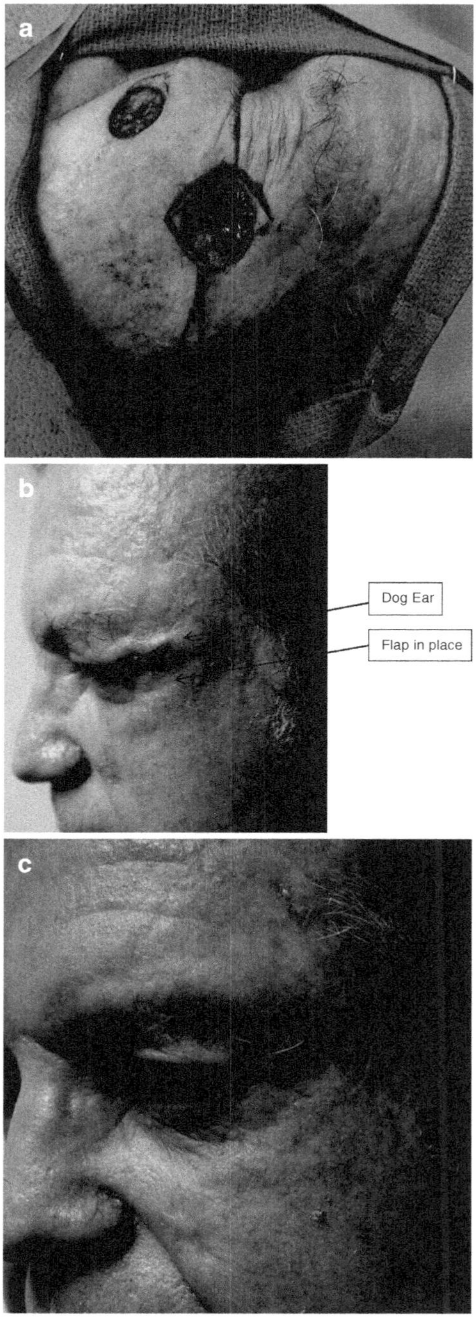

Fig. 23.17 (a) Rhomboid flap for upper cheek defect repair. Note that the flaps cannot be transposed onto the lids and that the optimal flap places tension such that appropriate lid closure is facilitated. The tension vector is depicted by the double-headed, black arrow. A "dog ear" will form as the flap rotates and may be excised after 3 weeks for optimal aesthetic result. (b) Rhomboid flap with resultant "dog ear." (c) Final result after dog ear excision. Note that the eyelid has good position. (d) Final result after dog ear excision. Note that the eyelid has good position

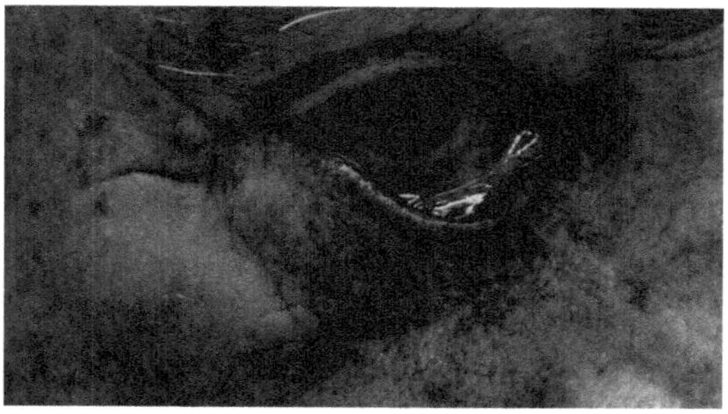

Fig. 23.18 Infraorbital cheek defect closed with skin graft. Insufficient lower lid support and skin graft contracture led to ectropion in this patient

degree of undermining are determined by the size of the defect (see Fig. 23.20a–d).

If the defect is oblong, the advancement should be made in the direction that will require the least amount of movement and dissection as well as create the least amount of tension. For example, if the defect is oblong with a horizontal axis, an advancement which moves tissue from inferior to superior will be easier than one which moves tissue from lateral to medial (see Fig. 23.21a–d).

Defects of the Forehead

The forehead is a broad, mobile, loose plane which borders the hairline, temporal sideburns, and brow and is not divided into subunits [15, 16]. Brow position is an important aesthetic feature and should not be deformed. The majority of MSTL in the forehead are horizontal due to force vectors generated by the underlying frontalis muscle. However, MSTL of the glabella are vertical because of the underlying corrugator muscles' orientation.

Compared to split thickness skin graft (STSG) donor sites, forehead skin is relatively thick and STSG's placed in this area have suboptimal color and texture match to the native forehead [16] (see Fig. 23.22).

Defects of the midline forehead ≤3 cm, which cannot be approximated with sutures, will heal satisfactorily via wound contracture and do not distort the brow or hairline [15, 16]. Similar defects are an unintended consequence

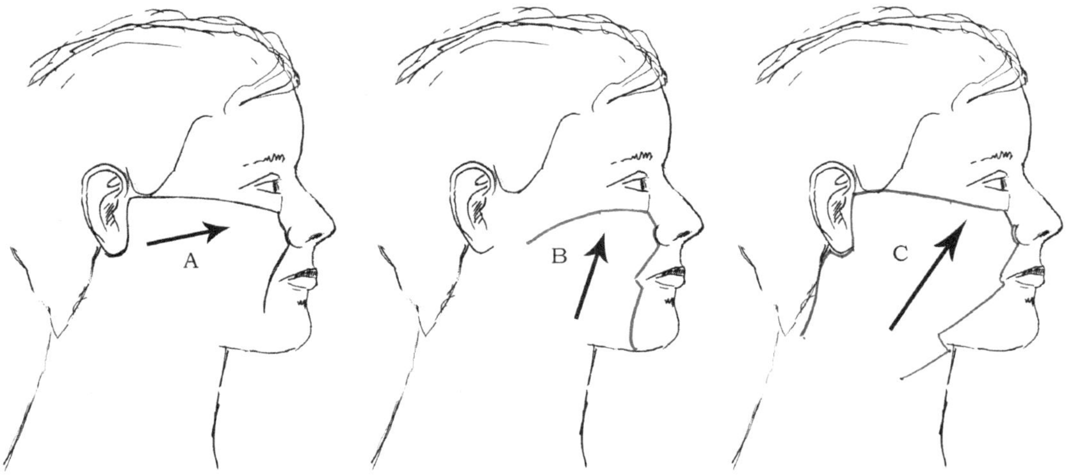

Fig. 23.19 Flap variations for mesial cheek advancement (**a**) Blood supply: inferior; advancement: lateral to medial; dog ear: along nasolabial fold. (**b**) Blood supply: infero-lateral; advancement: inferior to superior; dog ear: in cheek. (**c**) Blood supply: inferior; advancement: inferior to superomedial; incisions may extend to clavicle

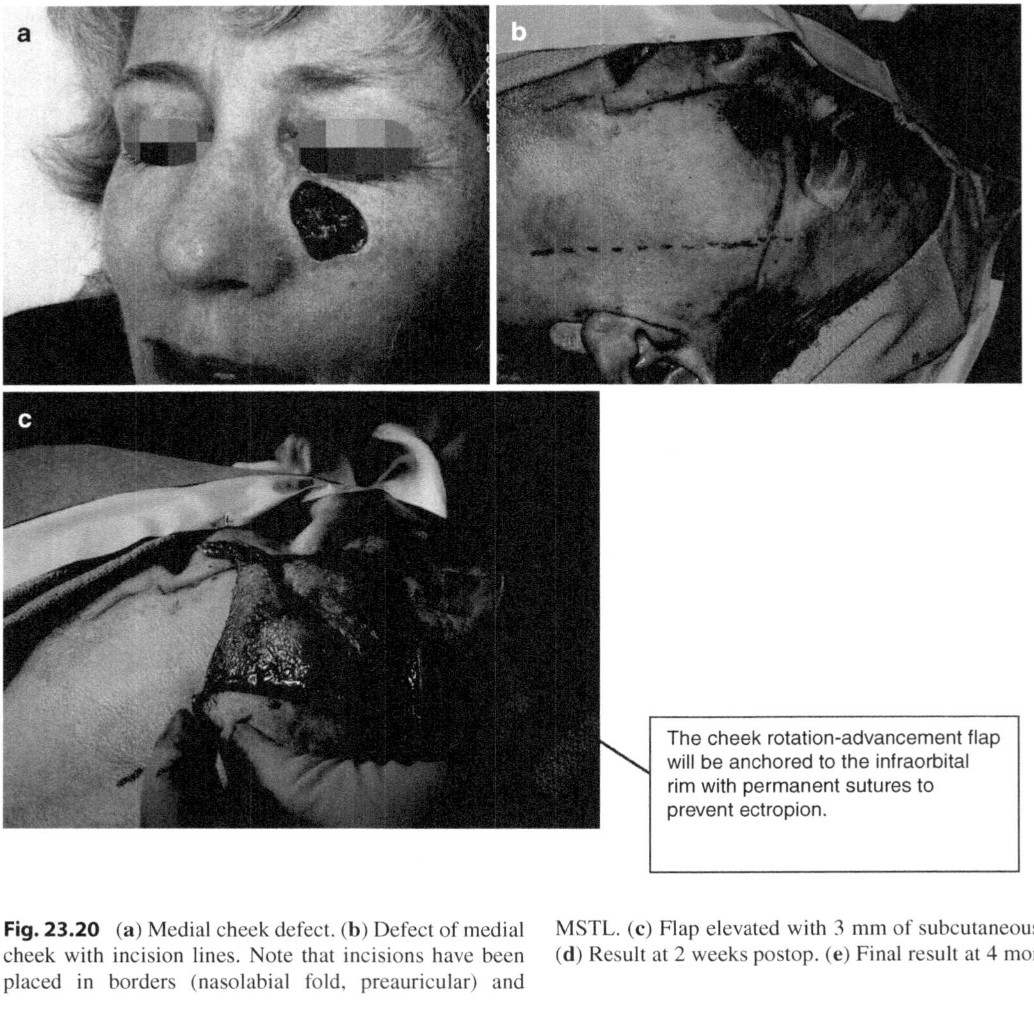

Fig. 23.20 (**a**) Medial cheek defect. (**b**) Defect of medial cheek with incision lines. Note that incisions have been placed in borders (nasolabial fold, preauricular) and MSTL. (**c**) Flap elevated with 3 mm of subcutaneous fat. (**d**) Result at 2 weeks postop. (**e**) Final result at 4 months

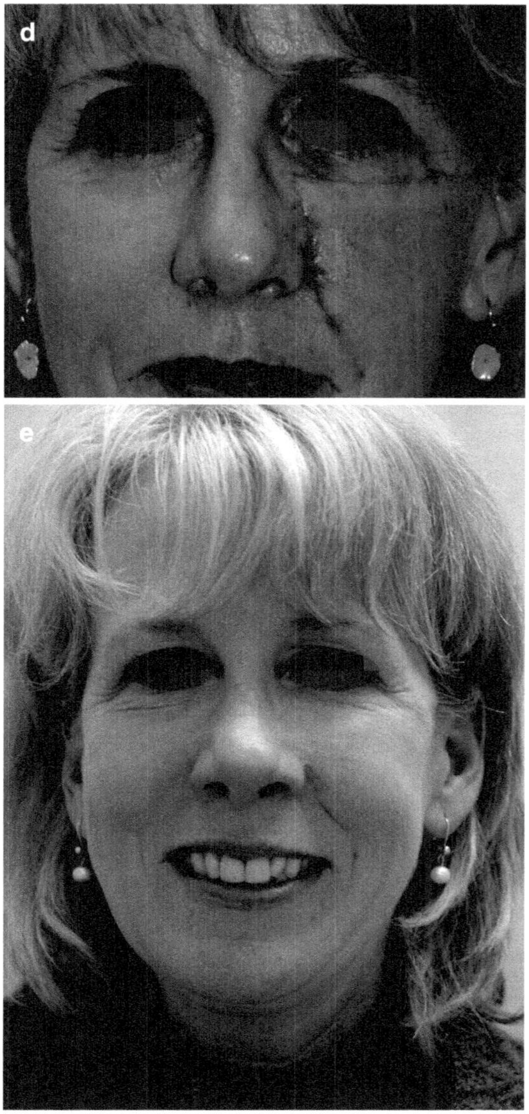

Fig. 23.20 (continued)

which arise when paramedian forehead flaps are used for nasal reconstruction (see Fig. 22.19 in Chap. 22).

Defects adjacent to the eyebrow can cause brow distortion if wound edge approximation or wound contracture places tension on the brow. Lagophthalmos and corneal exposure may result if scar formation occurs such that the brow is pulled superiorly.

Forehead defects ≤5 cm may be addressed with opposing rotation-advancement flaps. The flap incisions should be placed as close to MSTL as possible. To avoid de-animating the forehead, dissection should be conducted above the frontalis muscle (see Figs. 23.23a–d and 23.24a–c).

Larger defects of the forehead may be addressed with skin expansion, skin grafting, or free-tissue transfer. For the most part, skin grafts are a suboptimal choice even when they heal well. The disparity in texture, color match, and thickness are very apparent. Nonetheless, for select patients (elderly, poor candidates for surgery, etc.), skin grafts can prove useful.

Tissue expansion is a method of increasing the supply of soft tissue available for reconstruction by using an expandable prosthesis to create tension within the skin. Because the underlying skull provides a firm base for expansion, the forehead and scalp are excellent areas for skin expansion [17]. Unfortunately, skin expansion is a multi-staged procedure and requires much patience on behalf of both patient and surgeon.

Tissue expansion begins with insertion of a silicone prosthesis through an incision in the skin. First, a space equivalent to the size of the expander base diameter of the prosthetic is undermined and the prosthetic is placed in the resulting pocket. If the base of the expander is not flat and smooth, "knuckles" of prosthetic may be produced. These "knuckles" may cause pressure on the overlying tissue and result in subsequent exposure of the prosthetic [17]. After the initial implantation wounds have healed, saline is injected into the prosthesis through a fill port. Serial injections, administered over several months, increase the volume of the expander. The expander, supported by underlying bone, generates tension on the overlying soft tissue which slowly creates a reactive increase, or expansion, of the overlying soft tissue. The expansions can be uncomfortable and some patients may have significant difficulty with expansion. The expansion should be continued until the height of the expanded skin is equal to the width of the defect (see Fig. 23.25a, b).

Large defects of the forehead and scalp may require multiple expanders to generate significant tissue for closure. However, in most cases, large defects of the forehead have a better final appear-

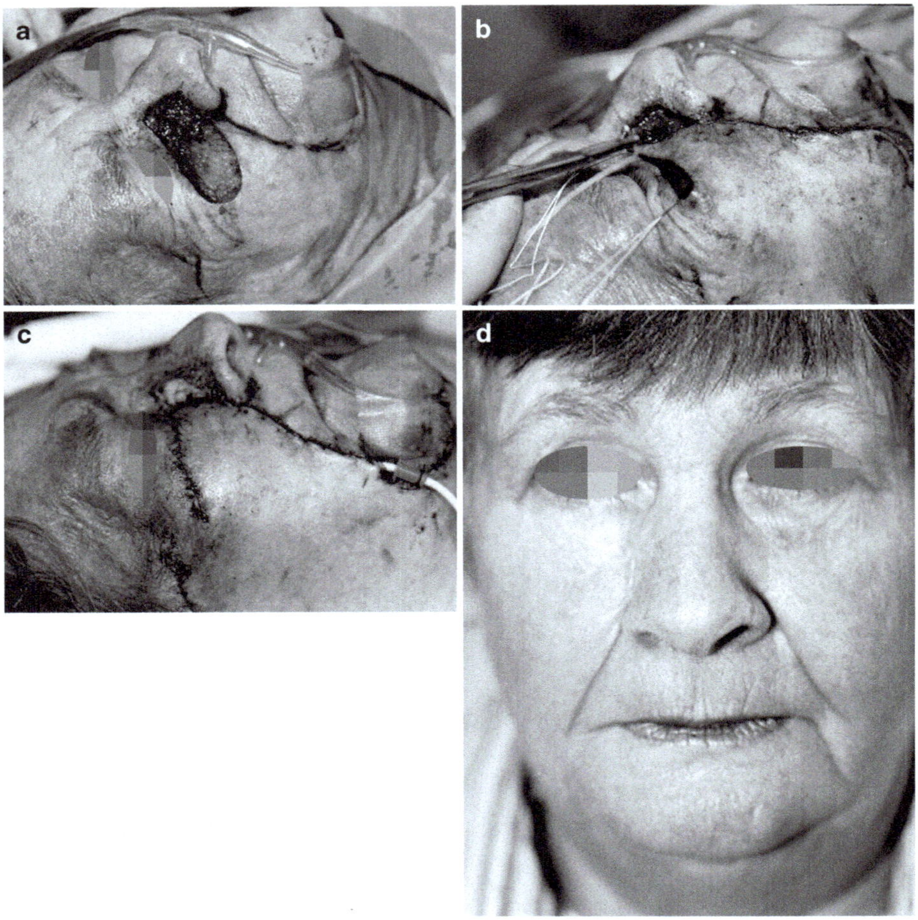

Fig. 23.21 (**a**) Defect with a horizontal axis. Tissue will be advanced from inferior to superior, with an incision placed beneath chin to close the horizontal defect. Note: The nasal sidewall will not be repaired with the cheek advancement flap because it is a separate unit. A full-thickness skin graft will be used to repair the nasal sidewall defect. (**b**) Cheek advancement flap is elevated. Note the sutures securing the flap to the infraorbital rim to support the weight of the flap and prevent tension on the lower lid. (**c**) The flap has been sutured in place and a full-thickness skin graft has been applied to the nasal sidewall. (**d**) Final result

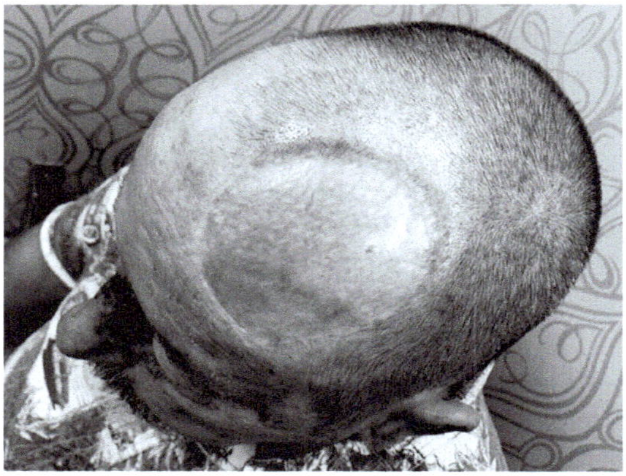

Fig. 23.22 Post-operative appearance after split-thickness skin graft to forehead and scalp

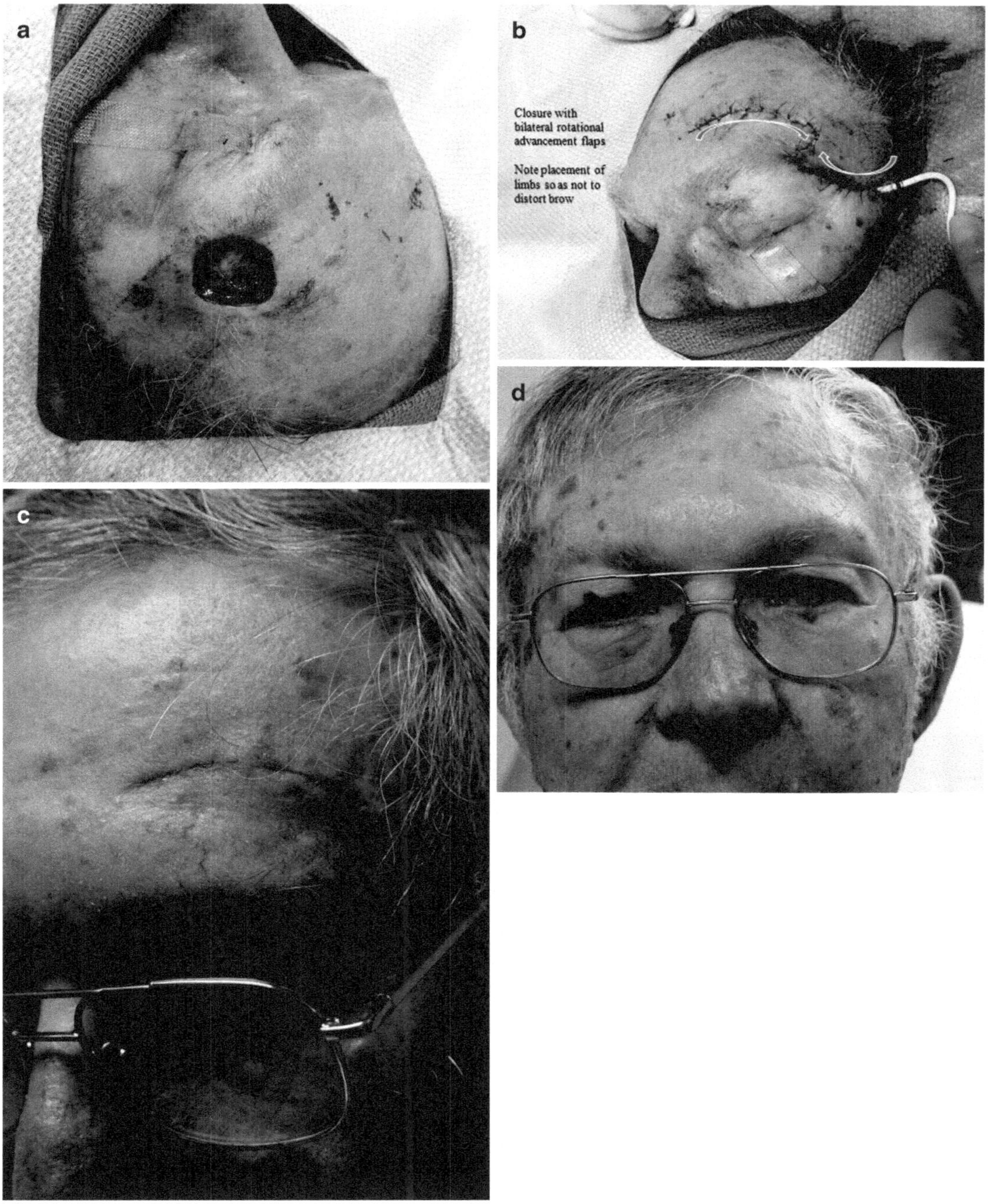

Fig. 23.23 (**a**) 3 cm defect of the left lateral forehead. (**b**) Bilateral rotation-advancement flaps after flap elevation and repair of the defect. Note that most of the incision is contained within MSTL. (**c**) Appearance at 3 months. (**d**) Final appearance at 6 months

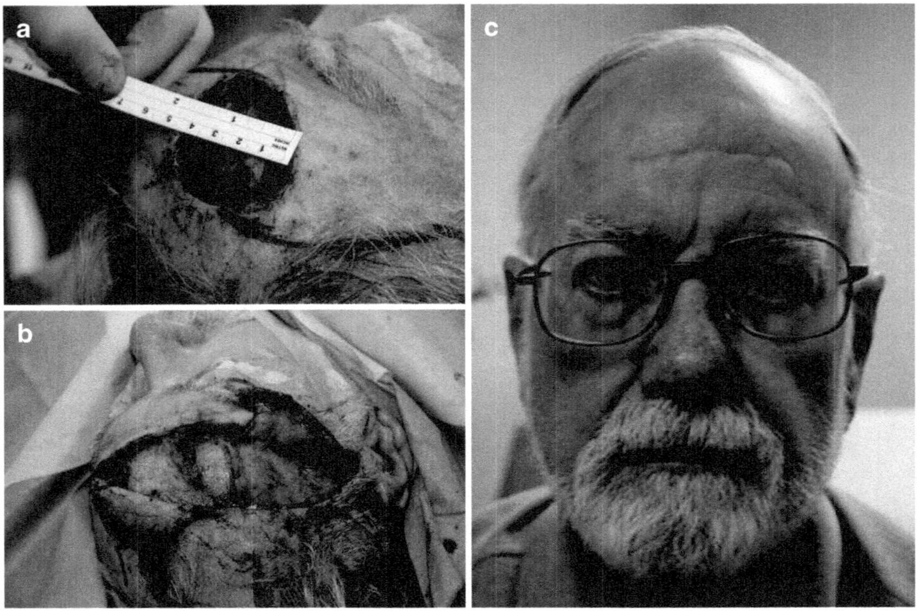

Fig. 23.24 (**a**) 4.5 cm defect of the right forehead. (**b**) Skin flaps elevated prior to advancement and rotation. Dissection is above the frontalis muscle. (**c**) Final appearance at 6 months

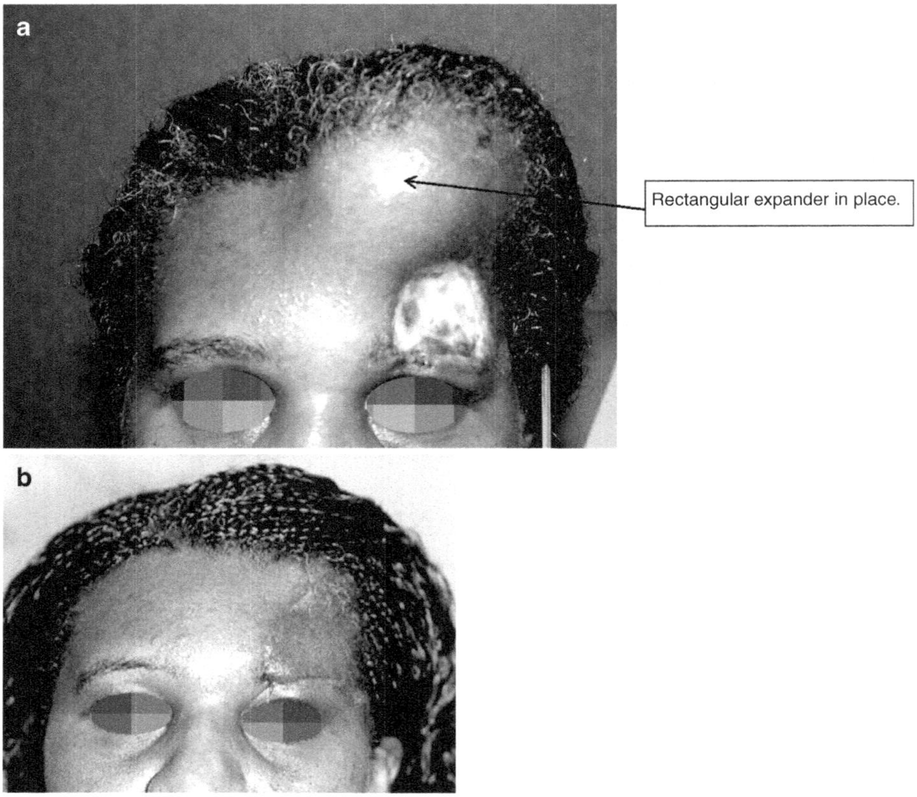

Fig. 23.25 (**a**) Delayed reconstruction with tissue expansion. The expander was placed beneath the superior, left forehead. This patient previously had a STSG placed over a left supra-brow defect. (**b**) Appearance at 1 month. Note: The hyperpigmentation will resolve over time

ance when reconstructed with skin expansion and local flaps when compared to reconstruction with free-tissue transfer.

If the patient is not a candidate for tissue expansion, free-tissue transfer is an acceptable alternative. Free-tissue transfer provides substrate which is significantly thick, but color and texture match is frequently suboptimal. There are relatively few free flap donor sites suitable for the "blush" area which provide reliable pedicles and acceptable aesthetics [18] (Fig. 23.26a–c).

Reconstruction of the Scalp

The scalp comprises multiple layers which include skin, subcutaneous tissue, muscular-aponeurotic tissue, a loose areolar plane, and pericranium [19]. Normally, only the skin and subcutaneous tissue are excised during resection of melanomatous lesions. It is therefore possible to apply a skin graft [20]. Skin grafts placed on scalp defects, however, become depressed over time and do not grow hair. They resemble areas of baldness and may distress patients with an otherwise normal hair distribution. Additionally, skin grafts on the scalp, especially if applied to the pericranium, may be quite thin and become unstable over an extended period of time. Skin grafts covering bare pericranium are notoriously unstable due to a relative paucity of underlying subcutaneous tissue.

Direct closure of scalp defects can be difficult, especially in the elderly. With advancing age, the scalp becomes thinner and tighter. Defects wider than two centimeters may prove very difficult to close and often create long "dog ears" which require subsequent excision. Even with significant undermining, advancement of the scalp may prove difficult and elliptical excision of "dog ears" may frustrate alternative efforts [21]. Scalp defects of 2–7 cm may be reliably closed with "Yin-Yang" flaps, which are a type of rotation-advancement flap. The flaps are designed to oppose each other at the center of the defect. They may be oriented in any direction, as long as the movement does not deform the donor area. After elevation of the flap, the surrounding scalp is widely undermined using a knife handle—the target tissue plane separates easily and is relatively avascular. Because melanoma excisions are rarely larger than 5 cm, "Yin-Yang" flaps provide adequate coverage for most excision-related defects [22, 23]. Rotation-advancement flaps, such as the Yin-Yang flap, can be an effective method for closing large defects secondary to melanoma excision (see Fig. 23.27a–d).

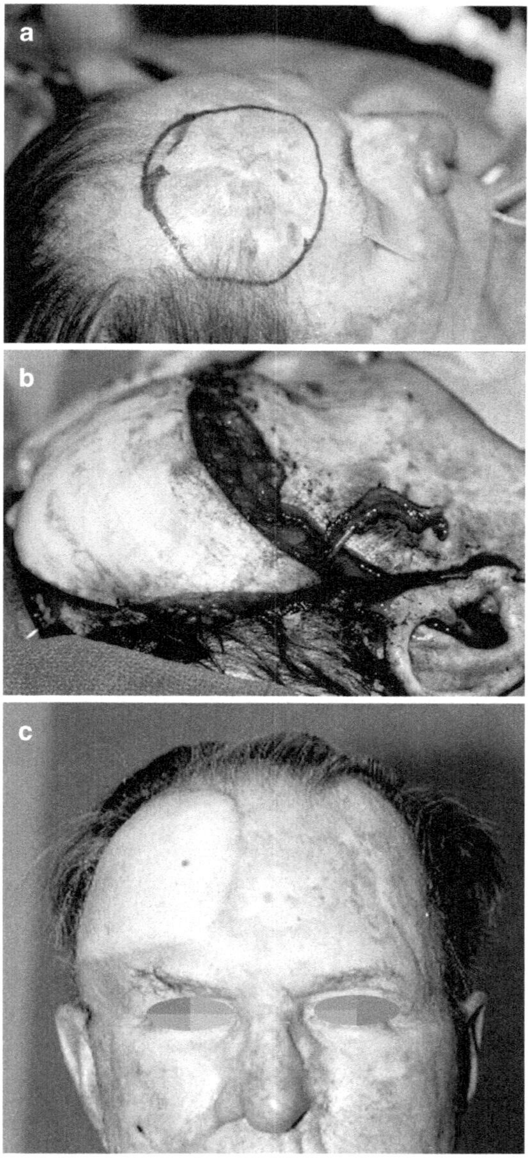

Fig. 23.26 (**a**) Patient will undergo 6 cm excision of this right forehead lesion. (**b**) Reconstruction using a Deep Inferior Epigastric Perforator (DIEP) free flap. The recipient vessels are the superficial temporal vessels. (**c**) Final result at 6 months after flap thinning via liposuction

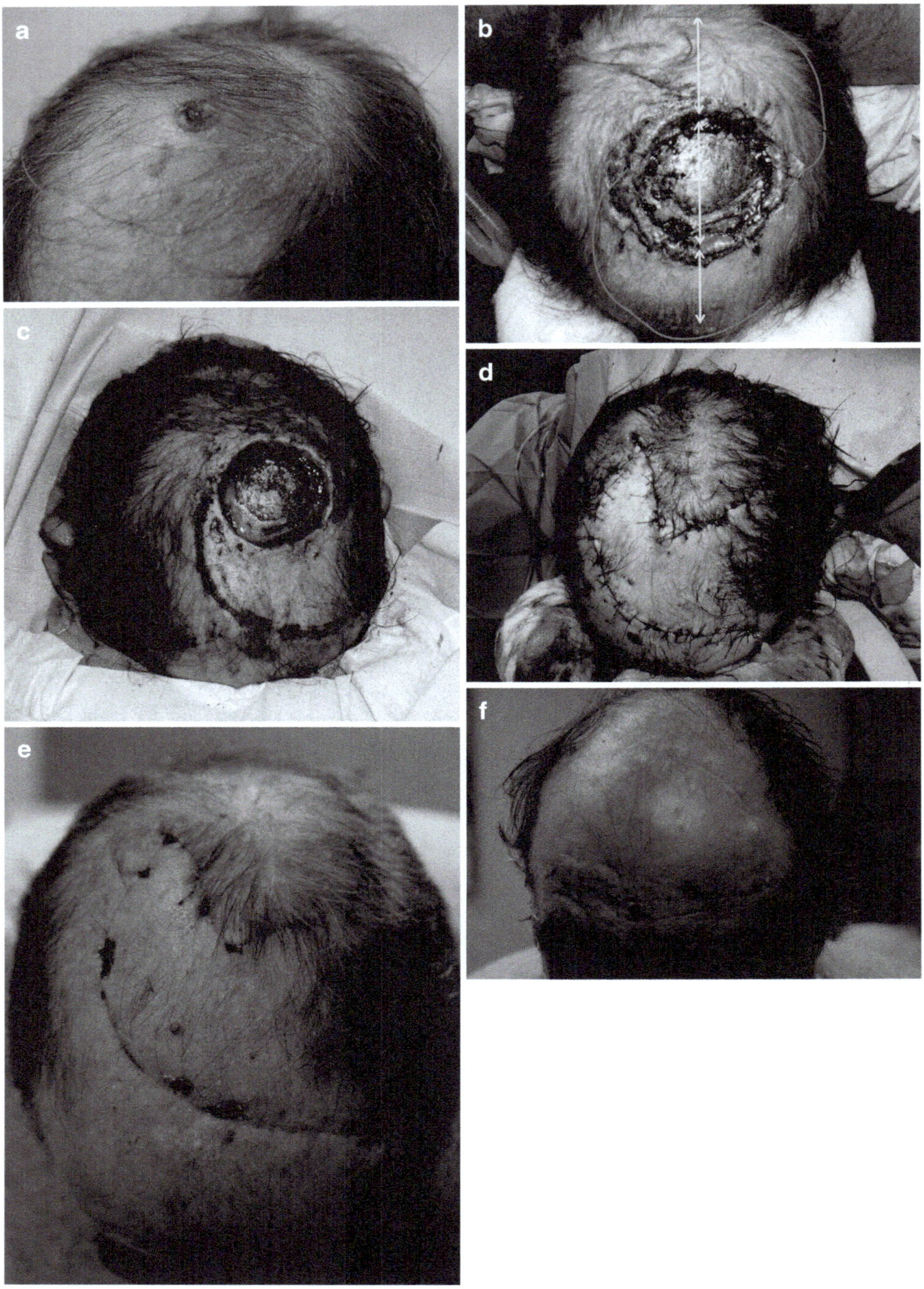

Fig. 23.27 (**a**) 2.5 mm thick melanoma of the scalp, requiring 5 cm excision. (**b**) Designing the "Yin-Yang" flaps. The length of the white lines should be equal. The flaps are raised in the plane between the galea and pericranium. After elevation, a large radius of tissue must be undermined in the plane above the periosteum to allow appropriate flap advancement. (**c**) Actual incision design on this patient: note that flaps are each as wide as the defect. To reduce tension, wide subgaleal undermining is used. The galea can also be "stripped" to release it and a Borrow' triangle added. (**d**) Intraoperative view after advancement of the Yin-Yang flaps. (**e**) Post-operative appearance following suture removal at 2 weeks. (**f**) Final appearance at 6 months

Alternative techniques for scalp closure include scalp expansion, the use of scaffolds, such as Integra, and free-tissue transfer. However, the excision of melanoma lesions generally results in smaller secondary defects and such techniques, which are often employed to cover large defects, are not necessary.

References

1. Bricca GM, Brodland DG, Ren D, Zitelli JA. Cutaneous head and neck melanoma treated with Mohs micrographic surgery. J Am Acad Dermatol. 2005;52(1):92–100.
2. Rawlani R, Rawlani V, Qureshi HA, Kim JY, Wayne JD. Reducing margins of wide local excision in head and neck melanoma for function and cosmesis: 5-year local recurrence-free survival. J Surg Oncol. 2015;111(7):795–9.
3. Zenga J, Nussenbaum B, Cornelius LA, Linette GP, Desai SC. Management controversies in head and neck melanoma: a systematic review. JAMA Facial Plast Surg. 2017;19(1):53–62.
4. Pirgousis P, Fernandes R. Reconstruction of subtotal defects of the lower lip: a review of current techniques and a proposed modification. J Oral Maxillofac Surg. 2001;69(1):295–9.
5. Eskiizmir G, Baker S, Cingi C. Nonmelanomatous skin cancer of the head and neck: reconstruction. Facial Plast Surg Clin North Am. 2012;20(4):493–513.
6. Knabel MR, Koranda FC, Olejko TD. Surgical management of carcinomas of the lower lip. J Dermtatol Surg Oncol. 1982;8(11):979–83.
7. Harrison CA, MacNeil S. The mechanism of skin graft contraction: an update on current research and potential future therapies. Burns. 2008;34(2):153–63.
8. Urushidate S, Yokoi K, Higuma Y, Mikami M, et al. New way to raise the V-Y advancement flap for reconstruction of the lower lip: bipedicled orbicularis oris musculocutaneous flap technique. J Plast Surg Hand Surg. 2011;45(2):66–71.
9. Lisa EI, Byrne PJ. Lip reconstruction. Facial Plast Surg Clin North Am. 2009;17(3):445–53.
10. Roldan JC, Teschke M, Fritzer E, Dunsche A, Harle F, Wiltfang J, Terheyden H. Reconstruction of the lower lip: rationale to preserve the esthetic subunits of the face. Plast Reconstr Surg. 2007;120(5):1231–9.
11. Baker SR. Local flaps in facial reconstruction. 3rd ed. Philadelphia, PA: Saunders Elsevier; 2014.
12. Bray DA. Clinical applications of the rhomboid flap. Arch Otolaryngol. 1983;109(1):37–42.
13. Al-Shunnar B, Manson P. Cheek reconstruction with laterally based flaps. Clin Plast Surg. 2001;28(2):283–96.
14. Baker SR. Local cutaneous flaps. Otolarngol Clin North Am. 1994;27(1):139–59.
15. Murillo W, Fernandez W, Caycedo D, Dupin C, Eileen B. Cheek and inferior eyelid reconstruction after skin cancer ablation. Clin Plast Surg. 2004;31:49–67.
16. Temple C, Ross D. Scalp and forehead reconstruction. Clin Plast Surg. 2005;32(3):377–90.
17. Antonyshyn O, Gruss JS, Zuker R, Mackinnon SE. Tissue expansion in head and neck reconstruction. Plast Reconstr Surg. 1988;82(1):58–68.
18. McCombe D, Donato R, Hofer S, Morrison W. Free flaps in the treatment of locally advanced malignancy of the scalp and forehead. Ann Plast Surg. 2002;48(6):600–6.
19. Horowitz JH, et al. Galeal-pericranial flaps in head and neck reconstruction. Anatomy and application. Am J Surg. 1984;148(4):489–97.
20. Molnar JA, DeFranzo AJ, Marks MW. Single-stage approach to skin grafting the exposed skull. Plast Reconstr Surg. 2000;105(1):174–7.
21. Hoffman JF. Management of scalp defects. Otolaryngol Clin N Am. 2001;34(3):571–82.
22. Ransom ER, Jacono AA. Double-opposing rotation-advancement flaps for closure of forehead defects. Arch Facial Plast Surg. 2012;14(5):342–5.
23. Ahuja RB. Geometric considerations in the design of rotation flaps in the scalp and forehead region. Plast Reconstr Surg. 1988;81(6):900–6.

Reconstruction Options for Trunk and Extremity Melanoma

24

Oren Tessler, Alex M. Lin, Shukan Patel, and Charles L. Dupin

Basic Principles

Melanoma is a malignant tumor comprised of the pigment-containing cells known as melanocytes. The most proven risk factors for development of the disease are prolonged sun exposure and being fair-skinned (Fitzpatrick type I–II) [1]. In 2017, the incidence rate in the United States was 20.2 per 100,000 people, with ~9730 deaths annually (Fig. 24.1) [2]. There are four major histopathologic subtypes of melanoma and their relative incidences are: lentigo maligna (10–40%), superficial spreading (30–60%), nodular (15–35%), and acral lentiginous (5–10%) [3, 4]. In addition to the histopathologic subtypes, patient age and the total amount of sun exposure also impact the relative incidence of melanoma. Specifically, lentigo maligna is more commonly found in the elderly patient with chronic sun exposure [5].

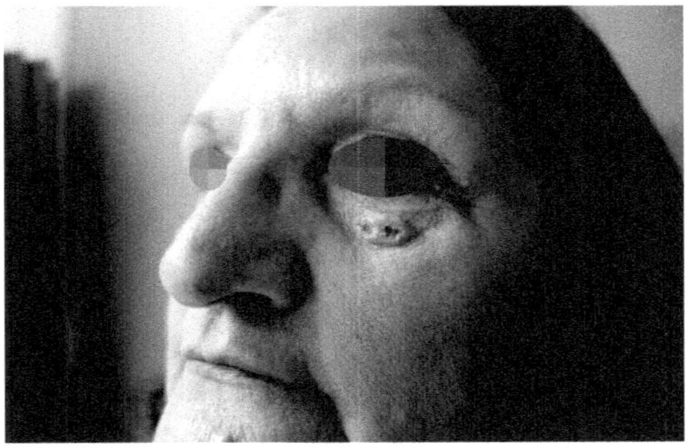

Fig. 24.1 Patient presenting with a periorbital melanoma

Anatomical Distribution of Melanoma

There is a significant gender difference in the anatomical location of primary melanoma. In females, superficial spreading melanoma occurs more frequently on the lower extremities, while in males, superficial spreading melanoma more frequently occurs on the trunk, especially on the back [6, 7]. In terms of head and neck predilection, the frequencies are roughly similar when

O. Tessler, M.D., C.M., M.B.A.
Department of Surgery, University Medical Center, New Orleans, New Orleans, LA, USA
e-mail: otessl@lsuhsc.edu

A. M. Lin, M.S. (✉)
Frank H. Netter MD School of Medicine at Quinnipiac University, Hamden, CT, USA
e-mail: alex.lin@quinnipiac.edu

S. Patel, B.S., M.S., M.D.
Department of Plastics and Reconstructive Surgery, Louisiana State University Health Science Center – New Orleans, New Orleans, LA, USA
e-mail: spat23@lsuhsc.edu

C. L. Dupin, M.D.
Division of Plastic and Reconstructive Surgery, Department of Surgery, Louisiana State University Health Sciences Center, New Orleans, LA, USA
e-mail: cdupin@lsuhsc.edu

A. I. Riker (ed.), *Melanoma*, https://doi.org/10.1007/978-3-319-78310-9_24

comparing males and females. Therefore, precautionary guidance should vary appropriately, such as instructing men to remember sun protective clothing when engaging in shirtless outdoor activities. Women should be educated on the importance of sunscreen products for exposed areas when outside. Despite efforts at primary prevention, melanoma is still responsible for the majority of skin-cancer-related deaths in the United States [8]. Hence, it is important for healthcare providers to understand anatomic predilections in order to identify suspicious skin lesions using the "ABCDE" diagnostic tool.

Treatment and Assessment of Melanoma

The preliminary step in treatment and assessment of melanoma is a full-thickness excisional biopsy of suspicious lesions with a recommended 1–2 mm margin of normal tissue. The goal is to provide a specimen sufficient for the pathologist to determine the tumor thickness in millimeters. This measurement, known as the Breslow's depth, strongly correlates with survivability of the disease, with a linear correlation between increasing thickness and the possibility of systemic spread of disease. Additional pathologic findings important for melanoma staging include ulceration, mitotic rate, angiolymphatic invasion, tumor infiltrating lymphocytes, tumor regression, and Clark's level of histologic invasion. Pathologic confirmation of melanoma from a skin biopsy should then lead to a repeat procedure of wider excision of tissue with the removal of the lesion and appropriate surgical margins based upon current NCCN treatment guidelines. This may be coupled with a sentinel lymph node biopsy for tumors with a Breslow's depth of >1.0 mm [9].

Surgical Treatment/Wide Local Excision—Margins

The purpose of wide local excision (WLE) of malignant melanoma is to decrease the risk of local recurrence. Obtaining clean (negative) margins is important, especially in high risk areas like the hands and feet (acral lentiginous) and vermillion of the lips, where there are reported recurrence rates as high as 12% [10]. The recommended margins are determined by the Breslow's depth of invasion. For in situ melanoma, the excision requires 0.5 cm of clear margins. Invasive melanoma requires a 1-cm margin for lesions ≤1 mm in depth, a 1–2-cm margin for lesions 1–2 mm in depth, and a margin of at least 2 cm for lesions ≥2 mm in depth. These recommendations for negative surgical margins after wide local excision for primary cutaneous melanoma are continuously being examined, based upon multiple factors and evidence [11]. As reconstructive surgeons, we are continually trying to find the balance between pursuing an aggressive resection to minimize locoregional recurrence, while minimizing the resultant defect, which ultimately may require a complex wound reconstruction for the patient.

Reconstructive Considerations

The primary goal of melanoma treatment is disease eradication, and this often involves wide excision. The plastic surgeon often assists with the reconstructive challenges associated with a residual defect from the primary excision performed by the surgical oncologist. These patients may require tissue reconstruction in any part of the body, depending upon the location and size of this defect. In any reconstructive scenario where malignancy has occurred, the overriding oncologic principle is to successfully remove the primary melanoma with the appropriate surgical margins. This is often performed at the same operation, with the plastic surgeon performing the complex wound reconstruction. Function, as well as aesthetics, must be at the forefront of the plastic surgeon's mind when planning the reconstruction. As part of the preoperative discussion, the plastic surgeon should be aware of the negative impact a scar can have on the patient's self-image. Interestingly, it has been shown that patients care more about the overall contour of the scar than the length of incision regardless of its anatomical location [12]. This should be an important consideration as surgeons navigate through the reconstructive ladder. The guiding principle is to implement the simplest reconstructive options first, moving upwards in complexity as the need exists. Typically, viable options for reconstruction are guided by the size of the defect and its anatomical location.

Trunk

Primary Closure

Fortunately, most excisions of a melanoma of the abdomen leave enough tissue with appropriate laxity for simple primary closure. One can imagine the ease of primary closure in a patient yielding copious amounts of soft tissue supplying enough laxity for such a simple repair. Up to a 15-cm diameter circular excision on the lower abdomen can be closed. The upper abdomen has less laxity, but a resection bed of 4 cm in diameter has the possibility of being closed primarily. The surgeon must bear in mind that primary closure of a defect on the chest or the back may incur more tension upon primary closure due to lack of adipose distribution in these regions. Additionally, active range of motion in the postsurgical setting may result in the disruption of a strong suture line, regardless of the inherently thick nature of the skin on the back. This bears significant impact in patients with a tendency to scar poorly, as there are poorly defined relaxed skin tension lines in these areas. Thus, anterior chest, shoulders, and back incisions produce higher rates of hypertrophic, widened, and keloid scarring [13].

Skin Grafts

If the possibility does occur that an abdominal or back wound incurs too much tension for primary closure, a split, or full-thickness skin graft is an option. Skin grafts undergo secondary contraction that may be of benefit to reducing overall size of the reconstruction site. In the trunk area, care must be taken to avoid a step-off in depth between native skin and grafts as much as possible. There are different techniques for this, including tacking the skin edges to the underlying tissue, generating a gentle slope between native skin and the skin graft. Meshing of the grafts (normally 2:1 or 3:1 ratio) allows smaller donor sites to be used, but the final cobblestone appearance of the grafts can be unattractive after final healing. Typically, skin grafts of the trunk have a high viability rate, with graft failure being the result of a hematoma or seroma forming underneath the graft. A full-thickness, unmeshed skin graft may also be utilized, with the advantage of primary wound closure of the donor site. Appropriate bolster dressings must be properly applied either with a negative pressure device using a non-adherent contact layer (i.e., Xeroform) or with a suture strengthened traditional pressure bolster dressing. On the back (and in further sections of this chapter discussing extremities), one must be more cautious of direct graft shearing due to the motion applied to the graft or direct blunt injury to the graft. Using negative pressure devices with a contact layer directly applied to the graft protects the graft from shear forces and allows removal of the dressing within 5 days.

Flap Reconstructive Options of the Trunk

Rarely are melanoma defects of the trunk complex in nature. If more complex wounds are encountered along the abdomen, chest, or back, one may employ the use of local skin flaps along with some undermining of the surrounding skin edges. Local flaps such as a V-Y advancement flap, rhomboid, rotational or transposition flap can be easily applied to any region of the trunk. Other factors include local skin laxity and the amount of local undermining of the skin edges (Figs. 24.2a, b and 24.3a, b). Basic local flap principles of geometry apply to the trunk and allow for a wide range of options.

For managing melanoma defects, it is uncommon for the wide local excision to disrupt the deep abdominal fascia. However, in cases where there is a need for complex wound reconstruction within the chest or abdomen, it is best to approach the abdominal wall defect based upon four primary locations: zone 1A, upper midline defects with extension across the midline; zone 1B, lower midline defect with extension across

Fig. 24.2 Rotation flap. The edge is four to five times the length of the base of the defect triangle. A back cut or a Burow's triangle can be used if the flap is under excessive tension. (**a**) Pivot point and line of greatest tension. (**b**) Back cut. (**c**) Burow's triangle

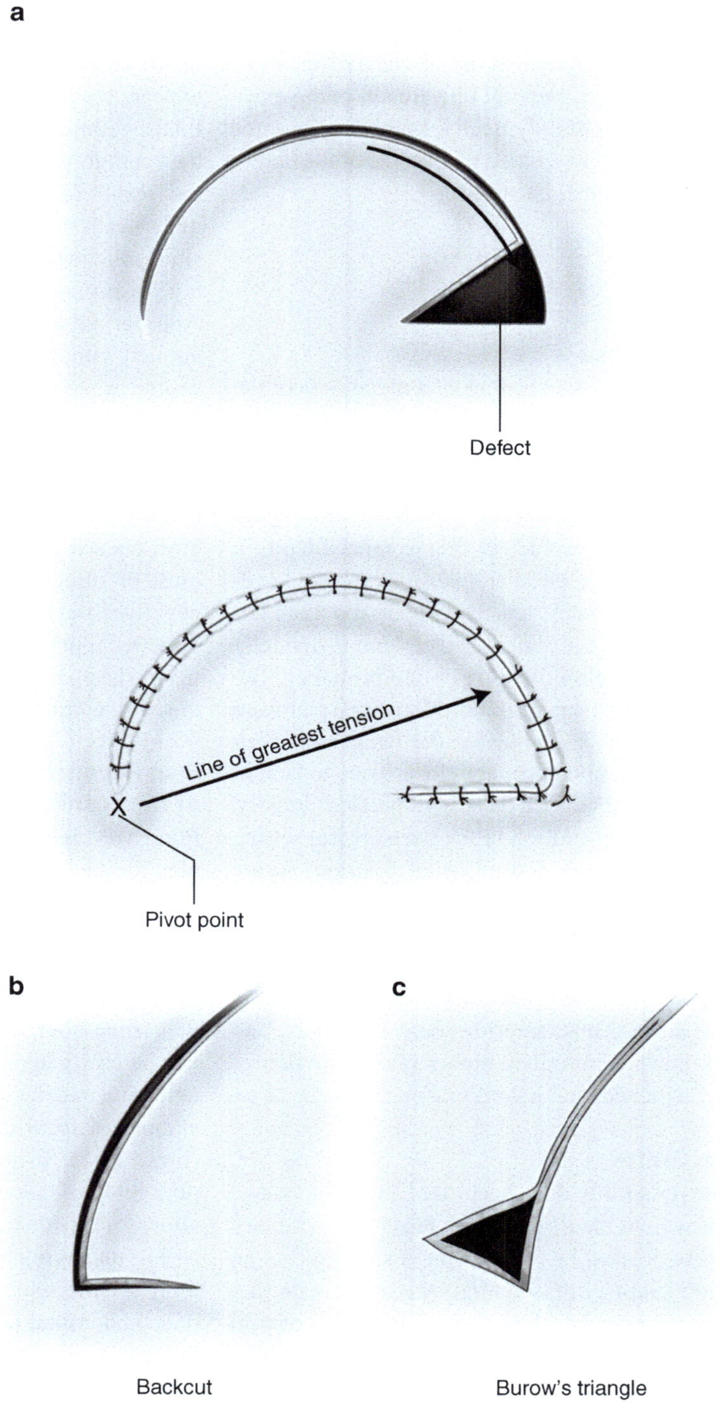

Fig. 24.3 Transposition flap. The secondary defect is often closed with a skin graft. A back cut can be used if the flap is under excessive tension

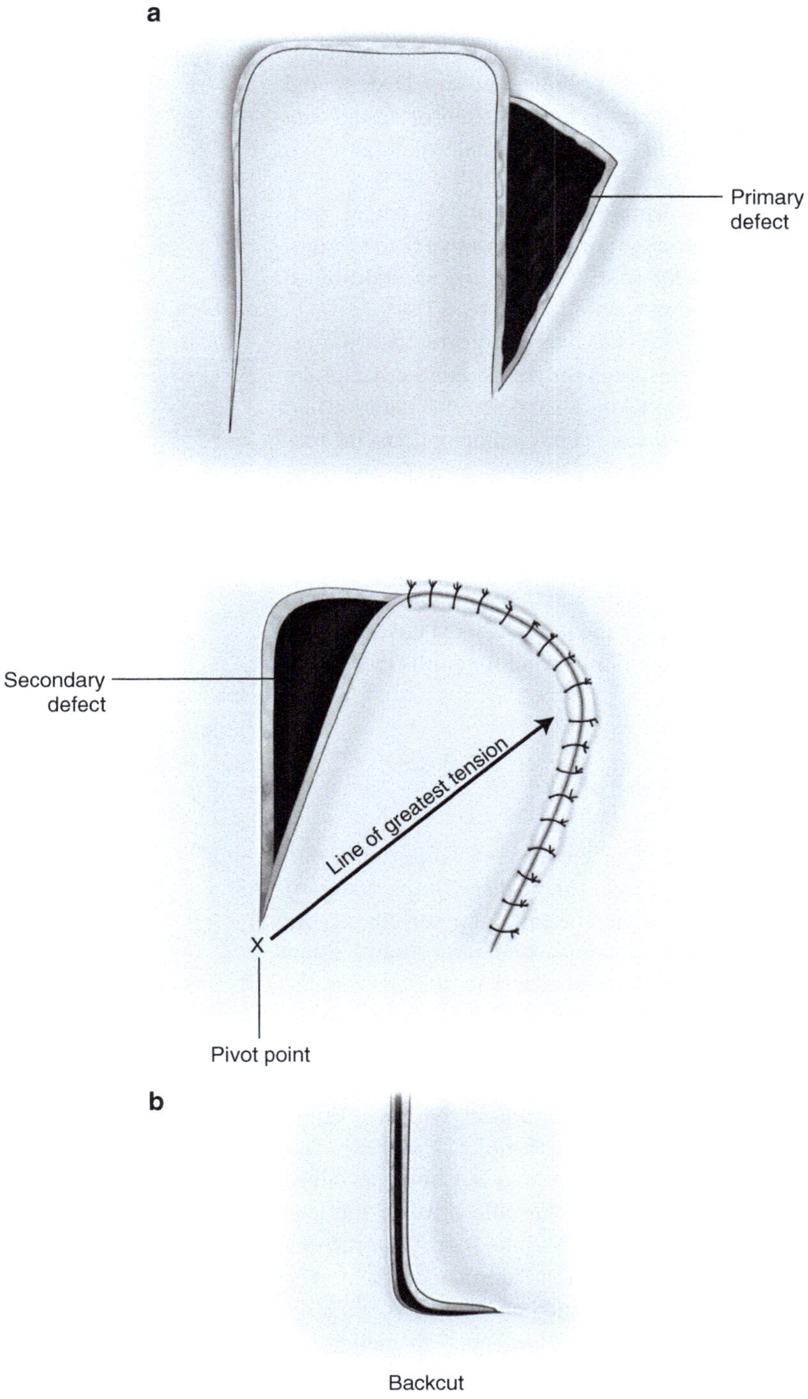

the midline; zone 2, upper quadrant defect; zone 3, lower quadrant defects. Specific local flap options for the abdomen include rectus abdominus and external oblique muscle. Distant and free flap options include the tensor fascia lata flap, latissimus dorsi flap, anterolateral thigh flap, and groin flap [14, 15]. These flap techniques are primarily used for abdominal wall defects where the surgical objective is to reestablish the abdominal wall integrity in addition to reconstructing a skin defect [16, 17].

For complex chest wall reconstructive options, the local flaps commonly used are the pectoralis major, latissimus dorsi, and serratus anterior flap [18, 19]. For distant and free flap options, the rectus abdominis and latissimus dorsi are the most common (Fig. 24.4a–c) [20]. As for reconstructive options of the back, a midline defect can often be closed using paravertebral and erector spinae muscle flaps [21]. A non-midline defect will often require the use of a local advancement flap because their arc of rotation limits these midline muscles.

Lower Extremity

The lower extremity is of great importance due to the obvious function of these limbs in regard to ambulation and bearing the weight of the body. Lower extremity melanoma more often occurs in females younger than 40, with important aesthetic concerns of visible scarring with certain clothing [6]. The majority of melanoma found in the extremities, specifically acral lentiginous melanoma, is found in the lower limbs (78%) versus the upper limbs (22%) [22]. The lower extremity can be divided into the thigh, upper third of the leg, middle third of the leg, lower third of the leg, and the foot. With respect to the distribution of melanoma of the lower extremities, melanoma occurs twice as often on the leg than on the thigh or foot. For melanoma found in the upper limbs, the majority of the tumor burden is along the shoulder, with equal distribution for the upper arm and forearm, while the least tumor burden is found on the hand [23].

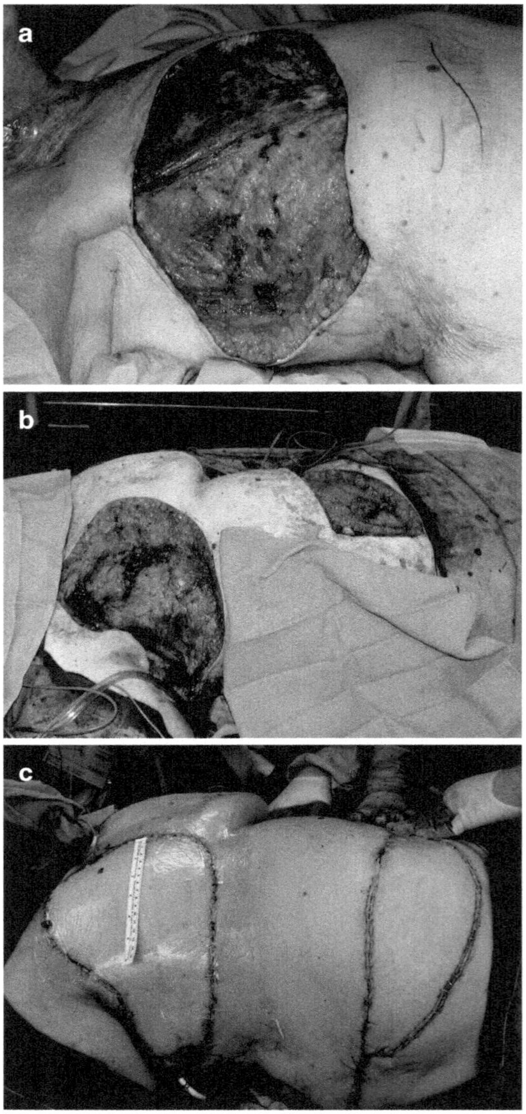

Fig. 24.4 (**a**) Patient presented with a large right chest wound to be closed with a unilateral left DIEP (Deep Inferior Epigastric Artery Perforator). (**b**) Chest wall defect with left DIEP raised. Donor site was closed with a combination of primary closure and V-Y advancement of the contralateral hemi-abdomen. (**c**) Chest wall defect with DIEP in place and donor site closed

Thigh

Primary Closure

The thigh is the most forgiving area of the lower extremity for reconstruction. It is the bulkiest area with the largest muscle volume and largest amount of skin. While primary closure in the thigh is feasible after excision of a melanoma, one should be aware that a defect with dimensions that could be easily closed primarily on the abdomen may be met with significant tension and difficulty when that same defect is replicated on the thigh.

Graft and Flap Reconstructive Options of the Thigh

Split thickness skin grafts to the thigh are viable options, yet these areas are usually used as skin graft donor sites in other situations, so donor skin can be harvested from the contralateral thigh or an abdominal region that is relatively discreet. A full-thickness skin graft is a reasonable alternative, with the donor site commonly utilized along the abdomen. Likewise, local flaps can be easily employed in this region with more than adequate bulk and mobility due to the inherent nature of the tissue in this anatomical region. Some of the commonly used local flap options of the thigh include flaps based off of the lateral femoral circumflex artery (tensor fascia latae, vastus lateralis, and rectus femoris), gracilis, and vertical rectus abdominus flap.

Additionally, any local perforator flap can be identified and mobilized based off of its vascular pedicle [24, 25]. These customized perforator flaps can be identified with various modes of imaging, including ultrasound and CT angiography. They provide adequate soft tissue bulk and breadth and closely match the defect with using similar tissue to reconstruct. Creating propeller island flaps that have tremendous freedom of movement enhances the arc of rotation of these flaps. Elaborate free flap reconstruction is rarely needed in this area; however, recipient vessels in this area may branch from various vessels such as the superior gluteal and lateral circumflex femoral artery [26]. A widely split latissimus dorsi muscle flap has been used for long, soft tissue defects in the lower extremities [27].

Melanoma of the Leg

Defects along the upper, middle, and lower leg may require a greater frequency of skin grafts, local flaps, or even free flaps for reconstruction. This is primarily due to the diminishing volume of tissue and skin laxity in the region compared to thigh, especially in the lower one-third of the leg. The anterior leg specifically has a paucity of soft tissue laxity due to the overlying tibial bone, with elderly patients found to have a less well-perfused vascular bed compared to the thigh and trunk. The primary goal of reconstruction within the leg is to restore or maintain function, in addition to providing adequate tissue coverage of large defects.

This provides a unique challenge to the reconstructive ladder, as skin grafts may be inferior to local and free flap reconstruction, in terms of restoring the patient's function. For example, defects of the heel and plantar surface of the foot require durable and adherent tissue in order to maximize functional restoration post-melanoma extirpation. As a reconstructive surgeon, this scenario often requires the surgeon to rely on his surgical judgment instead of sequentially working through the reconstructive ladder when choosing the best reconstructive options.

Flap Reconstructive Options of the Leg

The most common local flaps available for reconstruction of the leg are the gastrocnemius and soleus flaps. The gastrocnemius flap is the flap of choice for coverage of the knee and the upper one-third of the leg, while the soleus muscle is commonly utilized for the middle one-third of the leg [28, 29]. In the lower one-third of the leg, soleus muscle can be used for smaller-sized defects [30]. Larger defects within the lower one-third of the leg usually require microvascular free flaps. Other possible options include the gracilis, rectus abdominus, latissimus dorsi, anterolateral thigh, deep inferior epigastric perforator, and superficial inferior epigastric perforator flaps [31–33]. If individuals have contraindications for microvascular transplantation, some local fasciocutaneous flaps have been identified for reconstruction. These fasciocutaneous flaps consist of the anterior tibial, peroneal, and posterior tibial artery, saphenous flap, and reverse sural flap [34–36].

Melanoma of the Foot

Melanoma of the foot or toe is also frequently seen. The majority of melanoma found in the foot or toes is the acral lentiginous subtype, comprising >60% of cases [37]. This type of melanoma is more aggressive and has a poorer overall prognosis compared to the other subtypes [38]. They are commonly found in patients with darker skin types (Fitzpatrick type V and VI) and they tend to occur at an earlier age compared to the general population [39]. While skin laxity is present on the dorsal surface of the foot, subcutaneous tissue is minimal. For dorsal defects, a split thickness skin graft in this area usually fares quite well with good overall graft viability. The skin on the plantar surface of the foot is thick and densely adherent to the underlying fascia, making primary wound closure of an excision in this area difficult. Melanoma can also present on a toe or under a finger or toenail, with specific recommendations for the surgical management of these lesions. In the case of acral lentiginous melanoma that are >1.0 mm in Breslow's thickness, an amputation is usually indicated of the affected digit. The amputation is performed back to the closest interphalangeal joint in order to maximize digit functionality. For subungual primary melanoma >1.0 mm in Breslow's thickness, the surgical recommendation is also an amputation of the distal phalanx, with the addition of a sentinel lymph node biopsy [40].

Flap Reconstructive Options of the Foot

In terms of reconstructive options for the foot, it is best to categorize them based upon four distinct anatomical locations: (1) The Achille's tendon area, the ankle and foot dorsum; (2) The plantar forefoot; (3) The plantar midfoot; and (4) the plantar hindfoot.

For the ankle and foot dorsum, the flap reconstructive options consist of an extensor digitorum brevis muscle flap and the lateral supramalleolar flap [41–44]. The extensor digitorum brevis muscle flap is good for covering the defects on the anterior ankle, proximal dorsum, and lateral malleolus if there is strong anterograde blood flow from the lateral tarsal artery. The lateral supramalleolar flap is used for deep wound defects found on the lateral malleolus and the anterior ankle.

For the plantar forefoot, local flap techniques are useful for reconstruction of deep wound defects along the distal third of the foot. A well-known option is a neurovascular island flap from the adjacent toe [45]. This flap is effective for defects up to 2–3 cm in diameter. For defects up to 4–5 cm in diameter, one can advance the forefoot skin and fascia in a V-Y fashion, known as the V-Y plantar flap. In the midfoot region, the neurovascular island flap is also a good option for 2–3 cm defects. The most useful option for small wound defect in this region is the V-Y advancement flap (Fig. 24.5b, c). Additional local flap options for small defects are the bilobed flap, rhomboid flap, and the transposition flap (Fig. 24.6). One can also consider the suprafascial plantar flaps, specifically, a medially dissected plantar flap to preserve sensation in this region. If a regional muscle flap is required, a pedical abductor hallucis flap or an abductor digiti minimi flap can be used for medial and lateral coverage, respectively.

Lastly, the flap reconstruction of the hindfoot is one of the greatest challenges to the reconstructive surgeon [46]. The hindfoot is a very specialized location. Reconstruction of this area should provide adequate soft tissue coverage for safe weight bearing along with maintaining normal ankle function for the patient. For this situation, the reconstructive options can be extensive. These include intrinsic muscle flaps, medial plantar artery flap, heel pad flaps, sural artery flap, and free flaps [47, 48]. There are three intrinsic foot muscle flaps for hindfoot reonstruction: abductor hallucis, abductor digiti minimi, and flexor digitorum brevis. Abductor hallucis is used for small defects found on the heel and medial malleolus.

Abductor digiti minimi is useful for lateral calcaneal defects. Flexor digitorum brevis is used for heel pad reconstruction because the muscle has sufficient bulk to provide adequate padding. The medial plantar artery flap is also a useful alternative for heel pad reconstruction. However, the transverse arch of the midfoot

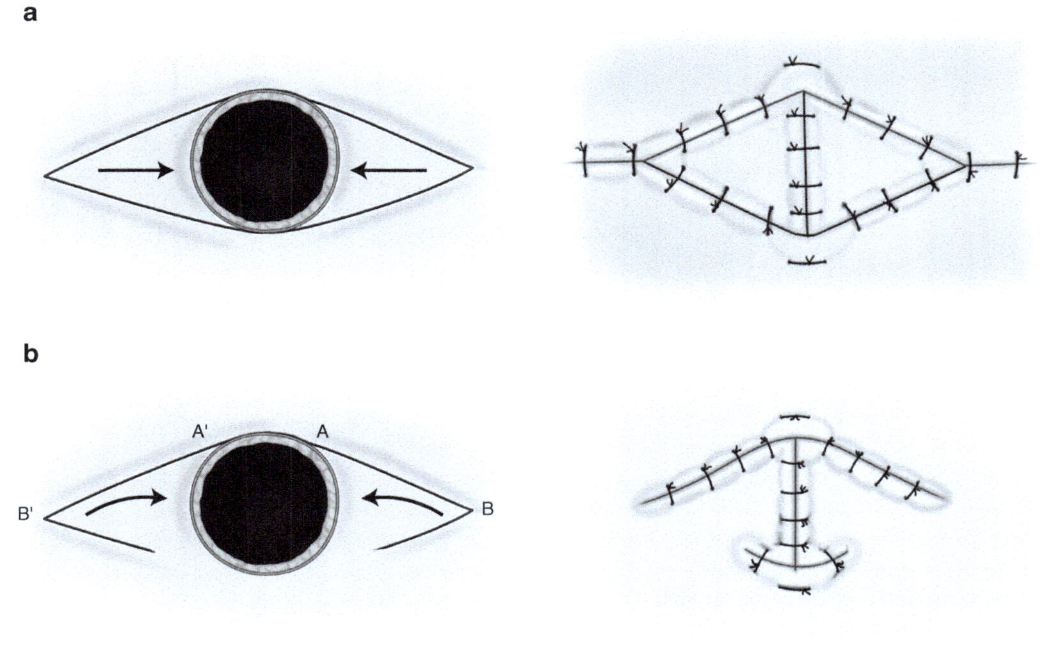

Fig. 24.5 Closure of a tissue defect following circular excision. (**a**) Sliding triangular subcutaneous pedicle flaps can be advanced to close the circular defect; the triangular defect is closed in a V-Y fashion. (**b**) Transposition flaps based on a skin pedicle and rotated towards each other can also be used. Circular defects can also be closed by other flaps or by purse string suture

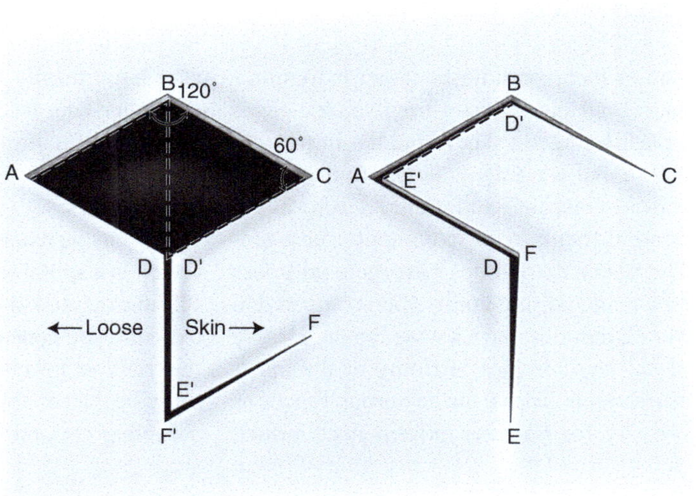

Fig. 24.6 Planning a rhomboid flap. The rhomboid defect must have 60- and 120-degree angles. The flap is planned in an area of loose skin so that direct closure of the wound edges is possible. The short diagonal BD (which is the same length as each side) is extended its own length to point E. The line EF drawn parallel to CD and is of the same length. After the flap margins have been incised, the flap is transposed into the rhomboid defect

Fig. 24.7 Skin graft placed superior to right ankle

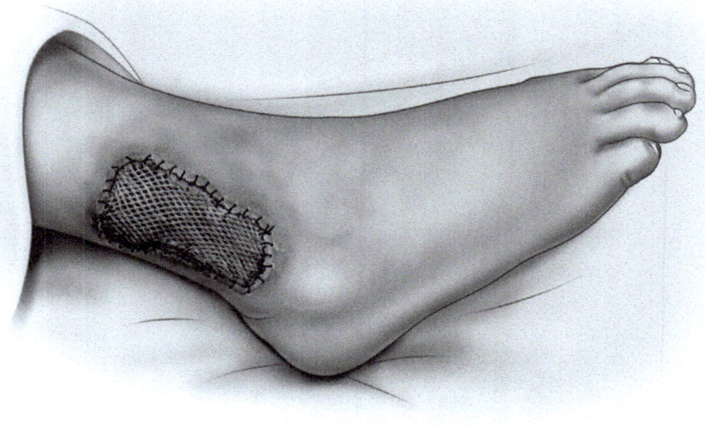

must be maintained because a skin graft is required for coverage at the donor site (Fig. 24.7). For patients with large heel defects and limited ambulation, a suprafascial heel pad flap should be considered. Free flaps are commonly reserved for wounds greater than 6 cm. Free flaps that have been proven successful in the past are latissimus dorsi, gracilis muscle, radial forearm flap, lateral arm flap, the parascapular fascia flap, and the anterolateral thigh flap [49–51].

Upper Extremity

Resection of melanoma in the upper extremities may lead to intriguing reconstructive challenges for the plastic surgeon. The shoulder, in particular, has skin that is tightly adherent to the underlying fascia, muscle, and bone. Even 2 cm wounds are difficult to close without excess tension. The upper extremities have generally less soft tissue bulk and skin laxity when compared to the lower extremities, have a wide range of active motion, and the complex anatomy of the upper extremities stems from their dexterous functions and necessity for fineness movements. Further, these areas are widely visible and aesthetic considerations become a factor.

Primary Closure

Primary closure in this region may not be met with much difficulty. Generally, laxity can be comparable to the lower leg but naturally differs based on the body habitus of each patient. However, in regard to the hand, primary closure in this area may be deceptive. The dorsum of the hand, with fingers extended, may appear to have enough laxity to close a wound primarily; however, when a fist is made, the tension across this wound will increase exponentially. Also, similarly to the plantar surface of the foot, the palmar skin is uniformly thick and densely adherent to the underlying fascia, making primary closure of this area difficult.

Skin Grafts

Following the reconstructive ladder, the next viable option is a split thickness skin graft, followed by a full-thickness skin graft. Skin grafts to the upper extremity are generally more exposed compared to the trunk or lower extremities. Postoperative care must be taken not to shear these grafts off the accepting wound bed. Aesthetic consideration should be undertaken to match skin color and type of the recipient site to the donor site; for example, a skin graft inlaid to the palm of the hand are generally full thickness and should be of light color and relatively hairless. In African–Americans, the color match is an important concern, with split grafts from the plantar surface of the foot as the best source of color-matched grafts. This varies from split-thickness skin grafts suitable for the proximal forearm region.

Local Flap Reconstruction for a Melanoma of the Hand

Local flaps for the hand are as numerous as they are intricate. Well-performing flaps for this region include the first dorsal metatarsal artery perforator flap, based on the recurrent cutaneous branch of the dorsal metacarpal artery, and the Kite flap, based on the first dorsal metacarpal artery [52, 53]. Melanoma of the fingers or fingertips, as seen in acral-lentiginous melanoma, is an indication for digit amputation to establish clear margins with resection of the tumor [54]. Importantly, most invasive melanoma of the fingers requires interphalangeal joint amputation to the middle phalanx proximal to the primary lesion and are not treated by fingertip/pulp excisions. For subungual melanoma, amputation is through the midportion of the middle phalanx or the proximal phalanx if the lesion is found on the thumb.

Several excellent local flap options exist for soft tissue defects of the finger post-amputation such as a Visor flap, Atasoy, Kleinert flap, and Kutler flap [55, 56]. The Volar V-Y advancement flap (Atatsoy, Kleinert Flap) provides excellent functional and cosmetic results if the distal defect is less than 1 cm. For transverse and oblique defects on the lateral aspect of the digit, the Kutler flap provides a vascularized and sensate skin coverage. Another flap that is useful for maintaining length following transverse digit amputation is the Visor flap [57]. Local flaps for the thumb, where sensation is paramount, include the Moberg and Littler flaps [58–61]. Reconstructive options for the fingers require extensive consideration of patient morbidity after surgery. Sensation is of great importance, so reconstruction with local flaps that bring their own cutaneous nerve supply is often chosen. Disability, interference with jobs or hobbies, and changes in quality of life should all be considered when determining whether revision amputation should be performed or reconstruction should be attempted.

Local Flap Reconstruction of the Arm and Forearm Melanoma

Local flaps for reconstruction of the arm and wrist itself are numerous as well, taking advantage of the regional vascularity. The safety of local flap reconstruction following melanoma excision of the extremities has been well established [62]. A radial forearm flap based on the radial artery can serve as a flap for soft tissue coverage of defects from the hand distally, to the forearm proximally, reaching to ~25 cm above the elbow [63–65]. A posterior interosseous flap based on the posterior interosseous artery has similar indications as well [66, 67]. Free tissue transfer to the upper extremity is relatively flexible, in terms of free flaps that a surgeon can use for reconstruction.

A general guideline for the best choice of tissue flap is that a bulky flap should not be used in a region of the arm where thin skin and lack of adipose tissue is present. Conversely, a thin flap, such as the tensor fascia lata flap, should not be attempted to cover a large defect in an upper arm defect requiring extensive replacement of subcutaneous tissue. From an aesthetic perspective, while there are multiple local rotation and transposition flap options as well as free perforator flaps available to the upper extremities, it is important to match the reconstructive donor to recipient in terms of contour, texture, and skin color. Therefore, a thin flap is more suited for reconstruction for the forearm, while a thicker flap is optimal for coverage of a more proximal arm defect (Fig. 24.8a, b).

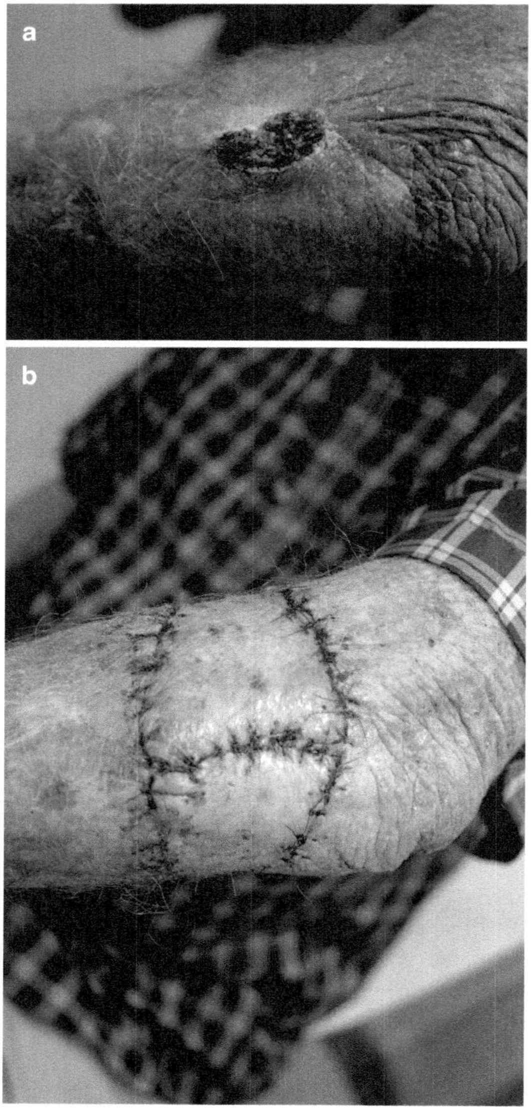

Fig. 24.8 (**a**) Patient presented to the clinic with a melanoma of the left forearm. (**b**) Post-operative image of reconstruction of arm and forearm with opposing V-Y advancement flaps

References

1. Elwood JM, et al. Pigmentation and skin reaction to sun as risk factors for cutaneous melanoma: Western Canada Melanoma Study. Br Med J (Clin Res Ed). 1984;288(6411):99–102.
2. Melanoma of the Skin At a Glance. American Cancer Society. 2017. https://cancerstatisticscenter.cancer.org/#/cancer-site/Melanoma%20of%20the%20skin.
3. Katalinic A, Kunze U, Schafer T. Epidemiology of cutaneous melanoma and non-melanoma skin cancer in Schleswig-Holstein, Germany: incidence, clinical subtypes, tumour stages and localization (epidemiology of skin cancer). Br J Dermatol. 2003;149(6):1200–6.
4. McGovern VJ, et al. The classification of malignant melanoma and its histologic reporting. Cancer. 1973;32(6):1446–57.
5. Swetter SM, et al. Increasing incidence of lentigo maligna melanoma subtypes: northern California and national trends 1990–2000. J Invest Dermatol. 2005;125(4):685–91.
6. Anderson WF, et al. Divergent cancer pathways for early-onset and late-onset cutaneous malignant melanoma. Cancer. 2009;115(18):4176–85.
7. Borges SZ, et al. Distribution of clinical-pathological types of cutaneous melanomas and mortality rate in the region of Passo Fundo, RS, Brazil. Int J Dermatol. 2007;46(7):679–86.
8. Linos E, et al. Increasing burden of melanoma in the United States. J Invest Dermatol. 2009;129(7):1666–74.
9. Pavri SN, et al. Malignant melanoma: beyond the basics. Plast Reconstr Surg. 2016;138(2):330e–40e.
10. Urist MM, et al. The influence of surgical margins and prognostic factors predicting the risk of local recurrence in 3445 patients with primary cutaneous melanoma. Cancer. 1985;55(6):1398–402.
11. Wong JY, Sondak VK. Unanswered questions about margin recommendations for primary cutaneous melanoma. J Natl Compr Cancer Netw. 2012;10(3):357–65.
12. Cassileth BR, Lusk EJ, Tenaglia AN. Patients' perceptions of the cosmetic impact of melanoma resection. Plast Reconstr Surg. 1983;71(1):73–5.
13. Crockett DJ. Regional keloid susceptibility. Br J Plast Surg. 1964;17:245–53.
14. Sharma RK, Verma GR, Biswas G. Reconstruction of a major abdominal and chest wall defect using latissimus dorsi and extended deep inferior epigastric artery flap. Ann Plast Surg. 1992;28(4):366–9.
15. Lv Y, et al. Abdominal wall reconstruction using a combination of free tensor fasciae lata and anterolateral thigh myocutaneous flap: a prospective study in 16 patients. Am J Surg. 2015;210(2):365–73.
16. Baumann DP, Butler CE. Soft tissue coverage in abdominal wall reconstruction. Surg Clin North Am. 2013;93(5):1199–209.
17. Baumann DP, Butler CE. Lateral abdominal wall reconstruction. Semin Plast Surg. 2012;26(1):40–8.
18. Tobin GR. Pectoralis major muscle-musculocutaneous flap for chest-wall reconstruction. Surg Clin North Am. 1989;69(5):991–1006.
19. Moelleken BR, Mathes SA, Chang N. Latissimus dorsi muscle-musculocutaneous flap in chest-wall reconstruction. Surg Clin North Am. 1989;69(5):977–90.
20. Miyamoto Y, et al. Reconstruction of full-thickness chest wall defects using rectus abdominis musculocu-

taneous flap: a report of fifteen cases. Ann Plast Surg. 1986;16(2):90–7.
21. Mericli AF, et al. Paraspinous muscle flap reconstruction of complex midline back wounds: risk factors and postreconstruction complications. Ann Plast Surg. 2010;65(2):219–24.
22. Bradford PT, et al. Acral lentiginous melanoma: incidence and survival patterns in the United States, 1986-2005. Arch Dermatol. 2009;145(4):427–34.
23. Green A, et al. Occurrence of melanomas on the upper and lower limbs in eastern Australia. Melanoma Res. 1996;6(5):387–94.
24. Ali RS, et al. The versatility of the anterolateral thigh flap. Plast Reconstr Surg. 2009;124(6 Suppl):e395–407.
25. Gravvanis AI, et al. Application of the pedicled anterolateral thigh flap to defects from the pelvis to the knee. Microsurgery. 2006;26(6):432–8.
26. Gurunluoglu R. The ascending branch of the lateral circumflex femoral vessels: review of the anatomy and its utilization as recipient vessel for free-flap reconstruction of the hip region. J Reconstr Microsurg. 2010;26(6):359–66.
27. Lin CH, Wei FC. Widely split latissimus dorsi muscle flaps for reconstruction of long soft-tissue defects in lower extremities. Plast Reconstr Surg. 2000;105(2):706–9.
28. McCraw JB, Fishman JH, Sharzer LA. The versatile gastrocnemius myocutaneous flap. Plast Reconstr Surg. 1978;62(1):15–23.
29. Anract P, et al. Knee reconstruction with prosthesis and muscle flap after total arthrectomy. Clin Orthop Relat Res. 2001;384:208–16.
30. Beck JB, Stile F, Lineaweaver W. Reconsidering the soleus muscle flap for coverage of wounds of the distal third of the leg. Ann Plast Surg. 2003;50(6):631–5.
31. Zenn MR, Levin LS. Microvascular reconstruction of the lower extremity. Semin Surg Oncol. 2000; 19(3):272–81.
32. Vranckx JJ, et al. The gracilis free muscle flap is more than just a "graceful" flap for lower-leg reconstruction. J Reconstr Microsurg. 2004;20(2):143–8.
33. Hong JP. The use of supermicrosurgery in lower extremity reconstruction: the next step in evolution. Plast Reconstr Surg. 2009;123(1):230–5.
34. Isenberg JS. When less is more: revascularization and sural artery fasciocutaneous flaps in ischemic limb salvage. J Reconstr Microsurg. 2003;19(4):235–40.
35. Rashid M, et al. A comparison of two fasciocutaneous flaps in the reconstruction of defects of the weight-bearing heel. J Coll Physicians Surg Pak. 2003; 13(4):216–8.
36. Sharma GN, Nepram SS. Sural artery flap: a dependable solution in lower leg and foot soft tissue reconstruction. Int Surg. 2001;86(3):144–50.
37. Virgili A, Corazza M. Guess what! Metastatic malignant melanoma of the leg from a warty acral amelanotic malignant melanoma. Eur J Dermatol. 2001;11(6):591–2.
38. Durbec F, et al. Melanoma of the hand and foot: epidemiological, prognostic and genetic features. A systematic review. Br J Dermatol. 2012;166(4): 727–39.
39. Albreski D, Sloan SB. Melanoma of the feet: misdiagnosed and misunderstood. Clin Dermatol. 2009;27(6): 556–63.
40. Heaton KM, et al. Surgical management and prognostic factors in patients with subungual melanoma. Ann Surg. 1994;219(2):197–204.
41. Leitner DW, Gordon L, Buncke HJ. The extensor digitorum brevis as a muscle island flap. Plast Reconstr Surg. 1985;76(5):777–80.
42. Masquelet AC, et al. The lateral supramalleolar flap. Plast Reconstr Surg. 1988;81(1):74–81.
43. Hierner EL, Corterier C, Hierner R. Lateral supramalleolar flaps for reconstruction in the ankle and foot. Oper Orthop Traumatol. 2013;25(2):122–30.
44. Furukawa M, et al. One-stage procedure using a digitorum brevis muscle flap for reconstruction of a surgical defect after excision of malignant melanoma in the heel. Osaka City Med J. 1985;31(2):135–44.
45. Morain WD. Island toe flaps in neurotrophic ulcers of the foot and ankle. Ann Plast Surg. 1984;13(1): 1–8.
46. Liu J, et al. Resection of malignant melanoma on heel and reconstruction of defect. Zhongguo Xiu Fu Chong Jian Wai Ke Za Zhi. 2010;24(11): 1350–3.
47. Jandali Z, et al. The free medial sural artery perforator flap: versatile option for soft tissue reconstruction in small-to-moderate size defects of the foot and ankle. Microsurgery. 2018;38:34–45.
48. Kang HG, et al. Soft tissue reconstruction of the foot using the distally based island pedicle flap after resection of malignant melanoma. Clin Orthop Surg. 2010;2(4):244–9.
49. Tan BK, Lim BH. The lateral forearm flap as a modification of the lateral arm flap: vascular anatomy and clinical implications. Plast Reconstr Surg. 2000;105(7):2400–4.
50. Attinger CE, Ducic I, Zelen C. The use of local muscle flaps in foot and ankle reconstruction. Clin Podiatr Med Surg. 2000;17(4):681–711.
51. Weinzweig N, Davies BW. Foot and ankle reconstruction using the radial forearm flap: a review of 25 cases. Plast Reconstr Surg. 1998;102(6): 1999–2005.
52. Bailey SH, Andry D, Saint-Cyr M. The dorsal metacarpal artery perforator flap: a case report utilizing a quaba flap harvested from a previously skin-grafted area for dorsal 5th digit coverage. Hand (N Y). 2010;5(3):322–5.
53. Adani R, et al. The "kite flap" for dorsal thumb reconstruction. Acta Chir Plast. 1995;37(3):63–6.
54. Lee KT, et al. Surgical excision margin for primary acral melanoma. J Surg Oncol. 2016;114(8): 933–9.

55. Rinker B. Fingertip reconstruction with the laterally based thenar flap: indications and long-term functional results. Hand (N Y). 2006;1(1):2–8.
56. Arpaci E, Unlu RE, Altun S, Ertas NM. Super Kutler flap: an alternative technique for reconstruction of fingertip defects. J Hand Surg Eur Vol. 2017;42(6):626–32.
57. Karamursel S, et al. Dorsal visor flap in fingertip reconstruction. Plast Reconstr Surg. 2001;108(4):1014–8.
58. Macht SD, Watson HK. The Moberg volar advancement flap for digital reconstruction. J Hand Surg Am. 1980;5(4):372–6.
59. Kandamany N, Naasan A. The composite Moberg flap for reconstruction of complex thumb tip injuries. Plast Reconstr Surg. 2014;133(2):235e–6e.
60. Shah R, Cavale N, Fleming A. A modification of the V-Y Moberg advancement flap for thumb reconstruction. J Hand Surg Eur Vol. 2007;32(3):357–8.
61. Meyer-Marcotty M, Kall S, Vogt PM. Covering palmar thumb tip defects with the Littler-Flap. Unfallchirurg. 2007;110(5):447–9.
62. Cuono CB, Ariyan S. Versatility and safety of flap coverage for wide excision of cutaneous melanomas. Plast Reconstr Surg. 1985;76(2):281–5.
63. Hegazi MM. The use of island radial forearm flap for local hand coverage. Ann Saudi Med. 1995;15(3): 219–21.
64. Zambacos GJ, Mandrekas AD. The reverse radial forearm flap in reconstruction of the hand. Plast Reconstr Surg. 2008;122(6):1979–80; author reply 1980.
65. Neumeister, M. (2017). Upper Extremity Reconstruction. In: F. Wei and S. Mardini, ed., Flaps and Reconstructive Surgery, 2nd ed. Edinburgh: Elsevier, pp.227–41.
66. Chmiel Z. Use of a fascia-cutaneous island flap based on the posterior interosseus artery of the forearm—a case report. Chir Narzadow Ruchu Ortop Pol. 1996; 61(1):17–21.
67. Ferreira MC, et al. Use of posterior interosseus artery flap in the repair of forearm and hand. Rev Hosp Clin Fac Med Sao Paulo. 1991;46(3): 137–40.

Sentinel Lymph Node Biopsy for Melanoma

25

Ann Y. Chung, Catalina Mosquera, and Jan H. Wong

Introduction

Intraoperative lymphatic mapping and selective sentinel lymphadenectomy (ILM and SLND) has dramatically altered the surgical management of the regional lymphatics in cutaneous melanoma. Once considered a standard component in the surgical management of patients with cutaneous melanoma, immediate complete lymph node dissection (CLND) or elective lymph node dissection (ELND) is now infrequently performed. Now commonly referred to as "sentinel lymph node biopsy," ILM and SLND is an operative technique that was developed in order to identify patients with cutaneous melanoma who might benefit from the early detection and surgical management of metastatic disease in the regional lymph nodes while avoiding the significant morbidity of CLND in individuals without regional lymph node metastases and who had little likelihood of benefit from that procedure.

The development of ILM and SLND as a reproducible operative technique to identify metastatic disease in clinically node-negative patients with cutaneous melanoma represents a surgical approach to understanding the underlying mechanism of the metastatic process in cutaneous melanoma. This chapter will highlight the rationale, the history, current status, and future of ILM and SLND.

A. Y. Chung, M.D. · C. Mosquera, M.D.
J. H. Wong, M.D. (✉)
Division of Surgical Oncology, Department of Surgery, East Carolina University Brody School of Medicine, Greenville, NC, USA
e-mail: chungan@ecu.edu; mosquerac@ecu.edu; wongj@ecu.edu

Surgical Management of Melanoma in the Pre-ILM and SLND Era

The evolution of the surgical management of melanoma reflected the prevailing understanding of the natural history and biology of melanoma of the time. More than a century and a half ago, William Norris published "Eight Cases of Melanosis, with Pathologic and Therapeutic Remarks on that Disease" [1] and noted that local recurrences occurred following minimal excisions and advocated for a wide excision of the tumor along with surrounding "healthy" tissue.

The removal of a secondary deposit of melanoma of the groin was reported in The Lancet in 1851, but it was the British surgeon, Herbert Snow, who advocated that the optimal approach to prevent the progression of cancer was "anticipatory excision" [2]. In 1892, Snow wrote that "the danger lies in the diffusion of malignant particles from this primary focus; these always implicate the nearest lymph glands….Palpable enlargement of these glands is unfortunately but a late symptom….by the time it occurs there is almost always implication of deeper organs or tissues. We thus see the utter futility of operative measures which are addressed to the primary lesion only" [3]. In 1907, William Handley [4],

A. I. Riker (ed.), *Melanoma*, https://doi.org/10.1007/978-3-319-78310-9_25

on the basis of a single autopsy examination of a patient with advanced melanoma demonstrated lymphatic permeation surrounding the primary tumor and advocated for a "wide local excision" of 2 inches along with excision of the lymphatic glands. This recommendation, wide excision and immediate lymphadenectomy, formed the basis for the surgical management of clinically localized melanoma for the next 50 years.

The Elective Lymphadenectomy Controversy

The management of the regional lymphatics has been one of the longest standing controversies in the management of patients with melanoma who are without clinical evidence of metastasis in the regional lymph nodes. The rationale for the performance of ELND, first articulated by Snow [2] in 1892, is based upon the hypothesis that melanoma metastasizes in a sequential and orderly fashion from the primary tumor, initially to the regional lymph nodes and then subsequently to distant sites. Therefore, the early surgical excision of this disease, when the tumor burden is microscopic, may prevent the untimely progression of disease to distant sites and improve survival. A number of observational studies have documented that when melanoma metastasizes, it most commonly does so, at least initially, to the regional lymph node basin. In the majority of these reports, patients who underwent ELND and were found to have microscopic disease, when compared to individuals who underwent a therapeutic lymphadenectomy for clinically detectable disease appeared to enjoy an improved survival [5–10]. Observational studies showed that survival is considerably better following regional node dissection for clinically negative, but pathologically positive, nodes than for clinically positive and pathologically positive nodes in cutaneous melanoma. Thus, wide excision and ELND was considered the standard surgical management of melanoma confined to the primary site and regional lymphatics.

However, it became increasingly apparent that cutaneous melanoma was a heterogeneous disease and only a minority of patients (~20%) who were clinically node-negative would be found at the time of ELND to have microscopic metastatic disease. Those who were node-negative were subjected to a morbid procedure with little likelihood of therapeutic benefit, raising justifiable concern over routinely performing ELND in clinically node patients with melanoma [11, 12]. A need for a rational approach to identify individuals who were most likely to benefit from an aggressive surgical approach was recognized.

Prognosis in Cutaneous Melanoma and Elective Lymphadenectomy

The introduction of microstaging of the primary tumor provided an approach in which clinicians could more accurately predict overall prognosis and the risk of regional lymph node metastases. By doing so, they could more selectively manage patients with cutaneous melanoma. Although the prognostic significance of depth of invasion had been previously recognized [13, 14], it was Clark and coinvestigators who, in 1969, defined five anatomic levels of invasion of the dermis and subcutaneous fat. They noted the correlation between an increase in Clark's level of invasion with an overall worse prognosis [15]. They also noted that in addition to the level of invasion, the histologic subtype also had prognostic relevance. Clark suggested that ELND be restricted to patients with level III, IV, or V lesions because these were the lesions most likely to harbor clinically occult metastatic disease. He later commented that the "evaluation of therapy might be meaningless unless correlated with the level of invasion."

A year later, Breslow reported that tumor thickness reliably predicted outcome and suggested that tumor thickness may be helpful criteria for selecting patients for ELND [16]. Breslow suggested that tumors thicker than 1.50 mm had a sufficient risk of nodal metastases in order to justify immediate node dissection and were most likely to benefit from ELND. Other characteristics of the primary tumor that were associated with poorer outcomes included the anatomic site of the primary [17], the presence or absence of ulceration [18], and histologic subtype [15]. Patients with "intermediate" thickness melanoma were routinely offered ELND, while "thin" and "thick" melanomas were felt not likely to benefit from ELND and generally underwent wide excision alone.

Prospective Randomize Trials Evaluating the Survival Benefit of Elective Lymphadenectomy

To address this ongoing controversy, a series of prospective, randomized trials were initiated in an attempt to resolve the long-standing question as to the value of ELND for cutaneous melanoma. The conflicting evidence from observational studies were the impetus for four prospective, randomized trials [19–22] that were initiated beginning in 1967 [22] with the last, the Intergroup Melanoma Trial, beginning enrollment in 1982 [23]. These trials were designed to address the benefit of ELND in clinically node-negative patients with cutaneous melanoma, failed to demonstrate a statistically significant benefit for ELND [20, 22, 23]. There was, however, a certain subsets of patients undergoing ELND who appeared to have an improved survival [20, 23].

These trials were subject to a number of criticisms that included the anatomic site of the primary [22], the absence of the utilization of lymphoscintigraphy [20], as well as a preponderance of females [22]. Despite the utilization of well-recognized prognostic criteria to enroll patients who were most likely to benefit from ELND, only 87/395 (22%) patients were found to have regional metastatic disease. Due to the small numbers of patients who could potentially benefit from ELND (patients with lymph node metastases without distant metastatic disease), the number of patients was insufficient to reject the null hypothesis, raising the possibility of a type II statistical error.

Observational data suggests four biologic subgroups of melanoma patients. The first and largest group were those patients with disease confined the primary site with neither regional nor distant metastatic disease. A second, much smaller group, consisted of individuals with disease confined to the primary site and regional lymph nodes at diagnosis. A third group consisted of individuals with disease apparently confined to the primary site and regional lymph nodes at diagnosis. This group had clinically occult metastatic disease, with a small, fourth group of patients without disease in the regional lymph nodes. The latter group had clinically occult, hematogenously disseminated metastatic disease. Thus, if ELND was to have a therapeutic benefit, it could only be in the second group of patients, specifically in those with disease confined to the regional lymphatics and without occult distant metastatic disease.

It became apparent that in order to address the controversy surrounding the value of ELND, a method was needed to identify the ~15–20% of clinically node-negative patients who would be found on complete lymphadenectomy to be pathologically node-positive. This was the group of patients that could potentially benefit from ELND, while excluding the much larger population of patients who were node-negative and had minimal, if any, potential for a survival benefit from ELND. In an effort to resolve this dilemma arose the operative approach of ILM and SLND.

The Sentinel Node Hypothesis

The concept that carcinomas frequently metastasize to lymph nodes in proximity to the primary tumor was generally well accepted. However, the idea that a malignancy might have a specific pattern of lymphatic drainage, to a specific node, or limited number of nodes had rarely been considered. Random biopsy of clinically negative nodes was rightfully regarded as unlikely to accurately stage a regional node basin. Furthermore, clinical observations had noted that nodes that were geographically in proximity to the tumor were not necessarily the nodes with metastatic disease.

We hypothesized that if melanoma would metastasize to lymph nodes, it would do so in an orderly manner based not on the geographic proximity to the primary, but instead, upon the anatomy of the dermal lymphatics. Drainage of a specific area of the skin would be to what we referred to as a "sentinel" lymph node(s). If this hypothesis of the dermal spread of melanoma was correct, then the sentinel lymph node would be the most likely node to harbor occult metastatic disease, if there was metastatic disease in the regional lymph node basin. The corollary of this hypothesis was that if the sentinel lymph node was negative, the likelihood of metastatic disease in any of the other lymph nodes within the regional lymph node basin was negligible.

If a method could be developed to identify the sentinel lymph node(s), which is most likely to harbor metastatic, this could be excised and examined. Only those individuals who were found to have metastatic disease within the sentinel lymph node, and thus could potentially benefit from an immediate completion lymphadenectomy, would then undergo the procedure. This would spare a majority of those patients the morbidity of a complete lymph node dissection. This led us to explore intraoperative approaches that would allow us to reproduce the lymphatic drainage of cutaneous melanoma and identify the node(s), presumably at greatest risk for harboring metastatic disease.

Feasibility of Lymphatic Mapping in an Animal Model

Lymphangiographic studies of the skin have demonstrated fine, dermal lymphatic channels that coalesce to form a number of major lymphatics trunks that eventually drain to the regional lymph nodes [24]. Although lymphangiographic studies had been utilized to characterize lymph nodes in Hodgkin's disease and lymphoma [25], the utility of radiopaque techniques was deemed too insensitive to detect micrometastatic disease in cutaneous melanoma. For this reason, an operative technique was necessary in which the sentinel node(s) could be excised and examined microscopically to confirm the presence or absence of metastatic disease. In the late 1980s, we began studies of the dermal lymphatics at the University of California, Los Angeles (UCLA), to test the feasibility of operative mapping of the dermal lymphatics in an attempt to identify the sentinel lymph node.

In contrast to several lymph nodes within a nodal basin in humans, most rodents and mammals have a single large lymph node within the groin or axilla. The node(s) accepts the lymphatic drainage of the extremity or trunk, before draining into larger ducts. However, the cat has a lymphatic anatomy somewhat analogous to that of humans, with three distinct lymph nodes in the groin [26]. Thus, we utilized the cat in order to examine the hypothesis of site-specific lymphatic drainage of the skin.

We studied several potentially effective lymphatic mapping dyes, with isosulfan blue dye proving to be the most useful mapping dye. Isosulfan blue was developed as an adjunct to lymphangiography, with a rapid visualization of the dermal lymphatics upon injection between the web spaces of the digits. The dye is easily visualized, turning the lymph node a light blue in color. By carefully elevating skin flaps in the groin, blue-filled lymphatic channels could be identified that led directly to a lymph node (Fig. 25.1).

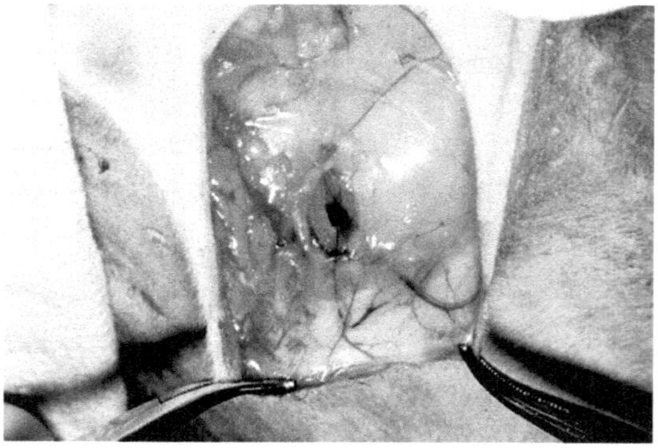

Fig. 25.1 Intraoperative demonstration of the dermal lymphatics following intradermal injection of isosulfan blue in the medial thigh of a feline model. The blue lymphatic channel was easily visualized and drained to a blue-stained lymph node. (From Wong JH, Cagle LA, Morton DL. Lymphatic drainage of skin to a sentinel lymph node in a feline model. Ann Surg 1991:214;637–641. Reprinted with Permission)

The anatomy of the cat allowed identification of medial, mid-, and lateral lymph nodes. If the sentinel node hypothesis were valid, then it would be anticipated that injection of a mapping dye in a specific area of skin would reproducibly drain to a specific lymph node. A predictable pattern of drainage was noted for each location, with the injection of isosulfan blue in the lateral thigh or abdomen uniformly draining to the lateral lymph node. Injection of isosulfan blue in the medial aspect of the thigh uniformly drained to the middle lymph node. Injection of isosulfan blue in the perineum and lower abdomen uniformly drained to the most medial lymph node, thus providing compelling evidence that the lymphatics of the skin was reproducible and would drain to a "sentinel" lymph node (Fig. 25.2). The feline model initially utilized to examine the feasibility of an operative technique for selective lymphadenectomy supported the potential utility of ILM and SLND in cutaneous melanoma [27].

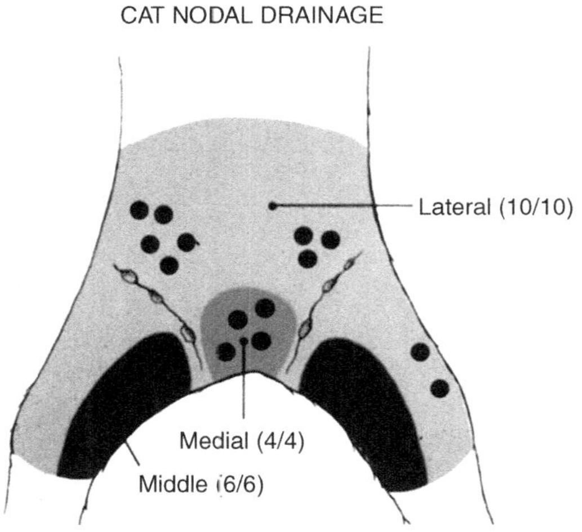

Fig. 25.2 A schematic representation of the injection sites in the feline model. A reproducible pattern of drainage emerged by injection into the medial aspect of the thigh, which led to drainage to the middle lymph node; and the perineum and lower abdomen which drained to the medial lymph node. (From Wong JH, Cagle LA, Morton DL. Lymphatic drainage of skin to a sentinel lymph node in a feline model. Ann Surg 1991:214;637–641. Reprinted with Permission)

Intraoperative Lymphatic Mapping and Selective Lymphadenectomy in Cutaneous Melanoma

Based upon these feline studies, we embarked on developing an operative technique to map the lymphatics in patients with cutaneous melanoma diagnosed with a primary, intermediate-thickness melanoma. We wished to validate our hypothesis that when cutaneous melanoma cells metastasize to the regional lymph nodes, it would most likely drain to the sentinel lymph nodes. We utilized cutaneous lymphoscintigraphy [28] to identify the lymphatic basin potentially at risk for harboring occult metastatic disease. We also utilized a radioactive sulfur colloid to aid in the identification of the sentinel lymph node, by marking on the skin the approximate site of the uptake of radioactive colloid in the regional node.

The identification of a sentinel lymph node proved to be extremely challenging. Initially, an incision over the presumed site of the sentinel node, as determined by preoperative lymphoscintigraphy. The incision was carried down through the subcutaneous tissue, and with blunt dissection, blue lymph nodes were identified and individually harvested. It was the recognition that careful elevation of the proximal flap allowed for the identification of afferent lymphatic channels that could be traced to a blue-stained node that provided a reproducible technique to identify the sentinel lymph node (Fig. 25.3).

With experience, we developed a standardized technique in which approximately 0.5–1.0 mL of isosulfan blue was injected intradermally in four sites around the biopsy site. To facilitate the migration of the dye, the injection site was gently massaged. Flaps were carefully developed, and based upon preoperative lymphoscintigraphy, a meticulous dissection of the subcutaneous fat was performed over the anticipated site of the afferent lymphatics. Once a blue afferent lymphatic channel(s) was identified, it was followed to the blue-stained node(s) by gently separating and dividing the overlying fat of the blue lymphatic channel. The sentinel lymph node(s) was removed, and a completion node dissection was

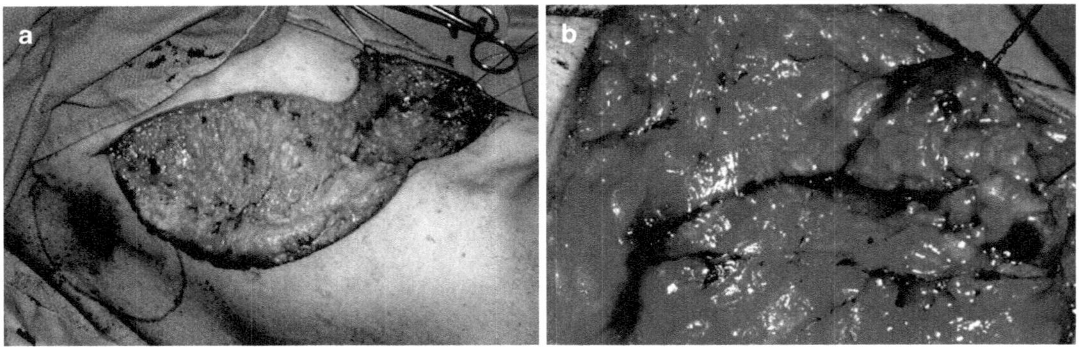

Fig. 25.3 Intraoperative view of an incontinuity dissection of a melanoma of the right scapula with intraoperative lymphatic mapping and an axillary sentinel node dissection. Panel (**a**) Injection of isosulfan blue at the primary site and elevation of skin flaps allowed the identification of an afferent lymphatic channel that drained to a sentinel lymph node. Panel (**b**) Close-up blue lymphatic channel and blue-stained sentinel lymph node

performed in the usual fashion [28] with all non-sentinel nodes examined by routine hematoxylin and eosin staining.

In our original report, we identified sentinel lymph node(s) in 197 of 237 lymphatic basins. Forty specimens (21%) were found to have occult metastatic disease detected either by hematoxylin and eosin stains or immunohistochemical staining. In the 197 successful ILM and SLND, 259 sentinel nodes were analyzed, of which 47 had occult metastatic disease. Only 2 nodes of the 3079 non-sentinel nodes were found to have occult metastatic disease. Of the 40 patients who were found to have metastatic disease, the sentinel node identified 38 of them (false negative rate of 5%).

These results were first reported in 1990 at the Annual Meeting of the Society of Surgical Oncology in Washington, DC, and subsequently published in the Archives of Surgery [29]. This seminal article provided the proof-of-principle concept of the overall validity of the sentinel lymph node hypothesis. Instead of wide excision alone, or wide excision with ELND, we proposed a selective approach to the management of the regional node basin in intermediate-thickness melanoma, in which only patients with metastatic disease in the sentinel lymph node would be subjected to an immediate completion node dissection.

External Validation of ILM and SLND Beyond UCLA

It was apparent that if ILM and SLND were to become the procedure of choice to identify occult micrometastatic disease, our results would need to be reproduced and validated beyond the confines of UCLA. Melanoma surgeons from Roswell Park Memorial Institute, New York University, the University of South Florida, Moffitt Cancer Center, and the M.D. Anderson Cancer Center were invited to UCLA to observe how we performed ILM and SLND. The expectation was that they would be able to then return to their home institutions to successfully perform these procedures as part of a multicenter clinical trial to determine the therapeutic utility of this approach.

On a single operative day, we demonstrated, in nine patients, the technical details that we had developed and were later to be published [29] on the conduct of ILM and SLND. We emphasized the need to utilize preoperative lymphoscintigraphy to not only localize the lymphatic basin at risk, but also to identify the approximate location of the sentinel node(s) within the basin and marking of the overlying skin by nuclear medicine physicians. We demonstrated the meticulous and careful elevation of the skin flaps, along with identification and careful dissection of the afferent, blue-stained lymphatic channels.

Our initial results as to the accuracy of ILM and SLND in cutaneous melanoma and the identification of occult lymph node metastases were subsequently confirmed at several other institutes [30–34]. Subsequently, multiple other institutions participated in the Multicenter Selective Lymphadenectomy Trial, confirming that ILM and SLND is technically feasible and accurate.

Radioguided Sentinel Lymphadenectomy

It became evident that mastering ILM and SLND with isosulfan blue as the sole mapping agent was technically challenging. The technical challenges were formidable, whereby we estimated that 60 cases would need to be performed in order to become proficient. Additionally, a completion lymph node dissection was also necessary to be proficient in during this period of learning [29]. Given the relative infrequency of melanoma, this was a procedure that in all likelihood would only be learned and performed in high-volume melanoma centers.

Krag and colleagues [35] at the University of Vermont began utilizing radiocolloid for intraoperative lymphatic mapping as an adjunct to isosulfan blue. First, verifying the utility of radiocolloid in a feline model, they used technetium-99 sulfur colloid to map 10 patients and found it to be equally sensitive to isosulfan blue in the identification of the sentinel lymph node(s) [35]. The use of a radiocolloid to facilitate lymphatic mapping allowed, with the use of a gamma-detecting probe, identification of the sentinel node. It also allowed confirmation that all sentinel nodes had been removed when there was no longer significant radioactivity detected in the lymphatic nodal basin. In a larger experience of 121 patients, Krag and coworkers [30] were able to demonstrate the successful identification of the sentinel node in 97.6% of patients. Additionally, when combined with isosulfan blue, there was a 100% concordance of blue nodes that were radioactive. The addition of a radiocolloid to intraoperative lymphatic mapping with isosulfan blue, and the development of a handheld gamma probe made identification of the node substantially easier. This procedure was thus made more widely applicable beyond high-volume melanoma centers. With the addition of radioguided techniques, sentinel node identification rates in excess of 90% were readily achievable, even with minimal operative experience. Others soon duplicated these results [36], and dual agent mapping was widely adopted as the technique of choice in ILM and SLND.

Microstaging of the Sentinel Lymph Node

One of the benefits of ILM and SLND was the feasibility of examining the sentinel lymph node(s) in greater detail. The standard pathologic examination of a lymph node involves bisection of the lymph node with a single section from the two faces of the bisected nodes examined with hematoxylin and eosin staining. In a typical 1 cm lymph node, <1% of the node is effectively examined by the pathologist. It was presumed that this section was representative of the histology of the node, but had the potential of missing small deposits of metastatic disease. Although the ability to more thoroughly examine lymph nodes at multiple levels and with multiple sections was readily available, the routine use of this technology was not considered economically tenable. Furthermore, it is considered labor intensive considering that the yield of positive nodes is considerably low in most cases. However, the ability to identify the node(s) at greatest risk for harboring metastatic disease provided a feasible approach to a more detailed analysis and more accurate staging of the regional lymphatics.

The potential value of identifying previously occult metastatic disease might not be insignificant. Approximately 25% of node-negative melanoma patients will go on to develop metastatic disease. Although some of the patients likely had hematogenous dissemination of disease, it was not unreasonable to presume that some of these patient's might have had occult, lymph node only metastatic disease. One could further hypothesize that standard lymph node analysis would miss a positive lymph node which may be the source for distant metastatic disease. The accurate identification of early metastatic disease provides relevant prognostic information, but also allows for an intervention (lymphadenectomy) that might improve survival. To identify this potentially relevant micrometastatic disease, multiple sections at multiple levels of the lymph node became the standard pathologic analysis of the sentinel lymph node(s).

Routine hematoxylin and eosin staining is able to identify a single metastatic cell in a background of 10^4 lymphocytes, while the addition of immunohistochemical staining can identify a single metastatic cell in a background of 10^5 lymphocytes. More sensitive molecular assays utilizing reverse transcriptase, polymerase chain reaction detection of messenger RNA for tyrosinase [37, 38] were developed to stage sentinel lymph nodes and held the promise of identifying high and low risk melanoma patients. Early observational studies suggested that molecular staging has prognostic relevance [39].

ILM and SLND became quickly recognized as a multidisciplinary approach to staging of cutaneous melanoma that required not only surgical expertise, but a commitment from nuclear medicine physicians and pathologists as well. It is important to have accurate lymphoscintography and pathology to perform multilevel analysis of the sentinel lymph node utilizing appropriate immunostains in order to maximize the identification of metastatic tumor cells. The identification of any metastatic disease in the lymph node, even isolated tumor cells, was considered both clinically relevant and an indication for a completion lymphadenectomy. The ability to identify patients with occult metastatic disease provides the opportunity to perform a complete lymphadenectomy only in those patients who it could be potentially therapeutic.

Management of the Patient with a Positive Sentinel Lymph Node

The generally accepted management of the patient with a positive sentinel lymph node is to perform a completion lymphadenectomy, as originally advocated by Morton and coworkers [29]. Observational data from the John Wayne Cancer Institute suggests that patients undergoing a completion lymphadenectomy had significantly improved melanoma-specific survival when compared to sentinel node-positive patients who were observed [40] Data from the Multicenter Selective Lymphadenectomy Trial-I (MSLT-1) demonstrated that patients who underwent a sentinel node biopsy had on average 1.4 positive nodes, compared to 3.3 positive nodes in the observation arm. Since the number of positive nodes is an important prognostic characteristic, these data support a survival advantage in patients with an intermediate-thickness melanoma who are sentinel node-positive and undergo a completion lymphadenectomy [41, 42].

The Prognostic and Therapeutic Value of the ILM and SLND

Despite continued debate over the utility of ILM and SLND [43], ILM and SLND was widely adopted in the surgical management of intermediate-thickness melanoma. In 1999, just 7 years following the description of ILM and SLND, Cascinelli, president of the World Health Organization (WHO) Melanoma Program, declared intraoperative lymphatic mapping to be the standard of care for melanoma. He made this statement during his presentation of the abstract, "An Overview on Sentinel Lymph Node Dissection" at the 9th International Congress on Anti-Cancer Treatments held in Paris. Sentinel node staging rapidly became the standard of care for patients with intermediate-thickness melanoma.

Several reports have since validated that the status of the sentinel lymph node was one of the most powerful, if not the most powerful, predictor of outcome in early stage melanoma [44, 45]. This provided the opportunity to re-examine the question of the therapeutic value of an immediate completion node dissection in patients who were sentinel node-positive. This was also the impetus for two, prospective, randomized trials utilizing sentinel node staging as a key component in the randomization schema.

The Sunbelt Melanoma Trial

The Sunbelt Melanoma Trial was designed to address the efficacy of high-dose interferon alfa-2b in patients with histologically positive sentinel lymph nodes who underwent a completion lymphadenectomy. Secondly, this trial wanted to determine the significance of molecular staging by RT-PCR of melanoma-specific mRNA [46]. This six arm trial began enrollment in 1997, following the approval of high-dose interferon alfa-2b in the adjuvant setting by the US Food and Drug Administration. The approval was for select patients with resected, high-risk melanoma on the basis of the results of ECOG 1684 clinical trial published in 1996 [47].

Seventy institutions participated in the Sunbelt Melanoma Trial and randomized 218 patients with one positive sentinel lymph node following complete lymphadenectomy to observation or high-dose interferon alfa-2b. There were a total of 556 patients who were sentinel node-negative by routine histology, but RT-PCR positive. This group was randomized to either observation or a complete lymphadenectomy, with or without high-dose interferon alfa-2b. Interim analysis of the prognostic value of RT-PCR, as conducted in this trial, failed to provide additional prognostic information beyond the currently accepted histologic prognostic characteristics [48].

The Sunbelt Melanoma Trial failed to demonstrate a benefit with the use of adjuvant, high-dose interferon alfa-2b in patients who were sentinel node-positive by molecular staging. This was true whether they underwent observation only, immediate completion lymphadenectomy or patients with one positive sentinel lymph node following completion axillary node dissection. The Sunbelt Melanoma Trial provides evidence that a complete lymphadenectomy in either routine histologically positive sentinel nodes or RT-PCR positive sentinel node patients with melanoma ≥1.0 mm in thickness does not improve either disease survival or overall survival. However, this trial failed to address whether a complete lymphadenectomy identified by either routine hematoxylin and eosin or immunohistochemical staining was beneficial, when compared to wide excision alone.

The Multicenter Selective Lymphadenectomy Trials (MSLT-I and MSLT-II)

In January of 1994, Morton initiated the Multicenter Selective Lymphadenectomy Trial (MSLT-1), comparing wide excision with ILM and SLND to wide excision alone. This was for patients with American Joint Commission on Cancer Stage I and II cutaneous melanoma, with a Breslow's tumor thickness between 1.0 and 4 mm. The primary aim of this study was to determine the therapeutic benefit of lymphatic mapping and sentinel node biopsy and immediate completion node dissection in sentinel node-positive patients. Second, to determine the true accuracy of this technique in a multicenter clinical trial. The primary endpoint of the trial was to determine whether immediate complete node dissection would improve melanoma-specific survival when compared to patients who underwent wide excision alone and lymphadenectomy at the time of nodal recurrence during observation.

To assure surgical quality control, participating surgeons were required to perform 30 ILM and SLND with a completion node dissection, as well as successful identification of the sentinel node in ≥85% of cases. Further, each surgeon needed to show that no metastases were identified in non-sentinel nodes when the sentinel node was negative [49] before they could begin enrolling patients in the trial. The trial complete the targeted accrual in 2002, with the final report published in 2014 [42].

In this prospective, international, multicenter trial, the validation of the sentinel hypothesis and the prognostic significance of the sentinel node status were re-confirmed. [42] On multivariate analysis, sentinel node status was the most powerful predictor of disease recurrence or death from melanoma. An interim analysis of MSLT-I demonstrated that patients who underwent ILM and SLND had significantly fewer positive nodes compared to those in the observation arm (mean 1.1 nodes in the biopsy group versus 3.3 in the observation group) [41] indicating that the sentinel nodes were the most likely source for metastasis to other regional nodes. There were no significant, treatment-related differences identified in the 10-year melanoma-specific survival. However, subgroup analysis demonstrated an improved, 10-year distant disease-free survival and melanoma-specific survival for patients with nodal metastases identified by ILM and SLND.

Subgroup analysis suggested an improved overall survival in patients who were found to be node-positive by ILM and SLND, when compared to patients who underwent a complete lymphadenectomy at the time of regional recurrence. However, this group of sentinel node-positive patients represented only a minority of the entire study population. MSLT-1, in essence, suffered from the same statistical problems of the original prospective, randomized trials in which only a minority of patients undergoing immediate lymphadenectomy could potentially benefit from the surgical procedure.

In order to address these concerns and to determine whether sentinel node biopsy alone may indeed be therapeutic, Morton proposed the Multicenter Selective Lymphadenectomy Trial II (MSLT-II). This is a randomized trial comparing sentinel lymphadenectomy and complete lymph node dissection with sentinel lymphadenectomy alone in combination with ultrasound surveillance. Eligible patients are those diagnosed with a primary cutaneous melanoma and identified to have either molecular or histopathological evidence of metastases in the sentinel node [50]. All subjects receive sentinel lymphadenectomy, and if the subject is found to be sentinel node-positive, they are then randomized to receive either completion lymphadenectomy or observation with nodal ultrasound and completion lymphadenectomy at the time of ultrasound or clinical node recurrence.

The primary outcome measure is melanoma-specific survival, with secondary outcomes measuring disease-free survival and recurrence over 10 years of follow-up. Sixty-four participating institutions completed accrual in 2014. The study was designed to determine whether immediate completion lymphadenectomy in sentinel node-positive patients improves melanoma-specific survival. It will also reveal whether a completion lymphadenectomy might be avoided in patients with sentinel lymph node metastases. The results were recently reported [51]. Although immediate completion node dissection provided useful prognostic information, it failed to improve melanoma-specific survival in patients who were sentinel node-positive.

The Future of Sentinel Node Staging

In a little over 25 years, a simple, yet elegant, hypothesis has been thoroughly validated. When melanoma metastasizes, it does so in a defined manner that can reproduced with a simple operative technique. This procedure has dramatically altered the surgical management of cutaneous melanoma. Intraoperative lymphatic mapping and selective lymphadenectomy is an easily performed procedure that defines patterns of nodal metastases, and when negative, accurately reflects the status of the regional lymph node basin.

The maturation of the results for the MSLT-2 provides evidence that sentinel node metastases are indicators of a metastatic phenotype, but not determinants of survival. The hypothesis that the timely surgical resection of sentinel nodes can prevent the development of metastatic clones and potentially improve melanoma-specific survival no longer needs to be debated. The latter will show that surgical excision might be palliative, with little, if any, therapeutic benefit. The sentinel node status will likely remain the most powerful prognostic indicator in melanoma for the foreseeable future. It further provides relevant and important stratification criteria for any future adjuvant treatment trials for melanoma patients. Due to the sentinel lymph node identified as the initial site of metastases, it may provide insight into the tumor-host relationship and an improved understanding of the tumor microenvironment as well as the biology of the metastatic process [52].

References

1. Norris W. Eight cases of melanosis with pathological and therapeutic remarks on that disease. London: Longman, Brown, Green, Longmans, and Roberts; 1857.
2. Snow H. Twenty two years' experience in the treatment of cancerous and other tumours. London: Ballliere, Tindall, and Cox; 1898.
3. Snow H. Abstract of a lecture on melanotic cancerous disease. Lancet. 1892;2:872–4.
4. Handley W. The pathology of melanotic growths in the relation to their operative treatment. Lancet. 1907;927(96):1.
5. Balch CM, Soong SJ, Murad TM, Ingalls AL, Maddox WA. A multifactorial analysis of melanoma: III. Prognostic factors in melanoma patients with lymph node metastases (stage II). Ann Surg. 1981;193: 377–88.
6. Roses DF, Provet JA, Harris MN, Gumport SL, Dubin N. Prognosis of patients with pathologic stage II cutaneous malignant melanoma. Ann Surg. 1985; 201:103–7.
7. Callery C, Cochran AJ, Roe DJ, et al. Factors prognostic for survival in patients with malignant melanoma spread to the regional lymph nodes. Ann Surg. 1982;196:69–75.
8. Cohen MH, Ketcham AS, Felix EL, et al. Prognostic factors in patients undergoing lymphadenectomy for malignant melanoma. Ann Surg. 1977;186:635–42.
9. Morton DL, Wanek L, Nizze JA, Elashoff RM, Wong JH. Improved long-term survival after lymphadenectomy of melanoma metastatic to regional nodes. Analysis of prognostic factors in 1134 patients from the John Wayne cancer clinic. Ann Surg. 1991;214:491–9. discussion 9–501
10. Gumport SL, Harris MN. Results of regional lymph node dissection for melanoma. Ann Surg. 1974;179: 105–8.
11. Davis NC. Cutaneous melanoma. The Queensland experience. Curr Probl Surg. 1976;13:1–63.
12. Slingluff CL Jr, Stidham KR, Ricci WM, Stanley WE, Seigler HF. Surgical management of regional lymph nodes in patients with melanoma. Experience with 4682 patients. Ann Surg. 1994;219:120–30.
13. Allen AC, Spitz S. Malignant melanoma; a clinicopathological analysis of the criteria for diagnosis and prognosis. Cancer. 1953;6:1–45.
14. Lane N, Lattes R, Malm J. Clinicopathological correlations in a series of 117 malignant melanomas of the skin of adults. Cancer. 1958;11:1025–43.
15. Clark WH Jr, From L, Bernardino EA, Mihm MC. The histogenesis and biologic behavior of primary human malignant melanomas of the skin. Cancer Res. 1969; 29:705–27.
16. Breslow A. Thickness, cross-sectional areas and depth of invasion in the prognosis of cutaneous melanoma. Ann Surg. 1970;172:902–8.
17. Urist MM, Balch CM, Soong SJ, et al. Head and neck melanoma in 534 clinical Stage I patients. A prognostic factors analysis and results of surgical treatment. Ann Surg. 1984;200:769–75.
18. Balch CM, Murad TM, Soong SJ, Ingalls AL, Halpern NB, Maddox WA. A multifactorial analysis of melanoma: prognostic histopathological features comparing Clark's and Breslow's staging methods. Ann Surg. 1978;188:732–42.
19. Balch CM, Soong S, Ross MI, et al. Long-term results of a multi-institutional randomized trial comparing prognostic factors and surgical results for intermediate thickness melanomas (1.0 to 4.0 mm). Intergroup Melanoma Surgical Trial. Ann Surg Oncol. 2000;7:87–97.
20. Cascinelli N, Morabito A, Santinami M, MacKie RM, Belli F. Immediate or delayed dissection of regional nodes in patients with melanoma of the trunk: a randomised trial. WHO Melanoma Programme. Lancet. 1998;351:793–6.
21. Sim FH, Taylor WF, Ivins JC, Pritchard DJ, Soule EH. A prospective randomized study of the efficacy of routine elective lymphadenectomy in management of malignant melanoma. Preliminary results. Cancer. 1978;41:948–56.
22. Veronesi U, Adamus J, Bandiera DC, et al. Inefficacy of immediate node dissection in stage 1 melanoma of the limbs. N Engl J Med. 1977;297: 627–30.
23. Balch CM, Soong SJ, Bartolucci AA, et al. Efficacy of an elective regional lymph node dissection of 1 to 4 mm thick melanomas for patients 60 years of age and younger. Ann Surg. 1996;224:255–63. discussion 63–6
24. Kinmonth J. The lymphatics. Diseases, lymphography, and surgery. Baltimore: Williams & Wilkins; 1972.
25. Crispen JF, Jeffries PF. Lymphangiography: a simple method of dye infusion. JAMA. 1962;182:872–3.
26. Widschwendter P, Friedl TW, Schwentner L, et al. The influence of obesity on survival in early, high-risk breast cancer: results from the randomized SUCCESS A trial. Breast Cancer Res. 2015;17:129.
27. Wong JH, Cagle LA, Morton DL. Lymphatic drainage of skin to a sentinel lymph node in a feline model. Ann Surg. 1991;214:637–41.
28. Holmes EC, Moseley HS, Morton DL, Clark W, Robinson D, Urist MM. A rational approach to the surgical management of melanoma. Ann Surg. 1977; 186:481–90.
29. Morton DL, Wen DR, Wong JH, et al. Technical details of intraoperative lymphatic mapping for early stage melanoma. Arch Surg. 1992;127:392–9.

30. Krag DN, Meijer SJ, Weaver DL, et al. Minimal-access surgery for staging of malignant melanoma. Arch Surg. 1995;130:654–8. discussion 9–60
31. Reintgen D, Cruse CW, Wells K, et al. The orderly progression of melanoma nodal metastases. Ann Surg. 1994;220:759–67.
32. Ross M, Reintgen D, Balch CM. Selective lymphadenctomy. Emerging role of lymphatic mapping and sentinel node biopsy in the management of early stage melannoma. Semin Surg Oncol. 1993;9:219–23.
33. Thompson JF, McCarthy WH, Bosch CM, et al. Sentinel lymph node status as an indicator of the presence of metastatic melanoma in regional lymph nodes. Melanoma Res. 1995;5:255–60.
34. Karakousis CP, Velez AF, Spellman JE Jr, Scarozza J. The technique of sentinel node biopsy. Eur J Surg Oncol. 1996;22:271–5.
35. Alex JC, Weaver DL, Fairbank JT, Rankin BS, Krag DN. Gamma-probe-guided lymph node localization in malignant melanoma. Surg Oncol. 1993;2:303–8.
36. Albertini JJ, Cruse CW, Rapaport D, et al. Intra-operative radio-lympho-scintigraphy improves sentinel lymph node identification for patients with melanoma. Ann Surg. 1996;223:217–24.
37. Van der Velde-Zimmermann D, Roijers JF, Bouwens-Rombouts A, et al. Molecular test for the detection of tumor cells in blood and sentinel nodes of melanoma patients. Am J Pathol. 1996;149:759–64.
38. Wang X, Heller R, VanVoorhis N, et al. Detection of submicroscopic lymph node metastases with polymerase chain reaction in patients with malignant melanoma. Ann Surg. 1994;220:768–74.
39. Nicholl MB, Elashoff D, Takeuchi H, Morton DL, Hoon DS. Molecular upstaging based on paraffin-embedded sentinel lymph nodes: ten-year follow-up confirms prognostic utility in melanoma patients. Ann Surg. 2011;253:116–22.
40. Lee DY, Lau BJ, Huynh KT, et al. Impact of completion lymph node dissection on patients with positive sentinel lymph node biopsy in melanoma. J Am Coll Surg. 2016;223:9–18.
41. Morton DL, Thompson JF, Cochran AJ, et al. Sentinel-node biopsy or nodal observation in melanoma. N Engl J Med. 2006;355:1307–17.
42. Morton DL, Thompson JF, Cochran AJ, et al. Final trial report of sentinel-node biopsy versus nodal observation in melanoma. N Engl J Med. 2014;370:599–609.
43. Thomas JM, Patocskai EJ. The argument against sentinel node biopsy for malignant melanoma: its use should be confined to patients in clinical trials. Br Med J. 2000;321:3–4.
44. Gershenwald JE, Thompson W, Mansfield PF, et al. Multi-institutional melanoma lymphatic mapping experience: the prognostic value of sentinel lymph node status in 612 stage I or II melanoma patients. J Clin Oncol. 1999;17:976–83.
45. Jansen L, Nieweg OE, Peterse JL, Hoefnagel CA, Olmos RA, Kroon BB. Reliability of sentinel lymph node biopsy for staging melanoma. Br J Surg. 2000;87:484–9.
46. McMasters KM, Egger ME, Edwards MJ, et al. Final results of the Sunbelt Melanoma Trial: a multi-institutional prospective randomized phase III study evaluating the role of adjuvant high-dose interferon alfa-2b and completion lymph node dissection for patients staged by sentinel lymph node biopsy. J Clin Oncol. 2016;34:1079–86.
47. Kirkwood JM, Strawderman MH, Ernstoff MS, Smith TJ, Borden EC, Blum RH. Interferon alfa-2b adjuvant therapy of high-risk resected cutaneous melanoma: the Eastern Cooperative Oncology Group Trial EST 1684. J Clin Oncol. 1996;14:7–17.
48. Scoggins CR, Ross MI, Reintgen DS, et al. Prospective multi-institutional study of reverse transcriptase polymerase chain reaction for molecular staging of melanoma. J Clin Oncol. 2006;24:2849–57.
49. Morton DL, Thompson JF, Essner R, et al. Validation of the accuracy of intraoperative lymphatic mapping and sentinel lymphadenectomy for early-stage melanoma: a multicenter trial. Multicenter Selective Lymphadenectomy Trial Group. Ann Surg. 1999;230:453–63. discussion 63–5
50. Multicenter Selective Lymphadenectomy Trial II (MSLT-II). 2006. https://clinicaltrials.gov/ct2/show/NCT00297895. Accessed 18 Mar 2017
51. Faries MB, Thompson JF, Cochran AJ, et al. Completion dissection or observation for sentinel-node metastasis in melanoma. N Engl J Med. 2017;376:2211–22.
52. Cochran AJ, Morton DL, Stern S, Lana AMA, Essner R, Wen D-R. Sentinel lymph nodes show profound downregulation of antigen-presenting cells of the paracortex: implications for tumor biology and treatment. Mod Pathol. 2001;14:604–8.

Operative Techniques for Melanoma

26

Soraya A. Voigt, Catalina Mosquera, and Nasreen A. Vohra

Biopsy of a Cutaneous Lesion Suspicious for Melanoma

Shave Biopsy

A shave biopsy of a suspicious skin lesion is a simple procedure that allows for histologic evaluation of dermal tissue. Four techniques have been described depending on the instrument used to perform the excision. After proper skin preparation and injection of local anesthetic, the area of interest is stretched with the nondominant hand. Then with the use of a scalpel, razor blade, scissors, or a radiosurgical loop, the affected dermis is biopsied [1]. Proponents of shave biopsies highlight its time-saving nature. Moreover, as long as at least a 1 mm thick shave is obtained, the depth of the tumor, which is essential in planning the extent of surgery, can be accurately assessed. However, a superficial shave biopsy does not usually provide ample amount of the dermis, with some discouraging the use of a shave biopsy in cases where a melanoma is suspected. Positive deep margins can be seen in 22% of shave biopsy specimens, which may compromise the ability to properly stage patients prior to definitive surgery [2]. To this point, a recent study by Zager et al. found that when patients are diagnosed with a melanoma by shave biopsy and then proceed to wide local excision, only 3% have tumor upstaging and 2% potentially require a wider margin of excision. Moreover, only 1.3% of the cohort was recommended to undergo a sentinel lymph node biopsy after re-staging with the wide excision. In terms of locoregional recurrence rates, 2.3% of patients had developed locoregional disease, with 0.66% of these patients having their primary tumors upstaged after initial definitive wide excision [4]. In conclusion, it appears that while accurate staging of melanoma might be compromised at times with a shave biopsy, this rarely leads to a change in management, and if so, it likely is not causative for an adverse outcome in the vast majority of patients.

Incisional Biopsy

An incisional biopsy, as opposed to a shave, is indicated for larger, heterogeneous skin lesions, or for those that may require a more extensive surgical procedure based upon the location. An incisional biopsy allows for evaluation of the complete lesion, an accurate diagnosis, and determination of Breslow's depth prior to definitive excision. Incisional biopsies can be easily performed with the use of a scalpel blade or with a punch biopsy device, taken from the most elevated, darkly pigmented, or concerning tissue

S. A. Voigt, M.D. · N. A. Vohra, M.D. (✉)
C. Mosquera, M.D.
Division of Surgical Oncology, Department of Surgery, Brody School of Medicine at East Carolina University, Greenville, NC, USA
e-mail: johnsonso14@ecu.edu; vohran@ecu.edu; mosquerac@ecu.edu

A. I. Riker (ed.), *Melanoma*, https://doi.org/10.1007/978-3-319-78310-9_26

area [3]. While punch biopsies are limited in diameter with the largest punch tool at most practices being 6–8 mm, these are still widely used given the ease of performing them under local anesthesia and the high likelihood of obtaining an accurate Breslow's thickness. The primary disadvantage is the partial sampling nature of the biopsy, as this type of biopsy only removes a small portion of the skin lesion, which could lead to a potential misdiagnosis or inaccurate T-stage information [4]. It is particularly important when performing an incisional biopsy that the specimen be handled with fine forceps or skin hooks so that the specimen is not crushed, which will cause tissue artifacts on final pathology that are difficult to interpret. The area should include tissue that is thought to contain the neoplasm in the deepest area of skin penetration. For a lesion that is predominantly flat, a scallop shave biopsy is often an appropriate biopsy technique. This type of biopsy implies that the entire epidermis, dermis, and a portion of the subcutaneous tissue are removed, providing a full-thickness tissue biopsy for the dermatopathologist to examine [5].

Excisional Biopsy

Excisional biopsy remains the most definitive method of accurately determining lesion invasion [6]. If the size of the lesion is reasonable to excise completely with a local anesthetic only, a biopsy of the entire lesion can be safely performed in the office setting. Following proper skin preparation, the area of interest is marked. An ellipse is preferred to facilitate primary wound closure, with the long axis of the ellipse following the pathway of the lymphatic drainage. On the extremities, a longitudinal incision is preferred, while a lesion on the trunk, head, or neck should be planned for removal with an ellipse that is oriented parallel to the skin lines [7]. A field block using local anesthetic is placed just beyond the marked area. The skin is incised and dissection is carried down to include the subcutaneous fat [5].

Impact on Outcomes Depending on Biopsy Type

The most important consideration regarding the biopsy type in patients with potential melanoma is whether the type of biopsy leads to any significant differences in disease-free or overall survival. In a 2007 review of 471 patients that underwent excision for stage I and II melanoma, neither the diagnostic biopsy type (excisional wide with ≥2 mm margin, excisional narrow with <2 mm margin, incisional) nor the presence of tumor cells in the resected melanoma specimen influenced the disease-free or overall survival [8]. There have been some concerns regarding the manipulation of intact primary melanomas leading to disturbance of the tumor and possibly resulting in higher rates of nodal metastases. In a review of 1782 patients that underwent excisional, incisional, or shave biopsy, there were differences noted among the biopsy types regarding ulceration and regression of the tumor, with no differences appreciated in locoregional recurrence, disease-free survival, distant disease-free survival, or overall survival [9]. Thus, when used appropriately, incisional, excisional, and shave biopsies continue to play a central role in our daily clinical practice. The different techniques available will likely continue to be used at the physician's discretion depending upon anatomical factors and size of the lesion.

Definitive Excision of Primary Cutaneous Melanomas

Once a tissue diagnosis confirms a melanoma, complete excision with appropriate margins based on the Breslow's thickness of the lesion is indicated. Wide local excision of a primary cutaneous melanoma should be performed following the pathways of lymphatic drainage. In most cases, wide excision of a melanoma on the extremity can be performed using an elliptical area of resection. Dissection should include skin and all soft tissue down to the deep fascia [3]. Based on prospective data from several large clinical trials, current National Comprehensive Cancer Network Clinical Practice guidelines recommend wide excision of cutaneous melanoma based on the Breslow's depth of the lesion as indicated in Table 26.1 [10].

Wide Excision of Melanoma in Difficult Locations

Digits and Toes, Including Nailbeds

Management of an acral lentiginous melanoma can be challenging. Primary tumor excision from digits and toes follows the general recommendations for margins. This often requires a digit or toe amputation extending to the proximal mid-phalanx. Finger amputation should be performed proximal to the distal interphalangeal joint, with the goal of maintaining finger length as long as possible without compromising clinical margins [11].

When resecting a melanoma located on the great toe, attempt should be made to preserve the great toe metatarsal head as it provides important aspects of body balance and ambulation. For toe amputations, a racquet incision on the dorsum of the foot is made and extended proximally to the mid-phalanx, dissection is carried down until the metatarsal bone is identified and dissected in all its circumference. The bone is denuded and an amputation is performed with a double-levered osteotome. Hemostasis is achieved and the skin is closed with nonabsorbable vertical mattress stitches [12].

Table 26.1 Margins of excision based on Breslow's depth of the lesion

Breslow's thickness in millimeters (mm)	Recommended margins of excision in centimeters (cm)
Melanoma in situ	0.5
Less than 1	1
1.01–2.00	1–2
Greater than 2	2

Resection of Melanoma on the Heel

Wide local excision of melanoma of the heel involves dissection and excision down to the plantar fascia. Because the heel is a weight-bearing structure, reconstructive techniques require a durable repair. Either a full-thickness skin graft or a rotational flap is needed. A split-thickness skin graft is not appropriate for coverage of a defect on the heel [13]. The donor site for the rotational flap is the non-weight-bearing area of the heel with the flap elevated in the subfascial or supra-fascial location. The subfascial flap as shown in Fig. 26.1 can be based off of the medial or the lateral plantar vasculature, depending on the location of the primary melanoma. As shown in Fig. 26.2, the flap is rotated on to the defect on the heel and the donor site defect is covered with a full-thickness skin graft [14].

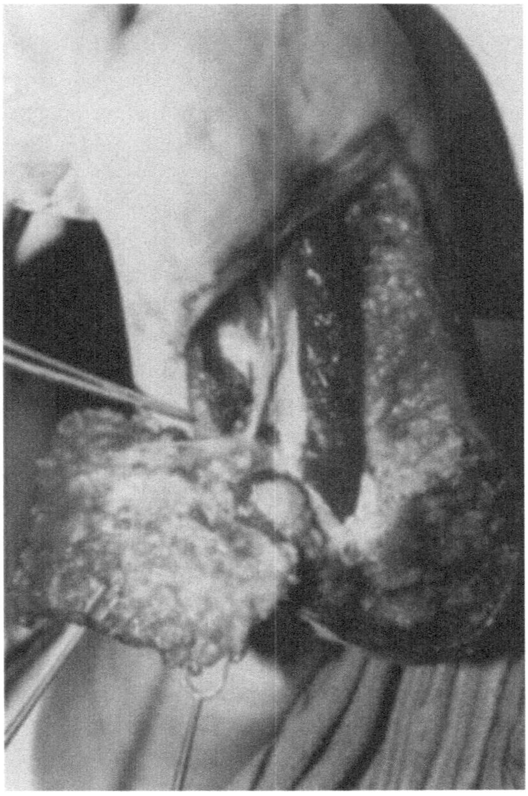

Fig. 26.1 Subfascial elevation of the plantar flap based on the medial plantar vasculature

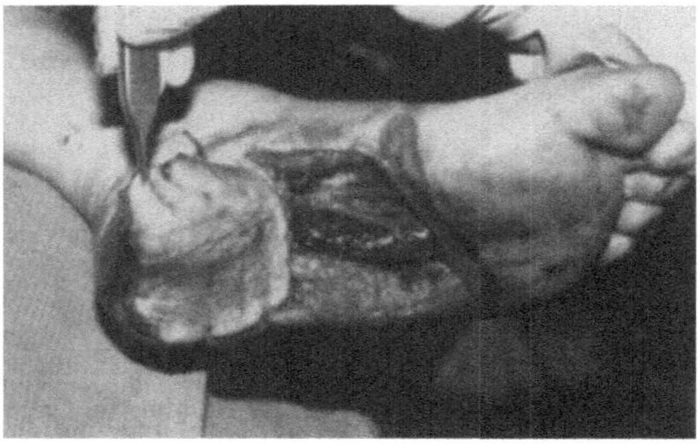

Fig. 26.2 Rotation of the medial plantar flap to cover the defect. The instep (donor site) is covered with a skin graft

Reconstructive Considerations for Closure of Defect After Wide Excision

The goal of reconstruction after melanoma excision is to maintain or restore similar tissue composition, function, and aesthetic appearance [15]. Depending on the anatomical region in question, resection of melanoma may require skin grafting or adjacent tissue transfer. Timing of this reconstruction is controversial, given the potential for positive margins at the time of melanoma resection, and thus some centers advocate for two stage operations. Karanetz and colleagues sought to determine the incidence of positive margins after melanoma resection and then assess the cost related to a potential two stage treatment. They found that in their prospective cohort, 2.7% of patients had positive margins on permanent pathology and the only variables associated with a positive margin were desmoplastic melanoma and a tumor location on the cheek. They also found that immediate reconstruction led to a mean cost savings of 38.5% at their institution [16]. Thus, immediate reconstruction appears to be a safe and cost-effective decision in a selected patient population. Some plastic surgeons are proponents of the square procedure in head and neck melanoma. This is a staged procedure in which the margins are excised first, followed by confirmation of negative margins on final pathology [17]. This technique results in high local control rates and allows the facial plastic surgeon to proceed with flap reconstruction, knowing that the risk of local recurrence is quite low in the setting of negative margins.

In order to reconstruct acquired defects, the main surgical options include: primary closure, skin grafting, adjacent tissue rearrangement with local skin flaps, regional muscle or fasciocutaneous flaps, free tissue transfer, and tissue expansion.

Skin Grafts

Skin grafts are indicated when the skin defect cannot be closed primarily. These are harvested from a donor site and transferred to the skin defect or the recipient site. Depending on the graft thickness, they can be classified as split-thickness graft, when only a portion of the dermis is harvested, or full-thickness graft which includes the entire dermis. Most patients undergoing melanoma excision are good candidates for full-thickness skin grafts. Split-thickness grafts may be more appropriate for larger defects. Full-thickness grafts have a better cosmetic outcome and greater mobility, but have a lower graft survival. In contrast, contractures are more frequent with thinner skin grafts.

Donor site considerations: A split-thickness graft can be harvested from any area of the body. Lower extremities, especially the thighs, and the trunk are more commonly used to harvest split-thickness skin grafts as these sites can be covered by clothing and provide a larger surface area. Full-thickness skin grafts are commonly obtained from the natural creases, blush zone, inner arm, inguinal crease, or abdomen (Fig. 26.3). It is common to use a full-thickness skin graft from the site of the sentinel node dissection, thereby allowing only one incision for both the node dissection and graft donor site and eliminate a third painful wound, the donor site. Relevant factors for donor site selection include: presence of hair follicles, skin color and pigmentation, thickness, texture, and defect size [18].

Recipient site considerations: Before an area is grafted, it is important to insure that the wound bed is hemostatic, well vascularized, and free of any infection. Hematoma formation underneath the skin graft may lead to failure of the graft, due to the hematoma preventing adherence of the graft to the wound bed. It also predisposes the wound to infection.

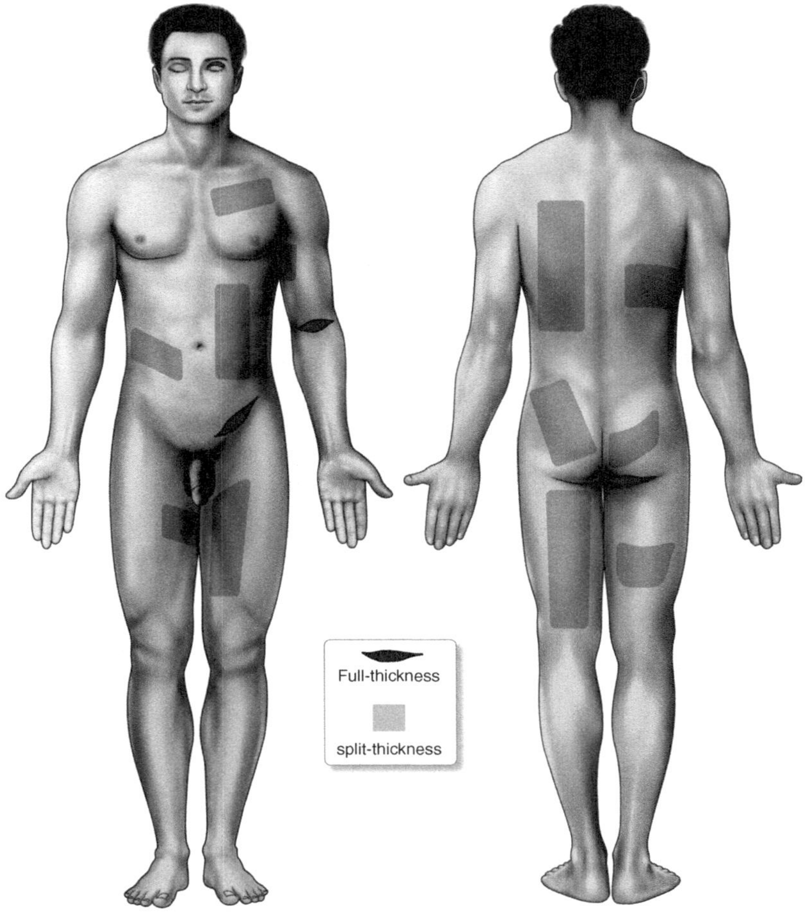

Fig. 26.3 Donor sites for full-thickness and split-thickness skin grafts

Placement of a Split-Thickness Skin Graft

Two skin harvesting methods are described, the freehand knife and the power-driven dermatome. In this chapter we will describe the latter, since the freehand technique has progressively fallen out of favor.

Once the donor site is chosen, markings are made to obtain a 15–20% longer graft compared to the skin defect. The dermatome should be properly set and selected thickness checked and corroborated. Commonly used skin thickness is between 0.012 and 0.018 in. with an average of 0.015 in. The blade and donor site are generously lubricated. Traction is applied by a surgical assistant on both ends of the donor site using towel clips or a tongue blade, while the surgeon positions the dermatome at a 30 ° angle against the skin and slowly advances through the donor site while simultaneously applying gentle pressure. At the end of the markings, the dermatome is lifted up, with the graft meshed, if necessary, to increase the total coverage area, as well as to allow evacuation of blood and fluid from under the graft. Upon grafting, care should be taking to place the external epithelium facing up and the shiny dermal side facing down. The graft is anchored to the site of the defect using an absorbable suture, such as a chromic suture.

Placement of a Full-Thickness Skin Graft

Once the donor site is chosen, markings are made slightly wider than the recipient site to account for primary contraction. Then with a scalpel, the skin including the dermis and some subcutaneous tissue is excised. Using fine tenotomy scissors, the skin is prepared for grafting by trimming off any fat or subcutaneous tissue from the underside of the skin. The graft should be secured peripherally with skin staples and with interrupted chromic sutures in between each of the skin staples. Several interrupted chromic sutures are also placed throughout the middle portion of the skin graft to the underlying fascial plane, thereby securing the entirety of the skin graft to the deep tissue. A bolster type of dressing is then placed over the entire skin graft, comprised of xeroform gauze, wet cotton balls, and secured with 2-0 silk ties. As mentioned previously, full-thickness skin grafts have better cosmetic outcome compared to split-thickness grafts, but also have a slightly higher graft failure rate. Complications include failure of the graft to remain viable due to compromised adherence secondary to hematoma, seroma, poorly vascularized wound bed, or infection [15, 19–21].

Local or Regional Flaps

A flap is a portion of vascularized tissue that is mobilized from a donor site to an adjacent or remote defect/recipient site. The purpose of a skin flap is reconstruction of tissue defects not amenable to primary closure.

Advancement Flap

As the name suggests, an advancement flap involves release of a portion of tissue to allow linear advancement of the tissue to cover a primary defect. Single pedicle advancement flaps are created by making two parallel incisions extending from the defect border, not exceeding a 2:1 length-to-width ratio. In the base of the flap, a Burow's triangle is created in each corner to allow for a smooth semicircular edge at closure as shown in Fig. 26.4, left panel.

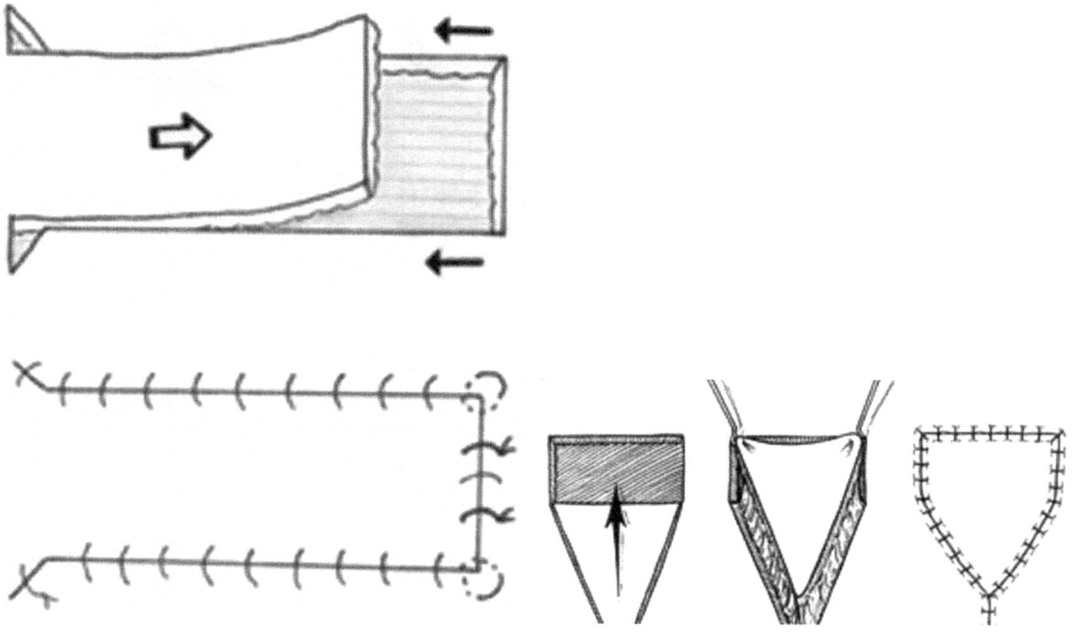

Fig. 26.4 Advancement flap techniques. Left panel shows a single pedicle advancement flap (Reproduced from Krishnan R, Garman M, Nunez-Gussman J, Orengo I. "Advancement flaps: a basic theme with many variations," *Dermatologic Surgery*. 2005;31(8 Pt 2):986–94, with permission of Wolters Kluwer). Right panel shows a V-Y advancement flap (Reproduced from Van Aalst, J. A., Mccurry, T. and Wagner, J. 2003. Reconstructive considerations in the surgical management of melanoma. Surg Clin North Am, 83, 187–230, with permission of Elsevier)

Bi-pedicle flaps are shaped by making opposite single pedicle advancement flaps, with the defect being perpendicular to the flaps and establishing an H-shaped wound. The V-Y advancement flap pushes a triangular flap into the defect and is closed in a straight line giving a Y-appearance when complete (Fig. 26.4, right panel) [15, 23, 44].

Limberg or Rhomboid Flap

The Limberg flap is a transposition flap used to repair rhombus-shaped defects. It is commonly used on the back after a wide excision since adequate mobilization of skin for primary closure can be difficult. To create this flap, the defect length is measured, followed by the creation of the first line which is extended along the short diagonal in order to match the defect side. A second line is drawn parallel to the defect and equal in length to the first line. The tissue is excised and the flap advanced as shown below (Fig. 26.5). A single rhomboid flap offers up to four potential flaps by creating a diagonal in each corner of the rhombus. A drawback of this flap is the more visible scar compared to other flaps given the use of diagonal incisions [15, 22].

Free Tissue Transfer

This technique is generally reserved for larger defects that cannot be reconstructed with local or regional flaps. The main considerations include the length and caliber of the vascular pedicle from the flap and assessment of the recipient vasculature to assure suitability [15]. Use of free flaps is quite uncommon in melanoma.

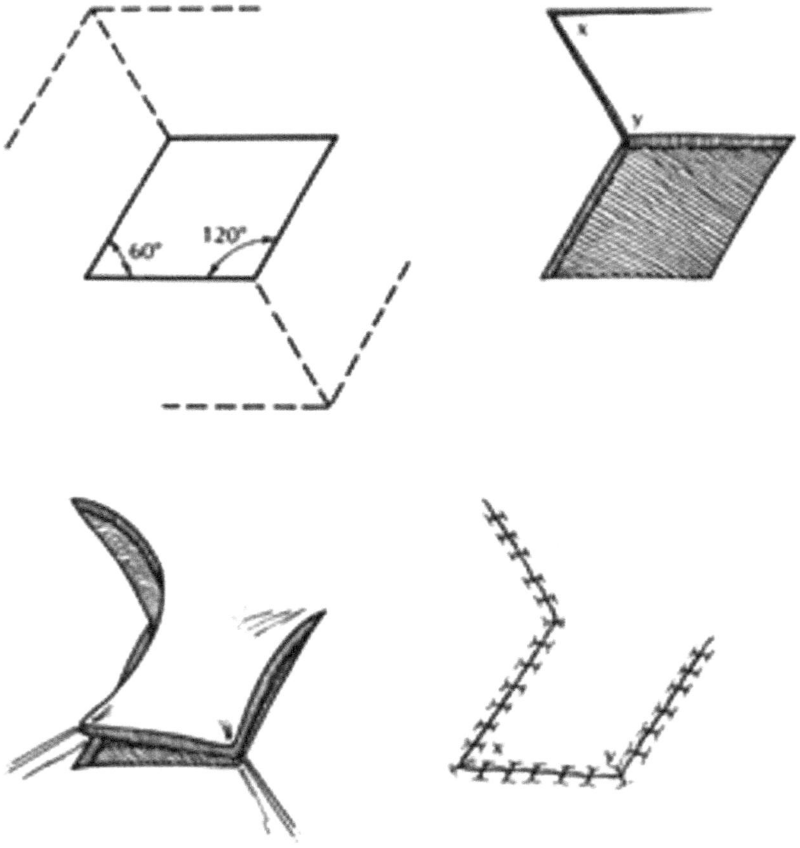

Fig. 26.5 Limberg or rhomboid flap technique. The rhomboid defect indicated by the shaded area is covered by rotating the skin flap with corners labeled X and Y. The defect resulting from rotating the flap is closed primarily. (Reproduced from Van Aalst, J. A., Mccurry, T. and Wagner, J. 2003. Reconstructive considerations in the surgical management of melanoma. *Surg Clin North Am*, 83, 187–230, with permission of Elsevier)

Tissue Expansion

Tissue expansion is generally reserved for secondary reconstructions in order to enhance aesthetic qualities of a previously grafted defect, or an unfavorable scar. The technique involves placement of an inflatable silicone expander under tissues that are adjacent to the defect. Serial expansion starts 2 weeks after the implants are placed and continues over 6–8 weeks. During this time, new skin is synthesized in response to the expansion. After enough excess tissue is obtained to close the secondary defect, the expanders are removed and the flaps are advanced to cover the defect [15].

Sentinel Lymph Node Dissection for Staging in Melanoma

Sentinel node dissection is an essential part of staging in cutaneous melanoma. It should be performed in patients with high-risk features for a thin primary melanoma between the Breslow's depth of 0.76–1.00 mm. In the United States, it is considered the standard of care for all primary melanoma's with a Breslow's thickness of >1.00 mm [21].

The technique involves the use of 1% solution of isosulfan blue dye and/or a radiotracer (Technetium Tc 99m Sulfur Colloid) [24]. Using sterile technique, a few hours before surgery, the radiotracer is circumferentially injected around the lesion in four different locations. The solution should be injected in the dermis rather than in the subcutaneous tissues and skin massaged to increase lymphatic flow. The draining lymphatic basin is identified using lymphoscintigraphy and the location of the lymph node is marked on the skin by the radiologist, facilitating intraoperative identification and resection of the node. Studies evaluating lymphoscintigraphy have shown that around 10% of patients with melanoma of the trunk have a dual lymph node drainage, thus making preoperative lymphoscintigraphy important in accurately assessing lymphatic drainage and staging [25].

In the operating room, 1–3 mL of isosulfan blue dye is injected intradermally around the primary melanoma prior to starting the sentinel node dissection. Using a sterile gamma probe, the tattooed "hot spot" should be verified and a survey of all pertinent lymph node basins and surrounding skin should be undertaken to pick up any additional basins or in-transit nodes. An incision is made over the tattoo and dissection is carried down to the subcutaneous fat. While dissecting, blue lymphatic channels may assist in locating the radioactive lymph node. After the node is circumferentially dissected and removed, radioactivity should be measured again to verify no remnant hot spots [21]. It is important to treat the node with care, to avoid tearing of its capsule which can lead to bleeding and potentially spread of cancer [24]. Currently, there is an effort to implement the use of immuno-targeted agents that can better determine tumor burden without the reliance of a sentinel lymph node biopsy. However, limitations to imaging resolution and sensitivity have slowed progress in this area [26] .

Completion Lymphadenectomy

Patients who have evidence of metastasis in the sentinel lymph node or have clinically positive lymph nodes are recommended to undergo a complete lymph node dissection of the respective nodal basin [27]. A thorough discussion regarding the risks and benefits of lymphadenectomy should be undertaken with the patient prior to surgery. Additionally, findings from the recently published MSLT-2 trial should be incorporated into the discussion about a completion lymphadenectomy after a positive sentinel node [28]. Briefly, the MSLT-2 trial was an international multicenter trial that randomly assigned patients with sentinel-node metastases detected by means of standard pathological assessment or a multimarker molecular assay to immediate completion lymph-node dissection or nodal observation with ultrasonography [28]. Immediate completion lymph-node dissection increased the rate of regional disease control and provided prognostic information but did not increase 3 year melanoma-specific survival among patients with melanoma and sentinel-node metastases at a median follow-up of 43 months [28]. For the patients enrolled in this trial, the Breslow's thickness of the primary melanoma ranged from 1.2 mm to 3.5 mm. It was also noted in this trial that presence on non-sentinel node metastases was a strong prognostic factor. The rate of lymphedema in patients who underwent completion lymphadenectomy was four times that of the observation group. When informing patients about the role of completion lymphadenectomy in intermediate thickness melanoma, discussion points should include the relatively short median follow-up, the additional information that can be gained from completion lymph node dissection, the type of follow-up surveillance required, and the substantial risk of lymphedema. Patients opting for observation should undergo periodic ultrasound examinations of the draining lymph node basin if possible.

Complete Axillary Node Dissection

The patient is placed in a supine position with the ipsilateral arm abducted. The extremity is prepped and draped to allow movement of the arm during the intervention. A transverse incision is made spanning the edge of the pectoralis muscle to the anterior border of the latissimus dorsi muscle. Alternatively a longitudinal incision can also be used. Dissection is carried down through subcutaneous tissue to the pectoralis major fascia. Superior and inferior flaps are raised, extending from the anterior nipple line to the latissimus dorsi muscle, exposing the thoracodorsal bundle. The anterior pectoralis muscle fascia is removed to expose the pectoralis major. The axillary vein is exposed by using sharp dissection of the thick axillary fascia and gentle sweeping of the axillary fat inferiorly. The pectoralis major is retracted to obtain access to the pectoralis minor. The extremity is flexed at the elbow and adducted to obtain access to the axillary apex. In order to facilitate access to the nodes medial to the pectoralis minor muscle, the muscle may be divided close to the coracoid process, avoiding injury to the thoracoacromial nerve and the lateral pectoral nerve. However, it is often not necessary, as palpation with the index finger is often adequate in order to feel for any hard, clinically suspicious lymph nodes in this area leading the clavicle. Axillary dissection is started at the apex of the axilla, and carried down following the axillary vein, ligating small tributaries off the axillary vein as necessary. Small arterial branches may also be ligated. The nodal tissue between the pectoralis major and minor is also included with the specimen. The intercostobrachial nerve crosses through this area, a sensory nerve innervating the upper inner aspect of the arm is often sacrificed to facilitate complete exposure and removal of the level 1 and 2 lymph nodes. The dissection is carried laterally and inferiorly to dissect the axillary contents along the chest wall. The long thoracic neurovascular bundle as well as the thoracodorsal neurovascular bundle are identified and preserved during dissection unless involved with disease. The specimen is removed and clips are placed in the superior and laterals borders to orient the specimen. The surgical field is irrigated. If the pectoralis major was divided, the muscle continuity is restored to obtain the natural axillary contour. A drain is placed anteriorly over the pectoralis major and another under the posterior flap. Drains are connected to bulb suction. The wound is then closed by approximating the skin in an interrupted intradermal layer and a continuous subcuticular layer.

A complete axillary node dissection can be divided into three levels:

- *Level I:* Nodal tissue lateral to the pectoralis minor (i.e., axillary vein superiorly, the pectoralis major medially, and the latissimus dorsi laterally)
- *Level II:* Nodal tissue underlying the pectoralis minor
- *Level III:* Nodal tissue medial to the pectoralis minor
- There is currently no evidence supporting a partial axillary lymph node dissection for melanoma in terms of comparable outcomes; however, a recent study showed a potential low frequency of melanoma metastases in level III, thus opening the field for further investigation [27, 29].

The incidence of lymphedema following nodal surgery is common in melanoma, with a significant increase after a therapeutic lymph node dissection and a borderline increased incidence for lower extremity versus the upper extremity [30]. Long-term studies have shown that peripheral vascular disease increases the risk of lymphedema in patients undergoing complete axillary lymph node dissection [31]. With respect to quality of life, patients undergoing complete axillary node dissection compared to those undergoing just sentinel lymph node dissection reported more problems and most pain long-term [32].

Inguinal Lymph Node Dissection

In patients with metastatic lymph nodes in the inguinal basin, a complete (inguinofemoral/superficial) lymph node dissection is indicated.

Superficial Inguinal Lymph Node Dissection

The patient is placed in supine position. The abdomen and extremity of interest are prepped and draped. An incision is created starting 2–3 cm cephalad and medial to the anterior superior iliac spine and continued caudally to a point 1–2 cm below the inguinal crease. The incision is then continued in the medial direction toward the femoral vein at which point it is gently curved caudally about 5 cm. Superior and inferior skin flaps are raised and extended until the borders of the femoral triangle are exposed (lateral border of the Sartorius muscle, medial border of the adductor longus, and the anterior iliac spine). Resection is started by dissecting the tissue between camper's fascia, the external oblique muscle, and the inguinal ligament. Dissection is carried down applying medial traction to the specimen, lateral to medial starting from the lateral border to the Sartorius muscle to the femoral sheath. The lateral femoral cutaneous nerve and the femoral nerve should be visualized and preserved under the Sartorius fascia. The saphenous vein is identified and ligated at the saphenous-femoral junction. Saphenous vein sparing approach has also been described with mixed reports regarding the reduction in morbidity [33, 34]. Dissection is continued by applying lateral traction on the specimen and incising the fascia in the medial border of the adductor longus. Resection is carried down to the femoral sheath were the lateral and medial dissection planes should join. The specimen is then divided at the apex of the femoral triangle. Attention is then turned to Cloquet's node which lays high in the femoral ring between the inguinal ligament superiorly, the lacunar ligament medially, Coopers ligament inferiorly, and the femoral vein laterally. Tissue within this space is retracted inferiorly and resected. This completes the superficial groin dissection. The femoral ring should then be obliterated. The Sartorius muscle may be transposed over the femoral sheath to protect the femoral vessels, and a two-layer interrupted closure is used to approximate the wound edges [35]. Skin is sutured and dressed with a light compressing dressing.

Indications for iliac and obturator (deep, pelvic) node dissection include the finding of a positive Cloquet's node intraoperatively or the detection of enlarged iliac or obturator nodes on preoperative CT scans, or fludeoxyglucose (FDG)-avid iliac or obturator nodes on a PET scan [35]. It has been shown that when palpable inguinal disease is present, up to 40% of patients are found to have pelvic nodal metastasis [36]. Controversy still persists regarding the exact indications for, and benefit of, pelvic lymphadenectomy [34].

Deep Iliac-Obturator Lymph Node Dissection

Dissection is started through a superficial inguinal node dissection incision. After the superior flap is created, an incision in made in the external oblique aponeurosis about 3–4 cm above the inguinal ligament. The underlying internal oblique muscle and the transversus muscles along with the transversalis fascia are divided but not the peritoneum. The deep inferior epigastric vessels arising just above the inguinal ligament form the external iliac artery and vein are ligated and the peritoneum and ureter are reflected medially and cephalad. Dissection is carried down to resect the tissue contained between the aortic bifurcation superiorly, the bladder medially, the femoral ring inferiorly, and the genitofemoral nerve laterally. Dissection should be carried so as to include lymphatic tissue between the external and internal iliac vessels and deep below the obturator nerve down to the obturator membrane overlying the obturator foramen. Layers should be anatomically closed once dissection is complete.

The main complication related to inguinal lymph node dissection, both deep and superficial, relates to the rate of wound infections. Some studies report up to 19% wound complication rate. Interestingly, this rate has been found to be higher among patients that undergo lymph node dissection for clinical disease compared to patients undergoing the procedure for a positive sentinel lymph node [37]. Authors hypothesize this might be due to surgeons wanting to leave a wider margin of disease-free tissue at the time of closure, and thus, compromising of the vascular supply at the wound edges. Rates of lymphedema were also higher among those with clinical disease at the time of lymphadenectomy.

Minimally Invasive Inguinal Lymph Node Dissection

In 2013, a prospective study compared the outcomes of minimally invasive lymph node dissection and open inguinal lymph node dissection for melanoma. They found that the minimally invasive approach required a longer operative time, however, the wound dehiscence rate, readmission rate, and postoperative length of stay were all lower in this group. Moreover, more lymph nodes were retrieved with the minimally invasive approach [38]. Another study comparing early outcomes found similar results with no significant difference in nodal yield or operative times but a shorter length of stay [39]. Since then, another study found that the procedure could be implemented easily among surgeons. They found that proficiency (assessed by scoring videos with the global operative assessment of laparoscopic skills (GOALS) tool) was correlated with fundamentals of laparoscopic surgery (FLS) scores.

Regardless, there was no association of FLS or GOALS with lymph node count, conversion rate, or complication rate [40]. There is even a case report of an inguinal lymphadenectomy performed robotically [41]. Most recently, a multicenter, prospective clinical trial (SAFE-MILND) sought out to determine safety and feasibility of minimally invasive inguinal lymph node dissection and they found that the technique was easily adopted and that lymph node retrieval rate met or exceeded current oncologic guidelines [42]. The adverse event was high at 71%, however, only 26% were grade 3 (graded per the NCI Common Terminology Criteria for Adverse Events Version 4.0) and the majority of these were wound infections. Overall, the data points at a promising and prominent role for minimally invasive inguinal node dissection as experience improves outcomes.

Neck Dissection

Cervical lymphadenectomy (neck dissection) is performed when a cervical sentinel lymph node is positive, or there is clinical evidence of disease in the cervical node.

There are 3 type of neck node dissections described:

- Radical neck dissection (RND).
- Modified radical neck dissection (MRND).
- Selective neck dissection (SND).

A radical neck dissection involves removal of cervical nodes contained between the inferior border of the mandible, the lateral border of the sternohyoid, the clavicle, and the trapezius as well as resection of the sternocleidomastoid muscle, the spinal accessory nerve and the internal jugular vein. This procedure is rarely used given the associated high morbidity. A modified radical neck dissection removes the same group of nodes as a radical neck dissection. However, the sternocleidomastoid muscle, the spinal accessory nerve, and the internal jugular vein are preserved. A MRND is indicated for clinically palpable nodal disease. Lastly, SND involves removal of specific lymph node groups based on the site, histology, and routes of lymphatic spread of the primary tumor. SND is the most commonly recommended type of node dissection [43].

Parotidectomy should be performed in two specific scenarios [44]:

1. If parotid lymphadenopathy is present without neck involvement, both neck dissection plus parotidectomy should be performed.
2. If neck disease is present without parotid involvement, parotidectomy should be considered only if the lymphatic drainage is likely to pass through the parotid gland.

An incision carried along the horizontal ramus of the mandible is recommended. Superior and inferior flaps are raised. The tail of the parotid is retracted superiorly gaining access to the retromandibular vein which is transected. Then, the facial artery and vein are identified, the facial artery is clamped, and the facial vein is ligated. Attention is given to preserve the lingual and hypoglossal nerves. Dissection is carried down to the submandibular nodes (located anteriorly and posteriorly to the submaxillary gland) and submental nodes (located between the two bellies of the digastric muscle, the symphysis of the mandible and the mylohyoid muscles). The submaxillary ganglion, submaxillary gland, and adjacent nodes are removed. The posterior digastric muscle fascia is incised and dissection continued along the digastric muscle anteriorly and posteriorly. The facial artery is transected under the posterior digastric muscle belly. Dissection is carried down to the sternocleidomastoid. The anterior fascia is incised from the sternocleidomastoid apex down to the clavicular and sternal heads. Dissection is carried circumferentially removing all fat and nodal tissue around the sternocleidomastoid muscle and spinal accessory nerve. Attention is then turned to the carotid sheath were the jugular vein, carotid artery, and vagus nerve should be identified. The Ansa cervicalis is transected. Dissection is carried inferiorly along the medial aspect of the jugular vein to excise the upper jugular and jugular chain nodes. The omohyoid muscle is identified and transected in the inferior aspect of the cervical dissection to obtain access to the lower jugular nodes located anteriorly to the jugular vein at the facial vein confluence. Attention is turned to the anterior border of the trapezius were the spinal accessory nerve is again identified. Tissue is resected circumferentially including all nodal tissue in the posterior cervical triangle. To finalize the dissection, lymphoid tissue is raised superiorly from the supraclavicular fossa and anteriorly from the posterior cervical region over the scalene muscles paying attention to preserve the integrity of the phrenic nerve. For skin lesions located above the mandible and medial to the crease behind the pinna, a preauricular incision in combination with the cervical incision will provide proper exposure for a parotid gland and parotid node excision [5].

References

1. Fewkes JL, Sober A. Skin biopsy: the four types and how best to do them. Prim Care Cancer. 1993;13:36–9.
2. Stell VH, Norton HJ, Smith KS, Salo JC, White RL Jr. Method of biopsy and incidence of positive margins in primary melanoma. Ann Surg Oncol. 2007;14(2):893–8.
3. Balch CM, Sober AJ, Adkins M. Textbook of oncology. 7th Philadelphia, PA: JB Lippincott; 2004.
4. Zager JS, Hochwald SN, Marzban SS, Francois R, Law KM, Davis AH, et al. Shave biopsy is a safe and accurate method for the initial evaluation of melanoma. J Am Coll Surg. 2011;212(4):454–60. discussion 60–2
5. Balch CM, Hunter, Peggy. Surgical approaches to cutaneous melanoma. Charles M. Balch; assistant editor PH, editor. Karger, Basel, New York; 1985.
6. Pavri SN, Clune J, Ariyan S, Narayan D. Malignant melanoma: beyond the basics. Plast Reconstr Surg. 2016;138(2):330e–40e.
7. Liegeois NJ, Johnson TM, Sober AJ. Cutaneous melanoma. 5th. St. Louis, MO: QMP; 2009.
8. Molenkamp BG, Sluijter BJ, Oosterhof B, Meijer S, van Leeuwen PA. Non-radical diagnostic biopsies do not negatively influence melanoma patient survival. Ann Surg Oncol. 2007;14(4):1424–30.
9. Martin RC 2nd, Scoggins CR, Ross MI, Reintgen DS, Noyes RD, Edwards MJ, et al. Is incisional biopsy of melanoma harmful? Am J Surg. 2005;190(6):913–7.

10. Coit DG, Thompson JA, Algazi A, Andtbacka R, Bichakjian CK, Carson WE 3rd, et al. Melanoma, Version 2.2016, NCCN clinical practice guidelines in oncology. J Natl Compr Cancer Netw. 2016;14(4):450–73.
11. Balch CM, Balch GC, Thompson JF. Biopsy and Definitive Excision of Primary Cutaneous Melanomas. In: Morita SY, Balch CM, Klimberg V, Pawlik TM, Posner MC, Tanabe KK. eds. Textbook of Complex General Surgical Oncology New York, NY: McGraw-Hill. http://accesssurgery.mhmedical.com.jproxy.lib.ecu.edu/content.aspx?bookid=2209&sectionid=168937390. Accessed April 09, 2018.
12. Steven G, Economou TS. Atlas of surgical techniques. Philadelphia: W.B. Saunders Company; 1996.
13. Nahabedian MY. Stretch JR, Tufaro AP. Cutaneous melanoma. Complex closures of melanoma excisions. 5th edn. St. Louis, MO: QMP; 2009.
14. Evans GR, Friedman J, Shenaq J, Mosser S. Plantar flap reconstruction for acral lentiginous melanoma. Ann Surg Oncol. 1997;4(7):575–8.
15. van Aalst JA, McCurry T, Wagner J. Reconstructive considerations in the surgical management of melanoma. Surg Clin North Am. 2003;83(1):187–230.
16. Karanetz I, Stanley S, Knobel D, Smith BD, Bastidas N, Beg M, et al. Melanoma extirpation with immediate reconstruction: the oncologic safety and cost savings of single-stage treatment. Plast Reconstr Surg. 2016;138(1):256–61.
17. Anderson KW, Baker SR, Lowe L, Su L, Johnson TM. Treatment of head and neck melanoma, lentigo maligna subtype: a practical surgical technique. Arch Facial Plast Surg. 2001;3(3):202–6.
18. Lewis JM, Zager JS, Yu D, Pelaez D, Riker AI, Dessureault S, et al. Full-thickness grafts procured from skin overlying the sentinel lymph node basin; reconstruction of primary cutaneous malignancy excision defects. Ann Surg Oncol. 2008;15(6):1733–40.
19. Yuen JC. Textbook of surgical oncology. Principles of skin grafting and flaps. Chapter 159. New York: McGraw-Hill Education/Medical; 2017.
20. Amir A. Ghaferi, Sabel MS. Operative management of melanoma (Current procedures: surgery). Chapter 28. New York: McGraw-Hill; 2010.
21. Robert MZ, Jr., Robert MZ, Sr. Zollinger's Atlas of Surgical Operations. 9th ed. New York, NY, 2011. McGraw-Hill Medical.
22. Judy Lee, Matthew White W. Local skin flaps in facial reconstruction. Current diagnosis and treatment in otolaryngology—head and neck surgery. Chapter 77. 3rd ed
23. Ravi Krishnan, Mary Garman, Janna Nunez-Gussman, Ida Orengo, Advancement Flaps: A Basic Theme with Many Variations. Dermatologic Surgery 31:986–994.
24. Faries MB, Morita SY, Balch CM, Suzanne Klimberg V, Pawlik TM, Posner MC, Tanabe KK. Textbook of general surgical oncology—sentinel lymph node biopsy for melanoma. McGraw-Hill Education: New York, NY; 2016.
25. Caprio MG, Carbone G, Bracigliano A, Acampa W, Mainolfi C, Molea G, et al. Sentinel lymph node detection by lymphoscintigraphy in malignant melanoma. Tumori. 2002;88(3):S43–5.
26. Cousins A, Thompson SK, Wedding AB, Thierry B. Clinical relevance of novel imaging technologies for sentinel lymph node identification and staging. Biotechnol Adv. 2014;32(2):269–79.
27. Tsutsumida A, Takahashi A, Namikawa K, Yamazaki N, Uhara H, Teramoto Y, et al. Frequency of level II and III axillary nodes metastases in patients with positive sentinel lymph nodes in melanoma: a multi-institutional study in Japan. Int J Clin Oncol. 2016;21(4):796–800.
28. Faries MB, Thompson JF, Cochran AJ, Andtbacka RH, Mozzillo N, Zager JS, et al. Completion dissection or observation for sentinel-node metastasis in melanoma. N Engl J Med. 2017;376(23):2211–22.
29. Nessim C, Law C, McConnell Y, Shachar S, McKinnon G, Wright F. How often do level III nodes bear melanoma metastases and does it affect patient outcomes? Ann Surg Oncol. 2013;20(6):2056–64.
30. Hyngstrom JR, Chiang YJ, Cromwell KD, Ross MI, Xing Y, Mungovan KS, et al. Prospective assessment of lymphedema incidence and lymphedema-associated symptoms following lymph node surgery for melanoma. Melanoma Res. 2013;23(4):290–7.
31. Friedman JF, Sunkara B, Jehnsen JS, Durham A, Johnson T, Cohen MS. Risk factors associated with lymphedema after lymph node dissection in melanoma patients. Am J Surg. 2015;210(6):1178–84. discussion 84
32. de Vries M, Hoekstra HJ, Hoekstra-Weebers JE. Quality of life after axillary or groin sentinel lymph node biopsy, with or without completion lymph node dissection, in patients with cutaneous melanoma. Ann Surg Oncol. 2009;16(10):2840–7.
33. Baur J, Mathe K, Gesierich A, Weyandt G, Wiegering A, Germer CT, et al. Morbidity and oncologic outcome after saphenous vein-sparing inguinal lymphadenectomy in melanoma patients. World J Surg Oncol. 2017;15(1):99.
34. Sarnaik AA, Puleo CA, Zager JS, Sondak VK. Limiting the morbidity of inguinal lymphadenectomy for metastatic melanoma. Cancer Control. 2009;16(3):240–7.
35. Balch CM, Balch GC, Thompson JF, Morita SY, Balch CM, Suzanne Klimberg V, Pawlik TM, Posner MC, Tanabe KK. Textbook of general surgical oncology—surgical management of metastatic melanoma (Stage III and IV disease). McGraw-Hill Education: New York, NY; 2016.
36. Glover AR, Allan CP, Wilkinson MJ, Strauss DC, Thomas JM, Hayes AJ. Outcomes of routine ilioinguinal lymph node dissection for palpable inguinal melanoma nodal metastasis. Br J Surg. 2014;101(7):811–9.
37. Sabel MS, Griffith KA, Arora A, Shargorodsky J, Blazer DG 3rd, Rees R, et al. Inguinal node dissection

for melanoma in the era of sentinel lymph node biopsy. Surgery. 2007;141(6):728–35.
38. Abbott AM, Grotz TE, Rueth NM, Hernandez Irizarry RC, Tuttle TM, Jakub JW. Minimally invasive inguinal lymph node dissection (MILND) for melanoma: experience from two academic centers. Ann Surg Oncol. 2013;20(1):340–5.
39. Dossett LA, Castner NB, Pow-Sang JM, Abbott AM, Sondak VK, Sarnaik AA, et al. Robotic-assisted transperitoneal pelvic lymphadenectomy for metastatic melanoma: early outcomes compared with open pelvic lymphadenectomy. J Am Coll Surg. 2016;222(4):702–9.
40. Zendejas B, Jakub JW, Terando AM, Sarnaik A, Ariyan CE, Faries MB, et al. Laparoscopic skill assessment of practicing surgeons prior to enrollment in a surgical trial of a new laparoscopic procedure. Surg Endosc. 2017;31:3313–9.
41. Sanchez A, Sotelo R, Rodriguez O, Sanchez R, Rosciano J, Medina L, et al. Robot-assisted video endoscopic inguinal lymphadenectomy for melanoma. J Robot Surg. 2016;10(4):369–72.
42. Jakub JW, Terando AM, Sarnaik A, Ariyan CE, Faries MB, Zani S Jr, et al. Safety and feasibility of minimally invasive inguinal lymph node dissection in patients with melanoma (SAFE-MILND): report of a prospective multi-institutional trial. Ann Surg. 2017;265(1):192–6.
43. Feig BW, Ching DC. The MD Anderson surgical oncology handbook—Cancers of the head and neck. 5th ed. Philadelphia: Lippincott Williams & Wilkins (LWW); 2011.
44. Ahmed OA, Kelly C. Head and neck melanoma (excluding ocular melanoma): United Kingdom National Multidisciplinary Guidelines. J Laryngol Otol. 2016;130(S2):S133–41.

27 Isolated Limb Infusion for Recurrent and Locally Metastatic Limb Melanoma

Hidde M. Kroon, Anna M. Huismans, Brendon J. Coventry, and John F. Thompson

Introduction and Historical Perspective

The treatment of patients with locally advanced or recurrent metastatic melanoma confined to a limb is often challenging, due to both the size and number of tumor deposits. Before the mid-1950s, amputation of the affected limb was often deemed necessary, but following the introduction of the isolated limb perfusion (ILP) technique by Creech et al., this mutilating procedure became unnecessary in the vast majority of patients [1]. During ILP, the blood circulation of the limb is temporarily isolated from the systemic circulation. With open surgical exposure, the femoral artery and vein (when treating a lower limb) or the axillary artery and vein (when treating an upper limb) are exposed and clamped, cannulated and connected to an extracorporeal circuit.

To achieve optimal isolation, minor vessels in the subcutaneous tissue and muscles are compressed using an external tourniquet [2, 3]. In this isolated circuit, the cytotoxic drug, typically melphalan, can be administered at a dosage of up to tenfold greater than could be tolerated systemically, without causing locally irreversible adverse effects [2–4]. The cytotoxic drug is typically circulated for 60–90 min, after which the limb is flushed to eliminate the remaining cytotoxic drug in the isolated limb. Following ILP, complete response (CR) rates of 7–91% (median 46%) and partial response (PR) rates of 0–44% (median 34%) have been reported. With this technique, it has been possible to avoid amputation of the affected limb in over 90% of cases [4–6].

Despite these generally satisfactory results, the ILP technique has some major disadvantages: It is a technically complex procedure and

H. M. Kroon, M.D., Ph.D. (✉)
Melanoma Institute Australia, The University of Sydney, Sydney, NSW, Australia

Department of General Surgery, Flinders Medical Centre, Adelaide, SA, Australia

Department of Surgery, Royal Adelaide Hospital, University of Adelaide, Adelaide, SA, Australia

A. M. Huismans, M.D., Ph.D.
Melanoma Institute Australia, The University of Sydney, Sydney, NSW, Australia

B. J. Coventry, M.D.
Department of Surgery, Royal Adelaide Hospital, University of Adelaide, Adelaide, SA, Australia
e-mail: brendon.coventry@adelaide.edu.au

J. F. Thompson, M.D.
Melanoma Institute Australia, The University of Sydney, Sydney, NSW, Australia

Sydney Medical School, The University of Sydney, Sydney, NSW, Australia

Royal Prince Alfred Hospital, Camperdown, NSW, Australia

Faculty of Medicine and Health Sciences, Macquarie University, North Ryde, NSW, Australia
e-mail: john.thompson@melanoma.org.au

A. I. Riker (ed.), *Melanoma*, https://doi.org/10.1007/978-3-319-78310-9_27

involves an invasive surgical approach. In the past, several attempts were made to design a simplified and less invasive alternative to ILP. Procedures such as direct intra-arterial infusion and "tourniquet infusion" with partial venous outflow occlusion have been investigated, but these techniques failed to achieve response rates comparable to those obtained following ILP [7–9].

In the early 1990s, Thompson and colleagues at the Sydney Melanoma Unit (now known as Melanoma Institute Australia) developed a simple, minimally invasive procedure that they called isolated limb infusion (ILI). Using the ILI technique, it proved possible to obtain the benefits of ILP without incurring its major disadvantages [10, 11]. ILI is essentially a low-flow ILP, performed via percutaneously placed catheters under hypoxic conditions (i.e., without oxygenation of the perfusate). This simplified technique, now in regular use at tertiary melanoma referral centers in Australia and at many other leading melanoma treatment centers around the world, produces response rates which are similar to those achieved following ILP [12–14]. To date, ILI with cytotoxic drugs, usually melphalan, with or without actinomycin D, has mainly been used as a stand-alone therapeutic procedure. Additionally, its simplicity and low morbidity offer great potential in the future for it to be used with other agents, or in combination with systemic therapies to control advanced limb melanoma.

Similarities and Differences Between Isolated Limb Infusion and Isolated Limb Perfusion

Both ILP and ILI involve vascular isolation and perfusion or infusion of an extremity with a high dose of cytotoxic agents under mild hyperthermia. Both ILI and ILP are usually performed under general anesthesia. Despite these similarities, both procedures have major differences also [3, 15, 16]. A major difference between the procedures is the lower flow rate and shorter circulation time of the cytotoxic agents in the isolated extremity during ILI. For ILP this is usually 150–1000 mL/min for 60 min whereas for ILI it is only 50–100 mL/min for 30 min. ILI is a hypoxic procedure, which leads to marked acidosis in the isolated circuit. In contrast, ILP involves full oxygenation of the perfusate by incorporating a membrane oxygenator in the external circuit. Scar tissue after a previous ILP or following groin or axillary lymph node dissection can make it technically difficult to obtain safe vascular access for a repeat ILP procedure, resulting in an increased risk of morbidity.

A repeat ILI, on the other hand, is normally straightforward because the catheters are radiologically placed percutaneously without dissection, are much smaller in diameter, and can be inserted via the contralateral groin. Additionally, blood transfusion, or more recently the use of autologous blood, is required for ILP to prime the perfusion circuit, but is not necessary for ILI. Infusion of 400 mL of normal saline into the limb is sufficient for ILI, due to the small volume of the circuit. Finally, ILP is a technically demanding procedure that requires complex and expensive equipment, occupies many hours of operating room time involving numerous surgical, anesthetic and nursing personnel, plus ancillary technical staff. In contrast to this, ILI is a much simpler, lower-cost procedure which requires much more modest equipment, less time in the operating room, and fewer personnel. The principal differences between ILI and conventional ILP are listed in Table 27.1.

Patient Selection for Isolated Limb Infusion

The primary indication for ILI and ILP is similar, namely extensive and/or unresectable in-transit metastases or locally recurrent melanoma of an extremity [16]. Limb melanoma deposits require an established vascular network supplying the tumor in order to be effective. Neither ILP nor

Table 27.1 Differences between isolated limb perfusion and isolated limb infusion

Isolated limb perfusion	Isolated limb infusion
Technically complex	Technically simple
Open surgical exposure of vessels for catheter insertion	Percutaneous vascular catheter insertion in radiology department
4–6 h duration	Approximately 1 h
Perfusionist and ancillary staff required	No perfusionist required and fewer total staff
Complex and expensive equipment needed	Equipment requirements modest
Magnitude of procedure excludes patients	Well tolerated by medically compromised, frail and elderly patients
Not possible in occlusive vascular disease	Can be performed selectively in occlusive vascular disease
Technically challenging to perform a repeat procedure	Not difficult to perform a repeat procedure
Systemic metastases normally a contraindication	Systemic metastases not a contraindication
Higher perfusion pressures predispose to systemic leakage	Low pressure system, effective vascular isolation with tourniquet
Limb tissues oxygenated, with normal blood gases maintained	Progressive hypoxia and acidosis
Hyperthermia (>41 °C can be achieved)	Usually not possible to raise limb temperature above 40 °C
General anesthesia (GA) required	Possible with regional anesthesia, GA preferred

ILI has proven effective prophylactically for microscopic, non-vascularized tumor deposits [17]. Due to its minimally invasive character, the ILI procedure can be offered to elderly and medically compromised patients who would not otherwise be considered suitable candidates for ILP [18, 19]. Patients in ILI studies have generally had a higher stage of disease, a higher average age, and more serious comorbidities than those in ILP studies [20, 21]. Of note, selected patients who cannot be treated safely and effectively with ILP because of occlusive vascular disease can be successfully treated with ILI. Finally, ILI can be offered as a minimally invasive, palliative treatment option for patients with stage IV disease. Many of these patients also have disabling limb disease that be effectively treated with ILI in order to avoid amputation, whereas the invasive ILP procedure would often not be considered under these circumstances [22, 23].

Technical Details of the ILI Procedure

The ILI technique as described below is currently used across Australia [15]. A schematic overview of the procedure is shown in Fig. 27.1. In the radiology department, standard radiological catheters with additional side-holes near their tips are inserted percutaneously into the major artery and vein of the disease-bearing limb, usually via the contralateral groin, using the Seldinger technique. For lower limb ILIs, the catheter tips are positioned in the popliteal artery and vein just above the knee; for upper limb ILIs, the catheter tips are positioned in the brachial artery and basilic vein, just above the elbow. Retrograde perfusion of tissues located more proximally to the catheter tips in the limb, but distal to the level of the tourniquet, occurs in a retrograde fashion via collateral vascular channels.

Due to the synergistic antitumor effects of hyperthermia and melphalan, strenuous efforts are made to maintain a warm limb preoperatively and to increase the limb temperatures to mild hyperthermia (ideally 38–39 °C) intraoperatively [2]. To achieve mild limb hyperthermia, precautions are necessary to avoid body and limb cooling in the preoperative period. These include the placement of a hot-air blanket or other warming device over the patient as soon as the vascular catheters have been inserted, especially during transport to the operating room. Intraoperatively, measures to

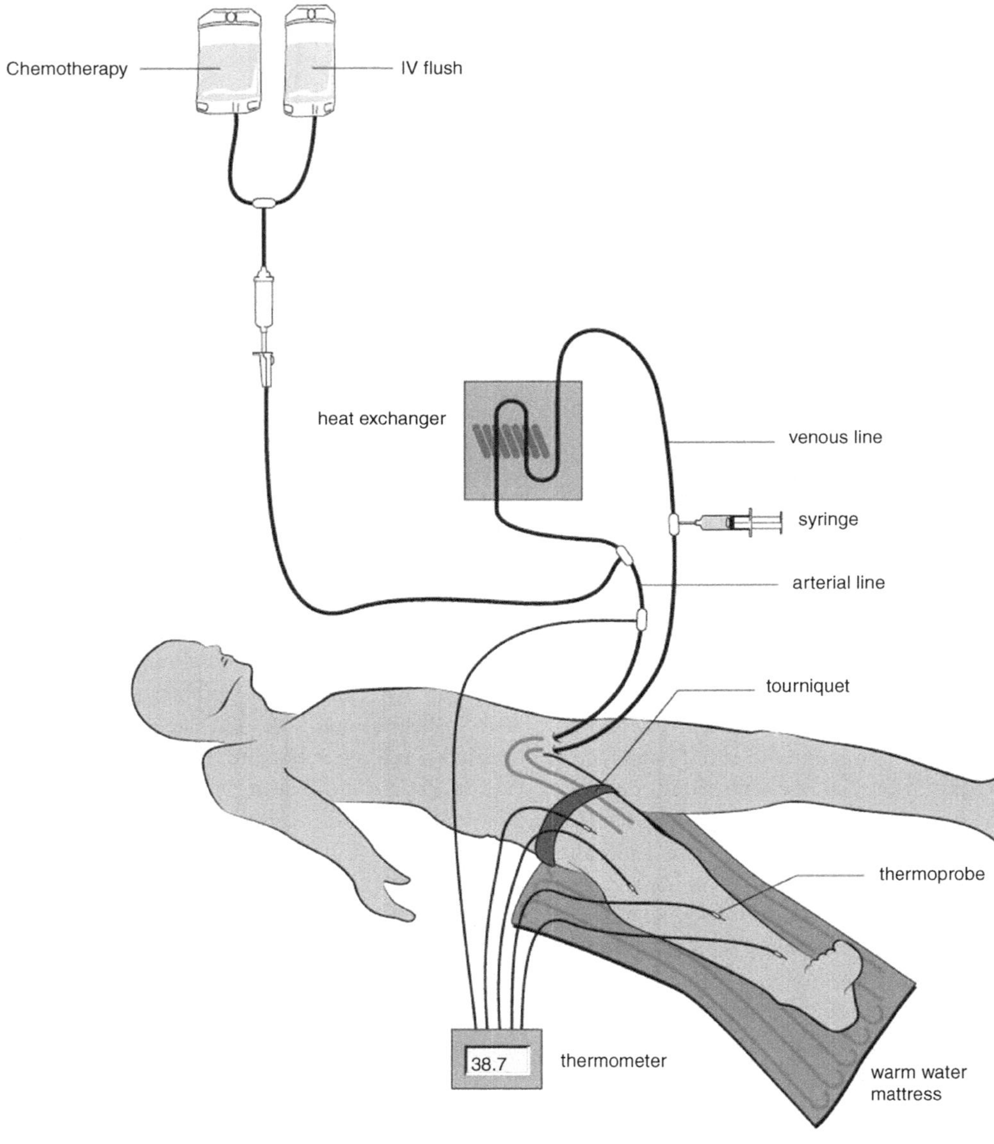

Fig. 27.1 Schematic illustration of the circuit used for isolated infusion of a lower limb

maintain limb temperature are employed, including an overhead radiant heater, placement of a hot-air blanket around the disease-bearing limb to form a cocoon, insulation of the circulation tubing, and incorporation of a blood-warming device in the extracorporeal vascular circuit (Fig. 27.2).

When in the operating room, the patient is given a general anesthetic, and heparin (3 mg/kg) is administered to achieve complete and full systemic heparinization. We then inject intra-arterial papaverine (30–60 mg) for optimal cutaneous vasodilatation, directly into the popliteal or brachial artery via the arterial catheter. This is done just prior to pneumatic tourniquet inflation around the proximal disease-bearing limb. If the foot or hand is not involved with tumor, it is excluded by wrapping an Esmarch bandage tightly around it, to prevent local toxicity.

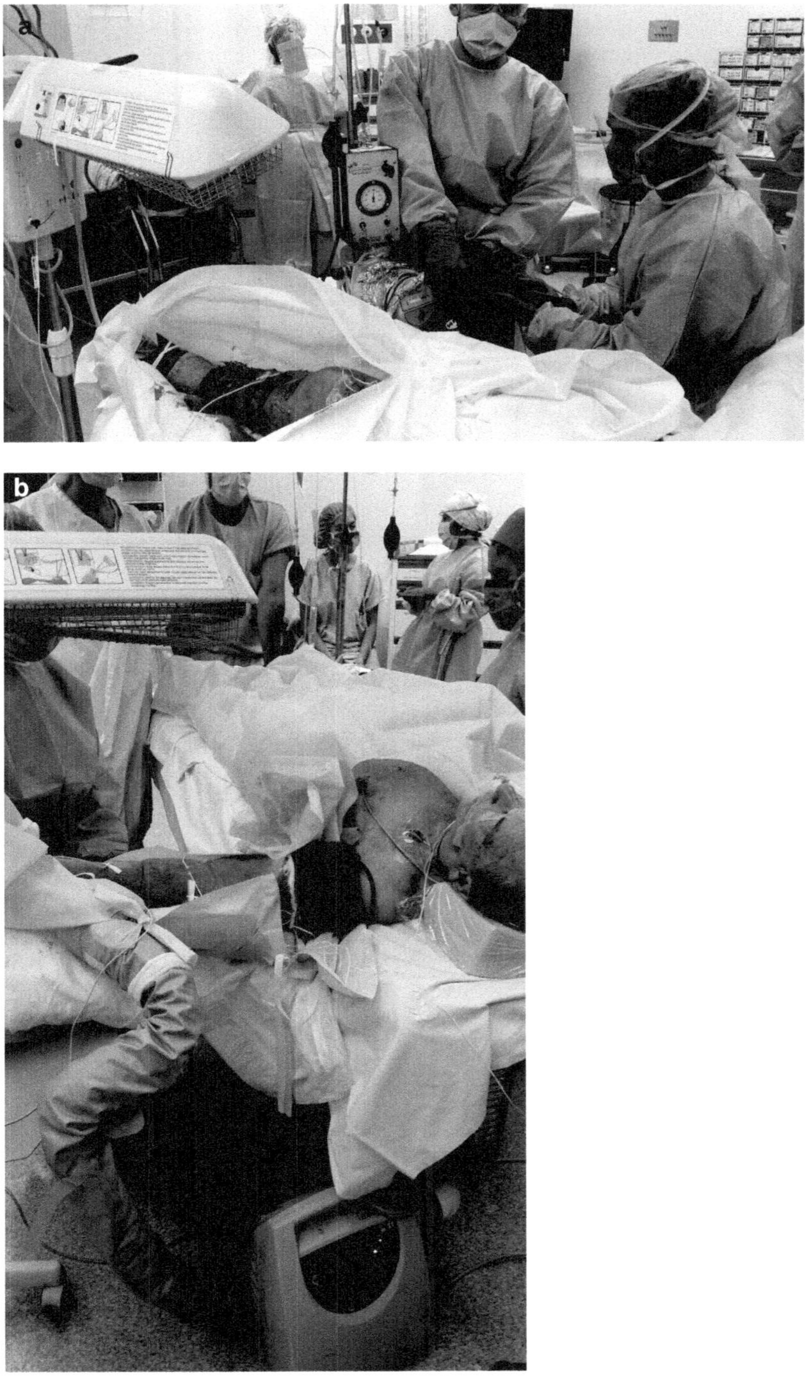

Fig. 27.2 (**a**) Photograph of a lower limb isolated limb infusion procedure. Note the Esmarch bandage around the foot to protect the acral (peripheral) region from developing postoperative toxicity. (**b**) Photograph of an upper limb isolated limb infusion procedure

To determine the appropriate drug dosage, the volume of limb tissue distal to the tourniquet and proximal to the Esmarch bandage (if used) is then calculated, based on preoperative volume measurements. These preoperative measurements, marked on the limb, assist the surgeon to calculate the volume of limb tissue that will be exposed to the infused drug/s. Preoperative limb volume measurements can be determined using several techniques. The simplest and most convenient is the water-displacement method, first described in antiquity by Archimedes, but employed for ILP by Wieberdink et al. [24]. Another method involves volume calculations based upon measurements of the patient's leg or arm circumference at 1.5 cm intervals up to the level of the tourniquet. This should encompass the entire region to be infused [25]. CT scan volumetric estimation can also be used [26].

Next, the cytotoxic drug solution is infused into the isolated limb via the arterial catheter. For the duration of the procedure (usually 30 min), the cytotoxic infusate is then circulated by repeated aspiration from the venous catheter and reinjection into the arterial catheter using a syringe attached to a three-way tap in the external circuit. Subcutaneous and intramuscular limb temperatures are monitored continuously during ILI, with blood samples from the isolated limb taken at regular intervals. This insures that the initial and subsequent cytotoxic drug concentrations, as well as the pH, O_2, and CO_2 levels are appropriate. These measurements are important to evaluate the increase in acidity and hypoxia of the isolated limb, as well as the uptake of the cytotoxic drugs into the tissues.

Melphalan is 1.5 times more potent in an acidotic environment, and up to three times more potent in an acidotic and hypoxic environment [27–30]. Drug leakage rates from the isolated limb into the systemic circulation are evaluated retrospectively by measurement of drug levels in systemic blood samples. Real-time intraoperative systemic leakage monitoring, as performed during ILP, is not necessary during ILI, since systemic leakage is invariably minimal [31]. Due to the low pressure of the circulating blood in the isolated limb circuit, influx of cytotoxic agent into the systemic circulation occurs only in a few patients at a very low concentration because of the much higher systemic blood pressure, and the efficiency of the pneumatic tourniquet. Great care is nevertheless required to ensure that the limb tourniquet is applied correctly to avoid leakage.

After 30 min of drug circulation in the limb, the procedure is terminated and the limb vasculature is flushed with 1 L of Hartmann's solution. Any residual heparin effect is reversed with intravenous (IV) protamine, after which the limb tourniquet is deflated to restore the normal limb circulation. Finally, the venous and arterial catheters are removed with pressure applied over vessel puncture sites. The risk of postoperative false aneurysm formation is reduced by routine use of an Angioseal™ device (St. Jude Medical, St. Paul, MN).

For patients with metastatic disease in the groin or axilla requiring both a regional lymph node dissection and an ILI, the dissection is undertaken immediately after the ILI, following heparin reversal, under the same general anesthetic. Postoperatively, limb toxicity and systemic toxicity are assessed clinically and biochemically each day, with serum creatinine kinase and lactate dehydrogenase levels acting as useful measures of muscle and tumor damage, typically peaking 3–4 days after ILI. The tumor response is assessed at regular intervals by noting the degree of regression, growth, or appearance of melanoma deposits. In some patients who achieve a CR following, this may not occur until 10–12 weeks after the procedure.

Drugs Used in Isolated Limb Infusion

The alkylating agent melphalan (L-PAM) remains the cytotoxic agent of choice for ILI procedures [16]. In most centers undertaking ILI, actinomycin-D is added to melphalan because good response rates are achieved without incurring increased toxicity [32, 33]. The normal melphalan dose that is administered for an ILI procedure is 7.5 mg/L of infused tissue, with a maximum dose of 100 mg for large limb volumes and a minimum dose of 15 mg for small limb volumes (usually upper limbs) [15]. The dose of actinomycin-D is usually 75 μg/L of infused tissue, with a maximum of 500 μg for larger limb volumes and a minimum of 200 μg for smaller limb volumes. Both drugs are mixed and infused in a warmed, heparinized normal saline solution. Infusion fluids containing albumin are not used because albumin binds melphalan, reducing melphalan uptake into the tissues by a factor of three [34].

The relationship between the infused melphalan dose in mg/L and outcome remains unclear [24, 32, 33]. Using a rat model, Roberts et al. demonstrated a dose-response effect where increasing the melphalan tissue concentration above a threshold of 25 μg/mL did not improve response rates. They did note that higher melphalan concentrations did cause more severe limb toxicity [35]. However, melphalan tissue concentrations in the limb during ILI vary between individual patients, making it challenging to estimate the correct dose for each patient. The factors determining the process of tissue uptake of melphalan are not yet fully understood [36, 37].

In an attempt to decrease toxicity without compromising outcome, Beasley et al. adjusted the melphalan dose according to ideal body weight (IBW) [37]. This adjustment was based on the observation that the strongest predictor of toxicity in patients undergoing conventional ILP was the ratio of estimated limb volume (Vesti) to steady-state limb drug volume of distribution (Vss). Hypothetically, patients with a weight greater than their IBW are likely to have a high Vesti/Vss ratio, since melphalan uptake is lower in fatty tissue as compared to muscle [38]. Beasley et al. reported that in their experience, dose adjustment according to IBW decreased the number of patients with grade III toxicity, but at the expense of a lower PR rate, while the CR rate was unchanged [37].

Although it might be argued that the achievement of a CR is clinically most important, any reduction in the PR rate due to the administration of a lower melphalan dose is still clinically relevant, since a PR following ILI greatly improves the quality of life in most patients. Moreover, in many cases a PR can be followed by systemic therapy, or other local therapies, to treat remaining lesions, including resection, CO_2-ablation, or intralesional injection of agents. Thus, ILI can serve as an induction therapy for achieving a disease-free limb [39].

A retrospective study conducted at the Melanoma Institute Australia to evaluate the results published by Beasley et al. could not replicate their outcomes. A correlation between larger limb volumes (and thus higher total melphalan doses) and toxicity was observed, but body mass index (BMI) was not correlated with toxicity [40]. Therefore, the effect of dose-adjustment according to IBW on limb toxicity and response rates remains uncertain. Clearly, more research is required to reduce toxicities of ILI and improve efficacy, focusing on optimizing melphalan (and other drug) effects in the individual patient.

Toxicity, Complications, and Side Effects Following Isolated Limb Infusion

ILI is generally a well-tolerated procedure. Typically, erythema and edema develop within 24 h. The skin overlying and surrounding tumor deposits often develops a dark gray hue at the time of ILI and then a ring of intense inflammation develops within 48 h [15]. Postoperatively, the daily serum creatine phosphokinase (CK) level reflects toxicity from damage to muscles and tissues. CK levels exceeding 1000 IU/L correlate with increased and potentially serious limb toxicity [33]. Therefore, patients with CK levels exceeding 1000 IU/L, or with clinically severe limb toxicity, can be treated with systemic corticosteroids (dexamethasone 4 mg IV every 6 h) until CK levels have fallen below this level and clinical signs of limb toxicity have subsided. Fasciotomy can be considered if signs of an impending compartment syndrome develop, but this is very rarely necessary [12, 33].

The peak limb toxicity is typically seen after 3–4 days, and patients are usually observed in the

Table 27.2 Systemic review of limb toxicity, assessed using the Wieberdink scale, following isolated limb infusion for melanoma with melphalan and actinomycin D [42]

Author, year	No. of patients	I (%)	II (%)	III (%)	IV (%)	V (%)
Mian et al. (2001) [62]	9	44	44	12	0	0
Kroon et al. (2008)	185	2	56	39	3	0
Marsden et al. (2008) [63]	13	0	46	38	16	0
Beasley et al. (2009) [13]	128	64	35[a]		1	0
Duprat Neto et al. (2014) [64]	31	0	40	50	10	0
Wong et al. (2013) [65]	79	80	20	20	0	0
Coventry et al. (2014) [66]	131	27	60	11	2	0
Total	576	33	46	19	2	0

[a]Beasley et al. and Wong et al. reported the combined toxicity for grades II and III

hospital until this peak has passed. Superficial desquamation of the skin from the infused limb often occurs after 2–3 weeks. Hair growth in the drug-exposed parts of the treated limb normally ceases for up to 3 months, and some residual pigmentation of the limb is common. If the foot or hand has not been excluded by an Esmarch bandage or pneumatic tourniquet, infused extremity toxicity can be appreciable with loss of the superficial layers of the epidermis of the sole and palm, leaving delicate and hypersensitive new skin exposed. Damaged plantar or palmar skin may take many weeks to regenerate and recover. Toenail or fingernail discoloration or loss can occur up to 3–4 months after the treatment. These effects are similar to those observed after conventional ILP [4].

The frequently used toxicity scale proposed by Wieberdink et al. for ILP is also applicable after ILI [24]. This scale grades regional limb toxicity as follows: No visible effect (grade I), slight erythema and/or edema (grade II), considerable erythema and/or edema with blistering (grade III), extensive epidermolysis and/or obvious damage to deep tissues with a threatened or actual compartment syndrome (grade IV), and severe tissue damage necessitating amputation (grade V). Alternatively, the "common terminology criteria for adverse events" version 3.0 (CTCAE v. 3.0) has been used to grade toxicity following ILI [41]. A systematic review showed that regional toxicity following ILI with melphalan and actinomycin-D was generally mild to moderate [42]. Slight erythema and edema was seen in 46% of patients (grade II toxicity) and was accompanied by blistering in 19% (grade III toxicity). In 2% of patients, clinical signs of an early compartment syndrome occurred (grade IV toxicity; Table 27.2). In those cases, a fasciotomy was indicated. Only one amputation due to severe regional toxicity (grade V toxicity) after ILI with melphalan and actinomycin-D has been reported.

The acute regional toxicity seen following ILI is similar to that following ILP. In large ILP series, 24% of patients experienced grade III toxicity or greater [6]. In ILI, however, grade III toxicity does not cause an increased hospital stay or greater long-term morbidity. In one study, the median hospital stay after ILI was 7 days. At 1 year, there were no symptoms of long-term morbidity in most patients, with only mild symptoms in the remainder, of which none were disabling [33].

Predictive factors for increased toxicity following ILI (Wieberdink grade III–IV) are: female gender, a high BMI, papaverine use, high peak and high final melphalan concentrations, a smaller rise in the CO_2 level in the infusate at the end of the ILI procedure, and a high peak CK level post-ILI [33, 41]. The increased toxicity for overweight patients might be explained by the fact that melphalan uptake in the skin and subcutaneous fat is lower compared to muscle and tumor, such that relatively higher concentrations and toxicity occur within muscle [38, 40].

As mentioned above, some centers adjust the drug dosage according to IBW in an attempt to decrease regional toxicity. The effect of this adjustment on the efficacy of ILI, however, remains unclear. An approach that has been used is to reduce the drug dose slightly (by an arbitrary 10%) when confronted with a large limb with an obviously high fat to muscle ratio. The advantage of the latter strategy is that patients with a high BMI, but without a fatty limb, receive the full, unadjusted melphalan dose. As yet, there are no formal studies that confirm or review the effect of this type of dose adjustment on toxicity or outcome.

Oncological Results of Isolated Limb Infusion for Melanoma

The primary goals of therapeutic ILI are to achieve a CR of limb disease and to avoid limb loss by amputation. Although a CR is optimal, achieving a PR or even stable disease (SD) can also substantially improve the patient's quality of life [42, 43].

Response Rates Following Isolated Limb Infusion

Since the introduction of ILI in the early 1990s, a multitude of studies reporting results following this procedure have been published [28, 42]. The range of reported response rates is wide, most likely due to the effects of small patient numbers and inclusion of "learning curve" results before mastery of the technique was achieved [12]. Furthermore, different institutions have used different protocols varying in small but potentially important ways [15]. A study performed at MIA showed that increased experience and small modifications that were made to the ILI protocol over a 14-year period resulted in a progressively improved effect on outcome [44].

Another possible explanation for the widely ranging results is that the response to the procedure is not assessed similarly in all studies [15, 25, 42]. Some tumor involution can usually be seen as soon as 7 days after the procedure. However, complete disappearance of tumor nodules may take weeks or even several months. Therefore, considerable time must elapse before the final response is determined. Some have assessed and reported the response exactly 3 months after ILI, while others have reported the outcome according to the World Health Organization (WHO) handbook for reporting results of cancer treatments, allowing a larger time window to detect the best identified response [45]. The WHO criteria define CR as the disappearance of all measurable disease, determined by two observations <4 weeks apart, and a PR as ≥50% decrease in total tumor size determined by two observations <4 weeks apart and no appearance of new lesions or progression of any lesion.

The results of the seven largest ILI studies using melphalan and actinomycin D to treat limb melanoma were combined and examined in a systematic review [42]. In this review of 576 patients, 33% experienced a CR and 40% a PR, with SD seen in 14% and progressive disease (PD) in 13%. Individual study results included in this systematic review are listed in Table 27.3. Overall, the results of ILI appear to be at the lower end of the spectrum of those reported after

Table 27.3 Systematic review of response rates following isolated limb infusion for melanoma with melphalan and actinomycin D [42]

Author, year	No. of patients	Response criteria	CR (%)	PR (%)	SD (%)	PD (%)
Mian et al. (2001)	9	Best response	44	56	0	0
Kroon et al. (2008)	185	Best response	38	46	10	6
Marsden et al. (2008)	13	Unknown	31	53	0	16
Beasley et al. (2009)	128	3 months	31	33	7	29
Duprat Neto et al. (2014)	31	Best response	26	53	21	0
Wong et al. (2013)	79	3 months	37	37	8	18
Coventry et al. (2014)	131	Best response	27	36	29	8
Total	576		33	40	14	13

CR complete response, *PR* partial response, *SD* stable disease, *PD* progressive disease

ILP. ILI, however, is often performed in considerably older and medically more compromised patients, in those who suffer from a higher stage of disease and in patients with a higher tumor burden at the time of treatment, sometimes even in a palliative setting in patients with Stage IV disease. All of these factors have been shown to be prognostic factors for an inferior response in some studies [12, 13, 19, 22, 32, 46]. The fact that the patient populations and tumor stage in ILI and ILP melanoma studies differ so substantially makes a simple comparison unreliable [47].

Disease-Free Survival and Overall Survival After Isolated Limb Infusion

Not all reports have included disease-free survival (DFS) rates following ILI. Patients treated at MIA who had a CR following ILI had a median DFS of 22 months and those with a PR had a median DFS of 9 months ($P = 0.012$) [32]. Beasley et al. reported a median DFS of 12 months following a CR [13]. Overall survival (OS) rates following ILI also vary widely, but can be substantial. In 2008, Kroon et al. reported a median OS after a CR of 53 months for patients treated at MIA [32]. More recently, Coventry et al. published results from a multicenter study and reported a median OS following a CR of 101 months [48]. In 2011, Raymond et al. reported that patients treated in the period 1995–2010 at Duke Medical Center had a median OS of 31 months after a CR [49]. These three studies all reported a less favorable OS for patients after a PR (range 27–41 months) and an even lower OS (range 13–33 months) for patients with SD or PD following ILI.

In a study conducted by Kroon et al., tumor infiltration beneath the deep fascia was associated with shorter OS compared to cutaneous or subcutaneous tumor growth only ($P = 0.029$) [32]. Other patient-related prognostic factors for longer OS were a thinner primary melanoma ($P = 0.038$), a lower number of melanoma nodules ($P = 0.010$), and a greater BMI ($P = 0.002$). The positive prognostic value of a higher BMI can be explained by the higher proportion of subcutaneous fat to muscle in these patients which, as already described, leads to a relatively higher melphalan concentration within the isolated limb skin and muscle compartments when standard drug dosages are used [38, 40]. The prognostic value of BMI for both increased toxicity and improved OS reveals the delicate balance between administering the highest tolerable melphalan dose for achieving an optimal response without incurring greater toxicity.

Elderly Patients

A multicenter Australian study examined the response rates following ILI for 148 elderly patients compared to 168 younger (<75 years) patients, and showed that ILI in elderly patients was effective and safe [18]. Older patients experienced less limb toxicity compared with younger patients (grade III/IV toxicity in 22% and 37%, respectively; $P = 0.003$). A CR was seen in 27% of patients ≥75 years and in 38% of patients <75 years ($P = 0.06$), while overall response (CR + PR) rates were 72% and 77%, respectively ($P = 0.30$). No difference in OS was seen, with a median follow-up of 40 months for both groups ($P = 0.69$).

Repeat Isolated Limb Infusion

At MIA, 48 patients received a repeat ILI after either progression or recurrence of disease following an initial ILI procedure [50]. The median interval between the two treatments was 11 months. Interestingly, the CR and OR rates obtained after the repeat procedures (23% and 83%, respectively) were not significantly different from the CR and OR rates obtained after the first ILI (35%; $P = 0.358$ and 75%; $P = 0.315$, respectively). There was a statistical difference, however, in the median duration of response, which was 6 months after the first ILI compared to 10 months after the repeat ILI treatment ($P = 0.014$). Toxicity was significantly increased following the second ILI, with five Wieberdink grade IV events occurring compared to only one grade IV toxicity after the initial ILI ($P = 0.027$). Despite the higher limb toxicity, a repeat ILI procedure can be of great value and should be considered if limb disease progresses, recurs, or fails to respond after an initial ILI.

Resection of Residual Disease After Isolated Limb Infusion

If a patient has a PR or SD following an ILI, surgical resection of residual disease, if possible, can be beneficial for OS and DFS, providing OS rates comparable to that of patients who have a CR after an ILI. A multi-institutional study compared 22 patients who underwent ILI plus surgical resection of residual disease (ILIRES), with patients who had a CR following ILI [39]. ILIRES patients had a similar OS (in the ILIRES group median OS not reached vs. 30.9 months; $P = 0.304$) and similar DFS (12.4 vs. 9.6 months; $P = 0.978$) compared with patients who had an ILI only. It must be borne in mind, however, that these results are only achievable in selected patients whose disease and limb is suitable for resection after ILI.

Upper Versus Lower Limb Isolated Limb Infusion

A multicenter study conducted in the USA compared upper and lower limb ILI [51]. Upper limb ILI was associated with lower regional toxicity compared to lower limb ILI (7% vs. 24% grade >3; $P = 0.005$), but no difference in CR rate was observed (28% vs. 32%). The blood gas analysis of the perfusate revealed that the mean base excess at 30 min (−13.9 vs. −9.1; $P < 0.001$) and the mean pH at 30 min (7.06 vs. 7.15; $P < 0.001$) were lower for upper limb compared to lower limb procedures. However, the mean ischemic time was longer in lower limb procedures (67.2 min) than in upper limb procedures (61.6 min; $P = 0.03$). From this study, it can be concluded that upper limb ILI has different physiologic sequelae despite the procedure being fundamentally similar to lower limb ILI. The upper limb appears to be relatively resistant to the toxic effects of the cytotoxic drugs used in ILI, which suggests the potential for further optimization of drug dosing for upper limb ILIs.

Patients with Distant Metastatic Disease

In the treatment of patients with symptomatic advanced limb melanoma, a major dilemma arises when systemic metastases are also present. ILI can be of palliative value in this select group of patients. At MIA, 37 patients had advanced symptomatic limb disease as well as distant melanoma metastases at the time of their ILI [22]. The OR was 76% (CR 22%; PR 54%) and DFS in the limb was 11 months. Limb salvage was achieved in 86% of these patients. Median OS was 22 months after a CR, 17 months after PR, and 4 months for those with SD or PD following ILI ($P = 0.002$). These OS rates were most likely a reflection of tumor biology. Since the introduction of more effective systemic therapies for melanoma, a potentially interesting approach for patients with systemic disease as well as symptomatic limb melanoma might be the combination of ILI with systemic treatment. This possible approach is discussed next.

Future Role of Isolated Limb Infusion in Melanoma Management

The simplicity and minimally invasive nature of the ILI procedure make this technique a useful model for testing new or alternative drugs and drug combinations, and for testing combinations of regional and systemic approaches for metastatic melanoma.

Isolated Limb Infusion with New Drugs and Drug Combinations

Temozolomide (TMZ) as an oral agent is believed to offer some clinical benefit to patients with systemic melanoma metastases, and the development of an intravenous formulation of the drug has generated considerable interest [52]. A USA-based multicenter, phase I clinical trial of ILI using intravenous TMZ showed limited toxicity, with efficacy even in some cases where melphalan had failed [53].

Isolated Limb Infusion in Combination with Systemic Therapies

With the use of new immune therapies, in addition to local therapies such as radiation therapy, injectable agents (rose bengal, viral agents, interleukins), and ablative therapies (cryotherapy, radiofrequency ablation), it is increasingly being appreciated that these combination therapies are capable of enhancing immune responses against melanoma [54, 55]. As a result, many potentially useful new treatment combinations are being considered, including ILI.

After a PR, or when new or recurrent lesions appear following ILI, simple local treatment of the remaining or recurrent lesions by excision (as indicated earlier), laser ablation, injection with agents such as rose bengal, viral agents, interleukin-2, or radiotherapy can be effective in controlling local cutaneous or subcutaneous disease [39, 54, 56]. Another approach that has been shown to be effective is the combination of ILI with doxorubicin plus external beam radiotherapy to obtain local disease control, making limb-sparing surgery feasible. Using this approach, a limb salvage rate of 82.5% was reported [57].

Until recently, response rates to systemic therapies for patients with metastatic melanoma were poor, with a median OS of 6–9 months [58]. Fortunately, this situation has changed dramatically in recent times, with the introduction of BRAF/MEK/KIT inhibitors, anti-cytotoxic T-cell leukocyte antigen-4 (CTLA-4) antibodies, and anti-programmed cell death receptor-1 (PD-1) pathway inhibitors [47, 59]. Although the majority of patients who entered clinical trials of these new therapies had stage IV disease, most protocols also allowed patients with unresectable stage III disease. Patients with localized in-transit metastases eligible for ILI, by definition, have unresectable AJCC stage IIIA/B disease and, therefore, trial results could potentially be extrapolated to this subset of patients.

However, this must be done with great caution because, to date, no randomized trial has been reported comparing ILI to systemic treatment. Although the response rates of the new agents are impressive, it is noteworthy that these are substantially lower than those achieved with ILI in patients with extensive limb disease [47]. Furthermore, ILI does not cause any systemic toxicity. However, the combination of two different methods of drug delivery could have great potential when systemic targeted therapies are administered in combination with regional chemotherapy by ILI. In addition, chemotherapy resistance to agents used for ILI might potentially be overcome by combining ILI with systemically administered immunological agents to increase clinical responses.

An interesting strategy in this regard has been described in a phase II study designed to test whether the systemic anti-vascular agent, alcohol dehydrogenase-1 (ADH-1), enhances the response following ILI with melphalan. In this study, an OR of 60% was achieved without increasing toxicity, compared with an OR of 40% achieved when melphalan alone was used at the same institution [60].

In a preclinical melanoma model, improved responses have also been observed when melphalan ILI was performed after systemic bevacizumab, a monoclonal antibody against vascular endothelial growth factor receptor (VEGF), theoretically expected to increase the entry of melphalan into tumor cells [61]. A clinical trial administering bevacizumab in combination with melphalan ILI is anticipated. Finally, the use of the systemic anti-CTLA-4 antibody ipilimumab, before or after melphalan ILI, is currently being investigated in phase I and II trials (NCT01323517, NCT02115243).

Conclusions

ILI is a safe, relatively simple and lower cost, minimally invasive alternative to conventional ILP. It results in satisfactory response rates and durations of response in patients with unresectable limb melanoma and avoids the need for amputation of the affected limb in most cases. The responses are obtained at a cost of mild to moderate regional toxicity, but systemic toxicity is avoided.

The ILI procedure is especially useful in elderly patients, patients with multiple comorbidities, and those with extensive limb disease. Although response rates may seem lower when compared to those achieved following ILP, it is important to remember that due to the higher tumor load and larger number of elderly and medically compromised patients included in ILI studies, the likelihood of a favorable response is lower. For this reason, results following ILP cannot simply be directly compared to results following ILI, as the patient populations in these studies are quite different. It is unlikely that a randomized trial directly comparing ILI and ILP will ever be conducted.

ILI provides an excellent model for testing new drugs, and new treatment regimens. Responses following ILI with melphalan (with or without actinomycin D) are still superior to those achieved by current systemic therapies, but response rates are likely to be improved further by combining ILI with other treatment modalities. Various strategies are currently being considered and investigated combining ILI with other local, regional, and systemic therapies.

References

1. Creech O Jr, Krementz ET, Ryan RF, Winblad JN. Chemotherapy of cancer: regional perfusion utilizing an extracorporeal circuit. Ann Surg. 1958;148:616–32.
2. Vrouenraets BC, Nieweg OE, Kroon BB. Thirty-five years of isolated limb perfusion for melanoma: indications and results. Br J Surg. 1996;83:1319–28.
3. Schraffordt Koops H, Lejeune FJ, Kroon BBR, Klaase JM, Hoekstra HJ. Isolated limb perfusion for melanoma: technical aspects. In: Thompson JF, Morton DL, Kroon BBR, editors. Textbook of melanoma. London: Martin Dunitz; 2004. p. 404–9.
4. Sanki A, Kroon HM, Kam PCA, Thompson JF. Isolated limb perfusion and isolated limb infusion for malignant lesions of the extremities. Curr Probl Surg. 2011;48:371–430.
5. Noorda EM, Vrouenraets BC, Nieweg OE, Van Coevorden F, Kroon BB. Isolated limb perfusion: what is the evidence for its use? Ann Surg Oncol. 2004;11:837–45.
6. Moreno-Ramirez D, de la Cruz-Merino L, Ferrandiz L, et al. Isolated limb perfusion for malignant melanoma: systematic review on effectiveness and safety. Oncologist. 2010;15:416–27.
7. Karakousis CP, Kanter PM, Lopez R, Moore R, Holyoke ED. Modes of regional chemotherapy. J Surg Res. 1979;26:134–41.
8. Bland KI, Kimura AK, Brenner DE, et al. A phase II study of the efficacy of diamminedichloroplatinum (cisplatin) for the control of locally recurrent and intransit malignant melanoma of the extremities using tourniquet outflow-occlusion techniques. Ann Surg. 1989;209:73–80.
9. Karakousis CP, Kanter PM, Park HC, Sharma SD, Moore R, Ewing JH. Tourniquet infusion versus hyperthermic perfusion. Cancer. 1982;49:850–8.
10. Thompson JF, Waugh RC, Saw RP, Kam PC. Isolated limb infusion with melphalan for recurrent limb melanoma: a simple alternative to isolated limb perfusion. Reg Cancer Treat. 1994;7:188–92.
11. Thompson JF, Kam PC, Waugh RC, Harman CR. Isolated limb infusion with cytotoxic agents: a simple alternative to isolated limb perfusion. Semin Surg Oncol. 1998;14:238–47.
12. Kroon HM, Coventry BJ, Giles MH, et al. Australian multi-center study of isolated limb infusion for melanoma. Ann Surg Oncol. 2016;23:1096–103.
13. Beasley GM, Caudle A, Petersen RP, et al. A multi-institutional experience of isolated limb infusion: defining response and toxicity in the US. J Am Coll Surg. 2009;208:706–15.
14. Cecchini S, Sarti D, Ricci S, et al. Isolated limb infusion chemotherapy with or without hemofiltration for recurrent limb melanoma. World J Clin Oncol. 2015;6:57–63.
15. Kroon HM, Huismans AM, Kam PCA, Thompson JF. Isolated limb infusion: technical aspects. J Surg Oncol. 2014;109:352–6.
16. Beasley G, Kroon HM, Ross M, Kam PCA, Thompson JF, Tyler D. Isolated limb infusion for melanoma (Chapter 27). In: Balch C, Houghton AN, Sober AJ, Soong SJ, Atkins MB, Thompson FJ, editors. Cutaneous melanoma. 5th ed. St. Louis, MO: Quality Medical Publishing Inc.; 2009. p. 541–60. ISBN: 978-1-57626-276-4.
17. Koops HS, Vaglini M, Suciu S, et al. Prophylactic isolated limb perfusion for localized, high-risk limb melanoma: results of a multicenter randomized phase III trial. EORTC Malignant Melanoma Cooperative Group Protocol 18832, the World Health Organization Melanoma Program Trial 15, and the North American Perfusion Group Southwest Oncology Group-8593. J Clin Oncol. 1998;16:2906–12.

18. Kroon HM, Coventry BJ, Giles MH, Henderson MA, Speakman D, Wall M, Barbour A, Serpell J, Paddle P, Smithers BM, Thompson JF. Safety and efficacy of isolated limb infusion chemotherapy for advanced locoregional melanoma in elderly patients: an Australian multicenter study. Ann Surg Oncol. 2017;24:3245–51.
19. Kroon HM, Lin DY, Kam PC, Thompson JF. Safety and efficacy of isolated limb infusion with cytotoxic drugs in elderly patients with advanced locoregional melanoma. Ann Surg. 2009;246:1008–13.
20. Madu MF, Deken MM, van der Hage JA, Jóźwiak K, Wouters MW, van Akkooi AC. Isolated limb perfusion for melanoma is safe and effective in elderly patients. Ann Surg Oncol. 2017;24:1997–2005.
21. Noorda EM, Vrouenraets BC, Nieweg OE, et al. Safety and efficacy of isolated limb perfusion in elderly melanoma patients. Ann Surg Oncol. 2002;9:968–74.
22. Kroon HM, Lin DY, Kam PC, Thompson JF. Isolated limb infusion as palliative treatment for advanced limb disease in patients with AJCC stage IV melanoma. Ann Surg Oncol. 2009;16:1193–201.
23. Takkenberg RB, Vrouenraets BC, van Geel AN, et al. Palliative isolated limb perfusion for advanced limb disease in stage IV melanoma patients. J Surg Oncol. 2005;91:107–11.
24. Wieberdink J, Benckhuysen C, Braat RP, et al. Dosimetry in isolation perfusion of the limbs by assessment of perfused tissue volume and grading of toxic tissue reactions. Eur J Cancer Clin Oncol. 1982;18:905–10.
25. Beasley GM, Petersen RP, Yoo J, et al. Isolated limb infusion for in-transit malignant melanoma of the extremity: a well-tolerated but less effective alternative to hyperthermic isolated limb perfusion. Ann Surg Oncol. 2008;15:2195–205.
26. Brys AK, Bhatti L, Bashir MR, et al. Computed tomography based limb volume measurements for isolated limb infusion in melanoma. Ann Surg Oncol. 2016;23:1090–5.
27. Siemann DW, Chapman M, Beikirch A. Effects of oxygenation and pH on tumor cell response to alkylating chemotherapy. Int J Radiat Oncol Biol Phys. 1991;20:287–9.
28. Kroon HM, Thompson JF. Isolated limb infusion: a review. J Surg Oncol. 2009;100:169–77.
29. Thompson JF, Ramzan I, Kam PCA, Yau DF. Pharmacokinetics of melphalan during isolated limb infusion for melanoma. Reg Cancer Treat. 1996;9:13–6.
30. Skarsgard LD, Skwarchuk MW, Vinczan A, Kristl J, Chaplin DJ. The cytotoxicity of melphalan and its relationship to pH, hypoxia and drug uptake. Anticancer Res. 1995;15:219–23.
31. Lindner P, Doubrovsky A, Kam PCA, et al. Prognostic factors after isolated limb infusion with cytotoxic agents for melanoma. Ann Surg Oncol. 2002;9:127–36.
32. Kroon HM, Moncrieff M, Kam PC, et al. Outcomes following isolated limb infusion. A 14-year experience. Ann Surg Oncol. 2008;15:3003–13.
33. Kroon HM, Moncrieff M, Kam PC, Thompson JF. Factors predictive of acute regional toxicity after isolated limb infusion with melphalan and actinomycin D in melanoma patients. Ann Surg Oncol. 2009;16:1184–92.
34. Wu ZY, Smithers BM, Parsons PG, Roberts MS. The effects of perfusion conditions on melphalan distribution in the isolated perfused rat hindlimb bearing a human melanoma xenograft. Br J Cancer. 1997;75:1160–6.
35. Roberts MS, Wu ZY, Siebert GA, Thompson JF, Smithers BM. Saturable dose-response relationships for melphalan in melanoma treatment by isolated limb infusion in the nude rat. Melanoma Res. 2001;11:611–8.
36. Cheng TY, Grubbs E, Abdul-Wahab O, et al. Marked variability of melphalan plasma drug levels during regional hyperthermic isolated limb perfusion. Am J Surg. 2003;186:460–7.
37. McMahon N, Cheng TY, Beasley GM, et al. Optimizing melphalan pharmacokinetics in regional melanoma therapy: does correcting for ideal body weight alter regional response or toxicity? Ann Surg Oncol. 2009;16:953–61.
38. Klaase JM, Kroon BB, Beijnen JH, van Slooten GW, van Dongen JA. Melphalan tissue concentrations in patients treated with regional isolated perfusion for melanoma of the lower limb. Br J Cancer. 1994;70:151–3.
39. Wong J, Chen YA, Fisher KJ, Beasley GM, Tyler DS, Zager JS. Resection of residual disease after isolated limb infusion (ILI) is equivalent to a complete response after ILI-alone in advanced extremity melanoma. Ann Surg Oncol. 2014;21:650–5.
40. Huismans AM, Kroon HM, Haydu LE, Kam PC, Thompson JF. Is melphalan dose adjustment according to ideal body weight useful in isolated limb infusion for melanoma? Ann Surg Oncol. 2012;19:3050–6.
41. Santillan AA, Delman KA, Beasley GM, et al. Predictive factors of regional toxicity and serum creatine phosphokinase levels after isolated limb infusion for melanoma: a multi-institutional analysis. Ann Surg Oncol. 2009;16:2570–8.
42. Kroon HM, Huismans AM, Kam PC, Thompson JF. Isolated limb infusion with melphalan and actinomycin D for melanoma: a systematic review. J Surg Oncol. 2014;109:348–51.
43. Jiang BS, Speicher PJ, Thomas S, Mosca PJ, Abernethy AP, Tyler DS. Quality of life after isolated limb infusion for in-transit melanoma of the extremity. Ann Surg Oncol. 2015;22:1694–700.
44. Huismans AM, Kroon HM, Kam PC, Thompson JF. Does increased experience with isolated limb infusion for advanced limb melanoma influence outcome? A comparison of two treatment periods at a single institution. Ann Surg Oncol. 2011;18:1877–83.
45. World Health Organization. WHO handbook for reporting results of cancer treatments (WHO offset publication no. 48). Geneva: World Health Organization; 1979.

46. Barbour AP, Thomas J, Suffolk J, et al. Isolated limb infusion for malignant melanoma: predictors of response and outcome. Ann Surg Oncol. 2009;16:3463–72.
47. Grünhagen DJ, Kroon HM, Verhoef C. Perfusion and infusion for melanoma in-transit metastases in the era of effective systemic therapy. Am Soc Clin Oncol Educ Book. 2015;35:e528–34.
48. Coventry BJ, Kroon HM, Giles MH, et al. Australian multi-center experience outside of the Sydney Melanoma Unit of isolated limb infusion chemotherapy for melanoma. J Surg Oncol. 2014;109:780–5.
49. Raymond AK, Beasley GM, Broadwater G, et al. Current trends in regional therapy for melanoma: lessons learned from 225 regional chemotherapy treatments between 1995 and 2010 at a single institution. J Am Coll Surg. 2011;213:306–16.
50. Kroon HM, Lin DY, Kam PC, Thompson JF. Efficacy of repeat isolated limb infusion with melphalan and actinomycin D for recurrent melanoma. Cancer. 2009;115:1932–40.
51. Beasley GM, Sharma K, Wong J, Miller M, Turley RS, Lidsky M, Masoud M, Dewhirst MW, Mosca PJ, Zager JS, Tyler DS. A multi-institution experience comparing the clinical and physiologic differences between upper extremity and lower extremity melphalan-based isolated limb infusion. Cancer. 2012;118:6136–43.
52. Ueno T, Ko SH, Grubbs E, et al. Modulation of chemotherapy resistance in regional therapy: a novel therapeutic approach to advanced extremity melanoma using intra-arterial temozolomide in combination with systemic O6-benzylguanine. Mol Cancer Ther. 2006;5:732–8.
53. Beasley GM, Speicher P, Augustine CK, et al. A multicenter phase I dose escalation trial to evaluate safety and tolerability of intra-arterial temozolomide for patients with advanced extremity melanoma using normothermic isolated limb infusion. Ann Surg Oncol. 2015;22:287–94.
54. Testori A, Faries MB, Thompson JF, et al. Local and intralesional therapy of in-transit melanoma metastases. J Surg Oncol. 2011;104:391–6.
55. Thompson JF, Agarwala SS, Smithers BM, et al. Phase 2 study of intralesional PV-10 in refractory metastatic melanoma. Ann Surg Oncol. 2015;22:2135–42.
56. Feldman AL, Alexander HR Jr, Bartlett DL, Fraker DL, Libutti SK. Management of extremity recurrences after complete responses to isolated limb perfusion in patients with melanoma. Ann Surg Oncol. 1999;6:562–7.
57. Hegazy MA, Kotb SZ, Sakr H, et al. Preoperative isolated limb infusion of doxorubicin and external irradiation for limb-threatening soft tissue sarcomas. Ann Surg Oncol. 2007;14:568–76.
58. Menzies AM, Long GV. Recent advances in melanoma systemic therapy. BRAF inhibitors, CTLA4 antibodies and beyond. Eur J Cancer. 2013;49:3229–41.
59. Menzies AM, Long GV. Recent developments in melanoma therapy. JAMA Oncol. 2016;2:1259–60.
60. Beasley GM, Riboh JC, Augustine CK, et al. Prospective multicenter phase II trial of systemic ADH-1 in combination with melphalan via isolated limb infusion in patients with advanced extremity melanoma. J Clin Oncol. 2011;29:1210–5.
61. Turley RS, Fontanella AN, Padussis JC, et al. Bevacizumab-induced alterations in vascular permeability and drug delivery: a novel approach to augment regional chemotherapy for in-transit melanoma. Clin Cancer Res. 2012;18:3328–39.
62. Mian R, Henderson MA, Speakman D, et al. Isolated limb infusion for melanoma: a simple alternative to isolated limb perfusion. Can J Surg. 2001;44:189–92.
63. Marsden J, Samarasinghe V, Duddy M, et al. Regional chemotherapy for inoperable limb cancer using isolated limb infusion. Br J Dermatol. 2008;159:10.
64. Duprat Neto JP, Mauro AC, Molina AS, et al. Isolated limb infusion with hyperthermia and chemotherapy for advanced malignancy: factors influencing toxicity. ANZ J Surg. 2014;84:677–82.
65. Wong J, Chen YA, Fisher KJ, et al. Isolated limb infusion in a series of over 100 infusions: a single-center experience. Ann Surg Oncol. 2013;20:1121–7.
66. Coventry BJ, Kroon HM, Giles MH, Henderson M, Speakman D, Wall M, Barbour A, Serpell J, Paddle P, Coventry AG, Sullivan T, Smithers BM. Multi-center experience outside of the Sydney Melanoma Unit of isolated limb infusion chemotherapy for melanoma. J Surg Oncol. 2014;109:780–5.

Surgery for Stage IV Metastatic Melanoma

28

David W. Ollila, Shachar Laks, and Eddy C. Hsueh

Introduction

The wise academic surgeon knows that the true sign of a mature, academic career is that your own publications serve as fodder for a point-counterpoint debate, with your latest manuscripts directly contradicting some of your earlier publications. Often, such drastic change in our thinking is a direct result of the data that it put forth in favor of a new or different approach. This chapter represents such a change for the two senior authors (DWO, ECH) from a staunch metastasectomy-first approach, which prevailed prior to 2011, to embracing the efficacious new drug therapies. In a relatively short time span (2011–2015), we have seven new Food and Drug Administration (FDA) approved drugs for advanced-stage metastatic melanoma patients [1–7].

The backdrop of improved overall survival in stage IV metastatic melanoma with the new agents needs to be balanced by the surgical literature that strongly suggests that complete metastasectomy also improves overall survival. Following complete resection of distant metastases, stage IV melanoma patients had a prolonged overall survival in several series [8–10]. It has also been observed that repeat metastasectomy of recurrent distant metastatic melanoma can prolong survival [11, 12].

This chapter will review the FDA-approved systemic therapy options, discuss the data for site-specific metastasectomy, critique the previous and current trials examining the role of metastasectomy, and discuss the concept of neoadjuvant therapy. We will also present our view for moving forward together as a team of systemic and locoregional therapists.

D. W. Ollila, M.D. (✉) · S. Laks, M.D.
Department of Surgery, University of North Carolina at Chapel Hill, Chapel Hill, NC, USA
e-mail: david_ollila@med.unc.edu; shachar.laks@unchealth.unc.edu

E. C. Hsueh, M.D.
Department of Surgery, Saint Louis University, St. Louis, MO, USA
e-mail: hsuehec@slu.edu

Systemic Therapy Options

Recent rapid succession of breakthroughs in melanoma therapy has dramatically changed the treatment paradigm for metastatic melanoma since 2011. The FDA approved ipilimumab, a cytotoxic T-lymphocyte 4 (CTLA-4) inhibitor, based on the results of a three-arm randomized phase III trial comparing a gp100 vaccine alone, ipilimumab alone, and the combination of vaccine with ipilimumab in 2011 [1]. Subsequently, vemurafenib, a BRAF inhibitor, was approved in the same year for patients with metastatic melanoma harboring a BRAF gene mutation [4, 13]. In 2013, the combination of a BRAF inhibitor, dabrafenib, and a MEK inhibitor, trametinib, was approved for BRAF mutation-positive metastatic

A. I. Riker (ed.), *Melanoma*, https://doi.org/10.1007/978-3-319-78310-9_28

melanoma patients [14]. Approval of two inhibitors of the programmed death 1 (PD-1) receptor, pembrolizumab and nivolumab, were granted in 2014 [15, 16]. Finally, in late 2015, talimogene laherparepvec (T-VEC), a modified herpes simplex virus type-1 was approved by the FDA for unresectable stage IIIB–IV melanoma patients [7]. In total, seven new drugs were granted FDA approval for metastatic melanoma in a 5-year time span.

Targeted Therapy

Mutations in the serine-threonine kinase BRAF were observed in ~50% of metastatic melanoma lesions, mostly of the valine to glutamine substitution in codon 600 (V600E) [17]. Vemurafenib and dabrafenib are the currently FDA-approved BRAF inhibitors that target these mutations for the treatment of melanoma. BRAF inhibitors have shown high rates of response (48–59%) in phase II and III trials, but with limited duration [4, 5, 13]. The lack of durability of response is due to the development of melanoma cell resistance mechanisms. Thus, clinical trials examined the combined treatment with BRAF and MEK inhibitors, hypothesizing that this may circumvent or attenuate the development of resistance by blocking the reactivation of the MAPK pathway induced by single-agent BRAF inhibitors [18, 19].

Combination of BRAF/MEK inhibition with dabrafenib (BRAF inhibitor) and trametinib (MEK inhibitor) was evaluated in a phase III study (COMBI-d) for previously untreated and unresectable stage IIIC or stage IV melanoma patients with BRAF V600E or V600K mutation randomizing patients to the combination of dabrafenib and trametinib or dabrafenib and placebo [20]. The median PFS was 9.3 months in combination group and 8.8 months in dabrafenib-only group (HR 0.75; $p = 0.03$). In a second phase III trial, combination of dabrafenib and trametinib were compared with vemurafenib orally as first-line therapy (COMBI-v) [21]. The combination also improved OS, PFS, and overall response rates (ORR) compared with the vemurafenib alone group. In the phase III coBRIM trial, patients with treatment-naïve BRAF V600 mutation-positive melanoma were randomized to receive vemurafenib and cobimetinib versus vemurafenib and placebo [22]. Median PFS was 9.9 months in the combination group and 6.2 months in the control group (HR 0.51; $p < 0.001$). The ORR was 68% in the combination group as compared with 45% in the control group ($p < 0.001$).

Checkpoint Inhibitors

In 2010, a major breakthrough in targeted immune therapy in melanoma occurred when Hodi et al. [1] published their phase III, prospective randomized trial of ipilimumab, a monoclonal antibody to the cytotoxic T-lymphocyte-associated antigen-4 (CTLA-4), in previously treated unresectable stage III or IV melanoma. Ipilimumab exerts its effect by binding and inactivating the CTLA-4 receptor, whose normal function is to promote immune tolerance. Thus, when bound, ipilimumab stimulates an antitumor T-cell mediated immune response. In this pivotal phase III trial, the patients treated with ipilimumab showed an improved median overall survival compared to peptide vaccine (10.1 vs. 6.4 months, $p = 0.003$) [1]. Following the significant results of this landmark clinical trial, the FDA granted approval in 2011 and opened the door to a flood of immune-based therapies [1].

Pembrolizumab, the first anti-PD-1 antibody to be approved by the FDA, is a highly selective, humanized monoclonal IgG4-kappa isotype antibody against PD-1. The results of the first phase I trial led to the FDA approval of pembrolizumab (in ipilimumab-refractory metastatic melanoma patients) in September 2014 [2, 15]. A randomized, controlled phase III study was performed (KEYNOTE 006) with treatment-naïve advanced melanoma assigned in a 1:1:1 ratio to two dosage schedules of pembrolizumab or ipilimumab [23]. Significant improvement in ORR were observed in both pembrolizumab treatment arms (33.7% for the every 2 week, 32.9% for the every 3 week regimen) compared with the ipilimumab group (11.9%) ($p < 0.001$ for both comparisons). As a direct result of this trial showing an improvement in OS, as well as fewer immune-related toxicities compared to ipilimumab, the FDA approved pembrolizumab as a first-line therapy for patients with metastatic melanoma.

Nivolumab, a fully human IgG4 monoclonal antibody, was the first anti-PD-1 antibody to be evaluated in humans in a phase I trial [24], producing a 31% response rate in previously treated metastatic melanoma patients [16]. Median duration of response and median OS were 22 months and 17.3 months, respectively. Two subsequent randomized trials comparing nivolumab with chemotherapy have been reported in ipilimumab-refractory patients and in untreated patients without BRAF mutation [3, 25]. Compared to dacarbazine as first-line therapy, nivolumab significantly improved 1-year OS rates, median PFS and ORR [3]. For ipilimumab refractory patients, nivolumab was also found to be superior to chemotherapy [25]. The FDA approved the usage of single-agent nivolumab in ipilimumab-refractory metastatic melanoma patients in December 2014.

Combination of Checkpoint Inhibitors

The success of CTLA-4 inhibition and PD-1/PD-L1 inhibition in the treatment of cancer has led to a greater appreciation of the complexity within the tumor microenvironment. Through much research worldwide, we have come to understand that the tumor microenvironment is a dynamic, interactive process that we are still yet to truly understand in the context of tumor immunology and immunotherapy. The observation that PD-1 inhibition is active in CTLA-4 inhibitor refractory patients confirms the complementary effects of dual checkpoint inhibition [15, 25]. In a randomized, double-blind three-arm study, treatment-naïve, unresectable stage III or IV melanoma patients were randomized in a 1:1:1 ratio to nivolumab, nivolumab plus ipilimumab, or ipilimumab alone [26]. The median PFS was 11.5 months in the combination group compared with 2.9 months in the ipilimumab group (HR 0.42; $p < 0.001$) and 6.9 months in the nivolumab group (HR for the comparison with ipilimumab, 0.57; $p < 0.001$). The ORR were 43.7% in the nivolumab group, 57.6% in the combination group, and 19% in the ipilimumab group.

Oncolytic Herpes Virus

Another novel agent recently approved by the FDA for the treatment of metastatic melanoma is talimogene laherparepvec (T-VEC), a modified herpes simplex virus type-1. In a phase III multicenter trial, 436 patients with unresectable stage IIIB-IV melanoma patients were randomized at a 2:1 ratio to intralesional T-VEC or subcutaneous GM-CSF [7]. Durable response rates (defined as a response lasting >6 months) was significantly higher in the T-VEC group (16.3%) compared with GM-CSF control group (2.1%; $p = 0.001$). ORR in the T-VEC arm was higher at 26.4% compared with 5.7% in the control arm. There was a trend for a longer median OS in the T-VEC arm at 23.3 months compared with 18.9 months in the control arm. However, it was not considered statistically significant ($p = 0.051$). The most common AEs with T-VEC were fatigue, chills, and pyrexia, with the most common grade 3/4 AE seen was cellulitis (2.1%). The results of yet another landmark article led to the FDA approval of T-VEC for intratumoral injection of cutaneous, subcutaneous, and nodal metastatic melanoma in those patients deemed unresectable.

Rationale for Complete Metastasectomy in Metastatic Melanoma Patients

Surgical resection for metastatic disease may seem counterintuitive, a local therapy for a systemic process. In fact, studies have shown that greater than 50% of stage IV melanoma patients have circulating tumor cells [27]. Historically, metastatic solid organ cancers were deemed uniformly fatal in most, if not all, patients with stage IV disease. We had little to offer such patients, often in the form of palliative systemic therapy that rarely provided an improvement in their overall outcome [28]. Nonetheless, progression of metastases is a complex process in which tumor cells must escape the primary lesion and gain access to the blood stream. These rogue cells must also avoid stimulating the host immune response, adhere to metastatic organ site endothelium, penetrate the basement membrane into the interstitial space, and promote appropriate angiogenesis and growth factors to allow for sufficient proliferation [29]. Hence, only a small percentage of circulating tumor cells have the capacity to successfully generate a metastatic deposit [30]. Thus, despite the systemic nature of stage IV disease, local therapy for resectable metastases may have curative potential if only limited oligometastatic disease exists.

Over the past half century, pulmonary metastasectomy for sarcoma [31] and hepatic metastasectomy for colorectal carcinoma [32] have paved the way for metastasectomy in other neoplasms. In each case, there are encouraging results showing significant long-term survival in select patients with stage IV disease. Pulmonary metastasectomy for sarcoma have demonstrated a 15–60% 5-year overall survival rate, with partial hepatectomy for colorectal carcinoma showing a 12–36% 10-year overall survival rate [31, 32]. Metastasectomy for melanoma has also shown improved survival in various settings [33]. In this chapter, we will discuss the available literature for a complete metastasectomy, removal of all clinical and radiographically identifiable metastatic deposits.

Palliative metastasectomy [34], the removal of only the symptomatic metastatic disease, or palliative surgery in stage IV melanoma patients is very important for symptom management, but does not improve overall survival. Skin, subcutaneous, and lymphatic metastases can cause horribly disfiguring, painful, and debilitating symptoms that can be quite difficult to control. Visceral metastases to the gastrointestinal (GI) tract can cause bleeding or obstruction that respond best to surgical resection or surgical bypass. Symptomatic brain metastases are resistant to radiation therapy and may be amenable to surgical resection. Metastasectomy remains an important part of the armamentarium in this setting. While understanding the principles of palliative surgery is important, the remainder of this chapter will address complete metastasectomy with the goal of improving overall survival.

Prognosis of Melanoma Patients with Stage IV Metastatic Disease

In 2017 the American Joint Committee on Cancer (AJCC) issued a revised 8th edition of TNM classification system that recognized the clinical and pathological features that are distinctive to melanoma and serve as prognostic markers [35]. The AJCC Melanoma Staging Committee recognized the variability of prognosis in stage IV metastatic melanoma based upon anatomic location. They divided stage IV melanoma into M1a for skin, subcutaneous, or distant lymph node metastases, M1b for pulmonary sites, and M1c for all other visceral metastases or any other distant site without (0) and with (1) elevated lactic dehydrogenase [35]. Balch et al. examined the outcomes of 7972 stage IV melanoma patients, demonstrating overall 1-year survival rates of 62% for M1a, 53% for M1b, and 33% for M1c melanoma ($p < 0.0001$) [36]. Given this framework, and understanding of the natural history in different metastatic patterns in melanoma, we will frame our discussion of metastasectomy along these lines, discussing outcomes of resection separately in M1a, M1b, and M1c groups.

The FDA approval of drugs with actual overall survival benefit has led several investigators to question the actual prognosis of stage IV patients in this current era of efficacious agents. Forschner and colleagues [37] examined 441 patients with stage IV melanoma from 2011 to 2014, 22.6% underwent metastasectomy, 58.5% received systemic therapy, and 18.9% had no therapy. Their metastasectomy patients had a 61% 3-year OS versus 23% for patients managed systemically ($p < 0.0001$) [37]. As would be expected, the 1-year OS was the best for patients with M1a disease (86.6%), followed by M1b (74.3%) and then M1c (51.6%). This modern day analysis in the era of effective therapies clearly demonstrates an improved prognosis of stage IV patients treated with either metastasectomy or efficacious systemic therapies.

Metastasectomy of Distant Skin, Soft Tissue, and Nodal Metastases (M1a)

Metastases to distant skin, soft tissue, and lymph nodes (M1a) are the second most common presentation of AJCC stage IV melanoma. Complete resection of M1a disease can be achieved in 70–80% of the study cohort [38–40]. M1a patients with nodal involvement had worse outcome compared with those having skin and soft tissue involvement [38, 41, 42]. Complete resection of skin and soft tissue metastases entails the removal of the metastatic deposit (Fig. 28.1) with a margin of normal-appearing tissue (<0.5 cm) [39]. Complete resection of nodal involvement often requires the complete dissection of all levels of the involved nodal basin, e.g., level I-III axillary dissection, superficial plus deep groin dissection, and a modified radical neck dissection (levels 1–5). Patients with M1a disease are associated with the most favorable outcome among the three subsets of stage IV melanoma. Median survival following resection of M1a disease ranges from 15 to >60 months with an 11–49% 5-year survival [11, 33, 38, 40–44]. Howard et al. reported the outcome of stage IV recurrence in patients enrolled in Multicenter Selective Lymphadenectomy Trial-1 (MSLT-1) [44]. Among the patients undergoing metastasectomy, 53% received adjuvant systemic therapy and 20% received preoperative systemic therapy. It is unclear whether perioperative systemic therapy contributed to the reported median survival of >60 months in this M1a metastasectomy cohort compared with 15–50 months reported in other historical series (Table 28.1).

Determining which patients should be offered T-VEC or surgical resection for their M1a disease is quite complex, often requiring a detailed discussion with the patient about the risks and benefits of each therapeutic option. In the absence of actual data that has examined the sequencing of therapy, the two senior authors (DWO, ECH) have utilized similar criteria to determine which patients should undergo a metastasectomy. If it is a single site of M1a disease, then surgical resection is recommended. If the patient has up to three sites of M1a disease, all less than approximately 2 cm, then surgical resection is also recommended. If a patient has ≥4 and/or multiple

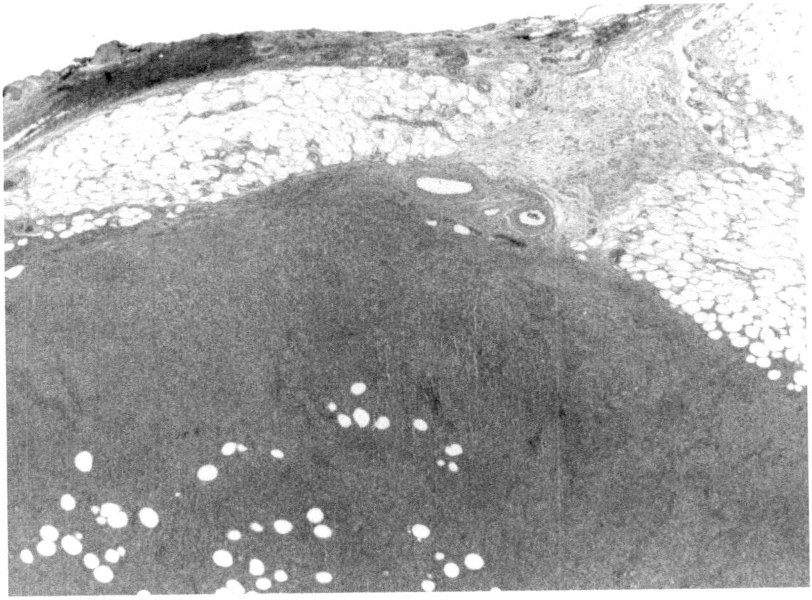

Fig. 28.1 Micrograph of in-transit metastasis (hematoxylin and eosin stain) with tumor-free surgical margins. (courtesy of P. Googe)

Table 28.1 Stage IV M1a metastasectomy survival data

Authors	Year	*N*	Median survival (mo)	5-year survival (%)	Sites
Feun et al [11]	1982	64	23		All
Overett and Shiu [38]	1985	20	15		LN
		12	25		SQ
Markowitz et al. [41]	1991	72	24	38	LN
		60	50	49	SQ
Gadd and Coit [43]	1992	199	20	11	All
Karakousis et al. [42]	1994	23	29	22	LN
		27	24	33	SQ
Barth et al. [8]	1995	281	15	14	All
Meyer et al. [40]	2000	45	18	20	LN
		30	17	18	SQ
Essner et al. [33]	2004	162	35		All
Howard et al. [44]	2012	26	>60		

lesions greater than 2 cm, then T-VEC injections are recommended as the initial therapy, with metastasectomy reserved for those patients whose lesion(s) have not completely responded to T-VEC therapy.

Metastasectomy of Pulmonary Metastases (M1b)

Complete metastasectomy for pulmonary metastases has the best prognosis of any stage IV patient with visceral metastases [36, 37, 45–47]. The data to support pulmonary metastasectomy is comprised mostly of single institution reports, with the largest reported series compiled in Table 28.2. Taken in aggregate, the median OS for complete pulmonary metastasectomy ranges from 16 to 40 months, with a 5-year overall survival range from 20 to 37% [11, 33, 44–54]. Furthermore, in the era of modern systemic treatment, including targeted and immune checkpoint therapies, patients undergoing a complete metastasectomy have 3-year survival rates of 41.7% [37] and 5-year survival rates as high as 39% [45–47].

Despite the impressive institutional data presented above, it is important to remember that this is a highly selected group of stage IV metastatic melanoma patients. In order to apply this information within the appropriate framework, it is important to identify which patients are most likely to benefit from metastasectomy. In 1996, Ollila et al. demonstrated the importance of tumor doubling time (TDT), defined as the time it takes for a pulmonary metastasis to double in size, in predicting outcomes from a pulmonary metastasectomy [57]. The updated analysis, published in 2010 with 20 years of pulmonary metastasectomies, identified that a TDT of >60 days ($p = 0.008$) was a good prognostic factor, warranting strong consideration for a complete metastasectomy [55]. TDT is easy to calculate and is a useful clinical gauge that provides insight into an individual patient's biology of progression. A TDT of at least 60 days seems to be a good prognostic factor and patients, if medically fit, should strongly be considered for a pulmonary metastasectomy.

In addition to TDT, other investigators have tried to determine which patients would benefit the most from a pulmonary metastasectomy. The addition of PET or fusion PET/CT (Fig. 28.2) to conventional imaging has been shown to be the most sensitive method to identify metastases in stage IV melanoma [52, 56]. This allows the surgeon to know that he/she is actually performing a complete metastasectomy because all possible known sites of metastatic disease have been identified within the detection limits of a modern fusion PET/CT [52]. Completeness of metastasectomy, disease-free interval, and number of metastatic lesions has all been shown to be important prognostic factors [33, 45, 46, 52, 53, 57].

Table 28.2 Stage IV M1b metastasectomy survival data

Authors	Year	*N*	Median survival (mo)	5-year survival (%)	Notes
Feun et al. [11]	1982	26	16		
Wong et al. [48]	1988	38	24	31	
Gorenstein et al. [49]	1991	54	18	25	Prognostic factors: antecedent nodal disease
Harpole et al. [50]	1992	84	20	20	Prognostic factors: # of lesions, DFI
Tafra et al. [45]	1995	106	23	27	CR in isolated lesions 39% 5-year survival Prognostic factors: # of lesions, TDT
IRLM [92]	1997	282	19	21	10-year survival was 14%
Dalrymple-Hay et al. [52]	2002	121	16	22	7-year survival was 13.5% Prognostic factors: # of lesions, DFI, PET usage
Essner et al. [33]	2004	364	28	21	Prognostic factors: antecedent nodal disease, DFI, # of lesions
Petersen et al. [53]	2007	249	19	21	CR has 19 months median survival vs. 11 months in PR Prognostic factors: DFI, # of lesions
Neuman et al. [54]	2007	26	40	29	Prognostic factors: # of lesions
Casiraghi et al. [47]	2011	27		37	All patients had CR
Younes [46]	2013	48	32	36	CR 35.6 median survival vs. 11.5 PR
Howard et al. [44]	2012	27	17.9		

DFI disease-free interval, *TDT* tumor doubling time, *IRLM* International Registry of Lung Metastases, *CR* complete resection, *PR* partial resection

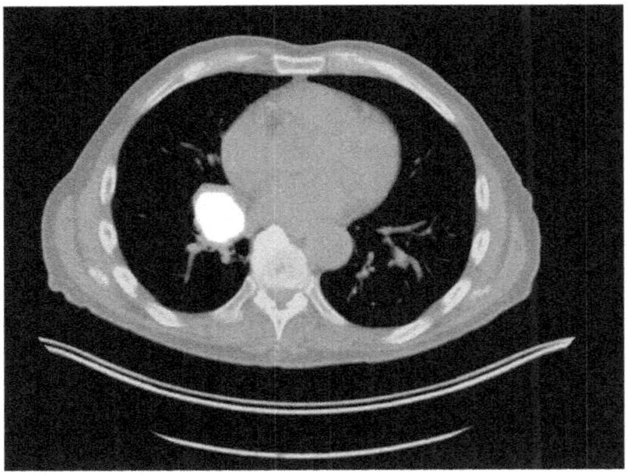

Fig. 28.2 Fusion PET/CT of pulmonary metastasis (courtesy of A. Khandani)

There has not been a clinical trial comparing pulmonary metastasectomy versus best medical therapy, and it is unlikely to ever be performed in this group of patients unless a novel clinical trial design is employed combining both the benefits of surgery and systemic therapy, such as metastasectomy followed by adjuvant therapy vs. neoadjuvant therapy followed by pulmonary metastasectomy. Nonetheless, the overwhelming institutional data presented above, and in Table 28.2, consistently shows improved outcomes of median survival, with an impressive 5-year overall survival in those patients undergoing complete metastasectomy. Using TDT, DFI, and number of pulmonary lesions, assists the surgeon in choosing which individual patient should be considered for a surgical approach to their pulmonary metastases.

Metastasectomy of M1c Disease

Gastrointestinal Metastases

Approximately 60% of patients with disseminated stage IV melanoma have evidence of gastrointestinal (GI) involvement [58]. The small bowel (Fig. 28.3) is the most common GI site occurring in approximately 75–90% of cases, followed by colon (20–25%) and stomach (3–16%) [58–60]. The most common presenting signs and symptoms include anemia, abdominal pain,

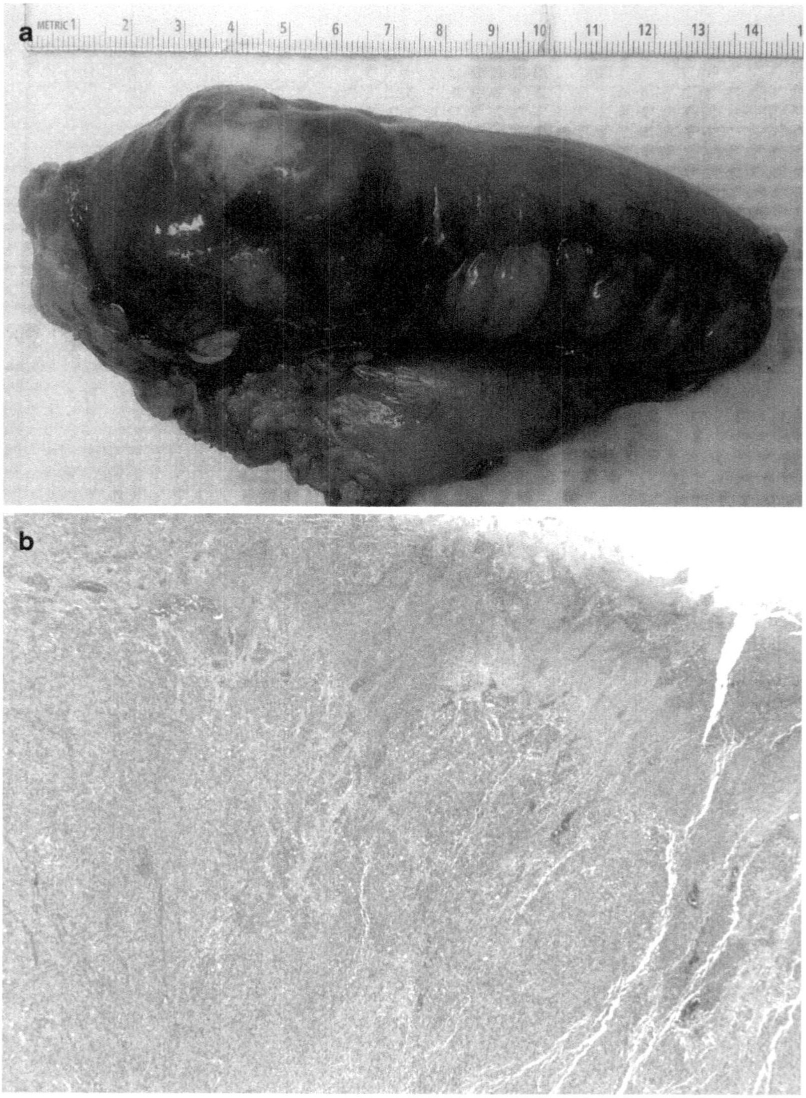

Fig. 28.3 (**a**) Partial small bowel resection for metastatic melanoma (courtesy of P. Googe). (**b**) Micrograph of small bowel metastasis (hematoxylin and eosin stain) with tumor-free surgical margins. (courtesy of P. Googe)

bleeding, obstruction, a palpable mass, and weight loss [59–63]. As fusion PET/CT (Fig. 28.4) is increasingly utilized, more asymptomatic GI metastases identified within the small bowel are being detected. As with other sites of stage IV melanoma metastases, complete resection of metastases is the best prognostic indicator [60, 62, 64, 65].

Median survival following complete resection of GI metastases ranged from 15 to 28 months, compared with 5 to 8 months for those who did not [34, 44, 59, 60, 62, 65, 66] (Table 28.3). Complete resection has been shown to have a 5-year OS as high as 41% in appropriately selected patients [34]. Median survival is no worse between patients with a single site versus multiple synchronous GI sites following complete resection of all disease sites. In some cases, multiple resections have been associated with longer median survival [34, 44, 65]. If a complete metastasectomy is not technically possible in a symptomatic patient, then a palliative procedure should be performed as this is very successful in alleviating symptoms in >90% of patients [34, 60–62, 65].

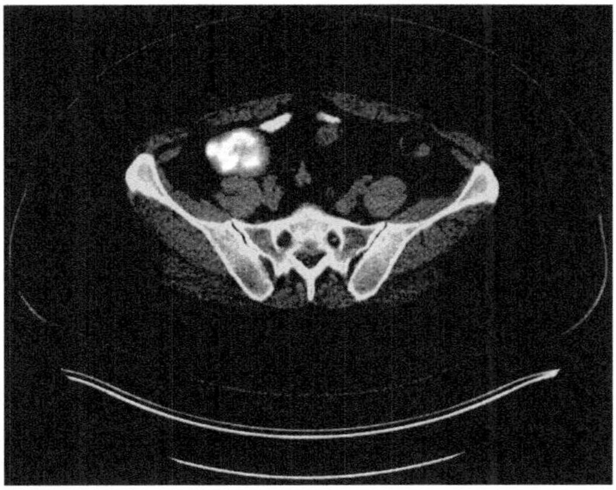

Fig. 28.4 Fusion PET/CT of small bowel metastasis (courtesy of A. Khandani)

Intra-Abdominal Solid Organ Metastases

The data concerning solid organ intra-abdominal metastases is limited to small institutional reports in highly selected patient populations. A variety of metastasectomy sites have been reported, such as within the liver, adrenal gland, gallbladder, pancreas, and spleen. Some reports indicate that as long as complete resection was obtained, there was a survival advantage for patients undergoing intestinal, solid organ, and combined metastasectomies [65]. In those patients with only liver metastases, complete metastasectomy is associated with a 38–44 month median survival, compared to 12–13 months for an incomplete

Table 28.3 Stage IV M1c gastrointestinal metastasectomy survival data

Authors	Year	*N*	Median survival (months)	5-year survival (%)	Notes
Klaase et al. [62]	1990	19		19	All patients symptomatic 9 of 19 had CR, of those 5 of 9 alive at 5 years
Gutman et al. [65]	2001	251 (135 surgical 116 medical)	11 vs. 5		Patients treated with CR, median survival 8 months Patients with second resection, 36 months median survival CR longest symptom-free survival at 10 months
Howard et al. [44]	2012	210 (108 surgical, 102 medical)	15 vs. 6.3	10.5 vs. 4.6 (4 year OS)	Patients with multiple resections had 21.2 months median survival vs. 13 months for single resections
Sosman et al. [66]	2011	20	21	31 (4 year OS)	All patients had CR
Ricaniadis et al. [59]	1995	68 (47 surgical, 21 medical)	27.6 vs. 5.1 (CR vs. PR)	28.3 vs. 0 (CR vs. PR)	
Ollila et al. [34]	1996	124 (69 surgical, 55 medical)	48.9 vs. 5.4 (CR vs. PR)	41% vs. 28% (CR vs. all surgical)	Most important prognostic factor was CR 67 of 69 surgical had symptom relief
Agrawal et al. [60]	1999	68	8.2	18%	In CR median survival 14.9 months and 35% 5-year OS Symptom relief in 90%

CR complete resection, *OS* overall survival, *PR* partial resection

resection [67, 68]. Adrenalectomy metastasectomies achieve symptom control in the majority of patients [69], with a median survival of 16–29 months for resected patients, compared to 5–9 months in non-resected patients [69–71]. Pancreatic metastasectomy has a median survival of 24 months [64, 72]. Metastasectomy for gallbladder disease achieves symptom relief in nearly all patients, and isolated long-term survivors as long as 13.8 years after resections have been reported [73], despite a poor median survival of only 16 months [74]. Symptomatic control of splenic metastases with splenectomy is also highly successful, with nearly all patients achieving symptom control after surgery. The overall median survival is 23 months in patients with a solitary resected lesion [75].

Howard et al. reported on the MSLT-I trial data in regard to metastasectomy data for M1c disease, including 108 patients treated with surgery as part of their treatment, versus 102 treated with systemic medical therapy alone [44]. Median survival and 4-year survival in the surgery group was 15 months and 10.5%, respectively, compared to 6.3 months and 4.6% in the systemic medical therapy group (HR = 0.424, $p < 0.001$). They also showed that patients who had multiple operations to treat their metastases had a longer (21.2 months) median survival and (25%) 4-year survival, compared to 13 months and 18% in patients undergoing only one operation ($p = 0.0218$). Survival was also better in patients with a single involved organ compared to two or three organs ($p = 0.0041$, $p = 0.0001$) [44].

Brain Metastases

In 2004, Fife et al. [76] reported on 686 melanoma patients with brain metastases treated with surgery and postoperative radiotherapy, surgery alone, radiotherapy alone versus supportive care alone. Median survival in these respective groups was 8.9, 8.7, 3.4, and 2.1 months, demonstrating the effect of surgery, with (HR 0.35) and without radiation (HR 0.44), versus palliative therapy ($p < 0.0001$) [76]. A comprehensive review of treatment options for brain metastases concluded that surgery with adjuvant whole brain radiation therapy was superior to whole brain radiation therapy. They also showed that stereotactic radiosurgery (SRS) had similar results to surgery when combined with whole brain radiation [77]. However, prospective trial data regarding SRS was lacking until 2016, when a prospective trial was performed in patients with one to three brain metastases, randomized to whole brain radiotherapy vs. SRS [78]. There was no significant difference in median overall survival for SRS alone (10.4 months) compared to SRS plus WBRT (7.4 months). The incidence of cognitive deterioration was comparatively less after SRS alone at 3 months, appearing to be a less morbid and most efficacious way to manage patients with one to three brain metastases.

Stage IV Metastasectomy Trials

Most of the peer-reviewed literature on metastasectomy for stage IV melanoma patients relies on highly selected, single institutional series. There is a paucity of evidence and prospective, randomized trials in support of metastasectomy. Additionally, there is a known inherent selection bias within any single institution series, with only the best operative candidates and most favorable biology chosen for surgery. Such critiques are justified against a metastasectomy-first approach to treatment, fueling the first international trial (Donald L. Morton, P.I.) to examine the role of upfront metastasectomy in stage IV patients. Trial eligibility (A Phase III, Randomized, Double-Blind, Placebo-Controlled Trial of Immunotherapy with a Polyvalent Melanoma Vaccine, Canvaxin™ plus BCG vs. Placebo plus BCG as a Post-Surgical Treatment for Stage IV Melanoma, NCT00052156), required all patients ($n = 496$) to have had a complete metastasectomy with tumor-free surgical margins. Although Onamelatucel-L (Canvaxin™) as an adjuvant therapy did not demonstrate an overall survival benefit, we identified an overall 5-year survival rate of 40% for the entire study cohort [79, 80]. This 5-year survival rate, with surgical metastasectomy, had never been achieved in any randomized stage IV melanoma trial. A prospective, multicenter trial for metastasectomy in stage IV melanoma patients was started by the Southwest Oncology Group (SWOG) [81]. Sixty-four patients met the standard of a complete metastasectomy with tumor-free surgical margins. Although the trial closed prior to reaching accrual goals, the median overall survival was 21 months, and OS at 3 and 4 years was 36% and 31%, respectively.

The medical oncology clinical trialists clearly took notice of these seemingly unexplainable survival rates. Based upon the improved survival in stage IV patients treated with ipilimumab [1], the Eastern Cooperative Oncology Group (ECOG) designed an adjuvant therapy trial, ECOG 1609, A Phase III Randomized Study of Adjuvant Ipilimumab (Anti-CTLA4 Therapy) Versus High-Dose Interferon a-2b for Resected High-Risk Melanoma. This trial compared high dose interferon alfa-2b versus low-dose ipilimumab (3 mg/kg), versus high dose ipilimumab (10 mg/kg). It included high-risk, surgically resected stage IIIb, IIIc, stage IC M1a and M1b patients. To be eligible for this trial, the patients had to have a curative intent lymphadenectomy or curative intent complete metastasectomy of stage IV disease with tumor-free surgical margins. The trial has closed to accrual and the results are anticipated in 2018.

Another adjuvant therapy trial is currently enrolling patients, SWOG 1404, High-Dose Recombinant Interferon Alfa-2B, Ipilimumab, or Pembrolizumab in Treating Patients With Stage III–IV High Risk Melanoma That Has Been Removed by Surgery. This trial is examining a PD1-inhibitor, pembrolizumab, in the adjuvant setting for patients with completely resected stage IIIb, IIIc, Stage IV M1a, M1b, or M1c melanoma. The trial will enroll 1240 subjects and is anticipated to close in late 2017 with results in 2020. Trial designs such as these combine the benefit of complete metastasectomy with our most efficacious systemic agents to date. These adjuvant trial designs require a relatively large number of patients and a longer follow-up, thus, an impetus for designing neoadjuvant therapy trials in this arena.

Neoadjuvant Therapy

Neoadjuvant therapy has improved resectability and local disease control in several types of solid tumors. Previously, due to the lack of efficacious systemic agent(s), neoadjuvant therapy has not been part of the treatment paradigm for patients with resectable metastatic melanoma. With the success of immune checkpoint inhibitors and targeted therapy for BRAF-mutated melanoma for the treatment of metastatic melanoma, several case series of salvage surgery following clinical response to modern systemic therapy have rekindled the interest of a neoadjuvant approach to the treatment of patients with resectable metastatic melanoma [82–86]. This will increase the number of patients receiving the benefits of both efficacious systemic therapy along with complete metastasectomy. By starting with a drug-first approach, the response to neoadjuvant therapy could serve as an important prognostic variable in metastatic melanoma patients, just as it does in breast and rectal cancer [87, 88]. Objective response to neoadjuvant therapy could also serve as a prognostic variable for stratification of care following complete metastasectomy.

In addition to assessing clinical response, the other important focus of neoadjuvant therapy is to determine the biologic and immunologic tissue response to therapy. We can also elucidate the mechanisms for resistance and immune escape within the tumor microenvironment. Gyorki et al. reported a higher percentage of CD4+,FOXP3+,T-regulatory cells in the tumor, compared to the peripheral blood in 23 patients undergoing surgery. All patients received induction or maintenance dose ipilimumab within 30 days of their surgery [89]. Tarhini et al. [90] published a study of neoadjuvant ipilimumab, followed by complete metastasectomy and then adjuvant ipilimumab. Although residual melanoma at definitive surgery was detected in all 33 enrolled patients, 5 patients had only microscopic disease, demonstrating a treatment effect of the ipilimumab. In a follow-up immunological analysis of the peripheral blood, they identified an increase in T-regulatory cell suppressive function, significantly associated with a decrease in PFS [91].

Currently, several trials are actively investigating the role of neoadjuvant therapy with various modern agents in stage IV metastatic melanoma patients: NCT02519322 (nivolumab versus nivolumab + ipilimumab), NCT02211131 (Talimogene Laherparepvec), NCT02303951 (NEO-VC; vemurafenib + cobimetinib), NCT02231775 (Combi-Neo; dabrafenib + trametinib), NCT02736123 (nivolumab versus nivolumab + ipilimumab).

Conclusion

While the recent breakthroughs in systemic therapy of melanoma are impressive, the decades of cumulative experience with complete metastasectomy in stage IV melanoma should not be ignored. As demonstrated in numerous systemic therapy trials of metastatic disease, complete response generally portends a good outcome, sometimes long-term. Similarly, complete metastasectomy conferred superior outcome compared with partial resection in patients with stage IV melanoma. While the modern melanoma systemic therapy can prolong survival, the rates of complete response are still <15%. The combination of systemic therapy and surgery in either the adjuvant or neoadjuvant setting will likely substanially improve patient outcomes as compared to just a drug or just a surgical approach. The paradigm for the treatment of metastatic melanoma is still shifting. Rational design of clinical trials examining both treatment modalities will define our future approach to the optimal management of patients with stage IV melanoma patients.

References

1. Hodi FS, O'Day SJ, McDermott DF, Weber RW, Sosman JA, Haanen JB, et al. Improved survival with ipilimumab in patients with metastatic melanoma. N Engl J Med. 2010;363(8):711–23.
2. Hamid O, Robert C, Daud A, Hodi FS, Hwu WJ, Kefford R, et al. Safety and tumor responses with lambrolizumab (anti-PD-1) in melanoma. N Engl J Med. 2013;369(2):134–44.
3. Robert C, Long GV, Brady B, Dutriaux C, Maio M, Mortier L, et al. Nivolumab in previously untreated melanoma without BRAF mutation. N Engl J Med. 2015;372(4):320–30.
4. Chapman PB, Hauschild A, Robert C, Haanen JB, Ascierto P, Larkin J, et al. Improved survival with vemurafenib in melanoma with BRAF V600E mutation. N Engl J Med. 2011;364(26):2507–16.
5. Hauschild A, Grob JJ, Demidov LV, Jouary T, Gutzmer R, Millward M, et al. Dabrafenib in BRAF-mutated metastatic melanoma: a multicentre, open-label, phase 3 randomised controlled trial. Lancet. 2012;380(9839):358–65.
6. Flaherty KT, Robert C, Hersey P, Nathan P, Garbe C, Milhem M, et al. Improved survival with MEK inhibition in BRAF-mutated melanoma. N Engl J Med. 2012;367(2):107–14.
7. Andtbacka RH, Kaufman HL, Collichio F, Amatruda T, Senzer N, Chesney J, et al. Talimogene laherparepvec improves durable response rate in patients with advanced melanoma. J Clin Oncol. 2015;33(25):2780–8. https://doi.org/10.1200/JCO.2014.58.3377.
8. Barth A, Wanek L, Morton D. Prognostic factors in 1521 melanoma patients with distant metastases. J Am Coll Surg. 1995;181:193–201.
9. Wong S, Coit DG. Role of surgery in patients with stage IV melanoma. Curr Opin Oncol. 2004;16(2):155–60.
10. Martinez SR, Young SE. A rational surgical approach to the treatment of distant melanoma metastases. Cancer Treat Rev. 2008;34(7):614–20.
11. Feun L, Gutterman J, Burgess M, et al. The natural history of resectable metastatic melanoma (Stage IV A melanoma). Cancer. 1982;50:1656–63.
12. Ollila DW, Hsueh EC, Stern SL, Morton DL. Metastasectomy for recurrent stage IV melanoma. J Surg Oncol. 1999;71(4):209–13.
13. Ascierto PA, Minor D, Ribas A, Lebbe C, O'Hagan A, Arya N, et al. Phase II trial (BREAK-2) of the BRAF inhibitor dabrafenib (GSK2118436) in patients with metastatic melanoma. J Clin Oncol. 2013;31(26):3205–11. https://doi.org/10.1200/JCO.2013.49.8691.
14. Flaherty KT, Infante JR, Daud A, Gonzalez R, Kefford RF, Sosman J, et al. Combined BRAF and MEK inhibition in melanoma with BRAF V600 mutations. N Engl J Med. 2012;367(18):1694–703.
15. Robert C, Ribas A, Wolchok JD, Hodi FS, Hamid O, Kefford R, et al. Anti-programmed-death-receptor-1 treatment with pembrolizumab in ipilimumab-refractory advanced melanoma: a randomised dose-comparison cohort of a phase 1 trial. Lancet. 2014;384(9948):1109–17.
16. Topalian SL, Sznol M, McDermott DF, Kluger HM, Carvajal RD, Sharfman WH, et al. Survival, durable tumor remission, and long-term safety in patients with advanced melanoma receiving nivolumab. J Clin Oncol. 2014;32(10):1020–30. https://doi.org/10.1200/JCO.2013.53.0105.

17. Davies H, Bignell GR, Cox C, Stephens P, Edkins S, Clegg S, et al. Mutations of the BRAF gene in human cancer. Nature. 2002;417(6892):949–54.
18. Su F, Viros A, Milagre C, Trunzer K, Bollag G, Spleiss O, et al. RAS mutations in cutaneous squamous-cell carcinomas in patients treated with BRAF inhibitors. N Engl J Med. 2012;366(3):207–15. https://doi.org/10.1056/NEJMoa1105358.
19. King AJ, Arnone MR, Bleam MR, Moss KG, Yang J, Fedorowicz KE, et al. Dabrafenib; preclinical characterization, increased efficacy when combined with trametinib, while BRAF/MEK tool combination reduced skin lesions. PLoS One. 2013;8(7):e67583. https://doi.org/10.1371/journal.pone.0067583.
20. Long GV, Stroyakovskiy D, Gogas H, Levchenko E, de Braud F, Larkin J, et al. Combined BRAF and MEK inhibition versus BRAF inhibition alone in melanoma. N Engl J Med. 2014;371(20):1877–88.
21. Robert C, Karaszewska B, Schachter J, Rutkowski P, Mackiewicz A, Stroiakovski D, et al. Improved overall survival in melanoma with combined dabrafenib and trametinib. N Engl J Med. 2015;372(1):30–9.
22. Larkin J, Ascierto PA, Dreno B, Atkinson V, Liszkay G, Maio M, et al. Combined vemurafenib and cobimetinib in BRAF-mutated melanoma. N Engl J Med. 2014;371(20):1867–76. https://doi.org/10.1056/NEJMoa1408868.
23. Robert C, Schachter J, Long GV, Arance A, Grob JJ, Mortier L, et al. Pembrolizumab versus Ipilimumab in Advanced Melanoma. N Engl J Med. 2015;372(26):2521–32. https://doi.org/10.1056/NEJMoa1503093.
24. Brahmer JR, Drake CG, Wollner I, Powderly JD, Picus J, Sharfman WH, et al. Phase I study of single-agent anti-programmed death-1 (MDX-1106) in refractory solid tumors: safety, clinical activity, pharmacodynamics, and immunologic correlates. J Clin Oncol. 2010;28(19):3167–75. https://doi.org/10.1200/JCO.2009.26.7609.
25. Weber JS, D'Angelo SP, Minor D, Hodi FS, Gutzmer R, Neyns B, et al. Nivolumab versus chemotherapy in patients with advanced melanoma who progressed after anti-CTLA-4 treatment (CheckMate 037): a randomised, controlled, open-label, phase 3 trial. Lancet Oncol. 2015;16(4):375–84. https://doi.org/10.1016/S1470-2045(15)70076-8.
26. Larkin J, Hodi FS, Wolchok JD. Combined nivolumab and ipilimumab or monotherapy in untreated melanoma. N Engl J Med. 2015;373(13):1270–1. https://doi.org/10.1056/NEJMc1509660.
27. Koyanagi K, Kuo C, Nakagawa T, Mori T, Ueno H, Lorico AR Jr, et al. Multimarker quantitative real-time PCR detection of circulating melanoma cells in peripheral blood: relation to disease stage in melanoma patients. Clin Chem. 2005;51(6):981–8. https://doi.org/10.1373/clinchem.2004.045096.
28. Das Gupta T, Brasfield R. Metastatic melanoma of the gastrointestinal tract. Arch Surg. 1964;88:969–73.
29. Leung AM, Hari DM, Morton DL. Surgery for distant melanoma metastasis. Cancer J. 2012;18(2):176–84.
30. Zetter BR. The cellular basis of site-specific tumor metastasis. N Engl J Med. 1990;322(9):605–12. https://doi.org/10.1056/NEJM199003013220907.
31. Digesu CS, Wiesel O, Vaporciyan AA, Colson YL. Management of sarcoma metastases to the lung. Surg Oncol Clin N Am. 2016;25(4):721–33. https://doi.org/10.1016/j.soc.2016.05.005.
32. Abbas S, Lam V, Hollands M. Ten-year survival after liver resection for colorectal metastases: systematic review and meta-analysis. ISRN Oncol. 2011;2011:763245. https://doi.org/10.5402/2011/763245.
33. Essner R, Lee JH, Wanek LA, Itakura H, Morton DL. Contemporary surgical treatment of advanced-stage melanoma. Arch Surg. 2004;139(9):961–6. discussion 6–7
34. Ollila D, Essner R, Wanek L, et al. Surgical resection for melanoma metastatic to the gastrointestinal tract. Arch Surg. 1996;131(9):975.
35. Amin MB, Edge S, Green F, Byrd DR, Brookland RK, Washington MK, et al., editors. AJCC cancer staging manual. 8th ed. New York: Springer; 2017.
36. Balch CM, Gershenwald JE, Soong SJ, Thompson JF, Atkins MB, Byrd DR, et al. Final version of 2009 AJCC melanoma staging and classification. J Clin Oncol. 2009;27(36):6199–206.
37. Forschner A, Eichner F, Amaral T, Keim U, Garbe C, Eigentler TK. Improvement of overall survival in stage IV melanoma patients during 2011-2014: analysis of real-world data in 441 patients of the German Central Malignant Melanoma Registry (CMMR). J Cancer Res Clin Oncol. 2017;143(3):533–40. https://doi.org/10.1007/s00432-016-2309-y.
38. Overett TK, Shiu MH. Surgical treatment of distant metastatic melanoma. Indications and results. Cancer. 1985;56(5):1222–30.
39. Essner R. Surgical treatment of malignant melanoma. Surg Clin North Am. 2003;83(1):109–56.
40. Meyer T, Merkel S, Goehl J, Hohenberger W. Surgical therapy for distant metastases of malignant melanoma. Cancer. 2000;89(9):1983–91.
41. Markowitz J, Cosimi L, Carey R, et al. Prognosis after initial recurrence of cutaneous melanoma. Ann Surg. 1991;214:70–707.
42. Karakousis C, Velez A, Driscoll B, et al. Metastasectomy in malignant melanoma. Surgery. 1994;115:295–302.
43. Gadd M, Coit D. Recurrence patterns and outcome in 1019 patients undergoing axillary or inguinal lymphadenopathy for melanoma. Arch Surg. 1992;127:1412–6.
44. Howard JH, Thompson JF, Mozzillo N, Nieweg OE, Hoekstra HJ, Roses DF, et al. Metastasectomy for distant metastatic melanoma: analysis of data from the first Multicenter Selective Lymphadenectomy Trial (MSLT-I). Ann Surg Oncol. 2012;19(8):2547–55.
45. Tafra L, Dale PS, Wanek LA, Ramming KP, Morton DL. Resection and adjuvant immunotherapy for mel-

anoma metastatic to the lung and thorax. J Thorac Cardiovasc Surg. 1995;110(1):119–28. discussion 29
46. Younes R, Abrao FC, Gross J. Pulmonary metastasectomy for malignant melanoma: prognostic factors for long-term survival. Melanoma Res. 2013;23(4):307–11. https://doi.org/10.1097/CMR.0b013e3283632cbe.
47. Casiraghi M, De Pas T, Maisonneuve P, Brambilla D, Ciprandi B, Galetta D, et al. A 10-year single-center experience on 708 lung metastasectomies: the evidence of the "international registry of lung metastases". J Thorac Oncol. 2011;6(8):1373–8. https://doi.org/10.1097/JTO.0b013e3182208e58.
48. Wong J, Euhus D, Morton D. Surgical resection for metastatic melanoma to the lung. Arch Surg. 1988;23:1091–5.
49. Gorenstein LA, Putnam JB, Natarajan G, Balch CA, Roth JA. Improved survival after resection of pulmonary metastases from malignant melanoma [see comments]. Ann Thorac Surg. 1991;52(2):204–10.
50. Harpole DH Jr, Johnson CM, Wolfe WG, George SL, Seigler HF. Analysis of 945 cases of pulmonary metastatic melanoma. J Thorac Cardiovasc Surg. 1992;103(4):743–8. discussion 8–50
51. Pastorino U, Buyse M, Friedel G, Ginsberg R, Girard P. Long term results of lung metastectomy: prognostic analyses based on 5206 cases. J Thorac Cardiovasc Surg. 1997;113:37–49.
52. Dalrymple-Hay MJ, Rome PD, Kennedy C, Fulham M, McCaughan BC. Pulmonary metastatic melanoma—the survival benefit associated with positron emission tomography scanning. Eur J Cardiothorac Surg. 2002;21(4):611–4. discussion 4–5
53. Petersen RP, Hanish SI, Haney JC, Miller CC 3rd, Burfeind WR Jr, Tyler DS, et al. Improved survival with pulmonary metastasectomy: an analysis of 1720 patients with pulmonary metastatic melanoma. J Thorac Cardiovasc Surg. 2007;133(1):104–10.
54. Neuman HB, Patel A, Hanlon C, Wolchok JD, Houghton AN, Coit DG. Stage-IV melanoma and pulmonary metastases: factors predictive of survival. Ann Surg Oncol. 2007;14(10):2847–53.
55. Lee JH, Gulec SA, Kyshtoobayeva A, Sim MS, Morton DL. Biological factors, tumor growth kinetics, and survival after metastasectomy for pulmonary melanoma. Ann Surg Oncol. 2009;16(10):2834–9. https://doi.org/10.1245/s10434-009-0583-5.
56. Finkelstein SE, Carrasquillo JA, Hoffman JM, Galen B, Choyke P, White DE, et al. A prospective analysis of positron emission tomography and conventional imaging for detection of stage IV metastatic melanoma in patients undergoing metastasectomy. Ann Surg Oncol. 2004;11(8):731–8. https://doi.org/10.1245/ASO.2004.01.023.
57. Newman EA, Sabel MS, Nees AV, Schott A, Diehl KM, Cimmino VM, et al. Sentinel lymph node biopsy performed after neoadjuvant chemotherapy is accurate in patients with documented node-positive breast cancer at presentation. Ann Surg Oncol. 2007;14(10):2946–52.
58. Patel J, Didolkar M, Pickren J, Moore R. Metastatic pattern of malignant melanoma. A study of 216 autopsy studies. Am J Surg. 1978;135:807–10.
59. Ricaniadis N, Konstadoulakis M, Walsh D, et al. Gastrointestinal metastases from malignant melanoma. Surg Oncol. 1995;4:105–10.
60. Agrawal S, Yao T, Coit D. Surgery for melanoma metastatic to the gastrointestinal tract. Ann Surg Oncol. 1999;6:336–44.
61. Branum G, Epstein R, Leight G, et al. The role of resection in the management of melanoma metastatic to the adrenal gland. Surgery. 1991;109:127–31.
62. Klaase JM, Kroon BB. Surgery for melanoma metastatic to the gastrointestinal tract. Br J Surg. 1990;77(1):60–1.
63. de la Monte S, Moore G, Hutchins G. Patterned distribution of metastasis from malignant melanoma in humans. Cancer Res. 1983;43:3427–33.
64. Wood T, DiFronzo L, Rose D, Haigh P, Stern S, Wanek L, et al. Does complete resection of melanoma metastatic to solid intra-abdominal organs improve survival? Ann Surg Oncol. 2001;8:658–62.
65. Gutman H, Hess K, Kokoysakis J, et al. Surgery for abdominal meatstases of cutaneous melanoma. World J Surg. 2001;25:750–8.
66. Sosman JA, Moon J, Tuthill RJ, Warneke JA, Vetto JT, Redman BG, et al. A phase 2 trial of complete resection for stage IV melanoma: results of Southwest Oncology Group Clinical Trial S9430. Cancer. 2011;117(20):4740–06.
67. Ryu SW, Saw R, Scolyer RA, Crawford M, Thompson JF, Sandroussi C. Liver resection for metastatic melanoma: equivalent survival for cutaneous and ocular primaries. J Surg Oncol. 2013;108(2):129–35. https://doi.org/10.1002/jso.23361.
68. Rose D, Essner R, Hughes T, et al. Surgical resection for metastatic melanoma to the liver: the John Wayne Cancer Institute and Sydney Melanoma Unit Experience. Arch Surg. 2001;136(8):950–5.
69. Collinson FJ, Lam TK, Bruijn WM, de Wilt JH, Lamont M, Thompson JF, et al. Long-term survival and occasional regression of distant melanoma metastases after adrenal metastasectomy. Ann Surg Oncol. 2008;15(6):1741–9. https://doi.org/10.1245/s10434-008-9836-y.
70. Flaherty DC, Deutsch GB, Kirchoff DD, Lee J, Huynh KT, Lee DY, et al. Adrenalectomy for metastatic melanoma: current role in the age of nonsurgical treatments. Am Surg. 2015;81(10):1005–9.
71. Romero Arenas MA, Sui D, Grubbs EG, Lee JE, Perrier ND. Adrenal metastectomy is safe in selected patients. World J Surg. 2014;38(6):1336–42. https://doi.org/10.1007/s00268-014-2454-x.
72. Sperti C, Moletta L, Patane G. Metastatic tumors to the pancreas: the role of surgery. World J Gastrointest Oncol. 2014;6(10):381–92. https://doi.org/10.4251/wjgo.v6.i10.381.
73. Dong XD, DeMatos P, Prieto VG, Seigler HF. Melanoma of the gallbladder: a review of cases seen at Duke University Medical Center. Cancer. 1999;85(1):32–9.

74. Katz SC, Bowne WB, Wolchok JD, Busam KJ, Jaques DP, Coit DG. Surgical management of melanoma of the gallbladder: a report of 13 cases and review of the literature. Am J Surg. 2007;193(4):493–7. https://doi.org/10.1016/j.amjsurg.2006.06.033.
75. de Wilt JH, McCarthy WH, Thompson JF. Surgical treatment of splenic metastases in patients with melanoma. J Am Coll Surg. 2003;197(1):38–43. https://doi.org/10.1016/S1072-7515(03)00381-8.
76. Fife KM, Colman MH, Stevens GN, Firth IC, Moon D, Shannon KF, et al. Determinants of outcome in melanoma patients with cerebral metastases. J Clin Oncol. 2004;22(7):1293–300. https://doi.org/10.1200/JCO.2004.08.140.
77. Bafaloukos D, Gogas H. The treatment of brain metastases in melanoma patients. Cancer Treat Rev. 2004;30(6):515–20. https://doi.org/10.1016/j.ctrv.2004.05.001.
78. Brown PD, Jaeckle K, Ballman KV, Farace E, Cerhan JH, Anderson SK, et al. Effect of radiosurgery alone vs radiosurgery with whole brain radiation therapy on cognitive function in patients with 1 to 3 brain metastases: a Randomized Clinical Trial. JAMA. 2016;315(4):401–9. https://doi.org/10.1001/jama.2016.9839.
79. Morton DL, Mozzillo N, Thompson JF, Kashani-Sabet M, Kelley M, Gammon G. MMAIT-IV Clinical Trial Group. Multicenter double-blind phase 3 trial of Canvaxin vs. placebo as post surgical adjuvant in metastatic melanoma. Society of Surgical Oncology 59th Annual Cancer Symposium, San Diego, CA; 2006.
80. Morton DL, Mozzillo N, Thompson JF, Kelley MC, Faries M, Wagner J, et al. MMAIT Clinical Trials Group. An international, randomized, phase III trial of bacillus Calmette-Guerin (BCG) plus allogeneic melanoma vaccine (MCV) or placebo after complete resection of melanoma metastatic to regional or distant sites. J Clin Oncol. 2007;25(18s):8508.
81. Sondak VK, Liu PY, Warneke J. Surgical resection for Stage IV melanoma: a southwest oncology group trial. J Clin Oncol. 2006;24(Suppl):4575.
82. Koers K, Francken AB, Haanen JB, Woerdeman LA, van der Hage JA. Vemurafenib as neoadjuvant treatment for unresectable regional metastatic melanoma. J Clin Oncol. 2013;31(16):e251–3. https://doi.org/10.1200/JCO.2012.45.3845.
83. Kolar GR, Miller-Thomas MM, Schmidt RE, Simpson JR, Rich KM, Linette GP. Neoadjuvant treatment of a solitary melanoma brain metastasis with vemurafenib. J Clin Oncol. 2013;31(3):e40–3. https://doi.org/10.1200/JCO.2012.43.7061.
84. Laks S, Brueske KA, Hsueh EC. Neoadjuvant treatment of melanoma: case reports and review. Exp Hematol Oncol. 2013;2(1):30. https://doi.org/10.1186/2162-3619-2-30.
85. Melnik I, Lotem M, Yoffe B. A new role of vemurafenib as a neoadjuvant treatment of axillary and brain melanoma metastases. Case Rep Oncol Med. 2013;2013:794239. https://doi.org/10.1155/2013/794239.
86. Klemen ND, Feingold PL, Goff SL, Hughes MS, Kammula US, Yang JC, et al. Metastasectomy following immunotherapy with adoptive cell transfer for patients with advanced melanoma. Ann Surg Oncol. 2017;24(1):135–41. https://doi.org/10.1245/s10434-016-5537-0.
87. Kaufmann M, von Minckwitz G, Mamounas EP, Cameron D, Carey LA, Cristofanilli M, et al. Recommendations from an international consensus conference on the current status and future of neoadjuvant systemic therapy in primary breast cancer. Ann Surg Oncol. 2012;19(5):1508–16. https://doi.org/10.1245/s10434-011-2108-2.
88. Landry JC, Feng Y, Cohen SJ, Staley CA 3rd, Whittington R, Sigurdson ER, et al. Phase 2 study of preoperative radiation with concurrent capecitabine, oxaliplatin, and bevacizumab followed by surgery and postoperative 5-fluorouracil, leucovorin, oxaliplatin (FOLFOX), and bevacizumab in patients with locally advanced rectal cancer: ECOG 3204. Cancer. 2013;119(8):1521–7. https://doi.org/10.1002/cncr.27890.
89. Gyorki DE, Yuan J, Mu Z, Zaidi B, Pulitzer M, Busam K, et al. Immunological insights from patients undergoing surgery on ipilimumab for metastatic melanoma. Ann Surg Oncol. 2013;20(9):3106–11. https://doi.org/10.1245/s10434-013-2999-1.
90. Tarhini AA, Edington H, Butterfield LH, Lin Y, Shuai Y, Tawbi H, et al. Immune monitoring of the circulation and the tumor microenvironment in patients with regionally advanced melanoma receiving neoadjuvant ipilimumab. PLoS One. 2014;9(2):e87705.
91. Retseck J, VanderWeele R, Lin HM, Lin Y, Butterfield LH, Tarhini AA. Phenotypic and functional testing of circulating regulatory T cells in advanced melanoma patients treated with neoadjuvant ipilimumab. J Immunother Cancer. 2016;4:38. https://doi.org/10.1186/s40425-016-0141-1.
92. The International Registry of Lung Metastases. Long-term results of lung metastasectomy: prognostic analyses based on 5206 cases. J Thorac Cardiovasc Surg. 1997;113(1):37–49.

29 Adjuvant Therapy of Melanoma

Elisabeth Eapen Paul and Sanjiv S. Agarwala

Introduction

There will be an estimated 87,100 newly diagnosed melanoma patients in the United States in 2017 and 9730 deaths from this disease [1]. Prognosis of melanoma is heavily dependent upon stage at diagnosis, and the 5-year survival rate decreases with advancing stage. Reported survival rates range from more than 90% for stage I, to 80% for stage II and 23–87% for stage III disease [2]. Stage IV melanoma has historically had a dismal prognosis and while the outlook for these patients is improving with recent major advances in immune and targeted therapies, there is still a need for effective postsurgical adjuvant therapies for patients with local regional disease, who are deemed at high risk for systemic relapse.

The challenges in developing an effective adjuvant therapy are several-fold. Who exactly is at "high-risk" for systemic relapse after surgery is controversial, and has evolved as new and more precise surgical staging techniques, such as sentinel lymph node mapping and more sophisticated imaging techniques have become available. Furthermore, for an adjuvant therapy to be clinically meaningful and acceptable to patients and physicians, it needs to be not only highly effective, but have a reasonable toxicity and cost. Needless to say, such a therapy does not yet exist. This chapter aims to summarize the historical and current developments in this field, illustrate some of these major challenges, and provide a glimpse into future developments in this area.

E. E. Paul, M.D. · S. S. Agarwala, M.D. (✉)
Department of Hematology and Oncology, University Health Network, Bethlehem, PA, USA
e-mail: Elisabeth.paul@sluhn.org

Defining High-Risk Melanoma

Although resection can cure patients with high-risk disease (Stage IIB–IIIC), those with nodal involvement (stage III) have the highest risk of tumor recurrence and death [3]. It is important to realize that the definition of stage III melanoma, and therefore of "high-risk," has evolved over the years.

The staging system in current use is the AJCC 7th edition from 2009 [4]. This staging system divides stage III melanoma into IIIA, IIIB, and IIIC and includes all melanomas with the presence of lymph node involvement and/or in-transit metastasis. The 7th staging and classification recommendation was based on a multivariate analysis of 30,946 patients with Stage I, II, and III melanoma and 7972 with stage IV; 3307 of these were stage III. Five-year survival within substages of stage III were found to be 78%, 59%, and 40% for stages IIIA, IIIB, and IIIC, respectively [4].

A. I. Riker (ed.), *Melanoma*, https://doi.org/10.1007/978-3-319-78310-9_29

In addition to lymph node involvement, tumor thickness has been shown to effect survival, with a 10-year survival of 92% for T1 tumors (≤1 mm), as compared to 50% in patients with T4 stage (thickness > 4 mm). Tumor ulceration also influences survival, and survival rates of ulcerated tumors are proportionately lower than non-ulcerated tumors of equivalent T category. Ulcerated tumors have similar survival rates to the tumors with one level higher T category. For instance, survival rates of T3b and T4a are similar at 68% and 71%, respectively. Likewise, mitotic rates of more than or equal to 1/mm^2 are associated with decreased survival and, along with ulceration, differentiates T1a from T1b.

The number of metastatic nodes is a well-established risk factor of stage III patients, and historically there has been a consensus of a correlation between decreasing survival and increasing number of nodes [5–14]. The second most significant risk factor is tumor burden, determined by clinically occult or clinically palpable nodal disease [15], which also follows intuitively. However, a novel finding in 2001 [15] showed that tumor ulceration was the third most significant risk factor in stage III patients, suggesting that nodal metastasis arising from an ulcerated primary were more likely to metastasize to distant sites than those arising from non-ulcerated primaries. These findings prompted the updated 6th AJCC staging system to replace the previous one, and emphasize the diversity of Stage III melanoma.

History is further complicated by the introduction of the widespread use of sentinel lymph node (SLN) biopsies, which pushed patients who would previously have been a stage II into the stage III category. Patients who have positive sentinel lymph nodes are automatically deemed stage III, and a regional lymph node dissection is usually offered, according to current US guidelines. Not surprisingly, these ongoing modifications of staging have confounded the interpretation of clinical trial data, in the adjuvant setting.

Adjuvant Therapy for Melanoma

Due to the limited treatment options for metastatic melanoma, particularly in the past, adjuvant treatment has been the focus of much research. Several agents have been studied through the years dating back to the 1960s, starting with BCG vaccines [16]. Subsequent treatments that have been investigated include other vaccines, chemotherapy, hormonal therapy, biological therapy, and combinations. None of these had been shown to show any statistically significant increase in overall survival, and are summarized in Table 29.1.

A major breakthrough came with the FDA approval of high-dose IFN-α-2b (HDI) in 1995. Since then, there has been a wealth of research on various regimens and schedules of interferons. As the treatment options for stage IV melanoma have steadily been expanding since 2011, with the FDA approval of Ipilimumab, the landscape of adjuvant treatment continues to rapidly change as several new agents recently approved for metastatic melanoma, are now being tested as adjuvant therapy.

Interferon in the Adjuvant Therapy of Melanoma

Interferons were discovered in 1957, and were purified and cloned in the 1980s [17, 18]. The mechanisms by which interferons exert antitumor effects in melanoma are not fully known. Both animal and human studies have suggested that these effects are immunomodulatory, rather than cytotoxic. Administration of HDI in the neoadjuvant setting has shown an increase in T lymphocytes and dendritic cells at the tumor site, which may correlate with clinical response, supporting the role of IFN-α-2b as an immunomodulator [19]. Specific pathways such as MEK/ERK in the MAPK (mitogen activated protein kinase) pathway, which play a role in tumor metastasis, have been shown to be downregulated by high-dose interferon (HDI) [20], and STAT3, which is a transcription factor impli-

Table 29.1 Selected phase II/III studies of agents in the pre-interferon era

Treatment arms	Study reference	Type of study	Follow-up time reporting	OS	DFS
DTIC BCG DTIC and BCG Obs	Veronesi et al. [63]	Randomized phase III	5 years median	NS	NS
DTIC BCG DTIC and BCG Obs	Agarwala et al. [64]	Follow-up of randomized phase III	Up to 30 years	NS	NS
DTIC Levamisole/placebo	Lejeune et al. [65]	Randomized phase III[a]	4 years median	NS	NS
CCNU (nitosurea) Obs	Fisher et al. [66]	Randomized phase III	3 years median	NS	NS
Corynebacterium Parvum BCG	Lipton et al. [67]	Pooled analysis	[b]	Significant[c]	Significant
GM-CSF Obs	Spitler et al. [68]	Phase II open label	NR[d]	Significant	NS
GM-CSF Obs	Grotz et al. [69]	Retrospective cohort study	34 month median	NS	NS
Iscador M rIFN-α-2b rIFN-γ	Kleeberg [70]	Prospective randomized phase III	8.2 years median	NS	NS
GM2/BCG BCG	Livingstone et al. [25]	Randomized phase III trial	5 years and 3 months	NS	NS

[a]Patients were first randomized to receive with DTIC or not. Then those not randomized to DTIC were randomized (blinded) to receive either Levamisole or placebo
[b]Median in Hershey study was 7.4 years for BCG population and 9.4 for *C. parvum*; Median in SECSG study was 4.2 years for BCG population and 4.9 for *C. parvum* population
[c]In patients younger than 60 years of age
[d]Not reported

cated in promoting metastasis and angiogenesis in cancer cells [21], has also been shown to be downregulated by HDI.

As noted, there have been a multitude of IFN-α-2b based trials in patients with surgically resected melanoma. The Eastern Cooperative Oncology Group (ECOG) in the United States pioneered the use of the aggressive high-dose regimen that included an intravenous induction phase of 4 weeks duration followed my maintenance therapy. This induction phase has been tested in isolation without the maintenance phase. Other regimens have looked at intermediate and lower doses in various schedules administered subcutaneously. Finally, a long-acting, pegylated version has also been the focus of a large adjuvant trial in Europe. The design and outcomes of these trials are discussed below and summarized in Table 29.2.

High-Dose IFN-α-2b Trials

ECOG 1684

This landmark trial established the role of HDI in high-risk melanoma patients and led to FDA

Table 29.2 Selected phase III studies of INF-α-2b/INF-α-2a in adjuvant setting

Study reference	Year of publication	Stage	Treatment arms	Dosing and scheduling	Follow-up time	DFS	OS	ELND[a]
NCCTG Creagan et al. [71]	1995	II–III[b]	INF-α-2b versus observation	*High dose* 20 MU/m² IM Three times a week for 4 months	6.1 years median	NS	NS	N
ECOG E1684 Kirkwood et al. [22]	1996	II–III[c]	INF-α-2b versus observation	*High dose* 20 MU/m² IV 5 days a week for 4 weeks followed by 10 20 MU/m² for 48 weeks	12.6 years median	S	S at 6 years/NS at 12 years	Y
ECOG E1690 Kirkwood et al. [24]	2000	II–III[c]	INF-α-2b HDI vs. low-dose INF-α-2b vs. observation	*High dose:* 20 MU/m² IV 5 days a week for 4 weeks followed by 10 20 MU/m² for 48 weeks *Low dose:* 3 MU/m² SC 2 days a week for 2 years	6.6 years median	S	NS	N
ECOG 1694 Kirkwood et al. [27]	2001	II–III[c]	INF-α-2b vs. GMK vaccine	*High dose:* 20 MU/m² IV 5 days a week for 4 weeks followed by 10 20 MU/m² for 48 weeks	2.1 years median	S	S	N
ECOG E2696 Kirkwood et al. [72]	2001	II–III (IV was also included)[d]	INF-α-2b and GMK given concurrently versus sequentially beginning 1 month after initiation of GMK versus GMK alone	3 arms: Induction dose given with GMK followed by maintenance versus GMK followed by maintenance versus GMK alone	2.4 years median	S	S	N
Grob et al. [34]	1998	II[e]	IFN-α-2a Obs	*Low dose:* 3 MU INF α-2a three times a week for 18 months	5 years	S	NS	N
Pehamberger et al. [35]	1998	II[e]	INF-α-2a Obs	*Low dose:* 3 mIU SC once a day for 3 weeks followed by 3 mIU SC three times a week for 1 year	41 months mean	S	[f]	N
Cascinelli et al. [32]	2001	III	INF-α-2a vs. observation	*Low dose* 3 MU three times a week for 3 years		NS	NS	Y

Table 29.2 (continued)

Study reference	Year of publication	Stage	Treatment arms	Dosing and scheduling	Follow-up time	DFS	OS	ELND[a]
AIM-HIGH Hancock et al. [33]	2004	IIB–III	INF-α-2a vs. observation	*Low dose* 3 MU three times a week for 2 years		NS	NS	N
EORTC 18952 Eggermont et al. [30, 73]	2005 (long term 2016)	IIB–III	INF-α-2b (10 MU for 1 year or 5 MU for 2 years) vs. observation	*Intermediate dose* 4 weeks of 10 MU 5 days per week followed by either 10 MU three times a week for 1 year or 5 MU three times a week for 2 years	4.65 years median (11 years long term follow-up)	NS	NS	N
DeCOG trial Mohr et al. [40]	2008	III	INF-α-2b Pulsed dose vs. standard regimen	*Pulsed dose* 20 MU/m^2 IV 5 days a week for 4 weeks (induction dose) Q12 weeks for three cycles vs. standard regimen	55.4 months median	NS	NS	N
Hellenic Cooperative Oncology Group Pectasides et al. [36]	2009	IIB–III	INF-α-2b	Induction 15 MU/m^2 IV 5 days a week for 4 weeks followed by either 10 MU flat dose three times a week for 48 weeks or observation	63 month median	NS	NS	N
Italian Melanoma Intergroup trial Chiarion-Sileni et al. [41]	2011	III	INF-α-2b	Four cycles of induction dose Q2 months vs. standard regimen		NS	NS	Y
E1697 Agarwala et al. [39]	2017	IIB–III	INF-α-2b	*Induction dose* 20 MU/m^2 IV 5 days a week for 4 weeks vs. Obs	7 years	NS	NS	N

[a]ELND—elective lymph node dissection performed for staging
[b]T2-4N0M0/TanyNanyM0
[c]T4N0M0/TanyNanyM0
[d]Included stage IV disease, but resected metastasis
[e]Breslow thickness > =1.5 mm
[f]Not reported

approval of the specific regimen used in this trial in 1995. Between 1984 and 1990, 287 patients with stage IIB-IIIC surgically resected melanoma were randomized to receive either IFN-α-2b at 20 $MU/m^2/d$ IV (intravenously), 5 days a week, for 4 weeks, followed by three times a week at 10 $MU/m^2/d$ SC (subcutaneously), for 48 weeks, or observation. Results of this trial [22] showed the 5-year RFS (Relapse-free survival) to be 37% in the IFN-α-2b group compared with 26% in the observation group, and this difference was found to be of statistical significance with a *P*-value of 0.0023. Overall survival (OS) was also found to be statistically significantly increased at 2.8 years in the observation group, compared with 3.8 years in the treatment group ($P = 0.0237$). Of note, this trial was performed in the pre-sentinel node era and all patients were pathologically staged with elective lymph node dissections.

Toxicity was substantial, mostly hepatic and hematological, and was largely reversible after dose reductions or drug discontinuation. There were two fatalities, both related to hepatotoxicity and liver failure. A total of 67% of patients had severe (Grade 3) toxicity at some point during 1 year of treatment and 9% had life-threatening toxicities.

The therapeutic effects of IFN-α-2b appeared to be time dependent, with the greatest impact evident in the early part of the year of treatment, which raised the issue of the high-dose induction during the first 4 weeks, being of critical importance to the therapeutic benefits observed. This observation has spawned trials looking at the role of IV induction only regimens (discussed later). A mature follow-up of the ECOG 1684 at a median of 12.6 years showed a persistent statistically significant improvement in RFS in the treatment group. However, the OS difference between the arm receiving IFN-α-2b and the observation arm was no longer statistically significant [23].

Intergroup E1690

The subsequent E1690 [24] trial was conducted to confirm the findings of the E1684 trial and also to assess the efficacy of low-dose IFN-α-2b (LDI), as compared to high-dose IFN-α-2b and observation. The patient population was similar to that in ECOG 1684; however, lymph node dissections were not required for the patients without clinically evident lymph node involvement. In this trial, 642 patients, accrued between February 1991 and June 1995, were randomized to receive either the same HDI regimen as E1684, LDI (3 MU/d TIW) for 2 years or observation [24].

With regard to RFS, this trial showed a statistically significant improvement for the HDI group when compared with the observation group, with the observation arm having a 28% higher risk of recurrence (HR 1.28, $P = 0.05$). There was no statistically significant RFS benefit identified for those receiving LDI when compared to observation (HR 1.19, $P = 0.17$). Neither HDI nor LDI had any statistically significant impact on OS when compared to observation. The negative result for OS in this trial for HDI led to some controversy regarding the benefit of this regimen and an ongoing debate as to whether this should be offered to all high-risk patients.

However, several factors may have accounted for this difference in OS between the E1684 and E1690 trials [24]. The demographics were slightly different, in that there were a higher percentage of node-positive patients in ECOG 1684 (89%) when compared to E1690 (75%). Elective lymph node dissection (ELND) was not required to enter the E1690 study, if there was no clinical evidence of nodal disease given that this was prior to the era of SLN biopsies, one can only assume that the number of node-positive patients may have been underestimated in E1690, when compared to E1684. A plausible factor that may have blunted any potential OS benefit in E1690 was the use of salvage therapies. These included IFN-α-2b in patients who relapsed, or had disease progression on the observation arm, as this drug was approved by the FDA during the conduct of this trial. In fact, a significantly larger proportion of relapsed patients from the observation arm, 31%, received an IFN-α-2b-containing salvage regimen, compared with only 15% of patients from the HDI arm ($P = 0.003$). Patients in the observation arm were also twice as likely to receive higher doses IFN-α-2b therapy at relapse, compared with those who failed on the HDI arm [24].

ECOG 1694

After the FDA approval of high-dose IFN-α-2b, the search for newer and better agents continued, particularly given the concern for substantial toxicities associated with HDI. The ganglioside GM2 is a well-defined melanoma antigen, and it had been demonstrated that administration of GM2 in combination with BCG induces immunoglobulin IgM anti-GM2 antibodies in the majority of patients, and that these antibody responses were correlated with improved RFS and OS in AJCC stage III melanoma patients [25, 26]. On the basis of this data, intergroup trial E1694 was initiated in order to determine whether GMK vaccine (GM2 coupled to keyhole limpet hemocyanin (KLH) and combined with the QS-21 adjuvant 22) was superior to high-dose IFN-α-2b with respect to RFS and OS [27].

Between June 1996 and October 1999, 880 patients were randomized to receive either 1 mL of GMK vaccine administered via a deep subcutaneous (SC) injection on days 1, 8, 15, and 22, then every 12 weeks until week 96; or high-dose IFN-α-2b, 20 MU/m^2/d IV 5 days/week for 4 weeks followed by 10 MU/m^2 SC TIW (three times a week) for 48 weeks. In 2000, the study was un-blinded showing that 39% of those treated with GMK and 25% of those treated with IFN-α-2b had experienced relapse ($P = 0.0015$). Results also showed a more than 50% increase in the hazard of death in the GMK patient population when compared to the IFN-α-2b patients. These results caused the study to be terminated based on P-values crossing protocol-specific lower boundaries. Of note, a trial performed by the European Organisation for Research and Treatment of Cancer (EORTC), EORTC18961, showed that this same GMK vaccine had a significantly detrimental effect on DFS and OS compared with observation [28]. This has been used as an argument to refute the conclusion that improved DFS and OS in ECOG E1694 was due to a beneficial effect of HDI, because HDI treatment in ECOG E1694 was not compared with observation or placebo, but rather to a vaccine which may be detrimental to OS or DFS [29].

Intermediate Dose IFN-α-2b

EORTC Trial 18592

Between 1996 and 2000, patients with stage IIB–IIIC disease were randomized to receive either intermediate dose interferon for 13 months, 25 month, or observation in the EORTC 18592 study [30]. The dosing regimen for the two treatment groups was IFN-α-2b, 4 MU 5 days a week followed by either 10 MU three times a week for 1 year or 5 MU three times a week for 2 years. No overall statistically significant survival benefit or DMFI (distant-metastasis-free interval) was demonstrated for stage IIB–IIIC patients. When subgroup analysis was performed, it showed that adjuvant IFN-α-2b appeared to have a greater effect at an earlier stage of disease. When the patient population with stage IIB disease treated with 25 months was compared to observation the HR was 0.54, with CI 0.3–0.98 and $P = 0.008$, showing a borderline significant effect. No other subgroup analysis showed any statistically significant benefit [30].

A post hoc meta-analysis of patients from EORTC 18891 and 18952 (discussed later) [31] utilizing IFN-α-2b/PEG-IFN-α-2b showed the interesting finding that the greatest risk reductions were observed in patients with ulceration and stage IIB/III-N1 disease, with estimated HR for RFS, DMFS, and OS of 0.69 ($p = 0.003$), 0.59 ($p < 0.0001$), and 0.58 ($p < 0.0001$), respectively. Moreover, efficacy of IFN-α-2b/PEG-IFN-α-2b was uniformly absent in patients without ulceration.

Low-Dose IFN-α-2b

Low doses of IFN-α-2b have the obvious advantage of lower toxicity and cost. In 2001, Cascinelli et al. published results from a randomized controlled trial which compared 3 MU subcutaneously of recombinant IFN-α-2a three times a week for 3 years versus observation [32]. All of the 424 patients who entered into the study had a complete lymphadenectomy for pathologically proven regional nodal spread of surgically resected melanoma (Stage III). The results of this trial showed no statistically significant benefit in RFS or OS on this low dose of interferon when compared to observation. The AIM-HIGH study performed in the UK randomized patients with surgically resected stage IIB–IIIC melanoma to receive either 3 MU three times per week for 2 years/until recurrence or observation. The results of this study were published in 2004 [33], and again, no statistically significant benefit was demonstrated for OS or RFS.

Grob et al. published findings from their low-dose interferon trial in 1998. In this trial, 489 patients were randomized to receive either 3×10^6 IU of interferon alpha-2a, three-times weekly for 18 months, or no treatment. A long-term analysis, after a median follow-up of 5 years, showed an improvement in the relapse-free interval ($p = 0.035$) but no statistically significant increase in overall survival ($p = 0.059$) in the treatment group when compared with observation [34]. Similarly, an Austrian study showed prolonged disease-free survival in patients treated with low-dose IFN-α-2a versus those who underwent surgery alone ($P = 0.02$) [35].

Abbreviated Courses of IFN-α-2b

Hellenic Cooperative Oncology Group Study

In 2009, Pectasides et al. published the results from the Hellenic Cooperative Oncology Group study [36]. This study was a prospective, randomized study comparing IV induction therapy versus a full year of high-dose IFN-α-2a, with primary endpoints of RFS and OS for patients with stage IIB, IIC, and III melanoma, within 56 days of curative surgery. Patients were randomly assigned to receive either IFN-α-2b, 15 MU/m^2/day IV × 5 days a week for 4 weeks versus the same regimen followed by IFN-α-2b 10 MU (flat dose), administered subcutaneously three times a week for 48 weeks. A total of 364 patients were enrolled, of whom 353 were evalable for the study endpoints. Approximately 30% of the treated patients were stage IIB or IIC, and roughly 60% were stage IIIA–IIIC, with most being stage IIIB. The authors proposed the hypothesis that the 1-month induction regimen would be considered as efficacious as the conventional 1-year regimen, if the relapse rate at 3 years from study entry were to be no more than 15% higher in the first group, compared to the group receiving a 10 MU flat dose. The results of this trial did not show any statistically significant difference in RFS or OS, and hence the question arose as to whether the current regimen of induction followed by maintenance phase could be substituted by just the induction phase.

Several concerns have been raised regarding the results of this trial [37]. Both the induction dose and the flat dose used in the Greek trial were lower than the doses used in the standard HDI. Furthermore, this study set their non-inferiority margin at 15%, when the 5-year RFS previously observed between IFN-α-2b and observation were 9% and 11% [22, 24], with even smaller differences in RFS observed at 3 years. It follows that a 15% difference between two active treatment arms is an unrealistic expectation, particularly when using lower doses compared to the initial trials [38].

ECOG 1697

The prospect of a shorter duration of IFN-α-2b has been one of great interest. As noted earlier, the results of the HDI trials appeared to show a benefit that was most pronounced in the early part of treatment during the induction phase. The ECOG 1697 trial was designed to test the hypothesis of whether or not induction therapy alone is sufficient for patients in the adjuvant setting. A total of 1420 patients with intermediate- and high-risk melanoma were randomized to receive either 4 weeks of high-dose IFN-α-2b IV 5 days per week, as in the E1684 trial induction phase, or observation. Those included in the trial were patients with T2bN0, T3a-bN0, T4a-bN0, and T1-4N1a-2a (micrometastasis to one or two nodes). This patient population is different than in previous ECOG trials, such as E1684 and E1690, in that it includes patients with stages IIA–IIIA, as compared to IIB–IIIC. Patients from these groups were selected for the study because they were considered to be at intermediate risk for recurrence and particularly likely to be motivated to pursue a shorter and potentially less toxic adjuvant therapy regimen.

This study enrolled patient starting in 1998 and was terminated in 2010 based on futility analysis. Results were analyzed in 2015 with a median follow-up of 7 years, and there was no significant benefit in RFS or OS observed in the treatment group. Only 4.6% of patients in the observation group had treatment-related grade 3 AEs versus 57.9% in the treatment group ($P < 0.001$). These results suggest that there is no benefit in treating surgically resected melanoma with adjuvant IFN-α-2b with induction treatment only, and that a benefit can only be seen if 4 weeks of induction is followed by a year of maintenance [39].

Pulsed Doses of Induction IFN-α-2b

In the DeCOG (Dermatologic Cooperative Oncology Group) trial, patients with stage III (AJCC 2002) resected melanoma were randomly assigned to receive either standard HDI regimen or three courses of IFN-α-2b 20 MU/m^2/day IV 5 days a week (induction dose) for 4 weeks repeated every 4 months [40]. The results of this trial did not show any statistically significant improvement in RFS or OS for those treated with pulsed treatments; however, advantages related to health-related quality of life and safety profiles seemed favorable.

Another trial which looked at pulsed doses of IFN-α-2b at induction doses was the Italian Melanoma Inter-group trial which conducted a randomized clinical trial to verify if a more intense, but shorter than the ECOG 1684 regimen, could improve survival without increasing the toxicity profile. Patients were randomly assigned to the two treatment groups: IFN-α-2b 20 MU/m^2/day IV 5 days per week × 4 weeks, repeated for three times on weeks 9–12, 17–20, and 25–28 (Dose-Dense/Dose-Intense, DD/DI, arm), or IFN-α-2b 20 MU/m^2/day IV 5 days/week × 4 weeks followed by 10 MU/m^2 SC three times per week × 48 weeks (HDI, arm).

The analysis of toxicity and drug delivery data, on the first 166 patients who entered this study and completed the treatment, was published in 2006 [41]. It showed that patients were able to tolerate significantly intensified treatment in the DD/DI arm, without a significant increase in the overall toxicity when compared to the standard HDI therapy. However, there did not appear to be any meaningful benefit from this study [42].

Pegylated IFN

Pegylated interferon (PEG-IFN-α-2b) is a pegylated derivative of recombinant IFN-α2-b, in which the protein moiety, which has a molecular weight of 19 kDa, is combined with a single linear PEG chain, with an average molecular weight of 12 kDa [43]. Pegylation does not appear to have a substantial effect on biological activity; however, it does reduce IFN-α-2b immunogenicity, as well as increase the elimination half-life from approximately 4–40 h [44, 45]. The slower elimination of PEG-IFN-α-2b allows for a more convenient weekly injection of this agent during the maintenance phase.

PEG-IFN-α-2b and EORTC 18991

The European Organisation for Research and Treatment of Cancer (EORTC) 18991 was a large, Phase III, randomized controlled trial, designed to assess the effect of long-term administration of PEG-IFN-α-2b in patients with resected Stage III melanoma. All patients participating in this trial had histologically documented stage III melanoma, following a complete regional lymphadenectomy, and were randomized to either observation or PEG-IFN-α-2b. Patients were enrolled between 2000 and 2003. Stratification factors included microscopic versus palpable lymph node involvement, number of lymph nodes involved, Breslow's thickness, ulceration, gender, and site.

Patients randomized to PEG-IFN-α-2b had a 13% decrease in risk of recurrence or death compared with those on observation at a median follow-up of 7.6 years, approaching, but not reaching, statistical significance ($P = 0.055$). This was in contrast to the initial results at 3.8 years median follow-up that had shown a statistically significant increase in RFS. There was no overall survival benefit observed at 3.8 years follow-up or 7.6 years. The benefits seen with regard to RFS were mostly driven by N1 patients, patients with one involved lymph node, and patients with ulceration of their primary tumor. In fact, this trial was important in that it showed that a lower tumor burden, as well as ulceration, was a predictive factor for response to PEG-IFN-α-2b.

Although this trial struggled to show statistically significant improvement in RFS, and showed no improvement in OS for PEG-IFN-α-2b patients, the subgroup analysis performed had more promising results. In the patient population with microscopic nodal involvement only, as well as ulceration, the median overall survival for the patients receiving PEG-IFN-α-2b was more than 8 years vs. 3.7 years in the observation group ($P = 0.006$). In contrast, no benefit in DMFS or OS was observed in those patients with bulky nodal disease. PEG-IFN-α-2b was FDA approved for adjuvant treatment of Stage III melanoma in 2011 [46].

EORTC 18991 was the largest adjuvant melanoma trial to date at the time follow-up results were published [47]. Conclusions from the long-term results of this trial were published in 2012, showing that there was a sustained improvement in RFS in those treated with PEG-IFN-α-2b. The benefit was greatest in those with a lower tumor burden and ulcerated primaries. These findings were important, not only with regard to validating the use of PEG-IFN-α-2b, but also for shedding light on tumor ulceration and the impact this has on the benefit of interferon therapy.

Naturally, PEG-IFN-α-2b has potential advantages in that it lacks a requirement for intravenous induction and requires injections only once a week, as compared to three times a week in the maintenance phase, for IFN-α-2b in the ECOG regimen. These are all factors that may presumably impact quality of life for patients as well as use of health-related resources and lead to greater patient acceptance. Bottomley et al. found that prolonged treatment with PEG-IFN-α-2b impaired global Health Related Quality of Life (HRQOL) as compared with patients on the observation arm of EROTC 18991 [48]. Social functioning, fatigue, and appetite loss were key factors that could account for the lower HRQOL in this patient population. Similarly, quality of life (QoL) has been found to be negatively effected in patients receiving IFN-α-2b [49]. Although the quality of life of patients on both regimens has been measured separately, there has been no head-to-head comparison between PEG-IFN-α-2b and IFN-α-2b to date.

Summary of Interferon Trials in the Adjuvant Setting for High-Risk Melanoma

Low-dose IFN-α-2b has not been shown to be beneficial when compared to observation, as evidenced by the European studies mentioned above [32, 33]. In addition, the E1690 trial [24] compared high-dose IFN-α-2b, low-dose IFN-α-2b, and observation, and here too, no statistically significant benefit in low-dose IFN-α-2b, with regard to RFS or OS, was demonstrated when compared to observation. Low dose remains approved for adjuvant use in resected melanoma in Europe. Intermediate dose IFN-α-2b did not show any statistically significant benefit for DMFS, DFS, or OS in the EORTC 18952 trial. The recently released results of ECOG 1697 fail to show any benefit in treating patients with the induction dose only when considering OS and RFS [39]. Repeated doses of induction doses or "pulsed therapy" of IFN-α-2b has also been tested in the two aforementioned European trials [40, 41], none of which showed any statistically significant benefit in OS or RFS.

The only regimen of IFN-α-2b that remains proven to give meaningful therapeutic benefit are IFN-α-2b as used in the ECOG 1684 trial, and PEG IFN-α-2b as used in the EORTC 18991. While PEG-IFN-α-2b is FDA approved for stage IIIA–IIIC only, IFN-α-2b is an option for those with stage IIB–IIIC. Arguments against the use of IFN-α-2b in the adjuvant setting have persisted [50], although, this has been tempered by the fact that there was no alternative treatment until 2015. In 2002, Lens et al. performed a systematic review of all trials to date, finding no evidence that there was a benefit in IFN-α-2b in the adjuvant setting for melanoma [51]. In contrast, Mocellin et al. conducted a systematic review and meta-analysis with results published in 2010 [52]. The meta-analysis included 14 RTC, and involved 8122 patients, and identified a statistically significant decrease in risk of death (HR 0.89, CI 95% 0.83–0.96 P = 0.002) and an improved DFS (HR 0.82, 95% CI 0.77–0.87, P = 0.001). The debate is likely to continue and there does appear to be somewhat of a "transatlantic divide," where HDI has been declared standard of care for high-risk melanoma and is widely used in the USA, while it is not used widely in Europe and the rest of the world [53].

Checkpoint Inhibitors

The checkpoint inhibitors have been a major breakthrough in treatment of metastatic melanoma, starting with the approval of ipilimumab in 2011. There are currently five checkpoint inhibitors that are FDA approved in the USA for the treatment of melanoma and other cancers: Ipilimumab [CTLA-4 inhibitor], the PD-1 inhibitors [Nivolumab and Pembrolizumab], and the PDL-1 inhibitors [Atezolizumab and Avelumab]. Of these, only the CTLA-4 and PD-1 inhibitors are FDA approved for melanoma, and only Ipilimumab is FDA approved in the adjuvant setting.

Cancer cells exhibit tumor antigens that can trigger the immune system, and these are processed and presented to cytotoxic T-cells by dendritic cells, potentially priming the immune system to fight the cancer cells. However, along with presenting the cytotoxic T-cell with the cancer antigen, the dendritic cells also transmit an inhibitory signal that downregulates the T-cell response. CTLA-4 (cytotoxic T-lymphocyte-associated protein 4) is a protein receptor on T-cells, which downregulates the immune system by transmitting an inhibitory signal to these cells, when dendritic cells stimulate these receptors.

Ipilimumab is a fully human monoclonal antibody, which blocks the inhibitory pathway at the CTLA-4 receptor, leading to an enhanced immune response. The PD-1 protein on the surface of activated T cells sends an inhibitory signal to the T cell as well, when PD-L1 or PD-L2 binds to it. Nivolumab and Pembrolizumab are both humanized monoclonal antibodies which inhibit PD-1, thus heightening the immune response. The above pathways work as "check points" and are intended to keep the human immune system from overreacting and causing a pathological or exaggerated immune response. Checkpoint inhibitors block these processes and aid the immune system in fighting cancer cells.

Ipilimumab in Adjuvant Therapy

EORTC 18071

In 2011, Ipilimumab was FDA approved for the treatment of metastatic melanoma based upon favorable results from a large, randomized, controlled trial [54–56]. This radically altered the landscape for advanced melanoma as being the first ever phase III, randomized, controlled trial to improve overall survival in patients with this disease. Not surprisingly, this agent very quickly moved into the adjuvant arena as part of clinical trials research.

EORTC 18071 was a double-blinded, Phase III trial, where 951 patients with stage III, surgically resected melanoma were randomly assigned to receive either 10 mg/kg of Ipilimumab or placebo every 3 weeks for four doses, then every 3 months for up to 3 years. Patients with lymph node metastasis less than or equal to 1 mm, or in-transit metastasis, were not included in this study. Complete regional lymphadenectomy was required within 12 weeks prior to randomization.

The primary endpoint of this trial was recurrence-free survival. Distant-metastasis-free survival, overall survival, and health-related quality of life were secondary endpoints. Recurrence-free survival was significantly longer in the Ipilimumab group when compared to the placebo, with a HR of 0.75 and 95% CI 0.64–0.9 and P = 0.0013. Median recurrence-free survival in the Ipilimumab group was 26.1 months compared with the placebo group at 17.1 months, with a 3-year recurrence-free survival of 46.5%

in the Ipilimumab group, compared to 34.8% in the placebo group.

Immune-related adverse events (AEs) were more frequent in the Ipilimumab group than in the placebo group, and the most common of these were GI, hepatic, and endocrine in nature. Five patients (1%) in the Ipilimumab group of patients died due to drug-related AEs, 3 of which were colitis, 1 myocarditis, and 1 with MOF (multisystem organ failure) and GBS (Guillain-Barre syndrome). In addition, AEs resulted in 40% of patients discontinuing treatment before maintenance therapy was started, and this rate is higher than that reported with advanced disease [56]. Most ir-AEs (immune-related adverse events) resolved within 4–6 weeks; however, for endocrinopathies, the median time to resolution was 31 weeks.

Based on the results of EORTC 18071, high-dose Ipilimumab (10 mg/kg) was FDA approved for the adjuvant treatment of surgically resected, stage 3 melanoma in 2015. However, its use is not without controversy, primarily because of the toxicity and the fact that the dose is significantly higher than the 3 mg/kg dose approved for metastatic melanoma. In November 2016, survival data was made available and showed a 65.4% overall survival in the ipilimumab group, versus 54.4% in the placebo group ($P = 0.001$). Additionally, there was a 48.3% distant-metastasis-free survival rate in the Ipilimumab group compared to 38.9% in the placebo arm ($P = 0.002$) [57]. This has certainly provided reassurance, but concern regarding the toxicity remains.

The Future of Adjuvant Therapy for High-Risk Melanoma

High-dose IFN remains a standard adjuvant treatment option for high-risk melanoma patients. An important, and as yet, unanswered question is whether ipilimumab is superior to IFN in a randomized trial. The intergroup E1609 trial comparing low-dose Ipilimumab (3 mg/kg) and high-dose Ipilimumab (10 mg/kg) with IFN-α-2b has completed accrual and the results of this trial are awaited with great interest. Of note, this trial is not powered to look for a difference between high- and low-dose ipilimumab.

PD-1 Inhibitors in Adjuvant Therapy

Given the superiority of PD-1 inhibitors over ipilimumab in a head-to-head comparison in metastatic melanoma, the role of these agents in the adjuvant setting needs to be addressed [58]. The fact that PD-1 inhibitors are significantly less toxic than ipilimumab is an obvious advantage in the adjuvant setting. Not surprisingly, several adjuvant trials are in progress looking at these agents in adjuvant therapy. The SWOG (Southwestern Oncology Group)-led intergroup trial, S1404, is randomizing patients with stage III, resected melanoma to either Ipilimumab (10 mg/kg) or IFN-α-2b (both considered standard of care and chosen at the discretion of the treating physician) versus pembrolizumab [59].

The CheckMate 238 trial, testing nivolumab versus Ipilimumab, will complete data collection in November 2018. Similarly, the EORTC 1352/KEYNOTE-054 trial, comparing pembrolizumab to placebo will complete data collection in August 2017. This trial allows un-blinding at progression, with crossover to pembrolizumab for patients receiving placebo. This trial may help to answer the question of whether delaying initiation of therapy at relapse is as good as upfront therapy in the high-risk setting.

Targeted Therapy Trials in Patients with *BRAF*$^{V600E/K}$ Positive Melanoma

A major breakthrough in the therapy for metastatic melanoma patients, whose tumors harbor the BRAF mutation, is MAP-kinase pathway therapy targeting BRAF and MEK [60]. Drugs approved include vemurafenib, dabrafenib, trametinib, and cobimetinib. These agents have also moved into adjuvant therapy trials. A Phase III, randomized, double-blinded trial comparing Vemurafenib (960 mg orally, twice daily for 52 weeks) to placebo in patients with stage IIC and stage III resected melanoma, positive for the *BRAF* ^{V600} mutation, completed final data collection in June 2016 and results are currently pending [61].

Similarly, the *BRAF*-inhibitor Dabrafenib, in combination with the MEK inhibitor, Trametinib, is being compared to placebo in a randomized double-blinded study for patients with high-risk, BRAF V600 mutation positive, melanoma after surgical resection. This study has also completed final data collection and the results are pending. Combination therapy with Dabrafenib and Trametinib has been shown to improve OS, when compared to dabrafenib alone in *BRAF* ^{V600} positive patients with metastatic melanoma [62].

We are entering into a new era of adjuvant treatment for stage III melanoma. For decades, IFN-α-2b and, more recently, PEG-IFN-α2b were the only treatment options for adjuvant therapy of melanoma. It is time to move the field forward, and it is hoped that the recently completed and ongoing trials outlined above will provide valuable information on new treatment options. For a summary of selected ongoing trials for adjuvant treatment of melanoma, see Tables 29.3 and 29.4.

Perhaps the true mark of success for us in melanoma therapy will be when our treatments for stage IV disease are good enough to cure all patients, and the entire concept of adjuvant therapy can be made obsolete. However, it will be a while before we can reach that goal, if ever, and until then, an effective way to prevent stage IV disease will continue to be a major, unmet clinical need.

Table 29.3 Selected ongoing phase III studies with checkpoint inhibitors ongoing/results pending

Study	Stage	Treatment arms
CheckMate 238	III B–C and IV[a]	Nivolumab vs. Ipilimumab
E 1609	III–IV[a]	*Arm A (high-dose Ipilimumab)* Ipilimumab 10 mg/kg Q3W for 4 weeks followed by 10 mg/kg Q90days for a maximum of four doses *Arm B (high-dose INF-α-2b)* INF-α-2b 20 MU/m^2 IV 5 days a week for 4 weeks followed by 10 20 MU/m^2 for 48 weeks. Arm C (low-dose Ipilimumab) Ipilimumab 3 mg/kg Q3W for 4 weeks followed by 3 mg/kg Q90days for a maximum of four doses
KEYNOTE-054	III	Pembrolizumab 200 mg Q3W for up to 1 year vs. Placebo
S1404	III and IV[a]	Arm A INF-α-2b 20 MU/m^2 IV 5 days a week for 4 weeks followed by 10 20 MU/m^2 for 48 weeks or Ipilimumab 10 mg/kg Q3W for 4 weeks followed by 10 mg/kg Q90days for a maximum of four doses Arm B Pembrolizumab 200 mg Q3W for up to 1 year

[a]Resected

Table 29.4 Selected ongoing phase III studies with targeted therapy for *BRAF* $^{V600E/K}$ positive high-risk melanoma

Study	Stage	Treatment arms
COMBI-AD	III	Dabrafenib 150 mg BID and Trametinib 2 mg QD PO for 12 months vs. Placebo
BRIM 8	IIC and III	Vemurafenib 960 mg PO BID for 52 weeks vs. Placebo

References

1. Siegel RL, Miller KD, Jemal A. Cancer statistics, 2017. CA Cancer J Clin. 2017;67(1):7–30.
2. Balch CM, et al. Multivariate analysis of prognostic factors among 2,313 patients with stage III melanoma: comparison of nodal micrometastases versus macrometastases. J Clin Oncol. 2010;28(14):2452–9.
3. Agarwala SS. An update on pegylated IFN-α2b for the adjuvant treatment of melanoma. Expert Rev Anticancer Ther. 2012;12(11):1449–59.
4. Balch CM, et al. Final version of 2009 AJCC melanoma staging and classification. J Clin Oncol. 2009;27(36):6199–206.
5. Buzaid AC, et al. Critical analysis of the current American Joint Committee on Cancer staging system for cutaneous melanoma and proposal of a new staging system. J Clin Oncol. 1997;15(3):1039–51.
6. Balch CM, et al. A multifactorial analysis of melanoma: III. Prognostic factors in melanoma patients with lymph node metastases (stage II). Ann Surg. 1981;193(3):377.
7. Balch CM. Cutaneous melanoma: prognosis and treatment results worldwide. In: Seminars in surgical oncology. Wiley Online Library; 1992.
8. Calabro A, Singletary SE, Balch CM. Patterns of relapse in 1001 consecutive patients with melanoma nodal metastases. Arch Surg. 1989;124(9):1051–5.
9. Gershenwald J, et al. The prognostic significance of microscopic tumor burden in 925 melanoma patients undergoing sentinel lymph node biopsy. Proc Am Soc Clin Oncol. 2000;19:551a.
10. Morton DL, et al. Improved long-term survival after lymphadenectomy of melanoma metastatic to regional nodes. Analysis of prognostic factors in 1134 patients from the John Wayne Cancer Clinic. Ann Surg. 1991;214(4):491.
11. Coit DG, Rogatko A, Brennan MF. Prognostic factors in patients with melanoma metastatic to axillary or inguinal lymph nodes. A multivariate analysis. Ann Surg. 1991;214(5):627.
12. Bevilacqua RG, et al. Axillary dissection in melanoma. Prognostic variables in node-positive patients. Ann Surg. 1990;212(2):125.
13. Drepper H, et al. The prognosis of patients with stage III melanoma prospective long-term study of 286 patients of the fachklinik hornheide. Cancer. 1993;71(4):1239–46.
14. Cascinelli N, et al. Prognosis of skin melanoma with regional node metastases (stage II). J Surg Oncol. 1984;25(4):240–7.
15. Balch CM, et al. Prognostic factors analysis of 17,600 melanoma patients: validation of the American Joint Committee on Cancer melanoma staging system. J Clin Oncol. 2001;19(16):3622–34.
16. Eilber FR, et al. Adjuvant immunotherapy with BCG in treatment of regional-lymph-node metastases from malignant melanoma. N Engl J Med. 1976;294(5):237–40.
17. Isaacs A, Lindenmann J. Virus interference. I. The interferon. Proc R Soc Lond B Biol Sci. 1957;147(927):258–67.
18. Pestka S. The human interferons—from protein purification and sequence to cloning and expression in bacteria: before, between, and beyond. Arch Biochem Biophys. 1983;221(1):1–37.
19. Moschos SJ, et al. Neoadjuvant treatment of regional stage IIIB melanoma with high-dose interferon alfa-2b induces objective tumor regression in association with modulation of tumor infiltrating host cellular immune responses. J Clin Oncol. 2006;24(19):3164–71.
20. Wang W, et al. Impact of IFNα2b upon pSTAT3 and the MEK/ERK MAPK pathway in melanoma. Cancer Immunol Immunother. 2008;57(9):1315–21.
21. Kortylewski M, Jove R, Yu H. Targeting STAT3 affects melanoma on multiple fronts. Cancer Metastasis Rev. 2005;24(2):315–27.
22. Kirkwood JM, et al. Interferon alfa-2b adjuvant therapy of high-risk resected cutaneous melanoma: the Eastern Cooperative Oncology Group Trial EST 1684. J Clin Oncol. 1996;14(1):7–17.
23. Kirkwood JM, et al. A pooled analysis of eastern cooperative oncology group and intergroup trials of adjuvant high-dose interferon for melanoma. Clin Cancer Res. 2004;10(5):1670–7.
24. Kirkwood JM, et al. High-and low-dose interferon alfa-2b in high-risk melanoma: first analysis of intergroup trial E1690/S9111/C9190. J Clin Oncol. 2000;18(12):2444–58.
25. Livingston PO, et al. Improved survival in stage III melanoma patients with GM2 antibodies: a randomized trial of adjuvant vaccination with GM2 ganglioside. J Clin Oncol. 1994;12(5):1036–44.
26. Livingston PO, et al. Characterization of IgG and IgM antibodies induced in melanoma patients by immunization with purified GM2 ganglioside. Cancer Res. 1989;49(24 Part 1):7045–50.
27. Kirkwood JM, et al. High-dose interferon alfa-2b significantly prolongs relapse-free and overall survival compared with the GM2-KLH/QS-21 vaccine in patients with resected stage IIB–III melanoma: results of intergroup trial E1694/S9512/C509801. J Clin Oncol. 2001;19(9):2370–80.
28. Eggermont AM, et al. Adjuvant ganglioside GM2-KLH/QS-21 vaccination versus observation after resection of primary tumor >1.5 mm in patients with stage II melanoma: results of the EORTC 18961 randomized phase III trial. J Clin Oncol. 2013;31(30):3831–7.
29. McMasters KM, et al. Final results of the sunbelt melanoma trial: a multi-institutional prospective randomized phase III study evaluating the role of adjuvant high-dose interferon alfa-2b and completion lymph node dissection for patients staged by sentinel lymph node biopsy. J Clin Oncol. 2016;34(10):1079–86.
30. Eggermont AM, et al. Long term follow up of the EORTC 18952 trial of adjuvant therapy in resected stage IIB–III cutaneous melanoma patients comparing intermediate doses of interferon-alpha-2b (IFN) with

observation: ulceration of primary is key determinant for IFN-sensitivity. Eur J Cancer. 2016;55:111–21.
31. Eggermont AM, et al. Ulceration and stage are predictive of interferon efficacy in melanoma: results of the phase III adjuvant trials EORTC 18952 and EORTC 18991. Eur J Cancer. 2012;48(2):218–25.
32. Cascinelli N, et al. Effect of long-term adjuvant therapy with interferon alpha-2a in patients with regional node metastases from cutaneous melanoma: a randomised trial. Lancet. 2001;358(9285):866–9.
33. Hancock BW, et al. Adjuvant interferon in high-risk melanoma: the AIM HIGH Study—United Kingdom Coordinating Committee on Cancer Research randomized study of adjuvant low-dose extended-duration interferon Alfa-2a in high-risk resected malignant melanoma. J Clin Oncol. 2004;22(1):53–61.
34. Grob JJ, et al. Randomised trial of interferon α-2a as adjuvant therapy in resected primary melanoma thicker than 1· 5 mm without clinically detectable node metastases. Lancet. 1998;351(9120):1905–10.
35. Pehamberger H, et al. Adjuvant interferon alfa-2a treatment in resected primary stage II cutaneous melanoma. Austrian Malignant Melanoma Cooperative Group. J Clin Oncol. 1998;16(4):1425–9.
36. Pectasides D, et al. Randomized phase III study of 1 month versus 1 year of adjuvant high-dose interferon alfa-2b in patients with resected high-risk melanoma. J Clin Oncol. 2009;27(6):939–44.
37. Hauschild A. Adjuvant interferon alfa for melanoma: new evidence-based treatment recommendations. Curr Oncol. 2009;16(3):3–6.
38. Agarwala SS, Gray RJ, Wong MK. Duration of high-dose interferon alfa-2b regimen for resected high-risk melanoma. J Clin Oncol. 2009;27(25):e82–3.
39. Agarwala SS, et al. Phase III Randomized Study of 4 Weeks of High-Dose Interferon-α-2b in Stage T2bNO, T3a-bNO, T4a-bNO, and T1-4N1a-2a (microscopic) Melanoma: A Trial of the Eastern Cooperative Oncology Group–American College of Radiology Imaging Network Cancer Research Group (E1697). J Clin Oncol. 2017;35:885–92.
40. Mohr P, et al. Intermittent high-dose intravenous interferon alpha 2b (IFNa2b) for adjuvant treatment of stage III malignant melanoma: an interim analysis of a randomized phase III study (NCT00226408). J Clin Oncol. 2008;26(15_suppl):9040.
41. Chiarion-Sileni V, et al. Intensified high-dose intravenous interferon alpha 2b (IFNa2b) for adjuvant treatment of stage III melanoma: a randomized phase III Italian Melanoma Intergroup (IMI) trial [ISRCTN75125874]. J Clin Oncol. 2011;29(15_suppl):8506.
42. Chiarion-Sileni V, et al. Tolerability of intensified intravenous interferon alfa-2b versus the ECOG 1684 schedule as adjuvant therapy for stage III melanoma: a randomized phase III Italian Melanoma Intergroup trial (IMI–Mel. A.)[ISRCTN75125874]. BMC Cancer. 2006;6(1):44.
43. Bukowski RM, et al. Treating cancer with PEG Intron. Cancer. 2002;95(2):389–96.
44. Glue P, et al. Pegylated interferon-α2b: pharmacokinetics, pharmacodynamics, safety, and preliminary efficacy data. Clin Pharmacol Ther. 2000;68(5):556–67.
45. Daud A, et al. Pharmacokinetic/pharmacodynamic analysis of adjuvant pegylated interferon α-2b in patients with resected high-risk melanoma. Cancer Chemother Pharmacol. 2011;67(3):657–66.
46. Herndon TM, et al. US Food and Drug Administration Approval: peginterferon-alfa-2b for the adjuvant treatment of patients with melanoma. Oncologist. 2012;17(10):1323–8.
47. Eggermont AM, et al. Long-term results of the randomized phase III trial EORTC 18991 of adjuvant therapy with pegylated interferon alfa-2b versus observation in resected stage III melanoma. J Clin Oncol. 2012;30:3810–8.
48. Bottomley A, et al. Adjuvant therapy with pegylated interferon alfa-2b versus observation in resected stage III melanoma: a phase III randomized controlled trial of health-related quality of life and symptoms by the European Organisation for Research and Treatment of Cancer Melanoma Group. J Clin Oncol. 2009;27(18):2916–23.
49. Trask PC, et al. Longitudinal course of depression, fatigue, and quality of life in patients with high risk melanoma receiving adjuvant interferon. Psycho-Oncology. 2004;13(8):526–36.
50. Chapman PB. Counterpoint: the case against adjuvant high-dose interferon-α for melanoma patients. J Natl Compr Cancer Netw. 2004;2(1):69–72.
51. Lens MB, Dawes M. Interferon alfa therapy for malignant melanoma: a systematic review of randomized controlled trials. J Clin Oncol. 2002;20(7):1818–25.
52. Mocellin S, et al. Interferon alpha adjuvant therapy in patients with high-risk melanoma: a systematic review and meta-analysis. J Natl Cancer Inst. 2010;102(7):493–501.
53. Kefford R. Adjuvant therapy of cutaneous melanoma: the interferon debate. Ann Oncol. 2003;14(3):358–65.
54. Hodi FS, et al. Improved survival with ipilimumab in patients with metastatic melanoma. N Engl J Med. 2010;2010(363):711–23.
55. Robert C, et al. Ipilimumab plus dacarbazine for previously untreated metastatic melanoma. N Engl J Med. 2011;364(26):2517–26.
56. Lebbé C, et al. Survival follow-up and ipilimumab retreatment of patients with advanced melanoma who received ipilimumab in prior phase II studies. Ann Oncol. 2014;25(11):2277–84.
57. Eggermont AM, et al. Prolonged survival in stage III melanoma with ipilimumab adjuvant therapy. N Engl J Med. 2016;375(19):1845–55.
58. Wolchok JD, Chiarion-Sileni V, Gonzalez R, Rutkowski P, Grob JJ, Cowey CL, Lao CD, Wagstaff J, Schadendorf D, Ferrucci PF, Smylie M. Overall survival with combined nivolumab and ipilimumab in advanced melanoma. New England Journal of Medicine. 2017 Oct 5;377(14):1345–56.

59. Grossmann KF, et al. SWOG S1404: a phase III randomized trial comparing high dose interferon to pembrolizumab in patients with high risk resected melanoma. Am Soc Clin Oncol; 2015
60. Chapman PB, et al. Improved survival with vemurafenib in melanoma with BRAF V600E mutation. N Engl J Med. 2011;364(26):2507–16.
61. Lewis KD, et al. BRIM8: A phase III, randomized, double-blind, placebo-controlled study of vemurafenib adjuvant therapy in patients with surgically resected, cutaneous BRAF-mutant melanoma at high risk for recurrence (NCT01667419). Am Soc Clin Oncol; 2014.
62. Robert C, et al. Improved overall survival in melanoma with combined dabrafenib and trametinib. N Engl J Med. 2015;372(1):30–9.
63. Veronesi U, et al. A randomized trial of adjuvant chemotherapy and immunotherapy in cutaneous melanoma. N Engl J Med. 1982;307(15):913–6.
64. Agarwala SS, et al. Mature results of a phase III randomized trial of bacillus Calmette-Guerin (BCG) versus observation and BCG plus dacarbazine versus BCG in the adjuvant therapy of American Joint Committee on Cancer Stage I-III melanoma (E1673): a trial of the Eastern Oncology Group. Cancer. 2004;100(8):1692–8.
65. Lejeune F, et al. An assessment of DTIC versus levamisole or placebo in the treatment of high risk stage I patients after surgical removal of a primary melanoma of the skin. A phase III adjuvant study. EORTC protocol 18761. Eur J Cancer Clin Oncol. 1988;24:81–90.
66. Fisher RI, et al. Adjuvant immunotherapy or chemotherapy for malignant melanoma: preliminary report of the National Cancer Institute randomized clinical trial. Surg Clin N Am. 1981;61(6):1267–77.
67. Lipton A, et al. Corynebacterium parvum versus bacille Calmette-Guérin adjuvant immunotherapy of stage II malignant melanoma. J Clin Oncol. 1991;9(7):1151–6.
68. Spitler LE, et al. Adjuvant therapy of stage III and IV malignant melanoma using granulocyte-macrophage colony-stimulating factor. J Clin Oncol. 2000;18(8):1614–21.
69. Grotz TE, et al. Adjuvant GM-CSF improves survival in high risk stage IIIc melanoma: a single center study. Am J Clin Oncol. 2014;37(5):467.
70. Kleeberg U, et al. Final results of the EORTC 18871/DKG 80-1 randomised phase III trial: rIFN-α2b versus rIFN-γ versus ISCADOR M® versus observation after surgery in melanoma patients with either high-risk primary (thickness >3 mm) or regional lymph node metastasis. Eur J Cancer. 2004;40(3):390–402.
71. Creagan ET, et al. Randomized, surgical adjuvant clinical trial of recombinant interferon alfa-2a in selected patients with malignant melanoma. J Clin Oncol. 1995;13(11):2776–83.
72. Kirkwood JM, et al. High-dose interferon alfa-2b does not diminish antibody response to GM2 vaccination in patients with resected melanoma: results of the Multicenter Eastern Cooperative Oncology Group Phase II Trial E2696. J Clin Oncol. 2001;19(5):1430–6.
73. Eggermont AM, et al. Post-surgery adjuvant therapy with intermediate doses of interferon alfa 2b versus observation in patients with stage IIb/III melanoma (EORTC 18952): randomised controlled trial. Lancet. 2005;366(9492):1189–96.

Radiation Therapy for Melanoma

30

Noelle L. Williams, Brittany A. Simone, Pramila R. Anné, and Wenyin Shi

Historical Perspective

Radiotherapy (RT) works by inducing DNA damage in cancer cells. There are several different methods of RT delivery including external beam radiotherapy (EBRT), stereotactic radiosurgery (SRS), stereotactic body radiotherapy (SBRT), brachytherapy, and particle therapy. RT indications in the treatment of melanoma vary, and are most commonly deemed palliative in nature. This frequently includes patients who develop symptomatic metastases or locally unresectable disease. In the case of oligometastatic disease, SRS and SBRT are increasingly utilized. While RT is seldom indicated for definitive therapy to regional nodal basins, adjuvant RT following surgical resection does appear to have an effect on the rate of local recurrence for high-risk patients (including those with multiple positive lymph nodes, one or more large lymph nodes over 3 cm, extracapsular extension, or recurrent disease) [1, 2].

Historically, melanoma has been deemed a radioresistant tumor, due to early in vitro studies demonstrating a broad shoulder in cell survival curves, indicating higher survival fraction at the low dose range due to a high repair capacity [3, 4]. Conflicting clinical experience with varying doses per fraction prompted a multicenter randomized phase III study through the Radiation Therapy Oncology Group (RTOG). This study (RTOG 8305) was one of many evaluating varying radiation dosing schemes. In this trial, 137 patients with metastatic melanoma received radiation in 8 Gy fractions, weekly for four doses, versus 2.5 Gy fractions daily for 20 fractions. There was no difference in the clinical response rate, however, short follow-up and non-standard fractionation patterns led to some difficulty in further interpreting this trial [5]. There have been multiple other retrospective studies evaluating various hypofractionated regimens, and this type of fractionation (2.5 Gy or higher per fraction) has become commonplace in the treatment of melanoma given its tolerability, convenience, and low risk of late effects.

There have been multiple advancements in the field of oncology, including technological RT developments in addition to an evolution of systemic therapy and immunotherapy, highlighting the importance of a multidisciplinary approach to treating melanoma. While RT historically has had a more limited role in the primary management of melanoma, there have been several recent intriguing developments, including the combination of RT with immunotherapy for patients with more advanced disease.

N. L. Williams, M.D. · B. A. Simone, D.O.
P. R. Anné, M.D. · W. Shi, M.D., Ph.D. (✉)
Department of Radiation Oncology, Sidney Kimmel Medical College, Thomas Jefferson University, Philadelphia, PA, USA
e-mail: Noelle.Williams@jefferson.edu; Brittany.Simone@jefferson.edu; Pramila.Anne@jefferson.edu; Wenyin.shi@jefferson.edu

A. I. Riker (ed.), *Melanoma*, https://doi.org/10.1007/978-3-319-78310-9_30

Radiotherapy Technological Advancements

EBRT has continued to see significant advancements with the evolution of high-resolution computed tomography (CT), magnetic resonance imaging (MRI), and advancements in radiation delivery techniques. Two-dimensional techniques have evolved into three-dimensional techniques with implementation of CT-planning scans. The development of inverse planning such as intensity-modulated radiotherapy (IMRT) and volumetric-modulated arc therapy (VMAT) has allowed for an even more precise method of RT delivery, while sparing normal tissues and decreasing associated toxicity [6].

SRS refers to a precisely delivered, single large dose of radiation achieved by multiple non-coplanar beams converging on a radiographically defined target [7]. For this type of RT delivery, there is a steep decline of the radiation dose just outside the target volume, thereby limiting the dose to normal critical structures (Fig. 30.1). Brain metastases occur in more than half of patients with advanced melanoma, with the majority of patients dying from central nervous

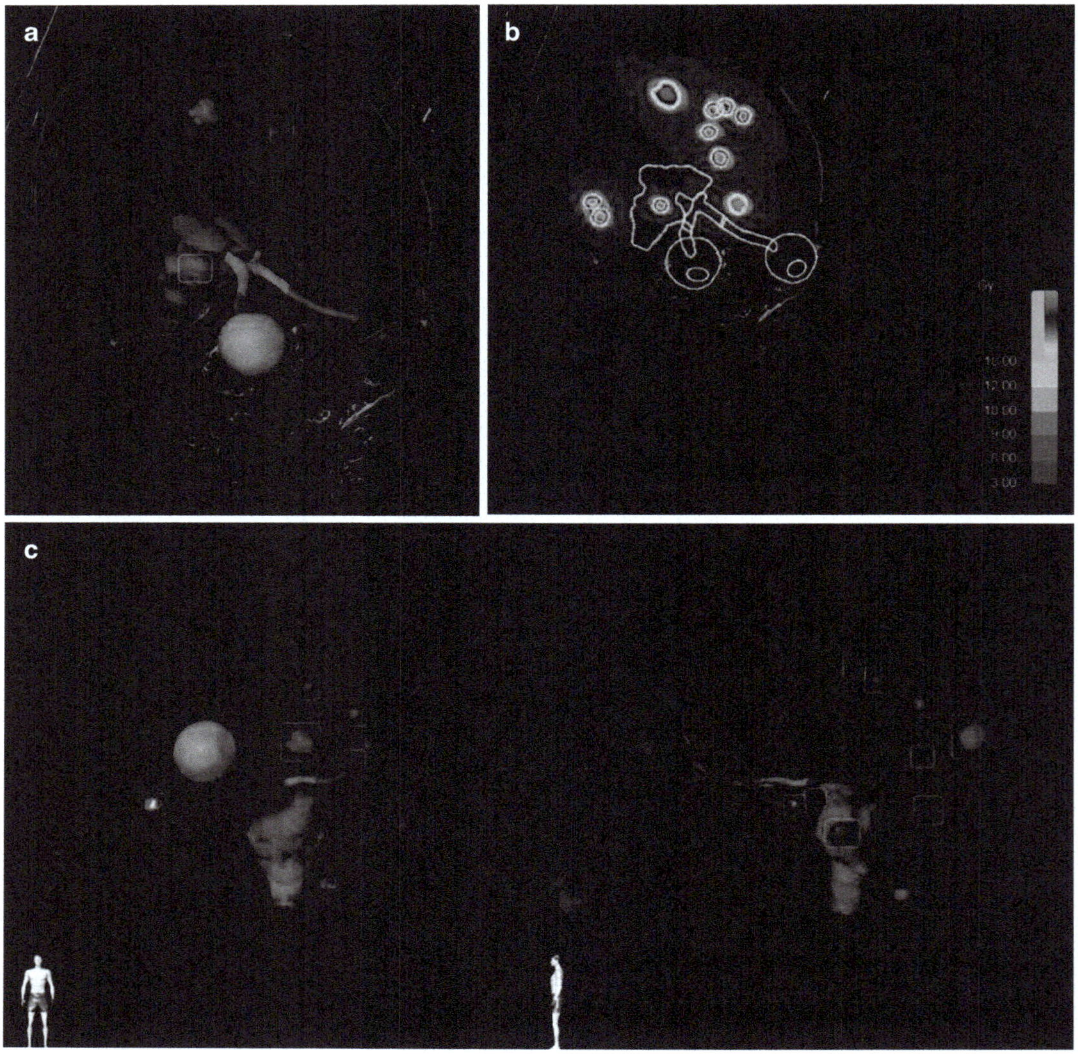

Fig. 30.1 Sample SRS plan for multiple brain metastases. (**a**–**c**) demonstrate different views of the multiple brain metastases being treated with SRS

system disease burden [8, 9]. Prior to the development of SRS, patients with brain metastases from melanoma were often treated surgically or with whole brain radiotherapy (WBRT). While WBRT may decrease the likelihood of neurologic death in these patients, overall survival following RT remains approximately 3–4 months, and has associated neurological side effects including cognitive decline [10]. SRS can alternatively be used for patients with a small number of metastases with current reports showing median survival times of approximately 5–6 months [11, 12].

SBRT is another example of a more recent advancement with applications in melanoma. SBRT refers to high dose per fraction, precise RT over approximately three to five treatment sessions (Fig. 30.2). This dose fractionation scheme is particularly useful for patients with oligometastatic disease, with several ongoing studies evaluating the optimal dose, timing, and fractionation schedules for such therapies, sometimes in combination with immunotherapy.

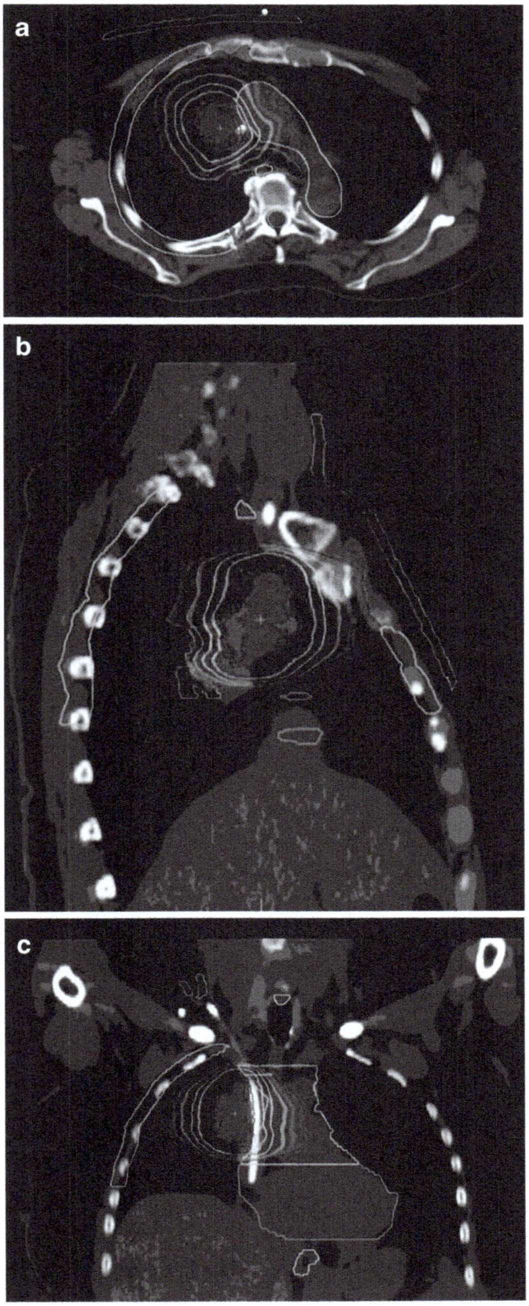

Fig. 30.2 Sample radiation SBRT plan of melanoma lung metastasis. (**a–c**) demonstrate different views of the lung metastasis being treated with SBRT

Adjuvant Radiation Therapy Following Excisional Surgery in Cutaneous Melanoma

The role for RT in patients following surgical excision for cutaneous melanoma is multifaceted. With respect to adjuvant RT to the primary lesion, this is typically offered to patients who have undergone surgery with wide local excision and have a risk factor present increasing their likelihood of local or regional recurrence. In the majority of patients who are appropriately staged and have only localized disease, the most common site of relapse is distant. Currently, adjuvant RT to the primary site is not considered standard of care for an average risk patient; however, it does play a role in the management of patients with desmoplastic neurotropic melanoma (DNM) as well as patients with lesions of the head and neck, where it may be quite difficult to achieve negative surgical margins on the primary resection. Additional risk factors that have been associated with increased propensity for local recurrence include tumor thickness >4 mm, ulceration, satellitosis, positive surgical margins, and mucosal origin [13].

The concept of using RT to increase local control following surgical excision of cutaneous melanoma dates back to the 1950s, when patients thought to be at high risk of relapse were treated with brachytherapy or orthovoltage X-rays to the primary site [14]. In 1981, Princess Margaret Hospital (Toronto, Ontario) published a retrospective experience with 37 patients who underwent surgical resection of head and neck melanoma followed by adjuvant RT [15]. This study provided insight into the importance of radiation dose fractionation, as they found patients who received fractions greater than 4 Gy had improved local control (71% versus 25%). There are several more recent retrospective analyses that have reported on local control rates associated with adjuvant RT after excisional surgery for melanoma. One such report from the Sydney Melanoma Unit suggested that there may be an advantage in local control in patients with microscopically positive margins and/or adverse pathologic features who were offered postoperative RT [16]. RT was delivered in a hypofractionated fashion to a total dose of 30–36 Gy in five to seven doses over 2.5 weeks. The recurrence rate observed at 6 months was 11% in this cohort of 174 patients receiving radiation, compared with surgical data from the same time period suggesting a recurrence rate of near 30%, that RT may have superior local control; however, because of the high rate of distant failure, no overall survival benefit has been noted for adjuvant RT in this setting [16].

With respect to patients with desmoplastic or neurotropic histology, data suggest that RT may offer a significant local control benefit. A retrospective analysis from Strom et al. examined 277 patients with non-metastatic desmoplastic melanoma who were treated with surgery with and without RT [17]. At a median follow-up of 43.1 months, RT was associated with improved local control (HR, 0.15; 95% confidence interval, 0.06–0.39 [$P < 0.001$]) and this was particularly evident in patients with adverse pathologic features (such as Breslow's depth > 4 mm, perineural invasion or positive resection margins). In the 164 patients who did not receive RT, the local recurrence rate was 17% compared with 7% in the 113 patients who received postoperative RT. While several other retrospective studies seem to show a local control benefit with adjuvant RT, one prospectively collected melanoma database from Arora et al. suggested that in the current era, local recurrence rates are considerably lower than historically reported (4% at 2 year median follow-up) [18]. Additional prospective data is needed to further clarify the role of adjuvant RT in desmoplastic or high-risk melanoma patients.

The role of adjuvant RT to the primary site in patients with a completely resected melanoma with neurotropic features is the question of a current clinical trial being run by Trans Tasman Radiation Oncology Group (www.ClinicalTrials.gov, NCT00975520). This is a two-arm, randomized controlled trial in which patients are treated with surgical excision alone or surgical excision followed by adjuvant radiation to a dose of 48 Gy in 20 fractions over 4 weeks. The primary outcome of this trial is time to local relapse with the hypothesis that RT will improve local control in this select patient cohort.

Definitive Radiation Therapy for Non-operable and Lentiginous Patients

Lentigo maligna (LM) and lentigo maligna melanoma (LMM) have slow growth rates and are associated with less potential for metastatic disease. While surgery is generally preferred for these lesions, the population most frequently presenting with LM and LMM is primarily elderly patients who may not be optimal surgical candidates. To compound this, many of these lesions appear in close proximity to critical structures, much like mucosal melanomas. Definitive RT has been used as a primary treatment modality for these patients with good long-term local control as well as acceptable cosmetic and functional outcomes [19–22]. A recently published pooled analysis of 8 studies with 349 patients with LM treated with definitive RT showed a 5% local recurrence rate [23]. A majority of the patients who recurred were successfully salvaged with further RT, surgery or other treatments.

Radiation Therapy in Mucosal Melanomas

Mucosal melanomas, while rare, are known to carry a worse prognosis than cutaneous melanomas. Local recurrence occurs in 29–79% of patients even with aggressive surgical interventions [24–26]. Therefore, the addition of a local treatment has been investigated and mixed results have been observed. A majority of the data pertains to head and neck mucosal melanomas with the addition of postoperative RT offering a local control benefit ranging from 15 to 30% [26–28]. In contrast, both Wu et al. and Patel et al. reported on the role of adjuvant RT in resected mucosal melanoma of the head and neck, showing no demonstrated benefit of local control with the addition of postoperative RT [29, 30]. However, they did demonstrate that postoperative RT was well tolerated in the modern era, in light of the fact that hypofractionated regimens are preferred in melanoma.

RT may be more relevant in the setting of unresectable mucosal melanoma. Many patients present with unresectable lesions, due to location and proximity to critical structures, particularly in the head and neck. In a retrospective series of 28 patients with mucosal melanoma of the nasal cavity and paranasal sinuses, definitive RT was given to a total dose of 50–55 Gy in 15–16 fractions and initial complete regression was observed in 22 out of 28 patients (79%). Local control of 49% at 3 years was observed in these patients [31]. A similar report on 31 patients from multiple institutions treated with definitive RT showed a local control of 58.1% [32]. The authors noted that there was an increase in the observed local control and survival in patients who received a hypofractionated regimen with a dose per fraction greater than 3 Gy [32]. The current literature suggests that in patients with unresectable mucosal melanoma, primary RT should be considered for patients with localized disease.

Adjuvant Radiation Therapy for Regional Nodal Metastases

According to National Cancer Center Network guidelines (www.NCCN.org), sentinel lymph node biopsy should be discussed with all patients who are clinically node negative and have lesions >0.75 mm in Breslow's thickness. Of those patients with positive sentinel nodes, approximately 20% will have additional positive non-sentinel nodes and therefore complete lymph node dissection becomes important in decreasing the risk of recurrence in these patients. Select patients with multiple positive nodes, large lymph nodes, extracapsular extension, and recurrence after prior lymph node dissection may be at increased risk for regional failure. This is the rationale for using adjuvant RT for regional nodal basins. The largest retrospective analysis was performed by Agrawal et al. in which 615 patients who met the "high-risk" criteria for nodal relapse were offered adjuvant RT [1]. In the patients who did elect RT, 10% local recurrence was noted at 5-year follow-up versus 41% in those patients who did not receive RT ($p < 0.0001$). The improvement in locoregional control must be carefully balanced with the morbidity that nodal RT can invoke. In this study, chronic lymphedema was significantly increased in patients receiving nodal RT after surgery as compared to those that received surgery alone (20% versus 13% at 5 years) [1].

The most robust data are from the only phase III trial run by the Australia and New Zealand Melanoma Trials Group and Trans-Tasman Radiation Oncology Group. In this trial, 250 high-risk patients with positive nodes were randomized following surgery to RT (48 Gy in 20 fractions) or observation. The criteria established for increased risk of regional recurrence were as follows: extracapsular extension, multiple positive nodes (>1 for parotid, >2 for neck and axilla, and >3 for groin location), and large lymph node (>3 cm for parotid, neck, and axilla, and >4 cm for groin location). After a mean follow-up of 73 months, lymph node recurrence in the RT arm was significantly lower as compared with observation (18% versus 33%), but no benefit was observed with respect to relapse-free or overall survival [33].

Radiation Therapy in Ocular Melanoma

Ocular melanoma is the most common primary intraocular malignant tumor in adults. Surgery for ocular melanoma typically consists of enucleation of the eye, which can be quite debilitating.

RT is a crucial part of the successful treatment of ocular melanoma while preserving the eye and vision. Local control is exceptionally good with RT delivered by either EBRT or episcleral plaque brachytherapy [34].

Preliminary experiences of episcleral brachytherapy used the high-energy isotope, 60 cobalt (Co^{60}) [35]. Currently, 125 iodine (I^{125}) is the most commonly used isotope, but other low-energy isotopes, such as iridium^{192}, cesium^{131}, protactinium^{103}, and ruthenium/rhodium^{106}, have also been used (ABS-OOTF 2014). The Collaborative Ocular Melanoma Study conducted a 12-year study that demonstrated relative equivalence of I^{125} plaque (85 Gy) compared with enucleation in the prevention of metastatic melanoma for medium-sized choroidal melanoma. Plaque brachytherapy was effective in sterilizing the gross tumor, with local control achieved in approximately 90% of patients; however, radiation-induced ocular injury necessitated enucleation in 5% of patients [36]. Radiation-induced ocular injury may be dose dependent, and therefore lower doses have also been investigated to reduce toxicity. Doses as low as 69 Gy are capable of achieving similar rates of local control, distant metastasis-free survival and overall survival as compared with 85 Gy [37]. Specific dose constraints for tumors close to the macula have been suggested in order to minimize the potential of visual acuity loss. For such tumors, a dose less than 70 Gy to the tumor apex should be considered [38].

In terms of EBRT, proton therapy is most commonly used for the treatment of ocular melanoma. As compared to plaque therapy, it has an advantage for treating larger tumors. For uveal melanoma, 60 Gy delivered in 4 daily fractions of 15 Gy is highly effective [39]. Based on an analysis of 2069 patients treated at Harvard Cyclotron Laboratory and Proton Therapy Center at Massachusetts General Hospital between 1975 and 1997, the 15-year local control rate was 95% and the rate of eye preservation of 84%. A meta-analysis of 8809 patients with uveal melanoma included 7457 patients treated with charged particle therapy and 1352 patients with brachytherapy or enucleation. The rate of local recurrence was significantly lower with charged particle therapy compared to brachytherapy (odds ratio 0.22). However, there was no advantage with respect to mortality or eye enucleation when comparing particle therapy and brachytherapy [40]. Dose reduction may be important for toxicity reduction with particle therapy as it is in brachytherapy. A prospective randomized trial of lower-dose (50 Gy) versus standard dose (70 Gy) proton radiation for small- to moderate-size uveal melanoma showed no differences in 5-year local or systemic recurrence or visual acuity loss, suggesting a lower dose may be acceptable moving forward [39].

Role of Palliative Radiation Therapy for Melanoma

RT is highly effective for symptom palliation for melanoma distant metastases. Palliative RT is effective for pain, tumor mass effect and related hemorrhage, and local irritation from skin or subcutaneous lesions [41]. New RT techniques, such as SRS and SBRT can achieve a high probability of local control with very limited toxicity, often preferred due to the relative radioresistant nature of melanoma.

Ablative doses of RT such as those used in SBRT or SRS can be quite effective in the treatment of patients with limited number of metastases. These techniques achieve a high probability of local control with very limited toxicity and are often preferred because of the relative radioresistant nature of melanoma. Patients with melanoma experience various sites of metastatic disease, including most commonly the brain, spine liver, and bone (Figs. 30.1, 30.2, and 30.3). Aggressive local treatment in patients who are considered oligometastatic may be particularly clinically meaningful [42]. Observed 5-year survival in patients with resectable metastases can be as high as 15–41% in the setting of just a few sites of distant metastases [43–46]. In two series of patients from Milano et al., patients with one to five metastases (mainly breast, lung, and colon primary) were treated with SBRT and the local control rate was reported to be 77% at 2 years [47]. Salama et al.

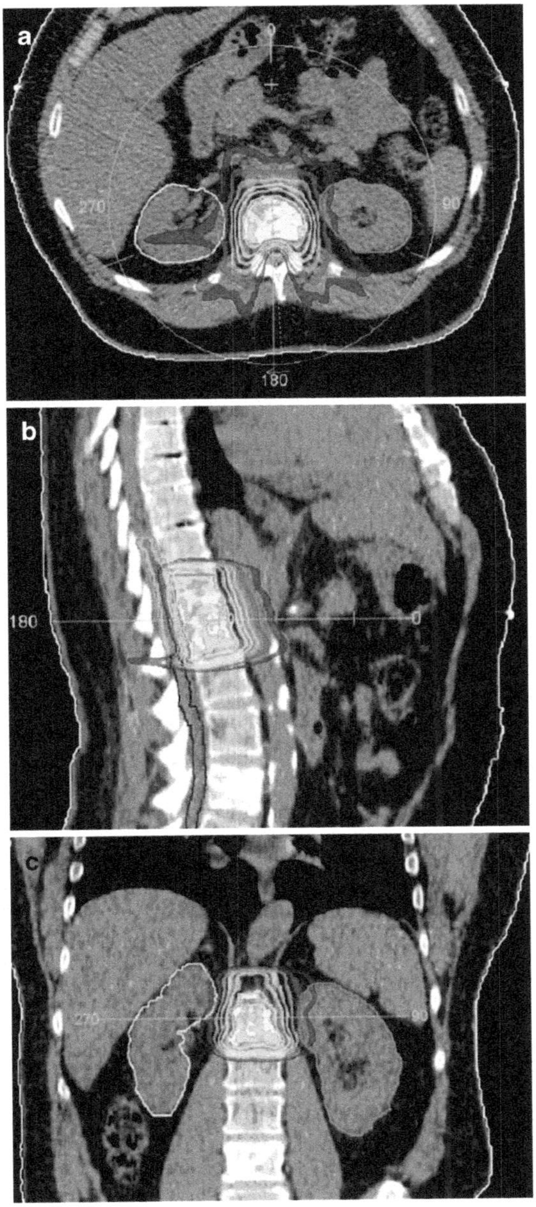

Fig. 30.3 Sample radiation plan of SBRT for melanoma spine metastasis. (**a–c**) demonstrate different views of the spine metastasis being treated with SBRT

reported on a similar protocol and demonstrated a 2-year local control rate of 52.7% [48]. SBRT for oligometastatic disease is a reasonable consideration for melanoma patients. There are currently eight open clinical trials investigating the use of SBRT in metastatic melanoma, most in combination with an immune checkpoint inhibitor (www.ClinicalTrials.gov). The potential elicited response following this combination of therapies continues to garner much interest. Specifically, there is increased curiosity in the possibility of utilizing local RT to produce "out-of field" tumor responses following a primed immune response after immunotherapy delivery. This concept of the so-called "abscopal effect" will be discussed further below.

Melanoma is the malignancy with the highest rate of brain metastasis, occurring in more than 50% of patients with advanced melanoma [8]. Intracranial disease progression is the cause of death in 20–54% of patients with disseminated melanoma [9]. Despite advances in systemic therapy, surgical and radiation techniques, the prognosis of patients with brain metastasis remains poor. The median survival of these patients is 4.4 months with a dismal 5-year survival rate of ~3% [49]. Overall survival can be extended by locoregional treatment. Surgery, WBRT, and SRS are all used in the treatment of brain metastasis, nonetheless, the best treatment remains controversial and many patients receive more than one treatment modality [50, 51]. Historically, WBRT is the de facto treatment for brain metastases because it is capable of controlling intracranial disease and delaying neurological decline [52]. The most commonly prescribed dose schedule is 30 Gy in 10 fractions. Melanoma is considered a less radiosensitive tumor, and the local control with WBRT is poor. The estimated local control rate with WBRT at 6 and 12-months are 37% and 15% [53]. The overall survival is unsatisfactory at 2–5 months [54]. Aside from having a dismal prognosis, WBRT is also associated with side effects, particularly high risk of neurocognitive decline [55, 56]. For patients with limited brain metastases, SRS can be used as an alternative to WBRT without compromising overall survival and with reduced neurocognitive impairment [11, 57–59]. SRS significantly improved the local control rate of melanoma brain metastases compared to those were treated with WBRT [60, 61]. The 12-month local control rate with SRS is about 65% [11, 59–61]. SRS also contributes to improved overall survival from 4 to ~6–8 months as compared to WBRT [11, 62, 63]. As a result, SRS alone should be considered the standard of care for patients with limited brain metastases (one to four brain metastases) and a size suitable for SRS (usually ≤4 cm in diameter). The maximum number of lesions that can be safely and effectively treated with SRS alone is currently unknown and is being examined in ongoing studies [64–66].

Bone metastases are common in patients with advanced melanoma. EBRT is a well-established treatment for vertebral metastases. Multiple prospective studies showed an improvement in pain levels by 50–90% [67–71]. However, conventional RT is limited by the low tolerance of the spinal cord and cauda equina, leading to a subtherapeutic dose delivery for tumor control, particularly for melanoma. Local control for bone/spine metastases treated with SRS/SBRT is also very favorable (70–90%) (Fig. 30.3) [72–77]. SBRT also has the advantage of better and more durable pain control for bone metastases. A large series of 500 patients (including melanoma) with spinal metastases received single fraction SBRT showed a long-term tumor control rate of 90%, and a long-term pain control rate of 85% [78].

Melanoma has a marked predilection for metastasizing to the liver. Liver metastases can occur in 15–20% of metastatic cutaneous melanoma [79, 80], and up to 95% of metastatic ocular melanoma [81, 82]. Only a small subset (~9%) of patients is eligible for resection [83, 84]. Treatment options for unresectable metastatic hepatic melanoma have historically been poor. Recent studies utilizing Yttrium-90 (90Y) radioembolization have led to encouraging results [83, 85–87]. This is a special form of radiation that was originally utilized for the treatment of hepatocellular carcinoma and other liver metastasis [88–90]. Existing experiences suggest it is an effective and safe option for managing hepatic metastases from melanoma, with a high response rate (partial response and stable disease) of ~80–90% [85–87, 91, 92] (Fig. 30.4). However, large randomized trials are warranted in order to validate radioembolization for melanoma liver metastases.

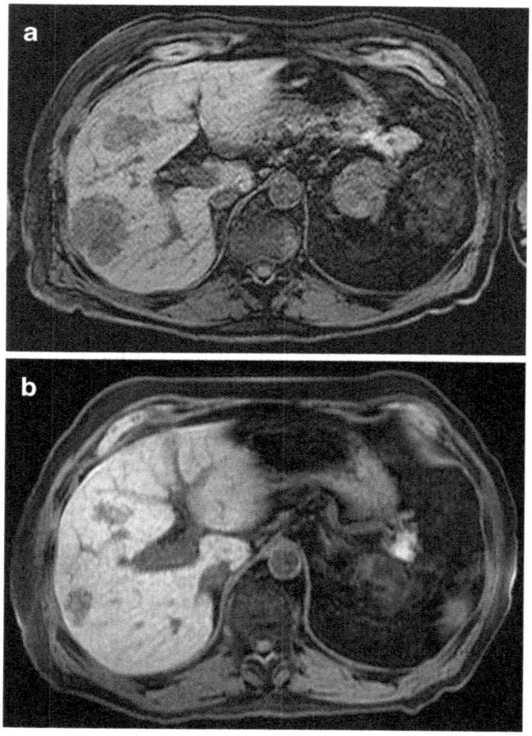

Fig. 30.4 A patient with liver metastases from uveal melanoma, treated with 90Y. (**a**) pre-treatment MRI (**b**) 6 months post-treatment MRI showed marked response

The Role of Radiation in Merkel Cell Carcinoma

Merkel cell carcinoma (MCC) is an entity separate from melanoma, although they share certain aggressive characteristics, making it relevant for discussion alongside melanoma [93]. MCC arises from dermal sensory cells and there is a demonstrated link between MCC and polyomavirus [94, 95]. Management of MCC is similar to the management of melanoma. Surgical excision is the preferred primary treatment with sentinel lymph node biopsy. With respect to margins, greater than 3 cm margins were historically encouraged at the time of wide local excision, given the possibility of satellite lesions. More recently, however, surgical margins of 2–3 cm and 2 cm deep (or down to the fascial plane) have been more generally accepted [96]. Even if not clinically involved, there is a high probability of microscopic nodal involvement in these patients (up to 30% in clinically node-negative patients). Due to this, the multidisciplinary management of regional nodes becomes crucial [97]. In those patients who have small (<1 cm) lesions and are node negative, without other risk factors such as positive margins, lymphovascular invasion or immunosuppression, observation only may be considered after resection of MCC [98]. Otherwise, patients should receive adjuvant RT to the primary site with or without treatment to the primary lymph node basin based upon sentinel lymph node biopsy involvement (or clinical concern for positive nodes if sentinel node biopsy was not performed) [96].

Based on a meta-analysis comparing surgery with or without the addition of RT, the use of local RT decreases the risk of local and regional recurrences in MCC [99]. The only randomized trial to evaluate the role of postoperative RT for MCC closed early due to poor accrual after the advent of the sentinel node biopsy, but in the patients that were randomized, there was an observed local control benefit to adding RT [100]. The group that underwent observation had a local recurrence rate of 16.7% versus 0% in the adjuvant RT group. In addition to local control, RT may offer a survival benefit in MCC, as evidenced by a large SEER database analysis that included 1187 patients who received adjuvant RT versus those who were observed. Patients receiving adjuvant RT had a median survival of 63 versus 45 months, in the observed patients ($p = 0.0002$) [101]. The dosing of RT for MCC is different from melanoma, as MCC tends to be more sensitive to RT than melanoma. Doses between 45 and 60 Gy offer adequate control after surgical intervention, whereas treatment of gross disease is typically done with 60–66 Gy [99, 102].

While MCC and melanoma share common surgical approaches including sentinel node mapping and biopsy as well as adjuvant RT in select cases, they do not share a similar systemic approach. Immunotherapy has made significant progress in the treatment of melanoma, but there is sparse literature on systemic therapy options in MCC [103]. Recently, the use of checkpoint inhibitors for the treatment of MCC have shown significant efficacy in the treatment of patients with metastatic MCC. Therefore, enrollment on clinical trials is highly encouraged, particularly for patients with metastatic disease.

Radiotherapy with Concomitant Agents

BRAF mutations occur in approximately 50% of patients and are associated with deregulated apoptosis. The development of BRAF inhibitors (i.e., vemurafenib, dabrafenib) has led to a significant improvement in overall survival among patients who harbor this mutation. Despite this achievement, very few prospective trials have investigated the combination of RT with BRAF inhibitors, thus leaving clinical questions in regard to toxicity and efficacy of combined treatment. Consensus Guidelines from the Eastern Cooperative Group (ECOG) were recently published, documenting severe toxicities reported in 27 publications in which patients received a BRAF inhibitor in combination with RT. Based on this review, recommendations for combination therapy include holding RT for at least 3 days before and after fractionated RT and at least 1 day before and after SRS. There were no fatal reactions documented with RT doses less than 4 Gy per fraction. Further prospective trials are necessary to further clarify the optimal timing of BRAF inhibition with RT [104].

In recent years, several studies have investigated combinations of RT with immunotherapy for patients with metastatic melanoma. Activated T-cells and antibodies targeting tumor-associated antigens have been detected in blood from cancer patients, suggesting an active host immune response against the tumor [105]. Moreover, tumor-infiltrating lymphocytes (TILs) in melanoma have prognostic significance, and when identified within nodal metastases, predict benefit in patients treated with neoadjuvant interferon-α-2b therapy [106–108]. RT promotes tumor cell death, releasing tumor debris and tumor antigens. Localized RT induces cell death and release of immunogenic factors via a process termed "immunogenic cell death" (ICD), which subsequently triggers the release of a number of endogenous damage-associated molecular patterns [109]. Released tumor antigens are thought to "prime" the host's immune response. For this reason, there has been growing enthusiasm for combining RT with immunotherapy agents such as checkpoint inhibitors targeted against cytotoxic T-lymphocyte antigen 4 (i.e., ipilimumab) and programmed death-1 (i.e., pembrolizumab). There are currently several open clinical trials evaluating various combinations of RT (EBRT, SRS, SBRT, or radiospheres) with immunotherapy (ipilimumab, nivolumab, atezolizumab) (www.ClinicalTrials.gov).

One of the largest prospective trials evaluating combination therapy was recently published. Hiniker et al. evaluated 22 patients with stage IV melanoma treated with palliative RT and four cycles of ipilimumab, with a primary objective of assessing safety and efficacy of this combination [110]. RT was delivered within 5 days following initiation of immunotherapy. The combination of treatments was well tolerated without unexpected toxicities. Three patients had an ongoing complete response at median follow-up of 55 weeks (range 32–65), and three had an initial partial response for a median of 40 weeks, suggesting further investigation into the combination of RT with immunotherapy in patients with stage IV melanoma [110]. The median progression-free survival for all 20 evaluable patients was 26 weeks (range 2–65; 95% CI 3–35.7). Similar responses have also been shown in the combination of RT with PD-1 or PDL-1 blockade in patients with advanced melanoma; however, prospective evaluation is needed [111]. Targeted molecular agents (BRAF, MEK, MET) hold similar promise as emerging therapies although have yet to be prospectively evaluated in combination with RT.

It is important to note that when evaluating patients for response following immunotherapy, there are several special considerations, including the following: (1) patients may have transient worsening (pseudo-progression) of their disease prior to improvement, (2) time to response may be longer, and (3) patients may not reach the criteria for an objective response, but they may still have clinically significant periods of disease stability [112]. For these reasons, the standard RECIST criteria, and modified WHO criteria, historically used for evaluation of response to cytotoxic therapies may not be applicable in the setting of immunotherapy. The immune-related response criteria were therefore developed for patients undergoing immunotherapy, and are important when these patients are treated with combination RT and immunotherapy as well.

Radiotherapy and the Abscopal Effect in the Era of Immunotherapy

First described in the 1950s, the abscopal effect refers to the infrequently reported phenomenon of tumor regression of a secondary site following RT to a separate primary site [113]. A more recent report investigating blood samples from melanoma patients with immunologic correlates of the abscopal effect, showed antigenic targets with increased antibody responses following RT [114]. The surprising response achieved by the patient in this report provided new insight in the mechanisms of combination therapy, with an underlying hypothesis that immunotherapy delivered in close proximity to SRS increases antigen release, primes the immune response and perhaps impacts distant control.

One recent report analyzed 21 patients with advanced melanoma treated with ipilimumab followed by RT and observed an abscopal response in 11 patients (52%) with the median time from RT to response of 1 month. Median overall survival for those patients who had an abscopal response was 22.4 months versus 8.3 months for those without a response. Larger prospective studies are required to bolster this small, but impressive, report [115]. Figure 30.5 demonstrates an example of the abscopal effect in a patient with multiple liver metastases from uveal melanoma following RT directed at a periportal lymph node. This patient did not receive systemic therapy or liver-directed therapy but had shrinkage of multiple liver metastases following the

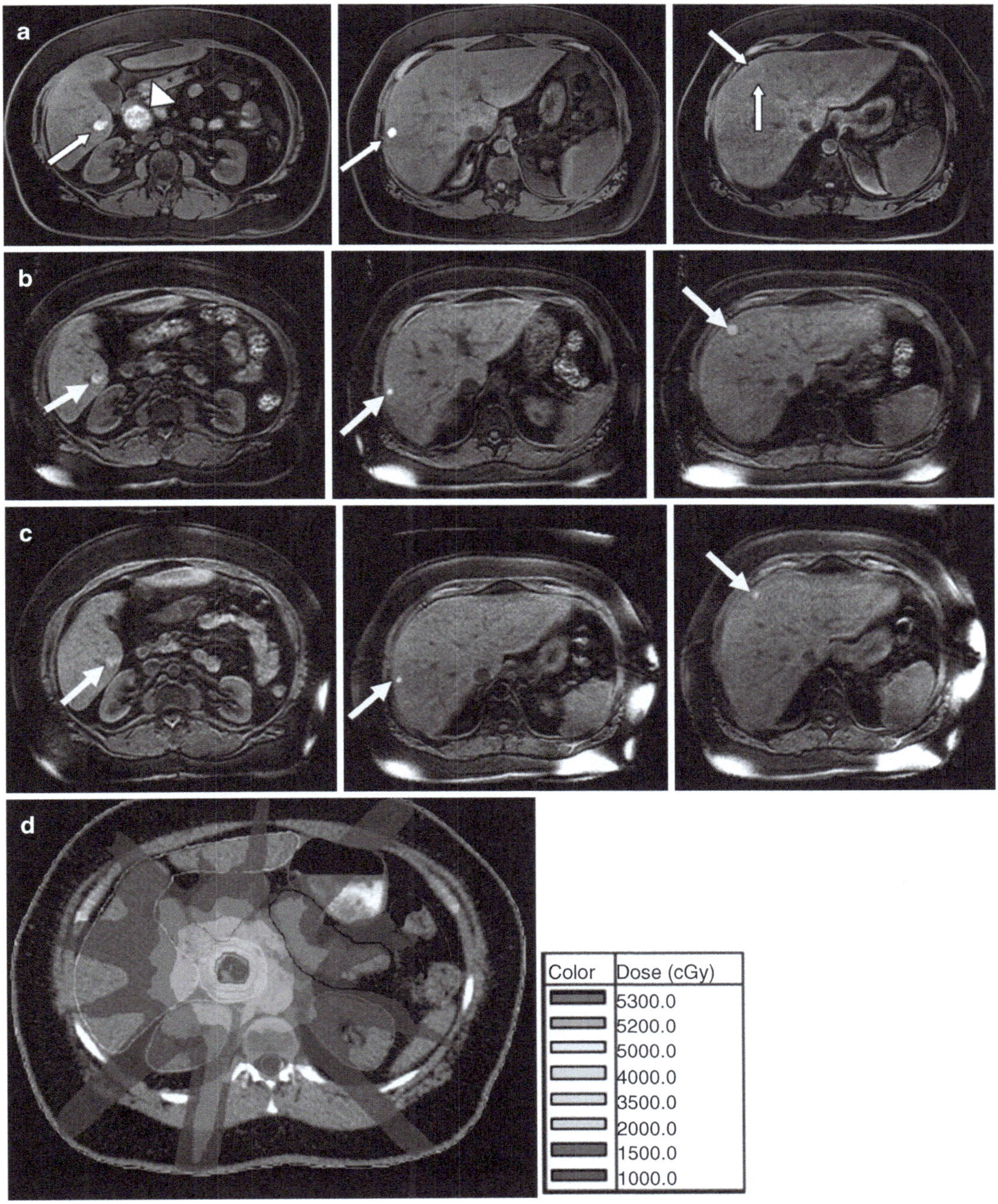

Fig. 30.5 A patient with metastatic uveal melanoma who received RT to a periportal lymph node (arrow head) with no systemic therapy or liver-directed therapy. Images depicted are initial (Panel **a**), 2 months post-RT (Panel **b**), and 10 months post-RT (Panel **c**). Response of the liver lesions outside of the primary radiation field (arrows) demonstrates an example of the abscopal effect. Image (**d**) shows the radiation plan showing conformal dose around the periportal lymph node with only low-dose radiation reaching parts of the liver. Images (**a**–**c**) courtesy of Takami Sato, M.D., Ph.D., and Donald G. Mitchell, M.D

periportal treatment. The abscopal effect from RT is rarely seen in metastatic uveal melanoma. She continues to have a durable response of lesions outside of the RT field 10 months post-treatment.

The Future of Radiotherapy for Melanoma

RT clearly has multiple roles in the overall management of melanoma. With additional data from randomized trials evaluating various fractionation schemes as well as combinations of RT with immunotherapy and other systemic agents, practice patterns will continue to evolve. There are currently several open clinical trials evaluating various combinations of RT with immunotherapy, and there is great enthusiasm for the potential synergism garnered with combination therapy. Initial reports combining RT with interferon unfortunately showed increased toxicity [116–118]. Newer immunotherapeutic agents have shown to be more safely tolerated concurrent with RT. Further advances in the management of patients with melanoma are assuredly in the near future. Despite these anticipated findings from large clinical trials, management of melanoma will continue to be multidisciplinary and collaborative by design.

References

1. Agrawal S, Kane JM 3rd, Guadagnolo BA, et al. The benefits of adjuvant radiation therapy after therapeutic lymphadenectomy for clinically advanced, high-risk, lymph node-metastatic melanoma. Cancer. 2009;115:5836–44.
2. Lee RJ, Gibbs JF, Proulx GM, et al. Nodal basin recurrence following lymph node dissection for melanoma: implications for adjuvant radiotherapy. Int J Radiat Oncol Biol Phys. 2000;46:467–74.
3. Dewey DL. The radiosensitivity of melanoma cells in culture. Br J Radiol. 1971;44:816–7.
4. Barranco SC, Romsdahl MM, Humphrey RM. The radiation response of human malignant melanoma cells grown in vitro. Cancer Res. 1971;31:830–3.
5. Sause WT, Cooper JS, Rush S, et al. Fraction size in external beam radiation therapy in the treatment of melanoma. Int J Radiat Oncol Biol Phys. 1991;20:429–32.
6. Noda SE, Lautenschlaeger T, Siedow MR, et al. Technological advances in radiation oncology for central nervous system tumors. Semin Radiat Oncol. 2009;19:179–86.
7. Barnett GH, Linskey ME, Adler JR, et al. Stereotactic radiosurgery—an organized neurosurgery-sanctioned definition. J Neurosurg. 2007;106:1–5.
8. Bafaloukos D, Gogas H. The treatment of brain metastases in melanoma patients. Cancer Treat Rev. 2004;30:515–20.
9. Sampson JH, Carter JH Jr, Friedman AH, et al. Demographics, prognosis, and therapy in 702 patients with brain metastases from malignant melanoma. J Neurosurg. 1998;88:11–20.
10. Fife KM, Colman MH, Stevens GN, et al. Determinants of outcome in melanoma patients with cerebral metastases. J Clin Oncol. 2004;22:1293–300.
11. Mathieu D, Kondziolka D, Cooper PB, et al. Gamma knife radiosurgery for malignant melanoma brain metastases. Clin Neurosurg. 2007;54:241–7.
12. Liew DN, Kano H, Kondziolka D, et al. Outcome predictors of gamma knife surgery for melanoma brain metastases. Clinical article. J Neurosurg. 2011;114:769–79.
13. Ballo MT, Zagars GK, Gershenwald JE, et al. A critical assessment of adjuvant radiotherapy for inguinal lymph node metastases from melanoma. Ann Surg Oncol. 2004;11:1079–84.
14. Dickson RJ. Malignant melanoma; a combined surgical and radiotherapeutic approach. Am J Roentgenol Radium Ther Nucl Med. 1958;79:1063–70.
15. Harwood AR, Cummings BJ. Radiotherapy for mucosal melanomas. Int J Radiat Oncol Biol Phys. 1982;8:1121–6.
16. Stevens G, Thompson JF, Firth I, et al. Locally advanced melanoma: results of postoperative hypofractionated radiation therapy. Cancer. 2000;88:88–94.
17. Strom T, Caudell JJ, Han D, et al. Radiotherapy influences local control in patients with desmoplastic melanoma. Cancer. 2014;120:1369–78.
18. Arora A, Lowe L, Su L, et al. Wide excision without radiation for desmoplastic melanoma. Cancer. 2005;104(7):1462.
19. De Groot WP. Provisional results of treatment of the melanose precancereuse circonscrite Dubreuilh by Bucky-rays. Dermatologica. 1968;136:429–31.
20. Farshad A, Burg G, Panizzon R, et al. A retrospective study of 150 patients with lentigo maligna and lentigo maligna melanoma and the efficacy of radiotherapy using Grenz or soft X-rays. Br J Dermatol. 2002;146(6):1042.
21. Panizzon R. Radiotherapy of lentigo maligna and lentigo maligna melanoma. Skin Cancer. 1999;14:203–7.
22. Schmid-Wendtner MH, Brunner B, Konz B, et al. Fractionated radiotherapy of lentigo maligna and lentigo maligna melanoma in 64 patients. J Am Acad Dermatol. 2000;43:477–82.

23. Fogarty GB, Hong A, Scolyer RA, et al. Radiotherapy for lentigo maligna: a literature review and recommendations for treatment. Br J Dermatol. 2014;170:52–8.
24. Meleti M, Leemans CR, de Bree R, et al. Head and neck mucosal melanoma: experience with 42 patients, with emphasis on the role of postoperative radiotherapy. Head Neck. 2008;30:1543–51.
25. Bachar G, Goldstein DP, Shah M, et al. Esthesioneuroblastoma: the Princess Margaret Hospital experience. Head Neck. 2008;30:1607–14.
26. Krengli M, Masini L, Kaanders JH, et al. Radiotherapy in the treatment of mucosal melanoma of the upper aerodigestive tract: analysis of 74 cases. A Rare Cancer Network study. Int J Radiat Oncol Biol Phys. 2006;65:751–9.
27. Moreno MA, Roberts DB, Kupferman ME, et al. Mucosal melanoma of the nose and paranasal sinuses, a contemporary experience from the M. D. Anderson Cancer Center. Cancer. 2010;116:2215–23.
28. Benlyazid A, Thariat J, Temam S, et al. Postoperative radiotherapy in head and neck mucosal melanoma: a GETTEC study. Arch Otolaryngol Head Neck Surg. 2010;136:1219–25.
29. Wu AJ, Gomez J, Zhung JE, et al. Radiotherapy after surgical resection for head and neck mucosal melanoma. Am J Clin Oncol. 2010;33:281–5.
30. Patel SG, Prasad ML, Escrig M, et al. Primary mucosal malignant melanoma of the head and neck. Head Neck. 2002;24:247–57.
31. Gilligan D, Slevin NJ. Radical radiotherapy for 28 cases of mucosal melanoma in the nasal cavity and sinuses. Br J Radiol. 1991;64:1147–50.
32. Wada H, Nemoto K, Ogawa Y, et al. A multi-institutional retrospective analysis of external radiotherapy for mucosal melanoma of the head and neck in Northern Japan. Int J Radiat Oncol Biol Phys. 2004;59:495–500.
33. Henderson MA, Burmeister BH, Ainslie J, et al. Adjuvant lymph-node field radiotherapy versus observation only in patients with melanoma at high risk of further lymph-node field relapse after lymphadenectomy (ANZMTG 01.02/TROG 02.01): 6-year follow-up of a phase 3, randomised controlled trial. Lancet Oncol. 2015;16:1049–60.
34. Munzenrider JE. Uveal melanomas. Conservation treatment. Hematol Oncol Clin North Am. 2001;15:389–402.
35. Stallard HB. Radiotherapy for malignant melanoma of the choroid. Br J Ophthalmol. 1966;50:147–55.
36. Melia BM, Abramson DH, Albert DM, et al. Collaborative ocular melanoma study (COMS) randomized trial of I-125 brachytherapy for medium choroidal melanoma. I. Visual acuity after 3 years COMS report no. 16. Ophthalmology. 2001;108:348–66.
37. Perez BA, Mettu P, Vajzovic L, et al. Uveal melanoma treated with iodine-125 episcleral plaque: an analysis of dose on disease control and visual outcomes. Int J Radiat Oncol Biol Phys. 2014;89:127–36.
38. Jones R, Gore E, Mieler W, et al. Posttreatment visual acuity in patients treated with episcleral plaque therapy for choroidal melanomas: dose and dose rate effects. Int J Radiat Oncol Biol Phys. 2002;52:989–95.
39. Gragoudas ES, Lane AM, Regan S, et al. A randomized controlled trial of varying radiation doses in the treatment of choroidal melanoma. Arch Ophthalmol. 2000;118:773–8.
40. Wang Z, Nabhan M, Schild SE, et al. Charged particle radiation therapy for uveal melanoma: a systematic review and meta-analysis. Int J Radiat Oncol Biol Phys. 2013;86:18–26.
41. Fogarty GB, Hong A. Radiation therapy for advanced and metastatic melanoma. J Surg Oncol. 2014;109:370–5.
42. Hellman S, Weichselbaum RR. Oligometastases. J Clin Oncol. 1995;13:8–10.
43. Sosman JA, Moon J, Tuthill RJ, et al. A phase 2 trial of complete resection for stage IV melanoma: results of Southwest Oncology Group Clinical Trial S9430. Cancer. 2011;117:4740–06.
44. Ollila DW, Essner R, Wanek LA, et al. Surgical resection for melanoma metastatic to the gastrointestinal tract. Arch Surg. 1996;131(9.; 979–80):975.
45. Agrawal S, Yao TJ, Coit DG. Surgery for melanoma metastatic to the gastrointestinal tract. Ann Surg Oncol. 1999;6:336–44.
46. Harpole DH Jr, Johnson CM, Wolfe WG, et al. Analysis of 945 cases of pulmonary metastatic melanoma. J Thorac Cardiovasc Surg. 1992;103:743–8. discussion748–50
47. Milano MT, Katz AW, Muhs AG, et al. A prospective pilot study of curative-intent stereotactic body radiation therapy in patients with 5 or fewer oligometastatic lesions. Cancer. 2008;112:650–8.
48. Salama JK, Hasselle MD, Chmura SJ, et al. Stereotactic body radiotherapy for multisite extracranial oligometastases: final report of a dose escalation trial in patients with 1 to 5 sites of metastatic disease. Cancer. 2012;118:2962–70.
49. Barth A, Wanek LA, Morton DL. Prognostic factors in 1,521 melanoma patients with distant metastases. J Am Coll Surg. 1995;181:193–201.
50. Andrews DW. Current neurosurgical management of brain metastases. Semin Oncol. 2008;35:100–7.
51. Thomas SS, Dunbar EM. Modern multidisciplinary management of brain metastases. Curr Oncol Rep. 2010;12:34–40.
52. Chu FC, Hilaris BB. Value of radiation theray in the management of intracranial metastases. Cancer. 1961;14:577–81.
53. Meyners T, Heisterkamp C, Kueter JD, et al. Prognostic factors for outcomes after whole-brain irradiation of brain metastases from relatively radioresistant tumors: a retrospective analysis. BMC Cancer. 2010;10:582.

54. de la Fuente M, Beal K, Carvajal R, et al. Whole-brain radiotherapy in patients with brain metastases from melanoma. CNS Oncol. 2014;3:401–6.
55. Chang EL, Wefel JS, Hess KR, et al. Neurocognition in patients with brain metastases treated with radiosurgery or radiosurgery plus whole-brain irradiation: a randomised controlled trial. Lancet Oncol. 2009;10:1037–44.
56. Brown PD, Jaeckle K, Ballman KV, et al. Effect of radiosurgery alone vs radiosurgery with whole brain radiation therapy on cognitive function in patients with 1 to 3 brain metastases: a randomized clinical trial. JAMA. 2016;316:401–9.
57. DiLuna ML, King JT Jr, Knisely JP, et al. Prognostic factors for survival after stereotactic radiosurgery vary with the number of cerebral metastases. Cancer. 2007;109:135–45.
58. Manon R, O'Neill A, Knisely J, et al. Phase II trial of radiosurgery for one to three newly diagnosed brain metastases from renal cell carcinoma, melanoma, and sarcoma: an Eastern Cooperative Oncology Group study (E 6397). J Clin Oncol. 2005;23:8870–6.
59. Clarke JW, Register S, McGregor JM, et al. Stereotactic radiosurgery with or without whole brain radiotherapy for patients with a single radioresistant brain metastasis. Am J Clin Oncol. 2010;33:70–4.
60. Powell JW, Chung CT, Shah HR, et al. Gamma Knife surgery in the management of radioresistant brain metastases in high-risk patients with melanoma, renal cell carcinoma, and sarcoma. J Neurosurg. 2008;109(Suppl):122–8.
61. Lo SS, Clarke JW, Grecula JC, et al. Stereotactic radiosurgery alone for patients with 1–4 radioresistant brain metastases. Med Oncol. 2011;28(Suppl 1):S439–44.
62. Choong ES, Lo S, Drummond M, et al. Survival of patients with melanoma brain metastasis treated with stereotactic radiosurgery and active systemic drug therapies. Eur J Cancer. 2017;75:169–78.
63. Feng R, Oermann EK, Shrivastava R, et al. Stereotactic radiosurgery (SRS) for melanoma brain metastases: a comprehensive clinical case series. World Neurosurg. 2017;100:297–304.
64. Yamamoto M, Serizawa T, Shuto T, et al. Stereotactic radiosurgery for patients with multiple brain metastases (JLGK0901): a multi-institutional prospective observational study. Lancet Oncol. 2014;15:387–95.
65. Rava P, Leonard K, Sioshansi S, et al. Survival among patients with 10 or more brain metastases treated with stereotactic radiosurgery. J Neurosurg. 2013;119:457–62.
66. Nichol A, Ma R, Hsu F, et al. Volumetric radiosurgery for 1 to 10 brain metastases: a Multicenter, single-arm, phase 2 study. Int J Radiat Oncol Biol Phys. 2016;94:312–21.
67. 8 Gy single fraction radiotherapy for the treatment of metastatic skeletal pain: randomised comparison with a multifraction schedule over 12 months of patient follow-up. Bone Pain Trial Working Party. J.R. Yarnold Radiother Oncol 1999;52:111–21.
68. Rades D, Stalpers LJ, Hulshof MC, et al. Effectiveness and toxicity of single-fraction radiotherapy with 1 x 8 Gy for metastatic spinal cord compression. Radiother Oncol. 2005;75:70–3.
69. Maranzano E, Bellavita R, Rossi R, et al. Short-course versus split-course radiotherapy in metastatic spinal cord compression: results of a phase III, randomized, multicenter trial. J Clin Oncol. 2005;23:3358–65.
70. Chow E, Harris K, Fan G, et al. Palliative radiotherapy trials for bone metastases: a systematic review. J Clin Oncol. 2007;25:1423–36.
71. Lutz S, Berk L, Chang E, et al. Palliative radiotherapy for bone metastases: an ASTRO evidence-based guideline. Int J Radiat Oncol Biol Phys. 2011;79:965–76.
72. Rule W, Timmerman R, Tong L, et al. Phase I dose-escalation study of stereotactic body radiotherapy in patients with hepatic metastases. Ann Surg Oncol. 2011;18:1081–7.
73. Lo SS, Teh BS, Mayr NA, et al. Stereotactic body radiation therapy for oligometastases. Discov Med. 2010;10:247–54.
74. Timmerman R, Paulus R, Galvin J, et al. Stereotactic body radiation therapy for inoperable early stage lung cancer. JAMA. 2010;303:1070–6.
75. Rusthoven KE, Kavanagh BD, Cardenes H, et al. Multi-institutional phase I/II trial of stereotactic body radiation therapy for liver metastases. J Clin Oncol. 2009;27:1572–8.
76. Hoyer M, Roed H, Traberg Hansen A, et al. Phase II study on stereotactic body radiotherapy of colorectal metastases. Acta Oncol. 2006;45:823–30.
77. Chawla S, Chen Y, Katz AW, et al. Stereotactic body radiotherapy for treatment of adrenal metastases. Int J Radiat Oncol Biol Phys. 2009;75:71–5.
78. Gerszten PC, Burton SA, Ozhasoglu C, et al. Radiosurgery for spinal metastases: clinical experience in 500 cases from a single institution. Spine (Phila Pa 1976). 2007;32:193–9.
79. Leiter U, Meier F, Schittek B, et al. The natural course of cutaneous melanoma. J Surg Oncol. 2004;86:172–8.
80. Cohn-Cedermark G, Mansson-Brahme E, Rutqvist LE, et al. Metastatic patterns, clinical outcome, and malignant phenotype in malignant cutaneous melanoma. Acta Oncol. 1999;38:549–57.
81. Becker JC, Terheyden P, Kampgen E, et al. Treatment of disseminated ocular melanoma with sequential fotemustine, interferon alpha, and interleukin 2. Br J Cancer. 2002;87:840–5.
82. Trout AT, Rabinowitz RS, Platt JF, et al. Melanoma metastases in the abdomen and pelvis: frequency and patterns of spread. World J Radiol. 2013;5:25–32.
83. Gonsalves CF, Eschelman DJ, Sullivan KL, et al. Radioembolization as salvage therapy for hepatic

metastasis of uveal melanoma: a single-institution experience. Am J Roentgenol. 2011;196:468–73.
84. Mariani P, Almubarak MM, Kollen M, et al. Radiofrequency ablation and surgical resection of liver metastases from uveal melanoma. Eur J Surg Oncol. 2016;42:706–12.
85. Eldredge-Hindy H, Ohri N, Anne PR, et al. Yttrium-90 microsphere brachytherapy for liver metastases from uveal melanoma: clinical outcomes and the predictive value of fluorodeoxyglucose positron emission tomography. Am J Clin Oncol. 2016;39:189–95.
86. Xing M, Prajapati HJ, Dhanasekaran R, et al. Selective internal yttrium-90 radioembolization therapy (90Y-SIRT) versus best supportive care in patients with unresectable metastatic melanoma to the liver refractory to systemic therapy: safety and efficacy cohort study. Am J Clin Oncol. 2017;40:27–34.
87. Memon K, Kuzel TM, Vouche M, et al. Hepatic yttrium-90 radioembolization for metastatic melanoma: a single-center experience. Melanoma Res. 2014;24:244–51.
88. Kennedy A. Radioembolization of hepatic tumors. J Gastrointest Oncol. 2014;5:178–89.
89. Memon K, Lewandowski RJ, Mulcahy MF, et al. Radioembolization for neuroendocrine liver metastases: safety, imaging, and long-term outcomes. Int J Radiat Oncol Biol Phys. 2012;83:887–94.
90. Dezarn WA, Cessna JT, DeWerd LA, et al. Recommendations of the American Association of Physicists in Medicine on dosimetry, imaging, and quality assurance procedures for 90Y microsphere brachytherapy in the treatment of hepatic malignancies. Med Phys. 2011;38:4824–45.
91. Piduru SM, Schuster DM, Barron BJ, et al. Prognostic value of 18f-fluorodeoxyglucose positron emission tomography-computed tomography in predicting survival in patients with unresectable metastatic melanoma to the liver undergoing yttrium-90 radioembolization. J Vasc Interv Radiol. 2012;23:943–8.
92. Klingenstein A, Haug AR, Zech CJ, et al. Radioembolization as locoregional therapy of hepatic metastases in uveal melanoma patients. Cardiovasc Intervent Radiol. 2013;36:158–65.
93. Tothill R, Estall V, Rischin D. Merkel cell carcinoma: emerging biology, current approaches, and future directions. Am Soc Clin Oncol Educ Book.2015:e519–26.
94. Kassem A, Schopflin A, Diaz C, et al. Frequent detection of Merkel cell polyomavirus in human Merkel cell carcinomas and identification of a unique deletion in the VP1 gene. Cancer Res. 2008;68(13):5009.
95. Feng H, Shuda M, Chang Y, et al. Clonal integration of a polyomavirus in human Merkel cell carcinoma. Science. 2008;319:1096–100.
96. Ramahi E, Choi J, Fuller CD, et al. Merkel cell carcinoma. Am J Clin Oncol. 2013;36:299–309.
97. Gupta SG, Wang LC, Penas PF, et al. Sentinel lymph node biopsy for evaluation and treatment of patients with Merkel cell carcinoma: the Dana-Farber experience and meta-analysis of the literature. Arch Dermatol. 2006;142:685–90.
98. Bichakjian CK, Lowe L, Lao CD, et al. Merkel cell carcinoma: critical review with guidelines for multidisciplinary management. Cancer. 2007;110:1–12.
99. Lewis KG, Weinstock MA, Weaver AL, et al. Adjuvant local irradiation for Merkel cell carcinoma. Arch Dermatol. 2006;142:693–700.
100. Jouary T, Leyral C, Dreno B, et al. Adjuvant prophylactic regional radiotherapy versus observation in stage I Merkel cell carcinoma: a multicentric prospective randomized study. Ann Oncol. 2012;23:1074–80.
101. Kim JA, Choi AH. Effect of radiation therapy on survival in patients with resected Merkel cell carcinoma: a propensity score surveillance, epidemiology, and end results database analysis. JAMA Dermatol. 2013;149:831–8.
102. Rush Z, Fields RC, Lee N, et al. Radiation therapy in the management of Merkel cell carcinoma: current perspectives. Expert Rev Dermatol. 2011;6:395–404.
103. Desch L, Kunstfeld R. Merkel cell carcinoma: chemotherapy and emerging new therapeutic options. J Skin Cancer. 2013;2013:327150.
104. Anker CJ, Grossmann KF, Atkins MB, et al. Avoiding severe toxicity from combined BRAF inhibitor and radiation treatment: consensus guidelines from the eastern cooperative oncology group (ECOG). Int J Radiat Oncol Biol Phys. 2016;95:632–46.
105. Nagorsen D, Scheibenbogen C, Marincola FM, et al. Natural T cell immunity against cancer. Clin Cancer Res. 2003;9:4296–303.
106. Hakansson A, Gustafsson B, Krysander L, et al. Tumour-infiltrating lymphocytes in metastatic malignant melanoma and response to interferon alpha treatment. Br J Cancer. 1996;74:670–6.
107. Mihm MC Jr, Clemente CG, Cascinelli N. Tumor infiltrating lymphocytes in lymph node melanoma metastases: a histopathologic prognostic indicator and an expression of local immune response. Lab Investig. 1996;74:43–7.
108. Moschos SJ, Edington HD, Land SR, et al. Neoadjuvant treatment of regional stage IIIB melanoma with high-dose interferon alfa-2b induces objective tumor regression in association with modulation of tumor infiltrating host cellular immune responses. J Clin Oncol. 2006;24:3164–71.
109. Chajon E, Castelli J, Marsiglia H, et al. The synergistic effect of radiotherapy and immunotherapy: a promising but not simple partnership. Crit Rev Oncol Hematol. 2017;111:124–32.
110. Hiniker SM, Chen DS, Reddy S, et al. A systemic complete response of metastatic melanoma to local radiation and immunotherapy. Transl Oncol. 2012;5:404–7.
111. Mohiuddin M, Park H, Hallmeyer S, et al. High-dose radiation as a dramatic, immunological primer in locally advanced melanoma. Cureus. 2015;7:e417.
112. Wolchok JD, Hoos A, O'Day S, et al. Guidelines for the evaluation of immune therapy activity in

solid tumors: immune-related response criteria. Clin Cancer Res. 2009;15:7412–20.
113. Mole RH. Whole body irradiation; radiobiology or medicine? Br J Radiol. 1953;26:234–41.
114. Postow MA, Callahan MK, Barker CA, et al. Immunologic correlates of the abscopal effect in a patient with melanoma. N Engl J Med. 2012;366:925–31.
115. Grimaldi AM, Simeone E, Giannarelli D, et al. Abscopal effects of radiotherapy on advanced melanoma patients who progressed after ipilimumab immunotherapy. Oncoimmunology. 2014;3:e28780.
116. Gyorki DE, Ainslie J, Joon ML, et al. Concurrent adjuvant radiotherapy and interferon-alpha2b for resected high risk stage III melanoma—a retrospective single centre study. Melanoma Res. 2004;14:223–30.
117. Nguyen NP, Levinson B, Dutta S, et al. Concurrent interferon-alpha and radiation for head and neck melanoma. Melanoma Res. 2003;13:67–71.
118. Conill C, Jorcano S, Domingo-Domenech J, et al. Toxicity of combined treatment of adjuvant irradiation and interferon alpha2b in high-risk melanoma patients. Melanoma Res. 2007;17:304–9.

Immuno-Oncolytic Virotherapy for Melanoma

31

Helene Woyczesczyk and Karim Essani

Abbreviations

AE	Adverse event
BSL	Biosafety level
CD	Cluster of differentiation
CRAds	Conditionally replicative adenoviruses
CTLA	Cytotoxic T-lymphocyte antigen
DC	Dendritic cell
DR	Durable response
FDA	FOOD and Drug Administration
GM-CSF	Granulocyte monocyte colony-stimulating factor
HMW-MAA	High molecular weight tumor-associated antigen
HSV	Herpes simplex virus
IFN	Interferon
IL	Interleukin
irPFS	Immune-related progression free survival
IT	Intratumoral
MAA	Melanoma-associated antigen
MHC	Major histocompatibility complex
MMP	Matrix metalloprotease
MV	Measles virus
NARA	Neutralizing anti-reovirus antibodies
NDV	Newcastle disease virus
NK	Natural killer
OPTiM	Oncovex (GM-CSF) Pivotal Trial in Melanoma
ORR	Overall response rate
OV	Oncolytic virus
PD	Programmed death receptor
Pfu	Plaque forming unit
PPE	Personal protective equipment
PPR	Progression prior to response
RECST	Response evaluation criteria in solid tumors
TAA	Tumor-associated antigen
TGF	Transforming growth factor
TNF	Tumor necrosis factor
TPV	Tanapox virus
Tregs	Regulatory T-cells
T-vec	Talimogene laherparepvec
VSV	Vesicular stomatitis virus
VV	Vaccinia virus
Wt	Wild type

H. Woyczesczyk · K. Essani, Ph.D. (✉)
Laboratory of Virology, Department of Biological Sciences, Western Michigan University, Kalamazoo, MI, USA
e-mail: karim.essani@wmich.edu

A Brief History

Oncolytic virotherapy, or the use of live virus particles to initiate tumor cell lysis, has been unknowingly involved with cancer regression for centuries, possibly even much longer, throughout history. The first claims were not firmly documented until the early 1900s [1]. It was then that physicians noted tumoral regression following inoculation with attenuated viruses, and by the early 1950s,

A. I. Riker (ed.), *Melanoma*, https://doi.org/10.1007/978-3-319-78310-9_31

the first clinical trials involving oncolytic viruses (OVs) began. This trial utilized a modified Herpes Simplex virus (HSV) to destroy cancer cells [2–5]. However, with the introduction of radiotherapy and chemotherapy around the same time, OV therapy was overshadowed as a treatment option until the 1990s when further research and clinical trials with OVs resurged [2, 6].

Over the last decade, OVs demonstrate great potential as a successful treatment for various cancers, with rapid progress towards their clinical use in humans. While adenovirus and HSV families were the first to be tested and introduced, viruses from the families *Poxviridae*, *Picornaviridae*, and *Rhabdoviridae* are all undergoing various stages of testing [7]. OV's ability to self-replicate within cancer cells, as well as their ability to serve as vectors for various immunostimulatory transgenes, provide them with an advantage that conventional drugs lack [8]. Specific to melanoma, OVs have been shown to serve as viable candidates for treatment, due to their ability to preferentially target and lyse tumor cells. OVs also have the ability to activate antitumor immune responses via the innate and adaptive arms of the human immune system [9]. The inclusion of gene promoters for melanoma biomarkers has been a recent tactic for designing OVs that specifically target melanoma cells [10, 11]. For melanoma patients with clearly unresectable disease, or in-transit or nodal metastases, oncolytic virotherapy has become a viable treatment option, either alone or in combination with other forms of therapy [12].

Experimental and Clinical Overview

Oncolytic virotherapy's task is two-pronged: To target cancer cells and to leave normal, post-mitotic cells unharmed by viral replication [1]. Oncoselectivity within OVs can be naturally occurring within a wild type (wt) virus or achieved through genetic engineering [6]. Oncoselectivity of wt viruses is a result of tumor cells' abnormally activated and regulated pathways, which may downregulate the antiviral response that is present in normal post-mitotic cells [12]. One common means by which genetically engineered oncoselectivity can be achieved is through thymidine kinase (TK) viral gene ablation. Through the deletion of TK, a gene required for viral replication, replication-handicapped viruses seek TK from their environment. Most solid tumors, which have been found to have surplus or aberrantly activated TK, are therefore targeted by the virus, while normal cells are left untouched [13]. This technique can be found in many OVs, including the first modified OV tested [3, 14]. Another example of this technique is found in JX-594, a vaccinia virus (VV)-derived OV, that has shown to preferentially replicate in cells with over-expression of TK [7] .

Oncoselectivity may also be enhanced through the insertion of tyrosinase and survivin gene promoters into the viral vector. Tyrosinase, the enzyme responsible for catalyzing the rate-limiting step in melanin production, is a melanoma biomarker commonly used for diagnosis. Survivin, responsible for apoptosis and cell cycle regulation, is commonly expressed in melanoma cells and contributes to chemotherapy drug resistance [11]. The resultant insertion of these gene promoters into a viral vector translates into increased oncoselectivity, as the modified virus will specifically target and replicate in melanoma cells. Two conditionally replicative adenoviruses (CRAds), AdTyrΔ24 and AdTyrΔ2Δ24, have been successfully tested in vivo, demonstrating melanoma oncoselectivity using tyrosinase gene promoters [10]. Recognizing that survivin is the fourth most commonly over-expressed gene in melanoma, the preclinical development of the anti-cancer vaccine, HIvax, a recombinant fowlpox virus encoding survivin epitopes, has been tested in human dendritic cells (DCs) and T-cells in vitro with promising results showing CD4+, CD8+, and IFN-γ activation [15]. However, successful OV therapy relies upon more than just oncoselectivity. Viral tumor regression tactics are multifaceted, with direct tumor cell infection, destruction of the tumor blood supply and activation of both innate and adaptive immune responses as key components of oncolytic virotherapy [16, 17]. Immune system activation is a key factor in the efficacy of an OV, with immunostimulatory genes, such as cytokines including granulocyte macrophage colony-stimulating factor (GM-CSF), Interleukin-2 (IL-2), IL-12, IL-18, and Interferon (IFN) commonly inserted to increase immunoreactivity [18–20]. VV JX-594 and HSV Talimogene laherparepvec (T-Vec) both utilize GM-CSF gene insertions and have each completed clinical trials for use in patients with advanced melanoma [12, 14].

Newcastle disease virus (NDV) [20, 21], HSV HF10 [22], and Tanapox virus (TPV) [23] have modified strains with the IL-2 gene inserted. Although these viruses have yet to advance to human clinical trials, murine studies have shown some promising results. Similarly, two CRAd strains include a functional IL-18 and IL-12 gene within their viral DNA, are currently still within the preclinical phases of study [24, 25]. Finally, ablation of viral immunoregulatory genes, which downregulate or suppress the host's immune response following infection, improve the immune response following inoculation. Recent Food and Drug Administration (FDA) approval of T-Vec has brought light to this method, with its ablation of the HSV *ICP47* gene, responsible for the suppression of antigen presentation and decreased major histocompatibility complex class-I (MHC-I) expression on the surface of infected cells. Through this gene's ablation, increased antigen presentation is achieved, resulting in a specific target and improved activation of the host immune response [8, 12, 26, 27]. Studies on another OV with immunoregulatory gene ablation involves TPVΔ2L, which removes a tumor necrosis factor (TNF)-neutralizing gene [28].

Targeting the tumor microenvironment, neovasculature or intermixed stromal tissue and cells is another key tactic in OV therapy [18]. Without proper vasculature and angiogenesis, tumor cells cease to replicate and die as a result of insufficient oxygen and nutrients delivered through local arterioles. By targeting growth factors known to stimulate angiogenesis in melanoma, such as vascular endothelial growth factor (VEGF), enhanced tumor regression has been achieved [18]. One CRAd expressing IL-18 showed marked melanoma regression within a murine melanoma model, achieving tumor regression fourfold over controls [24]. Immunohistochemistry analysis revealed VEGF suppression within virus-infected tumors [24]. In 2005, Kaufman et al. evaluated 12 patients following the monthly administration of a VV armed with cluster of differentiation (CD)80, a co-stimulatory molecule necessary for T-cell activation [29]. The study resulted in increased IL-10, CD8, and IFN levels within the tumor microenvironment and tumor regression noted in some patients [29].

Two emerging means by which OVs are tailored to enhance efficacy involve the targeting of melanoma signaling pathways and of tumor-associated antigens (TAAs) found on melanoma cells. Ras-activation has been reported in 20% of melanoma patients [18], making it an excellent target for OVs. One Influenza virus has demonstrated great potential in preliminary experimental mouse models [30]. The virus was designed on the principles that: (a) the NS1 gene has been shown to replicate in Protein Kinase-R (PKR)-deficient cells while leaving normal cells untouched, and (b) PKR is suppressed when Ras is activated [30]. The purpose of NS1 gene deletion for a melanoma-specific OV is understood within this context. In recent years, melanoma-associated antigens (MAAs) have been further explored for use in anti-cancer vaccines and immunotherapies [31].

One antigen of particular interest to OV researchers is High-Molecular-Weight Melanoma-associated antigen (HMW-MAA), which has been found to appear in over 90% of human melanomas [32, 33], and has been used as an insert into a viral vector in order to restrict tropism [33]. One retrovirus contains both a HMW-MAA and a matrix metalloprotease (MMP) cleavage site. MMPs are also over-expressed on cancer cell surfaces, and have successfully achieved melanoma-restricted replication in vitro and in vivo [33]. By using these same principles, a vesicular stomatitis virus (VSV) has been shown to demonstrate success in vivo, when the cDNA of three recognized TAAs were each inserted into a viral VSV vector. Having been used on established melanoma tumors in a mouse model, the recombinant viruses show promise [31].

Clinical Trials

Over the last decade, clinical trials have demonstrated varying degrees of success in OV therapy for the treatment of melanoma. Although other viruses, such as VV expressing CD80, have undergone clinical trials for the treatment of melanoma [29], JX-594, Reolysin, Cavatak, and T-Vec have completed the most extensive clinical testing for safety and efficacy as melanoma monotherapies. Table 31.1 illustrates the OVs that have completed clinical trials, as well as those still undergoing evaluation in melanoma patients.

VV's large genome makes it an appealing option for genetic modification for OV optimization, and as one of the first viruses to be used as a viable treatment option, the genome is understood quite well [5, 14]. JX-594, a Wyeth Strain VV with TK ablation and GM-CSF insertion, has provided robust results in clinical trials for the treatment of melanoma [7, 14]. In initial JX-594 trials, melanoma patients were first inoculated with wtVV before receiving intertumoral (IT) injections of JX-594. Results were noted with injections containing as little as 8×10^7 plaque forming units (pfu), with a standard dose of 10^8 pfu established for the study, which was <10% of

Table 31.1 Oncolytic virotherapy for treatment of melanoma

Virus		Modifications	Clinical trials as monotherapy	Clinical trials as combination therapy	References
Adenovirus		Adenoviral EA1 promoter ablation, tyrosinase promoter gene insertion	–	–	[10]
Coxsackie virus	CVA21 (*Cavatak*)	None	+	+	[14, 37, 38, 45]
Herpes Simplex virus	T-Vec (*Imlygic*)	ICP34.5 ablation, ICP37 ablation, GMCSF insertion	+	+	[12, 14, 16, 26, 39–41, 43, 46]
	HF10	IL-2 insertion	–	–	[22]
Influenza virus		NS1 ablation	–	–	[30]
Measles virus		Anti-CTLA-4 insertion	–	–	[51]
Newcastle disease virus		IL-2 insertion	–	–	[20, 21]
		Anti PD-1 insertion	–	–	[51]
Reovirus	(*Reolysin*)	None	+	+	[36, 47, 56]
		IL-12 insertion; IL-18 insertion, E1B ablation	–	–	[24, 25]
Retrovirus		MMP cleavage-site insertion, antibody recognizing HMW-MAA insertion	–	–	[32, 33]
Tanapox virus		TK ablation, IL-2 insertion	–	–	[23]
Vaccinia virus	JX-594 (*Pexa-Vec*)	TK ablation, GMCSF insertion	+	–	[7, 14, 34, 35]
		GMCSF insertion	–	–	[14]
		CD80 expression	+	–	[29]
Vesicular stomatitis virus		TAA cDNA insertion	–	–	[31]

Abbreviations: *CD* cluster of differentiation, *CTLA* cytotoxic T-lymphocyte antigen, *GM-CSF* granulocyte monocyte colony-stimulating factor, *HMWMAA* high molecular weight melanoma-associated antigen, *IL* interleukin, *MMP* matrix metalloprotease, *PD* programmed death receptor, *TAA* tumor-associated antigen, *TK* thymidine kinase the standard dose used in JX-594 clinical trials for liver tumors [34]. The ten participants received, on average, six prior forms of treatment including surgery, radiation, and chemotherapy. JX-594 treatment was generally well tolerated, with the most common adverse effects (AEs) documented as fatigue, pyrexia, myalgia, and anemia [34].

One participant exhibited stable disease following nine treatments of JX-594; this was noted in both injected and non-injected tumors. All patients' VV titers peaked on day 21, despite the 6-week duration of the study. Mean survival of patients following treatment was 7.1 months, with 5 noted to have stable disease. In one patient with biopsy samples at baseline, day 5, and day 43, no necrosis was seen at baseline, VV replication and slight tumor necrosis was noted in biopsy at day 5, and intense grade necrosis was documented at day 43 [34]. Transgene products were found in all ten participants [34]. Another 14-patient JX-594 trial completed in South Korea included two metastatic melanoma patients. Pyrexia, chills, and fatigue were again reported to be the most common AEs [35]. Stable disease was achieved in six out of seven patients assessed for non-injected tumor response and, of the ten patients assessed using CT scans, nine had either a durable response (DR) or stable disease.

Reolysin, a wt Reovirus Serotype 3-Dearing Strain, preferentially replicates in Ras-activated cells, present in 60% of metastatic melanoma cases [36]. One phase II study of Reolysin implemented an intravenous (IV) administration of the virus to 21 eligible participants with metastatic melanoma. Fatigue, nausea, and pyrexia were the most frequently reported AEs. Although one patient's tumor biopsy showed 75–90% tumor necrosis, only six patients achieved stable disease for more than 8 weeks, and the study did not proceed to the next stage. It must also be noted that all 21 participants were found to have neutralizing anti-reovirus antibodies (NARA) in their baseline serum samples, and that NARA presence did not prevent successful reovirus replication in all patients. Although the results were disappointing for utilizing Reolysin as a monotherapy, combinational therapies with the virus may prove to be more beneficial [36].

Cavatak, Coxsackievirus A21, began its first US clinical trials for melanoma in 2013. This study accrued 63 stage IIIc and IV melanoma over an 18-week period, with up to ten intratumoral (IT) Catavak injections administered into multiple lesions [37]. After evaluating the first 30 patients, the primary endpoint of ten patients achieving immune-related progression free survival (irPFS) following a single Cavatak injection was achieved [38]. As trials testing the efficacy of Cavatak as a monotherapy continue, combinatorial therapies may again prove to be even more beneficial [38].

T-Vec, arguably the most advanced OV method for the treatment of melanoma, is a modified HSV-1 expressing GM-CSF [39]. Compared to treatment with the cytokine alone, T-Vec elicits much greater treatment response rates. The immunostimulatory response resulting from viral infection in conjunction with the on-site expression of GM-CSF, have highlighted this effect in recent clinical trials [26, 39–41] and have generated much excitement due to its recent FDA approval for melanoma therapy in 2015 [8]. Originally isolated from a cold sore of a healthy volunteer donor, JS1, the HSV-1 strain used in T-Vec, was tested against other strains of the virus and determined to be the most effective in tumor cell replication and lysis [12]. HSV-1 serves as an effective vector for OV therapies due to the large genomic size, in addition to the numerous other nonessential genes for replication. This was helpful in introducing and inserting the human GM-CSF gene following viral gene ablation. T-Vec's ablation of *ICP34.5* and *ICP47* enhances tumor-selective replication, increases antigen presentation, and increases MHC class-I expression on HSV-infected cells [27]. HSV-1 infection leads to mild symptoms, and the ubiquity of the virus within human host populations serves as proof of the virus's ability to safely replicate within immunocompetent humans [12]. One reoccurring hurdle within OV therapy is the challenge of acquired viral-immunity. Despite an estimated global population exposure of 67% [42], HSV-1 is still able to replicate within people with preexisting exposure, thus, securing an OV that can be used for multiple dosing and in those with antibodies against the virus. However, one complication is that it has been found that patients lacking serological antibodies to the virus experienced more severe injection site reactions, such as erythema and ulceration. The virus has been shown to induce robust innate and adaptive immune responses, characterized by an increased presence of natural killer (NK) cells and IFN-γ, respectively [12]. This therapy is delivered via an intratumoral injection, thus, those patients with bulky, unresectable nodal or subcutaneous disease are optimal candidates for T-Vec treatment. The initial dose is 10^6 pfu/mL, with subsequent dosing at 10^8 pfu/mL, found to be safe and well tolerated in the phase I Oncovex (GM-CSF) Pivotal Trial in Melanoma (OPTiM). The total volume to be injected depends upon the tumor volume and the number of target lesions to be injected [12, 41]. The phase II OPTiM trial found that the quantity of immunosuppressive cell types commonly found in melanoma patients, such as CD4+ and regulatory T-cells (Tregs) was decreased following T-Vec treatment. Half of all patients enrolled in this trial experienced AEs ranging from pyrexia and fatigue to flu-like symptoms. However, severe reactions were extremely rare, with <1% of patients experiencing severe flu-like symptoms [12]. This study revealed an overall response rate (ORR) of 26% in patients with stage IIIC to IV melanoma [26].

In the OPTiM phase III clinical trial, which ultimately led to FDA approval of T-Vec for use in melanoma, 64% of injected lesions decreased in size by at least 50%, with 48% undergoing complete regression. A total of 34% of non-injected tumors shrank by greater than half, with a perceived systemic response of non-injected visceral lesions of 15%. Pseudo-progression, or progression prior to response (PPR) was noted in 48% of patients who experienced a DR in OPTiM, with the majority in this group developing new lesions [12, 40]. With this in mind, the number of patients who achieved a DR may be skewed, as a DR was noted 3 months earlier in patients without PPR, compared to those with a PPR. Nonetheless, the percentage of patients who achieved a DR was similar between those who had a PPR and those who did not [40].

T-Vec Administration and Use in the Clinic

T-vec currently shows most promise as an adjunct to immune checkpoint mediators and as a treatment for those awaiting surgery [12, 40].T-Vec, a biosafety level (BSL) 1 organism, does require some attention in preparing and administering in the clinical setting [41, 43]. Vials must be stored at a maximum temperature of −70 °C to protect the viability of the viral titer [41]. Healthcare providers who are pregnant or immunocompromised should not be allowed to prepare the agent [44]. Prior to patient administration, the vials must be thawed at room temperature within the confines of a sterile biosafety cabinet. Personal protective equipment (PPE) required for working with the BSL 1 agent includes gloves, gown, and a mask [43, 44].

A maximum injected volume is not to exceed 4 mL, and IT injected volume is dependent on the size of the lesion [41]. Prior to the intratumoral administration, a topical anesthetic or ice may be used to relieve injection-site pain. However, it must be noted that local anesthetic IT injection, such as lidocaine, has been shown to interfere with IT pH and may negatively impact the viruses' stability [41, 43]. Following injection, each site requires an occlusive dressing. Patient education should include proper dressing re-application in case of accidental removal, as well as instructions to seal soiled dressings in a plastic bag prior to disposal with common waste. The administration of acetaminophen and indomethacin can be used to treat flu-like AEs that have been reported with T-Vec [41]. In cases of accidental exposure of severe AEs, acyclovir is an effective antiviral therapy [41].

The cost of treatment with T-Vec is a common concern for many melanoma patients, with a full course of treatment considerably less than a comparable immunotherapy for melanoma treatment. For example, while a full course of treatment for an immune checkpoint inhibitor can cost well over $100,000, T-Vec has committed to maintaining the cost of the drug to around $65,000. Programs offering financial assistance are also available to patients for whom treatment co-pay costs remain too high [44].

Combination Therapies: Viral Oncolytics and Immune Checkpoint Inhibitors

When fighting metastatic melanoma, strength is in numbers. Clinical trials testing combination OV and immunotherapies have expanded within the past 5 years, often demonstrating higher response rates than either drug alone. Recently, T-Vec has been examined in combination trials with the immunotherapeutic drugs, ipilimumab and pembrolizumab. Ipilimumab has also been used with great success in combination with Cavatak [14, 45]. Reolysin was used in 2009 in combination with chemotherapeutic agents [46].

Anti-programmed cell death-1 (PD), an antibody checkpoint inhibitor, functions by blocking the interaction of programmed cell death-1 with its ligands, PD-L1 and PD-L2 [47]. Expressed on T-cells, B-cells, and macrophages, PD-1 receptor/ligand interactions mediate the immune response [47, 48]. When PD-L1 or PD-L2 bind to receptor PD-1, the T-cell response is suppressed. The expression of PD-L1 and PD-L2 is a common tactic to promote self-tolerance and immunosuppression among cancers, including melanoma [18]. Therefore, with the use of anti-PD-1, the receptor/ligand interaction can be intercepted and the downregulation of T-cells within the host will cease.

Cytotoxic T-lymphocyte antigen-4 (CTLA-4) is a receptor located on T-cells. Binding with ligands B7–1 and B7–2 results in an attenuated memory T-cell response, with an upregulation of CTLA-4 receptors in melanoma patients [48]. The boost of adaptive immune cells following immune checkpoint inhibitor administration makes the combination of immune checkpoint inhibitors, such as anti-PD-1 and anti-CTLA-4, a logical next-step in immunotherapeutic cancer treatment [47]. Pembrolizumab, nivolumab, and lambrolizumab, all PD-1 inhibitors, and ipilimumab, a CTLA-4 inhibitor, are FDA-approved monotherapies for the treatment of melanoma [18, 49].

Due to T-vec's mechanism of action of adaptive immune stimulation through the promotion of antigen presentation and T-cell priming within the tumor microenvironment, combination therapy with systemic immunotherapies, specifically CTLA-4 and PD-1, have recently been examined. One phase Ib trial that used T-vec in combination with ipilimumab revealed toxicity profiles to be consistent with ipilimumab treatment alone, with an overall immune response greater than that of ipilimumab alone [46, 50]. As pembrolizumab was found to improve T-cell tumor recognition ability [14], following T-Vec administration, the primed T-cells are better able to recognize tumor cells with the subsequent pembrolizumab dose. Compared to T-Vec's 26% ORR and pembrolizumab's 34% ORR, the combination therapy demonstrated a 57% ORR and 24% complete response rate. Clinical combination trials of T-Vec and ipilimumab, as well as T-Vec and pembrolizumab, are still ongoing [50].

In vivo data from one mouse study showed that the combination of Reolysin with a PD-1 inhibitor doubled the survival rate at 60 days, compared to Reolysin alone [47]. More importantly, this study identified the role that cytokines play in the antitumor response, finding that the addition of anti-PD-1 significantly increases the IFN-γ response. Similarly, it was found that this IFN- γ response resulted from NK cell, Treg and CD8+ T-cell expression, with the combination of the PD-1 inhibitor and Reolysin significantly enhancing NK cell activation compared to Reolysin alone.

Although classified as monotherapies, two recombinant measles viruses (MV) sought to incorporate the principle of OV and immune checkpoint inhibitor combination therapy into a single OV treatment by incorporating anti-CTLA-4 and anti-PD-1 into two MV vectors [51]. Tested in an immunocompetent mouse model, both viruses demonstrated enhanced melanoma tumor cell lysis compared to controls serving as monotherapeutic examples of the synergistic effects of immune checkpoint inhibitors and OV therapy [51].

Future of Viral Oncolytics for Treatment of Melanoma

Within the past decade, OV research and development has finally begun to be translated into viable treatment options for patients with melanoma, demonstrating a therapeutic alternative to, or combination with, other agents [18]. OV's ability to replicate oncoselectively, stimulate the immune system through viral infection and transgene expression, and work with other therapies are among the reasons that these OVs have had success in recent clinical trials [18]. In the next few years, the translation of successfully trialed OV's into FDA-approved therapies must continue along with the testing of OV's in combination with other therapies. Similarly, a continuous search for new OVs is one way to ensure a large bank of armed viruses ready to be used at the disposal of physicians if acquired viral-immunity occurs [52–54]. Zika virus has recently been reported to demonstrate strong OV qualities against glioblastoma cells in vitro [55], fowlpox has shown immunostimulatory effects in DCs and T-cells showing promise as an anti-cancer vaccine.

When combining OVs with immunotherapies, the role that increased adaptive and innate immunity has upon the success of viral infection must be further explored and understood to maximize efficacy of such therapies, with further refinements in oncoselectivity necessary [19, 53]. The standard treatment options of surgery, adjuvant chemotherapy and occasionally radiation therapy do not always provide the patient with optimal outcomes, with many still developing metastatic, and often, unresectable disease. Thus, oncolytic virotherapy now provides us with another tool to effectively treat such patients, either alone, or in combination with other known effective immunotherapy agents. The major limitation of OV technology is the development of an anti-OV immune response in patients following treatment with a select OV. This hopefully will be resolved in the near future by making OVs invisible to the human immune system using the basic principle of immune tolerance.

Acknowledgements We thank Dr. John Jellies, Dr. Cecil McIntire, and Susan McIntire for editorial comments.

References

1. Lin E, Nemunaitis J. Oncolytic viral therapies. Cancer Gene Ther. 2004;11:643–64.
2. Kelly E, Russell S. History of Oncolytic viruses: genesis to genetic engineering. Mol Ther. 2007;15:651–9.
3. Martuza R, Malick A, Markert J, Ruffner K, Coen D. Experimental therapy of human glioma by means of a genetically engineered virus mutant. Science. 1991;252:854–6.
4. Peters C, Rabkin S. Designing herpes viruses as oncolytics. Mol Ther Oncolytics. 2015;2:15010.
5. Kaufman HL, Kim DW, DeRaffele G, Mitcham J, Coffin RS, et al. Local and distant immunity induced by intralesional vaccination with an oncolytic herpes virus encoding GM-CSF in patients with III c and IV melanoma. Ann Surg Oncol. 2010;17:718–30.
6. Fukuhara H, Ino Y, Todo T. Oncolytic virus therapy: a new era of cancer treatment at dawn. Cancer Sci. 2016;107:1373–9.
7. Mastrangelo M, Maguire H, Eisenlohr L, Laughlin C, Monken C, McCue P, Kovatich A, Lattime E. Intratumoral recombinant GM-CSF-encoding virus as gene therapy in patients with cutaneous melanoma. Cancer Gene Ther. 1999;6:409–22.
8. Kee D, McArthur G. Immunotherapy of melanoma. Eur J Surg Oncol. 2017;43:594–603.
9. Chan W, Rahman M, McFadden G. Oncolytic myxoma virus: the path to clinic. Vaccine. 2013;31:4252–8.
10. Nettelbeck D, Rivera A, Balagué C, Alemany R, Curiel D. Novel oncolytic adenoviruses targeted to melanoma: specific viral replication and cytolysis by expression of E1A mutants from the tyrosinase enhancer/promoter. Cancer Res. 2002;62:4663–70.
11. Garg H, Suri P, Gupta J, Talwar G, Dubey S. Survivin: a unique target for tumor therapy. Cancer Cell Int. 2016;23(16):49. https://doi.org/10.1186/s12935-016-0326-1.
12. Grigg C, Blake Z, Gartrell R, Sacher A, Taback B, Saenger Y. Talimogene laherparepvec (T-Vec) for the treatment of melanoma and other cancers. Semin Oncol. 2016;43:638–46.
13. Conrad S, El-Aswad M, Kurban E, Jeng D, Tripp B, Nutting C, Eversole R, Mackenzie C, Essani K. Oncolytic tanapoxvirus expressing FliC causes regression of human colorectal cancer xenografts in nude mice. J Exp Clin Cancer Res. 2015;34:19.

14. Deng L, Fan J, Guo M, Huang B. Oncolytic and immunologic cancer therapy with GM-CSF-armed vaccinia virus of Tian tan strain Guang9. Cancer Lett. 2016;372:251–7.
15. Hoffmann P, Panigada M, Soprana E, et al. Preclinical development of HIvax: human survivin highly immunogenic vaccines. Hum Vaccin Immunother. 2015;11:1585–95.
16. Varghese S, Rabkin S. Oncolytic herpes simplex virus vectors for cancer virotherapy. Cancer Gene Ther. 2002;9:967–78.
17. Hermiston T, Kuhn I. Armed therapeutic viruses: strategies and challenges to arming oncolytic viruses with therapeutic genes. Cancer Gene Ther. 2002;9:1022–35.
18. Zhang T, Suryawanshi Y, Woyczesczyk H, Essani K. Targeting melanoma with cancer-killing viruses. Open Virol J. 2017;11:28–47.
19. Stephenson K, Barra N, Davies E, Ashkar A, Lichty B. Expressing human interleukin-15 from oncolytic vesicular stomatitis virus improves survival in a murine metastatic colon adenocarcinoma model through the enhancement of anti-tumor immunity. Cancer Gene Ther. 2011;19:238–46.
20. Zhao H, Janke M, Fournier P, Schirrmacher V. Recombinant Newcastle disease virus expressing human interleukin-2 serves as a potential candidate for tumor therapy. Virus Res. 2008;136:75–80.
21. Bai F, Niu Z, Tian H, Li S, Lv Z, Zhang T, Ren G, Li D. Genetically engineered Newcastle disease virus expressing interleukin 2 is a potential drug candidate for cancer immunotherapy. Immunol Lett. 2014;159:36–46.
22. Carew J, Kooby D, Halterman M, Kim S, Federoff H, Fong Y. A novel approach to cancer therapy using an Oncolytic herpes virus to package amplicons containing cytokine genes. Mol Ther. 2001;4:250–6.
23. Zhang T, Kordish D, Suryawanshi Y, Eversole R, Kohler S, Mackenzie C, Essani K. Oncolytic tanapoxvirus expressing interleukin-2 is capable of inducing the regression of human melanoma tumors in the absence of T cells. Curr Cancer Drug Targets. 2017;17:9.
24. Zheng J, Pei D, Mao L, Liu X, Sun F, Zhang B, Liu Y, Liu J, Li W, Han D. Oncolytic adenovirus expressing interleukin-18 induces significant antitumor effects against melanoma in mice through inhibition of angiogenesis. Cancer Gene Ther. 2009;17:28–36.
25. Lee Y, Kim J, Choi K, Choi I, Kim H, Cho S, Cho B, Yun C. Enhanced antitumor effect of Oncolytic adenovirus expressing Interleukin-12 and B7-1 in an Immunocompetent murine model. Clin Cancer Res. 2006;12:5859–68.
26. Andtbacka R, Kaufman H, Collichio F, et al. Talimogene Laherparepvec improves durable response rate in patients with advanced melanoma. J Clin Oncol. 2015;33:2780–8.
27. Liu B, Robinson M, Han Z, et al. ICP34.5 deleted herpes simplex virus with enhanced oncolytic, immune stimulating, and anti-tumour properties. Gene Ther. 2003;10:292–303.
28. Jeng D, Rahman MM, McFadden G, Essani K. Tumor necrosis factor inhibitors from poxviruses with an emphasis on Tanapoxvirus-2L protein. Recent Pat DNA Gene Seq. 2011;5:97–103.
29. Kaufman H, DeRaffele G, Mitcham J, et al. Targeting the local tumor microenvironment with vaccinia virus expressing B7.1 for the treatment of melanoma. J Clin Investig. 2005;115:1903–12.
30. Bergmann M, Romirer I, Sachet M, et al. A genetically engineered influenza a virus with ras-dependent oncolytic properties. Cancer Res. 2001;61:8188–93.
31. Pulido J, Kottke T, Thompson J, et al. Using virally expressed melanoma cDNA libraries to identify tumor-associated antigens that cure melanoma. Nat Biotechnol. 2012;30:337–43.
32. Martın F, Chowdhury S, Neil S, Phillipps N, Collins M. Envelope-targeted retrovirus vectors transduce melanoma Xenografts but not spleen or liver. Mol Ther. 2002;5:269–74.
33. Martin F, Neil S, Kupsch J, Maurice M, Cosset FL, Collins M. Retrovirus targeting by tropism restriction to melanoma cells. J Virol. 1999;73:6923–9.
34. Hwang T, Moon A, Burke J, et al. A mechanistic proof-of-concept clinical trial with JX-594, a targeted multi-mechanistic Oncolytic poxvirus, in patients with metastatic melanoma. Mol Ther. 2011;19:1913–192.
35. Park B, Hwang T, Liu T, et al. Use of a targeted oncolytic poxvirus, JX-594, in patients with refractory primary or metastatic liver cancer: a phase I trial. Lancet Oncol. 2008;9:533–42.
36. Galanis E, Markovic S, Suman V, et al. Phase II trial of intravenous Administration of Reolysin® (Reovirus Serotype-3-Dearing strain) in patients with metastatic melanoma. Mol Ther. 2012;20:1998–2003.
37. Viralytics starts enrollment in phase II CAVATAK melanoma trial. 2011. M2 Pharma.
38. Primary endpoint achieved in CAVATAK phase 2 melanoma trial. 2013. PR Newswire. http://libproxy.library.wmich.edu/login?url=https://search.proquest.com/docview/1433277955?accountid=15099
39. Lichty B, Breitbach C, Stojdl D, Bell J. Going viral with cancer immunotherapy. Nat Rev Cancer. 2014;14:559–67.
40. Andtbacka R, Ross M, Puzanov I, et al. Patterns of clinical response with Talimogene Laherparepvec (T-VEC) in patients with melanoma treated in the OPTiM phase III clinical trial. Ann Surg Oncol. 2016;23:4169–77.
41. Rehman H, Silk A, Kane M, Kaufman H. Into the clinic: Talimogene laherparepvec (T-VEC), a first-in-class intratumoral oncolytic viral therapy. J Immunother Cancer. 2016;4:53. https://doi.org/10.1186/s40425-016-0158-5.
42. Herpes simplex virus. In: World Health Organization. 2017. http://www.who.int/mediacentre/factsheets/fs400/en/. Accessed 7 Sep 2017.
43. Harrington K, Michielin O, Malvehy J, Pezzani Grüter I, Grove L, Frauchiger A, Dummer R. A practical guide to the handling and administration of talimogene laherparepvec in Europe. Onco Targets Ther. 2017;10:3867–80.

44. Orloff M. Spotlight on talimogene laherparepvec for the treatment of melanoma lesions in the skin and lymph nodes. Oncolytic Virother. 2016;5:91–8.
45. Gormley C, Agarwala SS. Intralesional combination shows early promise in melanoma. HEM/ONC Today. 2017;18(10):18–9. *ProQuest*. Web. 4 Sep. 2017
46. Puzanov I, Milhem M, Andtbacka R, Minor D, Hamid O, Li A, VanderWalde A, Kaufman H. Phase 1 results of a phase 1b/2, multicenter, open-label trial to evaluate safety and efficacy of talimogene laherparepvec (T-VEC) and ipilimumab (ipi) vs ipi alone in previously untreated, unresected stage IIIB-IV melanoma. J Immunother Cancer. 2013;1:P84.
47. Rajani K, Parrish C, Kottke T, et al. Combination therapy with Reovirus and anti-PD-1 blockade controls tumor growth through innate and adaptive immune responses. Mol Ther. 2016;24:166–74.
48. Webb E, Liu P, Baleeiro R, Lemoine N. Immune checkpoint inhibitors in cancer therapy. J Biomed Res. 2017. https://doi.org/10.7555/jbr.31.20160168.
49. Fellner C. Ipilimumab (Yervoy) prolongs survival in advanced melanoma: serious side effects and a hefty price tag may limit its use. PT. 2012;37:503–30.
50. Sosman J. Addice T-Vec to ipilimumab for advanced melanoma. NEJM J Watch. Oncology and Hematology. 2016.
51. Engeland C, Grossardt C, Veinalde R, et al. CTLA-4 and PD-L1 checkpoint blockade enhances Oncolytic measles virus therapy. Mol Ther. 2014;22:1949–59.
52. Christie JD, Byers ER, Essani K. Oncolytic Virotherapy: a brief overview. J Med Microb Diagn. 2016;5:e129. https://doi.org/10.4172/2161-0703.1000e129.
53. Suryawanshi Y, Zhang T, Essani K. Oncolytic viruses: emerging options for the treatment of breast cancer. Med Oncol. 2017;34(3):43. https://doi.org/10.1007/s12032-017-0899-0.
54. Thomas C, Ehrhardt A, Kay M. Progress and problems with the use of viral vectors for gene therapy. Nat Rev Genet. 2003;4:346–58.
55. Zhu Z, Gorman M, McKenzie L, Chai J, Hubert C, Prager B, Fernandez E, Richner J, Zhang R, Shan C, Wang X, Shi P, Diamond M, Rich J, Chheda M. Zika virus has oncolytic activity against glioblastoma stem cells. J Exp Med. 2017;214(10):2843–57.
56. Mahalingam D, Fountzilas C, Moseley J, Noronha N, Tran H, Chakrabarty R, Selvaggi G, Coffey M, Thompson B, Sarantopoulos J. A phase II study of REOLYSIN® (pelareorep) in combination with carboplatin and paclitaxel for patients with advanced malignant melanoma. Cancer Chemother Pharmacol. 2017;79:697–703.

Chemotherapy and Biochemotherapy for Melanoma

32

Chia-Yen Hung and John Wen-Cheng Chang

Introduction

Melanoma arises from normal human melanocytes that have undergone malignant transformation. Physiologically, melanocytes are responsible for melanin production in various tissues. In terms of embryology, precursor melanocytes originate from the neural crest and migrate to multiple locations (e.g., skin, meninges, mucous membranes, upper esophagus, and eyes) during fetal development. Therefore, melanoma typically arise within the epidermis and dermis of the skin, but can also arise from anywhere within this tissue. The most common location is the hair follicle, with melanocytes located in the dermal and epidermal layers. Epidemiologically, the incidence rates of melanoma show substantial variation worldwide [1]. The worldwide incidence of invasive melanoma is highest in Auckland, New Zealand, with an age-standardized rate (ASR) of 40.2/100,000 [2]. According to the 2012 GLOBOCAN statistics, the ASR of melanoma incidence is 8.6–13.8/100,000 persons for Europe and North America and lower in Asia at 0.4–0.5/100,000 persons.

C.-Y. Hung, M.D. (✉)
Hematology and Oncology Division, Internal Medicine Department, Mackay Memorial Hospital, Taipei, New Taipei, Taiwan

Division of Hematology and Oncology, Department of Internal Medicine, Chang Gung Memorial Hospital at Linkou, Taoyuan, Taoyuan, Taiwan
e-mail: eliza7301@hotmail.com

J. W.-C. Chang, M.D.
Division of Hematology and Oncology, Department of Internal Medicine, Chang Gung Memorial Hospital at Linkou, Taoyuan, Taoyuan, Taiwan

Locally Advanced Melanoma

Despite the increasing incidence of melanoma, most patients are diagnosed at an early stage with localized disease. Prompt diagnosis and further surgical intervention with curative intent is the treatment of choice for most early-stage melanoma patients. Moreover, many have tried to identify patients who have a higher potential to develop metastatic disease, and thus who may benefit from adjuvant therapy. For locally advanced melanoma, around 20–30% of patients with T2 or thicker primary melanomas were found to have stage III disease with regional lymph node involvement. This, in turn, is associated with up to a 30% risk of developing distant metastasis and mortality [3]. This group of patients are those that are recommended to discuss adjuvsnt therapy due to their high risk of developing a systemic recurrence of melanoma.

Prior to the utility of ipilimumab, an anti-CTLA4 inhibitor, as an adjuvant therapy, high-dose IFNα was considered by most to be the most effective therapy for high-risk melanoma, approved by the FDA in 1995. This approval was based upon three pivotal phase III clinical trials completed by the Eastern Cooperative Oncology

A. I. Riker (ed.), *Melanoma*, https://doi.org/10.1007/978-3-319-78310-9_32

Group (ECOG). These trials, namely E-1684, E-1690, and E-1694 examined the utility of IFN**α** in various clinical adjuvant settings for resected, stage 3 melanoma patients. ECOG 1684 involved 287 melanoma patients in stage IIB (depth > 4 mm) or stage III (subclinical or clinically positive regional lymph node involvement), who were randomized 1:1 to high-dose IFNα-2b (20 million units/m^2 intravenously for 5 days per week for 4 weeks, followed by 10 million units/m^2 subcutaneously 3 times weekly for 12 months) for 1 year versus observation only. The IFNα arm showed a superior relapse-free survival (RFS; median, 1.7 vs. 1 year, $p = 0.0023$) and overall survival (OS; median, 3.8 vs. 2.8 years, $p = 0.0237$) [4]. A similar result was found in ECOG 1694 with 880 patients with stage IIB and III melanoma, 1:1 randomized into groups of high-dose IFNα-2b for 1 year versus GM2-KLH vaccine (weekly ×4 cycles, then every 12 weeks × 8 cycles) [5]. Statistically improved RFS (hazard ratio [HR] 1.47, $p = 0.0015$) and an overall survival (HR 1.52, $p = 0.009$) advantage were noted in the high-dose IFNα group. However, ECOG 1690 revealed some different results, with 642 enrolled patients with stage IIB and III melanoma. This trial was a 1:1:1 randomized trial of three groups: high-dose IFNα for 1 year, low-dose IFNα for 2 years versus observation (OBS) [6]. The high-dose IFNα group had significantly higher RFS than the OBS group (HR 1.28, $p = 0.05$). However, the OS rates of the first two groups were similar, probably due to a substantial improvement of salvage therapy with IFNα-containing therapy after disease progression, with a longer median OS compared to that seen with ECOG 1684 (6 vs. 2.8 years).

The trial results indicate that patients with high-risk features, including primary T4 melanomas or regional nodal involvement, demonstrated RFS benefit with high-dose IFNα with treatment duration for 1 year [4–6]. A significant OS benefit was observed in studies E-1684 and E-1694, but not in E-1690. A pooled meta-analysis of 14 randomized control trials (RCTs) published from 1990 to 2008, enrolling ~8122 high-risk patients, among whom 4362 patients received high-dose IFNα, found that a survival benefit remained statistically significant (disease-free survival [DFS], HR 0.82, 95% CI 0.77–0.87; $p < 0.001$; median OS, HR 0.89, CI 0.83–0.96; $p = 0.002$) [7].

Numerous adverse events were seen with the adjuvant treatment of patients with high-dose IFNα, such as fatigue, myelosuppression, hepatotoxicity, fatigue, mild to moderate depression, congnitive impairment, and thyroid dysfunction (hypo- or hyper-thyroidism) [8]. Therefore, patients should undergo close monitoring throughout their therapy, with special attention to hematologic, liver, and renal function as well as neurologic and cognitive function.

Pegylated IFNα was developed in order to prolong the duration of the IFNα effect, along with a reduced dosing schedule when compared to the frequency of administration with high-dose IFNα. Pegylated IFNα was approved by the FDA in April 2011, based upon the results of a phase III study, EORTC 18991. This study randomized 1256 resected stage III melanoma patients into pegylated IFNα versus observation. A borderline survival benefit was noted, with a 7-year RFS rate of 39.1% and 34.6%, respectively, in the pegylated IFNα and observation groups (HR 0.87, 95% CI 0.76–1.00; $p = 0.055$). There was no difference observed in OS between groups ($p = 0.57$) [9]. The subgroup of patients with stage III-N1 disease and ulceration of the primary lesion showed the most significant survival benefit, with a prolonged distant metastasis-free survival (DMFS; HR 0.65, CI 0.41–1.04; $p = 0.02$) and OS (HR 0.59, CI 0.35–0.97; $p = 0.006$). As a result of this trial, pegylated IFNα was approved as an alternative adjuvant therapy for resected stage III melanoma.

In addition to interferon therapy, adjuvant biochemotherapy is an alternative option for high-risk, resected stage III disease. Biochemotherapy is defined as any regimen that includes both chemotherapy (either single or combined) and immunotherapy, typically IFN*a* and/or IL-2. The adjuvant use of biochemotherapy was evaluated in a randomized phase III study, SWOG S0008. In this trial, 432 high-risk, resected melanoma patients with stage IIIa-N2a through IIIc-N3 were randomly assigned to receive either 3 cycles of adjuvant biochemotherapy (BCT), comprising cisplatin, vinblastine, dacarbazine, IL-2, and IFN*a* every 21 days, or high-dose IFNα alone [10].

The trial had a median follow-up of 7.2 years, showing an improved RFS of 4 versus 1.9 years, in the BCT and IFN groups, respectively (HR 0.75, 95% CI 0.58–0.97; $p = 0.03$). However, OS, another co-primary endpoint, showed no significant difference (median, 9.9 vs. 6.7 years, HR 0.98, 95% CI 0.74–1.31; $p = 0.55$). Notably, the BCT group had a higher therapy completion rate with a shorter 9-week duration compared to the high-dose IFNα group (completion rate, 80 vs. 43%, $p < 0.001$). Grade 3 or higher toxicity was observed more frquently in the BCT group (76 vs. 64%), with the most common toxicities noted to be hematologic (leucopenia, neutropenia, or thrombocytopenia), gastrointestinal, metabolic (hypocalcemia), and hypotension. In contrast, more hepatotoxicity was noted in the high-dose IFNα group. Therefore, biochemotherapy seems to be a shorter alternative adjuvant therapy for high-risk melanoma patients, but with significant higher toxicity.

A large phase III trial, EORTC 18071, was completed, examining the utility of ipilimumab in the adjuvant setting for resected stage III melanoma patients. A total of 951 stage 3, resected treatment-naive patients were enrolled (excluding lymph node metastasis ≦ 1 mm or in-transit metastasis). Patients were randomized to receive ipilimumab (10 mg/kg every 3 weeks for a total of 4 doses, then every 3 months for up to 3 years) versus placebo [11, 12]. The study revealed a significant improvement in RFS of 26.1 (ipilimumab) versus 17.1 months in the placebo arm (HR 0.75, 95% CI 0.64–0.90; $p = 0.0013$). The 5-year RFS, with a median follow-up of 5.3 years, was 40.8% versus 30.3% (HR 0.76, 95% CI 0.64–0.89; $p < 0.001$). Of note, there was a 10% improvement in the 5-year OS rate of 65.4% versus 54.4% (HR 0.72, 95% CI 0.58–0.88; $p = 0.001$).

The most frequent and severe immune-related adverse events (irAE) were gastrointestinal, liver, and endocrine toxicity. A significant proportion of patients in the ipilimumab arm had either grade 3 or 4 irAE (41.6 vs. 2.7% in placebo arm), with 5 treatment-related deaths (3 for colitis, 1 for myocarditis and 1 for multiple-organ failure with Guillain-Barre syndrome). The median time to onset of irAE ranged from 4 weeks (dermatologic irAE) to 13.1 weeks (neurological irAE), with a median time to resolution of 4–8 weeks (with the exception of endocrine irAE of 54.3 weeks for complete resolution). However, in a risk-benefit ratio evaluation, the FDA approved the indication of ipilimumab in the adjuvant setting for high-risk melanoma patients in October 2015. Therefore, more evidence is still needed on whether increased toxicity is dose-related as shown in the EORTC 18071 trial, as well as finding the optimal dose is still an issue.

In summary, to prevent a locoregional recurrence or distant metastasis, some form of adjuvant treatment is recommended in high-risk melanoma patients with stage III disease. Feasible agents include conventional IFNα, pegylated IFNα, and the novel immune checkpoint inhibitor, ipilimumab, with recent FDA approval. No head-to-head study has been completed to compare the efficacy of newer agents until now. We will await the results of the SWOG S1404 study, which compares pembrolizumab to high-dose IFNα for completely resected, stage IIIA(N2)-IV melanoma patients. For clinicians, selection of an active adjuvant therapy in high-risk, resected melanoma patients depends on many factors, such as agent efficacy, duration, safety, patient preference, age, and comorbidities.

Metastatic Disease

Although 80% of the patients are diagnosed with only localized disease, about one-third of patients will unfortunately develop distant metastasis [13, 14]. An overall poor prognosis was noted along with a short median overall survival of 6–9 months following the diagnosis of distant metastasis, with a 5-year survival rate of <5% [14–17]. In the past, there was not an established standard of care for patients with stage 4 melanoma, with moderate to severe toxicity noted for such therapies as high-dose IL-2 and TNFα. Historically, cytotoxic chemotherapy was commonly utilized for patients who were not suitable candidates for high-dose IL-2, although such therapies were known to have minimal survival benefit.

The most commonly utilized cytotoxic chemotherapy agents in metastatic melanoma are dacarbazine and its prodrug, temozolomide. The other agents, including platinum, vinca alkaloids, taxanes, and nitrosourea, have all been shown to have a minimal clinical benefit. These agents demonstrated modest response rates of <20%, with relative short response durations in both first- and second-line settings. Dacabazine is generally considered to be the most active agent for metastatic melanoma, with an average response rate of around 8–20% and a median response duration of about 4–6 months [18, 19]. The typical treatment dose and schedule are 200 mg/m^2 intravenously for 5 days, or 850–1000 mg/m^2 intravenously over 1 h, every 2–4 weeks. Although Dacabazine had no phase 3 clinical trials to prove a survival benefit compared to no treatment, it was approved for metastatic melanoma by the FDA in the United States. Dacarbazine is usually tolerable with the major toxicity mainly associated with the gastrointestinal tract, including nausea, vomiting, and myelosuppression.

Temozolomide is an analog of dacarbazine that is metabolized in the liver by the enzyme, cytochrome P450, to (5-[3-methyl-triazen-1-yl]-imidazole-4-carboxamide (MTIC)), which is an active metabolite of dacarbazine as an alkylating agent. Notably, unlike dacarbazine, temozolomide can penetrate through the blood brain barrier and has shown efficacy with brain and central nervous system malignancies. In a phase III study of 305 patients with metastatic melanoma, temozolomide showed a nonsignificant overall survival benefit compared to dacarbazine, as well as progression-free survival (median OS, 7.7 months vs. 6.4 months; median PFS, 1.9 months vs. 1.5 months, respectively) [20]. Another EORTC study, involving 859 enrolled patients with metastatic melanoma, found no survival difference between the temozolomide and dacarbazine groups, with a median OS of 9.1 versus 9.4 months, and median PFS of 2.3 versus 2.2 months, respectively [21]. Unfortunately, the evidence for true efficacy of temozolomide is still lacking, clearly not definitive enough for FDA approval in the metastatic setting.

The nitrosoureas, namely fotemustine, carmustine (BCNU), lomustine (CCNU), and semustine (methyl CCNU), have shown objective response rates (ORR) of around 13–18% in metastatic melanoma patients. In the phase III study, a total of 229 patients with metastatic melanoma (with or without brain metastasis) revealed superior response rate of 15.2% in the Fotemustine group compared to 6.8% in the dacarbazine group. However, that study found a nonsignificant median time to progression (1.9 vs. 1.8 months) and overall survival (7.3 vs. 5.6 months) [22]. In the subgroup analysis, patients without brain metastasis at enrollment showed a significantly longer time to brain metastasis in the fotemustine group (22.7 vs. 7.2 months). A trend towards fotemustine was shown with respect to overall survival and time to progression with brain metastasis. Hematologic toxicity, especially neutropenia and thrombocytopenia, was more severe with fotemustine compared to dacarbazine.

Platinum, including cisplatin and carboplatin, demonstrates only modest activity in metastatic melanoma. The average response rate is around 15–20% (range 0–53%) with cisplatin at doses of 200 mg/m^2 [19]. One study found that cisplatin at a dose of 150 mg/m^2 combined with amifostine, a thiol derivative, protected the bone marrow and kidneys. The response rate was up to 53%, withthe median response duration of only 4 months [23]. Another randomized, phase II ECOG study comparing cisplatin (150 mg/m^2) plus amifostine and lower-dose cisplatin (125 mg/m^2) showed activity in both groups. However, both groups showed intolerable renal, gastrointestinal and ototoxicity, with amifostine failing to show improved clinical activity when combined with cisplatin [19].

In a phase 2 study, nanoparticle albumin-bound paclitaxel (nab-paclitaxel) shows response rates of 22% and 3%, respectively, in chemotherapy-naïve and previously treated melanoma patients [24]. A phase III study with 529 chemotherapy-naïve patients with metastatic melanoma, randomized to nab-paclitaxel and dacarbazine [25], found significant improvement of PFS, the primary endpoint, in the nab-paclitaxel arm (median PFS, 4.8 vs. 2.5 months, hazard ratio [HR] 0.79, 95% CI 0.63–0.99). However, the OS between nab-paclitaxel and dacarbazine was statistically insignificant (median OS, 12.6 vs. 10.5 months; HR 0.90, 95% CI 0.74–1.09; $p = 0.27$). Further subgroup analysis revealed that the nab-paclitaxel had similar activity in BRAF wild type and mutant type [25]. Vinca alkaloids have shown only modest activity, with a phase II study of patients with metastatic melanoma finding a complete response rate of 2.5%, with an ORR of 20%, mainly when applied as a combination therapy [26].

In addition to single chemotherapy agents, combining different chemotherapy agents with biochemotherapy, such as IL-2 or TNFα, has failed to show significant efficacy in previous studies. So far, no randomized trials have yet demonstrated the superiority of combination therapy over single chemotherapy agents. No phase III trials of combination regimens with different chemotherapy agents have confirmed a survival benefit with dacarbazine or temozolomide-based combination regimens. One such regimen, called the Dartmouth regimen, is comprised of dacarbazine 220 mg/m^2 and cisplatin 25 mg/m^2 (Days 1–3, every 3 weeks), carmustine 140 mg/m^2 (Day 1, every other cycle, every 3 weeks) and tamoxifen 10 mg BID taken orally. The trial found no significant improvement in overall survival compared to dacarbazine alone, with only a small increase in the response rate and greater toxicity [27].

Previous data has shown a modest activity with the combination of carboplatin and paclitaxel in the first- or second-line setting. A phase III study showed a response rate of 18% and OS of up to 11.3 months in the first-line setting [28]. The second-line setting had a response rate of 11% [29]. The phase III PRISM (Paclitaxel and carboplatin with vs. without sorafenib [second line] for advanced melanoma) study has found that the addition of sorafenib to carboplatin and paclitaxel failed to reveal any survival advantage [28, 29]. Combining carboplatin and paclitaxel with bevacizumab was found to be a potentially effective combination. A randomized, phase II BEAM (Bevacizumab Advanced Melanoma) trial enrolled 214 patients with previously untreated metastatic melanoma, randomized to receive either a combination regimen of carboplatin (area under curve [AUC], 5) and paclitaxel (175 mg/m^2) plus bevacizumab (15 mg/kg) (Day 1, every 3 weeks), or chemotherapy alone with carboplatin and paclitaxel [30]. At a median follow-up of 13 months, the median PFS was 5.6 versus 4.2 months (HR 0.78; $p = 0.1414$), with a median OS of 12.3 versus 8.6 months, respectively (HR 0.67, 95% CI 0.46–0.98; $p = 0.0366$). The subgroup analysis found a stronger survival benefit in more advanced patients with elevated serum lactate dehydrogenase (LDH). This phase II study showed a survival trend that was without statistical significance, with further studies needed in order to confirm the efficacy of this regimen.

Based on the theoretical addition, or even augmentation, by combining potential effective agents, we have studied the combination of biochemotherapy with various chemotherapy agents, namely dacarbazine, temozolomide, carmustine, cisplatin, vinblastine, and tamoxifen, combined with IL-2 or IFNα. The initial results of biochemotherapy with IL-2 or IFNα were promising, but multiple, randomized, phase III trials comparing biochemotherapy to chemotherapy alone failed to show a statistically significant survival benefit to biochemotherapy, despite the increased response rate or PFS [31–34]. Therefore, two systemic reviews, including 18 trials with over 2600 patients, showed no significant difference in overall survival despite higher response rates [35, 36]. Biochemotherapy, with one or more cytotoxic agents, plus IL-2 and/or IFNα cannot yet be viewed as a standard treatment. Many trials of combination regimens with different novel agents are still ongoing, and we will need to wait on such trials in order to address their efficacy in patients with metastatic melanoma. Other studies have focused on the introduction of maintenance with immunotherapy, in an attempt to prolong the efficacy of biochemotherapy.

Historically, melanoma was viewed as a relatively chemotherapy-refractory tumor due to the low response rates and insignificant survival benefit. However, melanoma management has advanced rapidly in the past decade, with the development of many novel agents, including immune checkpoint inhibitors (ipilimumab, nivolumab, and pembrolizumab) and targeted therapy (BRAF inhibitors [vemurafenib, dabrafenib and encorafenib] and MEK inhibitors [cobimetinib, trametinib, and binimetinib]), leading to major improvements in survival rates. However, conventional cytotoxic chemotherapy still has a role in treatment, often after failure of standard treatment options for metastatic melanoma, as well as in the palliative setting in certain circumstances. Although novel immune checkpoint inhibitors have been proven to improve survival and prognosis, they have also raised issues in patient management, such as the optimal agents of choice or the type of combination therapy, dose, and sequence. There are additional issues related to the immune-related toxicities which are different from those seen with cytotoxic chemotherapy. More studies are needed to resolve these new issues.

References

1. Garbe C, Leiter U. Melanoma epidemiology and trends. Clin Dermatol. 2009;27(1):3–9.
2. Sneyd M, Cox B. The control of melanoma in New Zealand. N Z Med J. 2006;119(1242):U2169.
3. Balch CM, Gershenwald JE, Soong SJ, Thompson JF, Atkins MB, Byrd DR, et al. Final version of 2009 AJCC melanoma staging and classification. J Clin Oncol. 2009;27(36):6199–206.
4. Kirkwood JM, Strawderman MH, Ernstoff MS, Smith TJ, Borden EC, Blum RH. Interferon alfa-2b adjuvant therapy of high-risk resected cutaneous melanoma: the eastern cooperative oncology group trial EST 1684. J Clin Oncol. 1996;14(1):7–17.
5. Kirkwood JM, Ibrahim JG, Sosman JA, Sondak VK, Agarwala SS, Ernstoff MS, et al. High-dose interferon alfa-2b significantly prolongs relapse-free and overall survival compared with the GM2-KLH/QS-21 vaccine in patients with resected stage IIB-III melanoma: results of intergroup trial E1694/S9512/C509801. J Clin Oncol. 2001;19(9):2370–80.
6. Kirkwood JM, Ibrahim JG, Sondak VK, Richards J, Flaherty LE, Ernstoff MS, et al. High- and low-dose interferon alfa-2b in high-risk melanoma: first analysis of intergroup trial E1690/S9111/C9190. J Clin Oncol. 2000;18(12):2444–58.
7. Mocellin S, Pasquali S, Rossi CR, Nitti D. Interferon alpha adjuvant therapy in patients with high-risk melanoma: a systematic review and meta-analysis. J Natl Cancer Inst. 2010;102(7):493–501.
8. Hauschild A, Gogas H, Tarhini A, Middleton MR, Testori A, Dreno B, et al. Practical guidelines for the management of interferon-alpha-2b side effects in patients receiving adjuvant treatment for melanoma: expert opinion. Cancer. 2008;112(5):982–94.
9. Eggermont AM, Suciu S, Testori A, Santinami M, Kruit WH, Marsden J, et al. Long-term results of the randomized phase III trial EORTC 18991 of adjuvant therapy with pegylated interferon alfa-2b versus observation in resected stage III melanoma. J Clin Oncol. 2012;30(31):3810–8.
10. Flaherty LE, Othus M, Atkins MB, Tuthill RJ, Thompson JA, Vetto JT, et al. Southwest oncology group S0008: a phase III trial of high-dose interferon Alfa-2b versus cisplatin, vinblastine, and dacarbazine, plus interleukin-2 and interferon in patients with high-risk melanoma--an intergroup study of cancer and leukemia group B, Children's oncology group, eastern cooperative oncology group, and southwest oncology group. J Clin Oncol. 2014;32(33):3771–8.
11. Eggermont AM, Chiarion-Sileni V, Grob JJ, Dummer R, Wolchok JD, Schmidt H, et al. Adjuvant ipilimumab versus placebo after complete resection of high-risk stage III melanoma (EORTC 18071): a randomised, double-blind, phase 3 trial. Lancet Oncol. 2015;16(5):522–30.
12. Eggermont AM, Chiarion-Sileni V, Grob JJ, Dummer R, Wolchok JD, Schmidt H, et al. Prolonged survival in stage III melanoma with Ipilimumab adjuvant therapy. N Engl J Med. 2016;375(19):1845–55.
13. Surveillance E, and End Results Program (SEER). [cited 2017 02/23]. https://seer.cancer.gov/statfacts/html/melan.html.
14. O'Day SJ, Kim CJ, Reintgen DS. Metastatic melanoma: chemotherapy to biochemotherapy. Cancer Control. 2002;9:1.
15. Balch CM, Soong SJ, Murad TM, Smith JW, Maddox WA, Durant JR. A multifactorial analysis of melanoma. IV. Prognostic factors in 200 melanoma patients with distant metastases (stage III). J Clin Oncol. 1983;1(2):126–34.
16. Balch CM. Cutaneous melanoma: prognosis and treatment results worldwide. Semin Surg Oncol. 1992;8(6):400–14.
17. Lotze MT, Kirkwood JM. Cutaneous melanoma. In: DeVita Jr VT, Rosenberg SA, editors. DeVita, Hellman, Rosenberg's cancer: principles & practice of oncology. 6th ed. Philadelphia: Lippincott, Williams & Wilkens; 2001. p. 2012–69.

18. Houghton AN, Legha S, Bajorin DF. In: Balch CM, Houghton AN, Milton CW, editors. Chemotherapy for metastatic melanoma. Philadelphia: JB Lippincott Company; 1992.
19. Atkins M. The role of cytotoxic chemotherapeutic agents either alone or in combination with biological response modifiers. New York: Marcel Dekker; 1997.
20. Middleton MR, Grob JJ, Aaronson N, Fierlbeck G, Tilgen W, Seiter S, et al. Randomized phase III study of temozolomide versus dacarbazine in the treatment of patients with advanced metastatic malignant melanoma. J Clin Oncol. 2000;18(1):158–66.
21. Patel PM, Suciu S, Mortier L, Kruit WH, Robert C, Schadendorf D, et al. Extended schedule, escalated dose temozolomide versus dacarbazine in stage IV melanoma: final results of a randomised phase III study (EORTC 18032). Eur J Cancer. 2011;47(10):1476–83.
22. Avril MF, Aamdal S, Grob JJ, Hauschild A, Mohr P, Bonerandi JJ, et al. Fotemustine compared with dacarbazine in patients with disseminated malignant melanoma: a phase III study. J Clin Oncol. 2004;22(6):1118–25.
23. Glover D, Glick JH, Weiler C, Fox K, Guerry D. WR-2721 and high-dose cisplatin: an active combination in the treatment of metastatic melanoma. J Clin Oncol. 1987;5(4):574–8.
24. Hersh EM, O'Day SJ, Ribas A, Samlowski WE, Gordon MS, Shechter DE, et al. A phase 2 clinical trial of nab-paclitaxel in previously treated and chemotherapy-naive patients with metastatic melanoma. Cancer. 2010;116(1):155–63.
25. Hersh EM, Del Vecchio M, Brown MP, Kefford R, Loquai C, Testori A, et al. A randomized, controlled phase III trial of nab-paclitaxel versus dacarbazine in chemotherapy-naive patients with metastatic melanoma. Annals of oncology : official journal of the European society for. Med Oncol. 2015;26(11):2267–74.
26. Quagliana JM, Stephens RL, Baker LH, Costanzi JJ. Vindesine in patients with metastatic malignant melanoma: a southwest oncology group study. J Clin Oncol. 1984;2(4):316–9.
27. Chapman PB, Einhorn LH, Meyers ML, Saxman S, Destro AN, Panageas KS, et al. Phase III multicenter randomized trial of the Dartmouth regimen versus dacarbazine in patients with metastatic melanoma. J Clin Oncol. 1999;17(9):2745–51.
28. Flaherty KT, Lee SJ, Zhao F, Schuchter LM, Flaherty L, Kefford R, et al. Phase III trial of carboplatin and paclitaxel with or without sorafenib in metastatic melanoma. J Clin Oncol. 2013;31(3):373–9.
29. Hauschild A, Agarwala SS, Trefzer U, Hogg D, Robert C, Hersey P, et al. Results of a phase III, randomized, placebo-controlled study of sorafenib in combination with carboplatin and paclitaxel as second-line treatment in patients with unresectable stage III or stage IV melanoma. J Clin Oncol. 2009;27(17):2823–30.
30. Kim KB, Sosman JA, Fruehauf JP, Linette GP, Markovic SN, McDermott DF, et al. BEAM: a randomized phase II study evaluating the activity of bevacizumab in combination with carboplatin plus paclitaxel in patients with previously untreated advanced melanoma. J Clin Oncol. 2012;30(1):34–41.
31. Rosenberg SA, Yang JC, Schwartzentruber DJ, Hwu P, Marincola FM, Topalian SL, et al. Prospective randomized trial of the treatment of patients with metastatic melanoma using chemotherapy with cisplatin, dacarbazine, and tamoxifen alone or in combination with interleukin-2 and interferon alfa-2b. J Clin Oncol. 1999;17(3):968–75.
32. Ridolfi R, Chiarion-Sileni V, Guida M, Romanini A, Labianca R, Freschi A, et al. Cisplatin, dacarbazine with or without subcutaneous interleukin-2, and interferon alpha-2b in advanced melanoma outpatients: results from an Italian multicenter phase III randomized clinical trial. J Clin Oncol. 2002;20(6):1600–7.
33. Keilholz U, Punt CJ, Gore M, Kruit W, Patel P, Lienard D, et al. Dacarbazine, cisplatin, and interferon-alfa-2b with or without interleukin-2 in metastatic melanoma: a randomized phase III trial (18951) of the European Organisation for Research and Treatment of Cancer melanoma group. J Clin Oncol. 2005;23(27):6747–55.
34. Eton O, Legha SS, Bedikian AY, Lee JJ, Buzaid AC, Hodges C, et al. Sequential biochemotherapy versus chemotherapy for metastatic melanoma: results from a phase III randomized trial. J Clin Oncol. 2002;20(8):2045–52.
35. Sasse AD, Sasse EC, Clark LG, Ulloa L, Clark OA. Chemoimmunotherapy versus chemotherapy for metastatic malignant melanoma. Cochrane Database Syst Rev. 2007;1:CD005413.
36. Ives NJ, Stowe RL, Lorigan P, Wheatley K. Chemotherapy compared with biochemotherapy for the treatment of metastatic melanoma: a meta-analysis of 18 trials involving 2,621 patients. J Clin Oncol. 2007;25(34):5426–34.

Therapeutic Cancer Vaccines for Melanoma

33

Kaitlin M. Peace, Garth S. Herbert, Timothy J. Vreeland, G. Travis Clifton, and George E. Peoples

Introduction

Melanoma has long been a prominent focus of investigation for cancer immunotherapy due to its intrinsically immunogenic nature, typically a consequence of a high mutational load. Furthermore, tumor infiltration by lymphocytes provides evidence of endogenous immune activity, as does the spontaneous regression described in some tumors. Conversely, the melanoma microenvironment promotes upregulation of immunosuppressive cells (myeloid-derived suppressor cells and regulatory T cells) and cytokines (such as IL-6, IL-10, TNFα, TGFβ, and VEGF) facilitating evasion of the immune response. The tumor microenvironment contains several targets for immunomodulation that are under active investigation. In this chapter, we will explore the development of immunotherapy for the treatment of melanoma, beginning with early, nonspecific immunomodulation through more recent advances in melanoma vaccines with specific discussion of several phase III clinical trials for peptide, viral, dendritic cell, and whole tumor cell-based vaccines.

Historical Perspective/Development of Melanoma Immunotherapy

The earliest attempt at immunotherapy occurred in the late nineteenth century by Dr. William Coley, who observed tumor regression in a sarcoma patient after an erysipelas infection. Dr. Coley then began inoculating cancer patients with a combination of *Streptococcus* and *Serratia* bacteria, known as Coley's toxin, again observing local regression of tumors [1]. Unfortunately, Dr. Coley's findings were met with great skepticism, and the advent of therapeutic radiation and chemotherapy would overshadow immunotherapy for cancer treatment in subsequent decades.

Interest was renewed in the 1950s when the work of Foley [2], Prehn, and Main [3] demonstrated the presence of tumor-specific antigens in a mouse sarcoma model. Throughout the following two decades, unique tumor-associated antigens (TAAs) would be identified in numerous cancer types, to include their discovery in melanoma by Morton and colleagues in 1967 using immunofluorescence techniques [4].

Melanoma TAAs are highly varied in terms of their composition and expression. Germ cell antigens, while typically silenced in somatic cells, are often expressed in cancer cells. In melanoma,

K. M. Peace · G. S. Herbert · G.T. Clifton
Department of General Surgery, San Antonio Military Medical Center, Fort Sam Houston, TX, USA
e-mail: kaitlin.m.peace.mil@mail.mil; garth.s.herbert.mil@mail.mil; guy.t.clifton.mil@mail.mil

T. J. Vreeland
Department of General Surgery, Womack Army Medical Center, Ft. Bragg, NC, USA
e-mail: timothy.j.vreeland.mil@mail.mil

G. E. Peoples (✉)
Cancer Insight, LLC, San Antonio, TX, USA

A. I. Riker (ed.), *Melanoma*, https://doi.org/10.1007/978-3-319-78310-9_33

germ cell antigens include NY-ESO-1 and members of the MAGE family. Other antigens are expressed in both melanoma cells and normal melanocytes, to include tyrosinase, gp100, MART-1, and gangliosides such as GM2. These antigens are variably immunogenic, with evidence of T cell recognition of MART-1 in up to 50% of patients and natural antibodies to GM2 in about 5% of patients [5]. All of these antigens serve as potential targets for directed immunotherapy via melanoma vaccines, as discussed later in the chapter.

Early attempts at immunotherapy for melanoma were nonspecific and aimed at augmenting the host immune response to tumor cells. Bacillus Calmette-Guerin (BCG), a nonspecific immune stimulant, was initially studied as an intratumoral injection for melanoma in the 1970s. While initial studies reported regression of 90% of the injected nodules and regression of distant nodules in 20% of patients [6], a randomized, controlled trial performed in the late 1970s found no difference in disease-free or overall survival among more than 700 stage I-III melanoma patients [7].

In the late twentieth century, interleukin 2 (IL-2), a T cell growth factor, was identified as having potent antitumor effects. It was approved for use after durable responses were seen in patients with metastatic renal cell carcinoma, another immunogenic malignancy. An evaluation of eight clinical trials involving treatment of metastatic melanoma revealed an overall objective response to high-dose systemic IL-2 in 16% of the 270 patients enrolled, although toxicities were severe [8]. IL-2 has also been evaluated as an intralesional injection to treat in-transit melanoma; a systematic review found a complete response in 78% of treated lesions; however, only half the patients responded overall, with varying responses among the six included trials [9].

Similarly, interferon alpha (IFNα) is another nonspecific immunotherapy that has been shown to have antitumor activity in high-risk, localized melanoma (stage IIB, IIC, III). In a large trial, 280 patients were randomized to either systemic recombinant IFNα-2b therapy or observation. A significant improvement in both relapse-free and overall survival was noted in the group receiving treatment, with prevention of relapse in 18–33% of patients [10]. However, a larger trial of 1256 patients with stage III melanoma demonstrated no difference in overall survival at 3.8 years of median follow-up. Of note, high toxicity levels were seen in 31% of patients, with discontinuation of IFNα-2b therapy due to side effects [11]. While still considered as a treatment option in the management of patients with advanced melanoma, IL-2 and IFNα have largely been supplanted by newer immunotherapies, mainly due to their limited efficacy but significant toxicity.

In the late 1980s, another advancement in melanoma immunotherapy was made with the use of adoptive cell transfer. Rosenberg and colleagues used autologous tumor-infiltrating lymphocytes (TILs) isolated from excisional biopsy specimens and administered in combination with cyclophosphamide after a non-myeloablative lymphodepletion of the patient. The hypothesis of this approach was an attempt to enhance antitumor immunity by allowing these antitumor lymphocytes to proliferate outside of the immunosuppressive tumor microenvironment. These T-cells would then be reintroduced to the patient in high enough numbers to effectively kill their tumor targets. Analysis of 86 metastatic melanoma patients treated with TIL therapy and high-dose IL-2 revealed an overall objective response rate of 34%, regardless of cyclophosphamide use [12]. In a trial of 93 heavily pretreated patients with metastatic melanoma, they demonstrated 3- and 5-year survival rates of 36% and 29%, respectively, with a 5-year survival of 93% in the 22% of patients who were complete responders [13]. Despite clear clinical benefits, access to TIL therapy remains limited due to time, costs, and technical requirements involved in production of TILs, as well as the inability of some patients to undergo the rigorous lymphodepletion regimen.

More recent research in cancer immunotherapy has led to the development of checkpoint inhibitors (CPIs) which have been very successful in the treatment of advanced melanoma. In general, many cancer types rely on the immune system's innate mechanism for preventing an excessive immune response and maintaining self-tolerance. This is partially controlled by several co-inhibitory molecules, such as CTLA-4 and PD-1, which can be upregulated by tumor cells facilitating immune escape. CPIs in the form of monoclonal antibodies directed at CTLA-4 (e.g., ipilimumab) and PD-1 (e.g., nivolumab and pembrolizumab) are able to preserve the antitumor immunity of endogenous cytotoxic T cells. A meta-analysis of 1861 patients with advanced melanoma treated with ipilimumab demonstrated an overall survival (OS) of 22% [14], and a phase III trial of nivolumab versus dacarbazine in 418 untreated stage III/IV melanoma was terminated early when 1-year OS was found to be significantly higher in the nivolumab arm (72.9 vs. 42.1%, $p < 0.001$) [15]. A randomized phase III trial comparing pembrolizumab given every 2 or 3 weeks to ipilimumab given every 3 weeks in 834 advanced melanoma patients demonstrated improved 1-year survival (74.1 vs. 68.4 vs. 58.2%, $p = 0.0005$), better response rates (33.7 vs. 32.9 vs. 11.9%, $p < 0.001$) and less grade 3–5 adverse events in the pembrolizumab arms versus the ipilimumab arm [16]. These trials ultimately led to FDA approval of these CPIs for metastatic and unresectable melanoma. Although there has been success with immunomodulators such as CPIs, IL-2, and IFNα, these therapies require that the patient have a de novo immune response to their tumor, resulting in limited overall response rates. Vaccines represent a mechanism by which this immune response can be generated in patients without a preexisting response or augment a weak and/or ineffective immune response.

Current Approach to Melanoma Vaccines

The aim of current melanoma vaccines is to induce an active immune response directed against melanoma cells. This involves one or more TAAs being supplied to, processed and presented by antigen presenting cells to prime the immune system against these antigens. In this chapter, we will review the strategies that have been developed to accomplish this goal in melanoma and explore specific examples of each strategy that have made it to phase III clinical trials. We will divide these vaccines by strategy, covering each of the following: peptide-based vaccines, viral vaccines, dendritic cell (DC) vaccines, and tumor cell vaccines. Table 33.1 includes a comprehensive list of the vaccines presented here with relevant details.

Peptide Vaccines

Peptide-based vaccines rely on antigen uptake and presentation by DCs in vivo to enable an immune response to one or more TAAs selected specifically for the cancer being treated. The response to the peptide is most commonly carried out via cytotoxic T cells, but antibody production may also be induced. The proteins or peptides selected are typically chosen because of common expression in a certain tumor type and for their immunogenicity. However, they often require the use of an immunoadjuvant to increase the likelihood of generating a robust active immune response. These peptide-based vaccines can be produced on a large scale at relatively low cost, and can therefore be administered to a large number of patients as an "off-the-shelf" therapy. Additionally, priming the immune system against only a small number of peptides results in much easier monitoring for an immune response to treatment. Shortcomings of this strategy include reliance on the patient's own dendritic cells to perform the crucial steps of uptake and presentation of the administered TAA, restriction of some peptide vaccines to certain HLA subtypes limiting the patient population that can be treated, and the possibility of immune escape due to a small number of antigens supplied.

Peptide-based vaccines can consist of a single immunogenic peptide, allowing the immune system to focus on one highly expressed TAA while simultaneously making evaluation of immune response to the vaccine straightforward. Alternatively, multiple peptides can be included in the vaccine to generate a response in patients with varied TAAs, potentially leading to multiple clones of T cells capable of attacking the tumors.

Table 33.1 Melanoma vaccines by category

Category	Vaccine name	Strategy	Study name	Vaccine description	Immunoadjuvant	Inclusion criteria	Year initiated	Number of patients	Results	References	NCT
Peptide	gp100	Peptide		gp100:209–217 peptide	Montanide ISA-51	Stage III/IV unresectable melanoma	1999	185	OS: 17.8 vs. 11.1 month, $p = 0.06$ PFS: 2.2 vs. 1.6 month, $p = 0.008$ response rate 16 vs. 6%, $p = 0.03$	[17–19]	NCT00019682
	GM2-KLH	Peptide	EORTC 18961	GM2 antigen combined with KLH to improve immunogenicity	QS-21	Adjuvant, NED stage II	1999	1314	Terminated after second interim analysis: 1.8 years median f/u, detrimental OS (HR = 1.66, $p = 0.02$) and futile RFS (HR = 1.00, $p = 0.99$). After 4 year f/u vaccinated patients had a decrease in RFS by 1.2% (HR = 1.03) and in OS by 2.1% (HR = 1.16) compared to controls	[20, 21]	NCT00005052
	Tyrosinase, gp100, MART-1	Multiple peptides	ECOG 4697		Montanide ISA-51; GM-CSF	Adjuvant, NED surgically resected stage IV or high risk stage III	1999	815	OS (HR, 0.93; 95% CI 0.71 to 1.21; $P = 0.598$), RFS (HR, 0.96; 95% repeated CI, 0.74 to 1.23; $P = 0.708$)	[22, 23]	NCT01989572
	Vitespen (HSPPC-96)	Multiple peptides	C-100-21 study group	Autologous tumor derived peptides complexed with gp96 (HSP)		Adjuvant; at least partially resectable stage IV	2002	ITT 322 PT 219	ITT OS no difference HR1.16, $p = 0.32$; PT M1a + M1b: HR = 0.45, $p = 0.03$	[24–26]	NCT00039000
	Seviprotimut-L (POL-103A)	Multiple peptides	MAVIS	Shed surface peptides from 3 allogenic melanoma cell lines	Alum	Adjuvant, NED surgically resected stage IIB, IIC, III	2012	Anticipated 1059	Currently enrolling, study start date April 2012, estimated completion Oct 2018	[26–28]	NCT01546571
	MAGE-A3	Protein	DERMA	recMAGE-A3	AS15	Adjuvant, NED, stage IIIB-C	2008	Anticipated 1351	Terminated for lack of efficacy	[26, 29, 30]	NCT00796445

Viral	Vaccinia melanoma cell lysates	Virus		Single allogeneic melanoma cell line (MM200) infected with vaccinia virus		Adjuvant, NED, resected stage IIB/III	1988	675	Median OS 88mo. Control vs. 151mo. Treated group (HR 0.81; 95% CI 0.64 to 1.02; P 0.068); median RFS was 43mo. Control group vs. 83mo. Treated group (HR, 0.86; 95% CI 0.7 to 1.07; $P = 0.17$)	[31–33]	
	Talimogene laherparepvec (T-VEC, oncovex)	Virus	OPTiM	Intralesional injection of herpes simplex virus type 1-derived oncolytic immunotherapy		Unresected stage IIIB to IV	2009	436	DRR: T-VEC (16.3%; 95% CI, 12.1–20.5%) vs. GM-CSF (2.1%; 95% CI, 0–4.5%]; odds ratio, 8.9; $P < 0.001$). Median OS: T-VEC 23.3 months (95% CI, 19.5 to 29.6 months) vs. GM-CSF 18.9 months (95% CI, 16.0–23.7 months) (hazard ratio, 0.79; 95% CI, 0.62–1.00; $P = 0.051$)	[34–36]	NCT00769704
Dendritic cell	DCaT-RNA	DC		Autologous tumor RNA loaded onto autologous DC		Adjuvant, NED resected uveal melanoma, monosomy 3	2014	Anticipated 200	Terminated for futility	[26, 37, 38]	NCT01983748

Table 33.1 (continued)

Category	Vaccine name	Strategy	Study name	Vaccine description	Immunoadjuvant	Inclusion criteria	Year initiated	Number of patients	Results	References	NCT
Tumor cell	Melacine	Tumor cell	S9035	Allogeneic melanoma vaccine	DETOX (detoxified Freund adjuvant)	Adjuvant, NED, stage II/III	1992	689	12.1 years median f/u, ITT no difference in RFS ($p = 0.58$) or OS ($p = 0.61$), subset analysis vaccinated and HLA-A2/Cw3+ 10 year RFS 66% vs. controls 54% ($p = 0.02$)	[42, 43]	
	Autologous DNP vaccine	Tumor cell		Intact tumor cells modified with the hapten, dinitrophenyl (DNP)	BCG	Adjuvant, NED, stage III, resectable	2000	214	5 year RFS 33% and OS 44%; patients who developed positive DTH to unmodified, autologous melanoma cells had a doubling of both RFS and OS ($p < 0.001$)	[26, 44, 45]	NCT00257465
	Canvaxin	Tumor cell	MMAIT	Allogeneic melanoma vaccine	BCG	Adjuvant, NED, stage III/IV	2002	1656	Terminated after interim analysis for futility: 5-year estimated survival 42.3% stage IV and 63.4% stage III	[46, 47]	NCT00052156; NCT00052130

NED no evidence of disease, *BCG* Bacillus Calmette-Guerin, *GM-CSF* granulocyte-monocyte colony-stimulating factor, *ITT* intention to treat, *PT* per treatment, *PFS* progression free survival, *RFS* relapse-free survival, *OS* overall survival, *HR* hazard ratio, *CI* confidence interval, *NCT* national clinical trial identifier

Lastly, the vaccine can consist of an entire protein, which allows the patient's own DCs to select the most immunogenic epitopes to be presented. We will discuss examples of each of the three separate strategies: single peptide vaccines, multiple peptide vaccines, and full protein vaccines.

Glycoprotein 100 (gp100)

gp100 is a melanosomal protein that induces a strong immune response, and a vaccine has been created based on a specific immunogenic peptide of gp100 (amino acids [aa] 209–217[210M]), administered with the immunoadjuvant Montanide ISA-51. Early clinical studies revealed that gp100 induced an effective immune response against melanoma cells in HLA-A0201-positive patients. In a phase II trial, gp100 was administered with high-dose IL-2 and improved objective response rates were demonstrated in comparison to prior reports of IL-2 alone [17]. This prompted the completion of a phase III trial randomizing 177 patients with stage III/IV melanoma to receive IL-2 alone or the gp100 vaccine plus IL-2. Patients in the vaccine group had a higher clinical response rate (16 vs. 6%, $p = 0.03$) and longer progression free survival (PFS) (2.2 vs. 1.6 months, $p = 0.008$) [18].

Subsequently, the gp100 vaccine was used as control in a landmark study of ipilimumab, a checkpoint inhibitor (CPI) that blocks the CTLA-4 receptor. Patients were randomized to receive either gp100 alone, gp100 with ipilimumab, or ipilimumab alone. Those treated with gp100 had the lowest median overall survival (OS) of the three groups, worse than those treated with ipilimumab and gp100 (6.4 vs. 10.0 months, $p < 0.001$) or ipilimumab alone (6.4 vs. 10.1 months, $p = 0003$) [19]. Although the results of this trial favored ipilimumab and led to its approval by the FDA, there was no placebo arm for comparison with the gp100 alone arm and IL-2 was omitted from this trial. Thus, research continues with gp100, particularly as a component of vaccines using multiple peptides.

GM2-KLH

GM2 is a ganglioside expressed in the majority of melanomas, with little to no expression in normal melanocytes and other tissues. It is known to induce the production of IgG and IgM antibodies in patients with melanoma and a favorable prognosis has been demonstrated in patients with serologic responses to GM2, though curiously, no T cell mediated responses have been observed. An initial phase III trial of a GM2 vaccine, made up of the ganglioside with BCG, randomized 122 stage III melanoma patients rendered disease-free by surgery to receive either the GM2/BCG vaccine or BCG alone. Of the 58 patients in the GM2/BCG group, the majority developed anti-GM2 IgM antibodies, while only 7 of the 64 patients in the control group developed antibodies. When the patients with preexisting antibody production were removed from the analysis, there was a 23% improvement in relapse-free survival (RFS) in the vaccine group ($p = 0.02$) [20]. This vaccine relies on the antibody response and further investigation into improving the GM2/BCG vaccine demonstrated optimal antibody production when recombinant GM2 was conjugated with keyhole limpet hemocyanin (KLH) and administered with QS-21 as an immunoadjuvant. A subsequent phase III trial was initiated comparing the GM2-KLH/QS-21 vaccine to observation, and a total of 1314 patients with stage II melanoma were randomized. Unfortunately, the trial was terminated after a median follow-up of 1.8 years, when the second interim analysis demonstrated futility of the vaccine with regard to RFS (hazard ratio [HR] 1.00, $p = 0.99$) and a detrimental OS outcome (HR 1.66, $p = 0.02$). On final analysis of the data, no detrimental effect was identified [21].

Tyrosinase, gp100, MART-1

This HLA-A2 restricted, multi-epitope vaccine targets immunogenic peptides known to be associated with melanoma. The combination includes peptides from the tyrosinase (aa 368–376), gp100 (aa 209–217), and MART-1 (aa 27–35) proteins emulsified in Montanide ISA-51. This multi-epitope vaccine was studied in a phase II trial that randomized 115 HLA-A2 patients to one of four arms: vaccine alone, vaccine combined with granulocyte-monocyte colony-stimulating factor (GM-CSF), vaccine combined with IFNα or vaccine with both GM-CSF and IFNα. There was a nonsignificant trend toward improvement in immune responses with the use of either GM-CSF or IFNα; however, the development of an immune responses to at least one of the vaccine peptides was associated with an improved median OS (21.3 vs. 13.4 months, $p = 0.046$) [22].

Results from the phase II study led to the development of a multicenter, placebo-controlled, phase III clinical trial aimed at evaluating RFS and OS in patients treated with GM-CSF with or without this multi-epitope vaccine. The trial enrolled 815 HLA-A2 positive patients with completely resected stage IV or high-risk stage III melanoma, and randomized them to receive GM-CSF alone, peptide vaccine alone, GM-CSF plus vaccine or placebo. There was no difference in OS (HR 0.93, 95% CI 0.71 to 1.21; $p = 0.598$) or RFS (HR 0.96, 95% repeated CI, 0.74 to 1.23; $p = 0708$) between vaccinated and unvaccinated patients. While the addition of GM-CSF to the vaccine improved the OS compared to patients who did not receive the combination by 17.3%, the difference was not significant ($p = 0.881$). A subset analysis revealed that patients with stage IIIC or M1a disease who received the vaccine, versus placebo, had an improved RFS (15.2 vs. 9.7 months, $p = 0.04$) and OS (91.1 vs. 39.1 months, $p = 0.128$) [23].

Vitespen (HSPPC-96)

Formerly known as Oncophage, vitespen (HSPPC-96) is a vaccine comprised of heat shock protein (HSP)-derived peptide complexes isolated from autologous tumor cells. HSPs are known to have high uptake by DCs without the need for an immunoadjuvant. Thus, this vaccine takes advantage of their natural immunogenicity, further showing a proof-of-principle with the completion of phase I and II trials of patients with both melanoma and renal cell carcinoma [24]. The first phase III trial was completed in patients with untreated stage IV melanoma, randomizing 322 patients to receive vitespen or the physician's choice (PC) of standard therapy for melanoma. Notably, 61 of the 215 patients in the vitespen arm were not inoculated because the vaccine could not be prepared for them, highlighting the challenges of using autologous proteins (rather than recombinant) in the creation of vaccines. Analysis demonstrated no improvement in OS in vaccinated patients in either the intention-to-treat population (HR = 1.16, $p = 0.32$) or the treated population (HR = 1.29, $p = 0.25$). Further exploratory analyses showed that patients with less disease burden (M1a and M1b) who received full treatment with vitespen (defined as 10 or more inoculations) had significant improvement in OS compared to similar patients in the PC arm (HR = 0.45, $p = 0.03$) [25]. A phase I/II trial was planned in which patients with stage III/IV melanoma would receive vitespen along with ipilimumab [26], in the hopes that combination with a CPI will enhance efficacy of the vaccine. Enrollment in this trial was not initiated due to operational issues, but there is still potential for future research into this combination.

Seviprotimut-L (POL-103A)

Seviprotimut-L is comprised of multiple surface peptides from three allogenic melanoma cell lines, given with alum as an immunoadjuvant. This vaccine is created using a variation of technology that allows for isolation and purification of shed surface peptides by culturing tumor cells in a specific culture medium. A similar polyvalent vaccine created using this technology was studied in a phase II trial in which 38 patients with resected stage III melanoma were randomized to vaccine or placebo. Vaccinated patients had significantly increased median time to progression (1.6 vs. 0.6 year, $p = 0.03$) and a nonsignificant increased median OS (3.8 vs. 2.7 year) [27]. A more recent phase II trial compared a trivalent and a quadrivalent vaccine, each produced in the same manner as Seviprotimut-L, to a null-vaccine used as a control. In this trial, 116 patients with stage II and III melanoma were randomized to either one of the vaccines or placebo. RFS was better among patients receiving the quadrivalent vaccine (HR = 0.632, $p = 0.095$) and the trivalent vaccine (HR = 0.407, $p = 0.0018$) compared to null vaccine [28]. Based on these findings, the phase III MAVIS trial of seviprotimut-L has started and is currently enrolling patients with

Stage IIB-III melanoma after complete resection. Patients are randomized to the vaccine or placebo; the trial is estimated to reach completion in October 2018 [26].

MAGE-A3

The MAGE-A3 protein is an ideal TAA, in the sense that it is expressed in very few normal adult tissues, but is expressed quite commonly in tumor cells with expression in up to 76% of melanomas [29]. The MAGE-A3 vaccine consists of a recombinant protein combined with one of two immunoadjuvants. Small preliminary studies showed MAGE-A3 to be immunogenic and induce antitumor activity in multiple malignancies [30], including melanoma. A small phase II trial attempted to identify the best immunoadjuvant to accompany MAGE-A3 in melanoma patients. Seventy-five patients were randomized to receive MAGE-A3 plus either AS15 or AS02. Patients receiving the AS15 immunoadjuvant (a combination of QS21, monophosphoryl lipid A, and CpG7909, a TLR-9 agonist, in a liposomal formulation) had improved immunologic response, longer median OS and higher PFS at 6 months [29]. Based on these results, MAGE-A3 was paired with AS15 in future trials. A phase III trial (the DERMA trial) was initiated to compare the vaccine to placebo. Investigators planned to enroll 1351 patients with stage IIIB-C melanoma for randomization. However, this trial was terminated early when evaluation of the primary endpoints revealed a lack of efficacy in the vaccine group compared to placebo [26]. Despite early enthusiasm for the specific nature of this ideal TAA, the disappointing trial outcome demonstrates the shortcomings of vaccines that rely on endogenous uptake and processing of a single protein and highlights the difficulty of generating an effective immune response to an administered protein.

Viral-Based Immunotherapy

Oncolytic viral vaccines take advantage of the natural immunogenicity of viruses to initiate an immune response. Lysis of tumor cells in response to viral infection leads to release of tumor antigens and priming of antigen presenting cells against those antigens. The virus may be modified by the addition of a plasmid coding for an immunoadjuvant or a cytokine, eliminating the need for separate administration of these therapies. The virus is then injected into the patient, where normal viral proteins induce a strong immune response and lead to the recruitment of antigen presenting cells. These cells are activated and subsequently process and present the viral proteins, to include the TAAs that have been selectively inserted into the virus. Thus, the immune system is primed against these TAAs and the tumors that express them.

Vaccinia Melanoma Cell Lysates (VCML)

This vaccine concept is based on early research demonstrating that viral infection of tumors can induce long-lasting immunity to the tumor, which is particularly true of the vaccinia virus in human melanoma studies. Vaccine production involves infection of an allogeneic melanoma cell line with the vaccinia virus, with subsequent administration of the lysed cells that contain immunogenic viral components, in addition to melanoma TAAs. A series of phase II trials comparing interventions to historical controls, first evaluated VCML alone, and later, VCML with or without cyclophosphamide pretreatment. Compared to historical controls, the trials demonstrated improved survival in patients treated with the VCML vaccine, regardless of pretreatment with cyclophosphamide [31, 32]. In light of the evidence from these trials, a randomized, multicenter, phase III trial was performed comparing VCML to no immunotherapy in 675 patients with stage IIB and III melanoma following surgical resection. At a median of 8 years follow-up, there was an improvement in OS in the vaccinated group compared to controls, but this result was not significant (151 vs. 88 months; HR 0.81, $p = 0.068$) [33], and no further trials using this technology have been initiated.

T-VEC (OncoVEX)

Talimogene laherparepvec (T-VEC) is a viral vaccine derived from herpes simplex virus type 1, which has been modified via the deletion of viral genes to attenuate the pathogenicity of the virus, and to insert a gene encoding human GM-CSF. This results in increased recruitment of antigen presenting cells and the induction of tumor-specific T cell responses. T-VEC is administered as an intralesional injection, and early trials confirmed replication and production of GM-CSF within the tumor. In a phase II trial, 50 patients with stage IIIC and IV melanoma were treated with intratumoral T-VEC injection. An overall response rate of 26% was demonstrated with regression noted in both injected and non-injected lesions, with durable responses found in some patients out to 31 months [34]. Based on these results, the phase III OPTiM study was developed to evaluate durable response rates and OS with T-VEC compared to GM-CSF alone in unresected, stage IIIB-IV melanoma patients. The trial enrolled 436 patients and when compared to GM-CSF alone, those treated with T-VEC had an improved durable response rate (16.3 vs. 2.1%; odds ratio [OR] 8.9, $p > 0.001$) and improved OS (23.3 vs. 18.9 months; HR 0.79, $p = 0.051$) with a mild toxicity profile. The beneficial effects on response rate and OS were most pronounced in pretreatment naive patients and those with stage IIIB, IIIC, and IV(M1a) disease [35]. In October 2015, the FDA approved T-VEC for use in unresectable cutaneous, subcutaneous and nodal melanoma lesions [36].

Dendritic Cell Vaccines

DCs are the body's most powerful and effective antigen presenting cells. Their function is to take up, process and present antigens to naïve T cells primarily in lymphoid organs. DC vaccines seek to enhance presentation of TAAs by priming the DCs in vitro to selected antigens. This may be accomplished by exposing the DCs to a single selected antigen, multiple TAAs, autologous tumor RNA, or to autologous tumor components and allowing the DCs to select which epitopes are presented. This strategy permits the investigators to directly load DCs, instead of hoping for successful in vivo uptake and processing of the antigen by the patient's DCs. As expected, the process of extracting, loading and re-introducing these cells to the patient can be expensive and time-consuming, limiting the broad applicability of this method of vaccine creation.

DCaT-RNA

The DC loaded with autologous tumor RNA (DCaT-RNA) vaccine uses a different approach in the production of DCs that present a wide range of TAAs specific to a patient's tumor. A sample of the patient's melanoma is obtained and tumor RNA is extracted and amplified. Autologous peripheral blood monocytes are matured into DCs through the addition of cytokines and loaded with the autologous tumor RNA via electroporation. This, in turn, leads to expression of multiple TAAs. These loaded DCs are then administered intravenously. Early clinical trials of this vaccine demonstrated minimal side effects and favorable OS rates (93% 2-year and 70% 4-year survival) when given to resected stage III/IV melanoma patients at high risk of recurrence [37]. Given these outcomes and the high rates of metastasis and recurrence in uveal melanoma, a multicenter, randomized, phase III trial enrolling patients with resected monosomy 3 (a marker of highly aggressive disease) uveal melanoma was begun utilizing the DCaT-RNA vaccine [26, 38]. This trial was subsequently terminated for futility.

TLPLDC

The tumor lysate, particle loaded, dendritic cell (TLPLDC) vaccine is a novel DC technology. This technology transforms the ability to efficiently produce a personalized DC vaccine by loading autologous tumor lysate into prepared yeast cell wall particles, which are naturally and efficiently phagocytized by isolated autologous DCs. The TLPLDC vaccine can be created in as little as 48 h using only a small amount of tumor (1 cm^3) with less DCs and reduced costs compared to previous DC vaccine technologies. TLPLDC achieves the same end as the dendritoma technology by administering the full range of tumor antigens from a given patient's tumor into the cytoplasm of the DC. The efficacy of TLPLDC has been confirmed in an ongoing basket trial enrolling patients with a variety of solid tumors, including melanoma [39]. Consequently, two trials have been initiated to further test the efficacy of the TLPLDC vaccine in melanoma. The first is a prospective, randomized, blinded, placebo-controlled, phase IIb trial of adjuvant TLPLDC in patients with fully resected stage III and IV melanoma to prevent recurrence. This trial has completed enrollment with120 patients randomized, and the first pre-specified interim analysis is pending. The second is a multicenter, phase I/IIa trial of TLPLDC in addition to standard of care CPI therapy in patients with metastatic melanoma. Both of these trials are estimated to reach their primary endpoints in 2018, with study completion in 2019 [26].

Dendritoma

This technology aims to harness the effective antigen presentation generated when DCs are fused with tumor cells. Typically, this is performed using established tumor cell lines, which limits the applicability to only patients expressing the TAAs found in those cell lines. It also requires time-consuming procedures for selection and expansion of the resulting fused cells. The dendritoma vaccine expands on this approach by using autologous DCs and tumor cells to form fused hybrid cells. This method does not require additional expansion and allows presentation of the full repertoire of TAAs expressed by that patient's tumor. Early in vitro human testing demonstrated that the dendritoma vaccine produces specific antitumor immunity via activation of autologous cytotoxic T cells that effectively lyse tumor cells [40]. A phase I/IIa trial of the dendritoma vaccine administered with IL-2 to 25 Stage IV melanoma patients was initiated based on this early research. Patients who received at least three inoculations had improved OS compared to those that received less than three (43.1 vs. 16.7%. $p = 0.02$). Patients with no evidence of disease prior to the initiation of therapy had the most significant improvement in 5-year OS compared to those with evidence of disease (80 vs. 14%, $p = 0.005$) [41]. While these results are encouraging, the multiple steps and expense of production limit the broader applicability of dendritoma technology.

Tumor Cell Vaccines

Tumor cell vaccines rely on the basic premise that the immune system is primed against tumors following cell lysis (similar to the oncolytic viral model), after which APCs take up tumor antigens and present encountered epitopes to the patient's T cells. These vaccines typically consist of allogeneic or autologous tumor cells that are inactivated (irradiated) and modified to increase their immunogenicity. After injection, the patient's immune system will select the most immunogenic epitopes from lysed cells in vivo, thus priming the immune system against tumor cells bearing those same epitopes.

Melacine

Melacine is a vaccine that is formulated from allogeneic tumor cells derived from two metastatic melanoma cell lines. The vaccine is created by culturing these cell lines and mechanically disrupting them to create an allogeneic cell-free lysate containing numerous melanoma TAAs. A phase I clinical trial demonstrated Melacine to be well tolerated and capable of inducing humoral and cell-mediated immunity, with regression of melanoma lesions in some patients [42]. A phase III clinical trial randomized 689 stage II/III resected melanoma patients to either vaccine or observation. At a median follow-up of 12.1 years, there was no difference in RFS ($p = 0.58$) or OS ($p = 0.61$). However, subset analysis limited to HLA-A2+ and/or HLA-Cw3+ patients revealed a significant advantage in vaccinated patients compared to controls in both RFS (10-year 66 vs. 54%, $p = 0.02$) and OS (10-year 75 vs. 63%, $p = 0.01$) [43]. These findings demonstrate the importance of identifying the appropriate target population for a vaccine and selecting patients with the appropriate biologic features. Additional trials using Melacine in this specific patient population will be required prior to FDA approval.

Autologous DNP Vaccine

The autologous dinitrophenyl (DNP) vaccine is another approach that takes advantage of the fact that autologous tumor cells are an ideal source of a wide variety of patient-specific TAAs, increasing the likelihood of generation of an effective immune response. This vaccine is created through irradiation of intact, autologous tumor cells and modification of those cells with DNP, a hapten capable of rendering the cells more immunogenic to the patient's immune cells. The autologous DNP vaccine was tested in stage III-IV melanoma patients after resection and lymphadenectomy. Early trial results demonstrated a 5-year RFS rate of 45% and OS rate of 58% with a positive association between the development of a delayed-type hypersensitivity (DTH) response and 5-year survival (71 vs. 49%, $p = 0.031$) [44]. In a phase II clinical trial with extended follow-up, the 214 enrolled stage III melanoma patients were noted to have a 5-year OS of 44% compared to 25% for similar patients undergoing conventional therapy. For those who developed a DTH response (47% of patients), the 5-year OS was double that of DTH-negative patients (59% vs. 29% respectively, $p < 0.001$). Development of DTH was noted to vary with the vaccination schedule, underscoring the importance of determining an optimal dosing schedule [45]. A phase III trial combining this autologous DNP vaccine (now called M-Vax) with IL-2 in stage IV melanoma patients is planned (NCT00477906) [26].

Canvaxin

Canvaxin is a polyvalent, irradiated, whole-cell vaccine derived from three allogeneic melanoma cell lines known to express greater than 20 common melanoma TAAs, including GM2, MAGE-A3, and MART-1. Phase II trials of adjuvant Canvaxin in patients with resected stage III melanoma demonstrated higher median OS in vaccinated patients versus controls (56.4 vs. 31.9 months, $p = 0.0001$). The vaccine therapy significantly reduced the relative risk of death (0.64, $p = 0.0001$) [46]. Based on these early results, two phase III clinical trials were initiated: one in patients with stage III melanoma that had been rendered clinically disease-free after surgery, and another in patients with stage IV melanoma (also rendered surgically disease-free). In both trials, patients were randomized to receive either Canvaxin and BCG as an immunoadjuvant, or placebo and BCG. BCG was given with the first two inoculations in each arm and omitted from subsequent inoculations. These trials were terminated for lack of efficacy following the second interim analysis. The 5-year OS rates were 59.1% in the Canvaxin group and 67.7% in the placebo group for stage III melanoma patients ($p = 0.04$) and 39.6% and 44.9%, respectively, for stage IV patients ($p = 0.245$) [47].

Combination Therapy

Overall, the results of vaccine trials have been disappointing; however, important lessons have been learned. In particular, several trials have shown vaccines to be more efficacious in patients with enhanced immune responses. Thus, maximizing the patient's immune response to vaccines is vital to the success of future vaccine trials. One strategy for improving the response to vaccine therapy is the combination of vaccines and other immunomodulators, such as CPIs. A full discussion of CPIs in melanoma is beyond the scope of this chapter, but their use has clearly revolutionized this field. The success of CPIs in melanoma has led to a great deal of excitement for immunotherapy in general, especially in the treatment of melanoma. Combination with CPIs is the next natural step for melanoma vaccines.

While the generation of tumor-specific T cells through the administration of a cancer vaccine has been frequently accomplished, these vaccines have, in general, had disappointing clinical efficacy. This is due, at least in part, to the highly inhibitory tumor microenvironment, leading to decreased effector cytokines and cytotoxic T cell inhibition. This T cell suppression is mediated in part by inhibitory receptors, such as PD-1 and CTLA-4. Blockade of these receptors by CPIs, to include nivolumab, pembrolizumab, and ipilimumab, can prevent T cell inhibition and help preserve antitumor function. Thus, vaccines direct the patient's immune response toward the melanoma cells, while CPIs help to counteract one of the tumor's defense mechanisms against immune attack, ultimately leading to a more robust and targeted immune response.

This combination therapy may not only increase the efficacy of vaccines, but also potentially decrease the overall toxicity of treatment through the ability to use a reduced dose or duration of CPI therapy. While single agent CPI therapy has reasonably low grade 3–4 toxicity of 15%, the response rate is approximately 20%. Combined therapy can increase the response rate to more than 50%, and as many as half of these patients will experience grade 3–4 toxicity [48]. There are currently 59 phase I-III clinical trials combining a melanoma vaccine with another therapeutic modality listed on the ClinicalTrials.gov registry, and there are likely many more combinations that are in the early stages of preclinical testing [26]. Many of these combinations have been successful in early clinical trials and, as discussed above, many vaccine trials are incorporating additional forms of immunotherapy in successive trials in an attempt to improve response rates while not dramatically increasing toxicity.

Future Insights

Cancer vaccines are very well tolerated with minimal toxicity, making them quite attractive as part of multimodal treatment of cancer. While many of these cancer vaccines have shown promise in early trials, only two cancer vaccines, T-VEC (listed above) and Provenge (a DC-based vaccine for prostate cancer), proved effective enough in Phase III trials to be granted FDA approval. Each of the different vaccine strategies has advantages, and there has been some level of success in each category. However, new strategies such as combination with CPI and the use of personalized vaccines will likely dominate vaccine research moving forward.

Personalized vaccines, which often involve sampling the patient's tumor and/or blood for the creation of the vaccine, have the benefit of priming a patient's own DC to their specific tumor. Advances in technology and improvement in the techniques involved in production of these personalized vaccines may lead to enhanced scalability of this particular approach to immunotherapy. This will provide a more specific vaccine for an individual patient, instead of relying on common TAAs. Along these lines, targeting "neoantigens" or mutated proteins expressed solely in tumors may prove to be an effective vaccine approach [49].

Another key factor necessary for the effective use of melanoma vaccines is to determine the correct patient population in which to administer these vaccines. Numerous studies have shown increased efficacy in patients with minimal disease (not surprising, given that immune mechanisms may not be able to overcome a large tumor burden), or only in specific subpopulations, but not the trial's broader target population. Results of many trials suggest that monotherapy with vaccines will likely provide the most benefit in the adjuvant setting, after standard of care surgery has reduced the overall burden of disease. More specific subgroups of patients (such as specific HLA types) that are likely to benefit most from therapy will vary according to the specific vaccine.

Finally, current studies on vaccine therapy in conjunction with CPIs will help inform future decision-making regarding the ideal treatment regimen and allow the extension of vaccines from the adjuvant to metastatic setting. This combination therapy may serve to maximize the effect of personalized vaccines, permitting an effective, durable response of a patient's T cells against their specific tumor. In such a way, we may be capable of optimizing the body's own defenses against cancer, to create a lasting antitumor response with minimal side effects.

References

1. Coley WB. The treatment of inoperable sarcoma by bacterial toxins (the mixed toxins of the streptococcus erysipelas and the Bacillus prodigiosus). Proc R Soc Med. 1910;3(Surg Sect):1–48.
2. Foley EJ. Antigenic properties of Methylcholanthrene-induced tumors in mice of the strain of origin. Cancer Res. 1953;13:835.
3. Prehn RT, Main JM. Immunity to Methylcholanthrene-induced sarcomas. J Nat Cancer Inst. 1957;18:769.
4. Morton DL, Malmgren RA, Holmes EC, Ketcham AS. Demonstration of antibodies against human

malignant melanoma by immunofluorescence. Surgery. 1968;64:233.
5. Ramirez-Montagut T, Turk MJ, Wolchok JD, Guevara-Patino JA, Houghton A. Immunity to melanoma: unraveling the relation of tumor immunity and autoimmunity. Oncogene. 2003;22:3180–7.
6. Morton DL, Eilber FR, Holmes EC, Hunt JS, Ketcham AS, Silverstein MJ, Sparks FC. BCG immunotherapy of malignant melanoma: summary of a seven-year experience. Ann Surg. 1974;180:635–43.
7. Agarwala SS, Neuberg D, Park Y, Kirkwood JM. Mature results of a phase III randomized trial of Bacillus Calmette–Guerin (BCG) versus observation and BCG plus Dacarbazine versus BCG in the adjuvant therapy of American joint committee on cancer stage I–III melanoma (E1673). Cancer. 2004;100:1692–8.
8. Atkins MB, Lotze MT, Dutcher JP, Fisher RI, Weiss G, Margolin K, Abrams J, Sznol M, Parkinson D, Hawkins M, Paradise C, Kunkel L, Rosenberg SA. High-dose recombinant interleukin 2 therapy for patients with metastatic melanoma: analysis of 270 patients treated between 1985 and 1993. J Clin Oncol. 1999;17(7):2105–16.
9. Byers BA, Temple-Oberle CF, Hurdle V, McKinnon JG. Treatment of in-transit melanoma with intralesional interleukin-2: a systematic review. J Surg Oncol. 2014;110:770–5.
10. Kirkwood JM, Strawderman MH, Ernstoff MS, Smith TJ, Borden EC, Blum RH. Interferon Alfa-2b adjuvant therapy of high-risk resected cutaneous melanoma: the eastern cooperative oncology group trial EST 1684. J Clin Oncol. 1996;14:7–17.
11. Eggermont AMM, Suciu S, Santinami M, et al. Adjuvant therapy with pegylated interferon alfa-2b versus observation alone in resected stage III melanoma: final results of EORTC 18991, a randomized phase III trial. Lancet. 2008;372:117–26.
12. Rosenberg SA, Yang JC, Sherry RM, et al. Durable complete responses in heavily pretreated patients with metastatic melanoma using T cell transfer immunotherapy. Clin Cancer Res. 2011;17(13):4550–7.
13. Rosenberg SA, Yannelli JR, Yang JC, et al. Treatment of patients with metastatic melanoma with autologous tumor-infiltrating lymphocytes and interleukin 2. J Natl Cancer Inst. 1994;86(15):1159–66.
14. Schadendorf D, Hodi FS, Robert C, et al. Pooled analysis of long-term survival data from phase II and phase III trials of ipilimumab in unresectable or metastatic melanoma. J Clin Oncol. 2015;33(17):1889–94.
15. Robert C, Long GV, Brady B, et al. Nivolumab in previously untreated melanoma without BRAF mutation. N Engl J Med. 2015;372(4):320–30.
16. Robert C, Schachter J, Long GV, et al. Pembrolizumab versus ipilimumab in advanced melanoma. N Engl J Med. 2015;372:2521–32.
17. Rosenberg SA, et al. Immunologic and therapeutic evaluation of a synthetic peptide vaccine for the treatment of patients with metastatic melanoma. Nat Med. 1998;4:321–7.
18. Schwartzentruber DJ, Lawson DH, Richards JM, Conry RM, Miller DM, Treisman J, et al. gp100 peptide vaccine and interleukin-2 in patients with advanced melanoma. N Engl J Med. 2011;364(22):2119–27.
19. Hodi FS, O'Day SJ, McDermott DF, Weber RW, Sosman JA, Haanen JB, et al. Improved survival with ipilimumab in patients with metastatic melanoma. N Engl J Med. 2010;363(8):711–23.
20. Livingston PO, Wong GY, Adluri S, et al. Improved survival in stage III melanoma patients with GM2 antibodies: a randomized trial of adjuvant vaccination with GM2 ganglioside. J Clin Oncol. 1994;12:1036–44.
21. Eggermont AMM, Suciu S, Rutkowski P, et al. Adjuvant ganglioside GM2-KLH/QS-21 vaccination versus observation after resection of primary tumor >1.5 mm in patients with stage II melanoma: results of the EORTC 18961 randomized phase III trial. J Clin Oncol. 2013;31:3831–7.
22. Kirkwood JM, Lee S, Moschos SJ, et al. Immunogenicity and antitumor effects of vaccination with peptide vaccine +/−granulocyte-monocyte colony-stimulating factor and/or IFN-alpha2b in advanced metastatic melanoma: Eastern Cooperative Oncology Group phase II trial E1696. Clin Cancer Res. 2009;15:1443–51.
23. Lawson DH, Lee S, Zhao F, et al. Randomized, placebo-controlled, phase III trial of yeast-derived granulocyte-macrophage colony-stimulating factor (GM-CSF) versus peptide vaccination versus GM-CSF plus peptide vaccination versus placebo in patients with no evidence of disease after complete surgical resection of locally advanced and/or stage IV melanoma: a trial of the Eastern Cooperative Oncology Group-American College of Radiology Imaging Network Cancer Research Group (E4697). J Clin Oncol. 2015;33:4066–76.
24. Srivastava P. Interactions of heat shock proteins with peptides and antigen presenting cells: chaperoning of the innate and adaptive immune responses. Ann Rev Immunol. 2002;20:395–425.
25. Testori A, Richards J, Whitman E, Mann GB, Lutzky J, Camacho L, et al. Phase III comparison of vitespen, an autologous tumor-derived heat shock protein gp96 peptide complex vaccine, with physician's choice of treatment for stage IV melanoma: the C-100-21 Study Group. J Clin Oncol. 2008;26(6):955–62.
26. National Institute of Health. ClinicalTrials.gov. http://clinicaltrials.gov. Accessed 31 May 2017.
27. Bystryn JC, Zelenuch-Jacquotte A, Oratz R, Shapiro RL, Harris MN, Roses DF. Double-blind trial of a polyvalent, shed-antigen, melanoma vaccine. Clin Cancer Res. 2001;7(2001):1882–7.
28. Polynoma. Prior Clinical Trials: Phase2 Studies. http://www.polynoma.com. Accessed 31 May 2017.
29. Kruit WH, Suciu S, Dreno B, Mortier L, Robert C, Chiarion-Sileni V, et al. Selection of immunostimulant AS15 for active immunization with MAGE-A3 protein: results of a randomized phase II study of the European Organisation for Research and Treatment of

Cancer melanoma Group in Metastatic Melanoma. J Clin Oncol. 2013;31(19):2413–20.
30. Vansteenkiste J, Zielinski M, Linder A, Dahabreh J, Gonzalez EE, Malinowski W, et al. Adjuvant MAGE-A3 immunotherapy in resected non-small-cell lung cancer: phase II randomized study results. J Clin Oncol. 2013;31(19):2396–403.
31. Hersey P, Edwards A, Coates A, et al. Evidence that treatment with vaccinia melanoma cell lysates (VMCL) may improve survival of patients with stage II melanoma. Cancer Immunol Immunother. 1897;25:257–65.
32. Berd D, Maquire HC, Mastrangelo MJ. Induction of cell- mediated immunity to autologous melanoma cells and regression of metastases after treatment with a melanoma cell vaccine preceded by cyclophosphamide. Cancer Res. 1986;46:2572–7.
33. Hershey P, Coates AS, McCarthy WH, et al. Adjuvant immunotherapy of patients with high-risk melanoma using vaccinia viral lysates of melanoma: results of a randomized trial. J Clin Oncol. 2002;20:4181–90.
34. Senzer NN, Kaufman HL, Amatruda T, et al. Phase II clinical trial of a granulocyte-macrophage colony- stimulating factor-encoding, second-generation oncolytic herpesvirus in patients with unresectable metastatic mel- anoma. J Clin Oncol. 2009;27:5763–71.
35. Andtbacka RH, Kaufman HL, Collichio F, Amatruda T, Senzer N, Chesney J, Delman KA, Spitler LE, Puzanov I, Agarwala SS, Milhem M, Cranmer L, Curti B, Lewis K, Ross M, Guthrie T, Linette GP, Daniels GA, Harrington K, Middleton MR, Miller WH Jr, Zager JS, Ye Y, Yao B, Li A, Doleman S, VanderWalde A, Gansert J, Coffin RS. Talimogene laherparepvec improves durable response rate in patients with advanced melanoma. J Clin Oncol. 2015;33(25):2780–8.
36. Food and Drug Administration. FDA approves first-of-its-kind product for the treatment of melanoma. http://www.fda.gov. Accessed 31 May 2017.
37. Wilgenhof S, Corthals J, Van Nuffel AM, et al. Long-term clinical outcome of melanoma patients treated with messenger RNA-electroporated dendritic cell therapy following complete resection of metastases. Cancer Immunol Immunother. 2015;64(3):381–8.
38. Schuler-Thurner B, Bartz-Schmidt KU, Bornfeld N, et al. Immunotherapy of uveal melanoma: vaccination against cancer. Multicenter adjuvant phase 3 vaccination study using dendritic cells laden with tumor RNA for large newly diagnosed uveal melanoma. Ophthalmologe. 2015;112(12):1017–21.
39. Greene J, Hale D, Schneble E, Yu X, Nichol P, Yin S, et al.. Initial phase I/IIa trial results of an autologous tumor lysate + yeast cell wall particles + dendritic cells vaccine (TLPLDC) in patients with solid tumors. CRI-CIMT-EATI-AACR - The Inaugural International Cancer Immunotherapy Conference: Translating Science into Survival; 2015; New York, NY, USA.
40. Holmes LM, Li J, Sticca RP, Wagner TE, Wei Y. A rapid, novel strategy to induce tumor cell-specific cytotoxic T lymphocyte responses using instant dentritomas. J Immunother. 2001;24(2):122–9.
41. Greene JM, Schneble EJ, Jackson DO, et al. A phase I/IIa clinical trial in stage IV melanoma of an autologous tumor-dendritic cell fusion (dendritoma) vaccine with low dose interleukin-2. Cancer Immunol Immunother. 2016;65(4):383–92.
42. Mitchell MS, Kan-Mitchell J, Kempf RA, et al. Active specific immunotherapy for melanoma: phase I trial of allogeneic lysates and a novel adjuvant. Cancer Res. 1988;48:5883–93.
43. Carson WE, Unger JM, Sosman JA, et al. Adjuvant vaccine immunotherapy of resected, clinically node-negative melanoma: long-term outcome and impact of HLA class I antigen expression on overall survival. Cancer Immunol Res. 2014;2(10):981–7.
44. Berd D, Maguire HC, Schuchter LM, et al. Autologous hapten-modified melanoma vaccine as postsurgical adjuvant treatement after resection of nodal metastases. J Clin Oncol. 1997;15(6):2359–70.
45. Berd D, Sato T, Maguire HC, et al. Immunopharmacologic analysis of an autologous, hapten-modified human melanoma vaccine. J Clin Oncol. 2004;22(3):403–15.
46. Morton DL, Hsueh EC, Essner R, et al. Prolonged survival of patients receiving active immunotherapy with Canvaxin therapeutic polyvalent vaccine after complete resection of melanoma metastatic to regional lymph nodes. Ann Surg. 2002;236(4):438–49.
47. SEC Archives. CancerVax announces results of phase 3 clinical trials of Canvaxin™ in patients with stage III and stage IV melanoma. http://www.sec.gov/archives. Accessed 1 June 2017.
48. Wolchok JD, Kluger H, Callahan MK, et al. Nivolumab plus ipilimumab in advanced melanoma. N Engl J Med. 2013;369:122–33.
49. Carreno BM, Magrini V, Becker-Hapak M, et al. A dendritic cell vaccine increases the breadth and diversity of melanoma neoantigen-specific T cells. Science. 2015;348(6236):803–8.

Adoptive Cell Therapy for Melanoma

34

Jane Mills, Phillip Darcy, and David E. Gyorki

Introduction

Melanoma has long been recognized as a strongly immunogenic cancer. The presence and density of a T cell infiltrate has been correlated with outcome [1]. The ability to harness this adaptive immune response for therapy has long been attractive to clinicians treating patients with metastatic melanoma. The development of therapies targeting immune checkpoints including CTLA4 and PD1 (discussed elsewhere) has seen immune therapies become first line treatment for many patients with metastatic melanoma. However, adaptive cell therapy predates the current era of immunotherapy and represents a very direct and individualized treatment modality where the antitumor response is exploited and expanded to develop a personalized approach to therapy.

J. Mills, M.B.B.S., B.Med.Sci., M.Epi.
Division of Cancer Surgery, Peter MacCallum Cancer Centre, Melbourne, VIC, Australia
e-mail: jane.mills@petermac.org

P. Darcy, B.Sc., Ph.D.
Research Division, Peter MacCallum Cancer Centre, Melbourne, VIC, Australia
e-mail: phil.darcy@petermac.org

D. E. Gyorki, M.B.B.S., M.D., F.R.A.C.S. (✉)
Division of Cancer Surgery, Peter MacCallum Cancer Centre, Melbourne, VIC, Australia

Department of Surgery, University of Melbourne, Parkville, VIC, Australia
e-mail: david.gyorki@petermac.org

Cellular and Molecular Principles in ACT

The human immune system is highly evolved to recognize, respond, and protect the host against a constant threat from infection and disease in the external environment (including the detection and elimination of malignant cells). The immune system may be broadly classified into two broad arms: the *innate* and *adaptive* immune systems. The adaptive immune system is capable of both specific antigen recognition and memory and it is these characteristics of antigen specificity and memory which make harnessing the adaptive immune system desirable for developing targeted cancer therapies.

The principal cells of the adaptive immune system relevant to ACT are T lymphocytes. The main focus of T cell-based therapies has been $CD8^+$ cytotoxic T cells, but it is now understood that $CD4^+$ T cells are also very important in tumor eradication [2–4].

T cells require three signals for activation of effector functions (Fig. 34.1):

1. MHC recognition: the TCR must ligate with the appropriate MHC receptor. $CD8^+$ T cells recognize MHC class I (MHC-I), expressed on all human nucleated cells. $CD4^+$ T cells recognize and bind MHC class II (MHC-II), expressed on the surface of professional antigen presenting cells (dendritic cells, macrophages, and B cells) [5].

A. I. Riker (ed.), *Melanoma*, https://doi.org/10.1007/978-3-319-78310-9_34

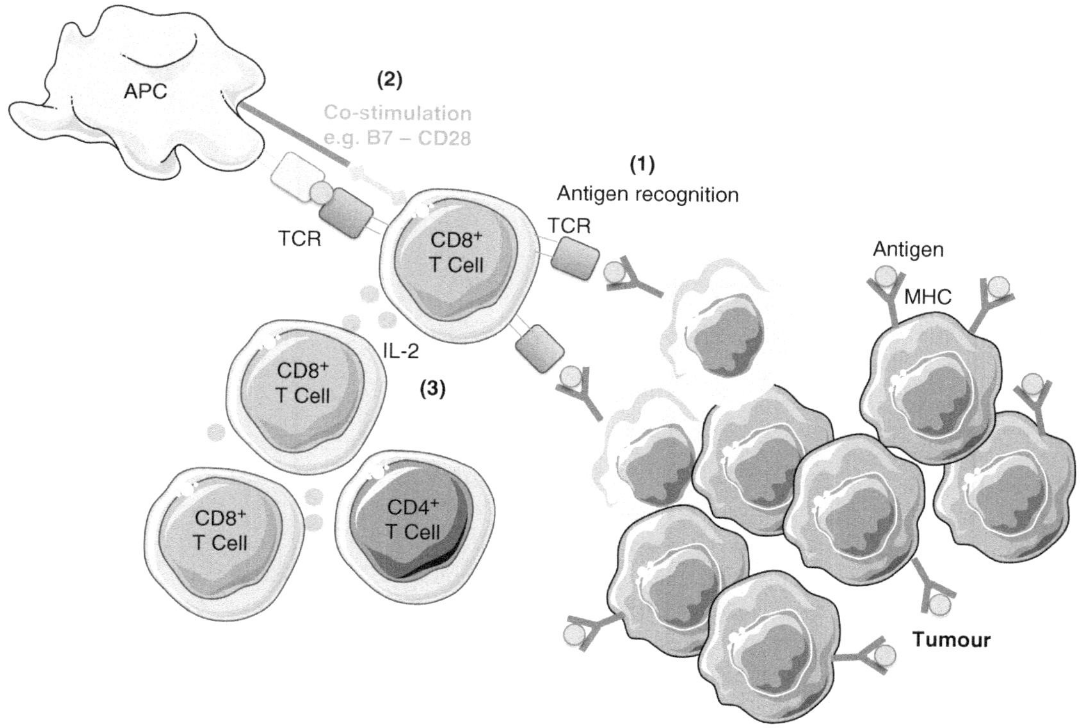

Fig. 34.1 Activation of T cells requires three signals [1]. Recognition of non-self antigen presented by MHC receptors [2]. Costimulation of T cells from antigen presenting cells (APCs). This results in activation of T cells which in-turn produce cytokines, including IL-2 [3]. This acts in a positive feedback manner, enhancing and sustaining the T cell response. (Adapted from [13])

2. Co-stimulation: the TCR-antigen-MHC complex interaction is not sufficient to reach a signalling threshold to induce a T cell response. It requires a second signal from the APC, of which the B-7 molecule is most important, engaging with CD28 molecule on the T cell. This results in TCR signal amplification, proliferation, and promotion of T cell survival. In the absence of co-stimulation, the T cell may be rendered anergic [6, 7].
3. IL-2: IL-2 is produced by activated T cells in a paracrine fashion. It encourages antigen-specific T cell proliferation and activates effector functions [8, 9].

To avoid excessive activation and resultant collateral tissue damage, there are multiple mechanisms in place to dampen the response and return homeostasis. These mechanisms include both humoral (e.g.,cytokines IL-12) and cellular components, including inhibitory co-stimulation, e.g., CTLA4 and PD1, and regulatory T cells (T_{reg}). These systems have been successfully exploited with novel immunotherapies (discussed elsewhere).

Adoptive cell therapy (ACT) involves the ex vivo identification and expansion of antitumor lymphocytes for the purpose of cancer therapy. The treatment has three primary components; non-myeloablative lymphodepletion (mainly using systemic chemotherapy), followed by expanded immune-cell infusion that is administered in combination with appropriate growth factors to promote T cell survival and expansion in vivo [10, 11].

Expansion in vitro allows optimization of T cell growth away from the potentially immunosuppressive tumor microenvironment [11]. This also allows for the optimization and modification of the host immune system to accept the immune graft and potentiate targeted immune cell proliferation and effector response.

Cells for use in adoptive cell therapy may be derived from:

1. Tumor-associated T lymphocytes (TIL)
2. Genetically modified autologous T cells targeted towards known tumor antigens, e.g., TCR and chimeric antigen receptor (CAR) directed therapies

Immune Evasion Mechanisms

A hallmark of cancer is the ability of a growing tumor to evade a host immune response [12]. Tumor cells may acquire genetic defects in antigen processing and presentation pathways, or develop reduced sensitivity to IFNγ or IFNα/β, thereby reducing sensitivity to immune-mediated elimination [13]. If tumor cells fail to express MHC-1 molecules, it renders them susceptible to eradication by NK cells. To avoid this, some tumor cells may lose the portion of MHC-1 capable of presenting antigenic peptide to T cells, retaining the residual molecule and thereby escaping elimination [5]. Genomic instability within tumor cells may result in tumor cell heterogeneity, with the loss or alteration of tumor-specific antigens that are no longer recognized by tumor-specific $CD8^+$ T cells.

Alternatively, cells may also evade innate immune detection by changes in genetic expression that result in the loss of ligands for NK cell recognition required for effector function. They may also suppress the production of cytokines that promote dendritic cell maturation and antigen presentation [13]. Tumor cells may evade apoptosis by upregulating antiapoptotic molecule expression (e.g., FLIP, BCL-2, BCL-XL). They can develop mutations that render them resistant to lysis by immune cells (e.g., mutations in receptors for TRAIL, DR5, and Fas), and may express ligands on the cell surface to reduce the cytotoxic actions or induce apoptosis of T cells (e.g., B7-H1, HLA-G, and HLA-E) [13]. Tumor cells may also influence cells of the innate immune system by inducing changes in the microenvironment through cytokine secretion (e.g., IL-10, VEGF). This, in turn, may induce antigenic tolerance of antigen presenting cells and inhibit NK cell mediated killing. IL-10 inhibits production of pro-inflammatory cytokines and hence limits immune cell recruitment [14]. Tumor cells may also secrete TGFβ and suppress T cell activation and effector functions, proliferation, and differentiation [5, 13, 14]. TGFβ may also downregulate $CD8^+$ expression of granzymes, perforin, and expression of Fas-L molecules, and hence impair effector functions [14].

Inflammation resulting from innate immune cell recognition of tumor cells may promote tumor initiation, promotion, and progression. TNFα may stimulate tumor cells to produce additional cytokines, e.g., IL-1 and IL-6, which act in a paracrine fashion to promote tumor growth, and increase resistance to the induction of apoptosis. Inflammatory cells produce reactive oxygen species (ROS) that may result in DNA mutations and promote tumorigenesis and drive tumor progression [5].

Melanoma-Associated Antigens Recognized by T Cells

The search and identification of tumor-associated antigens (TAAs) began after the discovery of endogenous tumor-reactive T cells. These T cells may be obtained from venepuncture with identification and culture of circulating T lymphocytes (CTL), or tumor infiltrating lymphocytes (TIL) that are obtained from the tumor itself [15].

Melanoma has been the signature tumor in the study and mapping of TAAs. The origin of the epitopes recognized by the T cell response are likely multifactorial. It is now known that melanoma has one of the highest rates of somatic mutations in human cancers. The initial methods of screening for mutations require tumor-reactive T cells obtained from expanding tumor-associated T cells. These were then tested against stable tumor cell lines in vitro that were more easily established compared to other tumor types [15].

Initial studies that examined the molecular landscape of TAAs in melanoma were first published in 1989 by Thierry Boon and colleagues [15–17]. They identified genes encoding antigens using a labor-intensive process of screening tumor DNA libraries that were generated from melanoma tumor cells. After this, they measured the cytokine response when combined with tumor-reactive T cell clones from peripheral blood [16]. MAGE-1 was the first tumor-specific T cell epitope to be identified [18]. Since this time, multiple other tumor-specific antigens have been identified using more sophisticated screening methods that are now available. These screening methods include SEREX, comparative proteome analysis (proteomics), and gene expression profiling (microarray) [17]. Other techniques include RT-PCR and whole genome sequencing of the tumor to identify antigen expression and mutational signatures of tumor cells to generate and identify reactive T cells [19].

Tumor antigens may be classified into five broad categories:

1. Tissue differentiation antigens, e.g., MART-1, gp100, CEA, CD19
2. Tumor-germline antigens, e.g., MAGE-1, NY-ESO-1
3. Normal proteins overexpressed by cancer cells, e.g., hTERT, EGFR, mesothelin
4. Viral proteins, e.g., HPV, EBV
5. Tumor-specific mutated antigens, e.g., ERBB2IP [15]

Adoptive cell therapy, using TCR targeting tumor-directed antigens and clinical trial outcomes, will be discussed later during this chapter.

Melanoma Is an Immunogenic Cancer

Melanoma, in particular, is recognized as a strongly immunogenic tumor, and combined with poor clinical outcomes and treatments with limited efficacy these attributes have made metastatic melanoma an ideal platform to study immune-based therapies. Approximately 3% of patients with melanoma present with metastatic disease with no known primary source, and this is thought to represent clinical evidence of immunoediting as a result of tumor clearance by the immune system [20]. In some patients, a small patch of depigmentation (vitiligo) at a previous pigmented site, which may be the location of the primary tumor, may be evident [21].

Evidence for the immunogenicity of melanoma also extends from a case report in renal transplant recipients. One patient received a donor kidney from a patient whom had localized melanoma 16 years previously. Upon receiving the donor organ and standard immunosuppression, this patient went on to develop metastatic melanoma. Despite cessation of immunosuppression and interferon therapy, this patient died 22 months after receiving the transplant [22]. The recipient of the second kidney also developed melanoma within the kidney but it did not metastasize, with the patient rendered disease free after resection of the donor kidney. This supports evidence for an immune equilibrium and tumor latency for melanoma in an immunocompetent individual. It also exemplifies the complex interaction between the same tumor and different host immune responses [21].

One explanation for the increased immunogenicity of melanoma is attributed to the high rates of somatic mutations frequently present. The Cancer Genome Atlas (TCGA) program has recently published a large dataset using a multiplatform analysis to clarify the genomic expression of melanoma. They identified over 228,000 mutations, with a median mutation rate of 16.8 mutations/Mb. This is the highest reported mutation rate for any cancer type [23]. In this paper, melanomas were classified into subgroups based on genetic expression. One subclass, designated the "immune subclass," were found to overexpress genes associated with immune cell subsets, signalling molecules, co-stimulatory and co-inhibitory immune checkpoint proteins, cytokines, chemokines and their receptors. Patients with melanomas expressing this subtype were found to have a more favorable prognosis than other subtypes. In addition, as identified in previous studies, patients in this same cohort with high-density immune cell infiltrates were also found to have significantly improved survival. There was a high concordance between TIL infiltrate and immune subtype. Immune cell infiltration was correlated with improved patient survival that was independent of the genomic subtypes examined. The presence of a dense immune infiltrate or an inflamed microenvironment correlates with a positive response to immunotherapy.

This chapter will now discuss the history and development, as well as results of clinical trials using ACT in melanoma. We will also discuss current strategies to optimize delivery and efficacy of ACT and outline future directions in this expanding field of immno-oncology.

History of ACT

The prognostic significance of the presence of a lymphocytic reaction within resected tumor specimens has been recognized for almost 100 years [24]. In 1954, Billingham and colleagues performed the first ACT using cells obtained from regional tumor-draining lymph nodes. However, successful lymphocyte growth in vitro was not achieved until 1980, when IL-2 was identified as an important growth factor in the activation and proliferation of T lymphocytes. In 1984, IL-2 was commercially produced and available for use in animals and humans [10].

The first successful studies in ACT utilized lymphokine-activated killer (LAK) cells (non-specific non-T and non-B lymphocytes) with high-dose IL-2. An initial study published in 1985 was the first to demonstrate tumor regression and the potential of immune therapy in human cancer therapy [10]. However, follow-up studies reported similar response rates to patients treated with high-dose IL-2 alone [25]. Hence, attention was turned to the use of tumor infiltrating lymphocytes (TIL) which had demonstrated superior tumor cell killing of established melanoma compared to LAK cells in murine models.

ACT using TIL has been chiefly pioneered and championed by Dr Steven Rosenberg and his team at the National Cancer Institute (NCI), in Bethesda, Maryland, USA. The protocol is summarized in Fig. 34.2. The Rosenberg group published their initial trial with ACT-TIL for metastatic melanoma in 1988. In this study, 86 patients with metastatic melanoma were treated with autologous TIL and high-dose, intravenous bolus IL-2. They achieved an objective response (OR) of 34% and five patients experienced a complete response (CR). Results were comparable to outcomes using IL-2 alone (OR 31%) and IL-2-based biochemotherapy (OR 35%) [25–27]. Since this initial ACT trial, TIL protocols have been modified to include lymphodepleting chemotherapy regimens. A recent report describes achieving an objective clinical responses in 52/93 patients (56%), with a complete response seen in 20/93 patients (22%) [28]. This technique has been reproduced in multiple centers with similar response rates [29–31].

Manipulation of the host prior to ACT transfer with non-myeloablative lymphodepletion techniques is an important component for most ACT protocols. It results in the elimination of other cells in vivo that might compete with infused TIL for critical cytokines, further allowing for a more effective function of these transferred cells [32]. Lymphodepletion usually involves the use of the chemotherapy regimen of cyclophosphamide and fludarabine. Total body irradiation (TBI), in addition to the chemotherapy agents, has been used in some protocols, demonstrating enhanced tumor response rates in earlier studies [28]. However, there was no difference noted in more recent studies [33]. Using these techniques, ACT has demonstrated high overall response rates ranging from 40 to 72%, with long-term, durable, and potentially curative complete response rates of up to 40% [10, 11]. In fact, in the 24% of patients from the National Cancer Institute who have achieved a complete response, there has only been a single recurrence after a median follow-up of over 5 years [28, 31].

ACT has several advantages over immunization and other immunotherapy strategies and represents an example of highly personalized cancer therapy. T cells exhibit chemotaxis and are able to home to tumor sites throughout the body, including the brain, as they are capable of crossing the blood–brain barrier [34]. If the cell transfer undertaken in ACT contains memory T cells, an enduring response may be obtained [34].

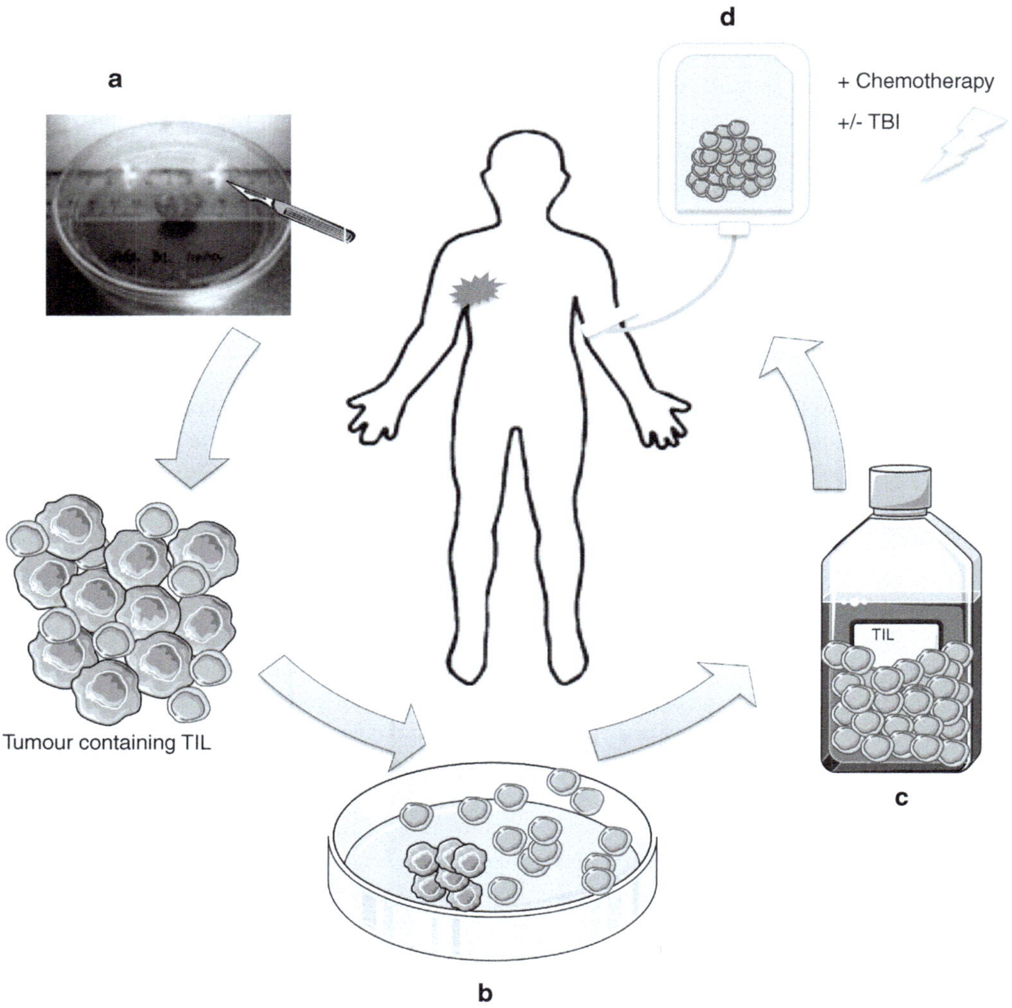

Fig. 34.2 Protocol for adoptive cell therapy using TIL: (**a**) Retrieval of tumor sample and partition into 2 mm^3 fragments; (**b**) Tumor fragments cultured in vivo in presence of IL-2 to promote TIL proliferation. (**c**) rapid expansion of TIL population in specialized flasks (**d**) reinfusion of expanded TIL population with administration of systemic IL-2 +/− total body irradiation

ACT only require a small population of antigen-specific tumor cells that can be expanded to large numbers for treatment [11].

ACT may be performed using various cell populations including:

1. Tumor-specific T cells (TIL or circulating tumor cells).
2. Genetically modifying peripheral blood T cells using tumor antigen-specific TCR or introducing chimeric antigen receptors (CAR) [32, 35].

Tumor Infiltrating Lymphocytes (TIL)

TILs are a subset of patient T lymphocytes that are located and expanded from tumor stromal cells. They are potentially a heterogeneous population capable of recognizing multiple tumor-specific antigens. However, they are incapable of eradicating the tumor due to inhibiting signals from other immune cells, tumor cells, and the surrounding tumor microenvironment. TIL can recognize and lyse autologous tumor cells, but are self-tolerant of antigens expressed on normal tissue [10].

After demonstrating successful elimination of metastatic tumor deposits in lung and liver using murine models [36], the first phase I clinical trial using TILs was performed in 1988 [10, 37]. This study examined 12 patients with advanced cancer of various tumor types and had resectable metastases from which TIL were grown. They also had remaining residual metastatic disease in order to evaluate for a clinical response to treatment. Patients were treated with a single preconditioning dose of cyclophosphamide and then transfused with varying numbers of TILs (10^9–10^{11} cells) and IL-2. However, results were modest with a tumor response reported in only one patient with melanoma and one patient with renal cell carcinoma. The results from this trial led to further trials and have since focused on optimizing the lymphodepletion regimen, modulating cytokine delivery and dose, and experimentation with the nature of reinfused TIL, such as exploring different subtypes and tumor antigen avidity [10, 38].

Advantage of Using TIL

TIL therapy capitalizes and enhances the patient's own adoptive immune system and specifically targets a unique and heterogeneous population of tumor antigens. They are HLA-matched for the patient, and may be tested for efficacy ex vivo prior to reinfusion [39]. The tumor antigens recognized by the cultured TIL are highly diverse. In a series of patients treated at the Surgery Branch of the NCI, 56 unique antigens were identified among the patients, with no overlap seen between patients. Tumor antigens recognized may include gp100, MART-1, TRP-2, tyrosinase, and NY-ESO-1 as well as other tumor antigens not yet identified. These unidentified antigens account for >90% of TIL and are thought to be the result of epitopes of mutant self-proteins (e.g., signalling and housekeeping genes). TIL exhibit self-tolerance therefore limiting collateral injury to normal tissues and have demonstrated the highest tumor response rates, including a significant complete response rate that is durable compared to other forms of immunotherapy [39].

Generating TIL

The generation of TIL involves resecting a tumor deposit and establishing multiple individual microcultures growing in vitro from single cell suspensions or 2 mm^3 tumor fragments in media containing IL-2. TIL cultures typically reach several million cells in 2–3 weeks and have the capacity to kill autologous tumor present within the individual cultures. A rapid expansion protocol (REP) using the T-cell stimulating antibody, OKT-3, is used to expand cell numbers and results in billions of cells available for patient transfusion. Response rates have correlated with total number of reinfused cells. The number of T cells infused may vary significantly between patients as they are often determined by the number of cells that can be manufactured during a REP [40], or a defined number of cells per kilogram of body weight. Using REP, the TIL are expanded more than 1000-fold, achieving typical numbers of ~50×10^9 [25]. However, as the T cells will continue to replicate and expand following infusion, the final cell number may be significantly higher than the initial number delivered and patient-specific [41].

Early Clinical Trials

The first clinical, phase II trial using TIL-based ACT for metastatic melanoma was performed in 1988 [26]. Twenty patients with metastatic melanoma received varying doses of TIL and high-dose IL-2 (720,000 IU/kg) given every 8 h as tolerated. Patients were pretreated with a single dose of cyclophosphamide 36 h prior to TIL transfusion. Eleven patients demonstrated objective tumor regression in multiple metastatic sites [26]. A subsequent trial involving 86 patients revealed an overall response rate of 34% [27]. Response rates did not vary among patients who had previously received treatment with IL-2 compared to patients who were IL-2 naïve [10, 27]. Since this time, ACT has been performed on many patients at multiple institutions and modifications to these original protocols have been made to enhance T cell engraftment, in vivo activity, T cell proliferation, and survival of transferred cells.

Modifications of ACT Protocols

Lymphodepletion

Lymphodepletion prior to reinfusion allows manipulation and optimization of the host microenvironment to support the transferred cells. Lymphodepletion was also associated with higher endogenous levels of cytokines IL-7 and IL-15, which are important for T cell survival [42]. These cytokines may improve expansion and activation of transferred T cells and suggest that endogenous immune cells may compete with the transferred cells for cytokines [10, 28]. Lymphodepletion enhances the activity of tumor-reactive $CD8^+$ T cells and reduces populations of host $CD4^+CD25^+FOXP3^+$ Regulatory T cells (T_{Reg}), which, in turn, may reduce the activation threshold of effector T cells [43, 44]. Additional explanations of enhanced activity following lymphodepletion include extravasation of enteric flora secondary to the chemotherapy and radiotherapy regimes employed resulting in stimulation of toll-like receptors [41, 42].

Total Body Irradiation (TBI)

When immunodepletion was intensified by adding radiotherapy to chemotherapy regimens, the objective tumor response improved even more. In a paper published in 2011 by Rosenberg and colleagues, a non-myeloablative, lymphodepleting chemotherapy regimen was given in combination with 2 versus 12 Gy of total body irradiation (TBI). The latter was given to enhance lymphocyte depletion prior to TIL infusion in patients with metastatic melanoma. The chemotherapy regimen consisted of 2 days of cyclophosphamide (60 mg/kg/day), followed by 5 days fludarabine (25 mg/m^2 per day). This was followed by TIL infusion or TBI for 2 or 12 Gy and TIL cell infusion. Patients receiving TBI also received 2 × 10^6/kg of autologous $CD34^+$ hematopoietic stem cells harvested from a granulocyte colony stimulating factor mobilized apheresis performed at least 1 week prior to starting cyclophosphamide. The median follow-up time for patients without TBI (43 patients), with 2 Gy TBI (25 patients), and with 12 Gy TBI (25 patients) was 90, 58, and 41 months, respectively. Objective tumor responses were seen in 56% of patients. Responses were seen in all tumor-affected organs (including brain, lung, liver). Complete tumor response was seen in 12% of patients without TBI; 20% of those treated with 2 Gy TBI, and 40% of patient treated with 12 Gy TBI. A total of 19/20 patients with complete response remain free of disease, with some ongoing responses lasting up to 82 months [28].

This trial was performed as sequential clinical studies comparing non-myeloablating chemotherapy alone to the addition of 2 and 12 Gy TBI. Subsequently, Goff et al. performed a follow-up clinical trial whereby patients with metastatic melanoma were randomly and prospectively assigned to preparative chemotherapy regimen alone or combined with 1200 cGy TBI. The objective and complete clinical response rates were then measured after treatment. They found the addition of TBI increased the rate of treatment toxicity and the need for ICU admission. There was no statistically significant change in complete response (CR) rates (24% for both groups, 12/50 vs. 12/51 in the TBI group) or overall survival (OS; median OS 38.2 months compared to 36.6 months in the TBI group). Although patients who received TBI had a greater proportion of partial responses (PR; 19/38 patients) than those who did not receive TBI (11/22), the duration of response was significantly shorter (median response duration 21 months vs. 10 months for TBI group) [40].

Selected Versus Unselected

In early clinical trials, TIL were "selected," meaning they were tested for antitumor recognition by coculture assays against autologous tumor or melanoma cell lines. It was only the cultures that demonstrated antitumor reactivity that were selected for REP expansion and clinical use. Using this protocol, TIL cultures were selected for expansion if they demonstrate IFNγ production when cocultured with the tumor target [45]. This additional selection requires additional time and prevented some patients from undergoing TIL therapy if the TIL cultures were unable to demonstrate adequate antitumor activity. Additionally, some patients did not receive treatment if rapid disease progression caused significant performance status decline during the growth of the TILs (4–6 weeks) [46].

More recent literature suggests that TIL grown for a shorter culture period ("young TIL") have characteristics (e.g., longer telomere lengths, and $CD27^+$) associated with higher proliferative potential and higher rates of tumor regression [33]. These "unselected" TIL spend less time in culture (10–18 days), and have shown similar efficacy rates in in vitro testing. This was confirmed in an initial pilot study of 33 patients, demonstrating a 58% objective tumor response rate [47]. Similar results have been achieved using these techniques at other institutions around the world [30, 38, 48].

High-Dose Versus Low-Dose IL-2

Original protocols, and indeed, most ongoing trials in TIL therapy, involve the administration of high-dose IL-2 to encourage T cell proliferation and persistence following cell transfer. Studies have been published examining the feasibility of utilizing lower doses of IL-2. Results from a pilot study by Ellebaek et al. in 2012 demonstrated complete and durable responses in patients with metastatic melanoma using ACT in combination with IL-2 delivered by subcutaneous low-dose injections of 2MIU/day [49]. The authors reported significantly reduced toxicity compared to the standard regimen.

N-Acetyl Cysteine

Activation induced cell death (AICD) is triggered by repetitive stimulation of the TCR and is an important regulatory process in developing peripheral tolerance and limits T cell self-reactivity. AICD may have a significant detrimental impact on the persistence of T cells in vivo. N-Acetyl cysteine (NAC) promotes accumulation of intracellular glutathione and has been demonstrated to increase the functional capacity and proliferative potential of T cells [50]. A recent publication by Scheffel et al. demonstrated improved persistence of transferred T cells, reduced tumor growth, and improved survival in murine models with the addition of n-acetyl cysteine (NAC) to TIL cultures during ex vivo expansion [51].

Limitations of TIL

The main limitations of TIL therapy to date relate principally to the technical expertise, labor intensity, biological and manufacturing facilities required for TIL production, and safe delivery of therapy to patients. Even when TIL therapy is available in highly select centers, production is limited in scale due to a number of key practical issues in T cell culture and expansion [48].

Current REP T cell expansion methods require large numbers of irradiated feeder cells. These feeder cells may be provided from the autologous patient or from multiple donors. When these feeder cells are obtained from multiple donors, however, there may be significant variations in potency between donors. This may be due to differences in co-stimulatory molecules present on individual T cells [48]. This, in turn, may impact the yield and quality of TIL for patient treatment. Currently, there is no commercially available standardized, artificial antigen presenting cell (APC) available for this use. There are several groups working on the development of such a product [52].

Obtaining TIL often requires an invasive procedure, with resection of accessible tumor. For patients who do not have an easily accessible tumor, such as a subcutaneous nodule or deposit, the complications of resection are potentially greater. Some studies have shown successful TIL generation, however, from smaller samples obtained using core biopsy [53, 54]. However, in some cases, a biopsy may not be achieved safely depending on the location of the tumor deposit, e.g., retroperitoneum, mediastinum, and pelvis. Alternatively, the adequate expertise to access these lesions, such as that from interventional radiology, may not be available in some institutions.

TILs are unable to be cultured in a moderate proportion (10–15%) of patients with melanoma, which limits this technology to a subgroup of patients. In addition, TIL production may take 6–8 weeks. During this time, patients may clinically deteriorate and miss the window for optimal therapy. Indeed, one-third of patients selected for this therapy were unable to complete treatment in one study [28]. Processes to reduce the time of TIL in culture need to be optimized in order to reduce the rate of attrition due to disease progression. Techniques to improve T cell persistence following ACT also require further investigation as this has been positively correlated on retrospective studies with improved patient tumor response [55].

Most TIL therapies to date involve the administration of IL-2. However, many of the adverse effects seen in patients undergoing ACT is attributed to the high dose of IL-2 administered in conjunction with current transfusion protocols. Several trials are investigating the clinical impact on performing ACT using low- and intermediate-dose IL-2, as well as other cytokines. Results to date have demonstrated reduced treatment toxicity, while maintaining partial and complete patient tumor responses [56, 57]. As a result of these limitations, TIL therapy is currently not FDA approved, and is only available in a few institutions in a clinical trial setting.

Predictors of Successful TIL Therapy

Initial protocols included identification, isolation, and expansion of tumor-specific cells capable of killing patient tumor in vitro; however, this step is no longer required. Instead, unselected and expanded TIL populations are reinfused, with these T cells known as "young TIL" [38, 58]. The omission of tumor-specific selection increased the number of patients eligible to receive this treatment, is clinically effective, and assists in reducing the time from resection to treatment. A reduced duration of TIL culture, as well as shorter doubling times, has been associated with improved tumor response rates [11]. Telomere length of TIL has also been demonstrated to positively correlate with tumor regression [11, 59]. Similarly, the number of $CD8^{+}CD27^{+}$ cells infused is correlated with a strong antitumor response. Both telomere length and expression of CD27 are markers of less differentiated cells [42].

The presence of regulatory T cells ($CD4^{+}CD25^{+}$ $FOX3^{+}$) has been demonstrated to reduce the tumor response in ACT [11]. Attempts have been made to reduce the number of regulatory T cells infused, or improving the ratio of $CD8^{+}$/T regulatory cells. Persistence of infused TIL in peripheral circulation at 1 month is highly correlated with a significant antitumor response [42]. Future directions of TIL therapy may be to combine treatment with checkpoint inhibitors to enhance T cell activation and increase tumor cell vulnerability to immune attack [60].

T Cell Engineering and Tumor Antigen Directed Therapy

As mentioned above, melanoma tumor cells are highly immunogenic. Tumor cells may produce tumor-specific antigens due to genetic mutations, impaired transcription, protein processing, and presentation that provide potential targets for immune-based therapies. T lymphocytes may be modified to express a desired T cell receptor (TCR) that is capable of recognizing tumor-specific antigens. The process by which foreign DNA is introduced into a cell by using viral vectors is known as transduction. These lymphocytes are isolated from a peripheral blood sample drawn from a patient, expanded ex vivo, and transfused back into the patient.

Tumor antigens may be classified into five broad categories:

1. Tissue differentiation antigens, e.g., MART-1, gp100, CEA, CD19, tyrosinase
2. Tumor-germline antigens, e.g., MAGE-1, NY-ESO-1
3. Normal proteins overexpressed by cancer cells, e.g., hTERT, EGFR, mesothelin
4. Viral proteins, e.g., HPV, EBV
5. Tumor-specific mutated antigens, e.g., ERBB2IP [15], β-catenins

When designing a targeted therapy, the overarching purpose is to maximize tumor elimination, minimize collateral damage to immediate and systemic normal tissues, and induce a durable response. Ideally, targeted tumor antigens should be:

1. Tumor specific, i.e., are only expressed by tumor cells and are not present on normal tissue
2. Immunogenic, i.e., are capable of generating a T cell response
3. High prevalence and level of expression on tumor cells [15]

As the initial hunt for tumor-specific antigens involved a disproportionate examination of melanoma tumors, many of the first antigens discovered were associated with pigment production and other constituent proteins overexpressed in tumor cells. However, TCR therapy was associated with significant toxicity due to "on target off tumor" activity. This phenomenon describes side effects due to activity against normal cells which express the target antigen. Targeting antigens involved in pigmentation resulted in severe skin rash, depigmentation, uveitis, and hearing loss [61]. Similarly, targeting CEA (which is overexpressed in many epithelial tumor cells), resulted in off-tumor activity in CEA-expressing normal cells scattered along the gastrointestinal tract resulting in severe colitis for some patients [62].

Tumor germline antigens, also known as cancer testis antigens, are expressed by some tumor cells and male germ cells in testis, but are not expressed in adult somatic tissues [63]. Epitopes of these antigens are not recognized by T cells in the testis, as these cells do not express MHC class I molecules. Therefore, these antigens are potential targets in ACT as theoretically "on target off tumor activity" is obviated. Since the initial identification of MAGE-A1 (Melanoma-Associated Antigen A1), multiple other genes in this family have been recognized and are clustered into three genetic groups, MAGE-A, -B, and -C, with their expression restricted to germ cells and tumors [64].

NY-ESO-1 is a germline antigen expressed by 10–50% of metastatic melanomas as well as other tumors including breast, prostate, thyroid, ovarian cancer, and up to 80% of synovial sarcomas. NY-ESO-1 was the first target for TCR-directed anticancer therapy to demonstrate antitumor activity in clinical trials. In a clinical trial using autologous T cells transduced with TCR directed against NY-ESO-1 in patients with metastatic melanoma or synovial sarcomas demonstrated objective clinical responses in 5 of 11 and 4 of 6 patients, respectively. In patients with metastatic melanoma, two patients demonstrated complete tumor response that persisted greater than 1 year. Unlike trials using T cells with MAGE-A, MART-1, and gp100 reactive TCRs, T cells with NY-ESO-1 directed TCR did not demonstrate on target tissue toxicities [65].

Several clinical trials have been performed examining the clinical effects of TCR targeting the MAGE-A family of antigens. However, despite tumor germline antigens theoretically restricted in activity to tumor cells, caution is warranted. Of note, clinical trials using TCR directed against these antigens have revealed significant side effects resulting from "on target off tumor" activity in tissues that was previously unrecognized to express these receptors [66]. In a clinical trial using a TCR-specific for MAGE-A3/A9/A12, 5/9 patients developed tumor regression. However, three patients developed severe neurologic side effects resulting in the death of two patients from previously unrecognized expression of MAGE-A12 in the brain [67]. In a second phase I clinical trial, patients were treated with a TCR targeting MAGE-A3 for melanoma or multiple myeloma, resulting in patient deaths from cardiotoxicity due to cross reactivity with the muscle protein titin [68]. These cases highlight an important note of caution when implementing TCR directed therapies, as these side effects can be difficult to predict prior to clinical trials and may have severe consequences for patients [66].

Oncogenic viruses are responsible for approximately 15% of the worlds' cancer burden. Oncogenic viruses may act directly (e.g., HPV, EBV, human herpesvirus 8, human T-cell leukemia virus, and merkel polyoma virus), or indirectly by producing chronic inflammatory state that may lead to tumorigenesis (e.g., hepatitis B and C) [69]. T cells specific for EBV have demonstrated complete tumor regressions in patients with nasopharyngeal tumors and lymphoma associated with EBV [70, 71]. There are no known associated viral targets in melanoma and therefore this strategy will not be discussed here further.

Limitations of TCR Therapy

TCR therapy with tumor directed antigens is an appealing form of immune-based cancer treatment. It has many cases of clinical success to date, however, it is not without significant limitations. In addition to the hurdles outlined above, TCR directed therapy relies on MHC presentation of antigen by tumor cells. Many tumors evade immune recognition by downregulating expression of MHC. A mis-pairing between endogenous and transduced TCRs has also been described, which may result in potential self-reactive TCRs [72]. There are also questions regarding the safety of retroviral transduction that have the potential to insert and enhance dormant oncogenes. They can also cause "off target on tumor" activity that results in tissue destruction when TCR targets are present in normal tissue or cross-react with other antigens as outlined above [63].

Chimeric T Cell Therapy

A chimeric antigen receptor (CAR) is a genetically engineered construct that combines the extracellular antigen binding domain with the intracellular signalling portion of a TCR (CD3ζ) and one or more co-stimulatory domains [45]. The "first generation" CARs linked CD3ζ or Fcγ signalling domains to the scFv recognizing tumor antigen. Second generation (incorporating CD28 or 4-1BB signalling domains) and third generation CARs (including additional CD28, 4-1BB, and/or OX-40) have subsequently been developed. These have all resulted in improvements in T cell proliferation, persistence, and cytokine/cytolytic function in vivo [73].

Although TCR-transduced T cells obtained from peripheral blood mitigates many of the limitations and risks of ACT associated with using TILs, this technique also has significant limitations. In particular, these T cells remain HLA-restricted. This means that the TCR is only activated when it recognizes non-self (MHC class I) or when it recognizes an antigen presented by the antigen presenting cell (APC) with the appropriate co-stimulation molecules (MHC class II). Many tumors may exploit this by down-regulating or eliminating MHC expression, or produce inhibitory molecules which, in turn, fail to provide the necessary co-stimulation required to incite a response [10, 11, 74].

In contrast, CAR are not HLA-restricted and do not require an APC consort with additional co-stimulation to produce an effective T cell response. CARs are able to not only target protein antigens, but also carbohydrate and lipid antigens, as well as other antigens that may be recognized by an antibody [63, 75]. CARs are, however, restricted to extracellular antigens and cannot induce a response to intracellular processed TCR antigens including MAGE and NY-ESO-1 tumor antigens [10, 76]. Monoclonal antibody therapies require a threshold of tumor antigen expression to be effective. In contrast, CAR T cells have demonstrated effective recognition and effector functions against antigens at low levels. This is because the avidity of the receptor can be modified and is greater than the avidity of a bivalent antibody. This has been demonstrated in osteosarcoma where the antigen, HER2, is expressed on up to 60% of tumors. This receptor is present at lower levels in other cancers, such as breast cancer, resulting in limited activity against HER2 directed monoclonal antibody therapies (such as trastuzumab). In contrast, CAR T cells directed against HER2 have shown significant activity against sarcoma cell lines in vitro [77].

CAR T cells have shown significant clinical success in hematological malignancies, such as lymphoma, leukemia and multiple myeloma. The most impressive clinical response rates to date have been in CAR targeting CD19, a protein expressed in most B cell malignancies, with some studies demonstrating complete remission rates of 50–90% [45, 78]. To date, success using this technology has been somewhat limited in solid malignancies. This is thought to be due to the interplay with the immunosuppressive tumor microenvironment, such as cytokine secretion, T cell trafficking to the tumor, inhibitory signals from other T cells and myeloid-derived suppressor cells [45, 73, 79]. Strategies to improve CAR therapy outcome include modifying T cells to express tumor-specific chemokine receptors, combining CAR therapy with anti-angiogenic agents and reducing T regulatory cells by combining CAR therapy with preconditioning lymphodepleting chemotherapy. Additionally, the combination of CAR T cells with checkpoint blockade with anti-CTLA-4 or PD-1 inhibitors is being examined in several clinical trials [45, 76, 80, 81].

Significant concerns were raised following the death of a patient treated with CAR T cells specific for HER2 antigen. This patient received non-myeloablative preconditioning chemotherapy followed by an intravenous infusion of 10^{10} autologous T cells transduced with a third generation CAR (containing CD28, 4-1BB, and CD3ζ signalling domains) and given in combination with IL-2. This patient developed severe respiratory distress within 15 min of receiving this infusion and despite aggressive resuscitation and supportive therapy the patient died 5 days later. Serum samples demonstrated high levels of inflammatory cytokines (IFNγ, GM-CSF, TNFα, IL-6, and IL-10) consistent with a cytokine storm. Authors speculated that this result was possibly due to the recognition of low levels of ERBB2 on lung epithelium [82].

A recent phase I/II clinical trial was conducted examining CAR T cell therapy directed against HER2 in patients with sarcoma. There was a total of 19 patients (16 with osteosarcoma, 1 with Ewing sarcoma, 1 with a primitive neuroectodermal tumor and 1 with desmoplastic small round cell tumor) with HER2 positive tumors treated with a dose-escalating protocol of T cells transduced with a second generation HER2-CAR. Four patients had stable disease for at least 3–14 months, with a median overall survival of 10.3 months (5.1–29.1 months). HER2-CAR T cells were detected 6 weeks post-infusion in 7/9 patients who received greater than $1 \times 10^6/m^2$ HER 2-CAR T cells, demonstrating persistence. Adverse effects were minimal, with only one patient on the highest dose of T cell infusion developed fever within 12 h of T cell infusion. This study demonstrates a safe dose of HER2-CAR T cells can be given to patients with cancer, and these cells demonstrate persistence in vivo [83].

Future of Adoptive Cell Therapy in Melanoma

In the modern era, there is an abundance of treatment options for patients with metastatic melanoma. The complexity of ACT and its limited accessibility to specialized melanoma centers has meant that its place in the therapeutic algorithm for patients with metastatic melanoma is not clearly defined. Future studies to better understand the patient subgroup who are most likely to respond, as well as to define the response rates in patients who have progressed following checkpoint inhibitor immunotherapy, are essential.

Furthermore, currently available methods of TIL culture involve open culture techniques requiring small cultures in plates, until established populations of TIL are transferred into flasks or bags for population expansion. This process often requires large volumes of media, multiple steps in handling with concomitant risks of contamination. It also requires highly skilled technicians and is time, space, and labor intensive. If this process can be transformed using closed system techniques and automated, it may better comply with regulatory requirements. This, in turn, may facilitate steps towards FDA approval, becoming more amenable to large-scale commercial production [48]. Several new devices are now available for T cell culture, such as the WAVE™ bioreactor (GE Healthcare) and G-REX rapid cell expansion systems, which may aid the transition to a commercially feasible large-scale manufacturing process [84, 85].

We still have many unanswered questions regarding optimal patient selection, despite many successes. Although the use of ACT is quite complex and costly, it offers a very effective therapeutic option for patients with metastatic melanoma, with among the highest rates of long-term disease control. As the tumor-immune interface becomes better understood, the combination of ACT with other immune therapies may be the key to increase the proportion of patients who benefit from these personalized therapies.

References

1. Schatton T, Scolyer RA, Thompson JF, Mihm MC. Tumor-infiltrating lymphocytes and their significance in melanoma prognosis. Methods Mol Biol. Totowa, NJ: Humana Press (Chapter 16). 2014;1102:287–324.
2. Hadrup S, Donia M, Thor Straten P. Effector CD4 and CD8 T cells and their role in the tumor microenvironment. Cancer Microenviron. 2012;6(2):123–33.
3. Friedman KM, DeVillier LE, Feldman SA, Rosenberg SA, Dudley ME. Augmented lymphocyte expansion from solid tumors with engineered cells for Costimulatory enhancement. J Immunother. 2011;34(9):651–61.
4. Rosenberg SA, Restifo NP. Adoptive cell transfer as personalized immunotherapy for human cancer. Science. American Association for the Advancement of Science. 2015;348(6230):62–8.
5. Delves PJ, Martin SJ, Burton DR, Roitt IM. Roitt's essential immunology. Chichester, West Sussex; Hoboken, NJ: Wiley Blackwell; 2011.
6. Acuto O, Michel F. CD28-mediated co-stimulation: a quantitative support for TCR signalling. Nat Rev Immunol. 2003;3(12):939–51.
7. Acuto O, Mise-Omata S, Mangino G, Michel F. Molecular modifiers of T cell antigen receptor triggering threshold: the mechanism of CD28 costimulatory receptor. Immunol Rev. 2003;192:21–31.
8. Cheng LE, Ohlén C, Nelson BH, Greenberg PD. Enhanced signaling through the IL-2 receptor in CD8+ T cells regulated by antigen recognition results in preferential proliferation and expansion of responding CD8+ T cells rather than promotion of cell death. Proc Natl Acad Sci U S A. 2002;99(5):3001–6.
9. Janeway CA, Travers P, Walport M, Capra JD. Immunobiology: the immune system in health and disease. London: Current Biology Publications; 1999.
10. Phan GQ, Rosenberg SA. Adoptive cell transfer for patients with metastatic melanoma: the potential and promise of cancer immunotherapy. Cancer Control. 2013;20(4):289–97.
11. Rosenberg SA, Restifo NP, Yang JC, Morgan RA, Dudley ME. Adoptive cell transfer: a clinical path to effective cancer immunotherapy. Nat Rev Cancer. 2008;8(4):299–308.
12. Hanahan D, Weinberg RA. Hallmarks of cancer: the next generation. Cell. 2011;144(5):646–74.
13. Vesely MD, Kershaw MH, Schreiber RD, Smyth MJ. Natural innate and adaptive immunity to cancer. Annu Rev Immunol. 2011;29(1):235–71.
14. Fourcade J, Zarour HM. Strategies to reverse melanoma-induced T-cell dysfunction. Clin Dermatol. 2013;31(3):251–6.
15. Ilyas S, Yang JC. Landscape of tumor antigens in T cell immunotherapy. J Immunol. 2015;195(11):5117–22.
16. Knuth A, Wölfel T, Klehmann E, Boon T. Meyer zum Büschenfelde KH. Cytolytic T-cell clones against an autologous human melanoma: specificity study and definition of three antigens by immunoselection. Proc Natl Acad Sci U S A. 1989;86(8):2804–8.
17. Stevanovic S. Identification of tumor-associated T-cell epitopes for vaccine development. Nat Rev Cancer. 2002;2(7):514–20.
18. van der Bruggen P, Traversari C, Chomez P, Lurquin C, De Plaen E, Van den Eynde B, et al. A gene encoding an antigen recognized by cytolytic T lymphocytes on a human melanoma. Science. 1991;254(5038):1643–7.
19. Molecular diagnostics for melanoma. 2016:1–711.
20. Katz KA, Jonasch E, Hodi FS, Soiffer R, Kwitkiwski K, Sober AJ, et al. Melanoma of unknown primary: experience at Massachusetts General Hospital and Dana-Farber Cancer Institute. Melanoma Res. 2005;15(1):77–82.
21. Gyorki DE, Callahan M, Wolchok JD, Ariyan CE. The delicate balance of melanoma immunotherapy. Clin Trans Immunol. 2013;2(8):e5–8.
22. MacKie RM, Reid R, Junor B. Fatal melanoma transferred in a donated kidney 16 years after melanoma surgery. N Engl J Med. 2003;348(6):567–8.
23. Akbani R, Akdemir KC, Aksoy BA, Albert M, Ally A, Amin SB, et al. Genomic classification of cutaneous melanoma. Cell. 2015;161(7):1681–96.
24. MacCarty WC. Longevity in cancer: a study of 293 cases. Ann Surg. 1922;76(2):238–45.
25. Hershkovitz L, Schachter J, Treves AJ, Besser MJ. Focus on adoptive T cell transfer trials in melanoma. Clin Dev Immunol. 2010;2010:260267.

26. Rosenberg SA, Packard BS, Aebersold PM, Solomon D, Topalian SL, Toy ST, et al. Use of tumor-infiltrating lymphocytes and interleukin-2 in the immunotherapy of patients with metastatic melanoma. A preliminary report. N Engl J Med. 1988;319(25):1676–80.
27. Rosenberg SA, Yannelli JR, Yang JC, Topalian SL, Schwartzentruber DJ, Weber JS, et al. Treatment of patients with metastatic melanoma with autologous tumor-infiltrating lymphocytes and interleukin 2. J Natl Cancer Inst. 1994;86(15):1159–66.
28. Rosenberg SA, Yang JC, Sherry RM, Kammula US, Hughes MS, Phan GQ, et al. Durable complete responses in heavily pretreated patients with metastatic melanoma using T-cell transfer immunotherapy. Clin Cancer Res. 2011;17(13):4550–7. http://eutils.ncbi.nlm.nih.gov/entrez/eutils/elink.fcgi?dbfrom=pubmed&id=21498393&retmode=ref&cmd=prlinks
29. Radvanyi LG, Bernatchez C, Zhang M, Fox PS, Miller P, Chacon J, et al. Specific lymphocyte subsets predict response to adoptive cell therapy using expanded autologous tumor-infiltrating lymphocytes in metastatic melanoma patients. Clin Cancer Res. American Association for Cancer Research. 2012;18(24):6758–70.
30. Itzhaki O, Hovav E, Ziporen Y, Levy D, Kubi A, Zikich D, et al. Establishment and large-scale expansion of minimally cultured "young" tumor infiltrating lymphocytes for adoptive transfer therapy. J Immunother. 2011;34(2):212–20.
31. Hinrichs CS, Rosenberg SA. Exploiting the curative potential of adoptive T-cell therapy for cancer. Immunol Rev. Royal Australasian College of Surgeons (RACS). 2014;257(1):56–71.
32. Rosenberg SA, Restifo NP. Adoptive cell transfer as personalized immunotherapy for human cancer. Science. Royal Australasian College of Surgeons (RACS). 2015;348(6230):62–8.
33. Donia M, Junker N, Ellebaek E, Andersen MH, Straten PT, Svane IM. Characterization and Comparison of 'Standard' and 'Young' Tumor-Infiltrating Lymphocytes for Adoptive Cell Therapy at a Danish Translational Research Institution. Scand J Immunol. Blackwell Publishing Ltd. 2012;75(2):157–67.
34. Fousek K, Ahmed N. The evolution of T-cell therapies for solid malignancies. Clin Cancer Res. 2015;21(15):3384–92.
35. Bernatchez C, Radvanyi LG, Hwu P. Advances in the treatment of metastatic melanoma: adoptive T-cell therapy. Semin Oncol. 2012;39(2):215–26.
36. Rosenberg SA, Spiess P, Lafreniere R. A new approach to the adoptive immunotherapy of cancer with tumor-infiltrating lymphocytes. Science. 1986;233(4770):1318–21.
37. Topalian SL, Solomon D, Avis FP, Chang AE, Freerksen DL, Linehan WM, et al. Immunotherapy of patients with advanced cancer using tumor-infiltrating lymphocytes and recombinant interleukin-2: a pilot study. J Clin Oncol. 1988;6(5):839–53.
38. Dudley ME, Gross CA, Somerville RPT, Hong Y, Schaub NP, Rosati SF, et al. Randomized selection design trial evaluating CD8+-enriched versus unselected tumor-infiltrating lymphocytes for adoptive cell therapy for patients with melanoma. J Clin Oncol. 2013;31(17):2152–9.
39. Wu R, Forget M-A, Chacon J, Bernatchez C, Haymaker C, Chen JQ, et al. Adoptive T-cell therapy using autologous tumor-infiltrating lymphocytes for metastatic melanoma: current status and future outlook. Cancer J. 2012;18(2):160–75.
40. Goff SL, Dudley ME, Citrin DE, Somerville RP, Wunderlich JR, Danforth DN, et al. Randomized, prospective evaluation comparing intensity of Lymphodepletion before adoptive transfer of tumor-infiltrating lymphocytes for patients with metastatic melanoma. J Clin Oncol. 2016;34(20):2389–97.
41. Sharpe M, Mount N. Genetically modified T cells in cancer therapy: opportunities and challenges. Dis Model Mech. 2015;8(4):337–50.
42. Rosenberg SA, Dudley ME. Adoptive cell therapy for the treatment of patients with metastatic melanoma. Curr Opin Immunol. 2009;21(2):233–40.
43. Gattinoni L, Finkelstein SE, Klebanoff CA, Antony PA, Palmer DC, Spiess PJ, et al. Removal of homeostatic cytokine sinks by lymphodepletion enhances the efficacy of adoptively transferred tumor-specific CD8+ T cells. J Exp Med. 2005;202(7):907–12.
44. Muranski P, Boni A, Wrzesinski C, Citrin DE, Rosenberg SA, Childs R, et al. Increased intensity lymphodepletion and adoptive immunotherapy--how far can we go? Nat Clin Pract Oncol. 2006;3(12):668–81.
45. Merhavi-Shoham E, Itzhaki O, Markel G, Schachter J, Besser MJ. Adoptive cell therapy for metastatic melanoma. Cancer J. 2017;23(1):48–53.
46. Goff SL, Smith FO, Klapper JA, Sherry R, Wunderlich JR, Steinberg SM, et al. Tumor infiltrating lymphocyte therapy for metastatic melanoma: analysis of tumors resected for TIL. J Immunother. 2010;33(8):840–7.
47. Dudley ME, Gross CA, Langhan MM, Garcia MR, Sherry RM, Yang JC, et al. CD8+ enriched "young" tumor infiltrating lymphocytes can mediate regression of metastatic melanoma. Clin Cancer Res. American Association for Cancer Research. 2010;16(24):6122–31.
48. Sim GC, Chacon J, Haymaker C, Ritthipichai K, Singh M, Hwu P, et al. Tumor-infiltrating lymphocyte therapy for melanoma: rationale and issues for further clinical development. BioDrugs. Royal Australasian College of Surgeons (RACS). 2014;28(5):421–37.
49. Ellebaek E, Iversen TZ, Junker N, Donia M. Adoptive cell therapy with autologous tumor infiltrating lymphocytes and low-dose Interleukin-2 in metastatic melanoma patients. J Transl Med. 2012;10:169.
50. Mantovani G, Macciò A, Melis G, Mura L, Massa E, Mudu MC. Restoration of functional defects in peripheral blood mononuclear cells isolated from cancer patients by thiol antioxidants alpha-lipoic acid and N-acetyl cysteine. Int J Cancer. 2000;86(6):842–7.
51. Scheffel MJ, Scurti G, Simms P, Garrett-Mayer E, Mehrotra S, Nishimura MI, et al. Efficacy of adop-

tive T-cell therapy is improved by treatment with the antioxidant N-acetyl cysteine, which limits activation-induced T-cell death. Can Res. American Association for Cancer Research. 2016;76(20):6006–16.
52. Ye Q, Loisiou M, Levine BL, Suhoski MM, Riley JL, June CH, et al. Engineered artificial antigen presenting cells facilitate direct and efficient expansion of tumor infiltrating lymphocytes. J Transl Med. 2011;9(1):131.
53. Ullenhag GJ, Sadeghi AM, Carlsson B. Adoptive T-cell therapy for malignant melanoma patients with TILs obtained by ultrasound-guided needle biopsy. Cancer Immunol Immunother. 2012;61(5):725–32.
54. Nguyen LT, Yen PH, Nie J, Liadis N, Ghazarian D, Al-Habeeb A, et al. Expansion and characterization of human melanoma tumor-infiltrating lymphocytes (TILs). Unutmaz D, editor. PLoS One. 2010;5(11):e13940–12.
55. Robbins PF, Dudley ME, Wunderlich J, El-Gamil M, Li YF, Zhou J, et al. Cutting edge: persistence of transferred lymphocyte clonotypes correlates with cancer regression in patients receiving cell transfer therapy. J Immunol. 2004;173(12):7125–30.
56. Ellebaek E, Iversen TZ, Junker N, Donia M, Engell-Noerregaard L, Met Z, et al. Adoptive cell therapy with autologous tumor infiltrating lymphocytes and low-dose Interleukin-2 in metastatic melanoma patients. J Transl Med. 2012;10(1):1.
57. Andersen R, Donia M, Borch T, Steensgaard E, Iversen T, Kongsted P, et al. Adoptive cell therapy with tumor infiltrating lymphocytes and intermediate dose IL-2 for metastatic melanoma. J Immunother Cancer. 2014;2(Suppl 3):1.
58. Besser MJ, Shapira-Frommer R, Treves AJ, Zippel D, Itzhaki O, Hershkovitz L, et al. Clinical responses in a phase II study using adoptive transfer of short-term cultured tumor infiltration lymphocytes in metastatic melanoma patients. Clin Cancer Res. 2010;16(9):2646–55.
59. Zhou J, Shen X, Huang J, Hodes RJ, Rosenberg SA, Robbins PF. Telomere length of transferred lymphocytes correlates with in vivo persistence and tumor regression in melanoma patients receiving cell transfer therapy. J Immunol. American Association of Immunologists. 2005;175(10):7046–52.
60. Russo A, Ficili B, Candido S, Pezzino FM, Guarneri C, Biondi A, et al. Emerging targeted therapies for melanoma treatment (review). Int J Oncol. 2014;45(2):516–24.
61. Johnson LA, Morgan RA, Dudley ME, Cassard L, Yang JC, Hughes MS, et al. Gene therapy with human and mouse T-cell receptors mediates cancer regression and targets normal tissues expressing cognate antigen. Blood. American Society of Hematology. 2009;114(3):535–46.
62. Parkhurst MR, Yang JC, Langan RC, Dudley ME, Nathan D-AN, Feldman SA, et al. T cells targeting carcinoembryonic antigen can mediate regression of metastatic colorectal cancer but induce severe transient colitis. Mol Ther. 2011;19(3):620–6.
63. Duong CPM, Yong CSM, Kershaw MH, Slaney CY, Darcy PK. Cancer immunotherapy utilizing gene-modified T cells: from the bench to the clinic. Mol Immunol. Royal Australasian College of Surgeons (RACS). 2015;67(2 Pt A):46–57.
64. Akers SN, Odunsi K, Karpf AR. Regulation of cancer germline antigen gene expression: implications for cancer immunotherapy. Future Oncol. 2010;6(5):717–32.
65. Robbins PF, Morgan RA, Feldman SA, Yang JC, Sherry RM, Dudley ME, et al. Tumor regression in patients with metastatic synovial cell sarcoma and melanoma using genetically engineered lymphocytes reactive with NY-ESO-1. J Clin Oncol. 2011;29(7):917–24.
66. Kershaw MH, Westwood JA, Slaney CY, Darcy PK. Clinical application of genetically modified T cells in cancer therapy. Clin Trans Immunol. 2014;3(5):e16.
67. Morgan RA, Chinnasamy N, Abate-Daga D, Gros A, Robbins PF, Zheng Z, et al. Cancer regression and neurological toxicity following anti-MAGE-A3 TCR gene therapy. J Immunother. 2013;36(2):133–51.
68. Linette GP, Stadtmauer EA, Maus MV, Rapoport AP, Levine BL, Emery L, et al. Cardiovascular toxicity and titin cross-reactivity of affinity-enhanced T cells in myeloma and melanoma. Blood. 2013;122(6):863–71.
69. Rooney CM, Leen AM, Vera JF, Heslop HE. T lymphocytes targeting native receptors. Immunol Rev. 2014;257(1):39–55.
70. Bollard CM, Gottschalk S, Leen AM, Weiss H, Straathof KC, Carrum G, et al. Complete responses of relapsed lymphoma following genetic modification of tumor-antigen presenting cells and T-lymphocyte transfer. Blood. American Society of Hematology. 2007;110(8):2838–45.
71. Louis CU, Straathof K, Bollard CM, Ennamuri S, Gerken C, Lopez TT, et al. Adoptive transfer of EBV-specific T cells results in sustained clinical responses in patients with locoregional nasopharyngeal carcinoma. J Immunother. 2010;33(9):983–90.
72. Bendle GM, Linnemann C, Hooijkaas AI, Bies L, de Witte MA, Jorritsma A, et al. Lethal graft-versus-host disease in mouse models of T cell receptor gene therapy. Nat Med. 2010;16(5):565–70. 1pfollowing570
73. Beavis PA, Slaney CY, Kershaw MH, Gyorki D, Neeson PJ, Darcy PK. Reprogramming the tumor microenvironment to enhance adoptive cellular therapy. Semin Immunol. 2015:1–9.
74. Kershaw MH, Westwood JA, Parker LL, Wang G, Eshhar Z, Mavroukakis SA, et al. A phase I study on adoptive immunotherapy using gene-modified T cells for ovarian cancer. Clin Cancer Res. American Association for Cancer Research. 2006;12(20 Pt 1):6106–15.
75. Westwood JA, Smyth MJ, Teng MWL, Moeller M, Trapani JA, Scott AM, et al. Adoptive transfer of T cells modified with a humanized chimeric receptor gene inhibits growth of Lewis-Y-expressing tumors in mice. Proc Natl Acad Sci U S A. 2005;102(52):19051–6.

76. Yong CSM, Dardalhon V, Devaud C, Taylor N, Darcy PK, Kershaw MH. CAR T-cell therapy of solid tumors. Immunol Cell Biol. 2017;95(4):356–63.
77. Ahmed N, Salsman VS, Yvon E, Louis CU, Perlaky L, Wels WS, et al. Immunotherapy for osteosarcoma: genetic modification of T cells overcomes low levels of tumor antigen expression. Mol Ther. 2009;17(10):1779–87.
78. Maude SL, Frey N, Shaw PA, Aplenc R, Barrett DM, Bunin NJ, et al. Chimeric antigen receptor T cells for sustained remissions in leukemia. N Engl J Med. 2014;371(16):1507–17.
79. Shou D, Wen L, Song Z, Yin J, Sun Q, Gong W. Suppressive role of myeloid-derived suppressor cells (MDSCs) in the microenvironment of breast cancer and targeted immunotherapies. Oncotarget. 2016;7(39):64505–11.
80. Rudolph M, Hebel K, Miyamura Y, Maverakis E, Brunner-Weinzierl MC. Blockade of CTLA-4 decreases the generation of multifunctional memory CD4+ T cells in vivo. J Immunol. 2011;186(10):5580–9.
81. Beavis PA, Henderson MA, Giuffrida L, Mills JK, Sek K, Cross RS, et al. Targeting the adenosine 2A receptor enhances chimeric antigen receptor T cell efficacy. J Clin Invest. American Society for Clinical Investigation. 2017;127(3):929–41.
82. Morgan RA, Yang JC, Kitano M, Dudley ME, Laurencot CM, Rosenberg SA. Case report of a serious adverse event following the administration of T cells transduced with a chimeric antigen receptor recognizing ERBB2. Mol Ther. 2010;18(4):843–51.
83. Ahmed N, Brawley VS, Hegde M, Robertson C, Ghazi A, Gerken C, et al. Human Epidermal Growth Factor Receptor 2 (HER2) -Specific chimeric antigen receptor-modified T cells for the immunotherapy of HER2-positive sarcoma. J Clin Oncol. 2015;33(15):1688–96.
84. Vera JF, Brenner LJ, Gerdemann U, Ngo MC, Sili U, Liu H, et al. Accelerated production of antigen-specific T cells for preclinical and clinical applications using gas-permeable rapid expansion cultureware (G-Rex). J Immunother. 2010;33(3):305–15.
85. Somerville RPT, Dudley ME. Bioreactors get personal. Oncoimmunology. 2012;1(8):1435–7.

Current Immunotherapy of Melanoma

35

Kimberly Loo, Clinton Wu, and Adil Daud

Introduction

Melanoma results from the malignant transformation of the melanocyte. This pigment producing cell, derived from the neural crest, resides in the epidermal–dermal junction in the skin but also in the eyes, mucous membranes, and a broad range of other tissues [1]. Over the last few years, it has been appreciated that the development of melanoma is often accompanied by an immune response [2]. Metastatic melanoma is currently treated and managed with two basic strategies. The first consists of targeting the oncogenic mutations driving tumor genesis [3]. The second, which is the subject of this chapter, is to exploit the immune system to control and eliminate the cancer.

K. Loo, B.S.
Department of Hematology/Oncology, Melanoma, University of California, San Francisco, San Francisco, CA, USA

C. Wu, B.S.
Department of Melanoma Oncology, University of California, San Francisco, San Francisco, CA, USA

A. Daud, M.B.B.S. (✉)
Department of Medicine, University of California, San Francisco, San Francisco, CA, USA
e-mail: adil.daud@ucsf.edu

Exploiting the Immune Response for Cancer Therapy

While we think of immunotherapy as a recent advance in medicine, the immune response has been exploited to treat cancer since ancient times. As early as 2600 B.C., the pharaoh Imhotep had court physicians apply a poultice followed by incision to treat a tumor he had developed. The idea of using infection to treat superficial tumors was common in the eighteenth and nineteenth centuries in Europe [4]. Indeed, the French physician, Dussosoy, published an observation that infection resulted in the disappearance of a breast cancer. The small pox vaccine (which may have previously been discovered in China) developed by Edward Jenner in 1796 brought immunotherapy to the forefront of modern medicine. William Coley, a New York surgeon who is considered the founder of modern cancer immunotherapy, published his experiments regarding surgical infection and bacterial inoculation resulting in regression of cancer in the late nineteenth century [5].

With the development of chemotherapy in the 1930s and the eventual success of chemotherapy for some cancers in the 1950s and 1960s, immunotherapy took a backseat during this time period. In 1957, Isaacs and Lindemann purified a protein from virally infected cells which appeared to "interfere" with, and prevent, subsequent viral infection [6]. This protein was called "interferon" and

A. I. Riker (ed.), *Melanoma*, https://doi.org/10.1007/978-3-319-78310-9_35

subsequently tested in clinical trials of cancer patients with moderate success. In 1982, Steven Rosenberg and coworkers at the Surgery branch of the NCI developed "lymphocyte activated killer" (LAK) cell therapy, which consisted of tumor lymphocytes grown in the lab, and transplanted back into patients with cancer, producing clinical regression of tumors and occasionally complete regression of all metastatic disease [7]. The Surgery branch also pioneered the therapeutic use of the cytokine, interleukin-2, for metastatic melanoma, also capable of inducing a long lasting, and sometimes, complete, tumor regression in a select group of treated patients [8].

More recently, a major advance was the discovery of the cytotoxic lymphocyte antigen-4 (CTLA-4) by Golstein and colleagues in France [9], followed by the demonstration by James Allison that inhibiting CTLA-4 resulted in regression of tumor in mice models [10–12]. This CTLA-4 antibody was eventually developed commercially by Bristol-Myers and was eventually approved for treatment in the USA in 2009 [13–15]. The concept of "taking off the brakes," or of inhibiting checkpoints that normally hold back the immune response, received an even bigger boost when the PD-1 protein was discovered in Japan by Tasuku Honjo and colleagues [16–18].

The first anti-PD-1 clinical trial showed impressive clinical responses in cancers that were generally considered to be responsive to immune therapy, such as melanoma and renal cell cancer. There were also other cancer types that were responsive to anti-PD-1 therapy, such as head and neck and lung cancer, not previously considered to be immune responsive [19–21]. There has much work over the last 2 decades that have definitively shown a pre-existing immune response that can be exploited therapeutically [22]. In other cancers that are associated with a weaker immune response, intratumoral therapy and other agents that might initiate an immune response could result in the specific activation of cytotoxic T-cells capable of becoming "unblocked" by immune checkpoint inhibitors.

The Immune System in Cancer

It is established that the host immune system plays a major role in controlling cancer, actively deleting and inhibiting the growth of cancer cells. This process has been called immunoediting, resulting in specific patterns of immune escape [23–26]. The immune system is composed of two major arms that are separated evolutionarily by millions of years [27]. The first arm of the immune system is the innate arm, which mobilizes rapidly in response to foreign microbes, viruses, and even cancer cells. This arm is comprised of macrophages, neutrophils, dendritic cells, and natural killer (NK) cells.

The second arm of the human immune system is the adaptive arm, responding specifically to a foreign invader with the proliferation of T-cells or by producing specific antibodies by our B-cells. It is currently thought that the release of tumor antigens upon cell death (apoptosis) or cell turnover are endocytosed by antigen presenting cells (APCs). The APCs then mature and migrate to the regional lymph nodes, expressing the tumor antigens on their cell surface in an MHC-restricted fashion. This, along with other co-stimulatory signals, provides the necessary presentation to naïve T-cells to properly and specifically recognize the tumor antigens, resulting in T-cell activation and proliferation.

A portion of this process is thought to be stimulated by the CTLA-4 antagonist, ipilimumab [28]. The activated T-cell then migrates to the tumor and upon antigen recognition, releases interferon, perforins, granzymes, and other cytolytic substances that either damage or destroy the cancer cell. Cancer cells can escape this attack by exploiting a variety of pathways, including the expression of the ligand for PD-1 (PDL-1), indoleamine deoxygenase (IDO), production of arginase and the loss of MHC class-1 molecules necessary for proper T-cell recognition [29]. In addition, the stroma surrounding the tumor microenvironment can adopt an immunosuppressive milieu, resulting in a diminished and suppressed immune response. This is partially caused by polarizing macrophages and APCs towards a suppressive phenotype, better known as a myeloid-derived suppressor cell (MDSC) [30–32]. Additionally, tumors actively utilize glucose and produce lactate which are also thought to be immune suppressive [33].

The status of the tumor microenvironment can be profiled utilizing a variety of laboratory techniques. The simplest and most widely used technique is immunohistochemistry (IHC) for the PDL-1 protein. This was first used in the initial clinical trials of PD-1 and shown to correlate with the response rate to therapy with an anti-PD-1 antibody [19]. The adaptive immune response can also be measured by IHC staining for CD3, CD4, CD8 T-cells, as well as NK cells, macrophages, and APCs [34, 35]. Recently, more sophisticated techniques allow for multiplex staining and fusion of images that can give a more detailed insight into the tumor microenvironment. A powerful technique used in many immunology laboratories is flow cytometry, which gives a very detailed picture of the functional status of T-cells and myeloid cells both within the tumor and peripheral blood [36–38].

Immunotherapy for Metastatic Melanoma

At present, immunotherapy forms the backbone of therapy for metastatic melanoma. For many years, it has been recognized that many melanoma tumors have immune infiltrates and occasionally subject to spontaneous remissions. Some of the earliest immunotherapies, such as interferon-gamma and interleukin-2, were shown to have modest clinical activity which results in their FDA approval for use in advanced melanoma. However, the last decade has shown us that the use of immune checkpoint blockade has significantly changed our paradigm of treatment options.

Checkpoint Inhibitors: Anti-CTLA4

The CTLA-4 protein, present on the surface of both CD4+ and CD8+ lymphocytes (as well as on suppressive regulatory T-cells, T-regs), is a critical negative regulator of immune activation [10–12, 28]. It prevents T-cell co-stimulation by the CD28 protein, required for T-cell activation, along with T-cell receptor binding with APCs in an MHC-restricted fashion. The inhibition of CTLA-4 therefore drives co-stimulation, and in effect, increases T-cell activation by engaging naïve T-cells circulating through the lymph nodes. Early trials examining the efficacy of the CTLA-4 antibody, ipilimumab, showed significant activity of this antibody in melanoma, as well as several other types of cancer [39]. Tremelimumab, developed by Pfizer, showed similar activity and confirmed the importance of this therapeutic target.

A pivotal Phase III trial of ipilimumab compared to a vaccine, gp100, as well as a combination of ipilimumab and gp100 showed that ipilimumab was superior to gp100 alone. Of importance, it also showed a longer overall survival of those patients treated with ipilimumab, confirming its benefit in melanoma. This trial also illustrates an important advantage of immunotherapy, showing its durability of benefit, previously exhibited with high-dose interleukin-2 and adoptive lymphocyte therapy, and so far appears to be true of checkpoint blockade as well [13].

Given the emergence of clinical trials that examine the targeting of the CTLA-4 pathway, the toxicity and adverse event profile sustained by patients exhibit a unique profile of immune-related adverse events (irAEs) in patients receiving ipilimumab at both the 3 and 10 mg/kg doses. In the phase 3 study of ipilimumab administered alone, or with gp100 (NCT00094653), approximately 60% of patients treated with ipilimumab alone exhibited irAEs, with a frequency of 10–15% of patients exhibiting grade 3 or 4 irAEs [13]. The immune-related AEs of anti-CTLA-4 therapies largely target the skin and gastrointestinal tract, but may range from mild to moderate side effects including rash, with the possibility of progressing to more severe side effects.

The most common side effect seen with patients treated with ipilimumab was diarrhea (warranting the administration of corticosteroids and or infliximab for resolution). Furthermore, dermatitis, colitis, and immune-related hypophysitis, hepatitis, pancreatitis, irodocyclitis, lymphadenopathy, neuropathies, and nephritis irAEs were reported with anti-CTLA-4 therapies [40]. Additionally, residual adverse events after treatment discontinuation have also been reported, including vitiligo, diarrhea, colitis, and endocrine irAEs that required hormone replacement therapy [13]. With this profile of immune-related toxicities, along with the increased propensity of patients to develop high-grade irAEs, providers administering anti-CTLA-4 therapies should closely monitor patients during each cycle of therapy, and beyond.

Checkpoint Inhibitors: Anti-PD-1

While PD-1/PDL-1 antibodies are referred to as checkpoint inhibitors along with anti-CTLA-4 antibodies, their mechanism of action is very different [41]. When activated effector T-cells attempt to kill cancer cells, they adaptively upregulate PDL-1 on their surface in an interferon-gamma dependent way. PDL-1 can bind to the PD-1 protein on the surface of T-cells and reduces their killing capacity. This downregulation of effector lymphocytes may be prevented by the use of PD-1/PDL-1 antibodies. The very first Phase I trial of the PD-1 antibody, nivolumab, showed an impressive response rate to treatment of patients with metastatic melanoma [42]. A second PD-1 antibody, pembrolizumab, also showed a remarkable degree of activity in a similar group of patients [43]. Both of these agents showed objective response rates in patients with melanoma of 20–40%, with a much lower frequency of grade 3–4 adverse events compared to ipilimumab (10–15%) [21, 43]. Subsequent phase III trials showed a durable clinical benefit with improved ORR, OFS, and OS from both pembrolizumab and nivolumab administered as first-line therapies when compared to ipilimumab (KEYNOTE-006 [44], CheckMate 067 trials [45], respectively) or to chemotherapy (Keynote 002) [43, 46–49].

In addition to the durable clinic benefit seen with anti-PD-1 therapies, the minimal adverse event profile compared to anti-CTLA4 therapies propelled the favorability of anti-PD1 therapies further. In a comparison between anti-PD1 therapy with pembrolizumab compared to anti-CTLA4 therapy with ipilimumab, 10.1% of patients receiving pembrolizumab every 3 weeks (which is the current standard of care regimen) experienced grade 3 to 5 adverse events, compared to 19.9% of patients receiving ipilimumab. Furthermore, the rate of permanent discontinuation of study drug due to treatment-related adverse events was lower in the pembrolizumab-treated groups, compared to those who received ipilimumab (6.9% vs. 9.4%, respectively). The most common adverse events among patients treated with pembrolizumab included fatigue, diarrhea, rash, and pruritis. The most common immune irAEs observed among patients receiving pembrolizumab were hypothyroidism, hyperthyroidism, colitis, and hepatitis. In comparing the two treatment groups, hypothyroidism and hyperthyroidism were more frequently seen in the pembrolizumab-treated group, compared to colitis and hypophysitis within the ipilimumab-treated group [44].

Checkpoint Inhibitors: Combination Therapies and Beyond

Given the antitumor activity seen with anti-CTLA4 and anti-PD1 agents as single agents, it made intuitive sense to next explore these agents in combination. Preclinical experiments confirmed that these agents were additive and possibly synergistic when given together or sequentially. The Phase I trial of this combination confirmed the higher rates of clinical activity of this combination, but also revealed a much higher rate of toxicity, with grade 3–4 adverse events noted in 55% of patients [50]. A phase III trial examining the combination of ipilimumab and nivolumab was rapidly launched, comparing the combination to ipilimumab alone or to nivolumab alone (CheckMate 067) [45]. In this trial, recently updated, the ipilimumab and nivolumab arm continues to outperform nivolumab, with both of the PD-1 arms showing a greater response rate when compared to ipilimumab alone. While the clinical benefits of objective response rates and progression-free survival has been clear, it comes with the cost to the patient of a higher degree of overall toxicity. Thus, efforts are underway to further identify those patients who will benefit the most from combination therapy, while elucidating if there is a subgroup of patients who will do just as well with PD-1 monotherapy.

Of note, combination therapies have exhibited an increased toxicity profile compared to that seen with monotherapy. In a phase 3 study (CheckMate 067, NCT01844505), treatment-related adverse events of any grade were reported in 95.5% of patients treated with nivolumab and ipilimumab, compared to 82.1% in the nivolumab alone group and 86.2% in the ipilimumab alone cohort. The most common adverse events reported in the combination therapy cohort were diarrhea, fatigue, and pruritus. Furthermore, grade 3, 4, or higher treatment-related adverse events occurred at a higher rate in the nivolumab-plus-ipilimumab-treated group (55.0%), versus the nivolumab alone (16.3%) and ipilimumab alone cohorts (27.3%). The most frequent treatment-related adverse events (grade 3 or 4) were diarrhea, colitis, and increased alanine aminotransferase levels. Given this, while the increased propensity for adverse events in the combination therapy group need to be closely monitored and managed, many of the select adverse events were modulated with the utilization of immune-modulatory agents, such as corticosteroids [45].

Other checkpoint inhibitors are being actively explored in the clinic and research laboratory. The inhibitory checkpoints TIM-3 and LAG-3 have a similar cell biology compared to PD-1, also expressed on CD8 T-cells. Antibodies to either protein have been generated and promising clinical data has been presented. A combination of LAG-3 and PD-1 antibody in melanoma appears to rescue some patients who have progressed on PD-1 alone or PD-1 combination therapy. The T-cell stimulatory proteins, OX-40 and 4-1BB can also be targeted by agonist antibodies and these agonist antibodies have also been tested in the clinic in Phase I trials with some efficacy. At present efforts are underway to combine these with PD-1 antibodies and to determine their spectrum of activity.

Indoleamine Deoxygenase (IDO) and Kynurenine

Many other potential mechanisms of tumor immunosuppression are exploited by several tumor types, including melanoma. One such mechanism that is moving to the center stage is the IDO pathway. The enzymes, IDO and tryptophan deoxygenase (TDO), convert tryptophan into kynurenine, which is an essential nutrient and stimulant for T-cells [51]. Kynurenine is an agonist of the aryl hydrocarbon receptor (AHR), identified as having a marked immune suppressive effect upon T-cells and APCs. It also has a stimulatory effect upon T-reg cells [52–55]. Many tumors, including melanoma, appear to increase the expression of IDO in response to T-cell infiltration. This increased IDO expression can be inhibited by enzymatic inhibitors. One of the first enzymatic inhibitors, epicadostat, has been explored in Phase I trials as a single agent. It showed minimal clinical when administered alone, however, in combination with either pembrolizumab or nivolumab, shows marked activity with objective responses in ~60% of patients treated.

In the preliminary reports of a small ($N = 11$ patients) Phase I/II trial of epicadostat (incb024360) in combination with pembrolizumab, the ORR was 57%, with a disease control rate (DCR) of 86% and which included two complete responders (CR) [56]. The most common adverse events of all grades were fatigue, diarrhea, rash, arthralgia, and nausea (majority were grade 1 or 2). The most commonly reported irAEs (grade 3 or above) were mucosal inflammation and rash. Unlike the combination of ipilimumab and nivolumab, the IDO/PD-1 combination does not appear to have as high an incidence of grade 3 or 4 toxicity.

Intratumoral Immunotherapy

While most of the immunotherapy agents discussed so far have been administered systemically, local immunotherapy approaches have a long history, as noted in the introduction. The advantage to the local delivery of immunotherapy directly to the tumor is that such agents can be delivered directly into the tumor microenvironment. This, in turn, may result in the maximal activation of the local immune response as well as minimizing the systemic toxicity that is seen with other agents. For example, systemic interleukin-12 (IL-12) is quite toxic when delivered intravenously, while intratumoral administration is noted to have minimal systemic side effects and a much higher overall antitumor response [57, 58]. In a phase II trial (OMS-I100), electroporation of a plasmid vector containing the full length IL-12 gene (pIL-12) in patients with stage IIIB-IV melanoma, regression of at least one non-treated lesion was seen in 54% of patients (13/24). The best overall response rate, as measured by RECIST criteria in 29 evaluable patients, was 31%, with 10% of patients achieving a complete response to therapy. The most common AEs reported were grade 1 or 2 pain at treatment site, with a single patient reporting grade 3 pain at the injection site. No grade 4 or higher AEs were reported [57]. Successful tumor regression and tolerable safety profiles of the intratumoral pIL-12 therapy suggests a tolerable and viable treatment option given as a monotherapy for patients with stage IIIB-IV melanoma. Furthermore, the induction of antitumor immune-related events presents the possibility of combining such an intratumoral approach with other systemic immunotherapies, such as with anti-PD1/PD-L1.

Continuing the groundbreaking work previously performed by Coley and others, a disabled virus with a granulocyte macrophage colony stimulating factor (GM-CSF) expression cassette, talimogene laherparepvec (T-VEC) has been tested intratumorally in melanoma patients. This approach was found to have significant activity, producing objective responses in both injected and non-injected melanoma lesions [59]. Following the single arm phase II trial, a phase III trial was carried out comparing T-VEC to subcutaneous GM-CSF alone. In this trial, progression-free survival was significantly longer compared to GM-CSF alone, with the OS trending toward improvement, but not found to be statistically significant in this study. In the phase III trial comparing T-VEC to GM-CSF in patients with unresected stage IIIB to IV melanoma, the most common AEs seen with T-VEC therapy were chills, fatigue, and pyrexia. No fatal treatment-related AEs were incurred, and the only grade 3–4 AE in more than 2% of T-VEC-treated patients was reported as colitis [60–62]. Given this, intratumoral therapy remains a viable and reasonable therapy for consideration, expanding the reach of patients to those with unresectable stage IIIB melanomas.

Adjuvant or Preventive Postsurgical Immunotherapy

It has been recognized for several decades that surgical resection of regionally advanced melanoma is often followed by either a local or systemic recurrence months, or even years, later. The use of interferon, a cytokine produced by the immune system and subsequently cloned and tested in humans, was explored in three major prospective randomized clinical trials [63]. The first, the ECOG 1684 trial randomized patients with high-risk node negative or node positive melanoma to either high dose interferon or observation alone. In this trial, the interferon arm was associated with a benefit in relapse-free survival (RFS) and overall survival (OS) [64]. The next trial, ECOG 1690 had three arms, two of which had interferon. Surprisingly, this trial failed to confirm the benefit of interferon in improving OS [65]. The next ECOG trial, 1694, showed a benefit of interferon in both RFS and OS, but the control arm here was the GMK vaccine, found to actually result in a worse outcome in this group of patients. Overall, it appears from a large meta-analysis of these and other interferon clinical trials that there is a benefit in RFS, with perhaps a modest benefit in OS, although much of this putative benefit lies within the interpretation of the data from the sum of the ECOG clinical trials [66].

Multiple trials have examined the utility and efficacy of so-called melanoma "vaccines," including killed, whole-cell, and melanoma lysate vaccines [67]. Unfortunately, none of them have shown clinical activity, with several possible reasons and conjecture as to their lack of benefit in patients with advanced melanoma. Although unclear, it appears that the presence of tumor antigens alone may not be sufficient for the full activation of the host immune system [68].

The discovery of the CTLA-4 protein, along with the development of a blocking antibody, ipilimumab, has led to several clinical trials in the adjuvant setting for patients with resected stage 3 disease. One of these trials, conducted by the EORTC, randomized 951 high-risk, node positive melanoma patients to either ipilimumab at a high 10 mg/kg dose level or to placebo [69]. This trial, with a recent update, showed a benefit in both RFS (26.1 vs. 17.1 months) and OS (add data here). The ipilimumab arm was associated with treatment-related deaths (1%) as well as a high (54%) incidence of serious or life-threatening toxicity. A more recent study, conducted by ECOG, showed that a lower ipilimumab dose of 3 mg/kg had similar clinical activity and better tolerability compared to the higher 10 mg/kg dose.

Recently, the PD-1 antibody, nivolumab, was compared to ipilimumab in a group of high-risk melanoma patients who had undergone complete resection [70]. The trial showed a marked benefit in RFS, with a notable lower incidence of grade 3–4 side effects (14.4 vs. 45.9%) for the nivolumab arm. Based on this trial, it is very likely that PD-1 antibodies will become the new standard first-line treatment for high-risk, resected patients with melanoma, replacing ipilimumab.

Biomarkers to Target Immunotherapy

The tumor microenvironment clearly determines the response to immunotherapy. Given the numerous treatment options, biomarkers of response to treatment have become increasingly important to elucidate the genetic, molecular and immune cell marker composition of metastatic melanoma tumors.

Several biomarkers have been proposed as candidates to help guide future clinical decision-making by optimizing options for frontline or second-line therapies. Several biomarkers are actively being studied as primary or secondary endpoints of ongoing clinical trials, including PD-L1 tumor expression, T-cell receptor (TCR) sequencing and peripheral blood markers [71].

PD-L1 IHC assays have been approved for use as complementary diagnostic tests in melanoma [3], yet the PD-L1 tumor positivity threshold requires further standardization among the different antibodies currently in use. For example, KEYNOTE-066 utilizes the Merck 22C3 antibody and denotes positive PD-L1 staining as $\geq$1% of cancer cells. Given this, 80.5% of patients in the study had PD-L1 positive tumors [44]. Conversely, the Checkmate 067 study showed a different level of PD-L1 tumor expression, performed using the Bristol-Meyers Squibb Dako 28–8 antibody, with a positivity threshold of $a \geq 5\%$ PD-L1 staining in $\geq$100 evaluable cancer cells. Here, 23.6% of patients in this study had PD-L1 positive tumors [45]. Given the variation in positivity between the two assays, PD-L1 tumor expression requires further research and standardization prior to its use as a sole predictor of response to monotherapy with anti-PD1 therapies.

Another active area of biomarker research lies in examining the tumor microenvironment. This provides a potent source of biomarkers that may help elucidate the optimal therapies given the tumor immune cell landscape. The microenvironment also serves as a predictor of response to immunotherapy in the metastatic melanoma setting.

The presence of cells within the tumor microenvironment expressing CD8, PD-1, and/or PD-L1 at the tumor invasive margin using IHC, together with TCR sequencing, has been proposed as a biomarker assay to elucidate the responsiveness of patients to anti-PD1 monotherapy. Tumor biopsies taken prior to anti-PD-1 treatment with high CD8 and PD-1/PD-L1 expression correlated to increased responsiveness to therapy, as well as a more clonal TCR repertoire [3].

Additionally, quantification of immune cell markers in the tumor microenvironment using FACS may provide another valuable biomarker to predict response to immunotherapies. Prior to anti-PD-1 treatment initiation, the presence of CD8+/CTLA4+/PD1+ tumor infiltrating lymphocytes (TILs) within the tumor microenvironment strongly correlated with an increased response rate (CR and PR) and PFS to anti-PD-1 monotherapy. A relative abundance of CD8+/CTLA4+/PD1+ TILs was significantly correlated with favorable responses (CR or PR) to anti-PD1 monotherapy, whereas those patients with CD8+/CTLA4+/PD1+ TIL counts below a relative abundance threshold of 20% were less likely to respond to anti-PD-1 monotherapy.[37]. Furthermore, those with a relatively low overall percentage of CD8+/CTLA4+/PD1+ TILs may derive clinical benefit from combination immunotherapy of nivolumab/ipilimumab [72].

Given this, the increased utilization of biomarkers will remain crucial in guiding clinical decision making, both in the first- and second-line therapy setting. For now, the propensity of various patients to exhibit debilitating adverse events, the varying dosing schedules and the emerging combinations of treatments remain at the forefront of tailoring clinical decision making. Further research and clinical trials are required to ascertain the efficacy of various treatment algorithms, coupled with biomarker profiles to identify the optimal treatment regimen for each individualized patient.

Conclusion

While the immune system is a very complex and multifaceted system, our improved understanding of the host immune system in response to cancer has allowed for the development of effective immunotherapies capable of producing long lasting responses to therapy. This durability of response is unique to immunotherapy and offers a compelling advantage to patients. In the years to come, we anticipate continuing advances and in using the lessons learned with melanoma in other diseases.

References

1. Mort RL, Jackson IJ, Patton EE. The melanocyte lineage in development and disease. Development. 2015;142(4):620–32.
2. Daud A. Current and emerging perspectives on immunotherapy for melanoma. Semin Oncol. 2015;42(Suppl 3):S3–S11.
3. Luke JJ, Flaherty KT, Ribas A, Long GV. Targeted agents and immunotherapies: optimizing outcomes in melanoma. Nat Rev Clin Oncol. 2017. [published online ahead of print: April 4, 2017];14(8):463–82. https://doi.org/10.1038/nrclinonc.2017.43.
4. Kucerova P, Cervinkova M. Spontaneous regression of tumour and the role of microbial infection--possibilities for cancer treatment. Anti-Cancer Drugs. 2016;27(4):269–77.
5. Říhová B, Šťastný M. History of immuno-therapy - from coley toxins to check-points of the immune reaction. Klin Onkol. 2015;28(Suppl 4):4S8–14.
6. Isaacs A, Lindenmann J. Virus interference. I. The interferon. Proc R Soc Lond B Biol Sci. 1957;147(927):258–67.
7. Grimm EA, Mazumder A, Zhang HZ, Rosenberg SA. Lymphokine-activated killer cell phenomenon. Lysis of natural killer-resistant fresh solid tumor cells by interleukin 2-activated autologous human peripheral blood lymphocytes. J Exp Med. 1982;155(6):1823–41.
8. Atkins MB, et al. High-dose recombinant interleukin 2 therapy for patients with metastatic melanoma: analysis of 270 patients treated between 1985 and 1993. J Clin Oncol Off J Am Soc Clin Oncol. 1999;17(7):2105–16.
9. Harper K, et al. CTLA-4 and CD28 activated lymphocyte molecules are closely related in both mouse and human as to sequence, message expression, gene structure, and chromosomal location. J Immunol. 1991;147(3):1037–44.
10. Krummel MF, Allison JP. CD28 and CTLA-4 have opposing effects on the response of T cells to stimulation. J Exp Med. 1995;182(2):459–65.
11. Krummel MF, Allison JP. CTLA-4 engagement inhibits IL-2 accumulation and cell cycle progression upon activation of resting T cells. J Exp Med. 1996;183(6):2533–40.
12. Krummel MF, Allison JP. Pillars Article: CD28 and CTLA-4 Have Opposing Effects on the Response of T Cells to Stimulation. The Journal of Experimental Medicine. 1995. 182: 459–465. J Immunol. 2011;187(7):3459–65.
13. Hodi FS, et al. Improved survival with ipilimumab in patients with metastatic melanoma. N Engl J Med. 2010;363(8):711–23.
14. Weber JS, et al. Phase I/II study of ipilimumab for patients with metastatic melanoma. J Clin Oncol Off J Am Soc Clin Oncol. 2008;26(36):5950–6.
15. Wolchok JD, et al. Development of ipilimumab: a novel immunotherapeutic approach for the treat-

ment of advanced melanoma. Ann N Y Acad Sci. 2013;1291:1–13.
16. Ishida Y, Agata Y, Shibahara K, Honjo T. Induced expression of PD-1, a novel member of the immunoglobulin gene superfamily, upon programmed cell death. EMBO J. 1992;11(11):3887–95.
17. Shinohara T, Taniwaki M, Ishida Y, Kawaichi M, Honjo T. Structure and chromosomal localization of the human PD-1 gene (PDCD1). Genomics. 1994;23(3):704–6.
18. Agata Y, et al. Expression of the PD-1 antigen on the surface of stimulated mouse T and B lymphocytes. Int Immunol. 1996;8(5):765–72.
19. Topalian SL, et al. Safety, activity, and immune correlates of anti-PD-1 antibody in cancer. N Engl J Med. 2012;366(26):2443–54.
20. Brahmer JR, et al. Phase I study of single-agent anti-programmed death-1 (MDX-1106) in refractory solid tumors: safety, clinical activity, pharmacodynamics, and immunologic correlates. J Clin Oncol Off J Am Soc Clin Oncol. 2010;28(19):3167–75.
21. Topalian SL, et al. Survival, durable tumor remission, and long-term safety in patients with advanced melanoma receiving Nivolumab. J Clin Oncol. 2014;32(10):1020–30.
22. Spranger S, Sivan A, Corrales L, Gajewski TF. Tumor and host factors controlling antitumor immunity and efficacy of cancer immunotherapy. Adv Immunol. 2016;130:75–93.
23. Mittal D, Gubin MM, Schreiber RD, Smyth MJ. New insights into cancer immunoediting and its three component phases--elimination, equilibrium and escape. Curr Opin Immunol. 2014;27:16–25.
24. Bui JD, Schreiber RD. Cancer immunosurveillance, immunoediting and inflammation: independent or interdependent processes? Curr Opin Immunol. 2007;19(2):203–8.
25. O'Sullivan T, et al. Cancer immunoediting by the innate immune system in the absence of adaptive immunity. J Exp Med. 2012;209(10):1869–82.
26. Matsushita H, et al. Cancer exome analysis reveals a T-cell-dependent mechanism of cancer immunoediting. Nature. 2012;482(7385):400–4.
27. Abbas AK, Janeway CA. Immunology: improving on nature in the twenty-first century. Cell. 2000;100(1):129–38.
28. Leach DR, Krummel MF, Allison JP. Enhancement of antitumor immunity by CTLA-4 blockade. Science. 1996;271(5256) 1734–6.
29. Pitt JM, et al. Resistance mechanisms to immune-checkpoint blockade in cancer: tumor-intrinsic and -extrinsic factors. Immunity. 2016;44(6):1255–69.
30. Gabrilovich DI, Nagaraj S. Myeloid-derived suppressor cells as regulators of the immune system. Nat Rev Immunol. 2009;9:162–74.
31. Fricke I, Gabrilovich DI. Dendritic cells and tumor microenvironment: a dangerous liaison. Immunol Investig. 2006;35(3–4):459–83.
32. Gabrilovich DI, Nadaf S, Corak J, Berzofsky JA, Carbone DP. Dendritic cells in antitumor immune responses: II dendritic cells grown from bone marrow precursors, but not mature DC from tumor-bearing mice, are effective antigen carriers in the therapy of established tumors. Cell Immunol. 1996;170(1):111–9.
33. Renner K, et al. Metabolic hallmarks of tumor and immune cells in the tumor microenvironment. Front Immunol. 2017;8:248.
34. Tumeh PC, et al. PD-1 blockade induces responses by inhibiting adaptive immune resistance. Nature. 2014;515(7528):568–71.
35. Feng Z, et al. Multispectral imaging of formalin-fixed tissue predicts ability to generate tumor-infiltrating lymphocytes from melanoma. J Immunother Cancer. 2015;3:47.
36. Broz ML, et al. Dissecting the tumor myeloid compartment reveals rare activating antigen-presenting cells critical for T cell immunity. Cancer Cell. 2014;26(5):638–52.
37. Daud AI, et al. Tumor immune profiling predicts response to anti-PD-1 therapy in human melanoma. J Clin Invest. 2016. [published online ahead of print: August 15, 2016];126(9):3447–52. https://doi.org/10.1172/JCI87324.
38. Loo K, et al. Partially exhausted tumor-infiltrating lymphocytes predict response to combination immunotherapy [Internet]. JCI Insight. 2017;2(14):93433. https://doi.org/10.1172/jci.insight.93433.
39. Hodi FS, et al. Immunologic and clinical effects of antibody blockade of cytotoxic T lymphocyte-associated antigen 4 in previously vaccinated cancer patients. Proc Natl Acad Sci U S A. 2008;105(8):3005–10.
40. Weber JS, Kähler KC, Hauschild A. Management of immune-related adverse events and kinetics of response with ipilimumab. J Clin Oncol. 2012;30(21):2691–7. https://doi.org/10.1200/JCO.2012.41.6750.
41. Homet Moreno B, Parisi G, Robert L, Ribas A. Anti-PD-1 therapy in melanoma. Semin Oncol. 2015;42(3):466–73.
42. Brahmer JR, et al. Safety and activity of anti-PD-L1 antibody in patients with advanced cancer. N Engl J Med. 2012;366(26):2455–65.
43. Hamid O, et al. Safety and tumor responses with Lambrolizumab (anti-PD-1) in melanoma. N Engl J Med. 2013;369(2):134–44. [published online ahead of print: June 2, 2013]. https://doi.org/10.1056/NEJMoa1305133.
44. Robert C, et al. Pembrolizumab versus ipilimumab in advanced melanoma. N Engl J Med. 2015;372(26):2521–32.
45. Larkin J, et al. Combined nivolumab and ipilimumab or monotherapy in untreated melanoma. N Engl J Med. 2015;373(1):23–34.
46. Ribas A, et al. Association of pembrolizumab with tumor response and survival among patients with advanced melanoma. JAMA. 2016;315(15):1600–9.
47. Robert C, et al. Anti-programmed-death-receptor-1 treatment with pembrolizumab in ipilimumab-refractory advanced melanoma: a randomised

dose-comparison cohort of a phase 1 trial. Lancet. [published online ahead of print: July 14, 2014]. 2014;384(9948):1109–17. https://doi.org/10.1016/S0140-6736(14)60958-2.
48. Ribas A, et al. Efficacy and safety of the anti-PD-1 monoclonal antibody MK-3475 in 411 patients (pts) with melanoma (MEL). [Internet]. J Clin Oncol. 2014;32(5s(suppl)):abstr LBA9000. http://meetinglibraryascoorg/content/133842-144. Accessed 20 Nov 2014
49. Daud AI, et al. Programmed death-ligand 1 expression and response to the anti-programmed death 1 antibody Pembrolizumab in melanoma. J Clin Oncol Off J Am Soc Clin Oncol. 2016;34(34):4102–9.
50. Wolchok JD, et al. Nivolumab plus ipilimumab in advanced melanoma. N Engl J Med. 2013;369(2):122–33.
51. Munn DH. Indoleamine 2,3-dioxygenase, tumor-induced tolerance and counter-regulation. Curr Opin Immunol. 2006;18(2):220–5.
52. Platten M, Litzenburger U, Wick W. The aryl hydrocarbon receptor in tumor immunity. Oncoimmunology. 2012;1(3):396–7.
53. Bessede A, et al. Aryl hydrocarbon receptor control of a disease tolerance defence pathway. Nature. 2014;511(7508):184–90.
54. Platten M, von Knebel Doeberitz N, Oezen I, Wick W, Ochs K. Cancer immunotherapy by targeting IDO1/TDO and their downstream effectors. Front Immunol. 2014;5:673.
55. Schulte KW, Green E, Wilz A, Platten M, Daumke O. Structural basis for aryl hydrocarbon receptor-mediated gene activation. Structure. 2017;25(7):1025–1033.e3.
56. Gangadhar TC, Hamid O, Smith D, et al. Preliminary results from a Phase I/II study of epacadostat (incb024360) in combination with pembrolizumab in patients with selected advanced cancers. J Immunother Cancer. 2015;3(Suppl 2):07. https://doi.org/10.1186/2051-1426-3-S2-O7.
57. Daud A, et al. Intratumoral electroporation of plasmid interleukin-12: efficacy and biomarker analyses from a phase 2 study in melanoma (OMS-I100). J Transl Med. 2015;13:2068.
58. Cha E, Daud A. Plasmid IL-12 electroporation in melanoma. Hum Vaccin Immunother. 2012;8(11):1734–8.
59. Harrington KJ, et al. Efficacy and safety of talimogene laherparepvec versus granulocyte-macrophage colony-stimulating factor in patients with stage IIIB/C and IVM1a melanoma: subanalysis of the phase III OPTiM trial. OncoTargets Ther. 2016;9:7081–93.
60. Andtbacka RHI, et al. Talimogene laherparepvec improves durable response rate in patients with advanced melanoma. J Clin Oncol Off J Am Soc Clin Oncol. 2015;33(25):2780–8.
61. Andtbacka RHI, et al. Patterns of clinical response with talimogene laherparepvec (T-VEC) in patients with melanoma treated in the OPTiM phase III clinical trial. Ann Surg Oncol. 2016;23(13):4169–77.
62. Ribas A, et al. Oncolytic virotherapy promotes intratumoral T cell infiltration and improves anti-PD-1 immunotherapy. Cell. 2017;170(6):1109–1119.e10.
63. Tarhini AA, Kirkwood JM. Clinical and immunologic basis of interferon therapy in melanoma. Ann N Y Acad Sci. 2009;1182:47–57.
64. Kirkwood JM, et al. Interferon alfa-2b adjuvant therapy of high-risk resected cutaneous melanoma: the eastern cooperative oncology group trial EST 1684. J Clin Oncol Off J Am Soc Clin Oncol. 1996;14(1):7–17.
65. Kirkwood JM, et al. High- and low-dose interferon alfa-2b in high-risk melanoma: first analysis of intergroup trial E1690/S9111/C9190. J Clin Oncol Off J Am Soc Clin Oncol. 2000;18(12):2444–58.
66. Kirkwood JM, et al. High-dose interferon alfa-2b does not diminish antibody response to GM2 vaccination in patients with resected melanoma: results of the Multicenter Eastern Cooperative Oncology Group Phase II Trial E2696. J Clin Oncol Off J Am Soc Clin Oncol. 2001;19(5):1430–6.
67. Hoshimoto S, et al. Assessment of prognostic circulating tumor cells in a phase III trial of adjuvant immunotherapy after complete resection of stage IV melanoma. Ann Surg. 2012;255(2):357–62.
68. Overwijk WW. Cancer vaccines in the era of checkpoint blockade: the magic is in the adjuvant. Curr Opin Immunol. 2017;47:103–9.
69. Eggermont AMM, et al. Adjuvant ipilimumab versus placebo after complete resection of high-risk stage III melanoma (EORTC 18071): a randomised, double-blind, phase 3 trial. Lancet Oncol. 2015;16(5):522–30.
70. Weber J, et al. Adjuvant nivolumab versus ipilimumab in resected stage III or IV melanoma. N Engl J Med. [published online ahead of print: September 10, 2017]. 2017;377:1824–35. https://doi.org/10.1056/NEJMoa1709030.
71. Loo K, Daud A. Emerging biomarkers as predictors to anti-PD1/PD-L1 therapies in advanced melanoma. Immunotherapy. 2016;8(7):775–84.
72. Loo K, et al. Novel T cell exhaustion marker to predict monotherapy PD-1 compared to combination CTLA-4 and PD-1 response in melanoma. J Clin Oncol. 2016;34(15 Suppl):9520.

Immune-Related Adverse Toxicities and Clinical Management

36

Michael Constantin Kirchberger and Lucie Heinzerling

Immunoregulatory molecules such as cytotoxic T-lymphocyte antigen-4 (CTLA-4) and programmed cell death-protein 1 (PD-1) or its ligand (PD-L1) can mediate immune evasion by tumors. Immune checkpoint inhibitors (ICPIs) target these molecules, thus reactivating cytotoxic T cells, and augmenting immunologic reactions against tumor cells. However, this immune activation not only unleashes antitumor immunity, but also leads to autoimmunity that can lead to a plethora of immune-related symptoms.

These unique side effects during treatment with ICPIs are named immune-related adverse events (irAEs) and can potentially involve every organ system of the body, ranging from mild to severe [1–3]. Even fatalities due to e.g. colitis, myocarditis, and Guillain-Barré syndrome have occurred [4, 5]. Overall, irAEs are frequent and occur in 70–90% of the patients treated with ICPIs [6–8]. Anti-PD-1 therapies, such as nivolumab and pembrolizumab, induce grade 3/4 side effects in 10–20% of patients, the anti-CTLA4 antibody, ipilimumab (3 mg/kg) in 27% [6, 9]. The incidence of irAEs when these antibodies are combined, such as with nivolumab and ipilimumab, occurs in ~54% of treated patients [9]. Therapy discontinuation due to side effects occurs in 8.6%, 15.1%, and 38.3% for anti-PD1, ipilimumab, and the combination, respectively [9]. The higher frequency of 54% grade 3/4 AEs in the adjuvant setting, which employed a higher dose of 10 mg/kg ipilimumab and continuous administration of treatment, induced fatalities in 1% of cases [4, 10, 11].

Organ systems most commonly affected are the skin, with manifestations such as a rash, pruritus, and xerosis, the gastrointestinal tract with colitis, the liver showing an autoimmune hepatitis, endocrinopathies of the thyroid and pituitary gland, the lung with pneomonitis, and the heart with myositis [6–9, 11–15]. The type of adverse events is similar between the checkpoint inhibitors; however, frequencies of induction of side effects in a specific organ can vary. For example, colitis being more frequently induced by ipilimumab than with anti-PD1 antibodies in 11.6 and 1.3% of cases, respectively [9].

When checkpoint inhibitors are used in a combined regimen, more than one organ system is involved with irAEs in about one-third of patients [16, 17]. Thus, when detecting one side effect, careful attention should be given to the occurrence of other side effects. Other ICPIs, such as anti-PD-L1 mAbs, may even improve toxicity profiles with lower incidence of grade 3/4 AEs in 5–9% of patients treated with atezolizumab and 5% grade 3 side effects in patients treated with avelumab [7, 18]. Table 36.1 shows an overview of the most common AEs under treatment with ICPIs. IRAEs occur frequently between 3 weeks

M. C. Kirchberger, M.D. · L. Heinzerling, M.D., M.P.H., Ph.D. (✉)
Department of Dermatology,
University Hospital Erlangen, Erlangen, Germany
e-mail: Lucie.Heinzerling@uk-erlangen.de

A. I. Riker (ed.), *Melanoma*, https://doi.org/10.1007/978-3-319-78310-9_36

Table 36.1 Grade 3 and 4 adverse events in different immune checkpoint inhibitor regimen

Organ system	Adverse events (%)	Ipilimumab (3 mg/kg 3-weekly)	Ipilimumab (10 mg/kg 3-weekly)	Nivolumab (3 mg/kg 2-weekly)	Pembrolizumab (2 mg/kg 2- and 3-weekly)	Ipilimumab + Nivolumab (3 mg/kg + 1 mg/kg every 3 weeks)
Cardiac	Cardiac adverse events	NR	NR	NR	1–2	NR
Neurological	Neurological adverse events	<1	NR	NR	0	NR
Endocrinopathies	Fatigue	1	2–3	0–1	0	4
	Hypothyroidism	0	0–1	0	<1	<1
	Hyperthyroidism	<1	NR	<1	0	1
	Hypophysitis	2	4–5	<1	<1	2
Pulmonary	Pneumonitis	<1	NR	<1	<1	1
Gastrointestinal	Diarrhea	3–6	10	0–2	1–3	9
	Colitis	7–9	7–8	<1	1–3	8
	Hepatitis	0–2	NR	2–3	1–2	19
Renal	Renal injury	<1	NR	<1	0	NR
Cutaneous	Pruritus	<1	2–3	<1	0	2
	Rash	1–2	1–2	<1	0	3
Miscellaneous	Myalgia	<1	NR	0	<1	NR
	Arthralgia	<1	NR	0	<1	<1

NR not reported
References: Robert et al. [15], Larkin et al. [9], Eggermont et al. EORTC 18071 [4], Robert et al. [13], and Weber et al. [33]

and 6 months after initiation of treatment [19, 20]. However, a delayed occurrence of irAEs after discontinuing treatment has been observed and requires long-term follow-up after discontinuation.

General Management of Adverse Events Associated with Immune Checkpoint Inhibitors

The successful management of AEs associated with ICPIs is based on education and good, open communication between the patient and the involved physicians. Before starting the treatment, a thorough history and physical exam is essential in order to establish potential risk factors that could favor the emergence of AEs, such as autoimmune disease or prior cardiac disease [21, 22]. Patients and their caregivers must be informed of the possible AEs under treatment with ICPIs, and that early communication of new symptoms or deterioration of already existing symptoms is necessary to mitigate potential severe or, sometimes, life-threatening consequences. Since there may be reluctance by the patient to report side effects for fear it would lead to treatment discontinuation, they should clearly understand that ICPIs are equally effective if treatment is discontinued due to side effects [23].

The most common AEs, such as gastrointestinal (diarrhea, abdominal pain, blood in the stool, hepatic), cutaneous (rash, pruritus), endocrine (fatigue, nausea, loss of vision), and pulmonary/cardiologic (shortness of breath, edema) should be carefully explained to all patients. A time-dependent manifestation of AEs has been reported [24, 25], but AEs can occur at any time, even months after the last treatment. However, the timing of the onset of AEs may be helpful to determine its etiology. In patients treated with nivolumab, the median onset of cutaneous irAEs was 5 weeks, gastrointestinal at 7 weeks, hepatic at 8 weeks, pulmonary at 9 weeks, endocrine at 10 weeks, and renal AEs at 15 weeks [23]. The median onset of irAEs is similar in the combined therapy with anti-CTLA-4 and anti-PD-1 monoclonal antibodies (mAbs) [24]. In patients treated with ipilimumab, the onset of cutaneous irAEs usually appears during the first few weeks of treatment [19], with gastrointestinal irAEs often developing between weeks 5 and 10, hypophysitis after 6 weeks, and liver toxicity between weeks 7 and 14 [25]. It must be mentioned that the sequence of checkpoint inhibitor therapy may influence the frequency of irAEs [19, 20, 26].

Algorithms for the general approach to AEs under ICPI are a useful tool for the management when symptoms occur [1–3, 24, 27–29]. Other etiologies to be included in the differential are progression of the tumor, infections and toxicity of other drugs. The mainstay of treating irAEs is immunosuppression with methylprednisolone (or equivalent). Steroid-refractory or steroid-dependent side effects should prompt escalation of immunosuppression with other immunosuppressants, such as infliximab for colitis [30], or mycophenolate mofetil for hepatitis [31]. The majority of irAEs responds well to corticosteroids and nearly all irAEs resolve under second-line immunosuppressive therapy. Exceptions include endocrinopathies which often require long-term hormone substitution and neurological side effects which often resolve with sequelae [1, 3]. The occurrence of irAEs with subsequent immunosuppressive therapy does not seem to affect clinical response rates or median time to response [23, 32]. ICPIs can be continued in grade 1 irAES and may be restarted after recovery from grade 2 or higher grade irAEs after assessing the risk/benefit ratio. A general approach to the management of irAEs, as well as the most common irAEs encountered, is depicted in Table 36.2.

Gastrointestinal Adverse Events

The most common gastrointestinal AEs are diarrhea/colitis (increase in the frequency of stools compared to baseline, abdominal pain and/or signs of colonic inflammation) that is observed in 8–19% of the patients treated with anti-PD-1 mAbs. It is seen in 23–33% of the patients receiving anti-CTLA-4 mAbs and in 44% of the patients undergoing dual therapy with anti-PD-1 and anti-CTLA-4 mAbs [9, 13, 15, 33, 34]. Intestinal

Table 36.2 Management of common immune-related adverse events (irAE)

irAE	Grade 1	Grade 2	Grade 3	Grade 4
General	S: Mild/asymptomatic P: Outpatient care Continue immunotherapy Immunosuppression not recommended	S: Moderate symptoms P: Outpatient care, monitor carefully Delay immunotherapy Screen for tumor progression or infections Corticosteroids may be necessary	S: Severe symptoms P: Hospitalization advised, consult organ specialist Discontinue immunotherapy and discuss resumption based on risk/benefit ratio Systemic corticosteroids (1–2 mg/kg/day), if no improvement within 2 days consider escalation of immunosuppression If symptoms resolve to grade 1, taper corticosteroids over 1 month Consider concomitant medication (e.g., prophylactic antibiotics)	S: Life-threatening symptoms P: Urgent hospitalization required Management as per grade 3 except for permanent discontinuation of immunotherapy
Gastrointestinal	S: Diarrhea: <4 bowel movements per day over baseline Colitis: asymptomatic P: Continue immunotherapy Symptomatic treatment such as oral fluid and anti-motility agents (loperamide)	S: Diarrhea: 4–6 bowel movements per day over baseline colitis: abdominal pain, blood in stool P: Delay immunotherapy, resume if symptoms improve to grade 1 If persists >5 days: 0.5–1.0 mg/kg/day methylprednisolone and continue until symptoms improve to grade 1, taper steroids over at least 1 month Sigmoidoscopy with biopsy, screen for infections	S: Diarrhea: ≥7 stools per day over baseline colitis: Severe abdominal pain, medical intervention indicated, peritoneal signs P: Discontinue immunotherapy Admit patient to hospital for intravenous hydration and 1–2 mg/kg/day methylprednisolone, if no improvement after 3 days, add infliximab 5 mg/kg i.v. (contraindication: sepsis, perforation) Sigmoidoscopy with biopsy, screen for infections If symptoms improve to grade 1, taper steroids over 1–3 months, infliximab may be re-administered at 2 and 6 weeks	S: Life-threatening, perforation P: Management as per grade 3 permanently discontinue immunotherapy

Table 36.2 (continued)

irAE	Grade 1	Grade 2	Grade 3	Grade 4
Hepatitis	S: ALT/AST ULN - 3× ULN and/or total bilirubin up to 1.5× ULN P: Continue immunotherapy Screen for hepatitis (A, B, C), CMV (PCR from EDTA), haemochromatosis, excessive alcohol intake	S: ALT/AST 3–5× ULN and/or total bilirubin 1.5–3× ULN P: Delay immunotherapy Rule out tumor progression Monitor liver function: if elevation persists, consider 1–2 mg/kg/day methylprednisolone	S: ALT/AST 5–20× ULN and/or total bilirubin >3× ULN P: Management as per grade 2 except that immunotherapy should be discontinued and corticosteroids initiated immediately If no improvement after 3 days, add mycophenolate mofetil 1 g BID Consider hepatic biopsy for differential diagnosis	S: AST/ALT >20× ULN and/or total bilirubin >10× ULN P: Management as per grade 3 except for 2 mg/day/kg methylprednisolone
Rash	S: <10% BSA P: Continue immunotherapy Symptomatic management with anti-histamines for pruritus and topical steroids	S: 10–30% BSA P: If rash persists despite management as per grade 1 or if intolerable, consider skin biopsy and delaying immunotherapy Consider 0.5–1 mg/kg/day methylprednisolone Consult dermatologist	S: >30% BSA P: 1 mg/kg/day methylprednisolone Skin biopsy Discontinue immunotherapy Exclude TEN/SJS	P: Management as per grade 3 Permanently discontinue immunotherapy
Pneumonitis	S: Asymptomatic, radiographic changes only P: Consider delaying immunotherapy Monitor for symptoms and screen for infectious diseases	S: Mild to moderate symptoms P: Delay immunotherapy Consider hospitalization and monitor symptoms daily 1–2 mg/kg/day methylprednisolone recommended, consider empiric antibiotics Consider bronchoscopy and lung biopsy If improving taper coticosteroids and resume immunotherapy if symptoms resolve completely	S: Severe symptoms P: Discontinue Immunotherapy Hospitalization 2–4 mg/kg/day methylprednisolone Add prophylactic antibiotics Bronchoscopy with lung biopsy/BAL Consider additional immunosuppression (e.g., infliximab, mycophenolate mofetil, cyclophosphamide, intravenous immunglobulin)	S: Life-threatening symptoms P: Urgent intervention required as per grade 3 Consider intensive care unit and intubation

(continued)

Table 36.2 (continued)

irAE	Grade 1	Grade 2	Grade 3	Grade 4
Nephritis	S: Creatinine > ULN and > 1–1.5× baseline Proteinuria 1+, <1.0 g/24 h P: Continue immunotherapy Hydration and cessation of nephrotoxic drugs Monitor creatinine weekly	S: Creatinine >1.5–3.0× baseline Proteinuria 2+, 1.0–3.4 g/24 h P: Delay immunotherapy, resume if improves to grade 1 0.5–1.0 mg/kg/day methylprednisolone Consider renal biopsy and rule out toxic or infectious etiology	S: Creatinine <3× baseline proteinuria ≥3.5 g/24 h P: Discontinue immunotherapy 1–2 mg/kg/day methylprednisolone	S: Life-threatening symptoms P: Management as per grade 3
Thyroid	S: Asymptomatic P: Monitor	S: Symptomatic P: Consider consulting endocrinology Hypothyreodism: Levothyroxine Hyperthyroidism: Nonselective beta-blocker (e.g., propanolol or atenolol), consider carbimazole and/or corticosteroids	S: Severe symptoms P: Consult endocrinology and consider hospitalization Management as per grade 2 except for 1–2 mg/kg/day methylprednisolone	P: Management as per grade 3
Hypophysitis	S: Asymptomatic Hyponatremia P: Diagnostic MRI fasting cortisol	S: Symptomatic P: Diagnostic MRI Fasting cortisol Substitute hydrocortisone 20 mg—10 mg—0		

S symptoms, *P* procedures, *BAL* bronchoalveolar lavage, *BSA* body surface area, *SJS* Steven-Johnson-Syndrome, *TEN* toxic epidermal necrolysis, *ULN* upper limit of normal

perforation due to autoimmune colitis may be fatal [4, 6]. Thus, careful assessment of gastrointestinal AEs without time delay is essential. For cases of diarrhea, the application of steroids should not be delayed. It is important to exclude other potential infectious causes, including bacterial (including Clostridium difficile) and viral pathogens as well as parasites.

Rectosigmoidoscopy and ileocolonoscopy can assess the full extent of inflammation and a biopsy can be performed for histopathologic assessment. Characteristic findings include a mixed inflammatory infiltrate in the lamina propria consisting of neutrophils, lymphocytes, plasma cells, and eosinophils. In contrast to inflammatory bowel disease, granulomas have rarely been described [35]. A less invasive procedure is confocal laser endomicroscopy (CLE), an imaging technique for real-time high-resolution visualization of the mucosa depicting cellular details [36]. In CLE the tissue is illuminated by laser and the reflected fluorescent light is detected potentially using contrast agents to enhance the images. An abdominal X-ray can exclude free air indicative of a bowel perforation. ICPI, treatment should be suspended and methylprednisolone (0.5–1 mg/kg/day or oral equivalent) should promptly be administered and symptoms should improve within days. Corticosteroids should be carefully tapered over 1 month to avoid recurrence. In severe and refractory cases, ICPI treatment must be stopped permanently, and immunosuppressive escalation with infliximab (5 mg/kg i.v.) may become necessary. However, some cases can be refractory to corticosteroids and infliximab [30]. The reactivation of CMV has to be considered, since reactivation can also occur simultaneously to autoimmune inflammation of another organ as reported in a patient with autoimmune colitis and CMV hepatitis [37]. Some centers use calprotectin in the feces as a marker for inflammation [38].

Subtitle: Autoimmune Hepatitis Grade 3/4 immune-related hepatitis is seen mainly through elevated transaminases in 14–20% of the patients that are treated with the combination of anti-CTLA-4 and anti-PD-1 mAbs, compared to 1–2% of patients treated with anti-PD1 monotherapy [9, 28]. Patients with autoimmune hepatitis are often asymptomatic. After exclusion of other etiologies (progressive disease, viral or toxic hepatitis), treatment with corticosteroids is started. Refractory cases may require therapy with mycophenolate mofetil (500–1000 mg/twice daily). Asymptomatic pancreatitis with elevations of lipase and amylase (grade 3/4) occurs in up to 15% of cases and the induction of exocrine pancreas insufficiency has been reported [1] as well as the development of diabetes mellitus. The latter can show a sudden onset with ketoacidosis [39].

Cutaneous Adverse Events

Cutaneous AEs occur very frequently in patients undergoing treatment with ICPIs but rarely lead to treatment stopdiscontinuation of treatment. Manifestations include erythema, palmoplantar erythrodysesthesia, photosensitivity, pruritus, rash, and urticaria. Another less common drug reaction with eosinophilia, systemic symptoms (DRESS), and bullous skin eruptions has been described [40, 41]. Less than 1% of patients display severe cutaneous AEs (grade 3/4). However, since Stevens-Johnson syndrome (toxic epidermal necrolysis) has been observed [42–44], bullous skin eruptions should be carefully worked up by a dermatologist [45]. Lichenoid skin reactions have been reported in 17–22% of patients undergoing therapy with anti-PD-1 mAbs, and can also involve the mucosa [45, 46]. Furthermore, occurrence of psoriasis, Grover's disease, and pityriasis lichenoides chronica-like reaction has been observed [46–48]. Sicca syndrome has also been reported under therapy with ICPIs [49]. Most cases of dermatitis are mild and can be managed with urea- or glycerin-containing creams or lotions. Topical corticosteroids and oral antipruritic agents are the pillars of managing cutaneous AEs. In grade 3/4 cutaneous AEs, skin biopsy should be performed to obtain the correct diagnosis, with administration of systemic corticosteroids when clinically appropriate.

Endocrine Adverse Events

During treatment with anti-CTLA-4 and anti-PD-1 mAbs, endocrine AEs of any grade occur in 5–10% of patients [8, 50]. Mostly, the thyroid gland is affected with hypothyroidism (4–8%) and/or hyperthyroidism (1–5%) [51, 52]. Acute thyroiditis (1%) and hypophysitis (1%) are observed less frequently. Patients may present with symptoms such as constipation, dizziness, fatigue, hair loss, headaches, loss of peripheral vision, tachycardia, and weight gain or loss [1, 2]. Type-1 diabetes mellitus (0.1%) can also occur, with associated symptoms such as increase in thirst, polyuria, and fatigue.

In cases of suspected thyroid AE, thyroid function tests, consisting of thyroid-stimulating hormone (TSH), thyroxine (free T4 or T4) and triiodothyronine (T3) are recommended. Antithyroid autoantibody titers of thyroid peroxidase and thyroglobulin should be assessed. Hormone replacement therapy is required in most cases of immune-related hypothyroidism, whereas immunosuppressive therapy often does not influence the outcome. Hyperthyroidism, if symptomatic may be treated with carbimazole and/or selective beta-blockers (e.g., propranolol). However, hyperthyroidism commonly resolves spontaneously with subsequent hypothyroidism [53, 54] and the subsequent need of hormone replacement with thyroxine.

Hypophysitis occurs in 1–4% of patients treated with anti-PD-1 mAbs or ipilimumab [9, 15] with a median onset at 11 weeks. Symptoms are unspecific and include fatigue, decrease in libido, vision changes, and confusion. It is important to exclude the development of a metastatic lesion to the brain. Hypophysitis can involve the anterior pituitary, notably the thyroid, adrenocortical and gonadal axes [55, 56]. For screening, changes in electrolytes can be used and testing of the pituitary axis is recommended (morning cortisol, ACTH, TSH, LH, FSH, prolactin, estradiol in women, and testosterone in men). An enlargement of the pituitary gland as seen with magnetic resonance imaging (MRI) scans may be observed, but not always present [50]. Subsequent hormone replacement with hydrocortisone is required in most cases.

Neurologic Adverse Events

Neurological adverse events are considered rare and occur in about 3% of patients treated with ICPIs [4, 9, 15, 33, 57]. Patients may present with apathy, ataxia, cognitive impairment, dizziness, headache, myoclonus, paralysis, seizures, speech disorders, or tremor. Early neurological consultation is strongly recommended and studies such as MRI, lumbar puncture, and nerve conduction studies can complement the exam as indicated. Neurological AEs can occur late during the treatment course, sometimes even after completion of treatment [58]. The median onset was at 13 weeks in an adjuvant ipilimumab trial [4]. The treatment with ICPIs should be withheld. Immunosuppression with corticosteroids is frequently required and leads to significant improvement of symptoms in most cases. Some patients develop permanent sequelae. Nevertheless, despite treatment with corticosteroids, plasmapheresis, intravenous immunoglobulin, therapy-refractory AEs have been observed [3]. Again, cerebral metastases and infectious etiologies should always be considered.

Although anti-PD-1 mAbs less frequently induce neurological AEs, the spectrum of symptoms is very similar. Less than 1% of patients have shown balance disorders, demyelination [59], dysgeusia or hypogeusia, Guillain-Barré syndrome, hyperesthesia, insomnia or hypersomnia, lethargy, memory disorders, myasthenia gravis [3], neuralgia, neuropathy (including facial nerve and abducens nerve paresis), optic neuritis, or seizures [60].

In patients treated with ipilimumab, peripheral neuropathies are the most common neurological AEs, occurring in 0.9% and 0.6% of patients, respectively [61]. Furthermore, aseptic meningitis [62], cerebral edema with seizures, chronic inflammatory demyelinating polyneuropathy [63], cranial peripheral neuropathy [64], enteric neuropathy, fatal Guillain-Barré syndrome [5], granulomatous CNS inflammation [2], meningoradiculoneuritis, myasthenia gravis [63, 65], necrotic myelopathy [66], Tolosa-Hunt syndrome [2], and transverse myelitis [63] have all been observed. Systemic diseases can also be accompanied by neurological symptoms as shown by a report on neurosarcoidosis [67] affecting the sella turcica and pituitary stalk.

Pulmonary Adverse Events

The most notable immune-related pulmonary side effect is pneumonitis. More uncommonly, sarcoidosis and pulmonary granulomatosis have been observed [68–72]. Immune-related pneumonitis under treatment with ICPIs is potentially life-threatening [73–76]. An incidence of up to 2% has been reported in patients treated with anti-PD-1 mAbs or ipilimumab [13, 15]. The time to onset ranged from 9 days to 19 months and 86% of the cases improved or resolved with drug holding and/or immunosuppression. Severe cases were reported in 28% of patients, and five patients died due to pneumonitis [14].

Patients can present with symptoms such as a dry cough, shortness of breath, and inspiratory crackles. A chest CT scan and spirometry with measurement of the carbon monoxide diffusing capacity are useful for diagnosis and follow-up. Immune-related pneumonitis can present with ground-glass lesions and disseminated nodular infiltrates in the lower lobes [71, 76]. To rule out infections prior to treatment with corticosteroids, a bronchoscopy with bronchoalveolar lavage is advised. Viral infections with pneumocystis jirovecii, influenza, metapneumovirus, syncytial virus, or other atypical infections with Chlamydia, Legionella pneumophilia, and Mycoplasma pneumonia should be excluded. If immune-related pneumonitis is confirmed, most cases can be managed effectively with high-dose corticosteroids, potentially given together with antibiotics if the infectious workup still has to be completed.

Renal Adverse Events

Adverse events affecting the renal system for patients undergoing treatment with ICPIs are rare. Nephritis, renal failure, and lupus nephritis have been observed in patients treated with ipilimumab [2, 77, 78]. Renal dysfunction occurred in less than 1% of the patients treated with nivolumab, but creatinine was elevated in up to 22% of patients [33]. The median time to onset of renal adverse events ranges from 6 to 10 weeks [27]. For grade 1 toxicity, monitoring creatinine at least once a week without interruption of ICPIs is recommended. For grade 2/3, most patients will recover to grade 1 after withholding ICPIs and administering methylprednisolone 0.5–1 mg/kg/day (or equivalent). A renal biopsy should be considered. In the case of grade 4 renal AEs, ICPIs should be permanently discontinued and high-dose corticosteroids administered.

Cardiologic Adverse Events

Despite absence of baseline cardiac symptoms and/or risk factors, cardiotoxicity may develop with a variable time to onset under treatment with ICPIs [22] and can manifest as myocarditis, heart failure, cardiomyopathy, heart block, and myocardial fibrosis [22, 79–81]. Patients with a history of cardiac conditions should be closely monitored (inlcuding creatine phosphokinase measurement before each infusion) for deterioration of heart function. Prompt and adequate management of cardiac toxicity, including the administration of steroids, is essential in order to avoid a potentially fatal outcome. Also myositis may occur in combination with cardiomyositis in about 1/3 of cases.

Other Adverse Events

Ocular AEs are rare and include conjunctivitis, iritis, and uveitis. Consultation with an ophthalmologist and therapy with corticosteroid eye drops appears to be sufficient in most cases. Deterioration of symptoms or vision loss [2] should lead to discontinuation of treatment and oral or intravenous corticosteroids.

Hematologic AEs include red cell aplasia, autoimmune neutropenia, hemophilia A, and pancytopenia and may be lethal [82–84]. Arthralgia and myalgia may be observed in patients treated with ICPIs [15, 33]. Mild symptoms are treated with paracetamol or nonsteroidal anti-inflammatories. If not sufficient, low dose corticosteroids are often effective (e.g. Prednisone 5 mg/day).

Biomarkers

Currently, we are unable to predict which patients will experience severe side effects. Predisposition to developing IRAEs may be associated with the patient's immunologic profile, such as their human leucocyte antigen (HLA) status [24]. Some irAEs like rash and vitiligo seem to be beneficial for overall survival [85, 86]. In addition, response, as well as occurrence of side effects, may be associated with the microbiota-dependent immunomodulatory effects [87]. Importantly, cessation of ICPI therapy after occurrence is not associated with decreased overall survival compared to patients who continue treatment.

Summary

Checkpoint inhibitors induce side effects in all organ systems. Before initiation of therapy, patients and involved physicians have to be properly educated, with early patient reporting of potential AEs to their treating physician.

Patients should understand and not be reluctant to stop their therapy, knowing that discontinuation due to side effects does not affect their long-term outcome. Baseline examinations and regular monitoring are essential to detect side effects early. Diagnostic workup with the exclusion of other causes (tumor progression, infection, CMV reactivation) is essential, and if irAEs are detected, adequate therapy with prompt use of corticosteroids is crucial. In case of steroid-refractory side effects, diagnostic efforts have to be broadened and if no other causes are detected, immunosuppressive therapy is then escalated.

Management of irAEs should be done as part of a multidisciplinary team and in cooperation with centers that are experienced in side effect management.

References

1. Hofmann L, Forschner A, Loquai C, Goldinger SM, Zimmer L, Ugurel S, et al. Cutaneous, gastrointestinal, hepatic, endocrine, and renal side-effects of anti-PD-1 therapy. Eur J Cancer. 2016;60:190–9. https://doi.org/10.1016/j.ejca.2016.02.025.
2. Voskens CJ, Goldinger SM, Loquai C, Robert C, Kaehler KC, Berking C, et al. The price of tumor control: an analysis of rare side effects of anti-CTLA-4 therapy in metastatic melanoma from the ipilimumab network. PLoS One. 2013;8:e53745. https://doi.org/10.1371/journal.pone.0053745.
3. Zimmer L, Goldinger SM, Hofmann L, Loquai C, Ugurel S, Thomas I, et al. Neurological, respiratory, musculoskeletal, cardiac and ocular side-effects of anti-PD-1 therapy. Eur J Cancer. 2016;60:210–25. https://doi.org/10.1016/j.ejca.2016.02.024.
4. Eggermont AMM, Chiarion-Sileni V, Grob J-J, Dummer R, Wolchok JD, Schmidt H, et al. Prolonged survival in stage III melanoma with Ipilimumab adjuvant therapy. N Engl J Med. 2016;375:1845–55. https://doi.org/10.1056/NEJMoa1611299.
5. Gaudy-Marqueste C, Monestier S, Franques J, Cantais E, Richard M-A, Grob J-J. A severe case of ipilimumab-induced guillain-barré syndrome revealed by an occlusive enteric neuropathy: a differential diagnosis for ipilimumab-induced colitis. J Immunother. 2013;36:77–8. https://doi.org/10.1097/CJI.0b013e31827807dd.
6. Hodi FS, O'Day SJ, McDermott DF, Weber RW, Sosman JA, Haanen JB, et al. Improved survival with ipilimumab in patients with metastatic melanoma. N Engl J Med. 2010;363:711–23. https://doi.org/10.1056/NEJMoa1003466.
7. Brahmer JR, Tykodi SS, Chow LQM, Hwu W-J, Topalian SL, Hwu P, et al. Safety and activity of anti-PD-L1 antibody in patients with advanced cancer. N Engl J Med. 2012;366:2455–65. https://doi.org/10.1056/NEJMoa1200694.
8. Topalian SL, Hodi FS, Brahmer JR, Gettinger SN, Smith DC, McDermott DF, et al. Safety, activity, and immune correlates of anti-PD-1 antibody in cancer. N Engl J Med. 2012;366:2443–54. https://doi.org/10.1056/NEJMoa1200690.
9. Larkin J, Chiarion-Sileni V, Gonzalez R, Grob JJ, Cowey CL, Lao CD, et al. Combined Nivolumab and Ipilimumab or Monotherapy in untreated melanoma. N Engl J Med. 2015;373:23–34. https://doi.org/10.1056/NEJMoa1504030.
10. Wolchok JD, Neyns B, Linette G, Negrier S, Lutzky J, Thomas L, et al. Ipilimumab monotherapy in patients with pretreated advanced melanoma: a randomised, double-blind, multicentre, phase 2, dose-ranging study. Lancet Oncol. 2010;11:155–64. https://doi.org/10.1016/S1470-2045(09)70334-1.
11. Bertrand A, Kostine M, Barnetche T, Truchetet M-E, Schaeverbeke T. Immune related adverse events associated with anti-CTLA-4 antibodies: systematic review and meta-analysis. BMC Med. 2015;13:211. https://doi.org/10.1186/s12916-015-0455-8.
12. Wolchok JD, Kluger H, Callahan MK, Postow MA, Rizvi NA, Lesokhin AM, et al. Nivolumab plus ipilimumab in advanced melanoma. N Engl J Med. 2013;369:122–33. https://doi.org/10.1056/NEJMoa1302369.
13. Robert C, Long GV, Brady B, Dutriaux C, Maio M, Mortier L, et al. Nivolumab in previously untreated melanoma without BRAF mutation. N Engl J Med. 2014;372:320–30. https://doi.org/10.1056/NEJMoa1412082.
14. Hamid O, Robert C, Daud A, Hodi FS, Hwu W-J, Kefford R, et al. Safety and tumor responses with Lambrolizumab (anti–PD-1) in melanoma. N Engl J Med. 2013;369:134–44. https://doi.org/10.1056/NEJMoa1305133.
15. Robert C, Schachter J, Long GV, Arance A, Grob JJ, Mortier L, et al. Pembrolizumab versus Ipilimumab in Advanced Melanoma. N Engl J Med. 2015;372:2521–32. https://doi.org/10.1056/NEJMoa1503093.
16. Bilen MA, Subudhi SK, Gao J, Tannir NM, Tu S-M, Sharma P. Acute rhabdomyolysis with severe polymyositis following ipilimumab-nivolumab treatment in a cancer patient with elevated anti-striated muscle antibody. J Immunother Cancer. 2016;4:36. https://doi.org/10.1186/s40425-016-0139-8.
17. Dasanu CA, Jen T, Skulski R. Late-onset pericardial tamponade, bilateral pleural effusions and recurrent immune monoarthritis induced by ipilimumab use for metastatic melanoma. J Oncol Pharm Pract. 2017;23(3):231–4. https://doi.org/10.1177/1078155216635853.
18. Kaufman HL, Russell J, Hamid O, Bhatia S, Terheyden P, D'Angelo SP, et al. Avelumab in patients

with chemotherapy-refractory metastatic Merkel cell carcinoma: a multicentre, single-group, open-label, phase 2 trial. Lancet Oncol. 2016;17:1374–85. https://doi.org/10.1016/S1470-2045(16)30364-3.
19. Weber JS, Dummer R, de Pril V, Lebbé C, Hodi FS, MDX010-20 Investigators. Patterns of onset and resolution of immune-related adverse events of special interest with ipilimumab: detailed safety analysis from a phase 3 trial in patients with advanced melanoma. Cancer. 2013;119:1675–82. https://doi.org/10.1002/cncr.27969.
20. Topalian SL, Sznol M, McDermott DF, Kluger HM, Carvajal RD, Sharfman WH, et al. Survival, durable tumor remission, and long-term safety in patients with advanced melanoma receiving nivolumab. J Clin Oncol. 2014;32:1020–30. https://doi.org/10.1200/JCO.2013.53.0105.
21. Gutzmer R, Koop A, Meier F, Hassel JC, Terheyden P, Zimmer L, et al. Programmed cell death protein-1 (PD-1) inhibitor therapy in patients with advanced melanoma and preexisting autoimmunity or ipilimumab-triggered autoimmunity. Eur J Cancer. 2017;75:24–32. https://doi.org/10.1016/j.ejca.2016.12.038.
22. Heinzerling L, Ott PA, Hodi FS, Husain AN, Tajmir-Riahi A, Tawbi H, et al. Cardiotoxicity associated with CTLA4 and PD1 blocking immunotherapy. J Immunother Cancer. 2016;4:50. https://doi.org/10.1186/s40425-016-0152-y.
23. weber. Safety profile of nivolumab (NIVO) in patients (pts) with advanced melanoma (MEL): a pooled analysis. ASCO Annual Meeting | Abstracts | Meeting Library; 2015.
24. Michot JM, Bigenwald C, Champiat S, Collins M, Carbonnel F, Postel-Vinay S, et al. Immune-related adverse events with immune checkpoint blockade: a comprehensive review. Eur J Cancer. 2016;54:139–48. https://doi.org/10.1016/j.ejca.2015.11.016.
25. Weber JS, Kahler KC, Hauschild A. Management of immune-related adverse events and kinetics of response with ipilimumab. J Clin Oncol. 2012;30:2691–7. https://doi.org/10.1200/JCO.2012.41.6750.
26. Maker AV, Yang JC, Sherry RM, Topalian SL, Kammula US, Royal RE, et al. Intrapatient dose escalation of anti-CTLA-4 antibody in patients with metastatic melanoma. J Immunother. 2006;29:455–63. https://doi.org/10.1097/01.cji.0000208259.73167.58.
27. Eigentler TK, Hassel JC, Berking C, Aberle J, Bachmann O, Grünwald V, et al. Diagnosis, monitoring and management of immune-related adverse drug reactions of anti-PD-1 antibody therapy. Cancer Treat Rev. 2016;45:7–18. https://doi.org/10.1016/j.ctrv.2016.02.003.
28. Spain L, Larkin J. Combination immune checkpoint blockade with ipilimumab and nivolumab in the management of advanced melanoma. Expert Opin Biol Ther. 2016;16:389–96. https://doi.org/10.1517/14712598.2016.1141195.
29. Champiat S, Lambotte O, Barreau E, Belkhir R, Berdelou A, Carbonnel F, et al. Management of immune checkpoint blockade dysimmune toxicities: a collaborative position paper. Ann Oncol Off J Eur Soc Med Oncol. 2016;27:559–74. https://doi.org/10.1093/annonc/mdv623.
30. Lankes K, Hundorfean G, Harrer T, Pommer AJ, Agaimy A, Angelovska I, et al. Anti-TNF-refractory colitis after checkpoint inhibitor therapy: possible role of CMV-mediated immunopathogenesis. Oncoimmunology. 2016;5:e1128611. https://doi.org/10.1080/2162402X.2015.1128611.
31. Cheng R, Cooper A, Kench J, Watson G, Bye W, McNeil C, et al. Ipilimumab-induced toxicities and the gastroenterologist. J Gastroenterol Hepatol. 2015;30:657–66. https://doi.org/10.1111/jgh.12888.
32. Horvat TZ, Adel NG, Dang T-O, Momtaz P, Postow MA, Callahan MK, et al. Immune-related adverse events, need for systemic immunosuppression, and effects on survival and time to treatment failure in patients with melanoma treated with Ipilimumab at Memorial Sloan Kettering Cancer Center. J Clin Oncol. 2015;33:3193–8. https://doi.org/10.1200/JCO.2015.60.8448.
33. Weber JS, D'Angelo SP, Minor D, Hodi FS, Gutzmer R, Neyns B, et al. Nivolumab versus chemotherapy in patients with advanced melanoma who progressed after anti-CTLA-4 treatment (CheckMate 037): a randomised, controlled, open-label, phase 3 trial. Lancet Oncol. 2015;16:375–84. https://doi.org/10.1016/S1470-2045(15)70076-8.
34. Garon EB, Rizvi NA, Hui R, Leighl N, Balmanoukian AS, Eder JP, et al. Pembrolizumab for the treatment of non-small-cell lung cancer. N Engl J Med. 2015;372(21):2018–28. https://doi.org/10.1056/NEJMoa1501824.
35. Gupta A, De Felice KM, Loftus EV, Khanna S. Systematic review: colitis associated with anti-CTLA-4 therapy. Aliment Pharmacol Ther. 2015;42:406–17. https://doi.org/10.1111/apt.13281.
36. Hundorfean G, Atreya R, Agaimy A, Heinzerling L, Kämpgen E, Schuler G, et al. Fluorescein-guided confocal laser endomicroscopy for the detection of ipilimumab-induced colitis. Endoscopy. 2012;44:E78–9. https://doi.org/10.1055/s-0031-1291603.
37. Uslu U, Agaimy A, Hundorfean G, Harrer T, Schuler G, Heinzerling L. Autoimmune colitis and subsequent CMV-induced hepatitis after treatment with Ipilimumab. J Immunother. 2015;38(5):212. https://doi.org/10.1097/CJI.0000000000000081.
38. Freie Vorträge. JDDG J Der Dtsch Dermatologischen Gesellschaft. 2015;13:1–19. https://doi.org/10.1111/ddg.12783.
39. Gaudy C, Clévy C, Monestier S, Dubois N, Préau Y, Mallet S, et al. Anti-PD1 pembrolizumab can induce exceptional fulminant type 1 diabetes. Diabetes Care. 2015;38:e182–3. https://doi.org/10.2337/dc15-1331.
40. Belum VR, Benhuri B, Postow MA, Hellmann MD, Lesokhin AM, Segal NH, et al. Characterisation and management of dermatologic adverse events to agents targeting the PD-1 receptor. Eur J

Cancer. 2016;60:12–25. https://doi.org/10.1016/j.ejca.2016.02.010.
41. Sibaud V, Meyer N, Lamant L, Vigarios E, Mazieres J, Delord JP. Dermatologic complications of anti-PD-1/PD-L1 immune checkpoint antibodies. Curr Opin Oncol. 2016;28:254–63. https://doi.org/10.1097/CCO.0000000000000290.
42. Carlos G, Anforth R, Chou S, Clements A, Fernandez-Peñas P. A case of bullous pemphigoid in a patient with metastatic melanoma treated with pembrolizumab. Melanoma Res. 2015;25:265–8. https://doi.org/10.1097/CMR.0000000000000155.
43. Naidoo J, Schindler K, Querfeld C, Busam K, Cunningham J, Page DB, et al. Autoimmune bullous skin disorders with immune checkpoint inhibitors targeting PD-1 and PD-L1. Cancer Immunol Res. 2016;4:383–9. https://doi.org/10.1158/2326-6066.CIR-15-0123.
44. Jour G, Glitza IC, Ellis RM, Torres-Cabala CA, Tetzlaff MT, Li JY, et al. Autoimmune dermatologic toxicities from immune checkpoint blockade with anti-PD-1 antibody therapy: a report on bullous skin eruptions. J Cutan Pathol. 2016;43:688–96. https://doi.org/10.1111/cup.12717.
45. Goldinger SM, Stieger P, Meier B, Micaletto S, Contassot E, French LE, et al. Cytotoxic cutaneous adverse drug reactions during anti-PD-1 therapy. Clin Cancer Res. 2016;22:4023–9. https://doi.org/10.1158/1078-0432.CCR-15-2872.
46. Hwang SJE, Carlos G, Wakade D, Byth K, Kong BY, Chou S, et al. Cutaneous adverse events (AEs) of anti-programmed cell death (PD)-1 therapy in patients with metastatic melanoma: a single-institution cohort. J Am Acad Dermatol. 2016;74:455–61. https://doi.org/10.1016/j.jaad.2015.10.029.
47. Mutgi KAJ, Milhem M, Swick BL, Liu V. Pityriasis lichenoides chronica–like drug eruption developing during pembrolizumab treatment for metastatic melanoma. JAAD Case Reports. 2016;2:343–5. https://doi.org/10.1016/j.jdcr.2016.06.012.
48. Uemura M, Faisal F, Haymaker C, McQuail N, Sirmans E, Hudgens CW, et al. A case report of Grover's disease from immunotherapy-a skin toxicity induced by inhibition of CTLA-4 but not PD-1. J Immunother Cancer. 2016;4:55. https://doi.org/10.1186/s40425-016-0157-6.
49. Cappelli LC, Gutierrez AK, Baer AN, Albayda J, Manno RL, Haque U, et al. Inflammatory arthritis and sicca syndrome induced by nivolumab and ipilimumab. Ann Rheum Dis. 2016:1–8. https://doi.org/10.1136/annrheumdis-2016-209595.
50. Ryder M, Callahan M, Postow MA, Wolchok J, Fagin JA. Endocrine-related adverse events following ipilimumab in patients with advanced melanoma: a comprehensive retrospective review from a single institution. Endocr Relat Cancer. 2014;21:371–81. https://doi.org/10.1530/ERC-13-0499.
51. Naidoo J, Page DB, Li BT, Connell LC, Schindler K, Lacouture ME, et al. Toxicities of the anti-PD-1 and anti-PD-L1 immune checkpoint antibodies. Ann Oncol. 2015;26:2375–91. https://doi.org/10.1093/annonc/mdv383.
52. de Filette J, Jansen Y, Schreuer M, Everaert H, Velkeniers B, Neyns B, et al. Incidence of thyroid-related adverse events in melanoma patients treated with pembrolizumab. J Clin Endocrinol Metab. 2016;101(11):4431–9. https://doi.org/10.1210/jc.2016-2300.
53. Orlov S, Salari F, Kashat L, Walfish PG. Induction of painless thyroiditis in patients receiving programmed death 1 receptor immunotherapy for metastatic malignancies. J Clin Endocrinol Metab. 2015;100:1738–41. https://doi.org/10.1210/jc.2014-4560.
54. Verma I, Modi A, Tripathi H, Agrawal A. Nivolumab causing painless thyroiditis in a patient with adenocarcinoma of the lung. BMJ Case Rep. 2016:bcr2015213692. https://doi.org/10.1136/bcr-2015-213692.
55. Okano Y, Satoh T, Horiguchi K, Toyoda M, Osaki A, Matsumoto S, et al. Nivolumab-induced hypophysitis in a patient with advanced malignant melanoma. Endocr J. 2016;63:905–12. https://doi.org/10.1507/endocrj.EJ16-0161.
56. Ishikawa M, Oashi K. Case of hypophysitis caused by nivolumab. J Dermatol. 2016;44(1):109–10. https://doi.org/10.1111/1346-8138.13437.
57. Rizvi NA, Mazières J, Planchard D, Stinchcombe TE, Dy GK, Antonia SJ, et al. Activity and safety of nivolumab, an anti-PD-1 immune checkpoint inhibitor, for patients with advanced, refractory squamous non-small-cell lung cancer (CheckMate 063): a phase 2, single-arm trial. Lancet Oncol. 2015;16:257–65. https://doi.org/10.1016/S1470-2045(15)70054-9.
58. O'Kane GM, Lyons TG, Colleran GC, Ahmad MW, Alken S, Kavanagh EC, et al. Late-onset paraplegia after complete response to two cycles of Ipilimumab for metastatic melanoma. Oncol Res Treat. 2014;37:757–60. https://doi.org/10.1159/000368316.
59. Tarhini A. Immune-mediated adverse events associated with Ipilimumab CTLA-4 blockade therapy: the underlying mechanisms and clinical management. Scientifica (Cairo). 2013;2013:1–19. https://doi.org/10.1155/2013/857519.
60. Yang JC, Hughes M, Kammula U, Royal R, Sherry RM, Topalian SL, et al. Ipilimumab (anti-CTLA4 antibody) causes regression of metastatic renal cell cancer associated with enteritis and hypophysitis. J Immunother. 2007;30:825–30. https://doi.org/10.1097/CJI.0b013e318156e47e.
61. Liao B, Shroff S, Kamiya-Matsuoka C, Tummala S. Atypical neurological complications of ipilimumab therapy in patients with metastatic melanoma. Neuro-Oncology. 2014;16:589–93. https://doi.org/10.1093/neuonc/nou001.
62. Thaipisuttikul I, Chapman P, Avila EK. Peripheral neuropathy associated with Ipilimumab: a report of 2 cases. J Immunother. 2015;38:77–9. https://doi.org/10.1097/CJI.0000000000000070.
63. Johnson DB, Saranga-Perry V, Lavin PJM, Bryan Burnette W, Clark SW, Uskavitch DR, et al. Myasthenia gravis induced by ipilimumab in patients with metastatic melanoma. J Clin Oncol. 2015;33:e122–4. https://doi.org/10.1200/JCO.2013.51.1683.
64. Abdallah A-O, Herlopian A, Ravilla R, Bansal M, Chandra-Reddy S, Mahmoud F, et al. Ipilimumab-

induced necrotic myelopathy in a patient with metastatic melanoma: a case report and review of literature. J Oncol Pharm Pract. 2016;22:537–42. https://doi.org/10.1177/1078155215572932.

65. Murphy KP, Kennedy MP, Barry JE, O'Regan KN, Power DG. New-onset mediastinal and central nervous system sarcoidosis in a patient with metastatic melanoma undergoing CTLA4 monoclonal antibody treatment. Oncol Res Treat. 2014;37:351–3. https://doi.org/10.1159/000362614.
66. Maurice C, Schneider R, Kiehl T-R, Bavi P, Roehrl MHA, Mason WP, et al. Subacute CNS demyelination after treatment with nivolumab for melanoma. Cancer Immunol Res. 2015;3:1299–302. https://doi.org/10.1158/2326-6066.CIR-15-0141.
67. Mandel JJ, Olar A, Aldape KD, Tremont-Lukats IW. Lambrolizumab induced central nervous system (CNS) toxicity. J Neurol Sci. 2014;344:229–31. https://doi.org/10.1016/j.jns.2014.06.023.
68. Vogel WV, Guislain A, Kvistborg P, Schumacher TNM, Haanen JBAG, Blank CU. Ipilimumab-induced sarcoidosis in a patient with metastatic melanoma undergoing complete remission. J Clin Oncol. 2012;30:e7–10. https://doi.org/10.1200/JCO.2011.37.9693.
69. Eckert A, Schoeffler A, Dalle S, Phan A, Kiakouama L, Thomas L. Anti-CTLA4 monoclonal antibody induced sarcoidosis in a metastatic melanoma patient. Dermatology. 2009;218:69–70. https://doi.org/10.1159/000161122.
70. Wilgenhof S, Morlion V, Seghers AC, Du Four S, Vanderlinden E, Hanon S, et al. Sarcoidosis in a patient with metastatic melanoma sequentially treated with anti-CTLA-4 monoclonal antibody and selective BRAF inhibitor. Anticancer Res. 2012;32:1355–9.
71. Barjaktarevic IZ, Qadir N, Suri A, Santamauro JT, Stover D. Organizing pneumonia as a side effect of Ipilimumab treatment of melanoma. Chest. 2013;143:858–61. https://doi.org/10.1378/chest.12-1467.
72. Berthod G, Lazor R, Letovanec I, Romano E, Noirez L, Stalder JM, et al. Pulmonary sarcoid-like granulomatosis induced by ipilimumab. J Clin Oncol. 2012;30:e156–9. https://doi.org/10.1200/JCO.2011.39.3298.
73. Nishino M, Chambers ES, Chong CR, Ramaiya NH, Gray SW, Marcoux JP, et al. Anti-PD-1 inhibitor-related pneumonitis in non-small cell lung cancer. Cancer Immunol Res. 2016;4:289–93. https://doi.org/10.1158/2326-6066.CIR-15-0267.
74. Steenbruggen TG, van den Heuvel MM, Blank CU, van Dieren JM, Haanen JBAG, Kok M. No hair loss, but colitis or pneumonitis: unique side effects of immune checkpoint inhibitors for cancer. Ned Tijdschr Geneeskd. 2016;160:A9873.
75. Sano T, Uhara H, Mikoshiba Y, Kobayashi A, Uchiyama R, Tateishi K, et al. Nivolumab-induced organizing pneumonia in a melanoma patient. Jpn J Clin Oncol. 2016;46:270–2. https://doi.org/10.1093/jjco/hyv199.
76. Nishino M, Sholl LM, Hatabu H, Ramaiya NH, Hodi FS. Anti–PD-1–related pneumonitis during cancer immunotherapy. N Engl J Med. 2015;373:288–90. https://doi.org/10.1056/NEJMc1505197.
77. Voskens C, Cavallaro A, Erdmann M, Dippel O, Kaempgen E, Schuler G, et al. Anti-cytotoxic T-cell lymphocyte antigen-4-induced regression of spinal cord metastases in association with renal failure, atypical pneumonia, vision loss, and hearing loss. J Clin Oncol. 2012;30:e356–7. https://doi.org/10.1200/JCO.2011.41.4359.
78. Fadel F, El Karoui K, Knebelmann B. Anti-CTLA4 antibody–induced lupus nephritis. N Engl J Med. 2009;361(2):211. https://doi.org/10.1056/NEJMc0904283.
79. Johnson DB, Balko JM, Compton ML, Chalkias S, Gorham J, Xu Y, et al. Fulminant myocarditis with combination immune checkpoint blockade. N Engl J Med. 2016;375:1749–55. https://doi.org/10.1056/NEJMoa1609214.
80. Mahmood SS, Fradley MG, Cohen JV, Nohria A, Reynolds KL, Heinzerling LM, Sullivan RJ, Damrongwatanasuk R, Chen CL, Gupta D, Kirchberger MC. Myocarditis in patients treated with immune checkpoint inhibitors. J Am Coll Cardiol. 2018. https://doi.org/10.1016/j.jacc.2018.02.037.
81. Tajmir-Riahi A, Bergmann T, Schmid M, Agaimy A, Schuler G, Heinzerling L. Life-threatening Autoimmune Cardiomyopathy Reproducibly Induced in a Patient by Checkpoint Inhibitor Therapy. J Immunother. 2018;41(1):35–8. https://doi.org/10.1097/CJI.0000000000000190.
82. Delyon J, Mateus C, Lambert T. Hemophilia a induced by ipilimumab. N Engl J Med. 2011;365:1747–8. https://doi.org/10.1056/NEJMc1110923.
83. Armand P, Nagler A, Weller EA, Devine SM, Avigan DE, Chen Y-B, et al. Disabling immune tolerance by programmed Death-1 blockade with Pidilizumab after autologous hematopoietic stem-cell transplantation for diffuse large B-cell lymphoma: results of an international phase II trial. J Clin Oncol. 2013;31:4199–206. https://doi.org/10.1200/JCO.2012.48.3685.
84. du Rusquec P, Saint-Jean M, Brocard A, Peuvrel L, Khammari A, Quéreux G, et al. Ipilimumab-induced autoimmune pancytopenia in a case of metastatic melanoma. J Immunother. 2014;37:348–50. https://doi.org/10.1097/CJI.0000000000000041.
85. Freeman-Keller M, Kim Y, Cronin H, Richards A, Gibney G, Weber JS. Nivolumab in resected and Unresectable metastatic melanoma: characteristics of immune-related adverse events and association with outcomes. Clin Cancer Res. 2016;22:886–94. https://doi.org/10.1158/1078-0432.CCR-15-1136.
86. Hua C, Boussemart L, Mateus C, Routier E, Boutros C, Cazenave H, et al. Association of vitiligo with tumor response in patients with metastatic melanoma treated with pembrolizumab. JAMA Dermatol. 2016;152:45. https://doi.org/10.1001/jamadermatol.2015.2707.
87. Vétizou M, Pitt JM, Daillère R, Lepage P, Waldschmitt N, Flament C, et al. Anticancer immunotherapy by CTLA-4 blockade relies on the gut microbiota. Science. 2015;350:1079–84. https://doi.org/10.1126/science.aad1329.

Management of Non-melanoma Skin Cancers: Basal Cell Carcinoma, Squamous Cell Carcinoma

37

Sheila Jalalat, Corin Agoris, Neil Alan Fenske, and Basil Cherpelis

Incidence and Trends for Nonmelanoma Skin Cancers

Non-melanoma skin cancer (NMSC) represents the most common malignancy in the United States, with incidence rates rising dramatically over the past two decades [1]. According to a recent study by Rogers et al. (2015), using US national claims and survey databases, there was a 100% increase in the incidence of NMSC from 1992 to 2012. The exact incidence of NMSC may be difficult to determine, as a majority of them are treated in private offices and precise data of these neoplasms are not routinely included in state cancer registries leading to significant under-reporting. Similarly, discrepancies in diagnostic accuracy and criteria such as differentiation between actinic keratosis (AK) and squamous cell carcinoma in situ (SCCIS) may also be a shortcoming in determining incidence. By and large, most reports describe that approximately 75–80% of NMSCs are basal cell carcinoma (BCC) and up to 25% are SCC [1]. However, recent reports describe the ratio of BCC to SCC closer to 1.0. This newer data represents a shift from the historical ratio of 4:1, as previously mentioned. Although BCC is more common in the younger population, there is a disproportionate rise in SCC in the aging population with chronic ultraviolet (UV) exposure, which is thought to account for the change in ratio. Nonetheless, NMSC poses a significant health concern and cost to society, and awareness of current trends is important for clinicians to recognize and treat patients appropriately.

S. Jalalat, M.D. · N. A. Fenske, M.D.
B. Cherpelis, M.D. (✉)
Department of Dermatology and Cutaneous Surgery, Morsani College of Medicine, University of South Florida, Tampa, FL, USA
e-mail: nfenske@health.usf.edu; bcherpel@health.usf.edu

C. Agoris, B.S., B.A.
Morsani College of Medicine, University of South Florida, Tampa, FL, USA
e-mail: cagoris@health.usf.edu

Risk Factors

There is significant overlap in risk factors among the various types of NMSC, distinctions among contributing risk factors including both genetic and environment exposures will be highlighted in the following discussion.

UV Exposure

- UV radiation
  - UV exposure has been well documented in the pathogenesis of NMSC through the mechanism of inducing DNA mutations [2]. The type of exposure is an important distinguishing factor between the development of SCC and BCC. Cumulative,

A. I. Riker (ed.), *Melanoma*, https://doi.org/10.1007/978-3-319-78310-9_37

chronic UV exposure in the early years of life increases the risk of individuals developing AKs and SCC. Whereas, periods of intense UV exposure and sunburns during an individual's lifetime increase the risk of BCC development [3, 4].

- Indoor tanning
  - Exposure to artificial sources of UV radiation has been shown to increase the risk of NMSC in individuals [5]. Those that were exposed were 2.5 times more likely to develop SCC and 1.5 times more likely to develop BCC than in unexposed controls [6].

Ionizing Radiation

- Studies have shown that dose-related exposure to ionizing radiation increases NMSC development years after exposure [7].
  - Occupations where radiation exposure is known, such as airline pilots, have shown to have an elevated risk of developing SCC and BCC [8].
  - Epidemiological studies report that patients are at enhanced risk of developing NMSC if they:
    - are exposed to radiation by atomic bombs
    - are bone marrow transplant recipients
    - have received radiotherapy
    - were treated with radiation for tinea capitis prior to the development of medications in the 1950s
    - were radiologic workers [7, 8]

Immunosuppression

- The development of NMSC in the immunosuppressed organ transplant population is characterized by decreased immunity, carcinogenic effects of medications, human papillomavirus (HPV) infection, and UV exposure. The incidence of SCC is 40–250 times greater than the general population, while BCC is 5–10 times greater; contributing to significant morbidity and mortality in this population. Age at transplantation, degree of immunosuppression required, and length of immunosuppression are significant risk factors contributing to development of NMSC. In addition, 70–90% of SCC lesions are found to contain various HPV strains [9, 10].
- Immunosuppressive drugs, used for purposes other than organ transplant, are found to be associated with increased risk of NMSC, particularly SCC. A study observing the effects of glucocorticoid usage reported that the length of exposure contributed to a twofold increase in SCC development [11].
- Individuals with human immunodeficiency virus (HIV) have been found to have increased rates of SCC [12]. An important clinical correlation is the increased prevalence of HPV-associated anogenital warts, which are at increased risk of developing into SCC.

Genetic

- *Individual phenotype*
  - Red hair color, fair skin pigmentation, decreased ability to tan, and freckling are all significant risk factors for development of NMSC [4].
- *Xeroderma pigementosum* is part of a group of disorders largely due to disorders of DNA repair. Sunlight exposure significantly increases the risk of developing NMSC and melanoma. Development of NMSC can be seen as early as 8 years of age in these individuals, and young adults are 4800 times more likely to have NMSC [13].
- *Oculocutaneous albinism* is part of a group of disorders in which there are varying degrees of pigmentation in an individual's skin, eyes, and hair. Individuals are predisposed to developing NMSC (SCC in particular) and cutaneous melanoma [14].
- *Epidermodysplasia verruciformis* results from HPV infection of the skin. Individuals are at risk of developing SCC at an earlier age than the general population [15].
- *Dystrophic epidermolysis bullosa* is a type VII collagen mutation that leads to scarring and

predisposes individuals to SCC due to associated chronic nonhealing wounds [16].

- *Nevoid basal cell carcinoma syndrome* is associated with a mutation in the PTCH gene. Individuals with this condition are usually children presenting with BCC. Other variable physical features include palmar pits, odontogenic cysts in the jaw, calcified falx cerebri, frontal bossing, and rib deformity among others [17].
- *Bazex syndrome* is a rare condition associated with primarily facial BCC. Presentation also includes follicular atrophoderma, hypotrichosis, localized hypohidrosis, milia, and epidermoid cysts [18].
- *Rombo syndrome* and Bazex share many of the same features and predispose individuals to BCC. People with this disease present with hypotrichosis, blepharitis, peripheral telangiectatic erythema, milia, and trichoepitheliomas [19].

Medications

- In general, immunosuppressive medications increase the risk of developing skin cancer. A large cohort study has described an increased incidence of NMSC among patients with systemically treated psoriasis, the majority of which were TNF-alfa inhibitors [20]. The study reported that NMSC rates, particularly SCC, were 42% higher among individuals ever exposed to a biologic [20]. Additionally, medications that are photosensitive, including but not limited to vandetanib, vemurafenib, and voriconazole, have all been shown to increase a person's risk of developing SCC [21, 22].

Chemical Exposures

- There have been multiple chemical compounds associated with the development of NMSC including polycyclic aromatic hydrocarbons, pesticides, asphalt, paraffin, and tar [23]. The correlation of arsenic exposure and development of SCC long after initial exposure has been well documented, usually resulting in the development of palmoplantar arsenical keratosis. Arsenic has also been associated with the development of BCC [24].

HPV

- HPV is known to infect epithelia of skin and mucosa leading to proliferative lesions commonly known as warts. Individuals with HIV or epidermodysplasia verruciformis and those who are immunosuppressed are at increased risk of HPV lesions developing into SCC [25].

Other Risk Factors

- Other risk factors for developing NMSC, predominately SCC, include tobacco use, thermal burns, bone infections, and chronic ulcers or skin damaged by severe inflammatory skin diseases [21, 26].

Education and Prevention of Nonmelanoma Skin Cancers

A focus on primary prevention by discussing the impact of sunlight exposure and by better educating the public in sun safe behaviors appears to have a positive effect in reducing the incidence of skin cancer [27]. In addition, reliable utilization of sunscreens has been shown to decrease the incidence of NMSC [28]. Although sun safety measures are vital, some patients require additional prophylaxis against developing skin cancers. Retinoids have been long used as prophylaxis against skin cancer development in solid organ transplant recipients and patients with multiple keratoacanthomas. They can also be used for those with nevoid basal cell carcinoma syndrome and those who develop multiple NMSCs due to their phenotype and harsh sun exposure history [29]. Other chemopreventive agents currently being explored include capecitabine, fluorouracil

(5-FU), difluoromethylornithine, and T4 endonuclease V [29–31]. Additional preventative agents that have been reported in the literature include polyphenolic antioxidants such as epigallocatechin gallate (found in green tea and grape seed extract), isoflavone, curcumin, silymarin, lycopene, vitamin E, beta-carotene, genistein, and selenium [21, 29]. Of recent news, oral nicotinamide (vitamin B3) has been shown to be safe and effective in reducing the rates of new NMSC and AK in high-risk patients by its protective effects against damage caused by UV radiation [32].

The main subtypes of cutaneous precancerous and cancerous lesions with corresponding treatments that will be discussed include AK, SCC, SCCIS, and BCC.

Actinic Keratoses

AKs represent a proliferation of atypical epidermal keratinocytes and are a known precursor to SCC. The overall likelihood of transformation for one lesion is less than 1%; however, the summative risk increases over time without intervention [33, 34]. Lesions are confined to the deeper portions of the epidermis and typically do not span the entire thickness. AKs are a common lesion seen in dermatology, making up 14% of dermatology visits [35]. AKs present on sun-exposed areas primarily in fair skinned individuals; areas include scalp, neck, dorsal surfaces of forearms and hands, and lower extremities. They develop as single or multiple scaly erythematous non-indurated macules with areas of adjacent skin showing signs of sun damage. Lesions are generally asymptomatic. Variants are the following:

- Classic: erythematous, scaled macules, papules, or plaques ranging from a few millimeters to 2 cm in diameter
- Hypertrophic: thick, hyperkeratotic scale on an erythematous base. Occasionally, they may develop cutaneous horns which may indicate a need for a biopsy to exclude the possibility of an underlying malignancy. It has been reported that approximately 9% of cutaneous horns have SCC at their bases [36]
- Atrophic: minimal surface change, pink slightly scaly macules or patches
- Pigmented: a subtype that is generally lacking associated erythema and has a hyperpigmented or reticulated appearance often resembling lentigines [21]
- Lichenoid: often identified histopathologically, however, clinically can present as more erythema surrounding the base of a lesion and associated tenderness or pruritus [21]
- Actinic cheilitis (solar cheilosis): classically presents on the lower vermilion lip of individuals with moderate to severe photodamage [21]

Squamous Cell Carcinoma

SCCIS, commonly known as Bowen's Disease, represents atypical keratinocytes that span the entire thickness of the epidermis. Lesions can either represent a progression of an AK or may arise de novo. Clinically, SCCIS presents as an erythematous scaly patch or slightly elevated or indurated plaque. The head and neck, followed by the extremities and trunk, are the most common sites for this type of skin cancer [21]. SCC represents the malignant proliferation of squamous keratinocytes, which normally are nondividing, fully differentiated cells. Malignancy can be due to progression of precursor lesions (AK or SCCIS) or may arise de novo. The natural course of SCC can vary from slowly enlarging to rapidly growing with associated symptoms such as pain and tenderness. High-risk SCC is more likely to metastasize [21]. Characteristics of high-risk SCC are outlined in Table 37.1.

Variants of SCC include:

- Keratoacanthoma (KA): papules that exhibit rapid enlargement, which, over a period of a few weeks, can evolve into a crateriform nodule with a keratotic core. As a natural progression, they may slowly regress over a span of several months leaving an atrophic cicatrix [21, 37]. Clinical presentations include

Table 37.1 High-risk NMSC [21, 95–100]

Location and size	Area L ≥ 2.0 cm; Area M ≥ 1.0 cm; Area H ≥ 0.6 cm
Depth of invasion	>0.2 cm (SCC only)
Histologic subtype	SCC: Sclerosing, basosquamous, small cell, poorly or undifferentiated, spindle cell, pagetoid, infiltrating, KA (centrofacial), single cell, clear cell, lymphoepithelial, sarcomatoid BCC: Basosquamous cell, infiltrative, micronodular, metatypical, morpheaform
Differentiation and borders	Poorly differentiated; ill-defined border; perineural involvement
Health risk factors	Immunosuppression, organ transplant patients, genetic propensity
Secondary factors	Site of burns, chronic inflammatory process, osteomyelitis, or previous radiation

Key: Area L: low risk for recurrenc
e: trunk, extremities
Area M: middle risk for recurrence: cheeks, forehead, neck, scalp
Area H: high risk for recurrence: "mask areas" of face (central face, eyelids, eyebrows, periorbital, nose, lips, chin, mandible, preauricular and postauricular skin/sulci, ear, temple), genitalia, hands and feet

solitary, multiple, grouped, KA centrifugum marginatum, giant, subungal, intraoral, multiple spontaneously regressing and generalized eruptive. KAs can be associated with genetic diseases, chemical exposure, immunosuppression, and HPV infection [38].

- Verrucous carcinoma: uncommon, well-differentiated variant of SCC commonly associated with HPV infection. Clinically, verrucous carcinomas present as large, exophytic verrucous tumors. They are considered a low-grade malignancy with rare metastatic risk [21].

Basal Cell Carcinoma

BCC represents a malignant proliferation of basal keratinocytes that reside in the deepest layer of the epidermis. Basal cells are known to be the stem cells of the epidermis and normally function to regenerate skin. BCC lesions arise de novo and present with a large variety of presentations [21]. It is important to consider that a confounding factor when classifying BCC subtypes is the variety of histopathologic patterns that are associated with clinical subtypes. Characteristics of high-risk BCC are outlined in Table 37.1. Common variants are noted below:

- Nodular: the most common subtype representing approximately 50% of all BCC. Lesions are typically described as a shiny, pearly papule with arborizing telangiectasia and, with time, developing a rolled border. Sites of predilection include the face, generally refraining from non-hair-bearing sites [21].
- Superficial: well-circumscribed erythematous macule, patch, or plaque with focal scale and slight induration. This type of BCC commonly favors the trunk and extremities.
- Morpheaform: a less common subtype, presenting as a slightly elevated to sometimes atrophic appearing area of induration that is light pink to white, often resembling a scar. Biologically, these are more aggressive and exhibit local destruction [21].
- Fibroepithelial: a rare variant of BCC that is a flesh colored, sessile papulonodule resembling a skin tag. This type of BCC often favors the trunk [21].

Treatment of NMSC

The treatment of NMSC encompasses a variety of modalities ranging from surgical to nonsurgical. Well-documented treatment approaches are described in this text, while complete guidelines developed based on consensus of existing literature can be found by the National Comprehensive Cancer Network [39]. Treatment of NMSC begins with a thorough evaluation of the patient, which includes history, physical examination and biopsy. When eliciting the history, the clinician must keep in mind risk factors that may contribute to the development of the lesion. A full skin examination is required as well as lymph node examination in higher risk patients. Although a physical examination will help guide a skin cancer diagnosis, proper biopsy technique is important to establish a diagnosis even in an experienced clinician as the type of skin cancer and depth of invasion can be categorized into low- or high-risk cancers. The exception includes suspected AKs, as they are often treated without an initial biopsy.

Surgical Treatment

Surgical approaches to NMSC include cryosurgery, electrodessication and curettage (ED&C), surgical excision, and Mohs micrographic surgery (MMS). The efficacy, as well as strengths and weaknesses including clearance and recurrence rates, cosmesis, cost and postsurgical complications of each treatment approach varies, and are discussed below.

Cryosurgery

Cryosurgery technique involves the use of liquid nitrogen to destroy cells via freeze-thaw cycles [40]. Most commonly used to treat AKs, well-defined superficial BCC and SCCIS [41]. Clinicians must confirm that the biopsy is sufficient to assess the extent of the lesion and whether or not it can appropriately be treated with cryotherapy. Clearance rates with cryotherapy are most favorable when used on small (<1.0 cm), well-defined, previously untreated tumors that are in areas that exclude the medial canthus, nasolabial folds, postauricular folds, or the hair-bearing scalp [42]. Ideal margin and temperature to achieve appropriate destruction of the tumor are freezing at least 0.3–0.5 cm around the cancer at −50 to −60 degrees Celsius. Skin cancers often require a repeated freeze-thaw cycles to increase the ideal destruction [43].

Actinic Keratoses

- Cryosurgery is a mainstay treatment for AKs. Although clinical experience plays a major role in determining duration of freeze, generally 5–7 s of freeze time with the open-spray technique will eliminate an AK. A shallow crust forms after the procedure and falls off within 2 weeks [21].

Squamous Cell Carcinoma In Situ

- Cryosurgery can be used to treat low-risk SCCIS under 2 cm [43]. The 5-year recurrence rate using cryodestruction was found to be 2.7% in a study, but has been reported to be as high as 10% in primary SCC measuring between 0.5 and 1.2 cm in diameter [41, 44].

Basal Cell Carcinoma

- There is limited evidence comparing cryosurgery to other surgical treatment modalities; however, evidence supports the use of cryosurgery for low-risk, superficial, BCC [45, 46]. A more common treatment modality for nodular BCC is use of ED&C rather than cryotherapy because margins can be felt with the curette as nonrecurrent skin cancer is softer than healthy skin [47]. In lesions with ill-defined borders, cryosurgery is generally contraindicated, and MMS is more appropriate [45].

Overall, cryosurgery is a quick and minimally invasive modality that offers good outcomes when used to treat low-risk lesions, especially in patients who wish to avoid invasive surgery. Local tissue reaction can lead to pain, post-inflammatory pigmentary changes, erythema, and scarring [42, 45]. A serious disadvantage to cryosurgery is the lack of margin control, which may ultimately result in the development of a recurrent carcinoma. The lesion that has been cryodestructed also has potential to become more extensive due to the lack of recognition within the fibrous scar [21]. For these reasons, most skin cancers are treated by excision or MMS which allows for margin control.

Electrodessication and Curettage

ED&C involves scraping lesional tissue with a curette, followed by application of an electric current to destroy remaining tumor cells. Use of ED&C is generally restricted to SCCIS, superficially invasive well-differentiated SCC <1 cm in diameter as well as superficial and nodular BCC. Due to the risk of metastases, excision or MMS is preferred for treatment of invasive SCC, rather than ED&C. Under local anesthesia, curettage begins typically with a 0.3–0.4-cm curette to scrape the bulk of the lesion. Removal of a bulk of the tissue is possible due to the ability to feel the softer "feel" of the skin cancer while curetting. This change in skin integrity is due to the decreased intracellular bonds of tumor cells compared with noncancerous tissue, allowing the skin to easily break apart. Electrodessication, or alternatively heat cautery, then follows and destroys any residual tumor cells at the base and rim of at least 0.2 cm around the lesion. Electrodessication also provides hemostasis as an added benefit [48, 49]. For adequate treatment, three cycles are often performed [50]. Treatment using ED&C is generally contraindicated in lesions that are invasive, as well as those with complex morphology [51]. Recurrence rates are approximately 4% [52–56]. One important drawback to this technique is that it does not provide a specimen for histological assessment, and therefore is not an ideal treatment for high-risk lesions that need margin control. Another drawback for lesions treated with ED&C is that sites are left to heal by secondary intention, causing a scar that is often hypopigmented and potentially hypertrophic compared to a lesion treated with standard excision and closed by primary intention.

Surgical Excision

Surgical excision involves the removal, usually in the form of an ellipse, around the lesion as well as an adequate, usually standard, normal tissue margin. Margins are commonly assessed postoperatively with formalin-fixed, paraffin-embedded tissue, though intraoperative frozen section can be performed as well [46]. This treatment modality is commonly performed for both SCC and BCC. The NCCN guidelines have reported that for low-risk BCC less than 2 cm in diameter, surgical excision with at least a 0.4-cm margin should result in complete removal in more than 95% of cases [50, 57]. The NCCN guidelines do not define a surgical excision margin recommendation for high-risk BCC due to the wide variability of tumor histology, location, and patient factors [50].

For a well-differentiated SCC, smaller than 2 cm, studies have shown that a minimum margin of 0.4 cm around the clinical border is appropriate, with a ~5-year local recurrence rate ranging from 5 to 8%. A 0.6–1.0-cm margin is required for tumors 2 cm and larger. The aforementioned are for sites that do not include the ears, eyelids, lips, nose, and scalp, as well as involvement of deeper tissue including subcutaneous fat [58].

MMS is favored, especially in higher risk lesions and/or sites, deep margin involvement and recurrences, particularly cases that involve large margins in areas such as the face, hands and feet which may compromise cosmetic units and functionality [47, 59]. Possible disadvantages of a standard surgical excision are similar in nature to other surgical procedures such as increased cost, postoperative pain, longer times out of work, poor wound healing, scarring, and infection [47].

Mohs Micrographic Surgery

MMS is a specialized technique that entails removing one thin layer of tissue at a time and intraoperatively reviewing the histologic specimen and margins for the presence of skin cancer. In doing so, 100% of the tumor margin can be assessed due to unique tissue preparation sectioning; this is in contrast to the less than 2% tumor margin assessed utilizing the standard histologic technique [60]. This allows the tumor to be excised while minimizing removal of surrounding normal tissue and offering superior results in areas where normal tissue salvage is desired [60]. Use of this technique is guided by a number of factors, most importantly risk stratification. Locations of tumors can be divided into three areas: low, medium, and high risk. High-risk areas include the ear, periauricular site, eyebrows, eyelids, nose, lips, chin, hands, nails, areola, genitalia, and ankles. Areas of medium-risk include head, neck, and pretibial surfaces. Low-risk sites include the trunk and extremities. Mohs is generally reserved for tumors arising in high- and medium-risk areas, aggressive tumors arising in low-risk areas as well as high-risk patients [61].

Overall, the unique technique of MMS can produce the highest cure rate with minimized scar outcome compared to other surgical treatments [60]. MMS remains the gold standard for the surgical management of NMSC. Rowe et al. reviewed over 10,000 cases of primary BCC treated with either standard surgical excision or MMS and revealed that long-term (>5 years) recurrence rates are 1.0% for MMS versus 10.1% for surgical excision [40]. Similar investigations have been documented for the treatment of SCC with recurrence rates of 3.1% for Mohs surgery versus 10.9% for surgical excision [41]. For high-risk primary NMSC, cryotherapy and ED&C are inappropriate treatment choices given the high recurrence rates [42, 43].

Non-surgical

Medical therapies, such as topical applications, have generally been reserved for lower risk lesions, most commonly for the treatment of AKs. On the other hand, while most patients with BCC and SCC are treated with surgical means, certain patient populations present with aggressive and widespread disease, which makes treatment by conventional modalities difficult [62]. As such, chemotherapy is typically reserved for patients with metastatic or locally advanced disease that may not be amenable to surgical and/or radiation therapies.

Topical Therapies for Actinic Keratoses

Cryotherapy is used in individuals with few lesions, whereas individuals with multiple lesions may benefit from field therapy with application of topical medication.

- 5-FU is a pyrimidine analogue that inhibits thymidylate synthase, an enzyme needed for DNA synthesis. The Food and Drug Administration (FDA) has approved 0.5 and 5% topical preparations for use. Both preparations demonstrate similar outcomes with approximately 50% of patients achieving complete clearance when applied twice daily for 2–4 weeks [63]. Adverse local skin reactions include erythema, erosions, and dryness [63].
- Imiquimod is an immune system modulator, specifically a toll-like receptor 7 (TLR-7) agonist that promote a Th1-type immune response. Preparations approved by the FDA include 2.5, 3.75, and 5%. Approximately 50% of patients achieve complete clearance with biweekly and triweekly applications for 16 weeks [64, 65]. Studies have not shown a statistically significant difference between treatment regimens [63]. Adverse local skin reactions are comparable to similar topical treatments including erythema, scabbing, or crusting and erosions or ulceration and are worse with prolonged regimens [64–66].
- Diclofenac is a nonsteroidal anti-inflammatory drug, shown to be effective by inducing cellular apoptosis [67]. Treatment consists of twice-daily application of 3% gel for 90 days. Although mixed results regarding clearance rates exist, diclofenac has been reported to be moderately efficacious with complete clearance of no more than 30% [68]. Overall, the therapy is well tolerated with rash, pruritus, and dry skin as the most commonly reported adverse effects. Effects on the nervous system, such as paresthesia and hyperesthesia, though less common, have also been associated with diclofenac use [69, 70].
- Ingenol mebutate is an agent that induces cell death and is one of the newest therapies, approved in 2012. Treatment consists of application of either 0.05 or 0.015% gel once daily for 2–3 consecutive days depending on the treatment site. Approximately 45% of patients

experience complete clearance [71]. Adverse events include local skin reactions including irritation, pain, and pruritus, most notable on day 3 and lasting up to 1 week after treatment [72, 73].

NMSC

As previously alluded to, SCC and BCC have traditionally been treated with surgical approaches. However, with a marked increase in research and expansion of medical management strategies for NMSC, tailoring to patient's preferences and comorbidities and considering alternative modalities has come to the forefront.

Topical Therapies for NMSC

- 5-FU has been approved for superficial BCC and SCCIS.
  - Superficial BCC: treatment regimen includes 5% solution applied twice daily for 3–6 weeks with complete clearance achieved in ~90% of individuals. Recurrence rates are ~10% [74].
  - SCCIS: treatment regimen includes 5% solution applied twice daily for 9 weeks yielding efficacy of 85%. A study found that 6 weeks is adequate to clear SCCIS in some patients; however, the authors concluded that a 9-week treatment plan is likely appropriate to keep recurrence rates low, and that modifications can be made based upon individual responses [75].
- Imiquimod 5% has been approved for superficial BCC and SCCIS.
  - Superficial BCC: treatment regimen includes topical solution applied daily for 6 weeks with 75–82% of individuals experiencing complete clearance. The recurrence rate for this type of treatment was found to be ~11% [76].
  - A few case studies have suggested imiquimod efficacy in nodular BCC 70–88% of participants experienced clearance, however, treatment with this modality is generally not accepted nor is it FDA approved for these types of skin cancers [76–78].
  - SCCIS: treatment regimen includes 5% solution applied twice daily for 8 weeks yielding efficacy of ~80% [75].
- Ingenol mebutate has shown limited evidence for use in superficial BCC [79].

There are currently no FDA approved treatment indications for intralesional therapy for NMSC as treatment regimens are variable and there is a limited research data on success.

- Therapies documented include methotrexate, bleomycin, 5-FU, and interferon.
  - Methotrexate injections have been studied to treat KAs. A small study was conducted using either 12.5 or 25 mg/mL until lesions are sufficiently infiltrated every 2 weeks. The study demonstrated ~90% efficacy after two treatments [80, 81].
  - Bleomycin injections have been studied in SCCIS, KA, and BCC using 0.5 mg/mL until lesions blanch. The frequency of injections varied in the study conducted. Treatment was found to have 100% efficacy; however, follow-up studies are necessary to confirm these results due to small sample sizes [80, 81].
  - 5-FU injections have been studied in BCC, KA, and SCC. 50 mg/mL was administered until lesion blanched, the average amount of weekly injections was 10. A small study conducted on BCC found 96% efficacy, while several publications on KA and SCC found similar efficacy of ~90% [80–82]. This treatment modality, and the use of methotrexate injections, may be useful in patients with multiple KA syndromes, as described previously in this chapter.
  - Recombinant interferon (INF), a type of cytokine involved in local cell signaling, has been studied in BCC, KA, SCC, and SCCIS. Treatment includes varying dosages given 3 times per week with an average of 3 weeks of use. Several reports support its use in BCC management and results are as follows: INF alpha-2b 76%,

INF beta 68%, INF gamma 22%. Fewer studies have been published for use in KA, SCC, and SCCIS, which have demonstrated ~90% efficacy; however, more studies are necessary to support these findings [80, 81].

Radiotherapy

Radiation therapy (RT) has been employed as a nonsurgical primary treatment option for NMSC and as an adjuvant treatment for high-risk tumors [31]. A disadvantage of RT as a primary treatment modality is that there is no histologic confirmation of tumor margins. As previously mentioned, patients may develop NMSC from the radiation treatment itself several years later after their treatment. Adjuvant RT is typically considered where there is a relatively high likelihood of residual tumor present, despite surgical treatment or in patients who are not optimal surgical candidates [31].

Systemic Therapy

Systemic therapy is typically recommended as an adjuvant treatment if surgical resection of BCC and SCC yields a histologic specimen with concerning characteristics such as positive margins, lymph node involvement, perineural or lymphovascular invasion, or if surgical and/or RT are deemed not possible in controlling the disease.

Chemotherapy

Chemotherapeutic (CRT) agents most commonly used include cisplatin alone or combined with 5-FU [83]. Given that these agents are nonselective, side effects of treatment can be quite significant. A few case studies report that SCC deemed to be unresectable might benefit from neoadjuvant RT and CRT. Therapies that have been documented in a series of case reports include cisplatin, bleomycin, methotrexate, 5-FU, and interleukin-22. Overall, there is limited evidence for their use in unresectable or metastatic SCC [84–87].

Targeted Therapies

EGFR receptor-focused therapies have been under recent investigational studies, as it is known that SCC tumors overexpress such receptors. Monoclonal antibodies including cetuximab, panitumumab, nimotuzumab and zalutumumab block the extracellular portion of the receptor, while small molecule tyrosine kinase inhibitors (TKIs) including gefitinib, erlotinib, lapatinib, and afatinib disrupt the intracellular signaling pathway. Currently, only cetuximab is FDA-approved for the treatment of head and neck SCC. In regard to BCC, hedgehog pathway inhibitors, including vismodegib and sonidegib, recently approved by the FDA for rare, unresectable BCC, have demonstrated appreciable response rates in the adjuvant and neoadjuvant setting [30, 88]. An overview of the pathway and currently approved inhibitors are discussed below.

Aberrant activation of the hedgehog-patched signaling pathway has been associated with the development of BCC. Critical components of this pathway include the PTCH gene, which when mutated, leads to production of an aberrant PTCH1 protein that normally binds and inhibits a seven-pass transmembrane G-protein receptor named Smoothened (SMO). Constitutive activation of SHH signaling by inactivating mutations in PTCH or activating mutations in SMO have been shown to lead to hereditary nevoid basal cell carcinoma syndrome. This complex pathway has been studied, leading to the discovery of Hedgehog pathway inhibitors like Vismodegib and Sonidegib, which bind SMO, preventing expression of transcription factors GLI1 and GLI2, inhibiting basal cell proliferation [21].

Vismodegib was approved in 2009; demonstrating a response rate of 30% for metastatic BCC and 43% for locally advanced BCC. The median duration of therapy for metastatic BCC is about 10 months. Common side effects reported include alopecia, dysgeusia, muscle spasms, weight loss, fatigue, decrease in appetite, nausea, and diarrhea [88].

Sonidegib, a more recent SHH inhibitor, has also proven to be efficacious. Support for the use of sonidegib over vismodegib for locally advanced BCC is due to an increased objective response rate of 47%. However, sonidegib is less promising than vismodegib in metastatic BCC, only demonstrating a 15.4% response rate. Side effects are generally more tolerable and include elevation in creatine phosphokinase and lipase, high blood pressure, weakness, and muscle spasms [89].

Immunotherapy

Recent advances in immunotherapy offer hopeful anticipation as a successful treatment of SCC. Therapies that block the circumvented "immune checkpoints" effect may thus heighten antitumor effects [90]. The CTLA-4 inhibitor, ipilimumab, and PD-1 inhibitors including nivolumab and pembrolizumab work through these pathways to help block the immunosuppressive effects of cancers [90].

In short, for systemic therapy, the bulk of evidence for oral therapy in NMSC appear to favor the neoadjuvant use of EGFR inhibitors for advanced SCC and adjuvant or neoadjuvant targeted hedgehog inhibitors for advanced BCC. Although data supporting adjuvant or systemic therapy in NMSC is limited, there are sufficient reports in the literature to suggest systemic agent benefit.

Other Treatments

Brachytherapy is becoming a more common method to treat SCC. Brachytherapy involves the direct application of a radioactive source to involved tissues. Given its recency and lack of long-term follow-up studies, long-term cure rate of brachytherapy is not yet known [91].

Photodynamic therapy is another treatment that involves the application of a photosensitizing agent on the skin followed by irradiation with a light source [92]. Currently, this treatment modality is approved by the FDA for the treatment of AKs, and rarely, for low-risk NMSC due to high recurrence rates [93, 94].

Conclusion

In summary, given the incidence of NMSC is increasing in prevalence, full recognition of these potentially life-threatening diseases is critical. As this chapter has described, surgical management is the mainstay treatment of NMSC. Appropriate and careful selection of the optimal surgical intervention is crucial, with careful consideration given to patient-specific factors, histologic features, as well as the risks versus benefits of the procedure. While a dermatologist primarily diagnoses as well as treats NMSC, a multidisciplinary team approach, especially in high-risk patients, is paramount for success.

References

1. Staples MP, Elwood M, Burton RC, Williams JL, Marks R, Giles GG. Non-melanoma skin cancer in Australia: the 2002 national survey and trends since 1985. Med J Aust. 2006;184(1):6–10.
2. Leffell DJ. The scientific basis of skin cancer. J Am Acad Dermatol. 2000;42(1 Pt 2):18–22.
3. Zanetti R, Rosso S, Martinez C, Nieto A, Miranda A, Mercier M, et al. Comparison of risk patterns in carcinoma and melanoma of the skin in men: a multi-centre case-case-control study. Br J Cancer. 2006;94(5):743–51.
4. Almahroos M, Kurban AK. Ultraviolet carcinogenesis in nonmelanoma skin cancer. Part I: incidence rates in relation to geographic locations and in migrant populations. Skinmed. 2004;3(1):29–35. quiz 35–6
5. Hemminki K, Zhang H, Czene K. Time trends and familial risks in squamous cell carcinoma of the skin. Arch Dermatol. 2003;139(7):885–9.
6. Karagas MR, Stannard VA, Mott LA, Slattery MJ, Spencer SK, Weinstock MA. Use of tanning devices and risk of basal cell and squamous cell skin cancers. J Natl Cancer Inst. 2002;94(3):224–6.
7. Lichter MD, Karagas MR, Mott LA, Spencer SK, Stukel TA, Greenberg ER. Therapeutic ionizing radiation and the incidence of basal cell carcinoma and squamous cell carcinoma. The New Hampshire Skin Cancer Study Group. Arch Dermatol. 2000;136(8):1007–11.

8. Ott C, Huber S. The clinical significance of cosmic radiation in aviation. Praxis. 2006;95(4):99–106.
9. Berg D, Otley CC. Skin cancer in organ transplant recipients: epidemiology, pathogenesis, and management. J Am Acad Dermatol. 2002;47(1):1–17. quiz 18–20
10. Comeau S, Jensen L, Cockfield SM, Sapijaszko M, Gourishankar S. Non-melanoma skin cancer incidence and risk factors after kidney transplantation: a Canadian experience. Transplantation. 2008;86(4):535–41.
11. Karagas MR, Cushing GL, Greenberg ER, Mott LA, Spencer SK, Nierenberg DW. Non-melanoma skin cancers and glucocorticoid therapy. Br J Cancer. 2001;85(5):683–6.
12. Clifford GM, Polesel J, Rickenbach M, Dal Maso L, Keiser O, Kofler A, et al. Cancer risk in the Swiss HIV Cohort Study: associations with immunodeficiency, smoking, and highly active antiretroviral therapy. J Natl Cancer Inst. 2005;97(6):425–32.
13. Kraemer KH, Lee MM, Andrews AD, Lambert WC. The role of sunlight and DNA repair in melanoma and nonmelanoma skin cancer. The xeroderma pigmentosum paradigm. Arch Dermatol. 1994;130(8):1018–21.
14. Summers CG. Albinism: classification, clinical characteristics, and recent findings. Optom Vis Sci. 2009;86(6):659–62.
15. Majewski S, Jablonska S. Skin autografts in epidermodysplasia verruciformis: human papillomavirus-associated cutaneous changes need over 20 years for malignant conversion. Cancer Res. 1997;57(19):4214–6.
16. Fine J-D, Mellerio JE. Extracutaneous manifestations and complications of inherited epidermolysis bullosa: part II. Other organs. J Am Acad Dermatol. 2009;61(3):387–402. quiz 403–4
17. Kimonis VE, Goldstein AM, Pastakia B, Yang ML, Kase R, DiGiovanna JJ, et al. Clinical manifestations in 105 persons with nevoid basal cell carcinoma syndrome. Am J Med Genet. 1997;69(3):299–308.
18. Bolognia JL, Brewer YP, Cooper DL. Bazex syndrome (acrokeratosis paraneoplastica). An analytic review. Medicine. 1991;70(4):269–80.
19. Castori M, Morrone A, Kanitakis J, Grammatico P. Genetic skin diseases predisposing to basal cell carcinoma. Eur J Dermatol. 2012;22(3):299–309.
20. Asgari MM, Ray GT, Geier JL, Quesenberry CP. Malignancy rates in a large cohort of patients with systemically treated psoriasis in a managed care population. J Am Acad Dermatol. 2017;76(4):632–8.
21. Bolognia J. Dermatology. 3rd ed. Philadelphia: Elsevier Saunders; 2012.
22. cancer.net. Skin cancer (Non-Melanoma): risk factors and prevention; 2016.
23. Yuspa SH. Cutaneous chemical carcinogenesis. J Am Acad Dermatol. 1986;15(5 Pt 1):1031–44.
24. Simeonova PP, LUSTER MI. Mechanisms of arsenic carcinogenicity: genetic or epigenetic mechanisms? J Environ Pathol Toxicol Oncol. Begell House. 2000;19(3):281–6.
25. Australian Cancer Network: CCA. Basal cell carcinoma, squamous cell carcinoma (and related lesions) – a guide to clinical management in Australia. Cancer Council Australia/Australian Cancer Network Sydney; 2008.
26. Freiman A, Bird G, Metelitsa AI, Barankin B, Lauzon GJ. Cutaneous effects of smoking. J Cutan Med Surg. 2004;8(6):415–23.
27. Iannacone MR, Wang W, Stockwell HG, O'Rourke K, Giuliano AR, Sondak VK, et al. Patterns and timing of sunlight exposure and risk of basal cell and squamous cell carcinomas of the skin--a case-control study. BMC Cancer. 2012;12:417.
28. Ulrich C, Jürgensen JS, Degen A, Hackethal M, Ulrich M, Patel MJ, et al. Prevention of non-melanoma skin cancer in organ transplant patients by regular use of a sunscreen: a 24 months, prospective, case-control study. Br J Dermatol. 2009;161(Suppl 3):78–84.
29. Wright TI, Spencer JM, Flowers FP. Chemoprevention of nonmelanoma skin cancer. J Am Acad Dermatol. 2006;54(6):933–46. quiz 947–50
30. Rudnick EW, Thareja S, Cherpelis B. Oral therapy for nonmelanoma skin cancer in patients with advanced disease and large tumor burden: a review of the literature with focus on a new generation of targeted therapies. Int J Dermatol. 2016;55(3):249–58. quiz 256, 258
31. Fu T, Aasi SZ, Hollmig ST. Management of high-risk squamous cell carcinoma of the skin. Curr Treat Options in Oncol. 2016;17(7):34.
32. Chen AC, Martin AJ, Choy B, Fernández-Peñas P, Dalziell RA, McKenzie CA, et al. A phase 3 randomized trial of Nicotinamide for skin-cancer chemoprevention. N Engl J Med. 2015;373(17):1618–26.
33. Marks R, Rennie G, Selwood TS. Malignant transformation of solar keratoses to squamous cell carcinoma. Lancet. 1988;1(8589):795–7.
34. Criscione VD, Weinstock MA, Naylor MF, Luque C, Eide MJ, Bingham SF. Actinic keratoses: natural history and risk of malignant transformation in the veterans affairs topical Tretinoin chemoprevention trial. Cancer. 2009;115(11):2523–30.
35. Gupta AK, Cooper EA, Feldman SR Jr, Fleischer AB Jr. A survey of office visits for actinic keratosis as reported by NAMCS, 1990–1999. National Ambulatory Medical Care Survey. Cutis. 2002;70(2 Suppl):8–13.
36. Yu RC, Pryce DW, Macfarlane AW, Stewart TW. A histopathological study of 643 cutaneous horns. Br J Dermatol. 1991;124(5):449–52.
37. Schwartz RA. Keratoacanthoma. J Am Acad Dermatol. 1994;30(1):1–19. quiz 20–2
38. Norgauer J, Rohwedder A, Schaller J. Human papillomavirus and Grzybowski's generalized eruptive keratoacanthoma. J Am Acad Dermatol. 2003;49(4):771–2.

39. NCCN. National Comprehensive Cancer Network Guidelines; 2017.
40. Network NCC. Basal cell carcinoma (version 1.2017).
41. August PJ. Cryotherapy of nonmelanoma skin cancer. Clin Dermatol. 1995;13(6):589–92.
42. Bahner JD, Bordeaux JS. Non-melanoma skin cancers: photodynamic therapy, cryotherapy, 5-fluorouracil, imiquimod, diclofenac, or what? Facts and controversies. Clin Dermatol. 2013;31(6):792–8.
43. Kuflik EG. Cryosurgery for skin cancer: 30-year experience and cure rates. Dermatol Surg. 2004;30(2 Pt 2):297–300.
44. Graham GF, Clark LC. Statistical analysis in cryosurgery of skin cancer. Clin Dermatol. 1990;8(1):101–7.
45. Kokoszka A, Scheinfeld N. Evidence-based review of the use of cryosurgery in treatment of basal cell carcinoma. Dermatol Surg. 2003;29(6):566–71.
46. Telfer NR, Colver GB, Morton CA. Guidelines for the management of basal cell carcinoma. Br J Dermatol. 2008;159(1):35–48.
47. Divine J, Stefaniwksy L, Reddy R, Padilla P, Hagele T, Patel NS, et al. A comprehensive guide to the surgical management of nonmelanoma skin cancer. Curr Probl Cancer. 2015;39(4):216–25.
48. Graham G. Electrodesiccation and curettage. In: Macfarlane D, editor. Skin cancer management. 1st ed. New York: Springer; 1988. p. 79–82.
49. Jackson R, Laughlin S. Electrodesiccation and curettage. In: Schwartz RA, editor. Skin cancer. 1st ed. New York: Springer. p. 292–5.
50. NCCN. Basal cell carcinoma (version 1.2017); 2017.
51. Jackson R. The treatment of skin cancer by electrodesiccation and curettage. J Surg Oncol. 1983;22(2):100.
52. Roenigk RK, Roenigk HH. Current surgical management of skin cancer in dermatology. J Dermatol Surg Oncol. 1990;16(2):136–51.
53. Honeycutt WM, Jansen GT. Treatment of squamous cell carcinoma of the skin. Arch Dermatol. 1973;108(5):670–2.
54. Motley R, Kersey P, Lawrence C. Multiprofessional guidelines for the management of the patient with primary cutaneous squamous cell carcinoma. Br J Plast Surg. 2003;56(2):85–91.
55. Rowe DE, Carroll RJ, Day CL. Prognostic factors for local recurrence, metastasis, and survival rates in squamous cell carcinoma of the skin, ear, and lip. Implications for treatment modality selection. J Am Acad Dermatol. 1992;26(6):976–90.
56. Silverman MK, Kopf AW, Grin CM, Bart RS, Levenstein MJ. Recurrence rates of treated basal cell carcinomas. Part 1: overview. J Dermatol Surg Oncol. 1991;17(9):713–8.
57. Wolf DJ, Zitelli JA. Surgical margins for basal cell carcinoma. Arch Dermatol. 1987;123(3):340–4.
58. Brodland DG, Zitelli JA. Surgical margins for excision of primary cutaneous squamous cell carcinoma. J Am Acad Dermatol. 1992;27(2 Pt 1):241–8.
59. Kimyai-Asadi A, Alam M, Goldberg LH, Peterson SR, Silapunt S, Jih MH. Efficacy of narrow-margin excision of well-demarcated primary facial basal cell carcinomas. J Am Acad Dermatol. 2005;53(3):464–8.
60. Narayanan K, Hadid OH, Barnes EA. Mohs micrographic surgery versus surgical excision for periocular basal cell carcinoma. Cochrane Database Syst Rev. 2014;12:CD007041.
61. Bogdanov-Berezovsky A, Cohen AD, Glesinger R, Cagnano E, Rosenberg L. Risk factors for incomplete excision of squamous cell carcinomas. J Dermatolog Treat. 2005;16(5–6):341–4.
62. Neville JA, Welch E, Leffell DJ. Management of nonmelanoma skin cancer in 2007. Nat Clin Pract Oncol. 2007;4(8):462–9.
63. Gupta AK, Paquet M, Villanueva E, Brintnell W. Interventions for actinic keratoses. Cochrane Database Syst Rev. 2012;12:CD004415.
64. Lebwohl M, Dinehart S, Whiting D, Lee PK, Tawfik N, Jorizzo J, et al. Imiquimod 5% cream for the treatment of actinic keratosis: results from two phase III, randomized, double-blind, parallel group, vehicle-controlled trials. J Am Acad Dermatol. 2004;50(5):714–21.
65. Szeimies R-MM, Gerritsen M-JPJ, Gupta G, Ortonne JP, Serresi S, Bichel J, et al. Imiquimod 5% cream for the treatment of actinic keratosis: results from a phase III, randomized, double-blind, vehicle-controlled, clinical trial with histology. J Am Acad Dermatol. 2004;51(4):547–55.
66. Korman N, Moy R, Ling M, Matheson R, Smith S, McKane S, et al. Dosing with 5% imiquimod cream 3 times per week for the treatment of actinic keratosis: results of two phase 3, randomized, double-blind, parallel-group, vehicle-controlled trials. Arch Dermatol. 2005;141(4):467–73.
67. Fecker LF, Stockfleth E, Nindl I, Ulrich C, Forschner T, Eberle J. The role of apoptosis in therapy and prophylaxis of epithelial tumours by nonsteroidal anti-inflammatory drugs (NSAIDs). Br J Dermatol. 2007;156(Suppl 3):25–33.
68. Metterle L, Russell JS, Patel NS. An overview of the medical management of nonmelanoma skin cancer. Curr Probl Cancer. 2015;39(4):226–36.
69. Wolf JE, Taylor JR, Tschen E, Kang S. Topical 3.0% diclofenac in 2.5% hyaluronan gel in the treatment of actinic keratoses. Int J Dermatol. 2001;40(11):709–13.
70. Gebauer K, Brown P, Varigos G. Topical diclofenac in hyaluronan gel for the treatment of solar keratoses. Australas J Dermatol. 2003;44(1):40–3.
71. Lebwohl M, Shumack S, Stein Gold L, Melgaard A, Larsson T, Tyring SK. Long-term follow-up study of ingenol mebutate gel for the treatment of actinic keratoses. JAMA Dermatol. 2013;149(6):666–70.
72. Anderson L, Schmieder GJ, Werschler WP, Tschen EH, Ling MR, Stough DB, et al. Randomized, double-blind, double-dummy, vehicle-controlled study of ingenol mebutate gel 0.025% and 0.05% for actinic keratosis. J Am Acad Dermatol. 2009;60(6):934–43.

73. Lebwohl M, Swanson N, Anderson LL, Melgaard A, Xu Z, Berman B. Ingenol mebutate gel for actinic keratosis. N Engl J Med. 2012;366(11):1010–9.
74. Arits AHH, Mosterd K, Essers BA, Spoorenberg E, Sommer A, De Rooij MJ, et al. Photodynamic therapy versus topical imiquimod versus topical fluorouracil for treatment of superficial basal-cell carcinoma: a single blind, non-inferiority, randomised controlled trial. Lancet Oncol. 2013;14(7):647–54.
75. Bargman H, Hochman J. Topical treatment of Bowen's disease with 5-Fluorouracil. J Cutan Med Surg. 2003;7(2):101–5.
76. Shumack S, Robinson J, Kossard S, Golitz L, Greenway H, Schroeter A, et al. Efficacy of topical 5% imiquimod cream for the treatment of nodular basal cell carcinoma: comparison of dosing regimens. Arch Dermatol. 2002;138(9):1165–71.
77. Schiessl C, Wolber C, Tauber M, Offner F, Strohal R. Treatment of all basal cell carcinoma variants including large and high-risk lesions with 5% imiquimod cream: histological and clinical changes, outcome, and follow-up. J Drugs Dermatol. 2007;6(5):507–13.
78. Williams HC, Bath-Hextall F, Ozolins M, Armstrong SJ, Colver GB, Perkins W, et al. Surgery versus 5% Imiquimod for nodular and superficial basal cell carcinoma: 5-year results of the SINS randomized controlled trial. J Invest Dermatol. 2017;137(3):614–9.
79. Siller G, Rosen R, Freeman M, Welburn P, Katsamas J, Ogbourne SM. PEP005 (ingenol mebutate) gel for the topical treatment of superficial basal cell carcinoma: results of a randomized phase IIa trial. Australas J Dermatol. 2010;51(2):99–105.
80. Chitwood K, Etzkorn J, Cohen G. Topical and intralesional treatment of nonmelanoma skin cancer: efficacy and cost comparisons. Dermatol Surg. 2013;39(9):1306–16.
81. Kirby JS, Miller CJ. Intralesional chemotherapy for nonmelanoma skin cancer: a practical review. J Am Acad Dermatol. 2010;63(4):689–702.
82. Kraus S, Miller BH, Swinehart JM, Shavin JS, Georgouras KE, Jenner DA, et al. Intratumoral chemotherapy with fluorouracil/epinephrine injectable gel: a nonsurgical treatment of cutaneous squamous cell carcinoma. J Am Acad Dermatol. 1998;38(3):438–42.
83. Jarkowski A, Hare R, Loud P, Skitzki JJ, Kane JM, May KS, et al. Systemic therapy in advanced cutaneous squamous cell carcinoma (CSCC): the Roswell Park experience and a review of the literature. Am J Clin Oncol. 2016;39(6):545–8.
84. Denic S. Preoperative treatment of advanced skin carcinoma with cisplatin and bleomycin. Am J Clin Oncol. 1999;22(1):32–4.
85. Guthrie TH, Porubsky ES, Luxenberg MN, Shah KJ, Wurtz KL, Watson PR. Cisplatin-based chemotherapy in advanced basal and squamous cell carcinomas of the skin: results in 28 patients including 13 patients receiving multimodality therapy. J Clin Oncol. 1990;8(2):342–6.
86. Sadek H, Azli N, Wendling JL, Cvitkovic E, Rahal M, Mamelle G, et al. Treatment of advanced squamous cell carcinoma of the skin with cisplatin, 5-fluorouracil, and bleomycin. Cancer. 1990;66(8):1692–6.
87. Santana AL, Felsen D, Carucci JA. Interleukin-22 and cyclosporine in aggressive cutaneous squamous cell carcinoma. Dermatol Clin. 2017;35(1):73–84.
88. Sekulic A, Migden MR, Oro AE, Dirix L, Lewis KD, Hainsworth JD, et al. Efficacy and safety of vismodegib in advanced basal-cell carcinoma. N Engl J Med. 2012;366(23):2171–9.
89. Migden MR, Guminski A, Gutzmer R, Dirix L, Lewis KD, Combemale P, et al. Treatment with two different doses of sonidegib in patients with locally advanced or metastatic basal cell carcinoma (BOLT): a multicentre, randomised, double-blind phase 2 trial. Lancet Oncol. 2015;16(6):716–28.
90. Honeychurch J, Cheadle EJ, Dovedi SJ, Illidge TM. Immuno-regulatory antibodies for the treatment of cancer. Expert Opin Biol Ther. 2015;15(6):787–801.
91. Cook J, Zitelli JA. Mohs micrographic surgery: a cost analysis. J Am Acad Dermatol. 1998;39(5 Pt 1):698–703.
92. Willey A, Mehta S, Lee PK. Reduction in the incidence of squamous cell carcinoma in solid organ transplant recipients treated with cyclic photodynamic therapy. Dermatol Surg. 2010;36(5):652–8.
93. Marmur ES, Schmults CD, Goldberg DJ. A review of laser and photodynamic therapy for the treatment of nonmelanoma skin cancer. Dermatol Surg. 2004;30(2 Pt 2):264–71.
94. Rhodes LE, de Rie M, Enström Y, Groves R, Morken T, Goulden V, et al. Photodynamic therapy using topical methyl aminolevulinate vs surgery for nodular basal cell carcinoma: results of a multicenter randomized prospective trial. Arch Dermatol. 2004;140(1):17–23.
95. Cherpelis BS, Marcusen C, Lang PG. Prognostic factors for metastasis in squamous cell carcinoma of the skin. Dermatol Surg. 2002;28(3):268–73.
96. Schmults CD, Karia PS, Carter JB, Han J, Qureshi AA. Factors predictive of recurrence and death from cutaneous squamous cell carcinoma: a 10-year, single-institution cohort study. JAMA Dermatol. 2013;149(5):541–7.
97. Jambusaria-Pahlajani A, Hess SD, Katz KA, Berg D, Schmults CD. Uncertainty in the perioperative management of high-risk cutaneous squamous cell carcinoma among Mohs surgeons. Arch Dermatol. 2010;146(11):1225–31.
98. Weinberg AS, Ogle CA, Shim EK. Metastatic cutaneous squamous cell carcinoma: an update. Dermatol Surg. 2007;33(8):885–99.
99. Kauvar AN, Arpey CJ, Hruza G, Olbricht SM, Bennett R, Mahmoud BH. Consensus for nonmelanoma skin cancer treatment, part II: squamous cell carcinoma, including a cost analysis of treatment methods. Dermatol Surg. 2015;41(11):1214–40.
100. Kauvar AN, Cronin T, Roenigk R, Hruza G, Bennett R. Consensus for nonmelanoma skin cancer treatment: basal cell carcinoma, including a cost analysis of treatment methods. Dermatol Surg. 2015;41(5):550–71.

Management of Non-melanoma Skin Cancers: Rare Subtypes

38

Michael Saco, Neil Alan Fenske, and Basil Cherpelis

Merkel Cell Carcinoma

Introduction

Merkel cell carcinoma (MCC), originally referred to as trabecular carcinoma by Toker [1], is a rare and highly aggressive form of neuroendocrine skin cancer [2, 3]. There is still ongoing debate regarding whether or not MCC truly originates from Merkel cells, specialized touch receptors in the skin [4]. Regardless of its derivation, however, early detection and treatment of MCC are paramount in management.

Epidemiology

The incidence of MCC in the United States increased from 0.22 per 100,000 in 1986 to 0.79 per 100,000 in 2011. Additionally, the mortality of MCC increased from 0.03 per 100,000 in 1986 to 0.43 per 100,000 in 2011 [3]. The increase in incidence has been attributed to multiple factors, including increased awareness of the clinical and histopathologic features of MCC resulting in more frequent and earlier diagnoses, as well as a greater proportion of individuals in the United States living into and past the eighth decade of life. Both incidence and mortality increased at a similar rate from 1986 to 2011, thus indicating a lack of improvement in MCC treatment options during this time period [3–5].

Clinical Features

MCC in the United States is slightly more prevalent in men and it presents with a mean age of onset of 74.9 years in a predominantly Caucasian population [3]. Clinically, the typical appearance of MCC is a solitary, asymptomatic, rapidly growing red-pink to violaceous-blue nodule, although the lesion may be skin-colored or yellowish-white and can sometimes be tender. Additionally, the lesion may grow slowly or may not have any noticeable change in size [6]. MCC is most commonly located on the head and neck region, followed by the extremities, all of which are areas of chronic sun exposure [7]. However, MCC can also arise in areas with less sun exposure, such as the trunk, buttocks, and genitalia [6].

Early detection and confirmatory biopsy of MCC are crucial in management. However, clinicians initially feel that more than half of lesions biopsied are benign, with the most common clinical impression listed being a cyst or acneiform lesion. Other diagnoses in the clinical differential include lipoma, dermatofibroma, pyogenic granuloma, basal cell carcinoma, squamous cell

M. Saco, M.D. (✉) · N. A. Fenske, M.D.
B. Cherpelis, M.D.
Department of Dermatology and Cutaneous Surgery, Morsani College of Medicine, University of South Florida, Tampa, FL, USA
e-mail: msaco@health.usf.edu; nfenske@health.usf.edu; bcherpel@health.usf.edu

A. I. Riker (ed.), *Melanoma*, https://doi.org/10.1007/978-3-319-78310-9_38

carcinoma, lymphoma, angiosarcoma, amelanotic melanoma, and adnexal tumors. MCC is rarely listed in the clinical impression of biopsied lesions, thus potentially explaining the frequent delay in diagnosis [6].

Risk Factors

Although Caucasian race represents a major risk factor for MCC, other variables that can increase the risk of MCC development usually do so by imparting some degree of immunosuppression. Namely, increasing age, chronic ultraviolet light exposure, solid organ transplantation, chronic lymphocytic leukemia (CLL), non-Hodgkin lymphoma (NHL) in men, ankylosing spondylitis, inflammatory bowel disease, Crohn's disease, and acquired immune deficiency syndrome (AIDS) have all been shown to increase the risk of developing MCC [5, 8–11]. Studies pertaining to human immunodeficiency virus (HIV) infection and the risk of developing MCC, however, have been conflicting [5, 8].

Merkel cell polyomavirus, first reported in 2008, is contained in approximately 80% of MCCs [12, 13]. Interestingly, Merkel cell polyomavirus has also been found in non-MCC cutaneous disorders and in normal-appearing skin of healthy individuals [14]. Research examining the role of Merkel cell polyomavirus in MCC pathogenesis is ongoing, but reports of monoclonal integration of Merkel cell polyomavirus DNA into the host genome suggest that Merkel cell polyomavirus integration is an early event and not a result of secondary infection of MCCs [15].

Pathology

On histopathology, MCC typically presents as a dermal nodule that can infiltrate into the subcutaneous fat and muscle. A grenz zone usually separates the dermal nodule from the overlying epidermis, but ulceration can sometimes be seen and epidermotropism has rarely been reported. Tumor cells appear as sheets and cords of small, monotonous, oval, darkly staining blue cells with round to oval nuclei, finely dispersed chromatin, small nucleoli, abundant mitotic figures, apoptotic cells, and scant cytoplasm [4, 16–19].

MCC can be difficult to distinguish from other poorly differentiated small blue cell tumors, such as melanoma, lymphoma, neuroblastoma, Ewing's sarcoma, retinoblastoma, and small cell carcinoma of the lung. Additionally, MCC can be mistaken for basal cell carcinoma given the basophilic appearance of the tumor. While presence of a grenz zone, a high mitotic rate, abundant mitotic figures, apoptotic cells, and absence of peripheral palisading of nuclei can help to distinguish MCC from basal cell carcinoma, immunohistochemistry is often needed to differentiate MCC from the other aforementioned small blue cell tumors [4, 16]. MCC is usually positive for cytokeratin 20 (CK20) and pancytokeratins AE1/AE3, as well as several neuroendocrine markers, such as synaptophysin, neuron-specific enolase, and chromogranin A. MCC is typically negative for S100, HMB-45, SOX-10, and Melan-A immunostains, thus differentiating it from melanoma. Positivity for CK20 and negative immunostaining for thyroid transcription factor 1 (TTF-1) strongly favors a diagnosis of MCC over small cell carcinoma of the lung, which is typically CK20 negative and TTF-1 positive [4, 17, 20, 21]. Increased p63 expression in MCC may be associated with a poorer prognosis, although results from different studies have not been consistently supportive of this association [4].

Treatment

Predicting survival and determining appropriate treatment for MCC begins with correct TNM staging [7, 22]. MCC has a high recurrence rate, with one study examining 240 patients showing locoregional recurrences in 30% of patients and distant metastases in 21% of patients [23]. Primary tumors ≤2 cm in diameter with no regional or distant metastases are associated with a five-year overall survival of 62.8%. The five-year overall survival drops to 54.6% in cases where the primary tumor is >2 cm in diameter in the absence of regional or distant metastases. The five-year overall survival rate decreases to less than 40% if the primary tumor has invaded fascia, muscle, cartilage, or bone; if there is regional lymph node metastasis; or if there is evidence of in-transit metastasis. Distant metastasis (i.e., spread beyond regional lymph nodes) portends a very poor prognosis and is associated with a five-year overall survival of 13.5% [7, 22].

Per the National Comprehensive Cancer Network (NCCN) guidelines [22], complete surgical excision of MCC remains the mainstay of treatment. Clinically apparent lymph nodes are defined as lymph nodes detectable through clinical inspection, palpation, or radiologic imaging. Ideally, in all cases of MCC, a sentinel lymph node biopsy (SLNB) should be performed for patients without clinically apparent lymph nodes, and a fine-needle aspiration (FNA) or core biopsy should be performed for patients with clinically apparent lymph nodes. If the FNA or core biopsy is negative, an open biopsy should be considered, with the results of the open biopsy being treated the same as the results of a SLNB. SLNBs, FNAs, core biopsies, and open biopsies should all include immunostaining with CK20 and pancytokeratins AE1/AE3 as part of their evaluations. Regardless of the method of surgical excision chosen, SLNB should be performed prior to definitive excision of the primary lesion given the importance of SLNB status in MCC staging, prognostication, and in potentially contributing to regional control. However, the impact of SLNB on overall survival is unclear [7, 22–26]. Per NCCN guidelines, the standard method for surgical excision is wide local excision (WLE) with 1–2 cm margins down to muscle fascia or pericranium when possible [22]. However, many experts feel that WLE should be performed with 2–3 cm margins given the propensity for lymphatic spread [27, 28]. Other methods of surgical excision, such as Mohs micrographic surgery, Mohs micrographic surgery with additional final margin assessment using permanent sections, and complete circumferential and peripheral deep margin assessment, may be considered for more extensive histologic margin assessment as long as they do not interfere with SLNB. In the setting of Mohs micrographic surgery, a debulked specimen of the central tumor should be sent for permanent sections to allow for accurate histopathologic staging [22, 29].

In instances where the SLNB, FNA, core biopsy, or open biopsy is positive, complete lymph node dissection (CLND) with brain MRI and PET/CT scans of the neck, chest, abdomen, and pelvis are recommended to evaluate the extent of lymph node and visceral organ involvement. If a PET/CT scan cannot be performed, CT or MRI with contrast is an acceptable alternative. Imaging can also be obtained whenever unresectable or metastatic disease is suspected based on the patient's history or physical exam [22].

In order to achieve a potentially better outcome, radiation therapy, whether treating the primary tumor site or draining nodal basin, is typically performed within a few weeks after surgery and should not be delayed. Adjuvant radiation to the primary tumor site is recommended in all cases of MCC. However, observation of the primary tumor site without adjuvant radiation can be considered in immunocompetent patients if the primary lesion is <1 cm and widely excised with no lymphovascular invasion or other risk factors identified. Conversely, in instances where complete tumor excision is not possible, surgery would result in significant morbidity, or the patient refuses surgery, radiation monotherapy of the primary tumor site may be considered for treatment [22, 30–34].

Radiation therapy to the draining nodal basin is recommended in all cases where neither a SLNB nor a CLND has been performed. Radiation therapy to the draining nodal basin is not required when the SLNB is negative, but it can be considered in patients with profound immunosuppression and in patients at risk for having a false negative SLNB. False negative SLNBs can be seen when SLNBs are performed incorrectly, SLN assessment is performed without immunostaining with CK20 and pancytokeratins AE1/AE3, and when there is anatomic distortion of lymphatic drainage patterns due to previous WLE. Additionally, the frequent presence of multiple SLN basins and aberrant lymphatic drainage patterns in the head and neck region increase the risk of obtaining a false negative SLNB in this anatomic region. Accordingly, if SLNB in the head and neck region is unsuccessful, radiation therapy to the draining nodal basin can be considered to treat potential subclinical disease. Radiation to the draining nodal basin is indicated when the SLNB is positive and a CLND is not performed. Of note, CLND is the preferred initial treatment for clinically apparent lymphadenopathy with MCC present on FNA, core biopsy, or open biopsy, followed by adjuvant radiation therapy if appropriate. In instances where a CLND is performed, adjuvant radiation therapy to the draining nodal basin is only indicated when multiple lymph nodes are involved or extracapsular extension is present [22, 30, 33, 34].

Chemotherapy for MCC is controversial and has not been shown to lead to improvement in overall survival [33, 34], although it may offer palliative benefit if the toxicities of the chemotherapeutic medications do not outweigh the palliative benefits. While some physicians advocate for chemotherapy if a patient has at least one clinically or radiologically visible lymph node shown to be positive for MCC, others only use palliative chemotherapy in patients with metastatic MCC. The most common chemotherapeutic regimen used is cisplatin or carboplatin with or without etoposide, but topotecan has been used in elderly patients. The cyclophosphamide, doxorubicin, and vincristine regimen has become less popular since it can cause significant toxicity [4, 22].

In a phase II, noncontrolled study, pembrolizumab, an anti-programmed death 1 (PD-1) monoclonal antibody, was given to adult patients with advanced MCC who had received no prior systemic therapy [35]. Out of 25 patients assessed, a 56% objective response rate, defined as percentage of patients who had either a partial or complete response confirmed radiologically, was found with pembrolizumab. Both patients positive and negative for Merkel cell polyomavirus responded to pembrolizumab. Moreover, whether or not the MCC being treated expressed PD-1 ligand (PD-L1) did not significantly affect response rate, despite the fact that pembrolizumab is a PD-1 inhibitor. The exact mechanism by which pembrolizumab treats MCC is still under investigation, and further research is needed to provide clarity [35].

Overall, given the complexity and aggressive nature of MCC, presenting the patient's case at a tumor board and enrolling the patient into a clinical trial are indicated if the patient has lymph node involvement detected either clinically or histopathologically, as well as in cases of distant metastatic disease [22].

Clinical follow-up visits for MCC patients are critical to monitor these patients since they are at high risk for recurrence. A total body skin exam and complete lymph node exam should be performed every 3–6 months for the first 2 years after diagnosis and then every 6–12 months thereafter. Imaging studies, as previously explained, should be performed based on clinical judgment. However, more frequent clinical monitoring and routine imaging should be considered in high-risk patients, such as immunosuppressed patients [22].

Ultimately, it is the job of the dermatologist to diagnose MCC promptly and to monitor these patients closely for recurrences. Although dermatologists can surgically treat MCC, this should be done in coordination with the surgical specialists on the treatment team in order to not interfere with performing the SLNB if indicated. Tumor boards allow for an excellent multidisciplinary approach to patient care, providing a platform for dermatologists, pathologists, surgeons, oncologists, and radiation-oncologists to work together to provide an individualized treatment plan for the patient.

Dermatofibrosarcoma Protuberans

Introduction

Dermatofibrosarcoma protuberans (DFSP) is a rare, locally aggressive sarcoma that is of intermediate malignancy. Although its derivation has been an issue of debate in the past, the current theory is that DFSP is of fibroblast origin. Its slow growth and nonspecific features often result in delays in diagnosis and treatment, making a high index of suspicion and adequate tissue sampling crucial in management [36–38].

Epidemiology

The overall incidence of DFSP in the United States steadily increased from 3.1 per million person-years in 1973–1977 to 3.5 per million person-years in 1978–1982 and then 4.2 per million person years in 1983–1987 [39]. Since then, the incidence has remained relatively steady, with the incidence rate from 2000 to 2010 calculated as 4.1 per million person-years [40]. Although the rate of local recurrence is relatively high, the 10-year relative survival is 99.1%. Older age and male gender have both been consistently associated with a higher all-cause mortality for DFSP [40, 41]. In one study [40], age was the strongest risk factor for increased all-cause mortality, with a statistically significant increased risk starting at 40 years of age and continuing to dramatically increase over time. Relative to the 19 years or younger group, the hazard ratios for all-cause mortality were 5.9 in the 40–59-year-old group, 30.9 in the 60–79-year-old group, and 168 in the 80 years or older group. The hazard ratio for all-cause mortality in the 20–39-year-old group was 1.7, which approached, but did not reach, statistical significance [40]. Other factors that have inconsistently been associated with a higher all-cause mortality for DFSP include African American race, tumor size ≥3.0 cm, and anatomic location on the limbs and head [40, 41].

Clinical Features

The majority of DFSP cases present between 20 and 59 years of age, but they can occur at any age, from birth to beyond the ninth decade of life. DFSP has a 1.14 times higher incidence in women than in men, and incidence among African Americans is almost twice as high as the incidence in Caucasians [40].

The most common anatomic location for DFSP is the trunk, followed by the proximal upper and lower limbs and, less commonly, the head and neck region. Although rare, DFSP can also occur in the genital region and on acral surfaces [37, 40, 42]. DFSP characteristically presents as a slowly growing, solitary, asymptomatic, indurated plaque that may be red-brown, violaceous, or skin-colored. As the plaque gradually enlarges over a period of months to decades, protuberant nodules develop within the plaque. The appearance of nodules within the plaque is often followed by accelerated growth, ulceration, bleeding, or pain. However, DFSP lesions may enlarge rapidly from onset. Other less common presentations of DFSP include the appearance of multiple primary lesions, a firm cutaneous nodule, a yellow sclerotic morpheaform plaque, a soft depressed plaque, and skin discoloration preceding the appearance of a clinically apparent mass. DFSP lesions are typically 1–5 cm in size, but lesions as large as 30 cm have been reported and satellite nodules can develop. While DFSP lesions are usually confined to the skin or subcutaneous tissue, they can be locally aggressive and invade underlying fascia, muscle, and bone [37, 41]. Although metastasis of DFSP is rare, when metastasis occurs, it is usually via hematogenous rather than lymphatic spread. Accordingly, lymph node metastases are unusual. The lungs are the most common site of metastasis, with soft tissue and bone representing two other commonly reported sites of metastasis [42, 43].

Clinically, DFSPs can be mistaken for keloids, dermatofibromas, lipomas, sarcoidosis, morpheaform basal cell carcinoma, desmoid tumor, morphea, or nodular fasciitis [37, 42].

Risk Factors

The cause of DFSP is currently unknown, and proposed predisposing factors, including a history of trauma, have been extensively debated, with no firm consensus having been reached [37, 39, 44].

Pathology

On histopathology, DFSP has the appearance of a well-differentiated fibrosarcoma. DFSP typically presents as a dense dermal spindle cell proliferation embedded in varying amounts of thin, delicate collagen fibers that destroys preexisting structures (e.g., adnexae) and infiltrates into the subcutaneous fat. The cells that comprise the proliferation are monotonous and have large nuclei, little pleomorphism, and a low to moderate number of mitotic figures. The deep dermal spindle cells are frequently arranged in cartwheel (cells radiating from a central acellular focus of collagen) or storiform/mat-like (cells arranged into irregular, interwoven fascicles) patterns. DFSPs frequently penetrate deep into the subcutaneous fat, resulting in a honeycomb pattern of tentacle-like strands of tumor cells invading into the fat, or a multilayered sandwich pattern of spindle cells oriented parallel to the skin surface. Furthermore, longstanding or recurrent DFSPs may invade into underlying fascia, muscle, and bone. Hemosiderin deposition, multinucleated giant cells, foamy histiocytes, and inflammatory infiltrates are uncommon. Angiolymphatic invasion and necrosis are rare, but dilated vascular spaces, hemorrhage, and cystic changes may occasionally be present. Small amounts of stromal mucin may be seen, typically just below the epidermis when present. Depending on the extent of tumor invasion into the epidermis, the epidermis may be ulcerated, atrophic, or normal in appearance [37, 42, 44].

The central portion of the DFSP is typically more cellular than the periphery. At the periphery of the lesion, irregular tentacle-like projections of tumor cells diffusely invade the dermis and subcutaneous tissue. Obtaining clear margins on excisions can be incredibly difficult because these peripheral extensions of neoplastic cells are significantly attenuated at their advancing edges and can potentially have a deceptively bland appearance that can be mistaken for normal collagen. Accordingly, the excision margins for DFSP are often inadequate and the recurrence rate is relatively high [37, 42, 44].

Immunostaining can be helpful in the histopathologic workup of DFSP. Classically, DFSP can be distinguished from a dermatofibroma since DFSP typically stains positively for CD34 and negatively for factor XIIIa, whereas the immunostaining pattern for a dermatofibroma is the opposite. Additionally, stromolysin-3 is typically strongly positive in dermatofibromas, but it is usually either negative or weakly positive in DFSPs [42, 45]. Of note, areas of fibrosarcomatous change within DFSP can be negative for CD34, and most or all of the tumor may be CD34 negative if there is a high proportion of fibrosarcomatous change within the DFSP lesion [44]. In cases with equivocal lesions despite adequate tissue sampling, additional immunostaining with apolipoprotein D, nestin, and cathepsin K can be used, as well as fluorescence in situ hybridization (FISH) or PCR for the characteristic translocation of collagen type I alpha 1 (COL1A1) on chromosome 17q22 with platelet-derived growth factor beta (PDGFB) on chromosome 22q13 to form the chimeric oncogenic fusion gene t(17;22)(q22;q13) [38]. The COL1A1-PDGFB fusion gene has been found in 72–100% of DFSP lesions, including those with and without fibrosarcomatous change, depending on the series examined [46].

Several histologic variants of DFSP exist. Pigmented DFSPs, also known as Bednar tumors, contain a variable number of melanin-containing dendritic cells, comprise 1–5% of all DFSPs, and do not appear to differ from the classic type of DFSP in terms of prognosis. Other histologic variants that may also have a different appearance clinically but do not seem to differ in terms of overall prognosis when compared to conventional DFSPs include myxoid, myoid, atrophic, sclerosing, and granular cell DFSPs, as well as giant cell fibroblastoma, a DFSP variant typically seen in the pediatric population [37, 42, 44, 46]. However, 10–20% of DFSP lesions can develop foci of fibrosarcomatous change (DFSP-FS) and, consequently, tend to possess a more aggressive biologic behavior. Fibrosarcomatous changes include a characteristic fascicular, frequently herringbone architecture, abundant cytologic atypia, increased mitotic rate (>5–10 mitoses per high-power field), hypercellularity, a compressive subcutaneous infiltration pattern, high p53 and Ki67 immunoreactivity, and focal or complete loss of CD34 expression [38, 43, 44, 46]. The designation of DFSP-FS is typically given if >5% of the surgical specimen possesses foci of fibrosarcomatous change [38]. Clinically, DFSP-FS is associated with a tumor size >4 cm, a median interval before diagnosis >5 years, and a much higher incidence of muscle invasion relative to DFSP without fibrosarcomatous changes [46]. In a 2014 systematic review [43], DFSP-FS, when compared with DFSP without fibrosarcomatous changes, was found to have a significantly higher rate of local recurrence (29.8 vs. 13.7%), metastasis (14.4 vs. 1.1%), and death from disease (14.7 vs. 0.8%). Interestingly, the rates of local recurrence, metastasis, and death from disease in DFSP-FS did not differ significantly based on the proportion of fibrosarcomatous change within the tumor [43].

The histopathologic differential diagnosis of DFSP includes fibrosarcoma, atypical fibroxanthoma, malignant fibrous histiocytoma, dermatofibroma, leiomyoma, leiomyosarcoma, and nodular fasciitis. These other lesions, however, typically differ from DFSP in terms of histopathologic architecture and/or immunostaining patterns. Superficial biopsy samples often lead to either misdiagnosis or an equivocal pathologic diagnosis, requiring repeat biopsies and delays in care. Accordingly, a punch or incisional biopsy, preferably of the deeper subcutaneous fat, is recommended in order to avoid sampling error. Moreover, biopsying only the periphery of a DFSP lesion may cause the lesion to be misdiagnosed as a benign neural tumor histopathologically since the aforementioned histopathologic description of the periphery of a DFSP lesion can be mistaken for a type of diffuse neurofibroma that can have a pattern of infiltration into the subcutaneous fat similar to that seen in DFSP [37, 38].

Treatment

Treatment of DFSP is primarily surgical, with every effort made to obtain clear surgical margins regardless of the approach chosen. Radiation is generally avoided as first line treatment for DFSP due to the risk of inducing sarcomatous change and a more aggressive cancer. If Mohs micrographic surgery, with or without obtaining an additional final margin for permanent section assessment, is chosen, debulking specimens should be examined to detect fibrosarcomatous transformation if present. Two other surgical options include complete circumferential and peripheral deep margin assessment (CCPDMA) and wide local excision (WLE) with at least 2 cm margins down to investing fascia of muscle or pericranium with clear histopathologic margins obtained when clinically feasible [38]. Reviews comparing Mohs surgery with WLE in terms of treatment of DFSP have shown that Mohs surgery results in a lower recurrence risk and smaller postoperative defects. However, no difference in all-cause mortality between patients treated with Mohs surgery and patients treated with WLE has been shown [41, 46–50]. Moreover, assessing Mohs frozen sections for clear margins may be more difficult than assessing permanent sections, so many surgeons who treat DFSP with Mohs surgery will send a final stage after clearing the tumor with Mohs surgery for permanent section assessment [42]. Interestingly, although the National Comprehensive Cancer Network (NCCN) guidelines recommend at least 2 cm margins when WLE is used for DFSP treatment, WLE using 3 cm margins appears to be associated with a significantly lower risk of recurrence when compared to WLE using <3 cm margins [50]. Margin assessment may require both H&E sections and CD34 immunostaining in order to increase the likelihood of achieving negative surgical margins. Irrespective of the surgical approach, extensive undermining and tissue movement to repair the surgical defect should be avoided or delayed until negative histopathologic margins are confirmed in order to prevent potential tumor seeding. An MRI with contrast may be needed for treatment planning if there is suspicion for extensive extracutaneous spread.

If clear margins cannot be obtained surgically, radiation therapy extending 3–5 cm beyond the surgical margin is the preferred adjuvant therapy [38]. If the DFSP lesion is positive for the t(17;22) translocation, imatinib mesylate represents a potential alternative to radiation therapy; however, tumors without this translocation may not respond to imatinib therapy [38, 51].

Dermatologists should examine these patients every 6–12 months, focusing on the primary excision site for any evidence of recurrence.

Although metastasis is rare, the history and physical should also include assessment for any signs or symptoms that would prompt a more in-depth workup to rule out metastases (e.g., hemoptysis or other pulmonary symptoms in the event of lung metastasis). In patients who have had extensive reconstruction, MRI with contrast may help detect early recurrence. In the event of recurrence, potential treatment options include resection with or without adjuvant radiation therapy, radiation monotherapy if radiation was not previously given and resection is not possible, and consideration of imatinib therapy for patients with unresectable disease with tumors positive for the t(17;22) translocation [38, 51, 52]. In patients with metastatic disease, a multidisciplinary consultation is warranted to coordinate treatment. Based on the specific clinical circumstances, potential treatment options include clinical trials, imatinib, chemotherapy, radiation therapy, or resection when possible [38, 51, 52].

Management of DFSP with fibrosarcomatous changes (DFSP-FS) is primarily surgical, but a full discussion pertaining to treatment of DFSP-FS requires in-depth knowledge pertaining to soft-tissue sarcomas that is beyond the scope of this chapter [53].

Dermatologists play an integral role in DFSP management, with initial diagnosis, margin-controlled surgical treatment, and continued monitoring for new lesions or disease recurrence. In cases with extensive lesions, a multidisciplinary approach that includes surgical oncologists and plastic surgeons performing the surgical excision and/or reconstruction can often benefit the patient. Depending on the clinical scenario, including radiation-oncologists and oncologists as members of the treatment team may be indicated.

Atypical Fibroxanthoma

Introduction

Atypical fibroxanthoma (AFX) is an uncommon, intermediate-grade, superficial fibrohistiocytic tumor. Although AFX has been considered a superficial variant of undifferentiated pleomorphic sarcoma (UPS, formerly known as malignant fibrous histiocytoma), some physicians consider AFX and UPS to be two completely separate lesions. As of yet, a consensus has not been reached, and the debate continues to be controversial [54, 55].

Epidemiology

In one study, the incidence rate of malignant fibrous histiocytoma (MFH) from 1992 to 2004 was 1.5 per 1,000,000 person-years, with a decline in the incidence of MFH starting in 2000 [56]. The decline in MFH incidence may be due to the restructuring of nomenclature from the term MFH (which included AFX) into AFX and UPS as separate entities. Data from this same study showed that MFH had a male:female ratio of 4.7 and a 5-year relative survival of 89%. The data also indicated that MFH affects predominantly Caucasians since approximately 97% of the MFH cases reported in the Surveillance, Epidemiology, and End Results (SEER) Program Registries were in Caucasian patients. MFH most commonly occurs in the head and neck region, and less commonly on the upper extremities, followed by the lower extremities and trunk. The incidence of MFH increased exponentially with age starting in the fourth decade of life, with more rapid increases noted during the fifth to sixth decades of life that continued to trend upward at a similar rate [56]. Given the controversy pertaining to how AFX should be classified resulting in some AFX lesions being classified as UPS and vice versa, determining the incidence of AFX is incredibly difficult. This task is made even more difficult by the fact that, although MFH is reportable to SEER, AFX is not [56].

Clinical Features

Demographic data pertaining to AFX is limited mostly to large case series. Approximately 80% of AFX cases occur on the head and neck (sun-exposed areas), while approximately 20% of cases occur on the limbs and trunk (non-sun-exposed areas). AFX can also occur in unusual anatomic locations, such as the ocular surface, the cornea, the eyelid, and the ethmoid sinus. In one case series, AFX lesions on the head and neck were found to have a median age of 69, while lesions on the limbs and trunk were found to have a median age of 39. In this same case series, AFX lesions were found predominantly in Caucasians, regardless of anatomic location [54, 57, 58]. Although the percentages have varied based on the case series, a consistent male predominance has been observed [54].

AFX typically presents as a solitary, red or pink, firm papule or nodule. The lesions are usually asymptomatic, but can sometimes ulcerate, bleed, or cause pain or pruritus. Lesion diameter is typically 1–1.5 cm, and most lesions are less than 2 cm in diameter. However, lesions as large as 10 cm in diameter have been reported. Extremity and trunk lesions are typically larger and have less defined borders; they may also grow more slowly and have a more nodular appearance relative to head and neck lesions [54, 57, 59]. Rare cases of metastatic disease have been reported in the regional lymph nodes, lungs, liver, and peritoneum, as well as cutaneous or subcutaneous metastatic disease. Local recurrence of the tumor is often seen in cases of metastatic disease. The estimated metastatic rate for AFX is approximately 0.5–4%. However, the true incidence of AFX is debatable since some of the tumors diagnosed as AFX may have actually been UPS lesions [54].

Since AFX has a nondescript appearance, the clinical diagnosis is rarely made preoperatively. The clinical differential diagnosis is broad and includes basal cell carcinoma, squamous cell carcinoma, pyogenic granuloma, and Merkel cell carcinoma. Pigmented AFX lesions can also mimic melanoma or pigmented basal cell carcinoma [54].

Risk Factors

Since AFX most commonly occurs on sun-exposed areas, ultraviolet radiation exposure likely plays a major role in the pathogenesis of AFX. Additionally, sites of chronic radiation dermatitis from prolonged therapeutic or occupational exposure are at increased risk for developing an AFX, typically more than 10 years after a site has been irradiated. Immunosuppression seen in chronic lymphocytic leukemia, transplant patients, and patients with HIV or AIDS represents another potential risk factor for developing AFX [10, 54, 60, 61].

Pathology

AFX is a dermal proliferation of pleomorphic spindle cells and epithelioid cells in varying proportions admixed with multinucleated giant cells within a collagenous matrix and background solar elastosis. Atypical mitotic figures with severe pleomorphism and hyperchromatism are frequently observed. The lesion can sometimes be contiguous with the epidermis, and occasionally, foam cells are present that can extend up to the epidermis. Conversely, the dermal proliferation may abut and be separated from the epidermis by a thin zone of collagen. The overlying epidermis is often thin and flattened or ulcerated [54, 61, 62].

On immunohistochemistry, AFX is typically positive for vimentin, alpha-1-antitrypsin, CD10, CD68, and procollagen 1. It is variably positive for CD99, CD117, LN-2 (CD4), CD31, CD34, SMA, and EMA. However, AFX is usually negative for HMB-45, S-100, Sox10, Melan-A, cytokeratins, and desmin [62, 63].

The histopathologic differential diagnosis includes similar-appearing spindle cell tumors, such as UPS, spindle cell squamous cell carcinoma, desmoplastic melanoma, and leiomyosarcoma. The majority of these tumors can be differentiated from AFX based on histopathologic features or immunohistochemistry [61]. Distinguishing between AFX and UPS is more controversial, with some physicians relying on histopathologic features over immunohistochemistry, while others favor immunohistochemistry over histopathologic features in order to determine the diagnosis. A recent study comparing

169 AFX patients with 7 UPS patients found that LN2 (CD74), CD10, and ezrin immunostains were unable to distinguish AFX from UPS [64]. Currently, AFX is differentiated from UPS by its dermal location and its pushing growth pattern, whereas UPS invades the subcutaneous fat and deeper structures underneath. Since AFX is rarely on the clinical differential prior to biopsy, most biopsies are superficial shave biopsies with the tumor transected at the base. Accordingly, differentiation between AFX and UPS is usually made postoperatively. However, development of recurrence or metastatic disease could potentially cause the diagnosis to be changed from AFX to UPS since AFX rarely metastasizes and UPS is an aggressive tumor [64].

Treatment

Although there are no standardized guidelines for staging or treating AFX, no imaging is typically required and the primary treatment is surgical [61]. The reported local recurrence rate after surgical treatment of AFX has ranged from 0 to 16%. Lower recurrence rates have typically been reported with Mohs surgery compared to wide local excision (WLE), although the numbers used in comparative studies are relatively small. Two centimeter WLE margins are typically required to achieve clear margins, so Mohs surgery has been recommended by some authors to especially be used for head and neck lesions and in other areas where tissue sparing is crucial. Not enough data are available to determine if Mohs surgery is associated with an improved mortality compared to WLE [54, 58, 59, 65–69]. Also, no strong data are available to support performing a sentinel lymph node biopsy in patients diagnosed with AFX [61]. Radiation therapy is typically used as adjunctive treatment for recurrent or metastatic disease. Metastatic disease treatment needs to be tailored to the patient, with some patients requiring radical neck dissections, radiation, parotidectomy, or systemic chemotherapy. Accordingly, patients diagnosed with metastatic AFX would benefit from a multidisciplinary approach to management, involving dermatology, surgical oncology, medical oncology, radiation oncology, and possibly plastic surgery [54]. Any patients diagnosed with AFX should have a total body skin examination performed at least every 6 months in order to check for recurrence at the surgical site, as well as for any new lesions and lymphadenopathy [54].

The rates of recurrence, metastasis, and mortality associated with AFX are much less substantial relative to the aforementioned rates seen in UPS [70]. Moreover, although the primary treatment for UPS is still surgical, treatment with radiation and/or chemotherapy may also be necessary. Further discussion regarding UPS treatment is beyond the scope of this chapter [62].

Sebaceous Carcinoma

Introduction

Sebaceous carcinoma is a rare and aggressive malignancy derived from the adnexal epithelium of sebaceous glands. Due to some differences in biologic behavior based on anatomic location, sebaceous carcinoma is separated into ocular/periorbital and extraocular/extraorbital types. Sebaceous carcinoma has been shown to have a high rate of recurrence after excision, and it also possesses the capacity for regional and distant metastasis [71, 72].

Epidemiology

The incidence of sebaceous carcinoma among Caucasians is almost three times the rate seen in other racial groups, and more than 75% of patients are 60 years of age or older at the time of diagnosis. One study showed a statistically significant 3.31% annual increase in the overall incidence of sebaceous carcinoma from 2000 to 2012, which was primarily due an increase in the incidence of sebaceous carcinoma among men during this time period [73]. The overall incidences per 100,000 person-years of sebaceous carcinoma were 0.32 in men, 0.16 in women, and 0.23 in men and women combined. From 2000 to

2012, five-year relative survival for all types of sebaceous carcinoma was 92.72% and 10-year relative survival was 86.98%. A higher all-cause mortality has been associated with male gender, African American race, and extraocular anatomic location [73]. Further studies should be performed to support extraocular anatomic location as a risk factor for higher all-cause mortality, especially since periocular sebaceous carcinoma has been shown to have a 3% higher rate of nodal and/or distant metastasis relative to extraocular sebaceous carcinoma [73, 74]. Data are lacking to determine whether periorbital sebaceous carcinoma has a greater risk of local recurrence than extraocular sebaceous carcinoma since most of the data pertaining to sebaceous carcinoma has historically focused on the periorbital rather than extraorbital subtype. However, certain histopathologic features that are associated with a higher risk of local recurrence, such as pagetoid spread and multicentricity, are more commonly seen in periorbital sebaceous carcinoma than in the extraocular subtype [72, 75].

Although most cases of sebaceous carcinoma are not associated with Muir-Torre Syndrome (MTS), up to 30% of patients with MTS present with a sebaceous carcinoma. Accordingly, sebaceous carcinoma can be used as one of the diagnostic criteria for MTS. As a result of the defects in DNA mismatch repair genes and the resultant microsatellite instability seen in MTS, patients with MTS have an increased incidence of developing colorectal carcinoma, genitourinary tumors, breast carcinoma, and hematologic disorders [72, 76].

Clinical Features

The most common anatomic location of sebaceous carcinoma is ocular, but extraocular sebaceous carcinomas as a whole are more common than ocular sebaceous carcinomas. Upper eyelids are the most common location for periorbital sebaceous carcinoma. Extraocular sebaceous carcinomas are most commonly located in the head and neck region since this is where the greatest number of sebaceous glands are located. Less common cutaneous locations for sebaceous carcinoma include the trunk, extremities, and genitalia [71–73, 77].

Clinically, sebaceous carcinomas are difficult to diagnose given the diversity of their presentations, often leading to a delay in diagnosis averaging between 1 and 2.9 years. Periorbital sebaceous carcinoma can be especially misleading, often easily mistaken for a chalazion, blepharoconjunctivitis, or keratoconjunctivitis. It most commonly presents as a painless subcutaneous eyelid nodule, but can also present with eyelid thickening or, rarely, as a pedunculated eyelid mass. Given the subtlety of the presentation of periorbital sebaceous carcinoma, an eyelid biopsy is warranted in cases of recurrent chalazion, eyelid thickening or eversion, loss of eyelashes, and eyelid ulceration in order to rule out this neoplasm. Extraorbital sebaceous carcinoma typically presents as a painless yellow or pink nodule, but can also present as flesh-colored or red papules, nodules, or plaques. Clinically, the differential diagnosis includes benign sebaceous lesions, basal cell carcinoma, squamous cell carcinoma, Merkel cell carcinoma, and amelanotic melanoma [72].

Regional lymph nodes are the most common sites of metastasis. Distant metastasis can involve the lung, liver, bone, or brain, with most reported cases of distant metastasis developing within the first 2 years after initial treatment [72]. Although reported rates of regional and distant metastasis were historically high, more recent data estimated that the rates of nodal and/or distant metastasis were 1.4% for extraorbital sebaceous carcinoma and 4.4% for periorbital sebaceous carcinoma [74]. The most significant predictor for increased mortality is development of metastatic disease, emphasizing the importance of prompt diagnosis and treatment [72].

Risk Factors

Age has been reported to be a likely risk factor for developing sebaceous carcinoma since most cases occur in patients 60 years of age or older. Sebaceous carcinoma has been associated with

MTS, a history of irradiation, immunosuppression, and familial retinoblastoma. Sebaceous carcinoma has also been reported to occur within nevus sebaceous lesions, albeit rarely. Prior associations with female gender and Asian race have not been substantiated in more recent studies, which instead support an increased incidence in Caucasian males [72, 73, 78].

Pathology

Sebaceous carcinoma presents as a lobular, unencapsulated, dermally based collection of sebaceous cells and undifferentiated cells. The cells have a characteristic "frothy" appearance due to lipid granules in the cytoplasm, which stain positively with Sudan black and oil red O. Cytologically, nuclear pleomorphism and hyperchromatism, as well as mitotic figures, are seen. Pagetoid spread and multicentricity, both features that may be associated with an increased risk of recurrence, are more commonly seen in periorbital sebaceous carcinomas than in extraocular sebaceous carcinomas. Intraepithelial spread is another histopathologic feature that can potentially lead to an increased risk of local recurrence. Poor prognosis has been associated with pagetoid spread, multicentric origin, poorly differentiated or undifferentiated lesions, and angiolymphatic or perineural invasion. Other high-risk features specific to extraocular sebaceous carcinoma include tumor thickness >2 mm, Clark level ≥ IV, and primary site on the lip or ear. In contrast, tumors involving the eyelid or tarsal plate are considered high-risk features for periocular sebaceous carcinomas [72, 79].

The histopathologic differential diagnosis for sebaceous carcinoma includes benign sebaceous lesions and neoplasms that exhibit pagetoid spread, such as melanoma and squamous cell carcinoma in situ. Although differentiation between sebaceous carcinoma and benign sebaceous lesions is often based on differences in histopathologic architecture and cytologic features, some cases can present a diagnostic challenge. In these scenarios, p53 and Ki-67 immunostains can be utilized, with sebaceous carcinoma more frequently showing overexpression of these markers than sebaceous adenomas. Differentiation between sebaceous carcinoma and other malignancies may require the use of immunohistochemistry, with EMA, Cam 5.2, adipophilin, and perilipin largely replacing fat stains like oil red O, which have a decreased sensitivity after formalin fixation [71, 72, 80].

Treatment

TNM staging differs based on whether the sebaceous carcinoma is of the periocular or extraocular subtype [72]. Unless patients are poor surgical candidates, surgery is the initial treatment of choice regardless of the patient's stage at the time of diagnosis. Wide local excision (WLE) with 5–6 mm margins is the standard treatment. Orbital exenteration is reserved for cases in which imaging shows unresectable orbital soft tissue invasion. WLE has been associated with a relatively high recurrence rate, ranging from 4 to 28% over the past two decades. Mohs surgery for the treatment of sebaceous carcinoma has been associated with relatively lower recurrence rates overall, with some of the larger series reporting recurrence rates ranging from 0 to 11%. However, additional data is needed to make a more accurate comparison between WLE and Mohs surgery in the treatment of sebaceous carcinoma. Due to the tendency for intraepithelial spread seen with sebaceous carcinoma, some physicians have advocated evaluation of a final peripheral margin with permanent sections. Additional tissue may be taken and sent for permanent sections to confirm clear margins if deemed necessary by the operating surgeon. The benefit of excising additional tissue must be weighed against the increased morbidity that may result, especially in vital areas such as the eyelid. Locally recurrent disease is typically treated with surgical re-excision and possibly adjuvant radiation. Unless patients are poor surgical candidates, radiation therapy is rarely used as a primary treatment modality, especially since radiation therapy performed near the eye can cause a multitude of issues, including permanent vision loss [72, 75,

78, 81–85]. Shielding of the eye can help reduce these complications.

Although there have been differing opinions regarding whether or not to perform a sentinel lymph node biopsy (SLNB) for sebaceous carcinoma, multiple authors have advocated performing a SLNB for periorbital sebaceous carcinomas >10 mm in diameter but not routinely for extraocular sebaceous carcinomas. A positive SLNB necessitates complete regional lymph node dissection and adjuvant radiation given the aggressive nature of this neoplasm [72, 74, 86–88].

As already mentioned, regional metastasis is typically treated with regional lymph node dissection followed by adjuvant radiation. Parotidectomy is included as part of the regional lymphadenectomy in cases of periocular sebaceous carcinoma. Given the potentially high morbidity associated with radiation therapy, radiation should be reserved for recurrent tumors, metastatic disease, or palliative therapy. Reports of chemotherapy used to treat metastatic sebaceous carcinoma are limited to a small number of case reports [72].

Little information is available regarding recommendations for imaging in cases of sebaceous carcinoma. A PET/CT scan should be considered in cases of a positive SLNB or palpable regional lymphadenopathy prior to performing a radical lymph node dissection. Advanced imaging can also be considered for both periocular and extraocular sebaceous carcinoma if the aforementioned histopathologic high-risk features are present or if tumor diameter is >2 cm. Routine dermatologic monitoring is imperative, with follow-up imaging to be performed at the discretion of an oncologist [72].

Given the association of sebaceous carcinoma with MTS, all patients diagnosed with sebaceous carcinoma should undergo immunohistochemistry to assess for loss of mismatch repair genes. Any cases with loss of mismatch repair genes should have genotyping for microsatellite instability and referral to a geneticist. However, in patients with a personal or family history of malignancy, a genetics referral is strongly recommended regardless of the results of the aforementioned tests. Patients who are diagnosed with MTS should be encouraged to follow up with their primary care physicians to ensure that they are up to date on screening for malignancies associated with MTS [72].

References

1. Toker C. Trabecular carcinoma of the skin. Arch Dermatol. 1972;105(1):107–10.
2. Youlden DR, Soyer HP, Youl PH, Fritschi L, Baade PD. Incidence and survival for Merkel cell carcinoma in Queensland, Australia, 1993–2010. JAMA Dermatol. 2014;150(8):864–72. https://doi.org/10.1001/jamadermatol.2014.124.
3. Fitzgerald TL, Dennis S, Kachare SD, Vohra NA, Wong JH, Zervos EE. Dramatic increase in the incidence and mortality from Merkel cell carcinoma in the United States. Am Surg. 2015;81(8):802–6.
4. Brummer GC, Bowen AR, Bowen GM. Merkel cell carcinoma: current issues regarding diagnosis, management, and emerging treatment strategies. Am J Clin Dermatol. 2016;17(1):49–62. https://doi.org/10.1007/s40257-015-0163-3.
5. Ma JE, Brewer JD. Merkel cell carcinoma in immunosuppressed patients. Cancers. 2014;6(3):1328–50. https://doi.org/10.3390/cancers6031328.
6. Heath M, Jaimes N, Lemos B, Mostaghimi A, Wang LC, Penas PF, et al. Clinical characteristics of Merkel cell carcinoma at diagnosis in 195 patients: the AEIOU features. J Am Acad Dermatol. 2008;58(3):375–81. https://doi.org/10.1016/j.jaad.2007.11.020.
7. Harms KL, Healy MA, Nghiem P, Sober AJ, Johnson TM, Bichakjian CK, et al. Analysis of prognostic factors from 9387 Merkel cell carcinoma cases forms the basis for the new 8th edition AJCC staging system. Ann Surg Oncol. 2016;23(11):3564–71. https://doi.org/10.1245/s10434-016-5266-4.
8. Lanoy E, Costagliola D, Engels EA. Skin cancers associated with HIV infection and solid-organ transplantation among elderly adults. Int J Cancer. 2010;126(7):1724–31. https://doi.org/10.1002/ijc.24931.
9. Lanoy E, Dores GM, Madeleine MM, Toro JR, Fraumeni JF Jr, Engels EA. Epidemiology of nonkeratinocytic skin cancers among persons with AIDS in the United States. AIDS. 2009;23(3):385–93. https://doi.org/10.1097/QAD.0b013e3283213046.
10. Brewer JD, Shanafelt TD, Call TG, Cerhan JR, Roenigk RK, Weaver AL, et al. Increased incidence of malignant melanoma and other rare cutaneous cancers in the setting of chronic lymphocytic leukemia. Int J Dermatol. 2015;54(8):e287–93. https://doi.org/10.1111/ijd.12564.
11. Engels EA, Frisch M, Goedert JJ, Biggar RJ, Miller RW. Merkel cell carcinoma and HIV infection. Lancet. 2002;359(9305):497–8. https://doi.org/10.1016/s0140-6736(02)07668-7.

12. Feng H, Shuda M, Chang Y, Moore PS. Clonal integration of a polyomavirus in human Merkel cell carcinoma. Science (New York, NY). 2008;319(5866):1096–100. https://doi.org/10.1126/science.1152586.
13. Kassem A, Schopflin A, Diaz C, Weyers W, Stickeler E, Werner M, et al. Frequent detection of Merkel cell polyomavirus in human Merkel cell carcinomas and identification of a unique deletion in the VP1 gene. Cancer Res. 2008;68(13):5009–13. https://doi.org/10.1158/0008-5472.can-08-0949.
14. Foulongne V, Dereure O, Kluger N, Moles JP, Guillot B, Segondy M. Merkel cell polyomavirus DNA detection in lesional and nonlesional skin from patients with Merkel cell carcinoma or other skin diseases. Br J Dermatol. 2010;162(1):59–63. https://doi.org/10.1111/j.1365-2133.2009.09381.x.
15. Tolstov YL, Pastrana DV, Feng H, Becker JC, Jenkins FJ, Moschos S, et al. Human Merkel cell polyomavirus infection II. MCV is a common human infection that can be detected by conformational capsid epitope immunoassays. Int J Cancer. 2009;125(6):1250–6. https://doi.org/10.1002/ijc.24509.
16. Ratner D, Nelson BR, Brown MD, Johnson TM. Merkel cell carcinoma. J Am Acad Dermatol. 1993;29(2 Pt 1):143–56.
17. Skelton HG, Smith KJ, Hitchcock CL, McCarthy WF, Lupton GP, Graham JH. Merkel cell carcinoma: analysis of clinical, histologic, and immunohistologic features of 132 cases with relation to survival. J Am Acad Dermatol. 1997;37(5 Pt 1):734–9.
18. Mott RT, Smoller BR, Morgan MB. Merkel cell carcinoma: a clinicopathologic study with prognostic implications. J Cutan Pathol. 2004;31(3):217–23.
19. Andea AA, Coit DG, Amin B, Busam KJ. Merkel cell carcinoma: histologic features and prognosis. Cancer. 2008;113(9):2549–58. https://doi.org/10.1002/cncr.23874.
20. Chan JK, Suster S, Wenig BM, Tsang WY, Chan JB, Lau AL. Cytokeratin 20 immunoreactivity distinguishes Merkel cell (primary cutaneous neuroendocrine) carcinomas and salivary gland small cell carcinomas from small cell carcinomas of various sites. Am J Surg Pathol. 1997;21(2):226–34.
21. Byrd-Gloster AL, Khoor A, Glass LF, Messina JL, Whitsett JA, Livingston SK, et al. Differential expression of thyroid transcription factor 1 in small cell lung carcinoma and Merkel cell tumor. Hum Pathol. 2000;31(1):58–62.
22. National Comprehensive Cancer Network. Merkel Cell Carcinoma (Version 1.2017). https://www.nccn.org/professionals/physician_gls/pdf/mcc.pdf. Accessed 26 Nov 2016.
23. Tarantola TI, Vallow LA, Halyard MY, Weenig RH, Warschaw KE, Grotz TE, et al. Prognostic factors in Merkel cell carcinoma: analysis of 240 cases. J Am Acad Dermatol. 2013;68(3):425–32. https://doi.org/10.1016/j.jaad.2012.09.036.
24. Iyer JG, Storer BE, Paulson KG, Lemos B, Phillips JL, Bichakjian CK, et al. Relationships among primary tumor size, number of involved nodes, and survival for 8044 cases of Merkel cell carcinoma. J Am Acad Dermatol. 2014;70(4):637–43. https://doi.org/10.1016/j.jaad.2013.11.031.
25. Gupta SG, Wang LC, Penas PF, Gellenthin M, Lee SJ, Nghiem P. Sentinel lymph node biopsy for evaluation and treatment of patients with Merkel cell carcinoma: the Dana-Farber experience and meta-analysis of the literature. Arch Dermatol. 2006;142(6):685–90. https://doi.org/10.1001/archderm.142.6.685.
26. Gunaratne DA, Howle JR, Veness MJ. Sentinel lymph node biopsy in Merkel cell carcinoma: a 15-year institutional experience and statistical analysis of 721 reported cases. Br J Dermatol. 2016;174(2):273–81. https://doi.org/10.1111/bjd.14240.
27. Lipsett PA, Ruan JH, Reeves M. A merkel cell carcinoma treatment algorithm. Arch Surg. 2009;144(6):582–5. https://doi.org/10.1001/archsurg.2009.91.
28. Ramahi E, Choi J, Fuller CD, Eng TY. Merkel cell carcinoma. Am J Clin Oncol. 2013;36(3):299–309. https://doi.org/10.1097/COC.0b013e318210f83c.
29. Kline L, Coldiron B. Mohs micrographic surgery for the treatment of Merkel cell carcinoma. Dermatol Surg. 2016;42(8):945–51. https://doi.org/10.1097/dss.0000000000000801.
30. Strom T, Carr M, Zager JS, Naghavi A, Smith FO, Cruse CW, et al. Radiation therapy is associated with improved outcomes in Merkel cell carcinoma. Ann Surg Oncol. 2016;23(11):3572–8. https://doi.org/10.1245/s10434-016-5293-1.
31. Kim JA, Choi AH. Effect of radiation therapy on survival in patients with resected Merkel cell carcinoma: a propensity score surveillance, epidemiology, and end results database analysis. JAMA Dermatol. 2013;149(7):831–8. https://doi.org/10.1001/jamadermatol.2013.409.
32. Frohm ML, Griffith KA, Harms KL, Hayman JA, Fullen DR, Nelson CC, et al. Recurrence and survival in patients with Merkel cell carcinoma undergoing surgery without adjuvant radiation therapy to the primary site. JAMA Dermatol. 2016;152(9):1001–7. https://doi.org/10.1001/jamadermatol.2016.1428.
33. Bhatia S, Storer BE, Iyer JG, Moshiri A, Parvathaneni U, Byrd D, et al. Adjuvant radiation therapy and chemotherapy in Merkel cell carcinoma: survival analyses of 6908 cases from the National Cancer Data Base. J Natl Cancer Inst. 2016;108(9):djw042. https://doi.org/10.1093/jnci/djw042.
34. Asgari MM, Sokil MM, Warton EM, Iyer J, Paulson KG, Nghiem P. Effect of host, tumor, diagnostic, and treatment variables on outcomes in a large cohort with Merkel cell carcinoma. JAMA Dermatol. 2014;150(7):716–23. https://doi.org/10.1001/jamadermatol.2013.8116.
35. Nghiem PT, Bhatia S, Lipson EJ, Kudchadkar RR, Miller NJ, Annamalai L, et al. PD-1 blockade with Pembrolizumab in advanced Merkel-cell carcinoma. N Engl J Med. 2016;374(26):2542–52. https://doi.org/10.1056/NEJMoa1603702.

36. McPeak CJ, Cruz T, Nicastri AD. Dermatofibrosarcoma protuberans: an analysis of 86 cases--five with metastasis. Ann Surg. 1967;166(5):803–16.
37. Gloster HM Jr. Dermatofibrosarcoma protuberans. J Am Acad Dermatol. 1996;35(3 Pt 1):355–74. quiz 75-6
38. National Comprehensive Cancer Network. Dermatofibrosarcoma Protuberans (Version 1.2017). https://www.nccn.org/professionals/physician_gls/pdf/dfsp.pdf. Accessed 26 Nov 2016.
39. Criscione VD, Weinstock MA. Descriptive epidemiology of dermatofibrosarcoma protuberans in the United States, 1973 to 2002. J Am Acad Dermatol. 2007;56(6):968–73. https://doi.org/10.1016/j.jaad.2006.09.006.
40. Kreicher KL, Kurlander DE, Gittleman HR, Barnholtz-Sloan JS, Bordeaux JS. Incidence and survival of primary Dermatofibrosarcoma protuberans in the United States. Dermatol Surg. 2016;42(Suppl 1):S24–31. https://doi.org/10.1097/dss.0000000000000300.
41. Criscito MC, Martires KJ, Stein JA. Prognostic factors, treatment, and survival in Dermatofibrosarcoma protuberans. JAMA Dermatol. 2016;152(12):1365–71. https://doi.org/10.1001/jamadermatol.2016.1886.
42. Bogucki B, Neuhaus I, Hurst EA. Dermatofibrosarcoma protuberans: a review of the literature. Dermatol Surg. 2012;38(4):537–51. https://doi.org/10.1111/j.1524-4725.2011.02292.x.
43. Liang CA, Jambusaria-Pahlajani A, Karia PS, Elenitsas R, Zhang PD, Schmults CD. A systematic review of outcome data for dermatofibrosarcoma protuberans with and without fibrosarcomatous change. J Am Acad Dermatol. 2014;71(4):781–6. https://doi.org/10.1016/j.jaad.2014.03.018.
44. Llombart B, Serra-Guillén C, Monteagudo C, López Guerrero JA, Sanmartín O. Dermatofibrosarcoma protuberans: a comprehensive review and update on diagnosis and management. Semin Diagn Pathol. 2013;30(1):13–28. https://doi.org/10.1053/j.semdp.2012.01.002.
45. Cribier B, Noacco G, Peltre B, Grosshans E. Stromelysin 3 expression: a useful marker for the differential diagnosis dermatofibroma versus dermatofibrosarcoma protuberans. J Am Acad Dermatol. 2002;46(3):408–13. https://doi.org/10.1067/mjd.2002.119656.
46. Llombart B, Monteagudo C, Sanmartín O, López-Guerrero JA, Serra-Guillén C, Poveda A, et al. Dermatofibrosarcoma protuberans: a clinicopathological, immunohistochemical, genetic (COL1A1-PDGFB), and therapeutic study of low-grade versus high-grade (fibrosarcomatous) tumors. J Am Acad Dermatol. 2011;65(3):564–75. https://doi.org/10.1016/j.jaad.2010.06.020.
47. Ratner D, Thomas CO, Johnson TM, Sondak VK, Hamilton TA, Nelson BR, et al. Mohs micrographic surgery for the treatment of dermatofibrosarcoma protuberans. Results of a multiinstitutional series with an analysis of the extent of microscopic spread. J Am Acad Dermatol. 1997;37(4):600–13.
48. Lowe GC, Onajin O, Baum CL, Otley CC, Arpey CJ, Roenigk RK, et al. A comparison of Mohs micrographic surgery and wide local excision for treatment of dermatofibrosarcoma protuberans with long-term follow-up: the Mayo clinic experience. Dermatol Surg. 2017;43(1):98–106. https://doi.org/10.1097/dss.0000000000000910.
49. Foroozan M, Sei JF, Amini M, Beauchet A, Saiag P. Efficacy of Mohs micrographic surgery for the treatment of dermatofibrosarcoma protuberans: systematic review. Arch Dermatol. 2012;148(9):1055–63. https://doi.org/10.1001/archdermatol.2012.1440.
50. Pallure V, Dupin N, Guillot B. Surgical treatment of Darier-Ferrand dermatofibrosarcoma: a systematic review. Dermatol Surg. 2013;39(10):1417–33. https://doi.org/10.1111/dsu.12299.
51. McArthur GA, Demetri GD, van Oosterom A, Heinrich MC, Debiec-Rychter M, Corless CL, et al. Molecular and clinical analysis of locally advanced dermatofibrosarcoma protuberans treated with imatinib: Imatinib Target Exploration Consortium Study B2225. J Clin Oncol. 2005;23(4):866–73. https://doi.org/10.1200/jco.2005.07.088.
52. Rutkowski P, Van Glabbeke M, Rankin CJ, Ruka W, Rubin BP, Debiec-Rychter M, et al. Imatinib mesylate in advanced dermatofibrosarcoma protuberans: pooled analysis of two phase II clinical trials. J Clin Oncol. 2010;28(10):1772–9. https://doi.org/10.1200/jco.2009.25.7899.
53. National Comprehensive Cancer Network. Soft Tissue Sarcoma (Version 2.2017). https://www.nccn.org/professionals/physician_gls/pdf/sarcoma.pdf. Accessed 6 Mar 2017.
54. Iorizzo LJ 3rd, Brown MD. Atypical fibroxanthoma: a review of the literature. Dermatol Surg. 2011;37(2):146–57. https://doi.org/10.1111/j.1524-4725.2010.01843.x.
55. Goldblum JR. An approach to pleomorphic sarcomas: can we subclassify, and does it matter? Mod Pathol. 2014;27(Suppl 1):S39–46. https://doi.org/10.1038/modpathol.2013.174.
56. Rouhani P, Fletcher CD, Devesa SS, Toro JR. Cutaneous soft tissue sarcoma incidence patterns in the U.S.: an analysis of 12,114 cases. Cancer. 2008;113(3):616–27. https://doi.org/10.1002/cncr.23571.
57. Fretzin DF, Helwig EB. Atypical fibroxanthoma of the skin. A clinicopathologic study of 140 cases. Cancer. 1973;31(6):1541–52.
58. Limmer BL, Clark DP. Cutaneous micrographic surgery for atypical fibroxanthoma. Dermatol Surg. 1997;23(7):553–7. discussion 7–8
59. Huether MJ, Zitelli JA, Brodland DG. Mohs micrographic surgery for the treatment of spindle cell tumors of the skin. J Am Acad Dermatol. 2001;44(4):656–9. https://doi.org/10.1067/mjd.2001.112381.
60. Colgan MB, Brewer JD, Weaver AL, Roenigk RK, Otley CC. Atypical fibroxanthoma in the setting of chronic lymphocytic Leukemia and other non-Hodgkin

lymphomas. Dermatol Surg. 2011;37(5):671–6. https://doi.org/10.1111/j.1524-4725.2011.01947.x.

61. Hollmig ST, Sachdev R, Cockerell CJ, Posten W, Chiang M, Kim J. Spindle cell neoplasms encountered in dermatologic surgery: a review. Dermatol Surg. 2012;38(6):825–50. https://doi.org/10.1111/j.1524-4725.2012.02296.x.
62. Henderson MT, Hollmig ST. Malignant fibrous histiocytoma: changing perceptions and management challenges. J Am Acad Dermatol. 2012;67(6):15–41. https://doi.org/10.1016/j.jaad.2012.04.013.
63. Shin J, Vincent JG, Cuda JD, Xu H, Kang S, Kim J, et al. Sox10 is expressed in primary melanocytic neoplasms of various histologies but not in fibrohistiocytic proliferations and histiocytoses. J Am Acad Dermatol. 2012;67(4):717–26. https://doi.org/10.1016/j.jaad.2011.12.035.
64. Hanlon A, Stasko T, Christiansen D, Cyrus N, Galan A. LN2, CD10, and Ezrin do not distinguish between atypical fibroxanthoma and undifferentiated pleomorphic sarcoma or predict clinical outcome. Dermatol Surg. 2017;43(3):431–6. https://doi.org/10.1097/dss.0000000000001000.
65. Davis JL, Randle HW, Zalla MJ, Roenigk RK, Brodland DG. A comparison of Mohs micrographic surgery and wide excision for the treatment of atypical fibroxanthoma. Dermatol Surg. 1997;23(2):105–10.
66. Ang GC, Roenigk RK, Otley CC, Phillips KP, Weaver AL. More than 2 decades of treating atypical fibroxanthoma at Mayo Clinic: what have we learned from 91 patients? Dermatol Surg. 2009;35(5):765–72. https://doi.org/10.1111/j.1524-4725.2009.01126.x.
67. Brown MD, Swanson NA. Treatment of malignant fibrous histiocytoma and atypical fibrous xanthomas with micrographic surgery. J Dermatol Surg Oncol. 1989;15(12):1287–92.
68. Seavolt M, McCall M. Atypical fibroxanthoma: review of the literature and summary of 13 patients treated with Mohs micrographic surgery. Dermatol Surg. 2006;32(3):435–41.; discussion 9–41. https://doi.org/10.1111/j.1524-4725.2006.32087.x.
69. Zalla MJ, Randle HW, Brodland DG, Davis JL, Roenigk RK. Mohs surgery vs wide excision for atypical fibroxanthoma: follow-up. Dermatol Surg. 1997;23(12):1223–4.
70. Hollmig ST, Kirkland EB, Henderson MT, Tang JY, Gladstone HB. The evolving conception and management challenges of malignant fibrous histiocytoma. Dermatol Surg. 2012;38(12):1922–9. https://doi.org/10.1111/j.1524-4725.2012.02538.x.
71. Nelson BR, Hamlet KR, Gillard M, Railan D, Johnson TM. Sebaceous carcinoma. J Am Acad Dermatol. 1995;33(1):1–15. quiz 6–8
72. Kyllo RL, Brady KL, Hurst EA. Sebaceous carcinoma: review of the literature. Dermatol Surg. 2015;41(1):1–15. https://doi.org/10.1097/dss.0000000000000152.
73. Tripathi R, Chen Z, Li L, Bordeaux JS. Incidence and survival of sebaceous carcinoma in the United States. J Am Acad Dermatol. 2016;75(6):1210–5. https://doi.org/10.1016/j.jaad.2016.07.046.
74. Tryggvason G, Bayon R, Pagedar NA. Epidemiology of sebaceous carcinoma of the head and neck: implications for lymph node management. Head Neck. 2012;34(12):1765–8. https://doi.org/10.1002/hed.22009.
75. Chang AY, Miller CJ, Elenitsas R, Newman JG, Sobanko JF. Management considerations in extraocular sebaceous carcinoma. Dermatol Surg. 2016;42(Suppl 1):S57–65. https://doi.org/10.1097/dss.0000000000000575.
76. Eisen DB, Michael DJ. Sebaceous lesions and their associated syndromes: part II. J Am Acad Dermatol. 2009;61(4):563–78.; quiz 79–80. https://doi.org/10.1016/j.jaad.2009.04.059.
77. Dasgupta T, Wilson LD, Yu JB. A retrospective review of 1349 cases of sebaceous carcinoma. Cancer. 2009;115(1):158–65. https://doi.org/10.1002/cncr.23952.
78. Hou JL, Killian JM, Baum CL, Otley CC, Roenigk RK, Arpey CJ, et al. Characteristics of sebaceous carcinoma and early outcomes of treatment using Mohs micrographic surgery versus wide local excision: an update of the Mayo Clinic experience over the past 2 decades. Dermatol Surg. 2014;40(3):241–6. https://doi.org/10.1111/dsu.124.
79. Day A, Abramson AK, Patel M, Warren RB, Menter MA. The spectrum of oculocutaneous disease: Part II. Neoplastic and drug-related causes of oculocutaneous disease. J Am Acad Dermatol. 2014;70(5):821.e1–19. https://doi.org/10.1016/j.jaad.2013.12.019.
80. Thosani MK, Marghoob A, Chen C-SJ. Current progress of immunostains in Mohs micrographic surgery: a review. Dermatol Surg. 2008;34(12):1621–36.
81. Spencer JM, Nossa R, Tse DT, Sequeira M. Sebaceous carcinoma of the eyelid treated with Mohs micrographic surgery. J Am Acad Dermatol. 2001;44(6):1004–9. https://doi.org/10.1067/mjd.2001.113692.
82. Yount AB, Bylund D, Pratt SG, Greenway HT. Mohs micrographic excision of sebaceous carcinoma of the eyelids. Dermatol Surg. 1994;20(8):523–9. https://doi.org/10.1111/j.1524-4725.1994.tb00137.x.
83. Snow SN, Larson PO, Lucarelli MJ, Lemke BN, Madjar DD. Sebaceous carcinoma of the eyelids treated by mohs micrographic surgery: report of nine cases with review of the literature. Dermatol Surg. 2002;28(7):623–31.
84. Brady KL, Hurst EA. Sebaceous carcinoma treated with mohs micrographic surgery. Dermatol Surg. 2017;43(2):281–6. https://doi.org/10.1097/dss.0000000000000943.
85. Eisen DB, Michael DJ. Sebaceous lesions and their associated syndromes: part I. J Am Acad Dermatol. 2009;61(4):549–60.; quiz 61–2. https://doi.org/10.1016/j.jaad.2009.04.058.
86. Everett JN, Raymond VM, Dandapani M, et al. Screening for germline mismatch repair mutations following diagnosis of sebaceous neoplasm. JAMA Dermatol. 2014;150(12):1315–21. https://doi.org/10.1001/jamadermatol.2014.1217.

87. Lee BA, Yu L, Ma L, Lind AC, Lu D. Sebaceous neoplasms with mismatch repair protein expressions and the frequency of co-existing visceral tumors. J Am Acad Dermatol. 2012;67(6):1228–34. https://doi.org/10.1016/j.jaad.2012.03.020.

88. Ho VH, Ross MI, Prieto VG, Khaleeq A, Kim S, Esmaeli B. Sentinel lymph node biopsy for sebaceous cell carcinoma and melanoma of the ocular adnexa. Arch Otolaryngol Head Neck Surg. 2007;1(8):820–6. https://doi.org/10.1001/archotol.133.8.820.

Management of Non-melanoma Skin Cancers: Merkel Cell Carcinoma

39

Isabel Prieto, Teresa Pérez-de-la-Fuente, M Susana Medina, Beatriz Castelo, Fernando Cassinello, David Esteban, and Nuria Rodriguez-Salas

Abbreviations

CLND	Complete lymph node dissection
CRT	Chemoradiotherapy
CTR	Clinical trials
DFS	Disease-free survival
H&N	Head and neck
IT	Immunotherapy
LTAg	Large tumor antigen
MCC	Merkel cell carcinoma
MCV	Merkel cell polyomavirus
NAFT	Nuclear factor of activated T cells
NK	Natural killer
OS	Overall survival
PD-1	Death protein-1
PD-L1	PD-1 ligand
RT	Radiation therapy
SEER	Surveillance, Epidemiology, and End Results
SLNB	Sentinel lymphatic node biopsy
sTAg	Small tumor antigen
UV	Ultraviolet light

I. Prieto, M.D., Ph.D. (✉) · D. Esteban, M.D.
Department of Radiation Oncology,
Fundación Jiménez Díaz, Madrid, Spain
e-mail: iprieto@fjd.es; david.esteban@genesiscare.es

T. Pérez-de-la-Fuente, M.D.
Department of Plastic Surgery,
Fundación Jiménez Díaz, Madrid, Spain
e-mail: tperezdelaf@fjd.es

M. Susana Medina, M.D.
Department of Dermatology,
Príncipe de Asturias University Hospital,
Madrid, Spain

B. Castelo, M.D., Ph.D. · N. Rodriguez-Salas, M.D., Ph.D.
Department of Medical Oncology,
Hospital Universitario La Paz, Madrid, Spain
e-mail: nuria.rodriguez@salud.madrid.org

F. Cassinello, M.D., Ph.D.
Department of Anesthesiology,
Fundación Jiménez Díaz, Madrid, Spain
e-mail: fcassinellop@gmail.com

Introduction

Merkel cell carcinoma (MCC) is a rare and very aggressive primary cutaneous carcinoma that is associated with a high risk of locoregional and distant spread and, hence, poor long-term survival. The therapeutic approach is often unclear, and considerable controversy exists regarding its pathogenesis and optimal management. An increasing number of cases over the past two decades and the discovery of the Merkel cell polyomavirus (MCV) by Feng et al. have focused much more attention on this aggressive malignancy [1–5].

MCC was recognized as an entity in the 1970s, when its pathologic criteria were defined and its distinct clinical behavior was described. In 1972, Toker et al. [1] described five patients with an unusual skin tumor in which trabeculae and cell nests in the dermis were the dominant histologic findings, and as a result he named it "trabecular carcinoma of the skin" [3, 4]. Owing to the discovery

A. I. Riker (ed.), *Melanoma*, https://doi.org/10.1007/978-3-319-78310-9_39

of electron-dense neurosecretory granules in the tumor cells, the disease was classified as a neuroendocrine carcinoma [5]. A few more years passed before the immunohistochemical differences between these tumors were more fully defined, and this time MCC was given the name that remains today.

Epidemiology

The overall age-adjusted incidence of MCC is 0.24 per 100,000 person-years in United States, which is higher than the 0.13 per 10,000 person-year estimated rate in Europe. Most series show a greater risk in males with a male-to-female ratio of 1.4:1–2.3:1 [6]. The mean age of patients at the time of initial diagnosis is above 70 years [7]. It presents more commonly in white males and in immunosuppressed patients. The role of ultraviolet light (UV) in the development of MCC is seen as having more of an immunosuppressive than a mutagenic or carcinogenic effect. According to the data from Surveillance, Epidemiology, and End Results (SEER) data for the time period of 1986–2001, there was a threefold increase in MCC cases [2, 8, 9]. The age-adapted incidence of MCC underwent a statistically significant annual increase of 8% during this period. In eastern England, MCC prevalence has risen threefold over the last 10 years and is now similar to the highest reported rates from Western Australia [10, 11].

This rapid increase is more dramatic than that of the increasing incidence of cutaneous melanoma worldwide. Causative factors implicated are a variety of environmental and population factors, such as a higher incidence of UV exposure and increasing numbers of immunosuppressed individuals within the population. Immunosuppression and immunodeficiency likely play an important role in the pathogenesis of MCC, with the incidence clearly higher in solid organ transplant recipients, most commonly those undergoing renal transplantation, as well as individuals with chronic lymphocytic leukemia (CLL), human immunodeficiency virus (HIV) infection, and acquired immunodeficiency syndrome (AIDS) [1, 3]. Patients with autoimmune diseases such as rheumatoid arthritis also are at an increased risk for developing MCC [11, 12].

The recent advancements in immunodiagnostic techniques may have also contributed to the increasing numbers of diagnosed cases [2]. Indeed, the American Cancer Society has predicted that the incidence of MCC will exceed that of cutaneous T-cell lymphoma, with similar data reported for Australia [1, 5]. The Danish study [13] by the Epidemiology Research Department (1978–2006) revealed an overall MCC incidence of 2.2 cases per million person-years, and warned of the possible association between MCC and other cancers, particularly squamous cell carcinoma.

Our Evolving Understanding of MCC Pathogenesis

Despite a marked improvement in our current understanding of the pathogenesis for MCC, the exact cellular mechanisms and genomic changes remain ill defined. There appears to be an association with various chromosomal abnormalities as well as perturbation along several cellular signaling and apoptotic pathways. Among the most viable hypotheses to possibly explain the development and malignant transformation of MCC the disease is the role of mast cells, specifically the hypermethylation of gene silencing of p14ARF, amino acid substitution in exon 10 of platelet-derived growth factor (PDGF) and, notably, the role of MCV [2, 14]. In this regard, recent evidence suggests that clonal integration of MCV is one of the main etiological mechanisms by which MCC develops. The most frequent factors and hypotheses related to the pathogenesis of the tumor seem to be as follows:

1. *The increasing evidence that sun exposure may also be a major independent etiological factor*. MCC most commonly develops in areas of the skin that are exposed to the sun, such as the head and neck (H&N) [15] (Fig. 39.1). The role of UV light in the development of this tumor is seen more as an

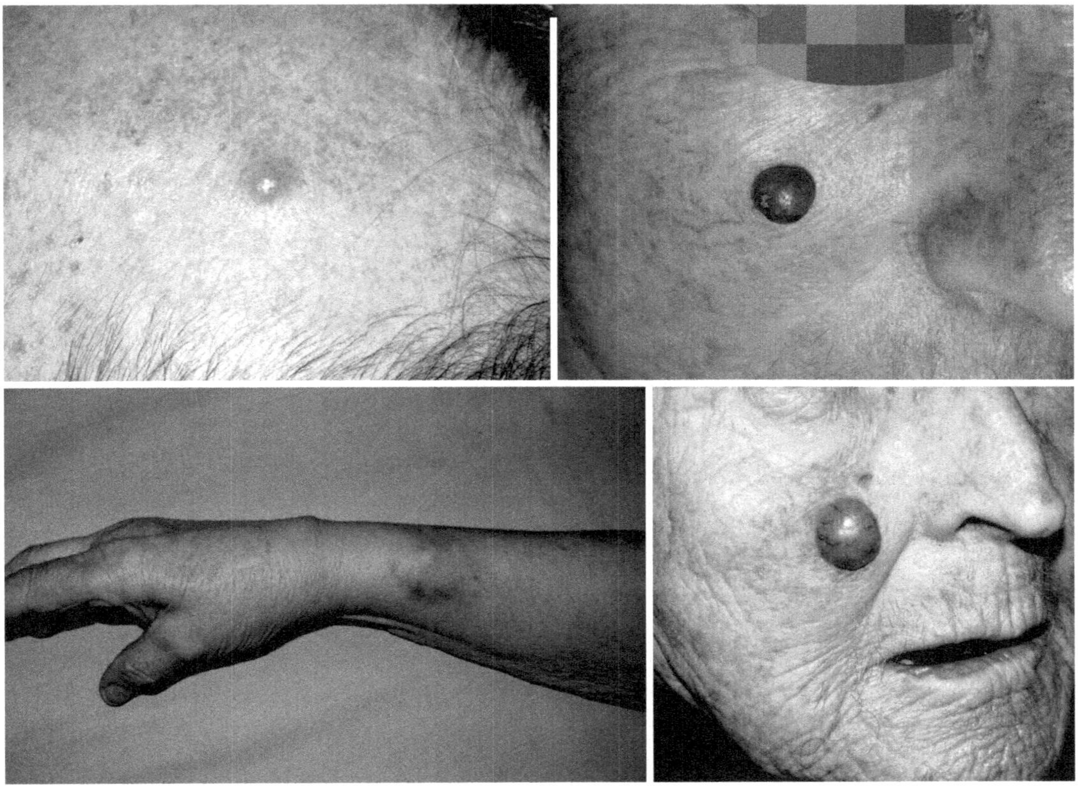

Fig. 39.1 Clinical appearance of MCC in sun-exposed areas

immunosuppressive effect, rather than as a mutagenic or carcinogenic effect. Pathogenetically, in addition to disturbed antigen presentation, the induction of immunosuppressive cytokines such as interleukin-1 and tumor necrosis factor-α, the isomerization of trans- to cis-urocanic acid, and the formation of reactive oxygen species are considered to be the main culprits [1].

2. *Multiple chromosomal abnormalities* have been found in MCC, with the most common abnormality identified as a deletion of the short arm of chromosome 1 (1p36), which is a structural aberration found in up to 40% of MCCs. Aberrations in other chromosomes, such as loss of heterozygosity in band 3p21 (an abnormality also reported in small-cell carcinoma), 10q23, and chromosome 13, have also been reported. [16, 17]. In MCC, the heterozygous loss of the long arm of chromosome 10 suggests that the tumor suppressor gene, PTEN, plays an important role in the transformation process of MCC. A recent study using MCC tissue microarrays to measure the exposure of various proteins (especially matrix metalloproteinases) revealed that PTEN could scarcely be identified in the samples examined, which could indicate inactivation of the second allele [5]. Other abnormalities also found in MCC include trisomy 1, 6, 11, 18, and the deletion of chromosome 7 [2, 18].
3. From a molecular perspective, the primary mechanisms of transformation promoting MCC are still relatively unknown. It has been suggested that the rapid growth seen in many cases of MCC is associated with *dysregulation of various normal growth factor receptors*. Mutations in the TP53 gene have been observed in 14–33% of MCC, mostly confined to MCV-negative cases [15, 19]. High expression of the bcl-2 proto-oncogene,

which is capable of inhibiting apoptosis, thereby promoting cell survival and contributing to tumor growth, was observed in 5 of 19 patients with MCC, although no relation between gene expression and survival was observed [20].

4. Finally, *the discovery by Feng* et al. [21] *in 2008 that MCV was identified in 8 of 10 MCC tumors has provided yet another important clue as to the pathogenesis of MCC*. MCV is most closely related to a lymphotropic polyomavirus found in African green monkeys, also unique in that it is the only polyomavirus known to naturally infect B-lymphocytes. Polyomaviruses are a group of icosahedral, double-stranded DNA viruses that encode a large tumor antigen oncoprotein known to cause tumors in animal models.

MCV infection usually occurs at a young age and establishes a clinically silent persistent infection [22]. MCV is thought to be part of the human skin microbiome and appears to be chronically shed from the skin in the form of assembled virions. The seroprevalence of antibodies specific to the capsid protein VP1 appears to increase with age, from approximately 40% in children up to over 80% in older individuals. In time, either due to prolonged sunlight exposure, viral genome replication in dermal cells, or infection of bystander Merkel cells, MCV genomes become integrated into the host genome [23]. The induction of matrix metalloproteinase through the normal aging process and prolonged UV exposure may favor active infection. Finally, immune downregulation by viral proteins allows MCV to establish a persistent infection [24].

It has been hypothesized that the rarity of MCV-positive MCC can be explained in terms of genomic instability. There are two likely distinct mutagenic steps that are believed to be required for MCC development. The first is the integration of MCV into the host genome, with the second being the prevention of autonomous viral replication by T antigen mutations [25, 26] (Fig. 39.2). The exact mechanism by which the MCV contributes to the development of MCC has yet to be identified. MCV may likely contribute to tumorigenesis via large T antigen (LTAg) inhibition of the tumor suppressor gene, Rb1, and enhanced oncoprotein gene stability and mTOR activation by small T antigen (sTAg) [27]. In MCC, MCV displays genomic integration and characteristic truncating mutations of LTAg, which render the virus replication-deficient but preserve the Rb binding site.

MCV-negative tumors exhibited a high mutation burden associated with a UV-induced DNA damage signature [15, 18, 26]. These expression levels were strongly correlated with unfavorable clinical outcomes, further providing important insights in the effort to develop novel targeted

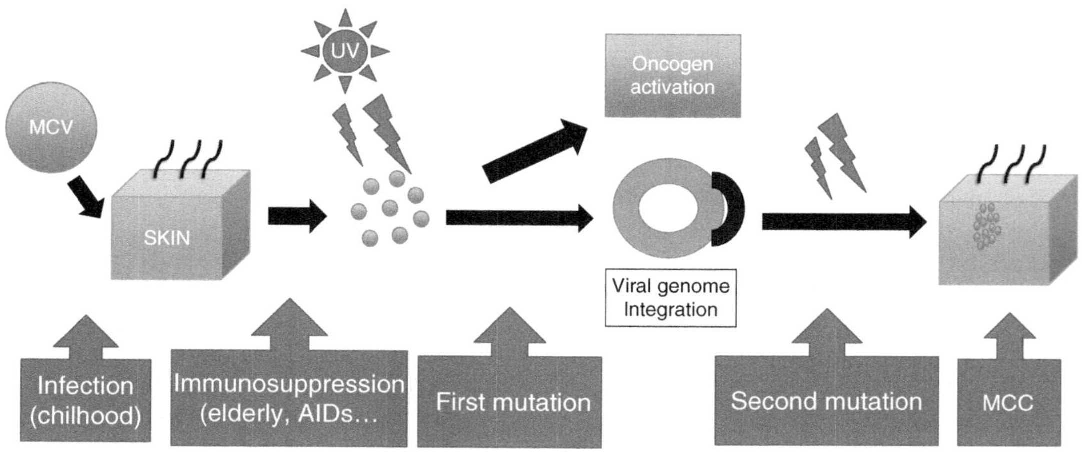

Fig. 39.2 Integration and replication of MCV into the host genome after sun exposition

therapies for MCC [28]. MCV DNA-positive MCCs tend to show better prognosis, with some studies reporting fewer regional lymph nodes at the time of diagnosis compared to MCV DNA-negative MCCs [29].

Gonzalez-Vela et al. found that MCV-negative tumors had higher mutational loads with UV signatures and more frequent mutations in TP53 and Rb compared to their MCV-positive counterparts [15]. Surprisingly, despite important genetic differences, both exhibited nuclear accumulation of oncogenic transcription factors such as the nuclear factor of activated T cells (NAFT), P-CREB, and P-STAT3, indicating commonly deregulated pathogenic mechanisms with the potential to serve as targets for therapy. A multivariable analysis identified P-CREB as an independent survival factor with respect to clinical variables and MCV status in our cohort of MCC patients [15]. Table 39.1 shows these differences between MCV-positive and -negative tumors.

Serological biomarkers that may help predict prognosis and identify those patients at a higher risk of early relapse is a focus of much research currently. Samimi et al. found that the major capsid protein (VP1) antibodies constitute a prognostic marker associated with a favorable prognosis when detected at high levels at baseline [30]. Conversely, the TAg antibodies were cleared in patients in remission, but showed higher titers in disease recurrence and were found to be a useful marker of disease progression when detected more than 12 months after diagnosis.

Table 39.1 Differences between MCV-negative and -positive tumors

	MCV-negative tumors	MCV-positive tumors
RB1, TP53 mutation	+ More frequent (almost exclusive)	– Less frequent
NOTCH1 and NFAT1 mutation	Nuclear accumulation	Nuclear accumulation
EGFR, *KIT*, and *PIK3CA* mutation	–	+
CADM1 expression	+	–
MAL expression	–	+

RB retinoblastoma, *NAFT* nuclear factor of activated T cells, *EGFR* epidermal growth factor receptor, *CADM1* cell adhesion molecule 1, *MAL* myelin and lymphocyte protein (also known as mal T-cell differentiation protein)

Current Surgical Management

The mainstay for the initial surgical management of MCC is wide local excision of the primary lesion with a minimum of 2-cm margins in all directions [31–33]. However, as with melanoma, there is a trend toward smaller surgical margins, with Gillenwater et al. comparing 1, 2 cm margins for MCC measuring < 1 cm in diameter, and found no statistical difference in locoregional control or survival [34]. Sattler et al. also failed to show a statistically significant difference in disease-free survival (DFS) or overall survival (OS) when comparing with margins of 1–3 cm [35].

Skin margins are determined by the tumor size, measured as the diameter of the lesion, and not Breslow's depth as with melanoma. As with melanoma, the excision extends down to the fascial plan (or galea for the scalp), with peripheral margins of at least 2 cm for lesions larger than 2 cm in diameter and 1 cm margins for lesions <2 cm in diameter [2]. For larger residual defects that cannot be closed primarily, we will often perform these operations with our plastic surgeons who will assist with the most aesthetic and durable form of tissue reconstruction, whether this be a local rotational flap or free flap depending upon the location of the defect (Fig. 39.3).

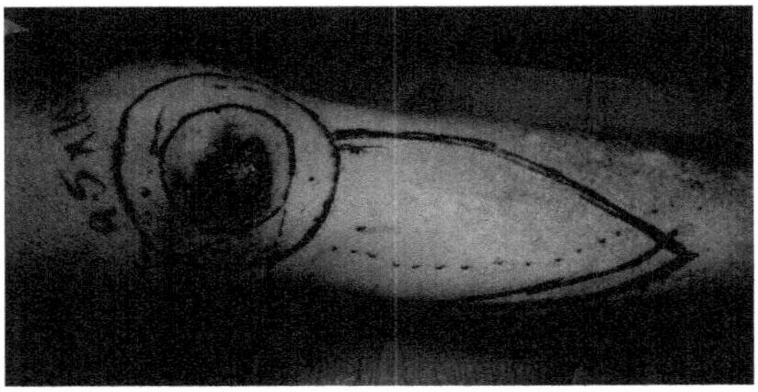

Fig. 39.3 Planning the surgical procedure and flap in MCC of the leg

In addition to the proper surgical excision of the primary MCC, concomitant sentinel lymph node biopsy (SLNB) is performed [36]. The SLN identifies those patients requiring further surgical management of the affected nodal basin, mainly a completion node dissection (axilla or groin), with the addition of adjuvant of radiation therapy (RT). Regional lymph node metastases occur early in the disease course and frequently, so it is thought that MCC spreads in a similar way to melanoma, with SLNB the best means of detecting subclinical nodal metastatic disease [36, 37]. Examination of the SLN's should be examined by both hematoxylin and eosin (H&E) and IHC staining, including delayed, rather than intraoperative CK20 immunostaining [38]. Allen et al. reported the largest single-institution series of MCC patients ($n = 251$) and showed that the incidence of positive sentinel lymph nodes was independent of tumor size [39].

Bichakjian et al. recommended performing SLNB as the standard of care approach for all clinically lymph node-negative MCC patients [20]. The authors make a strong argument for this regional staging, citing a fairly consistent SLN positivity rate of ~ 20–30% in clinically N0 patients. Clinically palpable lymph nodes, found to be positive by fine needle aspiration biopsy at presentation, is a strong indicator of poor outcome and reduces the 5-year overall survival rate to less than 50% [36]. Furthermore, the presence or absence of lymph node-positive disease is a strong predictor of OS and DFS in MCC, regardless of tumor size. Kachare et al. demonstrated that the early diagnosis of clinically occult nodal disease by SLNB is associated with a therapeutic advantage in MCC-specific survival [40]. Therefore, SLNB has become routine for patients with no clinical or radiological evidence of nodal disease [41]. Patients with a negative lymph node status confirmed by SLNB have better survival rates than patients.

Patients found to have a positive SLN should then undergo a completion lymph node dissection (CLND), adjuvant nodal radiation therapy (RT), or both. In the face of a positive SLN, further surgical management of the regional nodal basin with a CLND is considered the standard of care worldwide. However, therapeutic completion nodal dissection of the regional nodes appears to minimize, but not entirely eliminate, the risk of subsequent node recurrence and in-transit metastases [38, 39]. An emphasis on nodal disease in the current American Joint Committee on Cancer (AJCC) [42] staging system has evolved to include an approach for identification of micrometastatic nodal deposits. For similar reasons, the seventh edition of the TNM [43] staging system for MCC has replaced the Memorial Sloan Kettering Cancer Center system. The AJCC staging system separates those without or with nodal involvement into stage II and III disease, respectively, and thereafter depending on the presence of micrometastases or macrometastases. The staging system recognizes a distinction between micrometastases confirmed by SLNB or elective lymph node resection (3A), or macrometastases (3B) that include any detectable in-transit metastases. Implementing the AJCC system by pathological staging criteria of regional disease remains a challenge, as it suggests a greater proportion of patients would require SLNB or prophylactic neck dissection [36].

Surgical Management and Approach for Head and Neck MCC

MCC located in H&N should be given special consideration, as in this anatomical area outcomes are poorer than in MCC located elsewhere, possibly due to smaller margins, a less predictable draining pattern of the lymphatics and other intrinsic tumor-related factors [44, 45]. Bichakijian et al. margins smaller than 1 cm, showing similar local recurrence rates compared to larger margins of > 1-cm (9 vs. 10%, respectively) [20]. Recent studies have found that over-expression of TP53 (an oncogene associated with poorer prognosis) and P53 mutation can be related to ultraviolet B radiation exposure, resulting in aberrant protein P53 activation [15, 19]. In such cases, it is important to employ a good staging protocol at diagnosis so as to manage the neck properly. Narrow margins of the face, nose, eyelids, or lips in order to preserve optimal cosmetic outcome must be carefully balanced with the higher priority goal of successful locoregional control of the MCC. Such cases should be discussed and approached in a multidisciplinary fashion, involving the expertise of the facial plastic surgeons and others prior to proceeding to the operating room. Morand et al. report two cases of MCC in the nasal vestibule. One patient refused complete nose ablation, opting for primary RT in its place. The other patient was treated with Mohs surgery [46]. Snow et al. report three cases of MCC of the nose: one cutaneous and two originating in the nasal mucosa. The prognosis of the mucosal cases was poorer at 12 months of surveillance, which the authors suggest may be due to the greater access to internal vascular and lymphatic channels [47]. These studies should be viewed with caution, as such standardized approaches utilizing acceptable treatment guidelines remain the standard of care for all cases of MCC.

Regarding SLN mapping, Fritsch et al. reported that SLN-positive status was not an independent prognostic factor for predicting DFS due to different lymphatic pathways and behavior in the H&N [44]. However, the study by Sadeghi et al. did not show any difference between the H&N and other parts of the body in terms of the prognostic value for SLN status [48]. Protocols, anesthetic considerations, and a multidisciplinary approach must be considered, though each patient must be considered individually due to the aggressiveness required to achieve local and regional control [46].

The Role of Radiation Therapy in Treating MCC

The role of RT in MCC management has been widely described as an important part of the comprehensive management of MCC [36]. MCC is indeed sensitive to radiation therapy, shown to be effective at eradicating microscopic disease, both at the primary site and regional nodal basin. Bichakjian et al. [20] described a distinction between adjuvant RT to the primary site, RT to the regional lymph node basin, or both. Controversial results regarding this treatment strategy have been reported, and great heterogeneity has been seen. The question of whether primary MCC should be followed by adjuvant RT to the surgical bed will remain unanswered until higher level evidence becomes available. Based on what is known, after wide local excision of smaller primary lesions (<2 cm in the largest dimension) leaving clear margins, adjuvant RT to the primary site can most likely be omitted [38, 44, 49–52]. Retrospective studies of adjuvant radiotherapy suggest benefit on survival for tumor region in stage I and II, with significant improvement in local and regional control [53–56]. Although certainly not considered an optimal approach to managing the primary MCC, the use of RT as a definitive treatment to the primary MCC without surgical resection has been reported [36, 57].

As described previously, the most consistent predictor of survival for MCC patients to date is the presence or absence of MCC within the lymph nodes. Most studies examining this issue suggest that patients have a better outcome when the regional lymph node basin is both studied (with SLNB) and treated (surgically and with RT) [20, 44]. Current consensus guidelines from the NCCN recommend routine use of adjuvant nodal RT when the SLN is found to be positive, has not been performed or when patient presents with clinically positive regional nodes.

Controversy exists, however, when SLBN is found to be negative on final pathology. Lymph node recurrence is most often indicative of delayed manifestation of micrometastatic disease present at the time the primary tumor is treated [20]. Some authors recommend elective nodal RT in clinically negative nodes and/or in the absence of SLBN results [36, 58]. This point is also highlighted in a study by Kokoska et al. [59], which reported a recurrence rate of 0% (0 of 11 patients) when CLND was performed compared with 91% (20 of 22 patients) without CLND, finding a recurrence rate of 15% with RT and 90% without. However, because the morbidity of the nodal surgery could be unacceptable from the perspective of both the patient and the multidisciplinary tumor board, then RT to the lymph node basin has to be considered (Fig. 39.4).

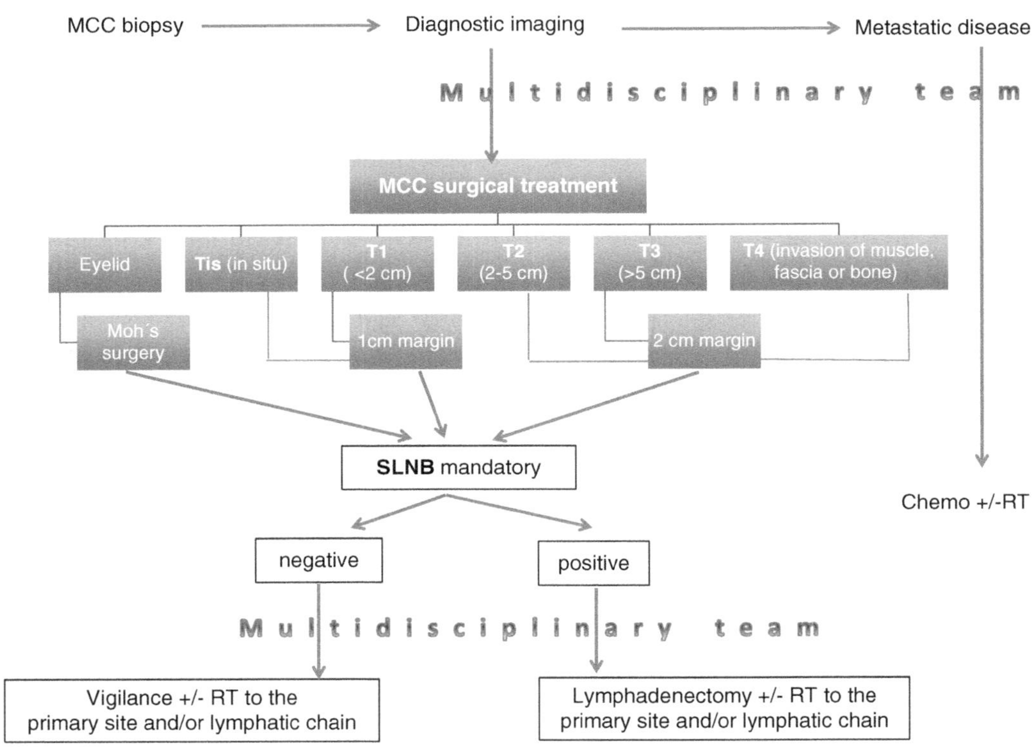

Fig. 39.4 MCC multidisciplinary decision algorithm. Recommended surgical margins, SLNB timing and multidisciplinary team interventions

Fang et al. reported that CLND and RT are equally effective in patients with micrometastatic disease [60]. However, it should be noted that more than half of the patients who underwent a CLND subsequently underwent adjuvant RT. A meta-analysis comparing resection and resection plus radiotherapy found that RT significantly lowered locoregional recurrence rates [20, 61]. For patients with extensive lymph node disease or extracapsular lymph node extension, adjuvant RT after CLND should be strongly considered [36].

Adjuvant Therapy for MCC: Chemotherapy and Immmunotherapy

The role of chemotherapy in the treatment MCC is mostly focused upon treating those patients with stage 4 metastatic MCC, and is therefore considered palliative in most cases. However, adjuvant chemotherapy and immunotherapy has been recently examined more closely, showing some promising results.

Adjuvant Chemotherapy Setting

Although no phase 3 clinical trials have demonstrated that adjuvant chemotherapy has an impact on OS, it may play a role in certain situations for those patients at a high risk of locoregional recurrence or distant metastasis, as in the presence of positive surgical lymph nodes, positive surgical margins, bulky mass, or rapidly expanding disease (evidence level 3) [62, 63].

From 1997 to 2001, the Trans-Tasman Radiation Oncology Group conducted a phase 2 clinical trial involving 53 patients with MCC and high-risk locoregional disease [63] High-risk locoregional MCC was defined as a relapse after initial treatment, surgically positive lymph nodes, primary tumor larger than 1-cm in diameter, gross residual disease after surgery, or occult primary tumor with positive nodes. Patients received locoregional RT with a planned treatment regimen with carboplatin-etoposide as a radiosensitizing agent. With a median follow-up of 48 months, the 3-year OS, locoregional control, and distant control were 76%, 75%, and 76%, respectively [63].

The most extensive data supporting chemoradiotherapy (CRT) come from another retrospective study of 4815 patients with MCC of the H&N region [64]. In this analysis, there were 1995 patients managed with surgery alone, 2330 with postoperative RT, 393 with postoperative CRT, and 97 with postoperative chemotherapy alone. OS rates with adjuvant RT (hazard ratio [HR] 0.80, 95% CI 0.70–0.92) or CRT (HR 0.62, 95% CI 0.47–0.81) were significantly improved compared to surgery alone. However, no benefit was observed with postoperative chemotherapy alone, producing a worse OS than surgery without adjuvant therapy (HR 1.74, 95% CI 1.10–2.75). In subset analyses, adjuvant CRT was associated with improved OS compared with adjuvant RT in patients with positive margins (HR 0.48, 95% CI 0.25–0.93), tumor size ≥3 cm (HR 0.52, 95% CI 0. 30–0.90), and male sex (HR 0.69, 95% CI 0.50–0.94). For patients with node-positive disease, there was a trend toward improved OS with CRT compared with RT alone (HR 0.67, $p = 0.07$). Further prospective trials are needed to confirm the observed benefit of CRT and also to determine their applicability to MCC occurring in other sites.

Adjuvant Immunotherapy

Checkpoint inhibitor immunotherapy (IT), such as pembrolizumab or nivolumab, is showing tremendous promise in patients with metastatic MCC. Another form of immunotherapy with ipilimumab, which blocks the CTLA-4 receptor and important negative regulator of T-cell-mediated anti-tumor response, is being evaluated in several clinical trials for MCC patients who have undergone definitive surgical resection (NCT02196961).

Advanced Disease

Chemotherapy

Although only 2% of MCC patients are diagnosed with advanced disease, approximately one-third will develop metastases at some point during the course of their disease [8]. There are no randomized trials or prospective studies examining the role of chemotherapy in MCC patients with distant metastases. However, there are studies looking at the role of chemotherapy in individual cases or small series of MCC patients, with variable response rates reported of short duration [65]. Due to morphological and immunohistochemical similarity with neuroendocrine tumors and small-cell lung carcinoma, similar chemotherapy treatment regimens have been previously used, including cyclophosphamide, methotrexate, 5-fluorouracil, cisplatin, etoposide, doxorubicin, procarbazine, dacarbazine, streptozotocin, and nitrogen mustards.

The most extensive results on the utility of chemotherapy in stage 4 MCC patients come from a retrospectively analyzed series of 103 patients with distant metastases [65]. Patients were treated with a wide range of chemotherapy regimens, with the combination of doxorubicin and cyclophosphamide obtaining a complete response rate of 38% and a partial response rate of 30%, achieving an improvement in DFS and OS [65]. Combinations containing cisplatin have led to a 55% overall response, and those based on cyclophosphamide and adriamycin had a 69% response rate [66, 67]. Schemes consisting of more than one drug are a reasonable option for patients with a good performance status, given the lack of effective therapies for metastatic MCC.

Immune Checkpoint Blockade

An improved understanding of the host immune system and tumor microenvironment has resulted in some promising new treatment modalities designed to stimulate the host immune system to selectively and robustly destroy metastatic MCC. Recently, such personalized, targeted approaches have focused upon the programmed cell death protein 1 (PD-1) pathway. The main checkpoint inhibitors that have been examined in recent, early phase clinical trials are:

Pembrolizumab: In a phase II study, 26 patients with metastatic MCC were treated with pembrolizumab (2 mg/kg every 3 weeks); no patients had received prior systemic therapy for their advanced disease. Objective responses were observed in 14 of 25 evaluable patients (56%), including four complete responses and ten partial responses. With a median follow-up of 33 weeks, only 2 of 14 patients (14%) had relapsed, and the 6-month rate of PFS was 67%. Responses were observed in 10 of 16 patients (62%) whose tumors were positive for the MCV and in four of the eight patients whose tumors were virus negative [68].

Nivolumab: A case report has also documented a response to nivolumab, another antibody targeting PD-1. The patient was started on off-label therapy with nivolumab, 3 mg/kg intravenously every 2 weeks, which was made available through a patient assistance program. Two weeks after completion of the fourth cycle of nivolumab, CT showed a marked reduction in tumor burden. The patient's pain resolved and he continues on nivolumab without any significant adverse events [69].

Avelumab: A monoclonal antibody that binds to the PD-1 ligand (PD-L1). At the 2016 American Society of Clinical Oncology meeting, results of a phase 2 clinical trial were presented for 88 patients with metastatic MCC treated with avelumab (10 mg/kg every 2 weeks). There were 28 objective responses (32%), 8 of which were complete (9%). Responses appeared to be durable, and the PFS and OS at 6 months were 40% and 69%, respectively. Immune-related toxicity was consistent with that seen with other PD-1 and PD-L1 checkpoint inhibitors [70]. Other immune-mediated strategies against MCC under evaluation are: paclitaxel+IL-2 (NCT02054884), cellular adoptive IT, activated NK cells (NCT02465957), and other immunostimulatory strategies, such as talimogene laherparepvec (T-VEC) (NCT02819843).

Somatostatin Receptor-Based Therapy

Like other neuroendocrine tumors, MCC possesses receptors for somatostatin. These receptors can be demonstrated in vivo by somatostatin receptor-based diagnostic imaging (indium-111) pentetreotide single-photon emission computed tomography or gallium-68 DOTATATE positron emission tomography scanning. Positive uptake on somatostatin receptor-based diagnostic imaging also identifies patients who might benefit from peptide receptor radioligand therapy with compounds such as lutetium-177 DOTATATE. Somatostatin analogues, such as octreotide, can be used [71]. Other analogues such as pasireotide or lanreotide are also being studied in ongoing clinical trials (NCT01652547 and NCT02351128).

Targeted Therapies

In parallel, efforts have shown cases the efficacy of targeted therapy inhibiting disease-driving mutations of BRAF [72]. The mammalian target of the rapamycin (mTOR) pathway is a master regulator of protein synthesis and is frequently found to be dysregulated in human cancers. Likewise, mTOR is found to be upregulated in MCC [73]. Rapamycin and its analogues are allosteric inhibitors via mTORC inhibition. Sirolimus, temsirolimus, everolimus, and deforolimus are also members of this family. Underscored by the clinical inefficacy of allosteric inhibitors, more potent inhibitors of the active site of mTOR kinase, such as PP242, WYE-354, Ku-0063794, and INK128, have been developed [74]. Based on its high potency, INK128 (MLN0128) is currently being used in an open-label dose-escalation study in patients with advanced solid tumors (NCT01058707). The surveillance pathway PI3K/AKT could also be targeted in MCC [73], and report of a single case that responded to idelalisib, a selective PI3Kδ inhibitor, has shown remarkable therapeutic efficacy in B-cell hematologic cancers, have been made recently. A standard dose of idelalisib (150 mg twice daily) was initiated. One week after the initiation of idelalisib, shrinkage of the liver lesion was visible on PET-CT. Repeat PET-CT performed 3 months later did not show tumor in patient's liver, suggesting a complete clinical response to idelalisib. The patient did not have substantial side effects. [75]. Imatinib mesylate failed in a phase II trial. Median progression-free survival was 1 month (95% CI: 1–2 months). Median overall survival was 5 months (95% CI: 2–8 months). One patient achieved a partial response and another had prolonged disease stabilization while receiving treatment. The majority of patients progressed rapidly within 1 to 2 cycles of treatment [76].

Other tyrosine-kinase inhibitors have been studied, revealing responses in individual cases to such as therapies as pazopanib [77]. Cabozantinib (XL184), another inhibitor of multiple receptor tyrosine kinases, is being used in a phase II trial in MCC (NCT02036476).

Future Directions

Newer approaches to advanced disease are required given the short duration of response seen with standard chemotherapy regimens. Patients with stage 4 MCC should be enrolled into a clinical trial whenever feasible. Efforts to identify novel targets are currently being evaluated in vitro and in vivo [78]. Decreased apoptosis is evident in MCC regardless of MCV status. YM-155 has been shown to downregulate surviving expression and promote apoptosis in MCC xenograft tumors. YM-155, a survivin suppressor, is cytotoxic to MCV-positive MCC cells in vitro at nanomolar levels. One MCV-positive MCC xenograft (MS-1) failed to significantly respond to YM155, which corresponds with in vitro dose-response activity. Combination treatment of YM155 with other chemotherapeutics resulted in additive but not synergistic cell killing of MCC cell lines in vitro. These results suggest that survivin targeting is a promising therapeutic approach for most but not all MCV-positive MCCs [79].

Molecularly targeted approaches based upon emerging data regarding the expression of various receptors and signaling pathways may eventually offer some benefit. For patients with distant metastatic disease, data suggest a high response rate with checkpoint inhibitors, such as pembrolizumab. Patients with advanced MCC should be referred for participation in PD-1 inhibitor-based IT trials whenever possible. Advances in the knowledge of the relationship between the immune system and MCC should open up an even wider range of possible treatments for MCC patients.

References

1. Toker C. Trabecular carcinoma of the skin. Arch Dermatol. 1972;105:107–10.
2. Wong HH, Wang J. Merkel cell carcinoma. Arch Pathol Lab Med. 2010;134:1711–6.
3. Becker J. Merkel cell carcinoma (symposium article). Ann Oncol. 2010;21(Suppl 7):vii81–5.
4. Hui AC, Stillie AL, Seel M, Ainslie J. Merkel cell carcinoma: 27-year experience at the Peter MacCallum cancer Center. Int J Radiat Oncol Biol Phys. 2011;80(5):1430.
5. Becker JC, Kaukzok CS, Ugurel S, Eib S, Bröker EB, Houben R. Merkel cell carcinoma: molecular pathogenesis, clinical features and therapy. J Dtsch Dermatol Ges. 2008;6:709–19.
6. Bobos M, Hytiroglou P, Kostopoulos I, Karkavelas G, Papadimitruou CS. Immunohistochemical distinction between Merkel cell carcinoma and small cell carcinoma of the lung. Am J Dermatopathol. 2006;28:99–104.
7. Albores-Saavedra J, Batich K, Chable-Montero F, Sagy N, Schwartz AM, Henson DE. Merkel cell carcinoma demographics, morphology, and survival based on 3870 cases: a population based study. J Cutan Pathol. 2010;37:20–7.
8. Reichgelt B, Visser O. Epidemiology and survival of Merkel cell carcinoma in the Netherlands. A population-based study of 808 cases in 1993–2007. Eur J Cancer. 2010;47:579–85.
9. Zhan FQ, Sharon Packianathan VS, Zeitouni NC. Merkel cell carcinoma: a review of current advances. J Natl Compr Cancer Netw. 2009;1:333–9.
10. Goon PKC, Greenberg DC, Igali L, Levell NJ. Merkel cell carcinoma: rising incidence in the east of England. J Eur Acad Dermatol Venereol. 2016;30(12):2052–5. https://doi.org/10.1111/jdv.13828.
11. Girschik J, Thorn K, Beer TW, Heenan PJ, Fritschi L. Merkel cell carcinoma in Western Australia: a population-based study of incidence and survival. Br J Dermatol. 2011;165:1051–7.
12. Christian WO, Bartus CL, Stephen M, Purcell SM. Merkel cell carcinoma: a review. Cutis. 2016;97:290–5.
13. Kaae J, Hansen AV, Biggar R, Boyd HA, Moore PS, Wohlfahrt J, et al. Merkel cell carcinoma: incidence, mortality, and risk of other cancers. J Natl Cancer Inst. 2010;102:793–801.

14. Brown JA, Smoller BR. Merkel cell carcinoma: what is it, what will it do and where will it go? What role should the pathologist play in reporting. J Cutan Pathol. 2009;36:924–7.
15. González-Vela C, Curiel-Olmo S, Derdak S, Beltran S, Santibañez M, Martínez N, et al. Shared oncogenic pathways implicated in both virus-positive and UV-induced Merkel cell carcinomas. J Invest Dermatol. 2016. pii:S0022-202X(16)32349-1.
16. Leonard JH, Williams G, Walters MK, Nancarrow DJ, Rabbitts PH. Deletion mapping of the short arm of chromosome 3 in Merkel cell carcinoma. Genes Chromosomes Cancer. 1996;15(2):102–7.
17. Leonard JH, Hayard N. Loss of heterozygosity of chromosome 13 in Merkel cell carcinoma. Genes Chromosomes Cancer. 1997;20(1):93–7.
18. Veija T, Sarhadi VK, Koljonen V, Bohling T, Knuutila S. Hotspot mutations in polyomavirus positive and negative Merkel cell carcinomas. Cancer Genet. 2016;209:30–5.
19. Van Gele M, Kaghad M, Leonard JH, Van Roy N, Naeyaert JM, Geerts ML, et al. Mutation analysis of p73 and TP53 in Merkel cell carcinoma. Br J Cancer. 2000;82:823–6.
20. Bichakjian CK, Lowe L, Lao CD, Sandler HM, Bradford CR, Johnson TM. Merkel cell carcinoma: critical review with guidelines for multidisciplinary management. Cancer. 2007;110:1–12.
21. Feng H, Shuda M, Chang Y, Moore PS. Clonal integration of a polyomavirus in Merkel cell carcinoma. Science. 2008;319:1096–9.
22. Bart H, Solis M, Kack-Kack W, Soulier E, Velay A, Kremer S. In vitro and in vivo models for the study of human Polyomavirus infection. Virus. 2016;8:292. https://doi.org/10.3390/v8100292.
23. Gossai A, Waterboer T, Michel A, Willhauck-Fleckenstein M, Farzan SF, Hoen AG. Seroepidemiology of human Polyomaviruses in US population. Am J Epidemiol. 2016;183(1):61–9.
24. Liu W, Margo M, You J. Merkel cell polyomavirus infection and Merkel cell carcinoma. Curr Opin Virol. 2016;20:20–7.
25. Donepudi S, DeConti RC, Samlowski WE. Recent advances in the understanding of the genetics, etiology, and treatment of Merkel cell carcinoma. Semin Oncol. 2012;39(2):163–72.
26. Wong SQ, Waldeck K, Vergara IA, Schröder J, Madore J, Wilmott JS, et al. UV-associated mutations underlie the etiology of MCV-negative Merkel cell carcinomas. Cancer Res. 2015;75(24):5228–34.
27. Hesbacher S, Pfitzer L, Wiedorfer K, Agermeyer S, Borst A, Haferkamp S, et al. RB1 is the crucial target of Merkel cel polyomavirus large T cell antigen in Merkel cell carcinoma cells. Oncotarget. 2016;7(22):329756–68.
28. Iwasaki T, Matsushita M, Nonaka D, Nagata K, Kato M, Kuwamoto S, et al. Lower expression of CADM1 and higher expression of MAL in Merkel cell carcinomas are associated with Merkel cell polyomavirus infection and better prognosis. Hum Pathol. 2016;48:1–8.
29. Sihto H, Kukko H, Koljonen V, Sankila R, Böhling T, Joensuu H. Clinical factors associated with merkel cell polyomavirus infection in Merkel cell carcinoma. J Natl Cancer Inst. 2009;101:938–45.
30. Samimi M, Molet L, Fleury M, Laude H, Carlotti A, Gardair C, et al. Prognostic value of antibodies to Merkel cell polyomavirus T antigens and VP1 protein in patients with Merkel cell carcinoma. Br J Dermatol. 2016;174:813–22.
31. Muller A, Keus R, Neumann N, Lammering G, Schnabel T. Management of Merkel cell carcinoma: case series of 36 patients. Oncol Rep. 2003;10:577–85.
32. Dancey AL, Rayatt SS, Soon C, Ilchshyn A, Brown I, Srivastava S. Merkel cell carcinoma: a report of 34 cases and literature review. J Plast Reconstr Aesthet Surg. 2006;59:1294–9.
33. Poulsen M. Merkel-cell carcinoma of the skin. Lancet Oncol. 2004;5:593–9.
34. Gillenwater AM, Hessel AC, Morrison WH, Burgess M, Silva EG, Roberts D, et al. Merkel cell carcinoma of the head and neck: effect of surgical radiation on recurrence and survival. Arch Otolaryngol Head Neck Surg. 2001;127:149–54.
35. Sattler E, Geimer T, Sick I, Flaig MJ, Ruzicka T, Berking C, et al. Sentinel lymph node in Merkel cell carcinoma: to biopsy or not biopsy. J Dermatol. 2013;40:374–9.
36. Prieto I, Pardo J, Olivera J, Medina MS, Jover R, Perez AM. Merkel cell carcinoma from 2008 to 2012: reaching a new level of understanding. Cancer Treat Rev. 2013;39:421–9.
37. Maza S, Trefzer U, Hoffmann M, Schneider S, Voit C, Krösin T, et al. Impact of sentinel lymph node biopsy in patients with Merkel cell carcinoma: results of a prospective study and review of the literature. Eur J Nucl Med Mol Imaging. 2006;3:433–40.
38. Ramahi E, Choi J, Fuller CD, Eng T. Merkel cell carcinoma. Am J Clin Oncol. 2013;36(3):299–309.
39. Allen PJ, Bowne WB, Jacques DP, Brennan MF, Busam K, Coit DG, et al. Merkel cell carcinoma: prognosis and treatment of patients of a single institution. J Clin Oncol. 2005;23:2300–9.
40. Kachare SD, Wong JH, Vohra NA, Zervos EE, Fitzgerald TL. Sentinel lymph node biopsy with improved survival in Merkel cell carcinoma. Ann Surg Oncol. 2014;21:1624–30.
41. Prieto I, Pérez de la Fuente T, Medina S, Castelo B, Sobrino B, Fortes JR, et al. Merkel cell carcinoma: an algorithm for multidisciplinary management and decision-making. Crit Rev Oncol Hematol. 2016;98:170–9.
42. www.cancerstaging.org
43. http://www.uicc.org/sites/main/files/private/TNM_Classification_of_Malignant_Tumours_Website_15%20MAy2011.pdf
44. Fritsch VA, Camp ER, Lentsch EJ. Sentinel lymph node status in Merkel cell carcinoma of the head and neck: not a predictor of survival. Head Neck. 2014;36:571–9.
45. Mogha A, Fautrel A, Mouchet N, Guo N, Corre S, Adamski H, et al. Merkel cell polyomavirus small T

antigen mRNA level is increased following in vivo UV-radiation. PLoS One. 2010;5:e11423.
46. Morand GB, Madana J, Da Silva SD, Hier MP, Mlynarek AM, Black MJ. Merkel cell carcinoma of the head and neck: poorer prognosis than non-head and neck sites. J Laryngol Otol. 2016;130(4):393–7.
47. Snow SN, Larson PO, Hardy S, Bentz M, Madjar D, Landeck A, et al. Merkel cell carcinoma of the skin and mucosa: report of 12 cutaneous cases with 2 cases arising from the nasal mucosa. Dermatol Surg. 2001;27:165–70.
48. Sadeghi R, Adinehpoor Z, Maleki M, Fallahi B, Giovanella L, Treglia G. Prognostic significance of sentinel lymph node mapping in Merkel cell carcinoma: systematic review and meta-analysis of prognostic studies. Biomed Res Int. 2014;2014:489536.
49. Gupta SG, Wang LC, Peñas PF, Gellenthin M, Lee SJ, Nghiem P. Sentinel lymph node biopsy for evaluation and treatment of patients with Merkel cell carcinoma. Arch Dermatol. 2006;142:685–90.
50. Veness MJ, Perera L, McCourt J, Shannon J, Hughes TM, Morgan GJ, et al. Merkel cell carcinoma: improved outcome with adjuvant radiotherapy. J Surg. 2005;75:275–81.
51. Median-Franco HU, Urist MM, Fiveash J, Heslin MJ, Bland KI, Beenken SW. Multimodality treatment of Merkel cell carcinoma: case series and literature review of 1024 cases. Ann Surg Oncol. 2001;8:204–8.
52. Frohm ML, Griffith KA, Harms KL, et al. Recurrence and survival in patients with Merkel cell carcinoma undergoing surgery without adjuvant radiation therapy to the primary site. JAMA Dermatol. 2016;152(9):1001–7.
53. Lebbe C, Becker JC, Grob JJ, Malvehy J, Del Marmol V, Pehamberger H, et al. Diagnosis and treatment of Merkel cell carcinoma. European consensus-based interdisciplinary guideline. Eur J Cancer. 2015;51(16):2396–403.
54. Mojica P, Smith D, Ellenhorn JD. Adjuvant radiation therapy is associated with improved survival in Merkel cell carcinoma of the skin. J Clin Oncol. 2007;25(9):1043–7.
55. Bhatia S, Storer BE, Iyer JG, Moshiri A, Parvathaneni U, Byrd D, et al. Adjuvant radiation therapy and chemotherapy in Merkel cell carcinoma: survival analyses of 6908 cases from the national cancer data base. J Natl Cancer Inst. 2016;108(9):djw042.
56. Kang SH, Haydu LE, Goh RY, Fogarty GB. Radiotherapy is associated with significant improvement in local and regional control in Merkel cell carcinoma. Radiat Oncol. 2012;7:171.
57. Harrington C, Kwan W. Outcomes of Merkel cell carcinoma treated with radiotherapy without radical surgical excision. Ann Surg Oncol. 2014;21(11):3401–5.
58. Foote M, Harvey J, Porceddu S, Dickie G, Hewitt S, Colquist S, et al. Effect of radiotherapy dose and volume on relapse in Merkel cell cancer of the skin. Int J Radiat Oncol Biol Phys. 2010;77:677–84.
59. Kokoska ER, Kokoska MS, Collins BT, Stapleton DR, Wade TP. Early aggressive treatment for Merkel cell carcinoma improves outcome. Am J Surg. 1997;174:688–93.
60. Fang LC, Lemos B, Douglas J, Iyer J, Nghiem P. Radiation monotherapy as regional treatment for lymph node-positive Merkel cell carcinoma. Cancer. 2010;116:1783–90.
61. Bichakjian CK, Coit DG, Wong SL. Radiation versus resection for Merkel cell carcinoma. Cancer. 2010;116:1620–2.
62. Satpute SR, Ammakkanavar NR, Einhorn LH. Role of platinum-based chemotherapy for Merkel cell tumor in adjuvant and metastatic settings. J Clin Oncol. 2014;5s:32.
63. Poulsen M, Rischin D, Walpole E, Harvey J, Mackintosh J, Ainslie J, et al. High-risk Merkel cell carcinoma of the skin treated with synchronous carboplatin/etoposide and radiation: a trans-Tasman radiation oncology group study--TROG 96:07. J Clin Oncol. 2003;21(23):4371–6.
64. Chen MM, Roman SA, Sosa JA, Judson BL. The role of adjuvant therapy in the management of head and neck Merkel cell carcinoma: an analysis of 4815 patients. JAMA Otolaryngol Head Neck Surg. 2015;141(2):137–41.
65. Voog E, Biron P, Martin JP, Blay JY. Chemotherapy for patients with locally advanced or metastatic Merkel cell carcinoma. Cancer. 1999;85(12):2589–95.
66. Tai PT, Yu E, Winquist E, Hammond A, Stitt L, Tonita J, et al. Chemotherapy in neuroendocrine/Merkel cell carcinoma of the skin: case series and review of 204 cases. J Clin Oncol. 2000;18(12):2493–9.
67. Iyer JG, Blom A, Doumani R, Lewis C, Anderson A, Ma C, et al. Response rate and durability of chemotherapy for metastatic Merkel cell carcinoma among 62 patients. J Clin Oncol. 2014;5s:32.
68. Nghiem PT, Bhatia S, Lipson EJ, Kudchadkar RR, Miller NJ, Annamalai L, et al. PD-1 blockade with Pembrolizumab in advanced Merkel-cell carcinoma. N Engl J Med. 2016;374(26):2542–52.
69. Mantripragada K, Birnbaum A. Response to anti-PD-1 therapy in metastatic Merkel cell carcinoma metastatic to the heart and pancreas. Cureus. 2015;7(12):e403.
70. Kaufman H, Russell JS, Hamid O, et al. Avelumab (MSB0010718C; anti-PD-L1) in patients with metastatic Merkel cell carcinoma previously treated with chemotherapy: results of the phase 2 JAVELIN Merkel 200 trial. J Clin Oncol. 2016;34(suppl):abstr 9508.
71. Cirillo F, Filippini L, Lima GF, Caresana G, Alquati P. Merkel cell tumor. Report of case and treatment with octreotide. Minerva Chir. 1997;52(11):1359.
72. Schrama D, Groesser L, Ugurel S, Hafner C, Pastrana DV, Buck CB, et al. Presence of human polyomavirus 6 in mutation-specific BRAF inhibitor-induced epithelial proliferations. JAMA Dermatol. 2014;150(11):1180–6.
73. Lin Z, McDermott A, Shao L, Kannan A, Morgan M, Stack BC Jr, et al. Chronic mTOR activation promotes cell survival in Merkel cell carcinoma. Cancer Lett. 2014;344(2):272–81.

74. Hafner C, Houben R, Baeurle A, Ritter C, Schrama D, Landthaler M, et al. Activation of the PI3K/AKT pathway in Merkel cell carcinoma. PLoS One. 2012;7:e31255.
75. Shiver MB, Mahmoud F, Gao L. Response to idelalisib in a patient with stage IV Merkel-cell carcinoma. N Engl J Med. 2015;373:1580–2.
76. Samlowski WE, Moon J, Tuthill RJ, Heinrich MC, Balzer-Haas NS, Merl SA, et al. A phase II trial of imatinib mesylate in Merkel cell carcinoma (neuroendocrine carcinoma of the skin): a southwest oncology group study (S0331). Am J Clin Oncol. 2010;33(5):495–9.
77. Davids MS, Charlton A, Ng SS, Chong ML, Laubscher K, Dar M, Hodge J, et al. Response to a novel multitargeted tyrosine kinase inhibitor pazopanib in metastatic Merkel cell carcinoma. Clin Oncol. 2009;27(26):e97.
78. Brunner M, Thurnher D, Pammer J, Heiduschka G, Petzelbauer P, Schmid C, et al. Expression of hedgehog signaling molecules in Merkel cell carcinoma. Head Neck. 2010;32(3):333.
79. Dresang LR, Guastafierro A, Arora R, Normolle D, Chang Y, Moore PS. Response of Merkel cell polyomavirus-positive Merkel cell carcinoma xenografts to a survivin inhibitor. PLoS One. 2013;8(11):e80543.

Index

A. I. Riker (ed.), *Melanoma*, https://doi.org/10.1007/978-3-319-78310-9

The manufacturer's authorised representative in the EU is Springer Nature Customer Service Centre GmbH, Europaplatz 3, 69115 Heidelberg, Germany. If you have any concerns regarding our products, please contact ProductSafety@springernature.com

Printed and bound by CPI Group (UK) Ltd, Croydon, CR0 4YY
05/10/2026
02228136-0002